PSYCHIATRIC MENTAL HEALTH NURSING

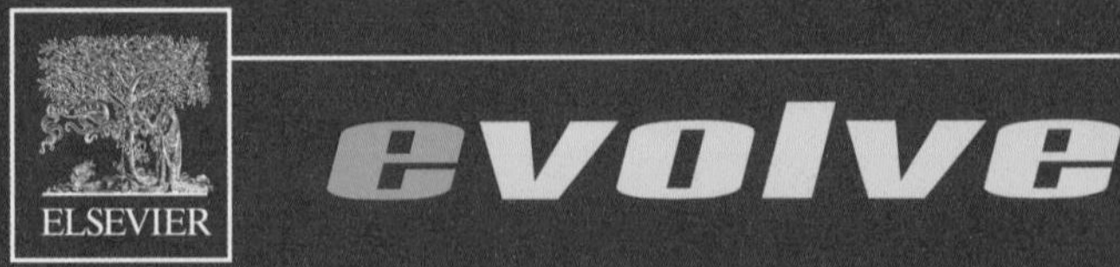

To access your Student Resources, visit:

http://evolve.elsevier.com/Fortinash/

Evolve Student Learning Resources for Fortinash/Holoday Worret: ***Psychiatric Mental Health Nursing***, 4th Edition offers the following features:

Student Resources

- **Case Study Critical Thinking Answer Guidelines**
  Check your responses with answer guidelines and rationales from the authors.
- **Chaper Outlines**
  For note-taking in or out of class.
- **Chapter Review Answers**
  Additional answer categories including rationales for the review questions at the end of each chapter.
- **Concept Map Creator**
  Walks you through the thinking process of creating individualized Concept Maps, from initial diagnoses to interventions to outcomes to a complete plan of care.
- **Online Resources**
  Direct links to websites of national organizations offering information and support for nurses and clients.
- **Practice Test**
  Interactive review questions for the NCLEX® examination with instant scoring and feedback at the click of a button.

http://evolve.elsevier.com/Fortinash/

PSYCHIATRIC MENTAL HEALTH NURSING

FOURTH EDITION

KATHERINE M. FORTINASH, MSN, APRN, BC

Clinical Specialist
Adult Psychiatric and Mental Health Nursing
Associate Faculty
Department of Health Sciences
Mt. San Jacinto College
Menifee, California
Lecturer and Consultant
San Diego, California

PATRICIA A. HOLODAY WORRET, MSN, APRN, BC

Clinical Specialist
Adult Psychiatric and Mental Health Nursing
Professor Emerita, Psychiatric and Mental Health Nursing
Nursing Education Department
Palomar College
San Marcos, California
Consultant
San Diego, California

MOSBY

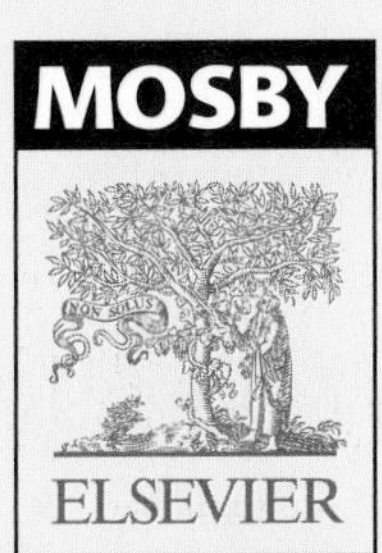

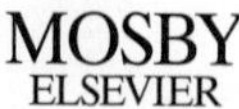

11830 Westline Industrial Drive
St. Louis, Missouri 63146

PSYCHIATRIC MENTAL HEALTH NURSING ISBN: 978-0-323-04675-6

NOTICE

Knowledge and best practice in this field are constantly changing. As new research and experience broaden our knowledge, changes in practice, treatment, and drug therapy may become necessary or appropriate. Readers are advised to check the most current information provided (i) on procedures featured or (ii) by the manufacturer of each product to be administered, to verify the recommended dose or formula, the method and duration of administration, and contraindications. It is the responsibility of the practitioner, relying on their own experience and knowledge of the patient, to make diagnoses, to determine dosages and the best treatment for each individual patient, and to take all appropriate safety precautions. To the fullest extent of the law, neither the Publisher nor the Authors assume any liability for any injury and/or damage to persons or property arising out of or related to any use of the material contained in this book.

The Publisher

ISBN: 978-0-323-04675-6

Executive Publisher: Tom Wilhelm
Senior Developmental Editor: Jill Ferguson
Publishing Services Manager: John Rogers
Senior Project Manager: Beth Hayes
Designer: Teresa McBryan

Printed in Canada

Last digit is the print number: 9 8 7 6 5 4 3 2 1

We dedicate this book to those who struggle with mental illness every day while striving to meet life's challenges in a complex world; their dignity and courage give us hope and make us humble.

And, to the families, friends, and nurses who support and care for them.

Contributors

Chapter Contributors

Merry A. Armstrong, DNSc, ARNP
Associate Professor
Intercollegiate College of Nursing
Washington State University College of Nursing
Spokane, Washington
Chapter 14 Substance-Related Disorders

Ann Wolbert Burgess, DNSc, APRN, BC, FAAN
Professor of Psychiatric Nursing
William F. Connell School of Nursing
Boston College
Chestnut Hill, Massachusetts
Chapter 22 Violence and Forensics in Clinical Practice: Abuse, Neglect, Anger, and Rape

Pauline Chan, RPh, MBA, BCPP, FCSHP, FASHP
Senior Pharmaceutical Consultant
Medi-Cal Pharmacy Policy Unit
California Department of Health Services
Sacramento, California
Chapter 24 Psychopharmacology

Ann Clarkin-Watts, MSW, LCSW
Private Practice
San Diego, California
Chapter 17 Eating Disorders

Nancy A. Coffin-Romig, DNSc, APRN, BC, CNS
Lecturer
School of Nursing
San Diego State University
Private Practice
San Diego, California
Chapter 23 Therapies in Clinical Practice

Dawn Marie Elders, MSN, NP-C, PHN
Oncology Nurse Practitioner
Pacific Oncology and Hematology Associates
Director of Eduction, Project Compassion
Escondido, California
Chapter 20 Crisis: Theory and Intervention

Robert L. Erb, Jr., PhD, RN, CS, CLNC
Advanced Clinician
Sharp HealthCare
San Diego, California
Chapter 8 Legal and Ethical Aspects in Clinical Practice

Chantal M. Flanagan, RN, MS, CNS
Associate Professor
Palomar College
San Marcos, California
Chapter 16 Disorders of Infancy, Childhood, and Adolescence

Candice A. Francis, EdD
Professor, Life Sciences
Palomar College
San Marcos, California
Chapter 6 Neurobiology in Mental Health and Disorder

Ruth N. Grendell, DNSc
Faculty
University of Phoenix
Professor Emerita
Point Loma Nazerene University
San Diego, California
Chapter 7 Cultural, Ethnic, and Spiritual Considerations
Chapter 25 Complementary and Alternative Therapies
Chapter 27 Mental and Emotional Responses to Medical Illness

Bonnie M. Hagerty, PhD, RN, CS
Associate Professor
School of Nursing
University of Michigan
Ann Arbor, Michigan
Chapter 11 Mood Disorders and Adjustment Disorders

Linda Hollinger-Smith, PhD, RN, FAAN
Senior Vice President for Research
Life Services Network
Hinsdale, Illinois
Chapter 5 Growth and Development Across the Life Span

Russell A. Kelley, MN, ARNP, BC
Instructor
Intercollegiate College of Nursing
Washington State University College of Nursing
Private Practice
Spokane, Washington
Chapter 15 Cognitive Disorders: Delirium, Dementia, and Amnestic Disorders

Shelly F. Lurie-Akman, APRN/PMH-BC, CTHY
Director of Specialized Treatment Services
Clifton T. Perkins Hospital Center
Jessup, Maryland
Faculty Associate
School of Nursing
Johns Hopkins University
Baltimore, Maryland
Chapter 19 Sexual Disorders

Pamela E. Marcus, RN, APRN/PMH-BC
Associate Professor of Nursing
Prince George's Community College
Largo, Maryland
Advanced Practice Nurse Psychotherapist
Private Practice
Upper Marlboro, Maryland
Chapter 9 Anxeity and Anxiety Disorders
Chapter 10 Somatoform, Factitious, and Dissociative Disorders
Chapter 13 Personality Disorders
Chapter 21 Suicide: Prevention and Intervention

Susan Fertig McDonald, MSN, RN, CS
Clinical Nurse Specialist
VA San Diego Healthcare System
San Diego, California
Chapter 4 Therapeutic Communication

Nancy Stark Napolitano, MSN, EdD, RN
Professor of Psychiatric Nursing and Health Science
Curriculum Content Expert, Psychiatric Nursing
Mt. San Jacinto College
Menifee, California
Chapter 18 Sleep Disorders

Kathleen L. Patusky, PhD, APRN-BC
Assistant Professor
School of Nursing
University of Medicine and Dentistry of New Jersey
Newark, New Jersey
Chapter 11 Mood Disorders and Adjustment Disorders

Diane L. Pavalonis, MBA, MSN, APRN, BC
Clinical Nurse Specialist
Western State Hospital
Staunton, Virginia
Chapter 12 Schizophrenia and Other Psychotic Disorders

Dona Petrozzi, MSN
Gradute Student
William F. Connell School of Nursing
Boston College
Chestnut Hill, Massachusetts
Chapter 22 Violence and Forensics in Clinical Practice: Abuse, Neglect, Anger, and Rape

Alwilda Scholler-Jaquish, PhD, APRN, BC
Associate Professor (Retired)
University of Nevada, Reno
Reno, Nevada
Chapter 28 Caring for Clients in the Community
Chapter 29 Caring for Persons With Severe and Persistent Mental Illness

Kathryn Thomas, PhD, APRN, FAACS
Clinical Sexologist, Private Practice
Instructor, School of Medicine
Department of Psychiatry and Behavioral Sciences
Johns Hopkins University
Adjunct Professor
Loyola College
Villa Julie College
Baltimore, Maryland
Chapter 19 Sexual Disorders

Feature Contributors

Teresa S. Burckhalter, MSN, RN, BC
Nursing Faculty
Technical College of the Lowcountry
Beaufort, South Carolina
Chapter review questions

Jean F. Fisak, MSN, APN, CNS-BC, RN
Psychiatric/Mental Health Clinical Nurse Specialist
Naval Medical Center
San Diego, California
Medication Key Facts boxes

Reviewers

Carole Schrumpf Dabbs, MSN, PhD, RN
Nursing Instructor
Northwest-Shoals Community College
Phil Campbell, Alabama

Teresa S. Fox, BSN, RN
Assistant Professor
Practical Nursing Program
Health Technology Division
Virginia Western Community College
Roanoke, Virginia

Mary Blessing Gilkey, MS, APRN, BC
Education and Health Care Consultant
Norfolk, Virginia

Beulah E. Hall, MSN, EdD, RN
Associate Professor, Nursing
Drexel University College of Health
Philadelphia, Pennsylvania

Ann Killian, MS, RN
Nursing Faculty
Brigham Young University–Idaho
Rexburg, Idaho

Sarah Magnuson-Whyte, MN, RN
Nursing Faculty
Pierce College
Puyallup, Washington

Linda Arcelia McDonald, MSN, RN
Associate Professor, Nursing
Southwestern College
Chula Vista, California

Jane Ellen Young, MSN, RN, FNP, MPH
Staff Nurse
Daybreak Behavioral Health Unit
Selby General Hospital
Marietta, Ohio

Roberta Waite, MSN, EdD, RN, CS
Assistant Professor
College of Nursing and Health Professions
Drexel University
Philadelphia, Pennsylvania

Preface

Psychiatric nurses are required to blend their broad base of scientific knowledge and interpersonal skills to meet the challenges of biologic and technologic advances in treating clients with mental disorders and their families. Even as the impetus continues to move toward biology and technology, the combination of psychotherapy and psychopharmacology remains the treatment of choice in the psychiatric setting.

Another challenge for psychiatric nurses is the managed care organizations that continue to influence the health care delivery system, resulting in the shift of client care from inpatient facilities to less costly alternatives for treatment. These include partial hospital programs, outpatient clinics, and community agencies. Ongoing advances in biology and technology and the changing health care environment strongly encourage psychiatric nurses to continue to deliver quality client care in the midst of emerging treatment complexities.

APPROACH AND INTENDED USE

The fourth edition of *Psychiatric Mental Health Nursing* is designed to help nurses successfully meet today's health care challenges by presenting the most current information from psychiatric mental health nursing, psychiatry, and the sciences. The balanced nursing and medical approach remains a distinguishing feature of this textbook. Although psychiatric nursing is thoroughly discussed as it relates to various well-regarded theorists, the text does not advocate any one specific nursing framework. This timely, state-of-the-art text is primarily intended to help students and practicing psychiatric nurses deliver professional nursing care for clients and their families, regardless of time, place, or circumstances.

As in past editions, this highly readable text provides clear, concise explanations and definitions of concepts and terminology that promote student understanding for a solid knowledge base. New content has been added to this edition in an ongoing effort to respond to the current health care climate and the needs of today's students and practicing nurses. Normal anxiety is presented to frame the discussion for anxiety disorders; a new chapter is devoted to sleep disorders; the clinical therapies chapter has been expanded, presenting the major theoretic bases for therapies and covering the therapeutic milieu and modes of therapy; and useful tools that enhance learning, promote documentation skills, and help students complete assignments in a timely manner—such as the concept map, process recording, and SOAP note, and standardized care plan—appear throughout the text.

STRUCTURE AND ORGANIZATION

The major organizing structure for the disorders chapters includes both the diagnoses of the North American Nursing Diagnosis Association International from *NANDA-I Nursing Diagnoses: Definitions and Classification* and the American Psychiatric Association from the *Diagnostic and Statistical Manual of Mental Disorders*. We strongly believe in the practicality and effectiveness of the collaborative efforts of nursing and medicine whenever possible. We contend that the use of current NANDA terminology most accurately describes the therapeutic services and contributions of nurses and also reflects contemporary nursing actions and responses. Application and use of refined diagnostic labels are essential to the evolution of the language and discipline of nursing.

This book is organized into six sections. *Part I, Foundations for Psychiatric Mental Health Nursing*, presents concepts that not only define nursing as an art and a science but also reveal the substantive changes and trends that currently shape and challenge the traditional professional nursing roles in the area of mental health. *Part II, Psychiatric Disorders*, focuses on major disorders described in the DSM-IV-TR. *Part III, Crisis and Aggression*, addresses the critical issues of crisis, violence, and suicide. *Part IV, Therapeutic Interventions*, emphasizes the major therapeutic modalities used to treat clients in the psychiatric setting. *Part V, Special Populations*, discusses psychiatric nursing care as it relates to the unique circumstances of grief and loss and acute, chronic, or life-threatening illness. *Part VI, Community Psychiatric Nursing*, describes current issues and concerns experienced by clients in different settings and treated by psychiatric nurses.

The most common psychiatric disorders are presented using a consistent, standardized format, with the nursing process featured as a distinct section in relevant chapters. The many features of this text are integrated within the discussion of the steps of the nursing process to demonstrate practical clinical application. Each clinical chapter begins with a disorder's history and theory, etiology and epidemiology, clinical description (including ***Clinical Symptoms* boxes** and ***DSM-IV-TR Criteria* boxes**), prognosis, and discharge criteria. Building on this knowledge, **The Nursing Process** begins with an **Assessment** section including ***Nursing Assessment Questions* boxes** that aid effective communication with specific questions that should be asked of the client. The **Nursing Diagnosis** section presents the most relevant *NANDA-I–approved nursing diagnoses* for a particular disorder, prioritized according to client needs from most urgent to least urgent. Prioritized *sample client outcomes* are presented in the **Outcome Identification** section. The **Planning** section promotes a consistent, collaborative plan of care. The **Implementation** section lists *specific nursing interventions with rationales* and features ***Additional Treatment Modalities* boxes** listing related treatment methods, ***Medication Key Facts* boxes** summarizing the most common psychopharmacologic interventions, and ***Client and Family Teaching Guidelines*** with important teaching points to support treatment compliance. The **Evaluation** section outlines criteria that determine client progress and response to treatment. Throughout the chapters, ***Case Studies*** depict effective nursing care strategies and encourage critical thinking, ***Clinical Alert* boxes** address issues critical to the safety or well-being of the client, and ***Research for Evidence-Based Practice* boxes** discuss implications of current research studies. Finally, ***Nursing Care Plans*** provide guidelines for care through an example clinical situation, with each plan including a brief case study, followed by assessment, diagnosis, goal setting, interventions with rationales, and evaluation.

TEACHING AND LEARNING PACKAGE

A complete ancillary package to enhance teaching and learning is provided for this text.

The **Companion CD** included with the textbook contains a variety of useful tools for additional study and review. A 150-term audio glossary provides definitions along with accurate pronunciations, interactive exercises reinforce key concepts, animations allow for a quick neurology review, and a bank of approximately 150 multiple-choice review questions will help in preparation for the NCLEX® examination.

The **Evolve Learning Resources** to accompany the fourth edition of *Psychiatric Mental Health Nursing* are available for both students and instructors. Students will find valuable resources such as chapter outlines for in-class or independent note-taking, rationales for the case study critical thinking questions, expanded answers to the textbook end-of-chapter review, supplemental review questions, and a concept mapping tool. In addition to the information available to students, instructors are able to access all of the components of the Instructor's Electronic Resource (CD-ROM).

The **Instructor's Electronic Resource (CD-ROM)** is available free to adopters of the textbook and includes the following resources, each corresponding to the 29 chapters of the textbook: (1) an *Instructor's Manual* including a chapter focus, objectives and key terms, critical thinking exercises, and enrichment activities; (2) *ExamView Test Bank* with more than 800 questions (including alternate item formats) organized by chapter and including objective, nursing process step, cognitive level, NCLEX category of Client Need, correct answer, rationale, and text page reference; (3) *PowerPoint slide presentations*, with more than 400 text and illustration slides; and (4) *Audience Response Questions*, in PowerPoint format for i>clicker and other systems, with multiple answer questions designed to stimulate student discussion and survey understanding of key concepts.

TERMINOLOGY AND LANGUAGE

We recognize the contributions of both men and women to the nursing profession. Whenever possible, we have attempted to use plural nouns and pronouns in place of the singular his or her. However, clarity sometimes has dictated the use of she for nurse and he for client.

We have chosen to use the term client instead of patient because we view individuals receiving treatment as significant participants in the reciprocal process of treatment. We also recognize that family can refer not only to blood relatives but friends and significant others. However, the term family is generally used for simplicity.

ACKNOWLEDGMENTS

Sincere thanks to all at Elsevier for help in completing this textbook. Special gratitude to those who worked closely and directly with us throughout the entire process, particularly Tom Wilhelm, Jill Ferguson, and Beth Hayes; your experience is greatly appreciated.

We thank our supportive and loyal families and friends for their patience and understanding while the book was being written.

We sincerely thank our contributors who join us in giving this textbook focus and meaning. We also acknowledge the following contributors to the third edition whose work continues to provide the basis for the content of the text: Donna Oradei Berger, Phillip R. Deming, Sandra S. Goldsmith, Charles Kemp, Richard C. Lucas, Kathleen Pace Murphy, Susan Selverston, James M. Turnbull, Joan C. Urbancic, Gwen van Servellen, Kathleen M. Walker, and Mary Magenheimer Webster.

Finally, the authors are grateful for the long-standing working relationship that perpetuates our texts. We acknowledge each other for enduring positive attitudes concerning the importance of comprehensive nursing education, particularly the role that psychiatric mental health plays in all aspects of nursing, and for our continued mutual desire to share this with other nurses.

We are proud to launch this new edition of our textbook and invite psychiatric nursing students and nurses at all levels to meet the challenges presented and to apply the concepts in clinical practice. We wish you well in your professional journey and feel confident that you will successfully meet these challenges while experiencing the satisfaction and wonder of psychiatric nursing.

Kathi Fortinash and Pat Holoday Worret

Contents

Part I

FOUNDATIONS FOR PSYCHIATRIC MENTAL HEALTH NURSING

Part V
SPECIAL POPULATIONS

Part VI
COMMUNITY PSYCHIATRIC NURSING

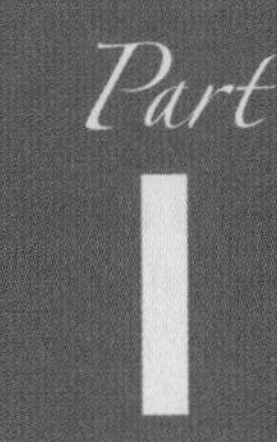

FOUNDATIONS FOR PSYCHIATRIC MENTAL HEALTH NURSING

Chapter 1 Principles of Psychiatric Nursing: Theory and Practice

PATRICIA A. HOLODAY WORRET

The doors of wisdom are never shut.
BENJAMIN FRANKLIN

OBJECTIVES

1. Discuss mental health as a right of all people.
2. Describe four core objectives of psychiatric mental health nursing.
3. Explain the objectives outlined in the levels of prevention of mental disorders.
4. Compare and contrast risk factors and protective factors related to mental health.
5. Describe indicators that identify mental health and mental disorder.
6. Discuss the significance of mind-body interaction in mental health or disorder.
7. Compare the prevalence of mental disorders today with the previous century and predicted prevalence of mental disorders in 2020.
8. Describe the underserved population of mentally disordered individuals and specific ways to improve their losses.
9. Explain advances in neuroscientific research since the "Decade of the Brain."
10. Discuss the effects of mental disorders on clients and the effects on their families.
11. Describe the pros and cons of the diagnoses of mental disorders.
12. Discuss the benefits and purpose of the therapeutic alliance and the nurse-client relationship.
13. Explain the reasons and purposes for a scope and standards of practice for psychiatric mental health nurses.
14. Name specific ways psychiatric mental health nurses advocate for their clients.

KEY TERMS

advanced practice level, p. 16
advocate, p. 16
attitude, p. 6
autodiagnosis, p. 15
basic practice level, p. 16
critical thinking, p. 15
eclectic, p. 4
etiology, p. 3
evidence-based, p. 12
extrinsic, p. 3
incidence, p. 3
indicators, p. 4
intrinsic, p. 3
label, p. 6
mental disorders, p. 2
mental health, p. 2
nurse-client relationship, p. 12
objective, p. 14
prevalence, p. 3
protective factors, p. 3
risk factors, p. 3
stigma, p. 10
subjective, p. 14
therapeutic alliance, p. 12

Mental health is the right of all people and is an essential element of every person's overall health regardless of race, age, gender, or socioeconomic status. Mental health is fundamental to daily functioning, productivity, and general well-being (Institute of Medicine [IOM], 2006; New Freedom Commission on Mental Health, US Department of Health and Human Services [USDHHS], 2003; USDHHS, 1999; World Health Organization Report [WHO], 1999b; Healthy people 2010, USDHHS, 1999; National Institutes of Mental Health [NIMH], 2006). This standard is ideal, but not all people enjoy mental health. In addition, experts predict that mental illness will increase in the early decades of the twenty-first century, posing a definite disadvantage for the people who live with **mental disorders** in this country and throughout the world.

Mental illness has always puzzled, fascinated, or frightened those who did not understand it. Throughout history, mental disorders interrupted the lives of many individuals, families, groups, and the public in general. In some eras, consequences for the disruptions were less than humane. Knowledge and understanding of mental disorders has grown remarkably over the past century and positively affected the perception and treatment of people who suffer with mental illnesses and their families. Humane individuals and professional advocates fought to stop mistreatment and intolerance of the mentally ill. Some of the professional advocates were psychiatric mental health nurses, who promoted mental health and provided interventions for people with mental disorders.

Now more than ever there is a need for skilled and educated psychiatric mental health (PMH) nurses. PMH nurses intervene for the purpose of assisting clients to (1) resolve mental, emotional, and dysfunctional aspects of life crises; (2) manage and alleviate distressing symptoms of mental disorders; (3) improve overall function; and (4) decrease the consequences of mental illness. This chapter describes and explores the topics of mental health, mental disorder, and other relevant associated topics that are significant for nurses, their clients, and society.

CORE OBJECTIVES

Psychiatric mental health is a nursing specialty, with the focus on clients (individuals, families, groups, community) in both theory and practice. Psychiatric mental health nursing (PMHN) utilizes fundamental principles of the art and science of the nursing profession and considers all aspects of client health during comprehensive interactions, as illustrated in Figure 1-1.

The primary goal for psychiatric nurses is client mental health. Four major objectives serve as guidelines toward achieving that goal:

- Promotion of mental health
- Prevention of mental disorders
- Treatment for clients with mental disorders
- Restoration of health

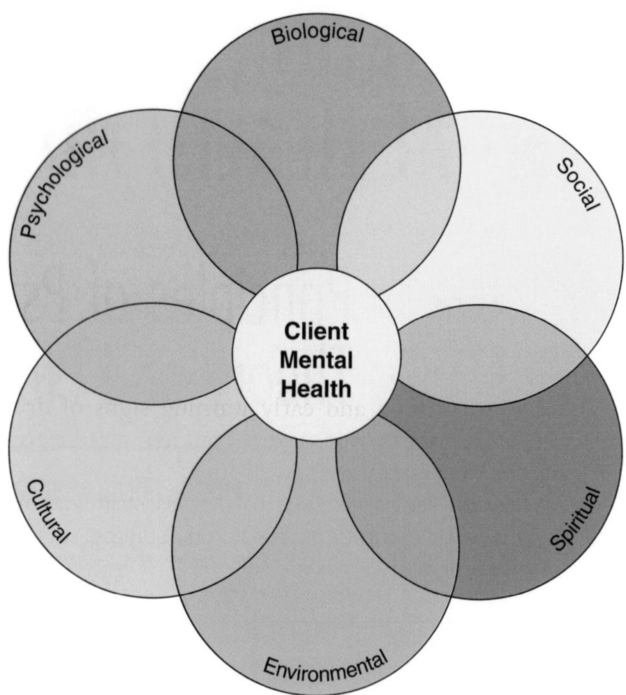

FIGURE 1-1 Comprehensive care model for psychiatric mental health nursing.

Nurses strive to achieve the first two proactive objectives when interacting with clients. However, nurses spend the majority of their time and resources on the second two objectives. Most psychiatric nursing interventions focus on the treatment of clients during or following a disruptive life crisis or an acute episode of a previously identified mental disorder, or by assisting them in their restoration of health and return to adequate function after disruption has occurred. There are several reasons why nurses emphasize the latter two objectives. Constraints in the current mental health care arena, such as economic and political influences, make it difficult for nurses to focus on promoting mental health and preventing mental disorders. Also, it is not possible to accurately predict who will develop mental disorders or when disorders will occur.

The public mental health model is a classic and effective standard that assists nurses in understanding and utilizing the four major PMHN objectives. The original prototype of this model with its levels of prevention was created in the 1960s (Caplan, 1964). The Institutes of Medicine reviewed the model and modified it slightly (IOM, 1994). It continues to be a useful tool that PMHN and several other disciplines frequently use.

LEVELS OF PREVENTION

The prevention of mental illness is paired with the core belief that mental health is every person's right. In each case, nurses and other health care providers consider the levels of prevention of mental disorders, and incorporate these when interacting with clients. Individual client situations and conditions determine the level of intervention.

Primary Prevention

Focus is on reducing the occurrences or **incidence** of mental disorders in the community. Emphasis is on promoting health and preventing disorders. Screening plays an important role in early identification of any disorder. Examples include the following:

- Teach normal childhood development criteria and discuss realistic expectations with young mothers in community.
- Assist new parents in learning parenting skills; help them practice and role-play.
- Hold seminars with parents or guardians on the topics of prevention and early warning signs of drug use, pairing behaviors, sexual conduct, and preparing for the "empty nest syndrome."
- Meet with senior citizens to discuss strategies for linking with community resources; staying socially and intellectually active.

Secondary Prevention

Focus is on reducing the **prevalence** of mental disorders through early identification of symptoms and early treatment of symptoms that occur. Examples include the following:

- Treat clients after making diagnoses of mental disorders. Treatment is any approved biologic or interactive type of therapy and takes place in any psychiatric setting (inpatient, clinic, day treatment center, home, school).
- Refer clients to other therapists for additional treatment (family therapy, couples therapy).

Tertiary Prevention

Focus has a dual purpose of (1) reducing residual effects of the disorder and (2) providing rehabilitation and restoration. Examples include the following:

- Lead ongoing outpatient therapy group of clients with the same situation (grief or loss) or same diagnosis to offer support, to monitor, and to evaluate members' progress.
- Continue to meet with family who has a member with a mental disorder. Assist and reinforce willingness to care for the member and help identify symptoms that recur.
- Conduct seminars and workshops to teach clients job skills and match potential employers with potential client employees.

RISK FACTORS AND PROTECTIVE FACTORS

The promotion of mental health and prevention of mental illness requires regular assessment and evaluation of risk factors and protective factors. **Risk factors** are predisposing internal characteristics and external influences that increase a person's vulnerability and potential for developing mental disorders. Risk factors include *biologic* (genetic predisposition, gender, age), *psychologic* (personality style, level of intelligence, skewed worldview, belief system, attitudes) or *sociocultural* (absent, neglectful or abusive family; parent with mental disorder; poverty; lack of social skills; rejecting cultural or ethnic group), or *environmental* (exposure to toxins, drugs, pollution). Some risk factors are fixed and unchanging, such as genetic inheritance, but other factors change over time and positively or negatively influence the outcome of a person's mental health or disorder.

Protective factors are characteristics that guard against risks and sometimes decrease the potential for developing mental disorders. They are either internal or external. Examples of *internal protective factors* are overall good health, high stress tolerance, resilience, average or better intelligence, adequate learned skills, competence and flexibility, and positive perception and attitude toward events. Examples of *external protective factors* include healthy, caring family/friends/culture; supportive teachers/boss; adequate income; and available age-appropriate resources, recreation, and hobbies. Sometimes altered factors influence a client's response and subsequently affect an outcome of mental health or disorder.

MENTAL HEALTH AND MENTAL DISORDER

Etiology

A frequently asked question, and one that nurses need to know is, "What causes mental illness?" At the present time, both the biologic and behavioral sciences agree on an integrative view of the **etiology**. Each person's mental status results from the convergence of an individual's (1) **intrinsic**, or internal, biology and constitution with (2) **extrinsic**, or external, psychosocial, cultural, and environmental influences. Both internal and external factors determine an individual's mental state. The human central nervous system, specifically the brain, is the most complex, sophisticated organ in the human body. It is the mediator of all thoughts, emotions, and behaviors. A mind and brain are one, and a healthy mind requires a healthy brain. Intact brain structure (anatomy) and function (physiology) are therefore necessary for mental health, but biology is only one factor that determines mental status. A person's interactions and experiences with the world also play a significant role in shaping the brain and influencing an individual's responses that result in mental health or disorder.

Nursing Perspectives

Many leaders in the nursing discipline maintain that health and illness depend on the interaction of internal and external factors. This concept has traditionally guided nursing theory and practice, particularly in psychiatric mental health nursing. Nurses held a holistic view of wellness and illness, in the belief that human well-being depends on a balance of intrinsic and extrinsic elements operating in unison. This thinking also guides principles for treating the whole person rather than separate aspects of the person. When human internal factors and a majority of external factors are intact and operate in unison, a person is healthy in body, mind, and spirit and will interact with the world accordingly. Although the current outlook on etiology agrees with this long-held nursing perspective, this was not always the case, as the following summary briefly explains.

Historical Aspects

During the twentieth century, psychiatry and psychology largely influenced ideas about mental health and disorders. Their perspectives and theories about causes and effects of mental illness differed widely at times and inspired scientific research, academic focus, government spending, and general opinions about mental health and disorders. Conclusions often varied from one experiment to another, and people often settled with the theory that was popular at the time—that is, *trend du jour*. All theories were supported by numerous research findings that explained and defended their theories for mental disorders, and each successive trend was followed by multiple new treatment methods that fit the accepted viewpoint. These cause-and-effect modes each lasted decades until it was clear that the popular theory and methods of treatment were no more effective at decreasing mental disorders than the previous major predictive trends.

Around the turn of the twentieth century, the mental health professions believed that biologic pathology was the cause of mental disorders. That theory existed unopposed for many years, as did the types of treatments. After decades, when the incidence and prevalence of mental disorders remained relatively unchanged, biologic theories grew less important, and innovative theories from psychology and sociology attempted to name causes and subsequent treatments for mental disorders. These social and interpersonal models and theories expanded abundantly and took the spotlight well beyond the middle of the century.

After several decades and extensive funding in this new direction, the industry and the government found that the focus on social/interpersonal models had also failed to significantly reduce incidence or prevalence of mental disorders. The pendulum again began to swing back toward biology. At the present time, biologic and behavioral theorists in the mental health professions agree that both models play an important role in determining a person's mental health or disorder. Now, more than any other time in history, mental health professionals are combining components from these models in order to (1) prevent disorders, (2) maintain mental health, (3) formulate effective treatment methods for mental disorders when they occur, and (4) restore health and function after episodes occur.

Although some nursing theorists emphasized one or the other model, a majority of nurses maintained the holistic approach. They continued to follow the theory that all aspects of health depend on a combination of factors. As a result, they often used combined, or **eclectic**, treatment methods with their clients.

Definitions

To effectively interact and treat clients in any psychiatric setting, nurses must first understand the meaning of *mental health* and *mental disorder*. Both terms are complex and not easily defined. Several elements regulate a person's mental, emotional, and behavioral responses that result in health or disorder. This wide variety of factors makes it difficult to form simple, conclusive, operational definitions. Specific **indicators**, however, are identifiable in both mental health and in mental disorders, as described later.

Mental Health

Mental health is not merely the absence of mental disorder. Mental health originates in a person's *biology* and then is demonstrated in the type, quantity, and quality of that individual's *perceptions, thoughts, emotions, and behaviors*. Box 1-1 presents several factors indicative of mental health. In addition, the presence or absence of several other factors that influence a person's state of mental health are presented in Box 1-2.

Mental Disorder

Subjective, arbitrary diagnosing of mental disorders has been replaced by more definitive criteria. Researchers have formally identified and classified specific indicators for mental disorders. When clients show symptoms that meet defined criteria for a specific psychiatric disorder, they are assessed, and, when applicable, diagnoses are assigned.

Diagnostic Indicators. The use of reliable and valid tools with specific criteria makes the practice of identifying and determining psychiatric diagnoses objective and standardized, with the result that treatments are more specific and procedurally governed. In past centuries, subjective medical or judicial decisions often determined who was mentally ill. People frequently misunderstood and feared those with mental disorders. Without specific criteria that identified mental disorders, severely mentally ill individuals were arbitrarily taken to prisons or sent into back wards of psychiatric institutions, where many were mistreated or literally forgotten and abandoned instead of being treated. That changed dramatically in the twentieth century with increased knowledge about mental illness, and the use of standardized diagnostic criteria.

Sets of criteria with defining features indicate the type of mental disorders and are categorized to form diagnoses. Each diagnosis outlines symptoms that describe a specific psychiatric disorder. At this time, standardized classifications of psychiatric diagnoses are described in the *Diagnostic and Statistical Manual of Mental Disorders* (DSM-IV-TR) (American Psychiatric Association, 2000) and in the *International Classification of Diseases* (ICD-10) (World Health Organization, 1992). Diagnostic descriptions of psychiatric disorders in the two texts are very similar.

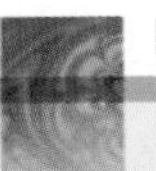

BOX 1-1

Indicators for Mental Health

- Intact anatomy and physiology of the brain and central nervous system
- Absence of signs and symptoms of mental disorder
- Freedom from excessive mental and emotional disability and pain
- Demonstrates mental and physical competence and skills
- Perceives self, others, and events correctly and realistically
- Recognizes own strengths, weaknesses, capabilities, and limitations
- Separates fantasy from reality
- Thinks clearly
  - Problem-solves
  - Uses good judgment
  - Reasons logically
  - Reaches insightful conclusions
- Negotiates each developmental stage
- Attains and maintains positive self-system
  - Self-concept
  - Self-image
  - Self-esteem
- Accepts self and others as uniquely different but humanly similar
- Appreciates life
- Finds beauty, joy, and goodness in self, others, and environment
- Is creative
- Is optimistic but realistic
- Is resilient
- Is autonomous
- Uses talents to fullest
- Involves self in purposeful, meaningful life work
- Engages in play
- Develops and demonstrates appropriate sense of humor
- Expresses emotions
- Exhibits congruent thoughts, feelings, and behaviors
- Accepts responsibility for actions
- Controls impulses and behavior
- Is accountable for own behaviors
- Respects societal rules and sanctions
- Learns from experiences
- Maintains wholesome values and belief system
- Copes with internal and external stressors in constructive and adaptive ways
- Returns to usual or higher function after crises
- Delays gratification
- Functions independently
- Maintains reasonable expectations concerning self and others
- Adapts to social environment
- Relates to others
  - Forms relationships
  - Maintains close, meaningful, loving, adaptive relationships
  - Works and plays well with others
  - Is intimate, appropriately and selectively
  - Responds to others in need
  - Feels and exhibits compassion and empathy toward others
  - Demonstrates culturally and socially acceptable interpersonal interactions
  - Manages interpersonal conflict constructively
  - Gives and receives gracefully
  - Learns from and teaches others
  - Functions interdependently
- Seeks self-actualization
- Attains self-defined spirituality

BOX 1-2

Influencing Factors for Mental Health or Disorder

- Inherited factors (genetic/familial)
  - Predisposition
  - Capacities
  - Limitations
- Pregnancy environment and experience (from conception to birth)
- Psychoneuroimmunologic factors
- Biochemical influences
- Hormonal influences
- Family
  - Composition
  - Birth position
  - Bonding
  - Members' mental health
- Developmental events
  - Completion of clearly defined stages
  - Resolution of developmental crises
- Cultures
- Subcultures
- Values
- Belief systems
- Perception of self
- Cognitive abilities
  - Capacity
  - Volition
- Personality traits and states
  - Competence
  - Resilience
  - Motivation
- Goals, aspirations
- Worldview
- Internal stressors
- External stressors
- Support system
  - Choice
  - Availability
  - Quality
- Demographic factors
- Geographic location
- Health practices and beliefs
- Spirituality/religion
- Negative influences
  - Internal/external
  - Mental disorders
  - Crime
  - Drugs
  - Psychosocial stressors
  - Poverty

Nurses can learn more about mental disorders by learning the defining criteria. The careful blending of psychiatric and the nursing content in this textbook offers a comprehensive representation of mental disorders and the most current nursing and medical treatment methods. This book combines psychiatric diagnoses according to the DSM classification with nursing diagnoses and all steps of the nursing process. Chapters in Part II of this text present thorough descriptions and discussions of the most common mental disorders. Also included in the chapters are three nursing taxonomies to use with clients who have psychiatric disorders or who are experiencing life crises. These three are the North American Nursing Diagnosis Association International taxonomy (NANDA-I, 2007-2008), the Nursing Interventions Classification (NIC) (Dochterman and Bulechek, 2004), and the Nursing Outcomes Classification (NOC) (Moorhead, Johnson, and Maas, 2004).

Symptoms alone do not determine mental disorders. In addition to client's symptoms, another indicator of mental disorders is the client's level of function, as measured by use of a standard assessment tool, such as the Global Assessment of Function (GAF) Scale (APA, 2000) (see Appendix C). The nursing taxonomies also include indicators of client function.

Diagnoses* Do Not *Define Clients. Many factors are considered when diagnosing mental disorders, and the primary consideration is the person who receives the diagnosis. With that in mind, an essential principle for PMH nurses, states that the client is an individual, separate from his or her disorder. Nurses never define the client by his or her diagnosis. Instead they continue to think of the client as a person who has been assigned a diagnosis. This simple but major shift in thinking greatly affects a nurse's **attitude** toward clients. The commitment to maintain a therapeutic attitude is vital and ultimately will affect client treatments, outcomes, and general well-being. The following communication between the registered nurse (RN) and staff members illustrates this principle, the nontherapeutic attitude.

NONTHERAPEUTIC

"There goes the peace and quiet. A polysubstance abuser has been on a 4-day binge and is coming over from the ER. She's also a bipolar manic. She is screaming and swearing at the staff one minute then joking and trying to seduce everyone in sight the next minute. Be prepared for her and watch her closely to make sure she doesn't bother the other clients. Put her alone in a room."

Note that the nurse identifies the client by her disorder. The following scenario illustrates an opposite effect, the therapeutic attitude.

THERAPEUTIC

"The emergency room just called. We will admit a 30-year-old female with a diagnosis of bipolar mania. She also has a history of polysubstance abuse and has been using drugs heavily for several days. She is exhibiting excessively labile mood swings and has been screaming, swearing, and acting seductively toward staff. We will admit her to a quiet area for now to reduce stimulation and temporarily separate her from the other clients who are vulnerable. Talk calmly with her and continue to observe her closely. Be sure she is well hydrated and monitor all of her other functions."

The nurse in the first scenario was judgmental, exhibited a lack of respect in her message to the staff, and placed a negative **label** on the client before meeting her. The nurse also undoubtedly influenced the staff by using unprofessional terms to describe the client. In contrast, note the communication of respect in the second scenario. The nurse describes the situation of a client who was being admitted because of her symptoms that were out of control, clearly communicating to staff that the client is a person with a diagnosis. Note also how the nurse considered treatment of the whole person, and not merely her psychiatric symptoms, by reminding staff to care for the client's almost certainly neglected physical needs.

These examples emphasize how attitudes of the nurse and the staff directly and indirectly affect our clients and client outcomes. Disrespectful labeling of clients by their diagnoses influences the way the nurse thinks about and approaches a client. When the nurse views the client as an individual who needs assistance, instead of as a troublesome diagnosis, the nurse will convey acceptance and respect. In turn, the client will usually perceive the nurse's interactions and interventions as facilitative and respond in the most cooperative way he or she is able at that time. Both client and nurse will benefit from the quality of this type of transaction. The nurse's role is important because the rest of the staff takes direction from the RN's demeanor and behavior. When the nurse models therapeutic interactions, he or she sets the tone for the staff to follow in providing total client care.

Unique Responses. *Individual* is the operative word when considering psychiatric diagnoses, and it implies each person's unique responses. Clients rarely exhibit symptoms that follow the textbook exactly. Nurses and others who regularly practice in psychiatric mental health settings know that two clients who have the same clinical mental disorder and diagnosis can express symptoms differently. This is due to each client's unique makeup, unique experience with, and unique responses to the disorder. Nurses keep their expectations open rather than fixed about client responses and behaviors. Nursing flexibility is a key for open, effective interactions. It requires a great deal of experience to be proficient at making diagnoses. Take caution that nurses do not label any person with a psychiatric diagnosis, unless they have advanced licensing permits. When first learning about psychiatric diagnoses, it is sometimes tempting to begin randomly assigning labels to those who are a challenge.

Mind and Body Interaction. Authors of *Mental Health: A Report of the Surgeon General* (USDHHS, 1999), the DSM-IV-TR (APA, 2000), and several other reports on mental health and illness emphasize that mind and body are inseparable when considering diagnoses and treatment of any client. Nurses agree with this concept in theory and practice. Mind and body are inextricably linked, and disruption of one will almost always cause dysfunction in the other, as illustrated by the following two examples:

> Courtney, a 35-year-old female, was enthusiastic and satisfied in her role as wife and mother of three. She and her husband and children were a closely knit family. Courtney helped manage her husband's business, volunteered in the children's school activities, was active in their church, and found time and energy to socialize with her many friends. On a routine annual visit, the physician told Courtney that she had a tumor in her breast; it was later diagnosed as cancer with metastasis. An extensive surgical mastectomy was performed, followed by chemotherapy. Courtney was surrounded by people who cared about her and helped her, but she began to stay in bed more each day, stopped attending to the needs of her home and family, quit her favorite activities, and started to reject her family's show of affection. She refused to see friends, and one day said she wanted to die, stating a well-organized plan. Courtney was diagnosed with clinical major depression and admitted to an acute care facility for her safety and for observation, medication, and interactive therapies.

This scenario demonstrates the interdependence of mind-body systems. Courtney's medical condition led to her diagnosis of major depression with suicide ideation and intent to harm herself. The next scenario further illustrates the point from another view:

> Jack was a 19-year-old male freshman in college. He managed to complete his academic work with good grades and still have time to see his high school girlfriend Myling, who attended the same college. During midterm exams Jack began acting suspicious, accusing Myling of going out with one of his friends when she said she was studying with classmates. He also started hallucinating, hearing voices that frightened him. Jack told Myling about the voices. His symptoms confused and worried her, and she refused to see him. Jack started to drink alcohol daily and use other drugs to escape and "feel better." He started to neglect personal hygiene, stopped eating regular meals, missed classes, and became more disorganized and unable to concentrate or complete his schoolwork. Jack's landlord found him in his rented room; Jack had not eaten or slept for several days. He had soiled his clothes and bed, and he was incoherent, rambling about the enemy who was trying to poison him. Jack was taken to an emergency room and diagnosed with an acute psychotic episode, dehydration, and malnutrition.

This example shows the bodily responses to an undeniable and debilitating mental disorder. When Jack's parents came to take him home, the physician told them Jack possibly had schizophrenia. In addition to supporting the psychiatric treatment regimen, they were told to continue monitoring his basic needs and functions—such as adequate food and fluid intake, rest, and elimination—because he was unable to care for himself at the time. Jack's mental disorder and responses to several major losses culminated in a notable disruption of his bodily functions, further emphasizing the inseparable connection between mind and body. Together, their delicate interaction equates to mental and physical health or disorder.

Statistical Reality

The number of mental disorders in the United States and in the world is notable. Several commissioned reports cited at the beginning of this chapter stated that mental health is a basic right, reserved for all people. Despite this widely agreed upon statement, approximately 26.2% of the adult population in the United States in any given year has a diagnosable mental disorder, and approximately 9% to 13% of those are in the category of seriously mentally ill (Kessler et al., 2005; Manderscheid and Henderson, 2002; NIMH statistics, 2006) (Figure 1-2). This means that more than one person in every four in the United States has a diagnosable mental disorder.

Global Predictions

A frequently quoted collaborative report conducted by the World Health Organization, the World Bank, and Harvard University describes the burden of mental illness on health and productivity in the United States and the world. The study, titled *The Global Burden of Disease* (WHO, 1999a), revealed that many earlier reports underestimated the impact of mental disorders on society. The study shows that mental illness accounts for over 15% of the burden of disease throughout the world. Earlier reports did not take into consideration the important factors of *death* and *disability* caused by mental disorders when figuring the burden of disease, but researchers factored both criteria into this more recent report. The results present a clearer picture of the damaging effects of mental disorders, which were previously unrecognized. The study findings in Figure 1-3 provide information and notable predictions for 2020. Note in the table that major depression will rank second among all noninfectious diseases, and researchers predict it will be a leading cause of disability or death by 2020.

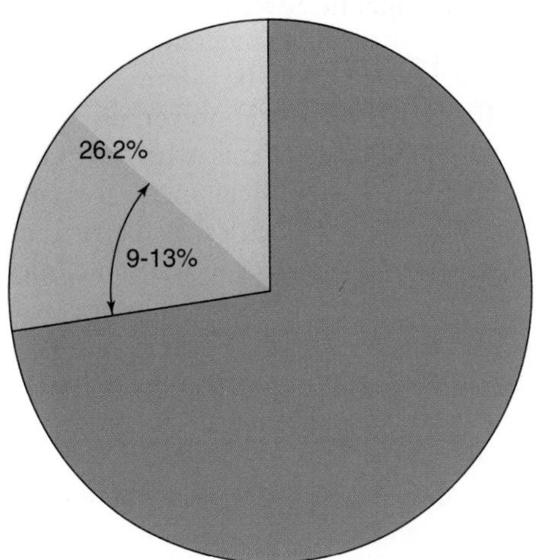

FIGURE 1-2 Approximately 26.2% of the adult population of the United States has a diagnosable mental disorder; 9% to 13% are seriously mentally ill (SMI). (From Kessler R et al: Prevalence, severity, comorbidity of 12 month survey replication, *Arch Gen Psychiatr* 6:617-627, 2005.)

Increasing Burden of Noncommunicable Diseases and Injuries

1999 Disease or injury	2020 Disease or injury
1. Acute lower respiratory infections	1. Ischemic heart disease
2. HIV/AIDS	2. Unipolar major depression
3. Perinatal conditions	3. Road traffic injuries
4. Diarrheal diseases	4. Cerebrovascular disease
5. Unipolar major depression	5. Chronic obstructive pulmonary disease
6. Ischemic heart disease	6. Lower respiratory infections
7. Cerebrovascular disease	7. Tuberculosis
8. Malaria	8. War
9. Road traffic injuries	9. Diarrheal diseases
10. Chronic obstructive pulmonary disease	10. HIV
11. Congenital abnormalities	11. Perinatal conditions
12. Tuberculosis	12. Violence
13. Falls	13. Congenital abnormalities
14. Measles	14. Self-inflicted injuries
15. Anemias	15. Trachea, bronchus and lung cancers

FIGURE 1-3 Change in rank order of disability-adjusted life years for the 15 leading causes (baseline scenario). (From World Health Organization: *The global burden of disease: a comprehensive assessment of mortality and disability from diseases, injuries, and risk factors in 1999 and projected to 2020,* vol 1, Geneva, 2000, WHO.)

Nursing Implications

Based on both present and predicted statistics for mental disorders here and in other chapters throughout this textbook, it appears essential that nurses have solid knowledge of all aspects of mental health and mental disorders, regardless of the discipline they choose for a career. PMHN curriculum and practicum are standard requirements for completing registered nursing programs, but nurses will use PMHN content throughout their careers. With the known fact that over 25% of the population has diagnosable mental disorders, nurses can plan to care for clients with diagnosed or undiagnosed mental disorders no matter which specialty they choose for employment.

The majority of acutely mentally disordered clients who require treatment will be admitted to psychiatric practices, programs, or units. However, unexpectedly, and frequently unannounced, clients with mental disorders appear in emergency rooms, in medical-surgical units, and in departments of obstetrics, pediatrics, neurology, and geriatrics; they also appear in walk-in clinics, client's homes, schools, prisons, physician's offices, and in all other areas where nurses work. Nurses need to be prepared to foster and support clients' mental well-being, in addition to recognize psychiatric impairment and dysfunction when and wherever it occurs.

A working understanding of both mental health and mental disorders enables nurses to identify the manifestations of each and effectively interact with clients who demonstrate all types of cognitive, emotional, and behavioral states. Within the scope of their education and level of practice, nurses use assessment skills and intervene with psychiatric symptoms when and where they arise, as well as other health care needs that accompany psychiatric episodes. Nurses must also understand when a client's condition or situation exceeds the nurse's scope of practice and when it is necessary to make appropriate referrals. The nurse's PMHN preparation, readiness, and skills will be used throughout his or her career.

Underserved Population

Significant statistics about mental illness have not improved overall mental health services for the mentally ill. Service for this population falls short of meeting their needs, especially for the poor and those referred to as *persistently mentally ill* or the *seriously mentally ill*—those with long term, chronic mental disorders. Figure 1-4 depicts the actual services provided to adults and children.

Major improvement in health care for the mentally ill is necessary and overdue. Consider the following research: "Improving the Quality of Health Care for Mental and Substance Use Conditions" (IOM, 2006), *Achieving the Promise: Transforming Mental Health Care in America* (USDHHS, 2003), *Mental Health: A Report of the Surgeon General* (USDHHS, 1999), and "Making a Difference" (WHO, 1999). The following suggests areas for improving the quality of care in mental health:

- More effective *resource allocation*, specifically adequate funding and improved use of funds
- Accelerated integration of *scientific research and treatment modalities*
- Increased efforts to reduce *stigma*

Resource Allocation. Adequate funding is necessary to meet client needs, and equally important is the allocation and use of available funds. As a sign of the times, funding for mental health varies and often terminates in a lack of funds for direct client care. On the national level, funding for mental health is unnecessarily complicated and differs from that of other health care segments. It therefore needs to be simplified and streamlined. Also the managed care and managed behavioral health care models that currently dominate and operate health care often dictate payment schedules that interfere with effective and appropriate treatment for clients with mental disorders. The needs of clients frequently go unmet as they try to find their way through the administrative maze to reach adequate services. Healthy, intelligent people often have problems with these systems, so it is easy to imagine and understand how difficult and frustrating it is for the mentally disordered population to get help.

In addition, governing bodies and laws are often out of step with the provision of services. There is a shortage of serious, active advocates on national, state, and city legislative levels to affect changes in the quantity and quality of care for this population. Also, each governing level separately mandates assistance and provisions for this group. Some states have instituted innovative means to accomplish that mandate. Consider, for example, the law recently enacted in California. After experiencing several years of inadequate funding for mental health programs, voters

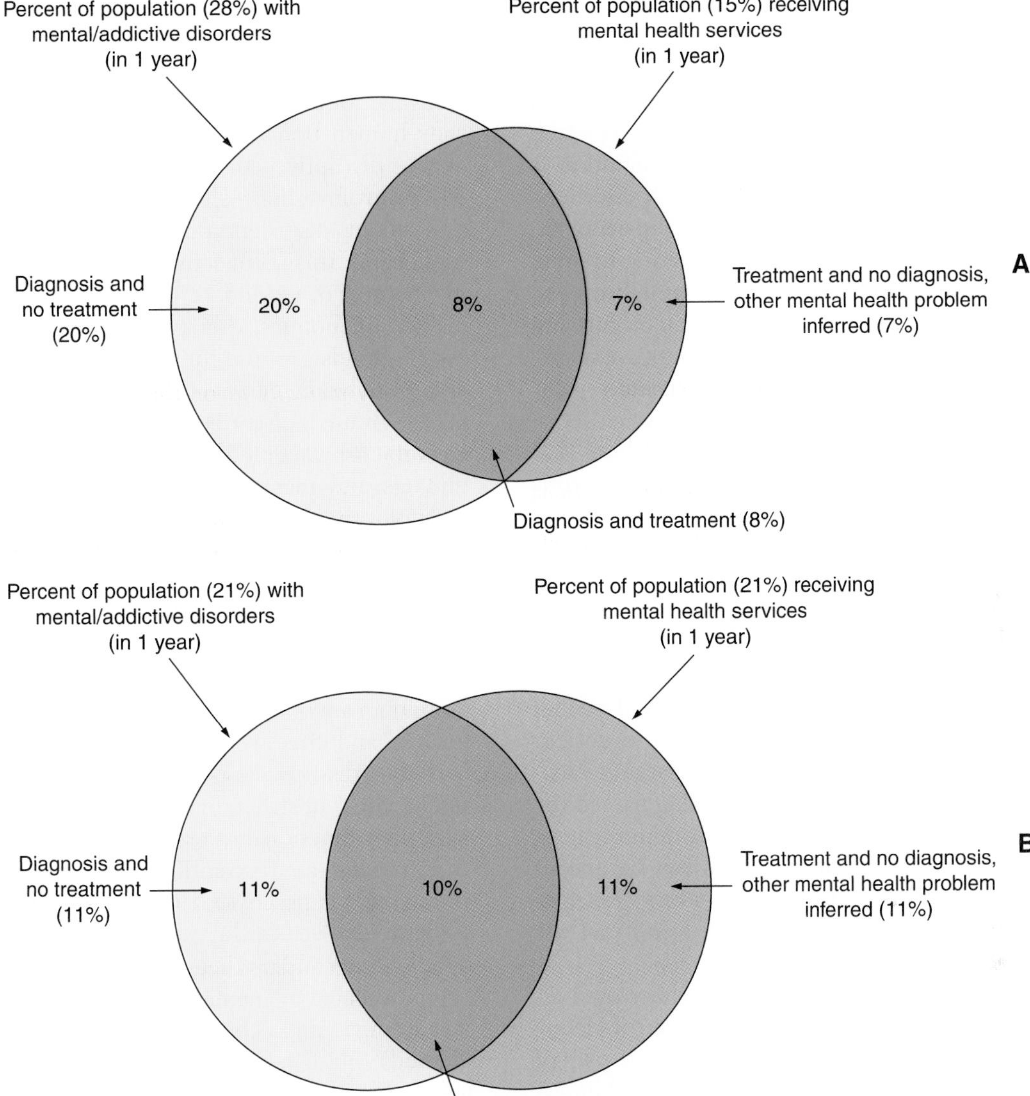

FIGURE 1-4 Annual prevalence of mental/addictive disorders and services for adults **(A)** and children **(B)**. (**A** from Regier D et al: The de facto US mental and addictive disorders service system: epidemiologic catchment area prevalence rates of disorders and services, *Arch Gen Psychiatry* 50:85, 1993; and Kessler RC et al: The 12 month prevalence and correlates of serious mental illness. In Manderscheid R, Sonnenschein M, editors: *Mental health, United States 1996,* Department of Health and Human Services Publication No. (SMA) 96-3098, Washington, DC, 1996, US Government Printing Office. **B** from Schaffer D et al: The NIMH diagnostic interview schedule for children: methods for the epidemiology of child and adolescent mental disorders study, *J Am Acad Child Adolescent Psychiatry* 35:865-877, 1996.)

actively took the matter into their own hands, changing state law that resulted in increased funding by imposing a special tax on the wealthy. In November of 2004, Proposition 63 was passed, morphing the state's Mental Health Services Act into law. One mandate states that those earning a million or more dollars annually will contribute 1% of their reported tax income toward care of the mentally ill. Funds for mental health increased significantly as a result and began the serious allocation of collected assets and increased authorization of treatments.

On the other hand, the National Institutes of Mental Health (NIMH) reported another aspect of funding in a retrospective review of several years of epidemiologic studies. The NIMH stated that even in times when health care providers increased traditional treatments, the number of mentally disordered persons remained fairly constant under current treatment modes (Kessler, 2005). The report suggests that continuing problems in the mental health care arena are due to more than insufficient funds or their allocation, and it emphasizes that some treatment methods require changes. In keeping with that suggestion, many changes are evolving as a result of current research in the neurosciences that will affect treatment methods.

Integration of Research and Treatment. The application of scientific findings to clinical practice is a primary goal for mental health research. However, in the midst of an explosion of research directed toward mental disorders, there remains a gap between current research and treatment modalities. Their effective integration is one solution for reducing prevalence of mental disorders. Researchers have made major discoveries in the neurosciences and imaging methods, particularly relating to brain structure and function, and their role in mental disorders. Innovative scientific research focusing on the origins and physiology of mental disorders has grown in the past several decades, having an impact on psychiatry and psychiatric nursing. Each year the neurosciences move closer to presenting conclusive findings regarding the causes and outcomes of mental disorders. That research will ultimately produce recommendations for the prevention of mental disorders and improvement of client treatment modalities.

Over the past half century, the methods of scientific research for defining mental disorders and determining etiologies and treatment methods have changed dramatically. We learned more about mental health and mental disorders during the last three decades of the twentieth century than any other time in history. Research blossomed in the 1990s, resulting in that era being named the "Decade of the Brain." Although serious work in the neurosciences began before that decade, few significant changes occurred to adequately ease the burden of mental disorders. Health care became a national priority at the turn of the century.

During the twenty-first century, there was increased effort to fund and launch research for the purposes of identifying biologic bases and effective treatments for mental disorders. Before this time, record costs for mental illness manifested in several forms, including the following:

- The loss of function and productivity weighed heavily on individuals with mental disorders, as well as on their families, and society.
- Clients were underserved and went untreated.
- Lives were lost as a result of mental illness.
- Treatment costs were at an all-time high and increasing annually.
- Public and private funds were spent on unsuccessful research.

Advances in Neuroscience. At the door to the new millennium, hopeful clinicians and clients looked forward with anticipation toward continued acceleration of progress that stemmed from the new information in neurosciences and related fields. Several discoveries are now helping to transform neuropsychiatry and are unlocking the secrets of mental disorders. Among these are human genome projects that opened avenues for further neurobiologic research that will influence psychiatric mental health (Schuler, 1996). Other innovative projects aimed at untangling the mysteries of mental disorders include studies from molecular biology, DNA research, brain mapping, stem cell research, and neurotransmitter tracking. In addition, several increasingly sophisticated computerized neuroimaging instruments such as magnetic resonance imaging (MRI), positron emission tomography (PET scans), among others enable researchers and clinicians to view human brain function during inactive periods and during disruptive episodes of specific mental disorders. The neuroimaging techniques provide pictorial information about disorders that previously were considered mysterious. Images of actual brain functions are presented in Chapters 6, 11, and 12.

Neurogenomics, the study of genes and the nervous system, holds promise for fueling a golden age of discovery in the neurosciences (Allen Brain Atlas, 2006; Gewin, 2005). Brain biology researchers work to find biologic answers for mental disorders. Their projects produce findings and recommendations that address prevention and point the way to innovative, effective treatment methods for costly mental disorders. Several new treatments will develop from this research (McGriffin, 2001).

Relevance for Clients and Caregivers. Research outcomes are promising for clients (individuals, families, and communities) who suffer from mental disorders. Clients, more than anyone continue to wait in hopeful expectation for new and effective interventions for the mental disorders that disrupt their quality of life and relationships, significantly obstruct or prevent growth, and interfere with their function and productivity.

Emerging neuroscientific developments are also encouraging for psychiatric nurses and other professionals who are involved in the care of clients with mental disorders. Current and predicted statistics related to numbers of people affected by mental illness each year make it evident that changes must continue toward perfecting treatment methods on all levels of care, to adequately meet client needs. Rapid scientific changes and evolving discoveries pose challenges for psychiatric mental health nurses and other care providers to keep pace. Nursing must commit to remaining current in scientific research and developments as well as integrating treatment methods that impact their client care. An ultimate goal is reduction of the large and growing numbers of mentally disordered individuals in this country and throughout the world.

Stigma. In addition to the issues of funding and integrating research and treatment, stigma remains a major obstacle for the mentally ill and another reason why their needs and those of their families are inadequately met (IOM, 2006; USDHHS, 1999). **Stigma** produces a negative attitude with a result that people with mental disorders are often ignored, mistreated, or alienated.

A heavy burden, or problem, exists for the mentally disordered population. The *primary burden* comes from experiencing and living with the symptoms of one or more mental disorders and the life disruption that follows. A *secondary burden* comes from the formal psychiatric diagnosis, which acts as a label and an identity for the client who then becomes known by his or her diagnosis. Some clients describe the diagnosis as a "brand" or a "scar" that marks them and changes their lives. Psychiatric diagnoses hold a negative connotation for people who do not understand mental disorders, resulting in stereotypes and judgments upon clients and their families. Some clients say they are not treated as individuals but as an outlying group, and they feel ashamed because of their psychiatric diagnoses.

Many other health disorders do not carry the stigma that is associated with psychiatric disorders. Through biologic research it is clear that major mental disorders are brain based disorders. They are therefore considered similar to other disorders of the body, such as those of the pancreas (diabetes), the heart (coronary artery disease), or the immune system (lymphoma). Most individuals believe there is little choice or control over getting one of these diseases. People do not choose to get major mental disorders either, but in those cases stigma is a frequent by-product. The general public often fears what it does not understand. Symptoms of mental illness often occur in ways that frighten or even repulse the inexperienced observer. When this occurs, the mentally ill suffer.

There are many reasons for the stigmatization of mental disorders. All forms of the media are primary sources for fueling this ongoing problem, which continues each year as giant film and television industries create tales of the mentally ill as violent and dangerous. They sensationalize unfortunate brain illnesses for economic purposes. The fact is that a very small percentage of clients are violent or dangerous, and the majority of people with mental disorders more often withdraw from interpersonal contact. Videogames, newspapers, magazines, and novels also portray the mentally ill in negative ways, at a heavy cost to innocent millions with mental disorders.

Reduction of Stigma. Many disciplines are working tirelessly to decrease this stigma. Nurses act as advocates for clients with mental disorders by helping to increase respect and reduce stereotypes, judgments, and labels that accompany mental disorders. Each national psychiatric nursing organization tries to reduce the stigma attached to mental disorders.

Several national organizations such as the National Association for Mental Illness (NAMI) strongly support and legislate for respect and acceptance of the mentally ill. Some methods include providing family and public education and personally involving the clients and families in their care and helping them take responsibility for their futures. NAMI lobbies in the legislature for changes in the treatment and care of this population. In addition, to decrease stigma, the American Psychiatric Association, states in their DSM-IV-TR that the diagnostic categories classify disorders and does not classify or stigmatize people (APA, 2000). Many religious organizations have taken on the cause of caring for the mentally ill. Exact statistics are not available, but these beneficent organizations provide a significant amount of daily basic care.

Psychiatric nurses who understand the stigma associated with mental disorders play an important role when intervening to prevent stigma or to minimize the outcomes. A major force in ending stigmas begins within the nursing profession in everyday encounters with clients and in interdisciplinary communication between nurses and other health care professionals. Nurses additionally have every opportunity through education to help change general public opinion about people with mental disorders. These opportunities exist in acute care facilities; outpatient settings; local, national, and international nursing and psychiatric organizations; and the governing bodies who make laws to protect our clients. When nurses reduce stigma, clients are treated fairly in health care systems and receive acceptance and respect. There is still much to do in this area.

Stigma and Diagnoses. Although formal diagnoses label clients, they also serve important functions. It may seem that changing or eliminating formal diagnoses for mental disorders is one way to avoid stigma, but it is not a practical solution. While diagnoses contribute to stigma, their positive aspects outweigh the negative. Diagnoses describe and classify mental disorders and also affect communication, treatment, funding, prognosis, and research.

Communication. Classifications of psychiatric disorders are clearly defined and organized into diagnostic categories making it easier to learn and understand the disorders and reasons for selecting treatment regimens. Each psychiatric diagnosis represents a specific set of symptoms that remains constant and thereby facilitates communication between and among staff members and other collaborative health team members. Staff members are able to state or write a diagnosis that conveys a general picture of a client's disorder without having to stop and explain symptoms each time. Mental health care providers are continually aware that each client will express symptoms in his or her own unique ways, but the diagnosis serves as an important communication tool. Diagnoses also help clients. Specific diagnoses provide clear explanations that help clients and their families to learn about their disorders, understand the symptoms, cooperate with treatment regimens, and form realistic expectations about prognoses.

Treatment. Diagnoses guide the treatment of a client. Each diagnosis alerts the staff to potential client needs and problems and helps staff members to plan symptom-specific treatment. While listening to morning report, the staff members will plan an initial approach, interaction, and treatment method for each client, based on their diagnoses. For example, a client with a diagnosis of major depression who is isolating and withdraws from engaging with others will receive treatment that is different from that of a client with a diagnosis of bipolar mania who is acting out physically and verbally in the psychiatric unit. Though psychiatric health care personnel use specific individual treatment plans, diagnoses provide an overall initial direction for interventions.

Nurses in PMHN learn that the goal of treatment for several mental disorders does not include expectations for a cure. Instead, a realistic expectation for clients is management of their symptoms with staff assistance. Successful treatment sometimes means that the client is able to return home at the same level of function he or she had before the current episode. Stabilization is often the main treatment goal for clients with any diagnosis that results in numerous acute, recurrent episodes. Diagnoses help to govern treatment levels and maintain realistic expectations.

Funding. Regardless of the type of psychiatric mental health setting, delivering services and providing client care depends on money. With the current managed care model controlling client care, it is important to note that client diagnoses dictate the type and amount of treatment, length of stay, discharge criteria, and aftercare provisions. Clients must meet specific criteria to receive funding, regardless of the source, and at this time the client's diagnosis is a major factor.

Prognosis. Each diagnosis carries a potential built-in prognosis that varies depending on several factors. Some of the factors are the client's age, the severity and persistence of symptoms, the rate of recurrent episodes, the client's individual resilience, available and sustained resources, and an adequate support system. Some psychiatric diagnoses carry a more favorable prognosis than others, as seen in the following examples:

Client A develops symptoms in her first episode of an adjustment disorder when her husband is sent to the Middle East with his military squadron during wartime.

Client B exhibits severe and persistent symptoms of disorganized type schizophrenia and has three acute episodes in 1 year.

The prognosis is more favorable for client A, whose symptoms and diagnosis will likely abate with the following interventions: supportive nursing care; identifying and ensuring a familial or other support system while her husband is away; temporary use of symptom-specific medications; temporary interactive or group therapy. The prognosis for client B, however, is less favorable because the diagnosis signifies a chronic course of illness with acute exacerbations and increasing frequency and severity of symptoms over time. This client requires ongoing care.

It is important to remain realistic but hopeful regarding client prognosis for any diagnosis, as well as to convey hope to clients and significant others when possible. Part II describes in more detail the prognosis for each psychiatric diagnosis.

Research. Diagnoses and the psychopathology they represent drive research. In the biology field, current research includes the neurobiology of specific disorders; detecting and identifying brain function that occurs with specific diagnoses; and genetic research probes for gene markers to identify mania, depression, or obsessive compulsive disorder. Researchers have discovered and altered medications by observing symptom modifications of specific diagnoses through neurotransmitter tracking. Neuroimaging detects altered brain structures in schizophrenia and brain function such as occurs with depression, anxiety, and drug use. Major research also continues within social and interpersonal fields. Researchers use different focuses and techniques to promote mental health, prevent and treat mental disorders with clients (individuals, families, groups, community, societies), and restore client function. Much of this research is also based on specific psychiatric diagnoses.

ROLE OF THE NURSE

Nurses are well positioned to formulate and implement changes that will ultimately benefit clients. Many changes that occur throughout a health care system begin with recommendations from nurses who work in close contact with clients throughout varied experiences providing them with primary, effective **evidence-based** care. Such is the case in the psychiatric setting, where many nurses have varied skills and practice methods but share common client-centered objectives. Psychiatric mental health nursing is a specialized area of the nursing practice that utilizes a wide range of theories and research on "human behavior as its science and the purposeful use of self as its art" (American Nurses Association, 2006).

Melding Science and the Art of Nursing

Effective nursing care of clients in any mental health setting depends on successfully integrating the science and the art of PMHN. With increased experience and practice, the art and science of nursing are inseparable. Although it is important for all nurses to be current in the basic and emerging sciences, it is equally if not more important for them to master the *art* of nursing and communication.

The word *art* is sometimes misunderstood. To some, art means creativity, being free and spontaneous, relying solely on feelings and intuition. Although elements of creativity will surface during client care, the art of interacting with clients in PMH nursing is built on sound education and thoughtful planning and intervention. For any art to become purposeful requires intention, commitment, time, and effort to learn its principles and guidelines and to practice the necessary skills. Meaningful creativity will naturally follow and be beneficial to clients.

The Therapeutic Alliance

A primary aspect of working with clients in any psychiatric setting is developing a **therapeutic alliance**. This alliance is a professional bond that exists between a nurse and a client and often plays a significant role in client well-being. The therapeutic alliance begins in the **nurse-client relationship** and is the cornerstone of nursing interventions in any psychiatric setting. The nurse-client relationship is not ordinary friendship but rather is guided by standards and objectives that are thoroughly described in later chapters.

Although a therapeutic alliance benefits the nurse by facilitating the interpersonal process, the alliance is primarily for clients. It serves as a vehicle for clients to freely discuss their needs and problems in the absence of judgment and criticism, gain insight, learn and practice new skills, effect life changes, heal mental and emotional wounds, and promote growth. The nurse must provide a safe environment for this relationship to occur.

The alliance begins with the nurse's

- Knowledge of principles that guide the formation and maintenance of the nurse client relationship and its inherent responsibilities
- Understanding the relational aspects of all nursing interventions and interactions
- Knowledge, understanding, and commitment to maintaining healthy boundaries
- Willingness to engage and interact with clients and guide them on their return to wellness
- Commitment to practice nursing interventions and interactions within prescribed reliable guidelines and to integrate time-tested interpersonal skills
- Inclusion of the client in the therapeutic process that focuses on the client's health
- Encouragement of client responsibility for his or her own health, within the client's capacity

Individuals who enter nursing for their life work must first like people, enjoy interacting with them, and sincerely want to help them. These altruistic and affective qualities, which are important for anyone who works with clients, are imperative for psychiatric nurses. Caring, however, is not enough. Altruism and its affective components must be accompanied by cognitive objectives, learned skills, and conscious motivation, intention, and direction. Nurses who enter helping relationships learn that intentions and motives for helping others are complex. Chapter 2 contains a section titled *Helping: The Concept and the Activity*, which clarifies this issue, guides the reader in the art of helping others, and offers direction for incorporating client-centered skills. Also, review the discussion of Johari's window in Chapter 4 (see Figure 4-2), which further clarifies the need to understand one's own intentions while helping others.

Commitment is necessary to actively and skillfully engage with clients, assisting them to meet their needs and solve their problems. The term *active* signifies the nurse's balanced participation in the client's process of overcoming obstacles to mental health. This includes giving assistance to clients who are unable to manage their own present situation because of the severity of their symptoms or a crisis event, but it does not imply taking charge of the clients' lives, leaving them to passively participate in their own care.

One of the more significant objectives for nurses is assisting clients to maintain their independence within their capacity to do so. This is especially important today when therapy and treatment time are dramatically short. New nurses sometimes miss the importance of encouraging clients to manage as many aspects of their own lives as possible, even when the outcomes do not appear perfect to the nurse. In their enthusiastic need to help others, nurses sometimes find it easier to do things and complete projects for the client, versus doing them with the client or waiting until the client acts on his or her own behalf. This encourages the client's dependence on others. Fostering independence is one of the client's main goals and ensures higher function when the client is on his or her own. Balance implies the nurse's careful assessment of each situation and encouraging clients to assume responsibility for their health whenever able. The skill-based therapeutic alliance makes this possible, as it becomes a partnership with its focus on clients and their goals, and both parties working together toward those goals.

Principles of the Nurse-Client Relationship

The therapeutic interpersonal relationship that develops between the nurse and the client is an important factor for effecting client change and growth. The following are principles and guidelines for developing and maintaining the relationship:

- The relationship is therapeutic rather than social.
- The focus remains on the client's needs and problems rather than on the nurse or other issues.
- The relationship is purposeful and goal directed.
- The relationship is objective rather than subjective in quality.
- The relationship is time limited rather than open ended.

Therapeutic vs. Social. A therapeutic relationship is formed to help clients solve problems, make decisions, achieve growth, learn coping strategies, let go of unwanted behaviors, reinforce self-worth, and examine relationships. The meetings between the nurse and the client are not for mutual satisfaction. Although the nurse can be friendly with the client, the nurse is not there to be the client's friend. Because boundaries define nurses and their roles and are important in any relationship, especially in a therapeutic relationship, trying to be a client's friend blurs boundaries and confuses roles. The nurse helps the client increase his or her awareness of boundaries and practice boundary setting. Box 1-3 gives some examples the nurse can use to assist clients in recognizing boundary violations.

Some social conversation is usual at the beginning of meetings and helps to establish or maintain rapport. Occasionally during meetings, superficial or social conversations briefly reappear, but the nurse must keep the majority of conversations focused and therapeutic. Table 1-1 compares therapeutic and social interactions.

Client Focus. Frequently during a session, a client redirects the focus away from self by changing the subject, talking about the weather, focusing on the nurse (nurse's appearance, personal problems, problems in the environment), or other issues. The nurse recognizes divergent tactics that are usually a form of resistance. The nurse confronts the diversion in a matter-of-fact way and refocuses the topic. Clients do this for one or more of several reasons: fear of being judged, resistance to discussing anxiety-producing material, boredom, repetition of material previously discussed with other therapists, or inability to stay cognitively focused because of a mental disorder.

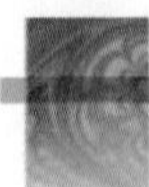

BOX 1-3

Signs of Unhealthy Boundaries

- Going against personal values or rights to please another
- Not noticing when someone displays inappropriate boundaries
- Not noticing when someone invades your boundaries
- Talking at an intimate level on the first meeting
- Falling in love with a new acquaintance
- Falling in love with anyone who reaches out
- Being overwhelmed by (preoccupied with) a person
- Acting on first sexual impulse
- Being sexual for your partner, not yourself
- Accepting food, gifts, touch, or sex that you do not want
- Touching a person without asking
- Taking as much as you can for the sake of getting
- Giving as much as you can for the sake of giving
- Allowing someone to take as much as they can from you
- Letting others direct your life
- Letting others describe your reality
- Letting others define you
- Believing others can anticipate your needs
- Expecting others to fill your needs automatically
- Falling apart so someone will take care of you
- Self-abuse
- Sexual and physical abuse
- Food abuse
- Loaning money you do not have
- Flirting; sending mixed messages
- Telling all

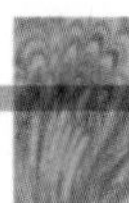

TABLE 1-1

Therapeutic vs. Social Interactions

THERAPEUTIC	SOCIAL
Offer client therapeutic assistance	Give and receive friendship equally
Focus on client's needs	Meet both person's needs
Discuss client's perceptions, thoughts, feelings, and behaviors	Share mutual ideas and experiences
Actively listen and use therapeutic communication skills and techniques	Give opinions and advice
Encourage client to choose subject for discussion	Randomly discuss topics at will or whim
Encourage client to problem-solve toward independence	Insist on helping as a friend; tolerate dependence
Keep no secrets that may harm client	Promise to keep secrets at any cost
Set goals with client	Recognize that goals of relationship are not important
Remain objective	Become subjectively involved
Maintain healthy boundaries	Accept blurred boundaries
Evaluate interactions with client	Avoid relational evaluations

Goal Direction. The primary purpose of a therapeutic relationship is helping clients to meet adaptive goals. Together the client and nurse determine problematic issues and collaboratively decide what the client needs and is able to achieve. Once goals are established, the nurse and the client agree to work toward those goals and put intentions into action, modifying strategies when necessary until the identified goals are achieved. The activities involved are usually many and varied, but each activity can be purposefully planned with the client's goals in mind.

Objective vs. Subjective. Nurses are therapeutic only when they remain objective. **Objective** refers to remaining free from bias, prejudice, and personal identification in interaction with the client and being able to process information based on facts. On the other hand, **subjective** refers to emphasis on one's own feelings, attitudes, and opinions when interacting with the client. When nurses act subjectively in relation to the client's problems or situations, they lose effectiveness in the relationship. With conscious intent to remain objective, the nurse will see situations and events realistically rather than identifying with the client or becoming overly and personally involved with the client's problems or needs. Of course, this approach does not imply that the nurse withdraws from feelings or constructs barriers to protect himself or herself by intellectualizing or avoiding responses. With knowledge, awareness, practice, and experience the nurse will be both objective and fully attentive to clients' situations and needs.

An example of *objectivity* versus subjectivity is the nurse's ability to remain empathic instead of becoming sympathetic when interacting with a client, even when having experienced a similar, painful situation. For example, consider a nurse who has lost a child in an accident and then encounters a client who is depressed and grieving the recent death of his or her own child. The nurse demonstrates objectivity by allowing and facilitating the client's full expression of thoughts and feelings and then responding in a warm, empathic way that remains client centered. This approach helps the client relieve pentup feelings in the normal grieving process, allows the client to feel understood, and helps the client to process and organize thoughts directed toward solving his or her own problems.

An example of *nontherapeutic subjectivity* is a nurse in the same situation who hears the client's expression of feelings and responds with excessive self-disclosure about his or her own similar experience. This approach represents a loss of therapeutic boundaries by identifying with the client's problem and becoming enmeshed in the situation by personalizing it. The client's response will most likely be negative. The client will probably stop sharing information because he or she feels unimportant and negated or because he or she worries that the nurse is fragile or the nurse is inept and cannot even manage his or her own problems, much less the client's problems. Clients compromised by their own conditions and situations cannot be burdened by the nurse's problems. Healthy nurses seek supervision or private therapy when personal problems arise and maintain fulfilling personal relationships outside of the work setting.

Time-Limited Interactions. Before establishing the relationship, the nurse sets necessary parameters by agreeing with the client on specific days and times when they will meet and the numbers of times meetings will take place. Such structure helps the client realize that this relationship has limits and is not open ended (e.g., the client cannot meet with the nurse whenever he or she wants and for as long as he or she wants). The principle of time-limited interaction is important for several reasons.

Sometimes clients have not learned during formative relationships that limits are important for all relationships and that without limits problems will occur. When participants define the amount of time they are willing and able to give, it eliminates anxiety-provoking guesswork. Individuals then decide how to make appropriate use of the time they have together. Also, all relationships have inevitable endings. Much grief is avoided if both the nurse and the client are certain of the boundaries of the relationship and enforce them together. The nurse-client relationship serves as a model for the client's subsequent relationships where he or she can successfully begin and appropriately end future alliances.

Stages of the Nurse-Client Relationship

The nurse-client relationship progresses through distinct stages. The nurse's knowledge and recognition of each stage facilitates the client's therapeutic progress.

Preorientation Stage. During this initial phase before the nurse and client ever meet, the nurse will accomplish several tasks. The first is to gather data about the client, his or her condition, and the present situation. Information is taken from all available sources (the client, client's chart, staff report, physician's report, input from family, or other reliable sources such as police and ambulance attendants).

From the information gathered, the nurse engages in a period of **autodiagnosis** regarding his or her thoughts, feelings, perceptions, and attitudes about this particular client. Judgmentalism, biases, or stereotyping sometimes arises that will influence the contact in a nontherapeutic way. For example, if the nurse learns information about a client that reminds him or her of a personal loved one or of a despised or feared person, the nurse's response to the client could be subjective, nontherapeutic, and ineffective if he or she does not recognize and examine the facts. The following is an example of a **critical thinking** tool:

Consider nurse A, whose father was dependent on alcohol and verbally abused her mother when he drank. What are some possible responses nurse A may demonstrate in the following situations if she fails to engage in autodiagnosis?

- A male client is admitted to the unit because of alcohol intoxication and wife abuse.
- A matronly female is admitted to the unit with major depression. Her husband drinks and abuses her, physically and emotionally.

Conscious efforts to examine each situation and put it in an objective perspective are important so that identification, judgmentalism, and stereotyping are avoided by the nurse.

Orientation Stage. After the nurse-client introduction, the relationship begins to grow. During this stage, participants become acquainted, build trust and rapport, and demonstrate acceptance of the process that develops when the client begins to work on his or her own important life issues.

The Contract. A contract is established in the orientation phase of the relationship. The contract is either formal or informal, written or verbal. Nurses most frequently use verbal, informal contracts with clients in acute care settings in which the client and nurse are continually together. It may become necessary for the nurse to write a more specific, formalized contract for clients who seek therapy outside of an acute care setting or when there is an expectation for a client behavior to continue (e.g., no self-harm contract).

Some contracts are short but still effective and efficient. For example, the nurse on an inpatient unit says to the client: "I will be your contact person while you are in (name the facility). I work Monday through Friday from 8 AM to 4 PM. Because of your schedule on this unit, it seems that the best time for us to meet is 9 AM. Is that a good time for you?" (nurse validates with client). If the client agrees, the contract is established.

In a community setting (e.g., home care, partial-day treatment program, halfway house), some nurses write a contract for the client, specifying dates, days, and times of meetings and phone numbers where the client can reach the nurse if she or he has questions between appointments. Some contracts specifically identify behaviors (expected outcomes) for the client to practice between meetings, as well as goals to achieve.

Regardless of the type of contract, the nurse will explain the purpose of the meetings, what is expected during the meetings, and the roles for both the nurse and the client. Together, the nurse and the client will determine long-term goals and short-term objectives for reaching those goals.

Dependability is important, and nurses must keep all appointments with clients. When circumstances prevent this, the nurse should contact the client to explain and set a new meeting time. Client dependability is also expected.

During the orientation stage, the nurse and the client together identify the client's strengths, limitations, and problem areas. Outcome criteria are established, and a plan of care is formulated. Clients' responses to this phase vary widely.

Working Stage. The orientation stage ends and the working stage begins when the client takes responsibility and actively engages in his or her own behavior changes. This means committing to working on problems and concerns that caused disruptions in the client's life versus merely discussing them.

Prioritizing clients' needs helps to determine those problems that will require immediate attention and promotes an organized way to manage the problems. A general principle is that safety and health problems are a main priority, above all others. For example, the nurse always determines first whether clients are free from danger to themselves or others and then addresses pertinent physical needs before traditional therapy begins. Within the established relationship, the nurse helps the client to modify behaviors that are socially unacceptable (e.g., hostile remarks, swearing, isolation, poor hygiene). The nurse helps the client to explore thoughts and feelings and change problematic behaviors in a safe environment where the client can practice new skills and the nurse can reinforce any positive outcomes the client achieves.

As nurses gain experience, they are able to recognize when clients are in the working phase. Sometimes clients repeatedly tell their "story," but resist making changes. Seasoned nurses are able to separate the provocative content from actual process and growth.

Termination Stage. In this stage, the relationship comes to a close. Termination actually begins in the orientation phase when the nurse first sets meeting times with the client. This lets the client know that the relationship is about to begin, but that it also has limits and will end. It avoids confusion on the part of the client, who occasionally may be unable or unwilling to recognize the boundaries of the relationship and may want to contact the nurse outside of the facility or after discharge. The nurse does not continue relationships after the client leaves treatment.

Termination generally occurs when the client has improved and has been discharged, but it also occurs if the client or nurse is transferred. When termination is anticipated, the nurse uses strategies to prepare for the event. Ending treatment is sometimes traumatic for clients who have come to value the relationship and the nurse's attention and assistance. Some methods that the nurse may use when preparing for termination include the following:

- Reduce the amount of time spent with the client in each session and increase the amount of time between sessions as the client's condition improves.
- Prepare for the client's postdischarge situation (plans for future) rather than focus on new or past problems.
- Have the client identify changes he or she has made toward growth; share perceptions of the client's growth.
- Help the client express feelings about ending the relationship; tell the client if the relationship has been pleasant.

When nurses recognize relationship stages and are aware of the strategies and responses during each stage, the course of the therapeutic process will run more smoothly. Thus, the nurse is not caught off guard or shocked by unexpected responses. When nurses are unaware of potential client responses, they take responsibility for what may seem like failure or they sometimes even abandon the relationship because it is unrewarding or unfulfilling. When the nurse has insight into client responses, however, he or she is prepared to use strategies to facilitate client growth.

Nurse as Advocate

The nurse acts as an **advocate** for clients concerning their rights and well-being, whether at the client's bedside or by being politically active in the wider community by joining professional associations or supporting consumers. Much work remains in the psychiatric mental health arena. That includes education of the public for purposes of promoting mental health, increasing understanding and preventing the not-so-mysterious mental disorders. It also includes acting in any capacity to help remove the stigma associated with mental illness and enforcing the laws already in place to achieve parity, or equality, of health care coverage for mental and physical illnesses. PMH nurses use their knowledge and skills to act as leaders and advocates in solving some of the major problems that affect clients and interfere with their quality of life.

NURSING STANDARDS OF PRACTICE

Each profession defines and develops its specific scope and standards of practice and determines a level of accountability to the people it serves. Individual state nurse practice acts, the nurse's level of education, and health care employers all define, differentiate, and govern the nursing clinical practice. In addition, nurses follow professional and personal codes of ethics and commit to evidence-based practice within their level of competence.

Many agencies, national associations, and organizations guide psychiatric mental health nursing practice. Included are the American Nurses Association (ANA) and other PMHN organizations that individually and specifically define the practice focus. Currently, the ANA offers certification for psychiatric mental health nurses at two levels: *basic level practice* and *advanced level practice.* Both level requirements begin with state licensure as a registered nurse (RN). They differ in type and extent of education, skills, competence, and privileges. The list of ANA practice standards appears in Appendix A.

Basic Level of Practice

The PMH nurse at the **basic practice level** and certification is a licensed registered nurse with a baccalaureate degree who has at least 2 years of working experience in psychiatric mental health settings (RN-PMH). This nurse is able to perform any function within the limits of the state RN license, and others functions within the specialty of psychiatric mental health nursing as specifically outlined in the *Scope and Standards of Psychiatric Mental Health Nursing Practice* (ANA, 2006). These include skills directed toward clients in psychiatric settings that relate to assessment, identification of nursing diagnoses, identification of outcomes, planning client care, intervening to treat actual and potential health problems using a variety of defined methods, and evaluating client responses and nursing care.

Advanced Level of Practice

The nurse at the **advanced practice level** (APRN-PMH) is a licensed RN who has been prepared at the psychiatric mental health nursing master's degree level or higher and

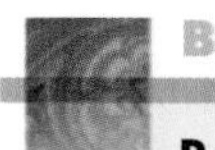

BOX 1-4

Roles of the Mental Health Team

Psychiatric Nurse

Nurses have the most widely focused position description of any of the member roles. This depends on their license and certification mandates, the policies of the psychiatric facility or care setting, and their experience. They interact with clients in individual and group settings; manage client care; administer and monitor medications; assist with numerous psychiatric and physical treatments; participate in interdisciplinary team meetings; teach clients and families; take responsibility for client records; act as a client advocate; interact with clients' significant others; and assess and intervene with clients' psychiatric, biologic, psychosocial, cultural, and spiritual problems.

Licensed vocational nurses provide direct client support. Registered nurses have expanded roles of unit management and decision making in addition to client interaction. Master's-prepared and doctoral-prepared nurses act as clinical specialists in individual, group, and family therapy, with expanded roles within psychiatric settings, or they act autonomously in private practice.

In some states, clinical nurse specialists prescribe medications and manage client caseloads. Teaching in nursing education requires a master's or doctoral degree. Graduate nurses frequently conduct psychiatric research or act as administrators of psychiatric settings.

Psychiatric Social Worker

This graduate-level position allows members to work with clients on an individual basis, conduct group therapy sessions, work with clients' families, and act as liaisons with the community to place clients after discharge. They emphasize intervention with the client in the social environment where he or she will live.

Psychiatric Technician

The licensed psychiatric technician has direct client contact in a psychiatric setting and usually reports to the registered nurse. Technicians observe and record symptoms and intervene under supervision. In some states, they administer medications under the supervision of a registered nurse.

Mental Health Technician

Some facilities call this position mental health counselor. It is an unlicensed position in which the member acts only under the supervision of an RN in assisting clients with activities of daily living, maintaining the schedule, and providing general support. Some mental health technicians have minimal education in psychiatry; others work in this position while accruing hours toward master's or doctoral degrees. They do not administer medications.

Psychiatrist

A psychiatrist is a licensed medical physician who specializes in psychiatry. Responsibilities include admitting clients into acute care settings, prescribing and monitoring psychopharmacologic agents, administering electroshock therapy, conducting individual and family therapy, and participating in interdisciplinary team meetings that focus on his or her clients.

Psychologist

A psychologist is a licensed individual with a doctoral degree in psychology. There are several different psychology tracks. Preparation is for assessment and treatment of psychologic and psychosocial problems of individuals, families, or groups (including those within industrial, educational, or environmental settings). Psychologists do not prescribe or administer medications. Many psychologists administer psychometric tests that aid in the diagnosis of disorders.

Marriage, Family, Child Counselor

These are licensed individuals who frequently work in private practice. They are prepared to work with individuals, couples, families, and groups, and they emphasize the interpersonal aspects of achieving and maintaining relationships.

Case Managers

This position is continuously changing. Nurses qualify for this position because of their diverse education. Case managers manage the delivery of individualized, coordinated care in cost-effective ways. Managed care and case management are not interchangeable concepts. *Managed care* is a system of cost-containment programs that direct, control, and approve access to services and costs within the health care delivery system. *Case management* is a process in the managed care strategy. Case managers need to know the various types of hospitalization and outpatient care settings, the coverage offered by different payers (insurance companies, health maintenance organizations, preferred provider organizations), and the impact of federal and state legislation. Case managers serve as a connection between agencies to provide the most favorable outcomes for the client.

who serves as a clinical specialist or a nurse practitioner. This nurse is able to perform all functions of the basic level nurse (RN-PMH) plus several advanced functions as outlined by the ANA (2006); this nurse functions autonomously to promote mental health or intervene with complex psychiatric mental health problems. The United States Congress and many individual states recognized the skill of the psychiatric mental health APRN by passing legislation that granted these nurses privileges to admit clients to inpatient facilities, write prescriptions for psychotropic medications, and obtain third party billing in their private practices.

Nurses who practice at either level perform holistic functions and collaborate with staff in other disciplines to meet the needs of their clients in a variety of settings. Roles other than that of the nurse are found in several PMH settings as illustrated in Box 1-4. As this chapter has described, nurses engage with clients in a wide variety of settings with the nursing focus on client mental health and well-being.

CHAPTER SUMMARY

- Psychiatric mental health nurses interact with and assist clients to (1) resolve the mental, emotional, and dysfunctional aspects of life crises; (2) manage and alleviate, or ease, painful symptoms of mental disorders; (3) improve overall function; and (4) decrease the personal and social consequences of mental illness, including the stigma attached to mental disorders. Nurses accomplish these goals in a variety of psychiatric settings and all other settings that employ nurses. Nurses must therefore learn and retain PMHN content and principles for use in any nursing discipline.

- Statistics regarding the increasing numbers of mental disorders throughout the world make it essential for continued funding and research into the etiology of mental disorders, diagnostic procedures that address all aspects of mental illness, and integration of research with treatments for mental illness. Nurses continue to integrate research findings into their practice. Science is important, but the art of nursing in the psychiatric arena is imperative.
- A primary focus of PMHN is the therapeutic alliance, which is evident in the nurse-client relationship. It provides a vehicle for clients to heal mental and emotional wounds and make significant changes in their lives.
- Nursing standards guide all aspects of nursing education and practice.
- Nurses are primary advocates for clients wherever needed: at the bedside and in several significant ways in local, state, national, and international communities.

REVIEW QUESTIONS

1 As a client with mental illness is discharged from a facility, the nurse invites the client to a birthday party for a staff psychologist. Select the correct analysis of this scenario.
1. The nurse's action helps the client to transition into community living.
2. The invitation will support development of the client's healthy self-esteem.
3. The nurse's action blurs the boundaries of a therapeutic relationship.
4. The nurse has demonstrated acceptance of persons with mental illness.

2 As a nurse terminates a therapeutic relationship with a client, the client gives the nurse a gift certificate to a local restaurant in appreciation of care received. Select the nurse's best action.
1. Acknowledge the effectiveness of the relationship and the client's thoughtfulness but decline the gift certificate.
2. Inform the client that accepting gifts violates policies and procedures of the facility and decline the gift.
3. Recognize the client's successful transition through the termination phase and accept the gift certificate.
4. Accept the gift certificate and invite the client to join the nurse for a meal at the restaurant.

3 Which statement(s) most clearly shows stigma with respect to mental illness? You may select more than one answer.
1. "Many mental illnesses are genetically transmitted. People cannot change their genes."
2. "If people with mental illness would use some self-discipline, they would not have so many problems."
3. "The main reason for mental illness is that mothers are working instead of staying home with their children."
4. "Many mental illnesses are brain disorders and produce changes evident in neuroimages."
5. "Most people with mental illness are just trying to collect government disability checks."

4 A psychiatric nurse practitioner works with clients in a community setting. Which intervention(s) would distinguish this nurse's practice from the basic practice level? You may select more than one answer.
1. Psychotherapy
2. Case management
3. Consultation
4. Milieu therapy
5. Prescription of pharmacologic agents

5 The parent of a 10-year-old asks the nurse to explain results of the child's psychologic testing. Select the nurse's best action(s). You may select more than one answer.
1. Give the phone number of the psychologist's office to the parent.
2. Read the psychologic testing results, and explain them to the parent.
3. Obtain the child's written consent to discuss the results with the parent.
4. Direct the parent to talk with the attending psychiatrist about the results.
5. Explain that the psychologist will discuss the results with the parent.

6 Select the example of tertiary prevention.
1. Helping a person with a long history of mental illness learn to manage money
2. Teaching school-age children about drug and alcohol abuse and dependency
3. Genetic counseling with a young couple expecting their first child
4. Restraining a psychotic client who has become aggressive and assaultive

Additional self-study exercises and learning resources are available to you on the ***Companion CD*** *at the back of the book and on the* ***Evolve website*** *at* ***http://evolve.elsevier.com/Fortinash/.***

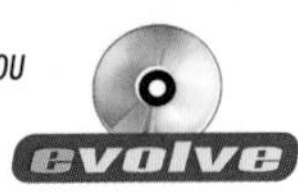

ONLINE RESOURCES

American Nurses Association: **www.nursingworld.org**

American Psychiatric Nurses Association: **www.apna.org**

Center for Reintegration, Inc.: **www.reintegration.com**

Family Diversity Projects: Nothing to Hide: Mental Illness in the Family: **nothingtohide.php**

FAQs educational requirements and schools: **www.allnursingschools.com**

Health Resources and Services Administration, Bureau of Health Professionals: **http://bhpr.hrsa.gov/nursing/**

Healthy People 2010: **www.healthypeople.gov**

International Society of Psychiatric–Mental Health Nurses: **www.ispn-psych.org**

Mental Health America: **www.nmha.org**

National Council on Disability; features full reports on public mental health system in the United States: **www.ncd.gov**

National League for Nursing: **www.nimh.nih.gov**

National Institute for Mental Health: **www.nln.org**

National Library of Medicine; with nursing and mental health information and articles through PubMed: **www.nlm.org**

Nothing to Hide: Mental Illness in the Family: **www.nothingtohide.php.**

World Health Organization: **www.who.int/nmh/en**

REFERENCES

Allen Brain Atlas. Seattle, 2006, Allan Brain Atlas Institute; www.brainatlas.org.

American Nurses Association: *Standards of clinical nursing practice*, Washington, DC, 1998, ANA Publishing.

American Nurses Association, American Psychiatric Nurses Association, and International Society of Psychiatric Mental Health Nurses: *Scope and standards of psychiatric mental health nursing practice*, Washington, DC, 2000, American Nurses Publishing.

American Psychiatric Association: *Diagnostic and statistical manual of mental disorders*, ed 4, text revision, Washington, DC, 2000, American Psychiatric Association.

Caplan G: *Principles of preventive psychiatry*, New York, 1964, Basic Books.

Gewin V: A golden age of brain exploration, *PLoS Biol* 3:e24, 2005.

Institutes of Medicine: *Reducing risks for mental disorders: committee on prevention of mental disorders*, Washington, DC, 1994, National Academies Press.

Institutes of Medicine: *Improving the quality of health care for mental and substance use conditions*, Washington, DC, 2006, National Academies Press.

Kessler RC et al: The 12 month prevalence and correlates of serious mental illness. In Manderscheid R, Sonnenschein M, editors: *Mental health, United States 1996*, Department of Health and Human Services Publication No. (SMA) 96-3098, Washington, DC, 1996, US Government Printing Office.

Kessler R et al: Prevalence, severity, comorbidity of 12 month survey replication, *Arch Gen Psychiatr* 6:617-627, 2005.

Link B et al: Public conceptions of mental illness: the labels, causes, dangerousness, and social distance, *Am J Public Health* 89:1328-1333, 1999.

Manderscheid R, Henderson M: *Mental health, 2002*, Rockville, Md, 2002, USDHHS.

Mazziotta J, Geffin D: *A decade of neuroscience information: looking ahead*, International Consortium for Brain Mapping (lecture synopsis), 2004: www.nimh.nih.gov/neuroinformatics/mazziotta.

McCloskey Dochterman J, Bulecheck GM: *Nursing interventions classification*, St. Louis, 2004, Mosby.

McGriffin P, Riley R, Plomin R: Toward behavioral genomics, *Science* 16:1232-1249, 2001.

Moorehead S, Johnson M, Maas M: *Nursing outcomes classification*, St. Louis, 2004, Mosby.

National Institutes of Mental Health: NIMH statistics, NIH Publication No. 06-4584, 2006; www.nimh.nih.govhealthinforamtion/statisticsmenu.ctm.

New Freedom Commission on Mental Health: *Achieving the promise: transforming mental health in America—final report.* DHHS pub No. SMA-03-3832. Rockville, Md, 2003, USDHHS.

Peek MC, Scheffer RM: An analysis of the definitions of mental illness used in state parity laws, *Psychiatr Serv* 53:1089, 2002.

Regier D et al: The de facto US mental and addictive disorders service system: epidemiologic catchment area prevalence rates of disorders and services, *Arch Gen Psychiatry* 50:85, 1993.

Schuler GD: A gene map of the human genome, *Science* 274: 540-546, 1996.

Schaffer D et al: The NIMH diagnostic interview schedule for children: methods for the epidemiology of child and adolescent mental disorders study, *J Am Acad Child Adolescent Psychiatry* 35:863-877, 1996.

Silver R et al: Nationwide longitudinal study of psychological responses to September 11, *JAMA* 288:10, 2002.

Toga A, Mazziotta J: *Brain mapping: the method*, ed 2, Philadelphia, 2002, Elsevier.

US Department of Health and Human Services: *Health data on older Americans*, Public Health Services, Centers for Disease Control and Prevention, National Center for Health Statistics, No. PHS93-1411, Hyattsville, Md, 1993, USDHHS.

US Department of Health and Human Services: *Mental health: a report of the Surgeon General*, Washington, DC, 1999, USDHHS, Substance Abuses and Mental Health Services Administration, Center for Mental Health Services, National Institutes of Health.

World Health Organization: *International classification of disease and related health problems*, revision 10 (ICD-10), Geneva, 1992, WHO.

World Health Organization: *Global burden of disease and injury*, Geneva, 1999a, WHO; www3.who.int/whosis/menu.cfm.

World Health Organization: *World health report, 1999: making a difference*, Geneva, 1999b, WHO; www.who.int/whr/1999.

World Health Organization (WHO): www.whoint/mipfiles/2008/NCDDiseaseBurden.pdf, p. 11.

Chapter 2 Clinical Practice: Rewards, Challenges, and Solutions

PATRICIA A. HOLODAY WORRET

There is a wisdom of the head and a wisdom of the heart.
CHARLES DICKENS

OBJECTIVES

1. Identify 10 rewards for working with clients in the psychiatric setting.
2. Discuss reasons for entering a professional helping relationship.
3. Name potential sources of fear related to entering a psychiatric setting and techniques for dispelling fear.
4. Describe the benefits for nurses who use autodiagnosis.
5. Discuss positive and negative aspects of use of power and control by nurses.
6. Write three scenarios describing synthesis of psychiatric nursing knowledge in any setting.
7. Discuss the effects a nurse's indifference has on clients, and list client responses.
8. Identify 10 challenges the nurse will encounter in the psychiatric mental health setting, and describe solutions.

KEY TERMS

altruism, p. 21
autodiagnosis, p. 22
burnout, p. 22
control, p. 22
helping, p. 21
indifference, p. 29
insight, p. 23
motives, p. 21
power, p. 22
realism, p. 21
vicarious learning, p. 23
vulnerable, p. 21

The clinical practice of psychiatric mental health (PMH) nursing is stimulating and has considerable potential for professional satisfaction and rewards. Registered nurses employed in a psychiatric setting continually utilize a wide variety of nursing skills in a challenging arena that is seldom routine or unexciting. A psychiatric mental health nursing specialty offers a dynamic balance between rewards and challenges.

REWARDS

Nurses who actively engage in the clinical practice of psychiatric mental health nursing for an extended time give multiple reasons why they choose that discipline. PMH nurses describe their professional involvement with clients as meaningful, purposeful, and amply rewarding. Nurses in this field will often plainly say it fits them.

Skilled and experienced registered nurses made the following responses about the intrinsic rewards they receive while working with clients and their families in the psychiatric setting.

- "In other clinical settings, there was never time to talk to clients or their families. I enjoyed the work, but the client load and lack of time forced me to focus 90% on the person's physical problems or illness and I never really get to learn the human side of the clients or help with those needs. I felt that my job was only partially done and that somehow I cheated the client. The PMH setting allows time for the human being."
- "It's a privilege to be paid for doing what I love to do, which is talking and working with clients in what I consider a purposeful, professional way, with a strong emphasis on interpersonal interactions. No other setting gives me so much opportunity to do just that."
- "Psychiatric nursing calls on all of my educational background. I thought I was going to only have conversations with clients all day long, but that's not so. My knowledge and skills from every area of nursing are constantly being challenged, causing me to

integrate information and data. For example, people are admitted with psychiatric diagnoses, but in addition may have a variety of medical problems, or are pregnant, or dying, or need surgical attention and are unable to communicate symptoms. Critical thinking is definitely necessary here. It is stimulating and satisfying."

- "Nurses frequently work with clients in other health care settings who have physical pain, but clients in the psychiatric setting often live with agonizing mental and emotional pain. I am glad to be part of the team that helps them find ways to ease the pain or to help clients just find meaning for it."
- "Intervening with a suicidal client who voluntarily stares death in the face is a constant challenge. Then, with watchful intervention a client will turn that corner and return from hopelessness. It is a very humbling experience to see life revisited and embraced, and is only one important reason why I stay."
- "Working with the clients often means working with their families. Frequently in this setting, a family member's mental disorder seriously disrupts the family's functioning. Its wonderful to see them change with intervention and education. It is especially rewarding to see them unite again."
- "Never a dull day! Each day brings unexpected events. Keeps me on my toes like no other position I ever held."
- "With experience, psychiatric nurses learn to see immense progress in even the smallest changes made by clients who struggle with severe and persistent mental disorders. To the untrained eye, or the uncaring individual, these changes seem insignificant, or worse are completely overlooked. But the experienced and astute nurses know that common daily routines are often difficult for these clients to meet. They recognize clients' efforts as sometimes being heroic for them, and we encourage them. What is more rewarding than to take part in a client's conquests in their daily personal struggles?"
- "To see clients reach the point where they identify their own solutions to problems, and gain insight that has potential for changing their lives, is very rewarding. When they stop defending themselves or blaming others for all their problems and begin to take appropriate responsibility, then their existence often takes on new meaning. I am glad to be a witness, especially knowing that my colleagues and I have played some small role in facilitating their progress."
- "It is good to observe a calm client who was admitted the previous day for violent behavior that was dramatically out of control. It's difficult for clients in turmoil over their disorders, but its rewarding to see them gain control and take actions toward managing their own wellness. Nurses help them do that."

Rewards are a natural consequence of joining clients on their journey to wellness. Like any other nursing discipline, not all events in the psychiatric setting are rewarding, but many are. When **realism** is tempered with optimism (seeing the glass half full instead of half empty) nurses will discover the rewards as they help clients become more resourceful and hopeful. With the focus on human behavior, each day presents a unique set of challenges when working with clients who have mental disorders. Some challenges and suggestions for solutions follow.

CHALLENGES AND SOLUTIONS

Challenge: Helping—The Concept and the Activity

Helping others includes activities that often define nursing. Nurses and clients benefit when nurses understand this complex concept. Nurses also need to know their own **motives** and behaviors associated with helping others before they enter any discipline of nursing, especially the psychiatric mental health area.

Nurses frequently identify *the desire to help others* as a core motivator for entering and maintaining employment in their profession. Clients in the psychiatric setting are often **vulnerable** because of altered thoughts and compromised emotions. This makes it essential for the nurses who work in the psychiatric setting to be mentally and emotionally healthy, as well as skillfully prepared for therapeutic interactions. Among several other aspects, this includes the nurse's awareness of his or her own reasons for choosing a helping profession. Frequent autodiagnosis by nurses and other health care providers will promote self-awareness and improve the quality of interactions.

Nurses have various reasons for working with clients within the helping professions. A nurse's motives directly or indirectly influence interactions between nurse and client, and they subsequently affect client outcomes. Some motives and reasons will promote health and benefit both client and nurse, but others are counterproductive. The following sections present examples of motivators for helping others and solutions for challenges that may arise while helping clients.

Altruism

Defined as having and showing compassion, generosity, goodwill, charity, kindness and benevolence toward others, **altruism** is a desirable and useful quality in the psychiatric setting and is a common reason why nurses help others. Often the world outside of the therapeutic environment shuns, alienates, or even abuses clients with mental disorders. Clients who are healing from mental and emotional wounds welcome the nurse's genuine altruism and unconditional positive regard. These qualities also promote client wellness.

Astute nurses, however, are constantly examining their own actions and motives, whenever interacting with clients. What seems like a kind gesture by the unskilled nurse is sometimes an obstacle to the client's improvement. A challenge occurs when inexperienced nurses want to be kind but instead let their feelings of goodwill toward a client cloud their judgment. For example, the nurse tells a client that he does not have to attend one of his scheduled activities, when client says he is "too tired to think today" and wants to go back to bed. The activity, however, is a priority in this client's individual treatment plan. In this case, the nurse's misplaced kindness is inappropriate. Instead, the client is encouraged to attend the meeting and engage in his own treatment.

Solutions. Recognize the client's avoidance, and focus on the client and his established plan of care. The nurse's warmth and generosity in wanting to help the client resulted in a nontherapeutic response. The next step for the nurse in the preceding situation is **autodiagnosis**, questioning why the treatment plan was manipulated. The answer may result in nurse-centered, rather than client centered reasons. Altruism is an excellent quality for nurses to have, when it is used with solid knowledge of specific therapeutic interventions, their rationale, and the use of critical thinking.

Satisfaction From Helping Clients

Nurses and all other professionals seek satisfaction from their life work. Satisfaction is usually a sign that the nurse engages in purposeful therapeutic activities with the clients and that both the nurse and client are benefiting. Without job satisfaction nurses frequently change their location of employment, describe **burnout**, or leave the profession entirely. Gaining satisfaction is one positive outcome from using educated efforts for the purpose of helping others.

A challenge occurs, however, if a nurse needs more than satisfaction and is helping others to fulfill his or her own need for love. At that point, there is a risk that the nurse-client relationship is nontherapeutic. To ensure that the professional relationship is not for the purpose of correcting an emotional deficit in the nurse's personal life, the nurse's sources of support, attention, and affiliation, need to exist separately from nurse-client relationships.

Solutions. First, a thorough understanding of boundaries, as described in Chapters 1 and 4, is essential to help prevent this problem. Second, recognize and identify the problem if it occurs. The nurse may personally become aware of the problem, or coworkers will recognize it. A work setting environment that fosters open, honest, professional interpersonal critiques among skilled nurses is a preventive factor for avoiding this problem. In addition, each nurse who works closely with clients consciously makes the effort to form and maintain healthy interpersonal relationships, personal supports, and sources of affection and affiliation outside of the employment environment.

Desire to Protect Others

Protecting others is an incentive and generates a nurse's desire to help clients. There are times when clients are at risk and require various levels of protection because of their symptoms and poor judgment related to their mental disorder or current life crisis. For example, a depressed client with suicidal thoughts and gestures definitely needs close observation and protection against self harm. A client with dementia who wanders and gets lost needs the protection of a closed unit and the staff needs to be alert to prevent inevitable harm to the client. In these situations, the nurse makes decisions that protect the client according to that person's needs.

A challenge will arise if the nurse fails to recognize when external protection is necessary and when to modify or remove it. With knowledge and experience, the nurse knows when clients are able to safely make their own choices and decisions. Often inexperienced nurses mistakenly think that making all decisions for clients is helpful and will prevent them from encountering negative consequences. This is usually counterproductive. Overprotective help makes clients dependent on the nurse and health care system and robs clients of opportunities to succeed in managing their own lives.

Solutions. Assess each individual condition, event, and situation and allow clients to make their own decisions whenever it is safe and they are able. Protect clients when they are not able to remain safe because of symptoms of their disorders or a current life crisis situation. Continually assess clients' readiness and willingness and encourage them to make their own decisions, remembering that some mistakes can also be learning tools. This helps clients to gain independence, to use learned skills, and negotiate their own way in the world. Increased self-esteem and self confidence are frequent outcomes for the clients who succeed in making beneficial decisions.

Power and Control

Nurses and other health care professionals recognize the imbalance of **power** and **control** between the nurse and the client in some psychiatric settings. Clients often perceive caregivers as being more knowledgeable or believe they themselves have little power or control over their own situations. This will manifest as client submission, aggression, or compliance.

Solutions. Avoid the need to be in control over unnecessary situations and events and avoid seeking importance or power from working with clients. Recognize and respect the potential imbalance of power and control in nurse-client interactions and relationships, and do not take advantage of it. Clients surrender various levels of control when admitted to any psychiatric setting, so purposefully act to preserve the dignity of all clients, regardless of their situation. This includes making sure clients control areas of their lives that do not interfere with their treatment. When a client perceives that the nurse is knowledgeable, this often has a positive influence on the client's compliance with necessary treatments. However, if clients refuse treatment, avoid forcing them to comply. If client's life is in danger, procedures will change.

In addition, the registered nurse (RN) supervises her or his treatment team and frequently reminds them of the dignity and rights of clients admitted to the health care setting. In the interest of safety, the use of chemical or physical restraints is necessary in some situations, and these include control issues. Nursing actions are guided by standards of practice and the facility policies and procedures. The RN also acts as a role model in all situations, sharing power and control with team members and with clients when appropriate. With few exceptions, most clients show improved function and report satisfaction when they are able to make decisions and have sufficient control over their own lives.

Insight From Helping

Throughout their clinical practice, nurses learn that increased **insight** and **vicarious learning** are frequent outcomes of interacting with clients. In the psychiatric setting, insight comes from various sources, which include the following:

- Therapeutic interactions with the client
- Reading client records
- Being involved in client therapies
- Interdisciplinary team meetings
- Specific client-focused interactions with other professionals
- Educational classes

Insight into clients' problems, needs, and outcomes is beneficial to both clients and nurses and is essential for growth. A potential challenge arises when nurses discover similarities between a client's problem and their own, or their family member or acquaintance. When this occurs, the focus may shift from the client to the nurse unless the nurse is aware of the similarity.

Solutions. Client outcomes are invariably distorted when the nurse identifies with clients' problems. Therefore, maintain focus on the client and the client's care and treatment plan. Cleary distinguish between the client's and nurse's problems by keeping them separate at all times. Nurses must avoid manipulating situations to get answers to their own problems. To make sure this does not happen, seek and maintain supervision over your practice, and discuss both successes as well as problems that arise. If a personal problem persists and interferes with nurse-client interactions, seek professional advice or therapy outside of the practice setting.

Various factors influence the decision to enter and remain in a helping profession. Psychiatric nursing is based on sound knowledge and practice, healthy self-awareness, an understanding of personal motivations, and open critiques with colleagues concerning interpersonal relationships and the act of helping clients. A primary objective for the entire interdisciplinary team is to maintain therapeutic interactions, interventions, and relationships that are beneficial for clients in their care. A therapeutic environment is maintained when nurses are able to openly discuss ideas with coworkers, including those activities and solutions to challenges that occur in the clinical setting.

The following are additional challenges that sometimes occur in the PMH setting and some suggestions for solutions. Discuss these and identify additional challenges and solutions for role-playing and rehearsing the actual clinical setting.

Challenge: Fear of the Psychiatric Setting

Fear of entering a psychiatric setting for the first time is a common response and comes from one or more sources. One source is *fear of the clients* or what they will do. Another source is *fear of failure*, and doubt about the nurse's own performance. A third source is the nurse's past or present *personal experiences* with someone who is mentally disordered or fear of the nurse's own stability. The challenge for nurses is to identify their fear, overcome it through gaining insight and understanding, and take action toward becoming effective communicators.

Fear of Clients

Frequently, a fear of clients comes from the nurse's preconceived thoughts and distorted images of people who have mental disorders. Frequent exposure to stories dramatized in television, films, news, literature, or video games designed to shock the viewer all influence how a nurse views the mentally ill. Mentally disordered individuals are stereotypically portrayed as frightening individuals who are out of touch with reality or as maniacal killers. Unfortunately, these thoughts and stereotyped images result in a fear of being injured. Stereotyping, as discussed in Chapter 1, not only creates a major problem for mentally disordered clients, their families, and the community, but it often creates major negative expectations by the inexperienced nurse. Unrealistic images and stereotyping have an effect on nurses, and the outcome is often observable when student nurses first enter the psychiatric mental health rotation or when graduate nurses are ready to begin a new position in a psychiatric setting.

Fear of Failure

When nurses have strong doubts about their own ability to interact with clients, the result is anxiety and avoidance. The most common doubt among nurses first entering the psychiatric setting is not knowing what to say or do. New nurses fear embarrassment or fear that clients will reject them. Imagined failure, rejection, or embarrassment is difficult to tolerate in any situation but is made worse in this setting because nurses want to appear competent when interacting with clients. For example, when fearful, the nurse may avoid approaching clients who require the nurse to initiate communication. As a result, both nurse and client fail to benefit from interactions. The nurse misses two opportunities in this case: the first is providing an empathic ear for the client and the second is increasing own experience while practicing communication skills.

Fear Based on Personal Experience

Some nurses have had negative experiences with relatives or people in their neighborhood who have mental disorders, and they enter nursing with a conditioned fear of clients with psychiatric disorders. In other instances, some nurses have gained skills and learned acceptance from interacting with a mentally disordered person. The term *general* is the key here, because no two clients are the same, even when they have the same diagnosis. Nurses grow personally and improve professionally when they see each client as an individual with individual needs, problems, and strengths and interact with them accordingly.

Some worry about their own stability in the psychiatric setting, generated from an excessive lack of confidence in own abilities or having personally experienced a psychiatric disorder. In either case, the nurse is encouraged to seek professional assessment and assistance before entering the PMH area rather than hide these facts and fears. Clients in this setting have a right to healthy responses and behaviors reflected in their nursing care. A client's progress will likely be interrupted if the nurse focuses on personal distractions rather than assists clients with their needs and opportunities for change and growth. In most cases, nurses facing these problems will meet their professional and personal objectives if they engage in facilitative supervision before and during a psychiatric clinical rotation.

Solutions

Enter the psychiatric setting with positive but realistic expectations for interacting with clients. Perfect performance is not a requirement. Being able to tolerate mistakes and rethink situations to determine successful alternatives is important. New nurses are frequently surprised when clients welcome them or when clients make efforts to help the nurse feel more at ease. Being honest and open with clients about the nurse's level of experience on initial encounter often gains the clients' trust and cooperation. This does not mean that the nurse emphasizes personal shortcomings, but when done openly, it lets clients know that this is a new rotation and the nurse is willing to learn.

Fear appears in many unintended ways, and sometimes a client perceives the nurse's fear as rejection. A relaxed facial expression and unimposing, open stance show interest and concern for the client. Reviewing and using other basic communication skills always helps.

Fear breeds avoidance, but knowledge and preparation stop fear and bring confidence. Being prepared before entering the psychiatric setting includes having knowledge and understanding of mental disorders. It is equally important to have knowledge of specific nursing interventions and the rationales for each intervention. Take time to learn specific theory and to practice therapeutic communication skills before entering the psychiatric setting. It is unreasonable, however, to think that the nurse will know everything at first encounter. Time and experience will increase knowledge and help improve skills, so it is necessary to take the first step toward gaining experience. This means taking some risks and seeking multiple opportunities to practice skills. Nurses who purposefully practice mastering these skills while focusing on the client and not on the self will succeed. Studies repeatedly reveal that clients improve in facilitative, genuinely caring, therapeutic environments. Additional suggestions include the following:

- Initiate the interaction. Approach clients for conversation, and do not wait for them to come to you. Clients have the right and sometimes refuse to talk to the nurse for many reasons. It is important that the nurse avoids taking this personally or focuses on oneself or one's own performance. That client may have another appointment or may be worried about disclosing information to someone he or she does not know. Regardless of the reason, continue on and talk to other clients. Make it a point to seek the client who refused, at another time.
- Approach each client on the unit using therapeutic communication techniques and open-ended questions and statements whenever possible.
- Make a conscious effort to avoid stereotyping. If this is a planned objective, it is easier to accomplish.
- Focus on the client rather than on the self and one's own performance. When thinking about what the client has to say and showing genuine concern, it is less probable that the nurse will worry about his or her own appearance or performance. The connection with a client and the result is usually rewarding to both client and nurse. The client becomes less threatening when the nurse interacts with him or her and sees the client as a human being instead of a psychiatric label to be feared.
- Learn basic communication techniques and skills and practice them at every opportunity.
- Challenge yourself by working with clients with varied diagnoses. Learn about the symptoms associated with each psychiatric diagnosis and learn specific interventions intended for these symptoms. The outcome is effective nursing care. Perfecting skills brings a sense of control in each situation that further reduces fear.
- Keep expectations about performance realistic. Nurses are not expected to be therapists by the end of the first few clinical experiences.
- Nurses become more skilled and confident each day as they practice and continue to learn about this specialty. Increased skill will be its own reward.
- Use positive self-affirmations such as "I am doing well and am exactly where I should be in the level of my performance."
- Review theory and policies about safety, confidentiality, and boundaries.
- Write specific objectives before each clinical day. These objectives will become the nursing plan and function as rehearsal tools for the actual clinical experience. An increase in confidence follows. Here are some examples of objectives:
  - Interact with a client who has major depression and use the following interventions:
    Ensure client safety by following the unit procedures (suicide assessment and precautions).
    Interact with the client, allowing time for answers.
    Create a safe environment for the client to interact.
    Encourage the client to express thoughts and feelings.
    When the client is able, help the client to join groups and activities.

Remember that the client with depression does not always want to socialize; continue to initiate contacts.

- Use the following therapeutic communication techniques with a depressed client:
  Silence
  Reflection
  Giving recognition
  Offering self
  Encouraging comparisons

Safety is always the most important nursing intervention and is the primary objective of the entire staff, the instructor, and the student nurse. The unit should also be safe for new nurses to practice their skills, or the inexperienced nurses will be reassigned to other units. Learning the agency policies and procedures is necessary, and selected policy and procedures are part of the orientation process for students and employees.

Challenge: Manage Stress

Our fast-paced world is stressful for individuals, young and old. It is doubly stressful for clients who live with mental disorders, their families, and caregivers. Mentally disordered clients and families have difficulty meeting daily demands: managing symptoms, caring for other family members needs, negotiating with agencies, and maintaining healthy social contacts outside the family.

Nurses also experience stress because of internal and external demands and circumstances related to helping clients in a health care environment. The nursing practice is full of responsibility. Clients, physicians, administrators, and colleagues depend on the nurse's educated decisions and actions, and they expect positive outcomes. Managed care and financial constraints are also a source of stress. The challenge for nurses is to realize and also teach clients that some stress is inevitable and then to manage stress for their clients and themselves.

Solutions

Some stressors are motivating and lead to positive activity and growth or change. Other stressors weaken health. The nurse must first recognize and identify stressors when they occur. The next steps are to modify, decrease, or eliminate harmful stressors when possible; accept those that cannot be changed; and manage the effects of stress. Nurses and other health care professionals realize the importance of learning and practicing techniques for relieving stress. Nurses practice the techniques themselves and teach clients techniques in any PMH settings. Many techniques are available for clients of all ages and states of health. Stress relief and management techniques appear in Chapter 25.

Challenge: Increase and Synthesize Knowledge and Skills

A challenge for nurses is to continually seek new ideas and skills that will improve their practice. State nursing boards require that nurses stay current in education for the purpose of ongoing licensure, but most nurses exceed this requirement. Learning continues throughout a dynamic career. In addition, content learned in basic nursing courses is not forgotten but instead is synthesized and incorporated into the nurse's specialty. Nurses continually draw from knowledge that was gained in several specialties. The following example illustrates how a registered nurse synthesized prior knowledge with data from a current clinical crisis to benefit both the client and the staff.

Tina, an emaciated and pregnant young woman, was admitted to the obstetrical unit from the emergency department of a large and busy health care facility. Workers found her screaming on the cold tile floor of the ladies bathroom in a fast-food restaurant. They determined that she was homeless and had been living on the street. Paramedics reported she was in active labor and seemed unable to contain her loud outbursts. She seemed very frightened, fought staff who tried to help her, and cursed at everyone around her during each contraction. Along with cursing, she gave loud commands to demons and witches who she said were all around her bed telling her they were going to take her baby to the devil. Laboratory results revealed no illicit drugs in Tina's body.

Sondra, the admitting registered nurse, realized the client was psychotic and began to use therapeutic interactive skills that she learned during a psychiatric affiliation. Tina responded positively with decreased outbursts and soon stated she was less frightened when Sondra stayed in the room and talked with her. Tina, saying she wanted her mother, told Sondra the phone number and asked the nurse to call her. Sondra helped Tina place the call. Tina's mother was relieved to learn that Tina was safe. Tina had run away from home after becoming pregnant and never contacted her mother until now. Tina's mother later reported to the staff that Tina was diagnosed as being mildly mentally retarded but had also demonstrated periodic delusions and hallucinations since she was a child. She had been able to live at home and function in the care of her family until she ran away.

The nurse and staff managed Tina's physical and obstetrical needs but also promoted a therapeutic environment by using learned psychiatric nursing interventions for the client's psychotic symptoms, averting a crisis. Tina calmed considerably when she felt accepted. She responded positively when the staff used specific psychiatric nursing interventions, and she cooperated with their instructions about labor and delivery. The staff modified directions so Tina could understand them. In addition, Tina's sense of security increased when her mother was encouraged to stay with her during labor. A psychiatric evaluation was ordered, and a postdelivery plan of care that included psychiatric interventions was prescribed.

Psychiatric nursing skills can be utilized in any health care setting, and nurses quickly learn that these valuable skills will enhance practice in all fields of nursing. This example represents a successful synthesis of skills from various nursing theory and practice areas. Tina benefited from the nurse's ability to use information from many sources and modify the client's care according to her imminent needs versus the scripted obstetrical protocol. All clients benefit from a nurse's abilities and willingness to synthesize theory and practice.

Solutions

Maintain an open cognitive stance regarding each situation in the clinical setting. Follow safe standards, procedures, and policies, but continually be aware of opportunities to improve your clients' experiences in the health care system, and assist them by being willing to synthesize information and practice components from all nursing areas.

Challenge: Set Priorities

Among the most important skills the nurse learns and practices is prioritizing. Identifying and determining priorities is essential in any psychiatric setting. The astute nurse begins to set priorities even before entering the psychiatric setting, then using data from the work environment, continues to modify priorities throughout the day. In relation to client care, the nurse prioritizes nursing diagnoses, expected client outcomes, and nursing interventions while being prepared to change each according to client responses and nursing evaluations. The following example illustrates a challenge and one nurse's choice of priorities:

Albert, a 65-year-old man, was admitted to the unit with a diagnosis of severe major depression. His wife died 5 months earlier and he completely dropped out of an active social life, refusing all invitations from friends. Albert had three grown children who cared for him, but each had their own families and jobs.

Within the past 2 weeks, Albert was eating very little food, stayed in his pajamas all day, was not bathing, and refused to go out of the house at all. The family called his physician and he was admitted to the psychiatric facility for evaluation and treatment. In the intake assessment it was clear that Albert was not an imminent suicide risk, but he made vague statements that resulted in the staff closely watching him on each shift. He began a regimen of antidepressants plus daily scheduled activities and therapy, and he received a copy of the unit introduction and unit rules. Staff explained the rules to Albert and why he was not allowed to go outside of the building for walks by himself at this time, to ensure his safety.

Albert continued to isolate himself for more than a week and did not attend any activities. Staff watched him closely on every shift. He began to dress himself in the morning without being asked and came to scheduled groups, participating occasionally, but he was still guarded when he talked about himself and his situation. In a few days his privileges were increased so that he was able to dine in the main dining room, but he still could not go outside alone.

Sam, his assigned RN for the day, kept the scheduled appointment to interact with Albert, who told Sam he felt "much better today." Albert was wearing a bright plaid shirt one of his daughters brought in, and Sam commented on the colors. Albert responded, "that is exactly how I feel today . . . bright and cheerful." Sam told Albert that he was saying the words he thought the nurse wanted to hear, but his words didn't seem genuine. Sam stayed with Albert for a long time, then told the unit manager and charted that Albert appeared more depressed, even though he was trying to mask it with forced but false cheerfulness.

Sam prepared for an important scheduled meeting that would focus on Sam's promotion to another position. He reported off the unit and was on time, but as he walked down the hall, Sam saw Albert's plaid shirt outside as Albert headed quickly for a busy intersection. Sam changed directions, told the receptionist at the front desk as he passed her to send more help, and ran after Albert. Sam caught up with Albert who resisted and seemed angry at first, but then held on to Sam tightly and started to cry, saying he had sneaked outside and was going to step into traffic in front of the first large speeding vehicle. He wanted to die. Sam and Albert walked back onto the unit and Sam stayed with Albert who was put on suicide precautions with close staff attendance.

In the preceding scenario, the RN's ability to place his personal agenda secondary to the client's acute need is a pointed example of the importance of prioritizing.

Solutions

Safety is always the first consideration when setting priorities. An established and organized plan is necessary for efficient functioning of any system. However, a set prioritized plan often needs modification depending on circumstances, and this is true of the psychiatric setting. Nurses set priorities and assess them continually, ready to respond when the situation demands changes. Often, making a change will interfere with the nurse's well-thought-out plan for the day, but clients' needs come first, and when the situation calls for it, necessary changes occur. Clear thinking and the ability to organize and manage are valued qualities, but flexibility is also a much needed characteristic in the psychiatric setting where the unpredictable usually happens. Prioritizing includes these steps:

- Obtain all relevant data.
- Analyze/organize the information.
- Identify immediate problems and needs, then prioritize.
- Intervene, beginning in order of importance as follows:
  - Safety
  - Health
  - Intrapersonal client needs and problems
  - Interpersonal client needs and problems
- Be flexible in the approach to client care.

With this sequence in mind, nurses continually reassess individual client responses to treatment, setting and modifying priorities in each step of the dynamic nursing process.

Challenge: Secrets and Promises

Keeping confidences is important in any meaningful relationship. In families and friendships, members often share private information or secrets. An important principle for nurses to learn and maintain is that the nurse-client relationship is a professional one, not a personal one. It is not a friendship. Nurses and other health care professionals do not keep secrets or make promises to clients when the secret will interfere with the client's treatment. Challenges occur when nurses fail to understand this principle and do not distinguish between professional and personal relationships. The following example illustrates this principle:

> Marilyn was in her fifth week of the psychiatric rotation in a registered nursing program. She felt comfortable on the psychiatric unit, having diligently studied the theory and practiced skills each day that she was assigned to the clinical setting. Marilyn established a contract with Sarah, a 15-year-old female client on the adolescent locked unit, and met with her each clinical day. Sarah's parents had admitted her because of her out-of-control behaviors that included polysubstance abuse, running away from home for weeks at a time, not attending school, and hanging out with friends who were many years older and who had past drug histories. Sarah said they were good friends because they gave her what she needed. She said she didn't get what she needed at home.
>
> One day Marilyn was preparing to leave the unit to attend a scheduled adjunctive therapy session. Sarah stopped her and quietly said she had a secret. Marilyn told Sarah that she was scheduled to attend a meeting and had 20 minutes to talk. The client continued to say she wanted to tell Marilyn but that the student had to promise not to tell anyone else. Marilyn was surprised that Sarah chose to confide in her, but maintained her composure remembering from class discussions and her reading what she had to do. She told Sarah that she couldn't keep any secret that may affect her care and that the physician and the staff who work as a team to help her would need to know. Then Marilyn continued with the next step. Instead of stopping there, she told the client that "her secret probably was very important or she wouldn't have brought it up" and then offered to talk with her about it for the next 15 minutes.
>
> Sarah cried as she told Marilyn that she had been sexually abused for 3 years by an uncle who came to her home often and frequently offered to stay with her and her younger sister when her parents went out for the evening. She said the uncle threatened to abuse her sister if she told, and that her parents would not believe her but would blame Sarah if they found out.
>
> Marilyn listened and responded therapeutically, using many of the communication skills she recently learned and encouraged the client to talk more about the situation. The student empathized with what Sarah had been through. Sarah said that her recent "craziness" and acting out made her scared for her life, and she was worried about her sister. Marilyn commented on Sarah's bravery in telling what had to be told. Sarah said she felt relieved.
>
> Marilyn reminded Sarah that she had to leave for the meeting but that she would be back the next clinical day and would get another nurse to be with her now. Marilyn reported the incident to the RN unit manager who assigned an RN to respond to the client's needs. Marilyn discussed this incident with her instructor, and the classmates processed this important learning experience in postconference, learning vicariously and gaining insight from Marilyn's experience.

Solutions

This example shows why it is important for nurses to explain the rationale for not keeping secrets before the client discloses information. Clients want to relieve the burden of their secret and will usually reveal information in the hope of getting help in a safe environment. The nurse's honesty often increases the client's trust and subsequent disclosure. When nurses forget or ignore this principle and encourage clients to give secret information that the nurse will share with the staff, the client feels betrayed and stops trusting the nurse and others. This causes a problem in the nurse-client relationship, and trust is often difficult to recover. Following these steps will assist the process:

- Describe the theory and rationale for avoiding making promises and keeping secrets with clients.
- Practice and role-play a situation where a client asks the nurse to keep a secret.
- Tell the client the rationale for not keeping secrets.
- Keep the communication open by recognizing the importance and meaning the secret holds for the client and by offering to discuss its content with the client.
- Share the content of all therapeutically significant information with the treatment team.
- Make a list of several potential significant "secret topics" that clients typically reveal. This will help avoid being caught off guard.

Challenge: Recognize Variations of Change

Unlike most physical sciences that are predictable and exact, psychiatry and psychology will sometimes seem elusive and ambiguous to the nurse. The definition, description, and categorization of psychiatric diagnoses in the *Diagnostic and Statistical Manual of Mental Disorders* (DSM-IV-TR) appear exact. Because of the complex nature of human beings, however, each client will express symptoms in unique ways.

Initially, a new nurse will think in absolutes, seeing symptoms as being totally present or totally absent (i.e., *all or none*). In reality, the client's symptoms change slightly or dramatically over hours or days (i.e., *more or less*). Because psychiatric symptoms are not always measured by laboratory values, charts, and graphs, beginning nurses sometimes overlook or miss them completely. Subtle changes are sometimes clues that more dramatic changes are coming, so the nurse will need to carefully note any increases or decreases in symptoms. The following clinical situation demonstrates this:

> Betty was admitted to the psychiatric acute care unit because she was jogging down the center of a busy two-way traffic boulevard and taunting motorists. She was wearing multiple layers of brightly colored clothes, high heels, and excessive jewelry. On admission she shouted out about the indignity of having to be in this facility against her will, which she termed a violation of her "personal, important rights." Betty was diagnosed with bipolar disorder, mania type.
>
> After several days of quiet surroundings, consistent unit routines, staff interventions, and medication (which she had stopped taking before admission), Betty calmed down. Staff reports and charting stated that she seemed ready to return home.

However, just before discharge, her contact staff person noted that Betty began to change her clothes every few hours and that the content of her conversation centered on "very important" things she was planning to accomplish when she got home. The nurse asked her if she had been taking her medication. Betty admitted she had been putting all medications in the toilet because she was getting too "normal" to accomplish her plans. Her health care provider postponed her discharge.

Solutions

Solutions to this challenge include the following:

- Be aware of even subtle changes in client's symptom pattern.
- Avoid absolute or black-and-white thinking.
- Be prepared for and accept an unpredictable course toward wellness.
- Avoid predicting client progress.
- Keep clients' expected outcomes hopeful but realistic.

Symptoms are *dynamic* and are more like shades of gray than black and white. Observe for fluctuation of symptoms rather than *static*, set patterns of behaviors and responses. For example, a client who is paranoid demonstrates mistrust by being loud and accusatory on admission. He then quiets down but remains guarded, suspicious, and controlled on subsequent days. The symptom of paranoia is the same, but the manifestations change depending on the client's internal stimuli, the unit environment, the present situation or events, and the client's personality style.

Also, write care plans reflecting a realistic appraisal of the client's symptoms, as seen in the following partial nursing care plan. Note that the correct realistic expectations indicate a reduction in symptoms (more or less) rather than a total absence (all or none).

- *Nursing diagnosis:* Disturbed thought processes *related to* an inability to process internal and external stimuli, secondary to bipolar disorder; psychosocial stressors that exceed the ability to cope; noncompliance with medication regimen; *as evidenced by* running into busy traffic, use of excessive colorful clothing and jewelry, screaming at motorists and staff, and grandiose statements of importance
- *Expected outcomes*

  Realistic: Client will verbalize that her thinking was disturbed and put her in danger (within 1 week).

  Unrealistic: Grandiose delusions will be absent in 1 week.

In some cases, it is unrealistic to expect a complete absence of symptoms. Interdisciplinary treatment plans aim at symptom reduction within reasonable time limits, with expectations that clients will achieve these objectives with assistance. Symptom "cure" is an unreasonable expectation for some clients.

Challenge: Avoid Evaluative Responses

Clients respond more favorably to interpersonal communication and treatment when they do not feel they are under a microscope, constantly being evaluated, or have to perform in a specific way to be accepted. For this reason, nurses avoid making evaluative responses of approval or disapproval that indicate the client is *good* or *bad*, *right* or *wrong*. Neutral recognition of the client's appearance, behavior, and progress is often more effective. The following example illustrates this principle:

Carlotta, a 47-year-old unmarried woman, was the main caregiver for her chronically ill mother in their home, and she had devoted her entire life to her mother for the past decade. The mother's condition finally required admission to a nursing home. Carlotta was hospitalized soon after that time for major depression. She was shy on the unit and demonstrated low self-esteem saying continually that her life was meaningless and there was nothing to live for. Carlotta's married sister visited and brought her clothes from home. Carlotta chose and wore only drab-colored clothing, failed to care for her hygiene unless encouraged, and refused to attend most group therapies.

One morning, 2 weeks after admission, Carlotta showered voluntarily and came out of her room in a pale yellow dress, ready for breakfast. Jonathan, an enthusiastic nursing student, saw her and replied loudly so that everyone turned toward her, "Wow, Carlotta, you sure look better today in that yellow dress than any day since I've been on this unit." Her face flushed, she turned around, and with drooped shoulders and head went to her room, changed back into her drab clothes and stayed there for the rest of the day, refusing meals and meetings.

Withdrawn or depressed clients reject praise for several reasons. One reason is it does not fit their present feeling and thinking states or their negative self-image. Praise is an evaluative comment of *approval* and conflicts with a depressed person's mind-set of "I am unlovable," "No one cares about me," or "I am unworthy." There is also some information in this scene showing that Carlotta experiences a high level of anxiety in social situations. The student nurse's praise that drew attention to the client had an additional negative impact on her.

Another reason depressed clients also recoil from excessive praise about their progress is because they fear external supports may be withdrawn when they are still feeling vulnerable and in need of help. They often sabotage their own progress and revert to old behaviors to cling to the support. Also, sometimes clients are not well enough to maintain the expected behaviors; they then feel even more unworthy and as if they let the staff down in addition to failing themselves.

Evaluative comments of *disapproval* are equally nontherapeutic and reinforce pathology. Clients may perceive either strong approval or disapproval as parental or authoritarian and reject them for that reason.

The nurse faces two challenges in this principle. The first comes with awareness and the conscious decision to avoid using strong evaluative comments and statements and to instead learn and practice using *neutral* statements. Neutral interactions show recognition, acceptance, and respect for the client without attaching requirements or qualifications. An example of a neutral statement for Carlotta is presented later.

The second challenge comes with overcorrecting and making the mistake by being indifferent. Giving neutral statements of recognition to the client is far from being indifferent. **Indifference** toward a client who is mentally or emotionally compromised is on the top-10 list of the *worst characteristics* of a nurse or therapist. Indifference will easily dampen client's spirit or decrease motivation and the client's will to engage in his or her own process of getting well. It is the opposite of effective psychiatric nursing practice.

Solutions

The following suggestions will help nurses to avoid making responses with evaluations:

- Give recognition.
- Avoid evaluative statements.
- Be neutral but not indifferent.
- Comment on client's behaviors and *not* on the client.

With these principles in mind, an example of a therapeutic response to the client is: "Good morning, Carlotta. You are already showered and dressed. I'll walk down to breakfast with you."

The neutral statement implies neither approval nor disapproval by the nurse, but it does offer recognition. In addition, the nurse offers her or his presence. Here, willingness to be with the client helps her feel accepted as she is, rather than how she dresses or performs. An evaluative statement usually closes communication, the clients withdraw or become defensive, and they feel unaccepted unless they meet certain criteria or act in a prescribed way.

There are exceptions to this principle. Well-timed and appropriately placed praise acts as an incentive for clients to repeat or continue a desired behavior. Behavior modification programs make specific use of praise, and with experience nurses learn when and how to praise. The nurse will also distinguish between cold indifference toward clients and the effective intervention of *extinguishing* that is used in behavior modification.

Challenge: Identify and Reinforce Strengths

Nurses invariably focus on disorders and the dysfunctional aspects of human behavior and its causes when first encountering clients and their families in the PMH setting. The theoretic content and clinical experiences in this specialty are always interesting, often fascinating, and sometimes dramatic. For that reason, nurses sometimes forget or overlook the healthy aspects and strengths of clients and their families. They occasionally fail to identify and reinforce strengths, which are the keys to client wellness and relative independence from the systems that treat them.

Nurses and all other members of the health care team help the client, family, and staff to identify client strengths and work with the clients to build strengths, increase competence, and reinforce reasons for seeking health and for living (Figure 2-1). Unless the client and family become invested in this pattern, the client is at risk for failure to succeed in overcoming life crises or learning to live with a recurrent mental disorder.

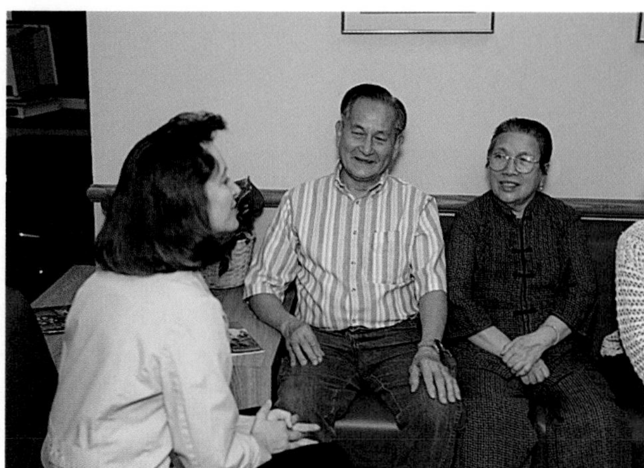

FIGURE 2-1 The nurse interacts with family members as they identify strengths and other positive aspects of their family unit. (From Wilson SF: *Health assessment for nursing practice,* ed 3, St. Louis, 2005, Elsevier.

For many reasons, clients and their families may not always be able to identify strengths at the beginning of an acute psychiatric episode. For example, sometimes family members are in shock or denial, or they are angry about the episode or the client's behavior. When clients are psychotic, severely depressed, under the influence of substances, or have low self-esteem, they are frequently unable to identify strengths. The family is often able to focus on only one thing at a time, and it is not always the client's strengths at that time. The nurse is able to assess client/family readiness for moving toward positive aspects of the current disruptive event and gives them time to understand and accept what has occurred.

At a time like this, nurses can recall Maslow's hierarchy of needs (Figure 2-2). Clients are usually not ready to self-actualize when their basic needs are unmet as a result of a disruptive episode of a severe mental disorder. When the time is right, however, the nurse will help clients and their families to identify and reinforce their strengths. When strengths are discussed, negative aspects of the situation are minimized and the client's courage, self-esteem, and motivation increase.

Be aware that the amount of time that is available for helping clients is short because of managed care and premature discharges. Thus, clients are often discharged well before the staff has time to intervene in all the areas they know are important for clients to maintain wellness. By discussing strengths much earlier in the treatment plan, the nurse will grasp the opportunity to help.

Solutions

Solutions to this challenge include the following:

- Assess client and family readiness for identifying strengths. Give objective input and encourage client.
- Help the client to name specific reasons and benefits for getting and staying well.
- If the client is unable to verbalize strengths, modify the plan, or use other methods: (1) have the client make a list after the meeting, and assign it as home-

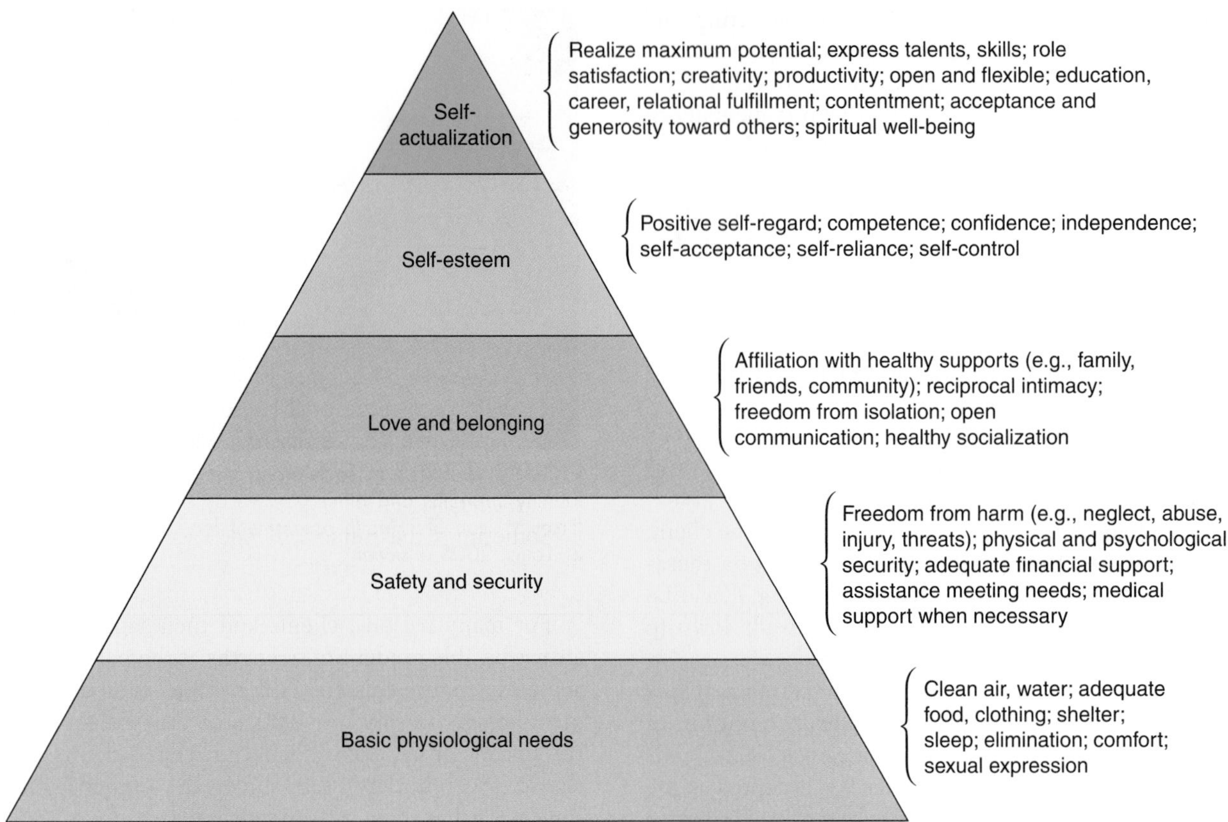

FIGURE 2-2 Maslow's hierarchy of needs. Basic needs must be met before clients can begin to self-actualize. (Redrawn from Maslow AH: *Motivation and personality,* Upper Saddle River, NJ, 1970, Prentice Hall.)

work before next meeting; (2) allow more time for the client to process the information; (3) have the client draw the "reasons" in art therapy or express strengths in recreational therapy or in other types of alternative therapy.

- Ask the client what another member of the family, clergy, or friend would say about him or her regarding his or her strengths.
- Have the client attend an interdisciplinary team meeting and hear what the physician and other staff members say are his or her strengths.
- Assign the task to clients in a process group to discuss each other's strengths.

Challenge: Make Observations vs. Inferences

It is sometimes difficult for the nurse who is new to the psychiatric setting to avoid inferences about a client's behavior. An *inference* is an interpretation of behavior that is made by finding motives and forming conclusions without having all of the information. When a nurse makes inferences, she or he interprets the client's behavior, decides on a cause, assigns a motive, and forms a conclusion. There is great potential for error and unfairness in this process.

Some dangers in drawing inferences are that the nurse is operating from his or her own experience and frame of reference that have little or no connection to the client's actual behavior. In addition, when the nurse makes an inference and forms a conclusion, this does not give the client the opportunity to problem-solve and share thoughts and ideas about important issues. A false conclusion will also misdirect treatment objectives.

Experienced nurses often interpret client behaviors and make correct inferences that lead to therapeutic conclusions. The difference is that experienced nurses take additional steps before reaching their final conclusions, as stated in the following paragraphs.

Solutions

Solutions to this challenge include the following:

- Respond through observation instead of inference.
- Validate interpretations with the client to reach mutual conclusions.
- Explore conclusions with the client.

To avoid making inferences, the nurse operates from an understanding of the importance of obtaining a client's viewpoint about situations and events that affect his or her own life instead of forming a personal opinion. Also, the nurse draws conclusions by responding to client behaviors without first interpreting them. This means that the nurse simply observes behaviors. For example, the nurse might say any of the following:

- "I saw your wife leave, Joe, and now you're crying."
- "Yesterday you sat alone, Mike, but today you joined the other children."
- "Janet, what you just said got a major reaction from the group."

Notice that the nurse does not offer any conclusions to these obviously significant situations. It will be difficult to withhold opinions, but it is a necessary tactic.

The client usually responds to the nurse's statement, and then communication, reasoning, and problem solving are able to begin. The experienced nurse continues beyond observation to interpretation. The critical difference is that the nurse immediately validates the interpretation with the client, and both form a mutual conclusion or at least are aware of the situation for future discussion. Here is an example of the entire process:

1. "I saw your wife leave, Joe, and now you're crying." *(Observation)*
2. "You said earlier that she was coming in today to discuss a divorce." *(Interpretation)*
3. "Is that the reason you're feeling sad now?" *(Validation)*
4. "This might be a good time for us to discuss your relationship." *(Offer to explore the situation)*

Notice that the nurse is not guessing but is reasoning based on prior information. Also, the client now has an opportunity to validate. The last important step is the nurse's willingness to be available to the client for processing this event through therapeutic communication.

Challenge: Offer Alternatives vs. Resolutions

Nurses sometimes feel inadequate before beginning to work in the psychiatric setting because they worry that they do not have answers for clients' problems. However, nurses are not responsible for solving client problems. Nurses actively listen and guide the client's process, versus provide answers.

Solutions

Solutions to this challenge include the following:

- Assist the client to express concerns and problems.
- Encourage the client to express feelings.
- Assist the client to problem-solve toward solutions.
- Avoid giving advice.
- Offer multiple alternatives or options only when the client is unable to do so.
- Facilitate choices.

The nurse engages in therapeutic communication with the client, facilitating the expression of thoughts and feelings. When the client is able to hear his or her own words, the problem-solving process has begun and the client starts to reach his or her own solutions.

Often clients will ask the nurse what he or she would do in the same situation. The client probably does not want the nurse's opinion as much as he or she wants the nurse to stay engaged. There is a relief in expressing problems openly to a willing listener. If the client asks, "What would you do?" or "What do you think I should do?" the nurse will reply, "I think it is more important for you to decide what works best for you. Let's talk about your ideas."

Telling the client what to do or how to do it negates the client's experience. This makes the client feel less worthwhile and childlike, as if the nurse is the parent telling her or him how to conduct his or her life. Also, the nurse's solutions may not fit the client's situation or lifestyle.

If for any reason the client is unable to come up with answers (depression, cognitive impairment or deficit, state of crisis), the nurse may then offer alternatives or options. This means offering assistance and giving some prompting without providing answers or advising. The nurse might say the following, for example:

- "Some things that have worked for other people in similar situations are . . . [*name several options*]. Do any of these seem reasonable for you?"
- "Have you considered . . . [*give several choices*]?"
- "What are some of the options you have for placement when you're discharged? Some that come to mind are . . . [*give several realistic and appropriate choices*]."

Sometimes the nurse will need to be more direct in helping the client when the client sees no solutions. For example, "You said you are a workaholic and can't relax since you got your own business." "What leisure activities have you enjoyed in the past?" "Which ones would you enjoy now if you had the time?" "What did you like most about [golfing, fishing]?" "Who do you trust to run the business while you take vacations?" "Since the business is open Monday through Friday, when could you find time to [golf, fish]?" Most clients know the solutions, they just need some assistance to bring these solutions into their awareness and take action toward change.

Challenge: Manage Your Own Frustration

Frustration occurs when expectations are unmet or a plan fails. Frustration is difficult to experience and tolerate. Nurses enter the PMH setting ready to interact with clients. They have diligently studied theory, practiced communication skills, and written specific and organized care plans, with expectations for successful outcomes.

Interventions, however, are not always successful, and clients may respond in unexpected ways. Some clients who originally consent to a plan of care change their minds about parts of the plan or choose not to cooperate. Nurses experience varying degrees of frustration with this type of reaction. In addition, some nurses lose confidence, think they have failed, or feel embarrassed, rejected, or even angry with clients who do not cooperate. The challenge is for the nurse to manage his or own responses, find meaning in the client's responses, and discuss the plan of care with the client.

Solutions

When frustration occurs in an exaggerated way, the nurse must step back, put the situation into realistic perspective, and review some basic principles of psychiatric mental health nursing. This will involve validating and discussing the situation with appropriate staff, the instructor, or coworkers. Also, review principles of care planning, recalling that plans must be:

- Client focused versus nurse focused and require client input.

- Goal directed (client's goals versus nurse's goals). If the nurse ignores the client's needs or objectives when making the plan, the goals usually fail.
- Objective versus subjective in approach. Keep an appropriate perspective and boundaries regarding the clients, their problems, and their own plans.

A nontherapeutic reaction to frustration for some beginning nurses is to abandon the plan and, in extreme cases, the client. When the nurse has insight into the need of all individuals to have some control over their lives (even though limited in many cases because of symptoms), the nurse begins to come closer to working *with* the client rather than *on* the client. When clients believe they have had sufficient input into their plan of care, cooperation usually increases relative to the client's capacity to engage. When the nurse collaborates with the client on a mutually formulated plan of care, frustration is minimized for both.

Some specific client-focused objectives for the nurse to use as a guideline are as follows:

- Maintain awareness of the client's capability and capacity to engage in his or her own care.
- Include the client in the plan of care.
- Assist the client toward understanding positive aspects of self-help.
- Encourage the client to engage in behaviors directed toward eliminating problems and maintaining health and well-being.
- Teach the client skills that will assist in making change possible.
- Encourage client's attempts to improve.
- Continually evaluate progress and reassess changes.

The nurse benefits from incorporating personal goals toward meeting the client's needs. These include the following:

- Be respectful of the client's need to maintain some control over his or her own life.
- Refrain from the need to complete your own agenda.
- Refrain from abandoning the client if frustration occurs (look for alternatives).
- Remain objectively involved in the problem-solving process.
- Lighten up. Use appropriate humor and relaxation techniques when needed to ease tension.
- Review the principles frequently.
- Get supervision (staff, instructor) to validate your own and the client's progress.

ADDITIONAL CLINICAL PRINCIPLES

Clinical experience is enhanced when the nurse integrates basic principles into practice. The previous sets of principles will be useful when interacting with clients in the PMH setting. The following is a list of additional principles that will facilitate the nurse-client relationship, the client's well-being, and nurse's actions.

1. *Accept the client's feelings, but it is not necessary to accept all of the client's behaviors.* Assist by setting limits on client behaviors that are self-defeating or that threaten the client or others in any way. Limits are not punishment but are external controls that are available when the client is unaware or unable to use his or her own internal controls. Clients need to learn that their actions result in consequences. Allowing them to do anything that is socially unacceptable not only impedes their progress and insight while under treatment, but it also interferes with acceptance by society when they are discharged. Set limits, and then follow through by discussing the incident with the client for the purpose of assessing the client's understanding, reinforcing any positive attempts, and encouraging and helping the client to continue the effective behavior.
2. *Avoid false reassurances, clichés, and global statements.* Give hope, but not false reassurances. New nurses are sometimes uncomfortable with the client's strong emotions and want to fix the situation or see the client cured. They say things like, "Don't worry, I bet your wife will come back to help you," "You'll be better in just a few weeks as soon as the medications take effect," "Everyone gets sick some time, and you'll get through this," or "There is a light at the end of every tunnel!" Statements with superficial content only serve to deny the client and the severe problems he or she is facing. Learn to tolerate the fact that all clients in the psychiatric setting are not cured of their mental disorders. Remember to remain hopeful but realistic.
3. *Avoid giving advice.* Advice often seems to be the perfect solution but does not always fit the client's situation as he perceives it or her or his way of addressing a problem. If clients are not able to assess their own situations, they will not be ready to make changes. Instead, help a client to identify and formulate alternatives and options and to select what the client believes will work in his or her unique situation. If the client is completely blocked and cannot think of any solutions, offer several options. When it is evident that a client is struggling for answers, some helpful statements are, "Have you ever tried. . ." (then offer two or three choices) or "In the past I knew some people with similar situations, and they were successful by doing. . ." (here, name two or three solutions for the client to choose).
4. *Avoid rescue fantasy.* When a nurse thinks he or she is the only one who can help a specific client, it is time to talk with a supervisor. Members of the health team collectively help clients to make changes toward wellness. No one staff member does this alone. Nurses who form the idea that they are special in a client's life may act outside or even against the treatment plan or may do the client favors that are actually nontherapeutic. Stay with the collective treatment plan prepared for the client, or discuss ideas with the entire health care team before acting on your own.
5. *Use simple, concrete, direct language with clients.* Avoid psychiatric jargon or language. Clients in the acute care setting in particular respond better to plainly spoken conversation than they do to language that they do

not understand. Clients with low self-esteem are embarrassed or ashamed and sometimes believe that they are not smart enough to understand what the nurse or physician is telling them when medical terminology is used. The client who is cognitively impaired cannot track long or complex sentences, particularly when they contain psychiatric terms or are abstract in content. Clients who have delusions often misinterpret content. Speaking plainly is most therapeutic.

6. *Avoid heroics!* When a staff member notices a client's behavior is becoming out of control or aggressive, that person should get help. Failing to act soon enough often leads to a client's loss of control over his or her own behavior, which could lead to unnecessary injury to the client or others. Use good discernment and judgment and be safe in all cases by getting help from other staff members instead of trying to intervene alone or change the client's behavior by yourself.
7. *Consider the clinical setting the client's laboratory.* Create a physically and emotionally safe, supportive environment for clients to practice newly learned skills. Encourage clients to discuss and role-play situations and events with the nurse, in individual therapy, or in supportive group therapy sessions. Often clients are able to solve many of their own problems when nurses make themselves available to discuss clients' ideas and let them practice new behaviors with the nurse's guidance.
8. *Encourage clients to take responsibility for their own actions, decisions, choices, and lives whenever they are capable.* Avoid fostering dependence. This often has to happen in stages, with a healthy mixture of nurturing, encouragement, limit setting, teaching, coaching, releasing control, and role modeling. There is no one absolute recipe, and the ingredients vary with each client. With genuine support from staff, most clients learn to structure their own lives within the parameters of their abilities and support groups.

CHAPTER SUMMARY

- Psychiatric mental health nursing is both challenging and rewarding.
- Understanding the concept of *helping* is essential to the nursing profession in any health care setting. This is particularly important in the practice of psychiatric nursing, where clients are mentally and emotionally vulnerable.
- Fear of entering the psychiatric setting is common and is based on several factors. Fears are manageable and are dispelled through (1) knowledge and understanding of theory governing psychiatric nursing and (2) actual practice and experience from working with clients with mental disorders.
- It is most important for nurses to recognize and identify the sources of stress for clients and themselves and to learn effective techniques to relieve, manage, or eliminate stress.
- Nurses will continually grow in knowledge in their field and synthesize information relating to the care of clients, which leads to effective nursing in the PMH setting.
- Setting priorities and modifying priorities are essential skills for nurses in all settings, but particularly in the PMH setting where unpredictability is the norm.
- Several other principles guide PMH nursing, such as the following:
  Expect and accept variations of change in client wellness.
  Avoid making evaluative statements.
  Make observations versus inferences.
  Offer alternatives versus resolutions.
  Manage your own frustration.
  Avoid giving advice and false reassurances.
  Avoid rescue fantasies and heroics.
  Speak plainly and openly with clients.
  Encourage clients to take responsibility for their lives within their capacity and facilitate learning skills to accomplish that.

REVIEW QUESTIONS

1 A beginning psychiatric nurse grew up with a mother who had schizophrenia. The nurse recalls feelings of anger and embarrassment about her mother's behavior in the community. Select the best way(s) for this nurse to cope with the memories. You may select more than one answer.

1. Recognize that the memories are unhealthy. The nurse should try to forget them while working with clients.
2. Reexamine the selection of psychiatric nursing as an appropriate area of practice. Explore other specialties.
3. The nurse should begin each new client relationship with the statement, "My mother had mental illness, so I know what you're going through."
4. Recognize that the memories may add sensitivity to the nurse's practice and discuss them with an experienced psychiatric nurse.
5. Seek ways to use the information and experience gained from childhood to help clients cope with their own illnesses.

2 Prioritize these outcomes for a client with mental illness. The client will:

1. Consume at least 50% of every meal within 3 days.
2. Identify his or her assets and strengths within 1 week.
3. Describe characteristics of healthy relationships with others within 1 week.
4. Contract with the team to report the incidence of suicidal thoughts within 24 hours.

3 A psychiatric nurse designs an hour-by-hour plan for working with clients for the day. Select the best analysis of this nurse's action.

1. The nurse has demonstrated goal-directed behavior.
2. The nurse is likely to feel rewarded at the end of the day.
3. The plan is likely to result in feelings of frustration for the nurse.
4. The plan will support development of the nurse's organizational skills.

4 **At shift change report, a group of nurses discuss a client who covers his head with underwear. Select the appropriate use of humor in this situation.**
1. "Well, this is a psychiatric hospital, and that's craziness for you. That's what we are all about."
2. "Another challenge for us! Does anybody have ideas of how to manage this behavior?"
3. "Let's all show acceptance of this client by wearing underwear on our heads too!"
4. Humor is not appropriate for this situation.

5 **A nurse is assigned to these four clients. Which client should receive the nurse's priority attention?**
1. A newly admitted client diagnosed with major depression whose assessment is incomplete
2. A client with schizophrenia who is having auditory hallucinations of a choir singing
3. A client who recently became unemployed and has a 10-year history of daily alcohol use
4. A client with disorganized schizophrenia who has difficulty completing activities of daily living

Additional self-study exercises and learning resources are available to you on the ***Companion CD*** *at the back of the book and on the* ***Evolve website*** *at* ***http://evolve.elsevier.com/Fortinash/.***

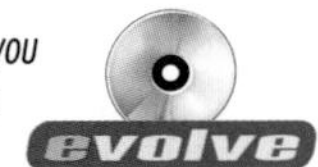

Chapter 3

The Nursing Process

KATHERINE M. FORTINASH

Nursing is a significant, therapeutic interpersonal process. It functions cooperatively with other human processes that make health possible for individuals.

HILDEGARD PEPLAU

OBJECTIVES

1. Define the six steps of the nursing process, and explain the nursing actions for each step.
2. Discuss the roles of critical thinking, expertise, and intuitiveness, and explain how nurses apply them to the nursing process.
3. Describe the parts of the mental status examination, and discuss how it adds to physical assessment findings.
4. Conduct a nursing assessment on a classmate using the mental status examination and parts of the psychosocial assessment.
5. Explain the role of assessment rating scales in helping nurses to assess clients' functions and status.
6. Describe the North American Nursing Diagnosis Association International (NANDA-I) taxonomy, and compare an actual diagnosis with a risk diagnosis.
7. Develop outcomes that accurately measure clients' achievable behaviors based on their nursing diagnoses.
8. Describe the Nursing Outcomes Classification (NOC) and its presentation of outcomes as "variable concepts that are measured along a continuum."
9. Explain the interchangeable role of client outcomes and behavioral goals in measuring client achievements.
10. Define evidence-based practice, and describe how its critical elements apply to nursing research and scientific reasoning.
11. Formulate nursing interventions that describe a course of action or therapeutic activity that mobilizes the client toward a more functional state.
12. Define the Nursing Interventions Classification (NIC) and its complementary relationship with NOC and NANDA-I.
13. Construct rationale statements that explain the reasons for each nursing intervention in terms that improve understanding and ensure nurses' accountability.
14. Evaluate clients' progress and achieved outcomes at various intervals along the continuum to ensure accountability for nurses' standards of care.
15. Document clients' progress and response to treatment using problem-oriented recording (SOAP notes) with consideration of charting purposes and standards.
16. List other methods of documentation used in the behavioral health care setting, such as the electronic method.
17. Describe and discuss the role that the Health Insurance Portability and Accountability Act (HIPAA) regulations have regarding discussing issues of client assessment and confidentiality.

KEY TERMS

assessment rating scales, p. 42
clinical pathway, p. 47
concept map, p. 48
critical thinking, p. 41
cyclic nature of the nursing process, p. 36
evidenced-based practice, p. 46
intuitive reasoning, p. 39
mental status examination, p. 36
NANDA diagnoses, p. 42
Nursing Interventions Classification, p. 52
Nursing Outcomes Classification, p. 44
psychosocial assessment, p. 36
SOAP note, p. 54
standardized care plan, p. 47
Standards of Care, p. 36

The nursing process is a familiar, long-standing, and problem-solving method that continues to provide nurses with a reliable, organized framework for delivering nursing care. It is designed to meet the needs of the client, the family, the community, and the environment. The nursing process provides nurses everywhere with a common language that unifies their knowledge base and distinguishes their discipline (Ankner, 2005). Though it is similar to the scientific method, the nursing process is unique to the nursing profession and is used throughout this text as the foundation for delivering quality care.

This chapter examines the six distinctive steps of the nursing process according to the American Nurses Association Standards of Clinical Nursing Practice (ANA, 2000) as they relate to psychiatric nursing. The six steps of the nursing process help nurses treat and evaluate clients' responses to health problems in a systematic and interactive way. The steps are as follows:

- Standard I. Assessment
- Standard II. Nursing Diagnosis
- Standard III. Outcome Identification
- Standard IV. Planning
- Standard V. Implementation
- Standard VI. Evaluation

HISTORY AND THEORY OF THE NURSING PROCESS

Nursing theorists agree that the nursing process is a simple, straightforward procedure in which a problem is identified, diagnosed, treated, and resolved. They believe that the nursing process is an ongoing, complex, cyclic method, in which the nurse is always collecting data, critically analyzing it, and incorporating it into the treatment plan according to the client's changing responses to health and illness. Figure 3-1 shows the **cyclic nature of the nursing process**. Nurses do not always perform the steps of the nursing process in order (beginning with assessment and ending with evaluation). This is because nurses may evaluate their assessment or even their plan of action at any given time. Kritek (1978) recognized long ago that the steps of the nursing process are interactive and continual, and they influence each other and the client at the same time. There are points throughout the process where the steps come together. The nurse is able to attend the client at any point throughout this interactive, changing process. For example, the nurse continues to assess the client while also planning interventions. The dynamic nature of the nursing process continues to guide and challenge both the new graduate and the seasoned nurse in making reliable clinical judgments and decisions.

STANDARDS OF CARE IN MENTAL HEALTH NURSING

The **Standards of Care** developed by the ANA, the American Psychiatric Nurses Association, and the International Society of Psychiatric-Mental Health Nurses refer to the professional activities the nurse performs during the steps of the nursing process (ANA, 2000). The standards of care are listed in Appendix A and are presented here as they apply to mental health nursing. They are the basis for the following:

- Certification criteria
- Nursing's legal definition (noted in the Nurse Practice Act in many states)
- National Council of State Boards of Nursing Licensure Examination (NCLEX-RN®)

Nurses working in the mental health setting use these standards as guidelines for clinical decision making with the goal of providing quality psychiatric-mental health care to all clients (ANA, 2000).

Standard I. Assessment

The nurse collects data from the mental status examination and the client's psychosocial state.

The **mental status examination** (MSE) and **psychosocial assessment** are essential parts of every nursing assessment, as well as the assessment of the client's physical health. The MSE is as important to psychiatry as the physical examination is to general medicine. The MSE helps the nurse to collect objective data about the client's appearance, behavior/activity, attitude, speech, mood and affect, perceptions, thoughts, sensorium, cognition, insight, and reliability. Psychosocial criteria assessed by the nurse include the client's stressors, coping skills, relationships, and cultural, spiritual, and work-related issues. The completion of the mental status examination sometimes involves several interviews, because the client is not always immediately responsive to all parts of the examination during the acute phase of illness. Patience and persistence are important in such instances.

The MSE may be administered to clients who are acutely ill on a daily basis (Sommers-Flanagan and Sommers-Flanagan, 2003). Nurses conduct the MSE in a variety of settings other than the mental health unit (see Assessment Settings, presented later in the chapter). Box 3-1 describes elements of the MSE and psychosocial criteria. Important components in nursing assessment include the following:

- Assess for behaviors or risk factors threatening the safety of client or others (suicide, self-harm, assault/violence, withdrawal from alcohol or other substances, allergic reactions, command hallucinations).
- Assess for physical pain or medical problems that may affect client functions or well-being.
- Establish trust, rapport, and respect.
- Display a calm, empathetic, nonjudgmental manner.
- Identify the current problem and relate that understanding to the client/family.
- Determine the client's current level of mental, emotional, and psychosocial functioning (include cognition, mood, affect, coping, relatedness, hygiene, and posture).
- Conduct a mental status examination (MSE) (see Box 3-1).
- Ask the client and family what outcomes they expect to get from treatment.

CLIENT DATABASE
• MENTAL STATUS
Cognitive, perceptual, affective, behavioral
• PSYCHOSOCIAL
Stressors, coping skills, relationships, cultural, value-belief, spiritual, sexual, occupational
• DEVELOPMENTAL
Growth, maturation
• PHYSIOLOGIC
Pain, nutrition, fluids
1. ASSESSMENT
• Mental status examination.
• Psychosocial status.
• Nurse-client interview.
• Assessment rating scales.
• History and physical.
2. DIAGNOSIS
• Identify problem.
• Formulate nursing diagnoses (risk and actual).
• Determine priority of nursing diagnoses.
3. OUTCOME IDENTIFICATION
• Construct descriptive client outcomes.
• Include time for outcome achievement.
4. PLANNING
• Determine priorities of care.
• Develop standardized care plan (with team).
• Select interventions based on evidence-based practice.
• Heighten awareness of client's special needs (e.g., culture ethnicity, spirituality, values/beliefs).
5. IMPLEMENTATION
• Implement interventions that:
– Promote health and safety
– Monitor medication and effects
– Strengthen coping skills
– Prevent relapse
6. EVALUATION
• Evaluate outcomes.
• Continue to work on unmet outcomes.
• Reassess as necessary.
• Revise plan as necessary.
DOCUMENTATION ("7th Standard of Care")
• Client safety, response to treatment plan and medications
• Legal, ethical, regulatory, quality assurance
• Case management, utilization review, peer review, research

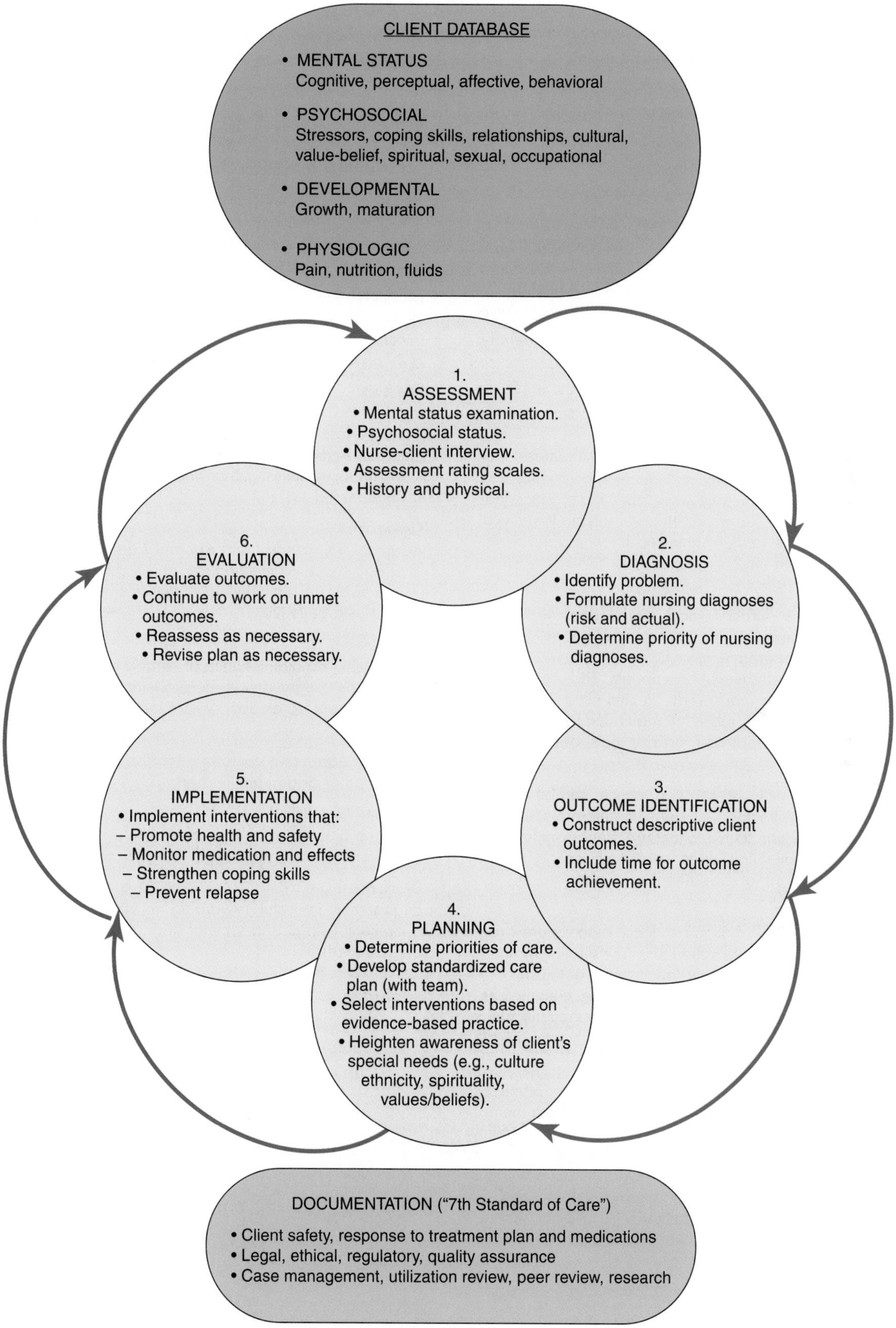

FIGURE 3-1 Cyclic nature of the nursing process (Standards of Care).

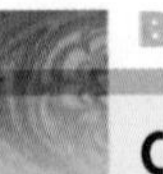

BOX 3-1

Components of Assessment: Mental Status and Psychosocial Criteria

MENTAL STATUS EXAMINATION

Appearance

Dress, grooming, hygiene, cosmetics, age, posture, facial expression

Behavior/Activity

Hypoactivity or hyperactivity, rigid, relaxed, restless or agitated motor movements, gait (way of walking) and coordination, facial grimacing, gestures, mannerisms, passive, combative, bizarre (odd repetitive gestures or abnormal movements)

Attitude

Interactions with the interviewer: cooperative, resistive, friendly, hostile, ingratiating

Speech

Quantity: Poverty of speech (few words), poverty of content (lack of content), voluminous (too many words)

Quality: Articulate (well spoken), congruent (makes sense), monotonous (monotone), talkative, repetitious, spontaneous, circumlocutory (circular), confabulation (fabrication), tangential (superficial), pressured (rapid, urgent), stereotypic (repetitive), disorganized (unstructured), fragmented (broken speech)

Rate: Slowed, rapid, normal

Mood and Affect

Mood (intensity, depth, duration): Sad, fearful, depressed, angry, anxious, ambivalent (opposing feelings), happy, ecstatic, grandiose (feeling of greatness)

Affect (intensity, depth, duration): Appropriate, sad, apathetic (indifferent), constricted (narrowed), blunted (little expression), flat (no expression), labile (changing expressions), euphoric (exaggerated happiness), bizarre (odd, abnormal)

Perceptions

Hallucinations (experiences an unreal presence; can be auditory, visual, tactile, olfactory), illusions (misinterprets reality; can be auditory, visual, tactile, olfactory), depersonalization (detachment), derealization (disconnects from reality), distortions (views objects out of proportion)

Thoughts

Form and content: Logical vs. illogical, loose associations (fragmented), flight of ideas (rapid thoughts), autistic (internally stimulated thoughts), blocking, broadcasting, neologisms (new words), word salad (mixed up words), obsessions (persistent thoughts), ruminations (re-thinking same thought), delusions (fixed belief), abstract (conceptual) vs. concrete (literal)

Sensorium/Cognition

Levels of consciousness, orientation (aware of person, place, time and situation), attention span, recent and remote memory (can recall current and past events), concentration; ability to comprehend and process information; intelligence, fund of knowledge (sufficient amount of knowledge), judgment (makes rational decisions), insight (aware of situation such as own illness and reason for hospitalization), ability to abstract and use proverbs (understands meanings of common sayings and expressions)

Judgment

Ability to assess and evaluate situations, make rational decisions, understand consequences of behavior, and take responsibility for actions

Insight

Ability to perceive and understand the cause and nature of own and others' situations; aware of his or her mental illness and effects/symptoms

Reliability

Interviewer's impression that individual reported information accurately and completely

PSYCHOSOCIAL CRITERIA

Stressors

Internal: Psychiatric or medical illness, including pain, perceived loss, such as loss of self-concept/self-esteem

External: Actual loss (e.g., death of a loved one, divorce, lack of support systems, job or financial loss, retirement, dysfunctional family system)

Coping Skills

Adaptation to internal and external stressors; use of functional, adaptive coping mechanisms and techniques; management of activities of daily living; ability to solve problems associated with daily life

Relationships

Attainment and maintenance of satisfying, interpersonal relationships congruent with developmental stage; includes sexual relationship as appropriate for age and status

Cultural

Ability to adapt and conform to prescribed norms, rules, ethics, and mores of an identified group

Spiritual (Value-Belief)

Presence of a self-satisfying value-belief system that the individual regards as right, desirable, worthwhile, and comforting

Occupational

Engagement in useful, rewarding activity, congruent with developmental stage and societal standards (work, school, recreation)

Modified from Fortinash KM, Holoday Worret PA: *Psychiatric nursing care plans,* ed 5, St Louis, 2007, Mosby.

- Recognize aspects of the client's behaviors, beliefs, vulnerabilities, or other areas needing modification to affect a positive outcome.
- Develop a treatment plan, prioritizing problems according to client needs.

The Nurse as the Primary Communicator

During assessment, the nurse is the primary instrument, or tool, used for communicating with the client. Nurses collect an enormous amount of data through interviewing, observing verbal and nonverbal behaviors, knowledge of functional and dysfunctional behaviors, and the individual's adaptation or maladaptation to life stressors. It is essential that nurses have a broad background and appreciation of the psychodynamics and psychopathology of human behavior to effectively assess the client's overall (holistic) health state. Although a broad base of knowledge is critical, the success of the interview relies heavily on the development of trust, rapport, and respect between the nurse and the client and the nurse and the family.

The nurse treats each client as an individual, avoiding stereotyping or biases that compromise quality care. The nurse is aware of the client's unique qualities, including age, sexuality, culture, ethnicity, religion, values and beliefs, and the ability to adjust to life stressors. The nurse also understands how these qualities influence the client's response to illness and treatment. The nurse-client interview allows the nurse to use the senses of sight, hearing, touch, smell, and knowledge and experience to explore key topics and concerns the client expresses while conducting a thorough (holistic) nursing history and assessment (Box 3-2). It is important to recognize that physical issues often present as impairment in mental functioning. Therefore, the nurse always conducts a complete assessment of the client both physically and mentally.

Managed Care and Nursing Assessment

Because of managed care regulations and payment issues, a holistic and thorough nursing assessment makes sure the nurse is less likely to miss critical symptoms, such as risk for suicide, risk for violence, other safety issues, or relapse potential. A comprehensive nursing assessment often takes longer than the number of days the client has for care; however, a complete assessment is necessary for recovery and to prevent relapse.

Health Insurance Portability and Accountability Act and Nursing Assessment

The Health Insurance Portability and Accountability Act (HIPAA) of 1996, guarantees the security and privacy of health information. The final HIPAA Privacy Rule became effective on April 14, 2003, for all health care providers. All client information that a facility keeps, files, uses, or shares in an oral, written, or electronic form is protected under the privacy rule that defines protected health information (PHI). The American Nurses Association *Code of Ethics* (ANA, 1982) also defines the importance of the confidentiality of client information. At the time of admission to a mental health facility, clients often sign a release of information document specifying what information will be released, for what purpose, to whom, and over what period of time. In compliance with HIPAA and the ANA code of ethics, client assessment data are shared only with authorized health care personnel caring for the client, and only the information related to the care and safety of the client is discussed. Nurses must make sure client assessment takes place in a private area to ensure confidentiality and never discuss the assessment, even with other caregivers, in open areas, such as elevators, stairways, hallways, or the hospital cafeteria, where others can hear it. Make sure written client information never leaves the designated charting area and that the information is placed in the client's medical record and not anywhere else. When nursing students or other health caregivers take notes during a report, they should shred the notes in the nursing station before leaving the area and make sure that the notes do not contain the client's name. (See Chapter 8 for more information on the HIPAA, client confidentiality, privileged information, and other legal issues.)

Intuitive Reasoning and Expertise in the Nursing Process

Intuitive reasoning occurs when a nurse applies insight into a situation without first performing a critical analysis. A "strong hunch" or a "gut feeling" is an example of intuitive reasoning that most nurses agree is compatible with scientific reasoning, since both are likely linked to practice and experience. A nurse cannot learn intuitive reasoning from school or books but rather through clinical practice. Benner's significant work, *From Novice to Expert: Excellence and Power in Clinical Nursing Practice* (2001), described the role of intuition in critical care nurses. She concluded that the nurses' reasoning based on both intuitiveness and science often reflected superior insight and sensible judgment when delivering nursing care. Fidaleo (2006), a psychiatrist and author specializing in suicidality, asserted that a gut feeling does not come out of nowhere. He noted that it generally comes from a client who transfers his or her pain to a nurse who approaches the client in a "neutral state," meaning that the nurse is open and accessible to the client's feelings and emotions. This type of intuitive reasoning is especially important when assessing clients who are suicidal, as in the following example:

> A client tells a nurse that the staff told him he is no longer suicidal and does not need close supervision. He says he is looking forward to some privacy and proceeds to enter his room. Although the client appears calm and self-assured, the nurse decides to follow him into the room. As the nurse quietly stands in the room, the client sits on his bed and begins to cry. The nurse sits down next to the client and the client confesses that he was thinking about taking a whole bottle of medication that he had been saving. When the nurse was later questioned about his nursing actions, he stated that he had a gut feeling that made him stay with the client at this particular time and he did not feel the client should be alone. The client admitted that it was the nurse's caring and concern that made him express his suicidal feelings and intentions at that moment.

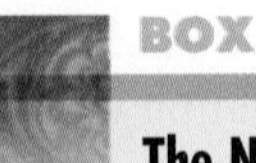

BOX 3-2

The Nurse-Client Interview: Sample General Questions

PRESENTING PROBLEM

Tell me the reason you are here (in treatment).

PRESENT ILLNESS

When did you first notice the problem?
What changes have you noticed in yourself?
What do you think is causing the problem?
Have you had any troubling feelings or thoughts?
If yes, describe them.

FAMILY HISTORY

How would you describe your relationship with your parents?
If troubling, what do you think was the cause?
Did either of your parents have emotional or mental problems?
If yes, describe the problem(s).
Were either of your parents treated by a psychiatrist or therapist?
Did their treatment include medication or electroconvulsive therapy (ECT)?
Did the treatment help them? (Minimally? Moderately? Greatly?)
How was your relationship with them following their treatment?

CHILDHOOD/PREMORBID HISTORY

How did you get along with your family and friends?
If you think there were problems, what do you think contributed to them?
How would you describe yourself as a child? (Quiet? Outgoing? Happy? Sad? Angry? Fearful?)
If childhood was troubled, what do you think may have caused it?

MEDICAL HISTORY

Do you have any serious medical problems?
If yes, describe them.
Are you taking any illegal substances?
Do you drink alcohol?
If yes, how often and how much?
How have these conditions affected your current problem?
Are you experiencing pain? *(If yes, complete a pain history and assessment.)*

PSYCHOSOCIAL/PSYCHIATRIC HISTORY

Have you ever been treated for an emotional or psychiatric problem? Have you been diagnosed with a mental illness? Substance abuse? Alcoholism?
Have you ever been a patient in a psychiatric hospital? Alcohol or drug rehabilitation facility?
Have you ever been in counseling/therapy for an emotional or psychiatric problem?
Have you ever taken prescribed medications for an emotional problem or mental illness? Did you ever have electroconvulsive therapy?
If so, did the medication or electroconvulsive therapy help your symptoms/problem?
How frequently do your symptoms occur? (About every 6 months? Once a year? Every 5 years? First episode?)
How long are you generally able to function well in between the onset of symptoms? (Weeks? Months? Years?)
What do you feel, if anything, may have contributed to your symptoms? (Nothing? Stopped taking medications? Began using alcohol? Street drugs?)

RECENT STRESSORS/LOSSES

Have you had any recent stressors or losses in your life?
Describe them and the effect they had on you.
What are your relationships like? (Poor? Fair? Good?)
How do you get along with people at work? (Well? Not well?)
If not well, what do you think is the reason?

EDUCATION

How did you do in school?
What were your grades like? (Poor? Fair? Good?)
Do you get along well with your teachers? Other students?
If not, what do you think was the reason?
How did you feel about school?
Were you active in school activities?
If not, what do you think prevented you from being involved?
Did you drink or use drugs while in school?
Did you get into trouble while in school?
If yes, what happened and how was it resolved?

LEGAL

Have you ever been in trouble with the law?
If so, describe the problem and how it was resolved.

MARITAL HISTORY

How do you feel about your marriage? *(If client is married)*
How would your describe your relationship with your spouse? (Poor? Fair? Good?)
How would you describe your relationship with your children? *(If client has children)*
How involved are you in your children's lives? (Minimally? Moderately? Greatly?)
What kinds of things do you do as a family?

SOCIAL HISTORY

Tell me about your friends, your social activities.
How would you describe your relationship with your friends? (Poor? Fair? Good?)
Do you and your friends support each other equally?

SUPPORT SYSTEMS

Who would you turn to if you were in trouble?
Do you feel you need someone to turn to now?

INSIGHT

Do you consider yourself different now from the way you were before your problem began? In what way?
Do you think you have an emotional problem or mental illness?
Do you think you need help for your problem?
What are your goals for yourself?

VALUE-BELIEF SYSTEM (INCLUDING SPIRITUAL)

What kinds of things give you comfort and peace of mind?
Will those things be helpful to you now?

SPECIAL NEEDS (INCLUDING CULTURAL)

How can staff help you during your treatment?
What kinds of things will be most helpful to you now?

DISCHARGE GOALS

How do you want to feel by the time you're ready for discharge?
What do you think you can do to help yourself reach that goal?
What things will you do differently from the way you did them before?

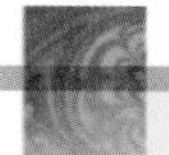

BOX 3-2

The Nurse-Client Interview: Sample General Questions—cont'd

DISCHARGE GOALS—cont'd
What things can you do to help prevent your symptoms from recurring and stay out of the hospital?
What are your goals for taking your medication each day as prescribed?
How will you manage your leisure time?
What activities do you plan to do each day? (Swimming, exercise, sports)
Are there community centers in your area that can help you with these activities?

CLIENT PARTICIPATION
Would you like to add anything to the topics we covered?
Contact staff any time with questions or concerns you may have.
Thank you for your contribution to this interview.

The critical analysis and skills that come from a broad background of knowledge and clinical practice reflect the level of expertise a nurse has. Both expertise and intuitive reasoning are necessary for making reliable clinical judgments, and both influence the phases of the nursing process. Expertise and intuition are worthwhile goals that nurses continue to pursue and develop throughout their professional lives.

Critical Thinking in the Nursing Process

Critical thinking is a concept that includes judgment, intuition, and expertise. Critical thinking skills develop over time and increase the nurse's expanding knowledge base. Like the nursing process, it is a circular, rather than a linear, method. The nurse generally selects a course of action based on knowledge, experience, and scientific principles. This requires hypothesizing many possible reasons for a problem; therefore, nurses do not make rapid or hasty diagnoses.

Whiteside (1997) has noted that productive memory, which is a blend of diagnostic reasoning and experience, is the basis for critical thinking and generally increases as one's knowledge and experience increase. Some examples of critical thinking are the following:

- The nurse hypothesizes alternative problem-solving methods in assessing clients when the usual methods fail.
- The nurse distinguishes meaningful data from irrelevant data, validates selected data through observations and communication, and retrieves the data when necessary.
- The nurse combines knowledge, experience, and judgment from nursing courses and other disciplines and applies her broad background to all aspects of the nursing process.

Assessment Settings

In psychiatric nursing, nurses often conduct mental status examinations in a variety of settings other than a mental health unit. This includes the emergency department, intensive care unit, medical surgical unit, home environment, school, correctional facility, community center, homeless shelter, or private practice. The nurse has many opportunities to observe the client and adjust assessment data according to the client's continued responses to the environment, treatment regimen, and progress made during hospitalization or outpatient setting.

Assessment Sources

Ideally, *the client is the primary source of information*. If the client is too ill to offer a complete or accurate health history, a reliable source, such as family members or friends, may be interviewed on the client's behalf. For example, clients who are extremely confused, delusional, hallucinating, unable to speak, or unconscious cannot be interviewed, so the nurse will rely on others. However, as soon as the client is able to respond, the nurse can approach the client for information. *Information given by anyone other than the client needs to be evaluated in terms of that person's relationship with the client.* For example, a person who is not familiar with the client's behavior, or who is not on good terms with the client, may not give accurate information about the client's problem. It is useful to check the information with other sources as much as possible. The *medical record* is also a source of information if the client has a written history. It is important to review the most current client information as soon as it is available because past records, although helpful, do not always completely describe the client's current response to mental illness. Many hospitals provide electronic charting, so nurses are able to access recent client information in a quick, efficient manner. *Laboratory studies* also provide useful information about the client's body chemistry, abnormal liver enzymes, and drug levels in the blood. Abnormal body chemistry sometimes results in personality and mood changes and violent behaviors (Table 3-1).

Consultation with the *client's physician* will also help to clarify information found in the medical record. Other *health team members* will also have observations about clients. Usually the staff is careful not to allow past negative experiences with a client influence current assessment. *Student nurses* are a significant help to staff, instructors, or psychiatrists in expanding the client's database. *Police officers* who transport clients with psychiatric problems to the emergency room have information

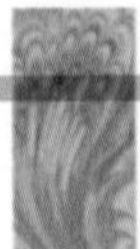

TABLE 3-1

Examples of Mood Changes Associated with Abnormal Body Chemistry

LABORATORY RESULTS	ASSOCIATED BEHAVIORS
Abnormal blood urea nitrogen (BUN) or electrolyte levels (related to kidney disease), abnormal liver enzymes	Agitation, depression, lethargy (sluggishness)
Abnormal glucose and insulin levels (related to diabetes)	Changes in mood and sensorium, possible agitation
Positive toxicology screen (prescription or illicit drugs)	Possible violence (see Chapter 14)

NOTE: Paradoxically, with elderly clients, behaviors such as agitation and irritability are also associated with such conditions as difficulty in urination, dehydration, fecal impaction, or pneumonia, which must be thoroughly explored before they become life threatening.

about the client's behavior as well. Regardless of the source of information, it is critical to confirm the database as much as possible. If the nurse cannot confirm or make sure information is true and correct, he or she should make sure to document that it is unverified information. Assessment based on good, verifiable data is the foundation for logical clinical judgments and the framework for the client's treatment plan.

Assessment Rating Scales

Several standardized **assessment rating scales** are used to assess and monitor a client's psychiatric diagnosis, mental functioning, or abnormal behaviors (Table 3-2). Usually a clinical nurse specialist, psychiatric nurse practitioner, psychologist, licensed social worker, or psychiatrist administers rating scales. Some scales are self-administered with guidance.

Standard II. Nursing Diagnosis

The nurse diagnoses the client from data analyzed in the assessment phase.

Nursing diagnoses are statements that describe a person's health state and responses to actual or potential health problems. They are based on reliable clinical judgments by the nurse following an extensive nursing assessment as described in the previous section.

It is critical for the nurse to select nursing diagnoses based on an accurate assessment of the client's immediate needs because the diagnoses are the basis for selecting therapeutic outcomes and interventions that will move the client toward wellness. Nursing diagnoses reflect an individual's biologic, psychologic, sociocultural, developmental, religious, spiritual, or sexual life process. Table 3-3 lists examples of the relationship of nursing diagnoses to life processes.

The North American Nursing Diagnosis Association International (NANDA-I) defines a nursing diagnosis as "a clinical judgment about an individual, family or community response to actual or potential health problems/life processes which provide the basis for definitive therapy toward achievement of outcomes for which the nurse is accountable" (NANDA-I, 2005, p. 229). This text uses **NANDA diagnoses** and terminology. NANDA's terms are used throughout the nursing profession to unite nurses with one common language regarding client diagnosis and care.

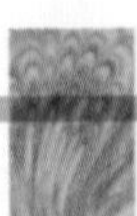

TABLE 3-2

Standardized Rating Scales*

SCALE	ASSESSMENT PURPOSE
Hamilton Anxiety Scale	Anxiety
Beck Inventory	Depression
Geriatric Depression Scale (GDS)	
Hamilton Depression Scale	
Mania Rating Scale	Mania
Brief Psychiatric Rating Scale	Schizophrenia
Overall psychiatric assessment	
Abnormal Involuntary Movement Scale (AIMS)	Extrapyramidal side effects
Mini-Mental State Examination (MMSE)	Cognitive disorders
Alzheimer's Disease Rating Scale	
Eating Disorders Inventory	Eating disorders
Body Attitude Test	
Brief Drug Abuse Screen Test (B-DAST)	Substance use disorders
Global Assessment of Functioning (GAF) Scale	Level of overall functioning

*Nurses and other mental health professionals can use these scales to help assess client status and plan client care. It is important to note that client responses may be subjective.

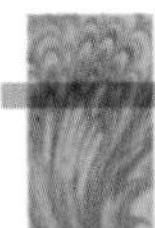

TABLE 3-3

Nursing Diagnosis Statements in Relationship to Life Processes

LIFE PROCESSES	NURSING DIAGNOSES
Biologic	Imbalanced nutrition: less than body requirements Readiness for enhanced nutrition
Psychologic	Chronic low self-esteem Readiness for enhanced self-concept
Sociocultural	Impaired social interaction Social isolation
Developmental	Delayed growth and development
Spiritual	Spiritual distress Readiness for enhanced spiritual well-being
Sexual	Sexual dysfunction Ineffective sexual pattern

Nursing Diagnoses: Actual and Potential

A nursing diagnosis is either an *actual problem* that the individual is currently experiencing or a *potential problem* that is called a *risk diagnosis*. An obvious example of a risk diagnosis is *risk for suicide*, in which there are *risk factors* that indicate an individual is at risk for suicide such as a history of suicide or verbal threats of suicide. These risk factors replace the etiology and defining characteristics

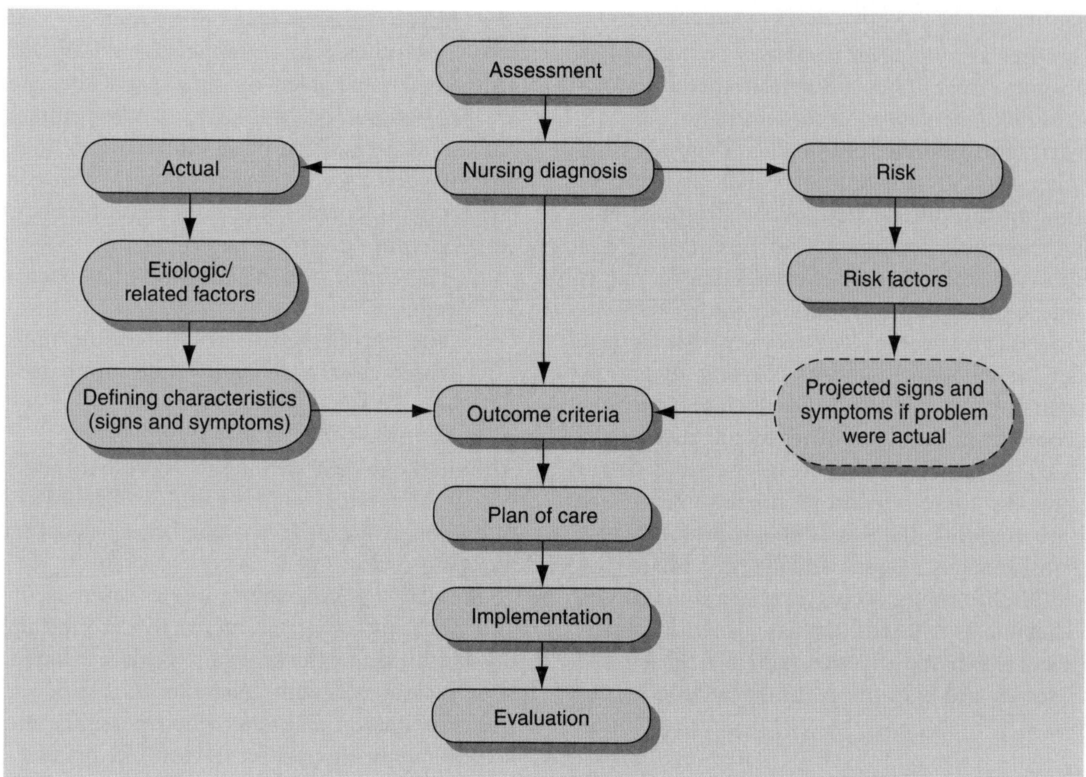

FIGURE 3-2 Nursing process depicting actual and risk diagnosis format of the six-step process.

BOX 3-3

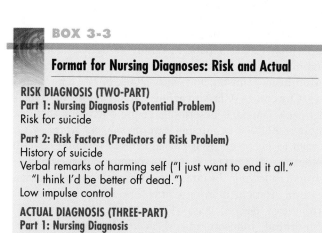

Format for Nursing Diagnoses: Risk and Actual

RISK DIAGNOSIS (TWO-PART)
Part 1: Nursing Diagnosis (Potential Problem)
Risk for suicide

Part 2: Risk Factors (Predictors of Risk Problem)
History of suicide
Verbal remarks of harming self ("I just want to end it all." "I think I'd be better off dead.")
Low impulse control

ACTUAL DIAGNOSIS (THREE-PART)
Part 1: Nursing Diagnosis
Posttrauma syndrome

Part 2: Etiology (Probable Cause)
Overwhelming anxiety secondary to:
- Rape or other assault
- Catastrophic illness
- War/disaster

Part 3: Defining Characteristics
Reexperience of traumatic event (flashbacks)
Repetitive dreams or nightmares
Intrusive thoughts about traumatic event
Excessive verbalization about traumatic event

that accompany an actual diagnosis. This is because in a risk diagnosis, the actual problem has not happened, so there are no defining characteristics. Also, etiology usually refers to probable cause, and because there cannot be a cause without an effect, there is no etiology, or cause, in a risk diagnosis. NANDA states that a nurse is able to change any actual diagnosis on the NANDA list to a risk diagnosis if the problem has not occurred yet. A risk diagnosis becomes an actual diagnosis if the problem happens. Box 3-3 lists examples of actual diagnoses and risk diagnoses. Figure 3-2 describes risk and actual diagnoses in the context of the nursing process. There is a complete list of NANDA-approved diagnoses on the inside back cover of this text.

DSM-IV-TR: Mental Disorders

In the medical model of psychiatry, "health problems" are the mental disorders in the *Diagnostic and Statistical Manual of Mental Disorders*, fourth edition, text revision (DSM-IV-TR) (APA, 2000). The client's diagnosis consists of five parts or axes:

Axis I	Psychiatric diagnosis
Axis II	Personality disorder or mental retardation
Axis III	Medical diagnosis
Axis IV	Psychosocial stressors
Axis V	Global assessment of functioning

The Global Assessment of Functioning (GAF) Scale measures a client's functional state at the time of admission and within the past year. The GAF is one of the tools nurses use to assess client functioning. Nursing diagnoses come from the medical diagnoses and their relationship to each other is discussed later. The complete DSM-IV-TR classification and GAF scale are in Appendix B and C, respectively.

Nursing Diagnoses and Medical Diagnoses Relationship

Nursing diagnoses are based on responses or needs that the nurse is able to treat. They differ from medical diagnoses in that *the medical diagnosis is the disease.*

In psychiatry, for example, the medical diagnosis is a mental disorder such as schizophrenia. The psychiatrist focuses mainly on the disease state of the diagnosis and works to find the cause, treatment, and cure, if a cure is possible. Although the nurse is knowledgeable about mental disorders and their treatments, *the nurse's main focus is on the client's responses to illness* such as risk factors, vulnerabilities, and coping abilities. Nursing diagnoses such as risk for suicide, disturbed thoughts, and ineffective coping come from these responses by the client.

Because a client can have many responses to a single medical diagnosis, there are more nursing diagnoses than there are medical diagnoses. Regardless of their special diagnostic focus, nurses and doctors share the common goal of developing accurate, relevant diagnoses that have a sensible assessment database, scientific principles, and evidence-based practice (EBP). *EBP is based on relevant research* and is in the planning section of the nursing process.

Standard III. Outcome Identification

The nurse predicts client behaviors (outcomes) resulting from nursing interventions.

Outcome statements are specific, measurable indicators that nurses use to evaluate the results of their interventions. They are measured along a continuum and describe the best health state that the client can realistically achieve. The nurse states outcomes in descriptive, measurable terms beginning with action verbs instead of using vague, nonspecific terms. *Timelines are most accurate in actual client situations and not in hypothetical cases.* There are examples of timelines later in this chapter and in other areas of the text.

The following are examples of correct outcomes (descriptive, with measurable timelines):

Client will do the following:

- Verbalize absence of suicidal thoughts and plans in 24 hours.
- Display absence of self-mutilating behaviors in 24 hours.
- Interpret environmental stimuli accurately in 36 hours.
- Contact staff when experiencing troubling thoughts and feelings in 24 hours.
- Interact socially with clients and staff in 36 hours.
- Bathe and dress self by 8:00 AM each day in 72 hours.

The following are examples of incorrect outcomes (nondescriptive, without timelines):

Client will do the following:

- Not be overwhelmed by suicidal feelings.
- Have no self-destructive tendencies.
- Not hear voices.
- Talk to other people on the unit.
- Have an acceptable appearance in the dining room.

Outcomes come from nursing diagnosis statements and are projections, or estimates, of what nurses expect to happen as a result of their interventions (i.e., *client's responses to illness will improve*). Table 3-4 shows examples of correct and incorrect outcomes based on nursing diagnoses. Outcomes illustrate the following:

- The actual nursing diagnosis has been resolved or reduced.
- The risk diagnosis has not become actual diagnosis (risk factors were resolved or eliminated).

Outcomes and Goals in Nursing Terminology

Although outcome statements represent the newer terminology in nursing, some health care facilities and schools of nursing continue to use outcomes or goal statements in planning care.

Behavioral goals is a term nurses often use interchangeably with outcome statements to describe the effectiveness of nursing interventions. Both are stated in observable, measurable, and realistic terms. They each specify a time for goal attainment, when possible, and list client achievements in positive terms. To present the reader with the most current nursing language, the authors will use the term *outcomes.* The correct outcome statements listed previously are also behavioral goals.

Nursing Outcomes Classification. In *Nursing Outcomes Classification*, the authors describe outcomes as "concepts that reflect a patient, family caregiver, family, or community actual state rather than expected goals" (Moorhead, Johnson, and Maas, 2004, p. 20). The **Nursing Outcomes Classification** (NOC) is the first standardized language describing client outcomes that are most responsive to nursing care or *most influenced by the actions or interventions of nurses.* NOC outcomes contain indicators that are rated along a 5-point Likert type continuum, allowing the nurse to measure a client's mental state in relation to an outcome. The Likert scale ranges from least desired state (1) to most desired state (5) (Moorhead, Johnson, and Maas, 2004). Table 3-5 illustrates NOC indicators for the depression level outcome with the Likert scale that measures a client state from severe (1) to none (5). Because clients demonstrate numerous responses during treatment, this rating method is beneficial in tracking many critical indicators over time.

NOC's Outcomes Continuum. Unlike goal statements, the NOC does not use short- and long-term outcomes in its classification system. The outcomes used throughout this text comply with NOC outcomes that are "variable concepts that are measured along a continuum" (Moorhead, Johnson, and Maas, 2004, p. 75). Outcomes reflect the client's actual health state at the time of achievement and are met at any place along the continuum. *Some outcomes are achieved in less time than others*, and the nurse continues to intervene with the client until the client reaches all outcomes at the highest possible level.

TABLE 3-4

Correct and Incorrect Outcome Statements

NURSING DIAGNOSIS	INCORRECT OUTCOME STATEMENT	CORRECT OUTCOME STATEMENT
Anxiety	Exhibits decreased anxiety; engages in stress reduction	Verbalizes feeling calm, relaxed, with absence of muscle tension and diaphoresis; practices deep breathing
Ineffective coping	Demonstrates effective coping abilities	Makes own decisions to attend groups; seeks staff for interactions vs. remaining isolated in room
Hopelessness	Expresses increased feelings of hope	Makes plans for the future (e.g., to continue therapy after discharge); states, "My kids need me to be well"

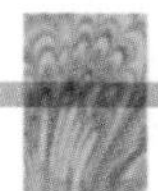

TABLE 3-5

NOC Indicators for Depression Level

Domain: Psychosocial Health (III)
Class: Psychologic Well-Being (M)
Scale(s): Severe to None (n)

Care Recipient:
Data Source:

Definition: Severity of melancholic mood and loss of interest in life events
Outcome Target Rating: Maintain at ____ Increase to ____

DEPRESSION LEVEL OVERALL RATING	SEVERE 1	SUBSTANTIAL 2	MODERATE 3	MILD 4	NONE 5	
Depressed mood	1	2	3	4	5	n/a
Loss of interest in activities	1	2	3	4	5	n/a
Negative life events	1	2	3	4	5	n/a
Lack of pleasure in activities	1	2	3	4	5	n/a
Impaired concentration	1	2	3	4	5	n/a
Inappropriate guilt	1	2	3	4	5	n/a
Excessive guilt	1	2	3	4	5	n/a
Fatigue	1	2	3	4	5	n/a
Feelings of worthlessness	1	2	3	4	5	n/a
Psychomotor retardation	1	2	3	4	5	n/a
Psychomotor agitation	1	2	3	4	5	n/a
Insomnia	1	2	3	4	5	n/a
Hypersomnia	1	2	3	4	5	n/a
Weight gain	1	2	3	4	5	n/a
Weight loss	1	2	3	4	5	n/a
Increased appetite	1	2	3	4	5	n/a
Decreased appetite	1	2	3	4	5	n/a
Recurrent thoughts of death or suicide	1	2	3	4	5	n/a
Indecisiveness	1	2	3	4	5	n/a
Sadness	1	2	3	4	5	n/a
Crying spells	1	2	3	4	5	n/a
Anger	1	2	3	4	5	n/a
Hopelessness	1	2	3	4	5	n/a
Loneliness	1	2	3	4	5	n/a
Low self-esteem	1	2	3	4	5	n/a
Decreased libido	1	2	3	4	5	n/a
Decreased activity level	1	2	3	4	5	n/a
Lack of spontaneity	1	2	3	4	5	n/a
Irritability	1	2	3	4	5	n/a
Recreational drug use	1	2	3	4	5	n/a
Increased alcohol use	1	2	3	4	5	n/a
Poor personal hygiene/grooming	1	2	3	4	5	n/a

From Moorhead S, Johnson M, Maas M: *Nursing outcomes classification (NOC)*, ed 3, St Louis 2004, Mosby.

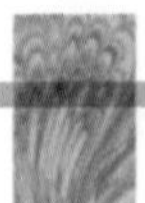

TABLE 3-6

Comparison of NANDA Diagnoses and NOC Outcomes

NANDA DIAGNOSIS	NOC OUTCOME
Impaired physical mobility	Mobility
Hopelessness	Hope
Deficient knowledge	Knowledge: Disease Process Knowledge: Medication Knowledge: Health Behavior Knowledge: Treatment Regimen
Constipation	Bowel Continence
Diarrhea	Bowel Elimination
Stress urinary incontinence	Urinary Continence
Reflex urinary incontinence	Tissue Integrity: Skin and Mucous Membranes Urinary Elimination
Interrupted family processes	Family Functioning Family Physical Environment Family Coping

Data from NANDA International: *NANDA nursing diagnoses, 2007-2008,* Philadelphia, 2007, Author; and Moorhead S, Johnson M, Maas M: *Nursing outcomes classification (NOC),* ed 3, St Louis, 2004, Mosby.

NOC's Relationship with NANDA-I and NIC. NOC outcomes appear appropriately in each care plan throughout this text to reflect how NOC outcomes are related to the language of NANDA diagnoses and the Nursing Intervention Classification (NIC) (Dochterman and Bulechek, 2004). The interventions sections of the care plans include NIC, and the implementation section of this chapter further describes NIC. Table 3-6 compares NANDA diagnoses and NOC outcomes.

Outcomes for Actual and Risk Diagnoses Including NOC Statements. Outcome statements for an actual diagnosis are the opposite of the defining characteristics (signs or symptoms) found in the assessment phase. This helps the nurse to establish areas that need improvement. Examples are as follows:

Nursing diagnosis: Self-care deficit: bathing/hygiene/dressing/grooming

Related to (etiology): Response to internal stimuli (auditory hallucinations)

As evidenced by (defining characteristics): Body odor, soiled clothing, disheveled appearance

Outcomes: Displays clean body/clothing and neat physical appearance

NOC: Self-Care: Activities of Daily Living (ADL)

Outcomes for a risk diagnosis come from the risk factors that replace the defining characteristics found in the actual diagnosis. Because clinical signs and symptoms are absent in a risk diagnosis, the outcomes come from the risk factors, as in the following example:

Nursing diagnosis: Risk for suicide

Risk factors: History of suicide attempts, verbalizes intent to commit suicide

Outcomes: Verbalizes absence of suicidal thoughts and plans, absence of suicidal gestures

NOC: Risk Control, Suicide Self-Restraint

Outcomes and Timeline Projections. Nurses often rely on their background of knowledge and practice and information about the client and the client's usual response to treatment to predict timelines for outcomes. Although it is useful to suggest a measurable timeline in actual client situations, outcomes do not always occur when expected. Sometimes other factors influence the outcomes, for example, when the client misses a dose of medication, receives a troubling phone call, has a discussion with a visitor, or when the discharge date is changed. Also, some concepts such as anxiety, hopelessness, powerlessness, or ineffective coping require the client's subjective perceptions and often resist measurability. Outcome statements such as "client appears less anxious" or "client seems more hopeful" or "client copes effectively" do not give measurable criteria for client achievement. Outcomes should be stated so that they clearly describe client behaviors and use the client's own words to describe feelings and thoughts, as appropriate. It is important to include some type of measurement tool or limits to predict client progress or problem resolution (refer to outcome examples listed above in this section).

Standard IV. Planning

The nurse plans client care with the client, physician, and interdisciplinary team.

Planning client care builds on the previous three phases of the nursing process and is crucial in the ultimate selection of nursing interventions that will help successful client outcomes. The planning phase consists of the total planning of the client's treatment to achieve quality outcomes in a safe, effective, timely manner. Nursing interventions with rationales are selected in the planning phase based on the client's identified risk factors and defining characteristics. The nurse's planning process includes the following:

- Meeting and working with clients, family members, and treatment team members
- Identifying priorities of care
- Coordinating and delegating responsibilities according to the treatment team's expertise as it relates to client needs
- Making clinical decisions about the use of psychotherapeutic, scientific principles using evidence-based practice

Evidence-Based Practice in Mental Health Nursing

Evidence-based practice (EBP) is a frequently used term in the psychiatric literature. It is practice based on evidence, and scientific principles based on relevant research. A critical element of EBP is to narrow the space between research and clinical practice so that clients are receiving the best available care. Care is most effective when it is based on evidence or when available evidence is not ignored (Geddes et al., 1998). A review of the EBP literature stresses the importance of including empirical methods in clinical practice when relevant, rather than using only intuitiveness, experience, fashion, or ideology,

RESEARCH for EVIDENCE-BASED PRACTICE

England M: Analysis of nurse conversation: methodology of the process recording, *Journal of Psychiatric and Mental Health Nursing* 12(6):661, 2005.

This study looked at effective nurse-client interactions between a nurse and a nursing home resident on the third day of the client's recovery from surgery. The interaction was recorded from memory in the form of a process recording, which is a therapeutic conversation between the nurse and the client that helps the client express feelings and experiences. The process recording was then divided into separate conversational pieces. It was found that one third of the conversation was oriented toward assessment and diagnosis, one half toward treatment of the client's experiences, and the rest toward planning and evaluation. It was noted that two thirds of the nurse's conversation was effective and consistent with the orientation phase of the nurse-client relationship. The client most often discussed issues of dependency, disorientation to time, unresolved grief, separation anxiety, and need for validation. The nurse responded by providing leadership, help, resources, and technical expertise. The nurse's approaches were evenly divided between making requests, giving information, and validating the client's experience. This study showed an inter-rater reliability of 0.98, which indicates that highly reliable methods were used. Findings indicated the valuable contribution that the nurse conversation makes to clinical practice and client care. This study also has implications for further refinement of the process recording and the nurse-client relationship.

because many research findings conflict with public beliefs about mental health (Wilson, 1997). Many health care facilities regularly promote research studies as part of their overall goal to provide quality, evidence-based practice for their clients. Advanced practice mental health nurses play a critical role in developing performance improvement projects for their discipline and including their findings in planning client care (Studor, 2002). The Research for Evidence-Based Practice box presents an example of research used in nursing practice. (See Chapter 4 for an example of a process recording.)

Interdisciplinary Standardized Care Plans

A current method used to plan and measure client care is the **standardized care plan** (Figure 3-3). This type of care plan generally features the NANDA diagnoses, client outcomes, and interventions that comply with nursing practice standards. The diagnoses are developed from DSM-IV-TR diagnostic categories in a standardized checklist format. Some facilities use variations of this format, but most follow the NANDA format and include all disciplines in the care planning process. The team works under the leadership of the nurse and the physician and uses client input to help achieve the best client outcomes.

Standardized care plans are popular for the following reasons:

- They reduce the need to create new care plans for each client.
- Nurses primarily identify, evaluate, and resolve the problems.
- Standardized guidelines for all disciplines encourage consistency of care.
- There is very little writing, so the nurse has more time to spend with clients.
- They satisfy managed care criteria for quality outcomes and length of stay.
- They promote safe, effective, evidence-based practice over time.

Standardized care plans do not prevent individualized treatment for each client, nor do they replace relevant documentation. They are updated and individualized as needed.

Clinical Pathways

A **clinical pathway** (also called the *critical pathway* or *care map*) is a standardized, multidisciplinary planning tool that monitors client care through projected caregiver interventions and expected client outcomes based on the client's DSM-IV-TR mental disorder. The pathway is mapped out along a continuum of chronologic targets, usually the number of days of the client's estimated length of stay (ELOS). Managed care regulations and payment issues make it necessary to determine the client's estimated length of stay based on the client's mental illness classification, which the designated related groups of mental illnesses (DRGs) recommends. Lengths of stay are modified depending on the client's resistance to treatment and relevant documentation that clearly describes the client's need for continued care.

The pathway projects the client's entire length of treatment from the day of admission through discharge. Figure 3-4 shows a pathway for a client with bipolar disorder (mania) with an 8-day length of stay. The upper columns list client outcomes. The lower columns are categories of care (processes). Evaluation of client progress is measured daily along the pathway timelines. Nursing is the primary supporter of the pathway, yet all disciplines are included in the planning and implementation, as noted in the example. A pathway may be extended to include the client's transfer to home care or other treatment facility. A pathway sometimes begins in a client's home or in a home care situation. In this case, the home care team develops the pathway.

Pathway Variances. Variances are actions that occur when a client's response "falls off" the pathway, meaning that the client did not respond to the interventions in the typical or expected way. This type of response requires separate documentation and investigation by the team. Variances are either positive or negative. Examples are:

Positive variance: A client responds more rapidly to treatment than expected and leaves the hospital before the estimated length of stay.

Negative variance: A client fails to achieve the desired state or condition on the projected time line, by date of discharge, so length of stay is prolonged.

Clinical pathways help to prevent complications while promoting timely lengths of stay, cost effectiveness, and interdisciplinary care. They also serve as a tool for communicating with other shifts. Although pathways are not

Date	Diagnoses (Etiology)	Outcome Criteria	Assessment (Defining Characteristics)	Interventions (Standards of Practice)
	Anxiety (Rank) Mild ___ Moderate ___ Severe ___ Panic ___ Etiology (R/T) ☐ Situational crisis ☐ Developmental/maturational crisis ☐ Threat to personal integrity ☐ Stressors that exceed coping mechanisms ☐ Traumatic event Describe ___________ ☐ Specific phobias: ☐ Being alone in a public space ☐ Being the focus of others' attention ☐ Other ___________ **Ineffective coping** Etiology (R/T) ☐ Situational crisis ☐ Inadequate support systems ☐ Personal vulnerability ☐ Threat to personal integrity ☐ Anxiety (Rank) Mild ___ Moderate ___ Severe ___ Panic ___	Client will: ☐ Identify own response to anxiety. ☐ Identify stimuli and events that precipitate anxiety responses. ☐ Identify and rank anxiety responses as: ☐ 1. Mild ___________ ☐ 2. Moderate ___________ ☐ 2. Severe ___________ ☐ 4. Panic ___________ ☐ Learn and practice effective anxiety-reducing techniques, stress management, and coping methods. ☐ Demonstrate improved: ☐ Vital signs/functions ☐ Behavioral symptoms ☐ Coping skills ☐ Request medication when needed to manage anxiety symptoms. ☐ Participate in group activities _____% of the time. ☐ Verbalize learned adaptive strategies to reduce anxiety to a manageable level by discharge. ☐ Identify signs/symptoms of increasing anxiety and describe ways to intervene to maintain anxiety at a manageable level by discharge.	Client reports: ☐ Apprehension ☐ Dread ☐ Increased somatic complaints ☐ Unfocused fears ☐ History of panic attacks ☐ Frequent urination Assess for increased: Pulse rate ___________ Respiration rate ___________ Blood pressure ___________ Observe for: ☐ Agitation ☐ Restlessness ☐ Selective inattention ☐ Hyperattentiveness ☐ Muscle tension ☐ Narrowing focus of attention	☐ 1. Provide safety and comfort to the client to establish trust. ☐ 2. Identify own anxiety and reduce it since anxiety is transferable. ☐ 3. Establish therapeutic relationship and verbal dialogue with client to determine level of anxiety. ☐ 4. Reduce environmental stimuli to promote a more calming milieu. ☐ 5. Assist client to recognize own anxiety to promote client awareness. ☐ 6. Help client to identify and rank precipitants to anxiety on a scale of 1 (least provoking) to 5 (most provoking). ☐ 7. Assist client to identify and rank level of anxiety as mild, moderate, severe, or panic. ☐ 8. Administer prescribed medications, as necessary, to reduce escalating or panic levels of anxiety. ☐ 9. Teach the client/family effective anxiety reducing strategies, stress management and assertive techniques, to help prevent/reduce anxiety responses. ☐ 10. Monitor and reduce the client's secondary gains resulting from client's anxiety to avoid overdependence on staff. ☐ 11. Engage client in educational and support groups to promote health and direct energy toward constructive activities. ☐ 12. Teach client/family about the therapeutic and nontherapeutic effects of medication to promote learning throughout hospitalization and at discharge.

☐ **Plan discussed with client/family** **Date:** ___________ **Time:** ___________

Comments: ___________

Signatures	Initials	Signatures	Initials

FIGURE 3-3 Interdisciplinary standardized care plan for behavioral health: the client with anxiety.

always the standard care plan method for all facilities, they reflect the changing trends in the current health care systems and continue to be developed and improved.

Concept Mapping

A **concept map** is a critical problem-solving plan that promotes the student's understanding of the relationships between ideas, concepts, or topics. Also known as a type of *algorithm*, the concept map featured in Figure 3-5 shows all the relevant elements of the client's holistic database (social, developmental, medical, nursing, pharmacology, laboratory, and teaching/learning needs). In this type of care map, the client is the focus of care. The student organizes all the elements of client care onto a large poster board or cardboard backdrop. The student presents the data on self-adhesive notes, cards, or paper, and arranges it in a logical structure that shows the relationships between the elements with lines or arrows. There is generally a brief case history of the client's status (diagnosis, objective data, subjective data, orders) and a summary statement at the end. This type of concept map takes the place of a lengthy written care plan

Clinical Pathway: Mania
DRG #430 - LOS - 8 Days

	Interval	Day of Admit	Day 2	Day 3	Day 4
	Location				
OUTCOMES	Physiologic	•Absence of pain •Takes adequate nutrition, fluids with assistance •Complies with lithium level evaluation	•Absence of pain •Demonstrates increased sleep/rest time •Demonstrates adequate elimination	•Absence of pain •Takes adequate nutrition/fluid with reminders •Demonstrates adequate elimination	•Absence of pain •Sleeping 4–6 hours •Demonstrates adequate elimination
	Psychologic	•Involved in stimulation-reducing activities with staff supervision	•Oriented to person and place	•Demonstrates reduction in: movement racing thoughts grandiosity/euphoria irritability	•Demonstrates increased attention span •Reality tests with staff •Oriented to person, place, time, and situation
	Functional Status/Role	•Tolerated orientation to the unit •Refrains from harming self/others with assistance	•Interacting with staff as told •Attends to hygiene/grooming needs with assistance •Refrains from harming self/others with assistance	•Engages in unit activities with staff supervision	•Maintains impulses with reminders •Complies with meds with reminders
	Family/Community Reintegration		•Identifies significant others to staff	•Attends community meetings with staff supervision	•Significant others involved in treatment/discharge planning
PROCESSES	Discharge Planning	•SW Assessment •Identify DC Placement •ELOS, contact family/SO •Nursing Assessment •Identify H/O chronicity •Med compliance, strengths, needs, knowledge deficit	•Team: Involved in D/C Planning Discuss with MD •UR notify managed care ( )	•SW eval completed •Treatment Team meeting #1 ( ) •Specific D/C plans, placement facility identified ( )	•Involve family/SO in DC plans •Review DC plans with patient
	Education	•Orient to unit •Inform of client's rights •Assess client's and family's/SO knowledge of disorder/meds	•Assist with symptom recognition and importance of compliance •Teach family/SO as needed	•Continue with symptom recognition •Continue assessing patient and family/SO learning needs	•Assist in linking symptoms with precipitating events
	Psychosocial/ Spiritual	•Assess: Safety ( ) •Mental status ( ) Spirituality ( ) •Legal status: Vol ( ) 72 hour hold ( ) •Revise Writ ( ) Payor ( ) Conservator ( )	•Continue to assess: Safety issues Mental status Spiritual needs Legal status	•Continue to assess: Safety issues Mental status (e.g. racing thoughts, grandiosity, euphoria, irritability) Spiritual/Legal needs	•Continue to assess: Safety issues Mental status (e.g. racing thoughts, grandiosity, euphoria, irritability) Spiritual/Legal needs
	Consults	•Physical exam within 24 hours	•Other consults as needed	•Other consults as needed	•Other consults as needed
	Tests/ Procedures	•Lithium level ( ) •Tegretol level ( ) •Drug screen ( ) •Thyroid function ( ) •CBC/SMAC ( ) •Other ( )	•Tests/Procedures as ordered	•Tests/Procedures as ordered	•Tests/Procedures as ordered
	Treatment	•Monitor: I&O •Sleep/Rest patterns •Level A ( ) •Reduce milieu stimulation •S&R yes( ) no( ) •Other	•Monitor: I&O •Sleep/Rest patterns •Level A ( ) •Reduce milieu stimulation •S&R yes( ) no( ) •Other	•Move to level B ( ) •Continue with treatment plan: Monitor: I&O Sleep/Rest Other	•Move to level B ( ) •Continue with treatment plan: Monitor: I&O Sleep/Rest Other
	Medications (IV & Others)	•Medications as ordered •See relevant protocols: Lithium •Other •Monitor side effects •Toxicity	•Medications as ordered •Continue to monitor side effects/toxicity	•Medications as ordered •Continue to monitor side effects/toxicity	•Medications as ordered •Continue to monitor side effects/toxicity
	Activity	•OT assessment •1:1 brief contacts •Reality orientation •Intervene to manage impulses: prevent harm to self/others	•Engage in stimulation-reducing activities as tolerated •Assist with hygiene, grooming, ADLs •Prevent harm to self/others during activities	•OT eval completed •Encourage hygiene, grooming, ADLs with reminders •Prevent harm to self/others during activities	•Engage in 2 groups per day •Increase group stimulation as tolerated •Prevent harm to self/others during activities
	Diet/Nutrition	•Offer adequate nutrition and fluids; normal salt intake	•Provide simple meals, finger foods, easy to carry drinks	•Encourage meals in client community as tolerated with staff supervision	•Encourage meals in client community as tolerated with staff supervision

FIGURE 3-4 Clinical pathway for a client with bipolar disorder (mania). *ADLs,* Activities of daily living; *DC,* discharge; *DRG,* designated related group; *ELOS,* estimated length of stay; *I&O,* intake and output; *OT,* occupational therapist; *SO,* significant others; *SR,* seclusion and restraint; *SW,* social worker; *UR,* utilization review. (Courtesy Sharp HealthCare Behavioral Health Services, San Diego, Calif.)

Continued

	Interval	Day 5	Day 6	Day 7	Day 8
	Location				
OUTCOMES	Physiologic	*Absence of pain *Takes adequate nutrition/fluid *Sleeps 4-6 hours *Lithium level in therapeutic range *Other drug level in therapeutic range	*Absence of pain *Sleeps 5-8 hours *Absence of drug toxicity	*Absence of pain *Sleeps 5-8 hours	*Absence of pain *Sleeps 5-8 hours *Able to manage food and activity requirements independently
	Psychologic	*Demonstrates more reality based thoughts *Able to focus on one topic x5-10 minutes	*Demonstrates enthymic mood *Able to focus on one topic x5-10 minutes	*Able to complete activities and unit assignments	*Able to complete activities and unit assignments independently *Able to plan and structure day
	Functional Status/Role	*Demonstrates less intrusive behaviors	*Able to interact with peers *Able to make simple decisions	*Demonstrates safe appropriate activities/behaviors *Independently complies with medical regimen	*Verbalizes need for ongoing medication compliance
	Family/Community Reintegration	*Identifies discharge needs	*Identifies discharge needs	*Identifies discharge needs *Able to identify supports and their appropriate use	*Able to utilize supports and lists ways to access them *States specific plans to manage symptoms, comply with medications, and aftercare
PROCESSES	Discharge Planning	*Assist client/family/SO to identify discharge needs *UR contact managed care as needed ( )	*Continue to problem-solve discharge needs with client, family/SO	*Treatment team meeting #2 ( ) *Transition to Day Treatment if indicated *Assist client, family/SO in finalizing discharge plans	*Discharge to least restrictive environment completed *UR inform managed care as needed ( )
	Education	*Teach client/family/SO about medication effects on symptom management *Instruct in medication, diet, exercise regimen	*Emphasize importance of compliance with meds after discharge *Teach about drug-to-drug effects on symptom management	*Develop aftercare plan to manage symptoms and contact supports	*Reinforce aftercare teaching plan with client, family/SO as needed
	Psychosocial/ Spiritual	*Continue to assess: Safety issues Mental status Spirituality Voluntary status	*Continue to assess: Safety issues Mental status Spirituality Voluntary status	*Continue to assess: Safety issues Mental status Spirituality Voluntary status	*Complete assessments confirm: Safety Mental status Spirituality Legal status
	Consults	*Complete consults as ordered *Arrange for aftercare consults as ordered	*Complete consults as ordered *Arrange for aftercare consults as ordered	*Complete consults as ordered *Arrange for aftercare consults as ordered	*Complete consults as ordered *Arrange for aftercare consults as ordered
	Tests/ Procedures	*Check lithium level for therapeutic range *Check other drug levels for therapeutic range as needed *Tests/Procedures as needed	*Check lithium level for therapeutic range *Check other drug levels within therapeutic range as needed *Tests/Procedures as needed	*Check lithium level for therapeutic range *Check other drug levels within therapeutic range as needed *Tests/Procedures as needed	*Confirm lithium level for therapeutic range *Confirm other drug levels within therapeutic range as needed *Tests/Procedures as ordered aftercare
	Treatment	*Move to level C ( ) *Continue with treatment plan I&O Sleep/Rest Other	*Move to level C ( ) *Continue with treatment plan I&O Sleep/Rest Other	*Transfer to open unit ( ) *Aftercare treatment instructions reviewed with client, family/SO as needed	*D/C with aftercare treatment instructions
	Medications (IV & Others)	*Medications as ordered *Contact managed care if any change in medication regimen	*Medications as ordered *Contact managed care if any change in medication regimen	*Medications as ordered *Review of medications with client, family/SO as needed	*D/C with medications and instructions as ordered
	Activity	*Encourage: Independent hygiene and grooming Independent ADLs Increased participation in groups	*Engage in all unit activities and groups *Encourage independent decision-making	*Reinforce active participation in all unit activities and groups; independent decision-making	*Confirm: Ability to complete activity assignments independently Ability to make decisions independently
	Diet/Nutrition	*Teach family/SO importance of adequate foods/fluids/salt intake	*Teach family/SO importance of adequate foods/fluids/salt intake	*Reinforce adequate nutrition fluids and normal salt intake	*Confirm client/SO/family knowledge of adequate foods/fluids/salt intake

FIGURE 3-4, cont'd Clinical pathway for a client with bipolar disorder (mania). *ADLs*, Activities of daily living; *DC*, discharge; *DRG*, designated related group; *ELOS*, estimated length of stay; *I&O*, intake and output; *OT*, occupational therapist; *SO*, significant others; *SR*, seclusion and restraint; *SW*, social worker; *UR*, utilization review. (Courtesy Sharp HealthCare Behavioral Health Services, San Diego, Calif.)

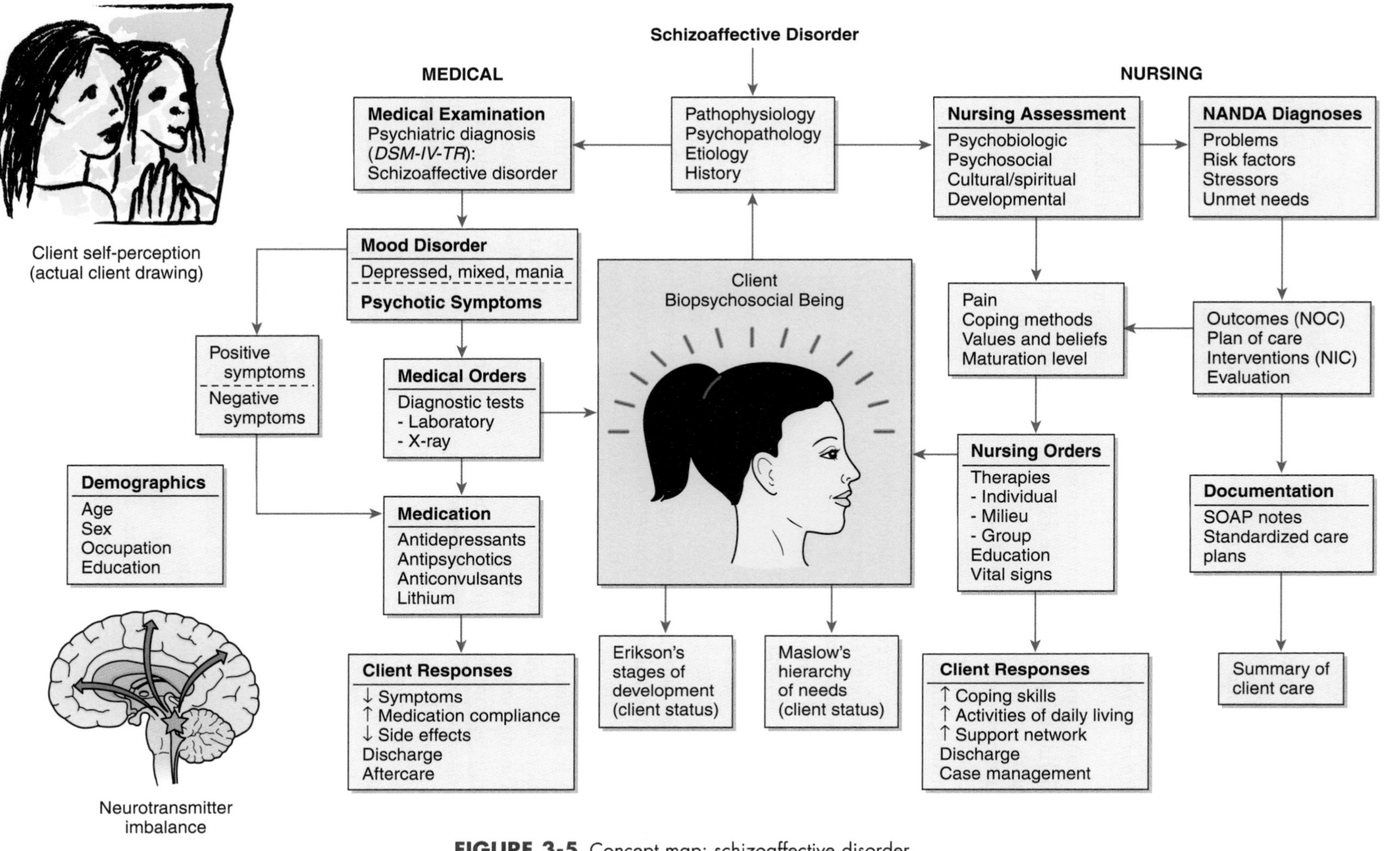

FIGURE 3-5 Concept map: schizoaffective disorder.

and some present it as a PowerPoint program. King and Shell (2002) list the following reasons that support concept mapping as a superior way to prepare students for the clinical experience:

- It allows students to combine complex, relevant data into manageable pieces.
- It requires students to understand the situation as a whole rather than relying on memory.
- It helps both students and instructors to make connections between concepts.

Standard V. Implementation

The nurse sets in motion the interventions prescribed in the planning phase.

Some general nursing considerations directed toward clients and families during this phase include the following:

- Promoting health and safety
- Monitoring medication schedules and effects
- Providing adequate nutrition/hydration
- Creating a nurturing, therapeutic environment
- Continuing to build trust, self-esteem, and dignity
- Participating in therapeutic groups and activities
- Developing client strengths and coping methods
- Improving communication and social skills
- Connecting family and community support systems
- Preventing relapse through effective discharge planning

Nursing Interventions

Nursing interventions (also known as *nursing orders* or *nursing prescriptions*) are critical action components of the implementation phase and the most powerful pieces of the nursing process. They make up the management and treatment approach to an identified health problem and are selected to achieve client outcomes and prevent or reduce problems. Nursing interventions describe a course of action or therapeutic activity that helps the client move toward a more functional state. Nursing interventions are not nondescriptive and weak and do not simply respond to physician orders. The following are examples of descriptive, action-oriented interventions:

- Engage the client gradually in interactions with other clients, beginning with individual contacts, progressing to informal gatherings, and eventually moving on to structured group activities.
- Teach the client/family that therapeutic effects of antidepressants sometimes take up to 2 weeks and that side effects often begin immediately.
- Praise the client for attempts to seek out staff and other clients for interactions and activities and for responding positively to others' attempts at socialization as well.

The following are examples of nondescriptive, weak, or vague interactions:

- Assist the client in talking to others.
- Teach client and family about medications.
- Praise the client for socializing.

The following are examples of interventions that repeat physician orders and lack definition:

- Monitor the client's progress.
- Check lithium levels.
- Notify social services.

Nursing Interventions Classification. In *Nursing Interventions Classification*, the authors define nursing interventions as "any treatment based upon clinical judgment and knowledge that a nurse performs to enhance patient/client outcomes" (Dochterman and Bulechek, 2004, p. 3). The **Nursing Interventions Classification** (NIC) is the first comprehensive, standardized classification of interventions for nurses. The NIC states that one should not change intervention labels and definitions so there is not confusion across settings. However, one is permitted to modify activities to provide individualized care. Box 3-4 lists the NIC definition and accompanying activities to achieve self-esteem enhancement. NIC interventions are linked to NOC outcomes, NANDA diagnoses, and other organizing structures to assure clear, consistent language for nurses in all practice settings and locations. NANDA, NOC, and NIC classification systems are the results of many studies conducted over time by groups of expert nurses using multiple research methods, including clinical field testing. Research continues to define and redefine evidence-based diagnoses, outcomes, and interventions.

Impact of Interventions on Etiologies and Risk Factors. Interventions have the greatest influence when focused toward etiologies (related factors) that accompany an actual diagnosis or when the nurse aims them at the risk factors of a risk diagnosis. Etiologies and risk factors change from client to client, even though the diagnosis is the same, so it is important to select interventions that target each client's specific etiologies, risk factors, and defining characteristics (signs and symptoms) (NANDA, 2005). The following examples illustrate the effect of interventions on two clients with the same diagnosis but different etiologies (related to):

1. *Nursing diagnosis:* Powerlessness related to loss of control over mental illness
   As evidenced by: Verbal statement that nothing will change the mental condition.
   Outcome: Client will gain some power and control over mental illness.
   Interventions: Teach the client that mental illness is treatable with medication and therapies.
2. *Nursing diagnosis:* Powerlessness related to inability to engage in social interactions
   As evidenced by: Statements of feeling powerless and incompetent in social interactions.
   Outcome: Client will demonstrate more control and competence in social interactions.
   Interventions: Discuss and role-model competent social interactions with client.

Rationale Statements. A rationale statement is the reason for the nursing intervention. Rationales are not always part of the written care plan in clinical practice, yet

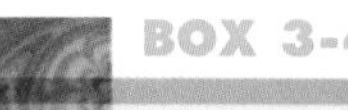

BOX 3-4

NIC Intervention: Self-Esteem Enhancement

Definition: Assisting a patient to increase his or her personal judgment of self-worth.

ACTIVITIES

- Monitor patient's statements of self-worth.
- Determine patient's locus of control.
- Determine patient's confidence in own judgment.
- Encourage patient to identify strengths.
- Encourage eye contact in communicating with others.
- Reinforce the personal strengths that patient identifies.
- Provide experiences that increase patient's autonomy, as appropriate.
- Help patient to identify positive responses from others.
- Refrain from negatively criticizing.
- Refrain from teasing.
- Convey confidence in patient's ability to handle situation.
- Assist in setting realistic goals to achieve higher self-esteem.
- Help patient to accept dependence on others, as appropriate.
- Help patient to reexamine negative perceptions of self.
- Encourage increased responsibility for self, as appropriate.
- Help patient to identify the impact of peer group on feelings of self-worth.
- Explore previous achievements.
- Explore reasons for self-criticism or guilt.
- Encourage the patient to evaluate own behavior.
- Encourage patient to accept new challenges.
- Reward or praise patient's progress toward reaching goals.
- Facilitate an environment and activities that will increase self-esteem.
- Help patient to identify significant effects of culture, religion, race, gender, and age on self-esteem.
- Instruct parents on the importance of their interest and support in their children's development of a positive self-concept.
- Instruct parents to set clear expectations and to define limits with their children.
- Teach parents to recognize children's accomplishments.
- Monitor frequency of self-negating verbalizations.
- Monitor lack of follow-through in goal attainment.
- Monitor levels of self-esteem over time, as appropriate.
- Make positive statements about patient.

From Dochterman JM, Bulechek GM: *Nursing interventions classification (NIC),* ed 4, St Louis, 2004, Mosby.

they are generally part of the overall discussion of treatment in team meetings. Rationales reflect nurses' accountability for their actions. Clear, descriptive rationale statements (in italics) follow the interventions in each chapter on disorders to help explain the selected interventions. Consider these examples:

- Listen actively to the client's expressed feelings *to show the client respect and dignity.*
- Engage the client in brief interactions during the day *to acknowledge the client's self-worth.*
- Praise the client for participating in activities *to reinforce healthy, functional behaviors.*

Standard VI. Evaluation

The nurse evaluates the client's outcomes.

Evaluation of the client's progress and the nursing activities involved are critical because nurses are accountable for the standards of care in each discipline. Evaluation of achieved outcomes occurs at various times during treatment, as stated in the outcomes section, with the client's health state and capability being the primary considerations. There are two steps in the evaluation phase:

1. *The nurse compares the client's current mental health state or condition with the outcome statement.* For example, is the client's anxiety reduced to a tolerable level? Can he or she sit calmly for 10 minutes, attend an activity for 15 minutes, or socialize with the staff for 5 minutes without distractions? Is there a significant reduction in pacing, fidgeting, or scanning? Did the client achieve these outcomes within the times initially projected? Also, the degree to which the client achieves outcomes is an evaluation of the effectiveness of nursing, though other factors have influence over outcomes.
2. *The nurse considers all of the possible reasons why the client did not achieve outcomes.* For example, sometimes it is too soon to evaluate the outcomes, and the plan of action needs to continue for a longer period of time. For instance, the client needed another 2 days of one-to-one interactions before attending group activities. Occasionally the interventions are too strong and frequent, or they are too weak and infrequent. Some outcomes are unattainable, impractical, or just not possible for a client, or sometimes they are not within the client's capabilities on a developmental or sociocultural level. What about the validity of the nursing diagnosis? Did the nurse develop it with a questionable or faulty database? Do he or she need more data? What were the conditions during the assessment phase? Was the assessment hurried? Did the nurse make conclusions too quickly? Were there any language, cultural, or other barriers to communication? The nurse will make recommendations based on the conclusions drawn from these questions. Often this includes a review of the previous steps of the nursing process. Informal evaluation of the client's progress takes place continually.

Documentation: The Seventh Standard of Care

It is mandatory for the nurse to record an evaluation of the client's changing condition, informed consents (for medication and treatment), response to medication, ability to engage in treatment programs, signs and symptoms (suicidal and homicidal tendencies being the most critical), client concerns (in the client's words as appropriate), and any other critical incidents that occur. The nurse documents according to facility standards. This can be in a narrative, a checklist, or an electronic (computerized) form. Although the entire mental health team is responsible for relating client progress, the nurse in charge is generally accountable for accuracy in record keeping. This is critical because documentation involves more than communicating client progress among team members. Documentation is important for legal issues such as confidentiality and privacy acts, insurance reimbursement accreditation, quality assurance, case management, utilization review, peer review, and research (see HIPAA information in the Assessment section of this chapter and Chapter 8; see managed care information in Assessment and Planning sections of this chapter and Chapter 28).

Problem-Oriented SOAP Charting

In an effort to reduce ineffective documentation, Dr. Lawrence Weed, a physician, developed the problem-oriented medical record (POMR) in 1968. The SOAP note evolved from the POMR in 1969 (Fitz, 2005; Weed, 1969). The **SOAP note** is a problem-solving method nurses commonly use in all health care settings to analyze relevant client problems and prevent long text. It is a form of *charting by exception* because the identified problem is an exception to the client's usual behavior.

SOAP is an acronym for *s*ubjective data (client statement), *o*bjective data (nurse's observations), *a*ssessment (nurse's analysis of S and O, which is often a problem statement or nursing diagnosis), and *p*lan (nurse's proposed actions). SOAP notes are generally based on problems or diagnoses formulated by the multidisciplinary team. SOAP notes then become part of the client's care plan. Although this promotes consistency in problem solving, it also restricts entries to only identified problems, therefore recorders need to be aware of other client issues that happen and report them as well. Two other letters were added later to the SOAP note: I (*i*nterventions, or nurse's response to problem) and E (*e*valuation of client outcomes). There are a number of similar problem-oriented methods, such as DAR (data, analysis, response) and PIE (problem, intervention, evaluation). Table 3-7 is an example of a SOAPIE note.

NURSING PROCESS IN COMMUNITY AND HOME SETTINGS

As trends in health care delivery continue to shift to community and home care settings, psychiatric nurses continue to rely on the nursing process to treat clients outside of traditional inpatient facilities. Areas of assessment include client safety, ability to manage symptoms, how clients use effective coping skills, how clients follow their medication regimen, and clients' use of support systems. The psychiatric home health nurse leads the team in identifying outcomes and developing treatment plans and interventions based on problems identified in the assessment phase. Community and home care are primary alternatives to hospitalization, and the nursing process plays a major role in helping nurses deliver effective care wherever it is needed. (See Chapter 28).

Psychiatric Case Management System

Psychiatric case management is a system that identifies candidates who are eligible for home care. A multidisciplinary team led by a registered nurse treats the clients on a health care continuum. The team relies on all available resources to meet treatment goals and achieve client out-

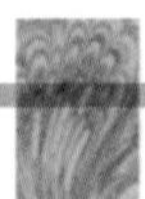

TABLE 3-7

Example of a SOAPIE Documentation Note

Admitting Diagnosis: Bipolar disorder, mania with psychotic features (persecutory delusions)

Identified Problem: Cognitive impairment (client believes people are planning to harm him)

S—Subjective data (client statement)	"I'm sure there are people here who are planning to hurt me; I see them talking and whispering together whenever I'm around."
O—Objective data (nurse's observation)	Client is hyperverbal; scans the environment; demonstrates worried affect (facial expression); is unable to attend activities for more than 5 minutes; cannot engage in one-to-one conversation for more than 2 minutes.
A—Assessment (nurse's analysis)	Disturbed thought processes (delusions of persecution) related to worsening of manic symptoms. Moderate anxiety because of belief that staff and other clients are planning to hurt him.
P—Plan (proposed action plan)	Reinforce client safety. Orient client to reality. Offer medications (as needed), and explain reason. Redirect client and remain with him as necessary. Alert staff of client's condition.
I—Interventions (response to problem)	Reassured the client that he will not be harmed on the unit: "You are safe on this unit. No one here will hurt you." Oriented client in a nonthreatening way: "I know you think this way now, but those people are staff as I am, and the others are clients." Administered 2 mg of haloperidol (Haldol), PO prn, as ordered. Informed client that medication will help clear up thoughts and reduce anxious feelings in time. Redirected client to other unit activities and remained with him until his symptoms were reduced and he felt safe on the unit. Alerted staff of client's delusions of persecution and anxious feelings. Continued to monitor client's response to treatment.
E—Evaluation (of client outcome)	Client's speech has slowed down to a normal pace; he no longer has a worried affect; is able to attend activities for 10 minutes; is able to engage in one-to-one conversation for 5 minutes; states that "thoughts are more subdued and less troubling, but still occur off and on." He believes medication has helped reduce anxiety about his thoughts and feels safe as long as staff members are close by and talk to him now and then. He no longer says others are talking about him and planning to harm him; he is spending more time on the unit arranging magazines and watching TV.

comes in a quality, cost-effective manner. At one end of the continuum is the highest degree of wellness within the client's capacity, and at the other end of the continuum is death, with varying levels of wellness and illness in between (Medina, 2002). Accurate placement of the client at the entry point on the continuum and a clear understanding of the team's best estimate for the final date of home care services are critical to the success of case management. (See Chapter 28).

CHAPTER SUMMARY

- The nursing process is a problem-solving method used by nurses to deliver care in all settings. The six steps are assessment, diagnosis, outcome identification, planning, implementation (interventions), and evaluation.
- The nursing process is an ongoing, cyclic approach to care in which data are continually analyzed and incorporated into a treatment plan. It is not a linear method.
- The mental status exam (MSE) and psychosocial assessment are foundations for the psychiatric nursing assessment. The client's history and physical exam are also relevant.
- The Health Insurance Portability and Accountability Act (HIPAA) of 1996 mandates the protection and privacy of a client's health information.
- Evidence-based research (relevant research), critical thinking, expertise, and intuitiveness are all elements used in the nursing process.
- Assessment includes collecting data that are subjective (client history) and objective (client mental state and behavior).
- Assessment rating scales are tools that help nurses evaluate and monitor client functioning and progress. An example is the global assessment of functioning scale.
- NANDA provides nurses with research-based diagnoses, a unique vocabulary that distinguishes the profession and defines the practice, a common language for nurses, and a way to ensure accountability for care.
- A nursing diagnosis consists of a problem or need, an etiology (related factors or probable cause), and defining characteristics (signs and symptoms; i.e., supporting data). A risk diagnosis consists of risk factors as supporting data and has no etiology.
- NOC and NIC are two nursing classification systems that present taxonomies for outcomes (NOC) and interventions (NIC) that complement the NANDA taxonomy and language.
- Outcome statements are highly specific, measurable, achievable indicators that come from nursing diagnoses. Outcomes evaluate client progress anywhere along a continuum.
- The planning phase consists of the total planning of the client's treatment approach and the nurse's selection of nursing interventions.
- Standardized care plans are for planning and measuring client care based on the nursing process. The team identifies and prioritizes client problems and works under the guidance of the nurse and psychiatrist to achieve the best client outcomes.
- A clinical pathway is an interdisciplinary, standardized format used to provide and monitor client care and progress. The pathway is a projection of the client's entire length of treatment beginning on the day of admission through discharge.
- The implementation phase involves the actual application of the interventions and rationale (reasons for interventions) developed in the planning phase.
- Evaluation of the client's expected outcomes as designated by the outcome criteria occurs at various levels along the health continuum.
- Documentation is often called the seventh step of the nursing process. The client's chart is a legal document that effectively communicates client outcomes, medications, treatments, responses, and unusual incidents. Insurance companies often use these data to justify the client's hospital stay, so documentation needs to be accurate, timely, and specific.
- A SOAP note is a problem-oriented recording based on problems or diagnoses developed by the interdisciplinary team. SOAP notes become part of the client's care plan and promote consistency in problem solving. The nurse should not restrict SOAP notes to only identified problems. SOAP is an acronym for subjective (S), objective (O), assessment (A), and planning (P). DAR (data, analysis, response) is a similar problem-oriented recording method.

REVIEW QUESTIONS

1 Select the most appropriate nursing diagnosis for the following etiology and defining characteristics: _________ *related to immature responses and manipulative behaviors as evidenced by unstable friendships and instigating conflict with peers*

1. Impaired social interaction
2. Powerlessness
3. Social isolation
4. Deficient knowledge

2 Which diagnostic documentation of a multi-axis diagnosis would the nurse expect in a psychiatric treatment setting?

1. I Chronic renal failure
   II 75
   III Major depression
   IV Loss of employment 2 months ago
   V None
2. I Schizophrenia, undifferentiated type
   II Death of parent last year
   III 60
   IV Paranoid personality disorder
   V Diabetes, type 1
3. I Episodic alcohol abuse
   II Antisocial personality disorder
   III 90
   IV Hyperlipidemia
   V Charges pending for simple assault
4. I Major depression
   II Dependent personality disorder
   III Hypertension
   IV Home destroyed by hurricane last year
   V 80

3 A client begins a new prescription for antipsychotic medication. In which part of the nursing care plan would a nurse record this item?
Monitor client twice a week for abnormal involuntary movements of face, eyes, and mouth.
1. Assessment
2. Diagnosis
3. Planning
4. Intervention
5. Evaluation

4 Which question would the nurse ask to assess a client's judgment?
1. On a scale of 1 to 10 where 10 is panic, how would you rate your anxiety level?
2. What events during your lifetime have caused the most sadness for you?
3. If you had fever and vomiting for three days, what would you do?
4. What is meant by the old saying, "An ounce of prevention is worth a pound of cure"?

5 After completing the nursing assessment of a new client, what is the nurse's next action?
1. Determine the goals and outcome criteria.
2. Implement the nursing plan of care.
3. Formulate the nursing diagnoses.
4. Design interventions to include in the plan of care.

Additional self-study exercises and learning resources are available to you on the ***Companion CD*** *at the back of the book and on the* ***Evolve website*** *at* ***http://evolve.elsevier.com/Fortinash/.***

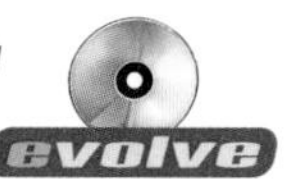

REFERENCES

American Nurses Association: *Code for nurses*, Kansas City, Mo, 1982, American Nurses Association.

American Nurses Association: *Standards of clinical nursing practice*, Kansas City, Mo, 2000, American Nurses Association.

American Psychiatric Association: *Diagnostic and statistical manual of mental disorders*, ed 4, text revision, Washington, DC, 2000, American Psychiatric Association.

Ankner GM: *The nursing process word search: advance for nurses*, Southern California, Nov 2005; www.advanceweb.com.

Benner P: *From novice to expert: excellence and power in clinical nursing practice*, Menlo Park, Calif, 2001, Addison-Wesley.

Dochterman JM, Bulechek GM: *Nursing interventions classifications (NIC)*, ed 4, St Louis, 2004, Mosby.

England M: Analysis of nurse conversation: methodology of the process recording, *J Psychiatr Ment Health Nurs* 12:661, 2005.

Fidaleo RA: Suicide assessment and interventions: a videotaped program for nurses and physicians, San Diego, Calif, 2002, *Sharp HealthCare*, updated 2006.

Fitz M: *The POMR (problem oriented medical record)*, Loyola University Chicago, Strich School of Medicine, update, Oct 2005.

Geddes J et al: Evidence-based practice in mental health, *Evidence-Based Mental Health* 1:4-5, 1998; www.evidbasedmentalhealth.com.

King M, Shell R: Teaching and evaluating critical thinking with concept maps, *Nurse Educator* 27:214-216, 2002.

Kritek PB: Generation and classification of nursing diagnosis: toward a theory of nursing, *Image J Nurs Scholarship* 10:73, 1978.

Medina, L: Clinical pathways: Sharp Home Health, *Home Care*, update 2002.

Moorhead S, Johnson M, Maas M: *Nursing outcomes classification (NOC)*, ed 3, St Louis, 2004, Mosby.

North American Nursing Diagnosis Association: *Nursing diagnoses: definitions & classification, 2007-2008*, Philadelphia, 2007, NANDA International.

Sommers-Flanagan J, Sommers-Flanagan R: *Critical interviewing*, ed 3, Hoboken, NJ, 2003, Wiley.

Studor Q: Sharp HealthCare Leadership Development sessions, Nov 2002.

Weed LL: *The problem oriented record (POMR), as a basic tool: medical records, medical education, and patient care*, Cleveland, Ohio, 1969, Cleveland Case Western Reserve University Press.

Whiteside C: A model for teaching critical thinking in the clinical setting, *Dimensions of Critical Care Nursing* 16(3):157-162, 1997.

Wilson GT: Treatment manuals in clinical practice, *Behav Residential Ther* 35:205-210, 1997.

Chapter 4

Therapeutic Communication

SUSAN FERTIG MCDONALD

It is the province of knowledge to speak and it is the privilege of wisdom to listen.
OLIVER WENDELL HOLMES

OBJECTIVES

1. Analyze the components of communication.
2. Discuss factors that influence communication.
3. Differentiate among social, intimate, collegial, and therapeutic communication.
4. Describe the characteristics of effective helpers.
5. Discuss the core qualities of the nurse and the various roles the nurse plays in interacting therapeutically with clients.
6. Explain the principles of therapeutic communication.
7. Compare and contrast the communication techniques that enhance and block therapeutic communication.
8. Examine therapeutic communication in the context of the nursing process.
9. Discuss three special communication challenges and their implications for the future.

KEY TERMS

boundary violations, p. 75
communication, p. 57
confidentiality, p. 78
congruent, p. 62
countertransference, p. 75
empathy, p. 67
feedback, p. 61
genuineness, p. 67
interpersonal communication, p. 64
intrapersonal communication, p. 64
medium, p. 61
message, p. 60
nonverbal communication, p. 62
positive regard, p. 67
receiver, p. 61
resistance, p. 75
sender, p. 60
stimulus, p. 60
therapeutic communication, p. 65
transference, p. 75
verbal communication, p. 62

Communication, the most powerful tool in psychiatric nursing, is the method used to activate the nursing process. Communication is the foundation for the nurse-client relationship, the domain of psychiatric nursing. Hildegard E. Peplau, a pioneer and educator in mental health nursing, first identified this concept (Peplau, 1952). Peplau believed that the therapeutic interaction between the nurse and the client occurs in the environment of the nurse-client relationship and passes through distinct but overlapping phases from orientation (admission) to resolution (discharge). As a way to educate nurses about the effects of the therapeutic interaction, Peplau developed the process recording, a time proven method that helps nurses examine the relationship between nurse and client through a written account of the interaction that the nurse records privately, directly after the interaction occurs (Table 4-1). Peplau (1991) believed that both the nurse and the client are equal participants in the therapeutic process, and the overall goal is to improve the client's health and wellness.

Communication is a dynamic, process in which two or more people share all types of information. Because we learn how to communicate at an early age, this seems like a relatively simple task. Instead, communication is a complex process that consists of a combination of verbal and nonverbal behaviors used in various ways to share information. Communication, therefore, requires much practice in order to be effective.

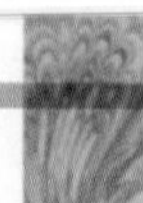

TABLE 4-1

Process Recording

NURSE'S COMMUNICATION (VERBAL AND NONVERBAL)	CLIENT'S COMMUNICATION (VERBAL AND NONVERBAL)	COMMUNICATION TECHNIQUES	
		CLIENT	NURSE
1. *(Verbal)* "Good afternoon, Joe. I'm Heather, a student nurse. I'll be here two evenings a week for about eight weeks. I'd like to spend some time talking with you about your hospital stay. How does that sound?" *(Nonverbal)* Open posture, eye contact, moderate voice tone, calm manner, good spatial boundaries.			1. Offering self and giving information, setting limits and boundaries, open-ended questioning (therapeutic techniques that build trust and rapport).
	1. *(Verbal)* "It sounds okay to me I guess, as long as we don't have to talk when I am scheduled for my patio breaks and the group activities. I'm making moccasins for my son. I really miss him." *(Nonverbal)* Closed posture, worried facial expression, shaky voice, restless, fidgeting in chair.	1. Agreeing to interact with condition that client's own needs are met. Revealing regard for client's schedule and his need to bring his son something positive from his hospital stay. May be anxious because of the effects of medication or may be nervous about revealing himself to a stranger.	
2. *(Verbal)* "I understand your need to participate in the activities and will not interrupt your schedule. How have things been going for you in the hospital?" *(Nonverbal)* Same as in #1.			2. Acknowledging and respecting client's expressed needs. Using open-ended questioning and listening skills to elicit client's perceptions and feelings about his hospital stay and progress.
	2. *(Verbal)* "Oh, so-so. I'm not sure I really belong here with the other patients. Their problems seem really serious. I just want to finish my moccasins and then go home." *(Nonverbal)* Same as in #1.	2. Expresses feeling fair ("so-so"), indicating he has not yet completely regained his mental health. Uses defense mechanism of denial and lack of insight with response, "I don't belong here with the other patients."	
3. *(Verbal)* "You don't think you need to be in the hospital? What brought you here?" *(Nonverbal)* Leaning slightly toward the client to show interest. Moderate voice tone, concerned facial expression.			3. Using reflectional restatement to repeat client's response, so he can think more about the content of his words. Using open-ended questions to elicit source of client's hospitalization.
	3. *(Verbal)* "Oh, I guess I just had too much energy and too many thoughts all at one time. I liked it when I had lots of energy, but all those thoughts were too much for me and I was confused. I feel better now and I just want to go home!" *(Nonverbal)* Began gesturing with arms in the air to show lots of energy. Tone seems to indicate episode was not serious.	3. Still denying problem. Appears to minimize seriousness of mental illness episode and repeats desire to go home.	

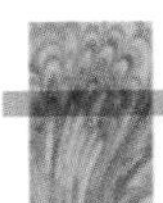

TABLE 4-1

Process Recording—cont'd

NURSE'S COMMUNICATION (VERBAL AND NONVERBAL)	CLIENT'S COMMUNICATION (VERBAL AND NONVERBAL)	COMMUNICATION TECHNIQUES	
		CLIENT	NURSE
4. *(Verbal)* "Tell me about the energy and the thoughts you were having." *(Nonverbal)* Eye contact. Concerned facial expression. Voice tone indicating interest.			4. Using exploration to determine more fully the client's experiences. Showing interest with nonverbal expressions.
	4. *(Verbal)* "Well, my doctor told me I had a manic episode so I must have skipped a few doses of my medication." *(Nonverbal)* No eye contact; gesturing with hands as if to dismiss the seriousness of his actions.	4. Client admits to having episode of mania, which is part of his bipolar disorder. Also admits to skipping his medication. Body language indicates action was not significant.	
5. *(Verbal)* "I see, so you're saying your manic episode happened because you stopped taking your medication?" *(Nonverbal)* Leaning forward to show interest. Slightly frowning to show concern and desire to understand client's admission.			5. Using consensual validation to determine congruence of nurse and client understanding.
	5. *(Verbal)* "Yeah, yeah, I guess I shouldn't have stopped my meds—but the side effects were bothering me." *(Nonverbal)* Slight eye contact, fidgeting in chair.	5. Admits to experiencing a manic episode and links it to stopping his medications. Shows some insight into why he stopped taking his medication and seems to understand the cause and effect of his illness and symptoms.	
6. *(Verbal)* "Joe, stopping medication because of side effects is very common, but it can also cause your symptoms to return. Perhaps we can talk about the side effects you were experiencing."			6. Providing information, acknowledging client's stated reasons for stopping medication. Uses refocusing to concentrate on a single important point. Suggests collaboration to work together to solve the problems the client is having with his medication.
	6. *(Verbal)* "Yeah, that would be okay. I know it was really dumb of me to stop them." *(Nonverbal)* Taking face in hands and shaking head from side to side.	6. Seems upset with self because of his behavior (stopping meds). Acting out his frustration by shaking his head and referring to himself as "dumb" when he actually is feeling inadequate.	

Continued

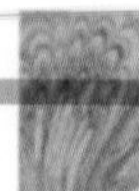

TABLE 4-1

Process Recording—cont'd

NURSE'S COMMUNICATION (VERBAL AND NONVERBAL)	CLIENT'S COMMUNICATION (VERBAL AND NONVERBAL)	COMMUNICATION TECHNIQUES	
		CLIENT	NURSE
7. *(Verbal)* "It sounds as if you recognize that stopping your medication may have resulted in your manic episode." *(Nonverbal)* Eye contact, empathetic tone and body language. *(Moment of silence)* *(Verbal)* "Joe, it's okay to question your actions. That is one way we all learn." *(Nonverbal)* Eye contact, sitting quietly next to client, empathetic demeanor.			7. Acknowledges insight and shows empathy for his distress. Gives client permission to express his feelings. Makes self available to the client by sitting quietly and not attempting to leave client during his time of need.
	7. *(Verbal)* "I guess so. It's just that I keep making the same mistake and then I end up in this stupid hospital, where I don't belong." *(Nonverbal)* Hanging head low toward chest and shaking head from side to side.	7. Seems to understand how stopping his medication worsens the symptoms of his mental illness, although he lacks insight as to how his thoughts and behaviors result in hospitalization.	
8. *(Verbal)* "Today we talked about the connection between the medication you take, your symptoms, and the problems you run into that prevent you from taking your medication. This may be a good point to end our time together today. The next time we meet, let's talk about the ways you might be able to handle the same situation differently in the future." *(Nonverbal)* Sitting back, open posture, offering eye contact.			8. Summarized what was discussed and terminated conversation by encouraging the formulation of a plan of action that suggests collaboration.
	8. *(Verbal)* "Okay, that's good because I need a cigarette now. Thanks for listening. I'll see you next time you're here." *(Nonverbal)* Gets up to begin his patio break. Gives very brief eye contact to the nurse. 9. *(Verbal)* "Okay Joe, I understand and I'll talk to you in a couple of days. Thanks for talking with me." *(Nonverbal)* Begins to stand slowly.	8. Client did well to remain throughout the entire interaction. Still has need to downplay his problems. Uses smoking to help cope. Agreed to talk to nurse again. Thanked the nurse for listening, which shows maturity and respect.	

Effective communication is a major factor in determining client satisfaction, treatment compliance, and recovery (Chant et al., 2002). Communication is critical to the successful outcome of nursing interventions, because without effective communication, a therapeutic nurse-client relationship is unlikely to happen. Therefore the nurse needs to understand and master the general principles of communication, as well as the specific principles and benefits of therapeutic communication.

COMMUNICATION PROCESS

Communication consists of several structural components: the stimulus, the sender, the message, the medium, the receiver, and feedback. Usually there is a **stimulus**, or reason for the communication to occur. The individual who initiates the transmission of information is the **sender**. Each transmission is both verbal and nonverbal. The information being sent and received, such as feelings or ideas, is the **message**. The method by which the mes-

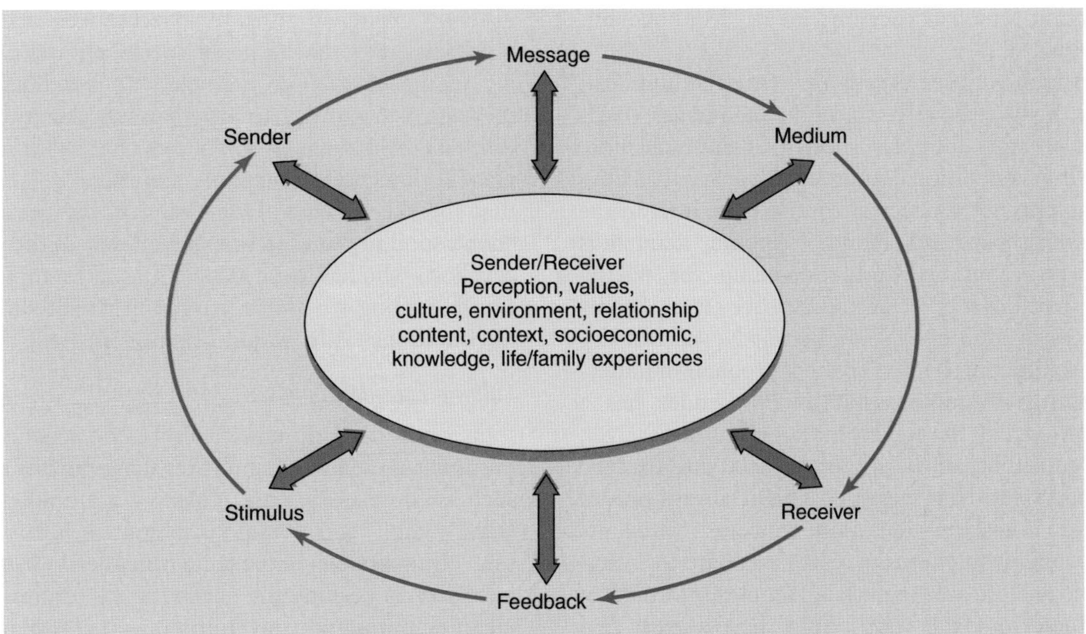

FIGURE 4-1 Model of the communication process.

sage is sent is the **medium**. The medium can be seen (visual), heard (verbal), felt (tactile), or smelled (scent). For example, a note or letter is *seen;* a shout, scream, or whisper is *heard;* body odor or the scent of perfume is *smelled;* a hug or pat on the back is *felt.*

The **receiver** both receives and interprets the message. In an ideal situation, the receiver will interpret the message exactly as the sender intends, producing effective communication. The **feedback** that the receiver gives back to the sender is how you measure the effectiveness of the message. Feedback is a continual process because it is a response to the message and provides a new stimulus to the sender, whereupon the original sender then becomes the receiver. In any interaction, the sender and receiver continually reverse roles. Figure 4-1 shows a model of the communication process.

FACTORS THAT INFLUENCE COMMUNICATION

Communication is a learned process influenced by several factors, including the environment, the relationship between the sender and the receiver, the content of the message, and the context in which the message takes place. Other factors include attitude, values, ethnic background, socioeconomic status, family dynamics, life experience, knowledge level, and the ability to relate to others.

Environmental factors that control the effectiveness of communication include time, location, noise, privacy, comfort, and temperature. Timing of the interaction is important. The phrase "counting to 10" describes a waiting or cooling off period necessary for some individuals to ensure that they are able to rationally discuss a hot topic or understand a critical concept. For example, the nurse chooses to wait for a better time to begin teaching a client about medications, because the client has just experienced an emotional outburst in the hallway and is unable to concentrate in that environment. A carefully chosen time will mean the difference between successful and unsuccessful client learning.

The location of the interaction is also instrumental in conveying the sincerity or importance of communication. For example, a man wishes to propose marriage to a woman and chooses a mutually predetermined, romantic place in which to do it. A carefully chosen location means the difference between a yes, maybe, and no answer. If the location is noisy and other people are present, messages in the conversation may not be heard, resulting in ineffective communication. Therefore, the type, quality, and perceived importance of the specific message conveyed depend in part on the general comfort of the environment.

The *relationship* between two people in a conversation greatly influences the communication. For example, a casual friend can give the same message to an individual as an intimate friend, but the receiver may react quite differently to each person according to the nature of each relationship.

The *context,* as well as the content, of the message also influences the receiver's response. The context or circumstances need to be appropriate to the type of interaction. Individuals need to feel safe in their environment in order to disclose highly personal information.

Attitude also affects interaction. Attitude determines how a person responds to another person and includes the person's biases, past experiences, and levels of openness and acceptance. Also, people from one socioeconomic class, ethnic background, or family background sometimes have difficulty communicating with individuals from a different background or class, possibly because of language, values, or knowledge barriers. For example, both eye contact and personal space vary greatly from one culture to another.

How a person is raised greatly influences communication as well. Each person's background encourages, models, and discourages different aspects of communication. For instance, if a traditional household teaches that boys are tough and do not cry, this discourages the boys in the family from expressing sad emotions. Another example is a teenager who is continually told to "shut up" for "talking too much" develops a quiet or nonassertive style of communication as an adult because of the way he was raised.

Knowledge differences often create a problem in understanding during communication. If the sender has a greater knowledge of the subject matter than the receiver, it is the responsibility of the sender to make sure that the receiver understands the message. This is always one of the challenges in teaching important concepts to students or clients. Some people have an ability to relate to a variety of people and are able to explain complex information in simple, understandable terms. Some have a great deal of difficulty doing this and are easily intimidated by others. Everyone has the ability to learn to communicate more easily and clearly and feel secure about it with knowledge about communication techniques, with practice, and with feedback about their efforts.

Perception is an individual's subjective experience that influences interpretation of the message. Because misperceptions create problems in communication, the sender needs to be certain that the receiver has a clear understanding of the message. Effective communication depends on understanding the message, interpreting the message, and providing feedback that supports the correct interpretation.

MODES OF COMMUNICATION

Written Communication

Written communication is primarily used to share information. The reader reads for knowledge, pleasure, and understanding. It is important that the nurse clearly expresses ideas in written form whether it is documentation in the medical record or in the form of statistical reports. Because more and more documentation is in the form of a computerized client record, the ability to navigate through and document within electronic records and templates is essential. The ability to write legibly, spell correctly, use proper grammar, and organize ideas clearly is critical for the nurse. As part of conducting an assessment and providing interventions, the nurse must have the ability to document a client's behavior in objective, descriptive, clear, and concise terms.

Verbal Communication

Verbal communication is the spoken words that encompass the symbols of language. Precise verbal communication is important because spoken words often mean different things to different people. Many words or phrases have slang meanings or have developed new meanings. Some words and phrases also have different meanings for different groups. Figures of speech, jokes, clichés, colloquialisms, and other terms or special phrases carry a variety of meanings. For example, "It is a blue Monday" means it is a sad day to a person who has the ability to think on an abstract level, but to a client with schizophrenia who interprets concretely and literally, it could mean that the sky is blue. "Don't rain on my parade" means "don't spoil my fun" to one person, but to the client with psychosis who has loose associations, it prompts the question regarding whether a parade is actually occurring or the question, "Why would I rain on a parade?"

Cultural Considerations

Individuals from different cultures or generations often misunderstand and misinterpret slang phrases and idioms such as "double dipping," "making good dough," "sick," "totally cool," and "let's go clubbing." It is easy to assume that other people understand intended meanings. It is necessary to periodically check their interpretation. This includes examining cues from nonverbal responses.

It is increasingly important for nurses to develop a greater sensitivity to the cultural aspects of communication. It is clearly a challenge to learn how to communicate effectively with psychiatric clients who not only have difficulty communicating in a clear, logical, or reasonable manner because of their mental disorder but who are also from another culture and use English as a second language. Chapter 7 further discusses issues of communication with those from cultural groups different from one's own.

Nonverbal Communication

Many communication theorists believe that **nonverbal communication** is the most important part of any message, composing about 93% of any communication. It includes elements that do not involve actual words. Nonverbal cues involve all five senses. They add to the meaning of verbal messages by performing several functions such as expression of feelings, the contradiction or validation of verbal messages, and the preservation of both the ego and the relationship. As a general rule, nonverbal behavior is more revealing and truthful than verbal communication. Actions really do speak louder than words. Therefore, it is important for the nurse to observe and consider the client's entire message, both verbal and nonverbal, before arriving at a conclusion.

To be an effective communicator, nonverbal cues need to be **congruent**, or consistent, with the verbal message. An example of congruent communication follows:

Verbal: "I became very worried when you did not arrive at 4:00 PM."

Nonverbal: Concerned facial expression, warm, friendly, outstretched welcoming hand.

Here is an example of incongruent or inconsistent communication:

Verbal: "I would like to get to know you better."

Nonverbal: Eyes looking away, detached, arms folded across chest.

Nonverbal communication includes facial expression, eye movements, body movements such as posture, gestures, touch, appearance, and the use of space, also known as proxemics (Arnold and Boggs, 2007). (See discussion of space and proxemics in the following paragraphs.)

Body Language

Body language, or cues, includes facial expressions, reflexes, body posture, hand gestures, eye movement, mannerisms, touch, and other body motions. Body posture and facial expressions, including eye movements, are two of the most important cues to determine how a person is responding to the message. When a client who is frowning, with clenched teeth and fists, narrowed eyes, and a red face, says, "I am always glad to see my mother," there is a contradiction between verbal and nonverbal cues that the nurse needs to address. A slumped or stooped posture sometimes means a client is depressed or, at the very least, feeling sad or dejected. A closed posture with arms folded often indicates that a client is withdrawing or possibly feeling some anger. An erect posture with shoulders back means that the client feels more confident or is trying to appear confident. The gait, or way an individual walks, also indicates the client's self-concept. The person who bounces along with shoulders back and head up high usually seems more upbeat than the individual who walks at a slow-moving pace with a slumped posture.

Nurses need to carefully observe hand gestures, as they also signal anger, restlessness, frustration, hopelessness, relaxation, or apathy. For example, the nurse needs to be aware of impending anger so that early interventions can be implemented to prevent a situation from becoming quickly out of control. The old saying "when in doubt, observe what people do, not only what they say" is especially important when dealing with psychiatric clients, because what they say and what they do are often dissimilar.

Paralinguistics

Paralinguistic (paralanguage) behavior includes any sound that is not a spoken word. It includes voice tone, inflection, word spacing, rate, emphasis or intensity, groaning, coughing, laughing, crying, grunting, moaning, and other audible sounds. Along with the silent cues, these audible nonverbal cues are important in assessing clients.

Space (Proxemics)

The use of space is another nonverbal cue. Each person has a comfort zone or space boundary that invisibly surrounds him or her when interacting with others. The boundary becomes larger or smaller, depending on the nature of the relationship. *Intimate space* is the closest distance between two individuals. *Personal space* is for close relationships within touching distance. *Consultive space* is farther apart than personal space, requiring louder speech. *Public space* is for public gatherings, such as where speeches are presented, and usually applies in a large hall or auditorium.

Space as a concept of boundaries and safety is important to understand because the nurse and client need to respect the distance each one needs. For example, if a client has a recent history of assault, the nurse is advised to stay a reasonable physical distance from the client for obvious safety reasons (Fox et al., 2004). For successful communication to occur, both parties need to feel safe. Some clients have problems with their boundaries and invade other clients' own safe zone. Clients who perceive this as threatening react aggressively to such boundary violations. At such times the nurse may need to help the client understand the appropriate distance by stating the boundary for the client in inches or feet, as needed. When the client violates the nurse's own comfortable space, the nurse will need to set a limit for the client after the initial intrusion. For example, the nurse can hold out an arm as a way to help the client assess boundaries.

Touch

Touch is a nonverbal message that involves both action and personal space. Touch typically conveys a message to the receiver that the sender wants to connect with him or her. Nurses have used touch to send messages of concern and empathy. One must be careful when deciding whether to touch a client with a psychiatric disorder. Not all clients want to be touched. Some perceive it as a threat and respond with aggression, or interpret it as an intimate move and respond by withdrawal or inappropriate sexual response. Touch as communication is detailed later in the chapter.

Appearance

Appearance nonverbally communicates a particular image, as well as a clue to one's mental status. Appearance refers to the way an individual uses clothing, makeup, hairstyle, jewelry, and other items such as hats, purses, or eyeglasses, as well as grooming and hygiene. These nonverbal cues often show how the person wishes to be viewed by others.

For example, a female nurse who comes to work wearing a revealing blouse, tight slacks, and high-heeled shoes looks more suitable for a social situation than a work situation. This image does not represent the nursing profession very well and may also confuse the clients as to the nurse's role. Another example is an individual who comes in for a professional job interview wearing jeans, a wrinkled knit shirt, and sandals, with his hair uncombed and his beard untrimmed. On first glance, the employer wonders if the candidate is serious about employment, because his appearance is too casual and sloppy, giving him an unfavorable image. The individual has forgotten the familiar saying "dress for success." A third example is an elderly woman who is admitted to the hospital wearing dirty, wrinkled clothing. A home health nurse finds her in a filthy apartment and she has not bathed in several weeks. On further assessment, she reveals that her husband died 2 months ago, and she was subsequently diagnosed with depression. Therefore her appearance is one result of her obvious unresolved grief response, which has caused her to stop taking care of herself. Try to interpret a client's nonverbal behavior while evaluating the verbal content, and incorporate this evaluation into the assessment of the client and the plan of care.

Finally, nurses need to be aware of their own nonverbal cues. For effective communication to occur, make sure nonverbal messages are congruent with verbal messages, and communicate genuine interest and respect.

TYPES OF COMMUNICATION

Intrapersonal Communication

Intrapersonal communication is essentially talking to yourself, or self-talk. During intrapersonal communication, individuals give themselves all types of positive and negative messages. Self-talk is useful if the messages are helpful or positive. Intrapersonal communication is either functional or dysfunctional.

For example, during a session with the nurse, a client identifies several problems she needs to work on, as well as realistic goals for her hospital stay. The client then tells herself that she is happy that she has finally accomplished a useful task and is now clear about what she needs to do before she leaves the hospital. In this situation, the client gives herself positive messages that assist in her recovery.

An example of dysfunctional self-talk occurs if this same individual persists in giving herself negative, self-defeating messages (e.g., "I can never accomplish anything," or "I will never reach my goals"). This type of self-talk stops or delays recovery.

In another example, a client with a diagnosis of schizophrenia continually hears many internal voices that tell him he is a "bad person," and that he must kill himself to "cleanse his soul." These internal voices, displayed through auditory hallucinations, are dysfunctional self-talk and may require medication. (See Chapter 12.)

Interpersonal Communication

Interpersonal communication occurs between two or more individuals and contains both verbal and nonverbal messages. As stated previously, it is a complex process consisting of a variety of factors affecting its outcome. The nurse communicates on an interpersonal level with a variety of individuals and groups throughout the day. The emphasis is on *therapeutic communication* and *collegial communication* when the nurse is at work. This chapter briefly discusses *social communication*, a form of communication used primarily away from work. The characteristics of social, collegial, and therapeutic communication are presented in Table 4-2.

Social Communication

Social communication occurs in everyday situations, usually away from the work setting. This type of interaction includes discussions regarding family relationships, social activities, vacations, school, and church. Much of this interaction is superficial and light, and it usually does not have a goal. The purpose of most social communication is to maintain relationships and for the enjoyment and mutual benefit of those involved.

Varying levels of intimacy exist in social communication. Communication between parent and child carries a level of intimacy that is different from communication between parent and teacher. Self-disclosure is common and occurs at varying levels, but superficiality is usually the standard, as there are no real expectations of help. When an individual expects help as the outcome of social communication, friends and family typically give help in the form of suggestions and advice. This type of help differs dramatically from the help a nurse gives to the client in a therapeutic relationship.

TABLE 4-2

Characteristics of Social, Collegial, and Therapeutic Communication

	SOCIAL	COLLEGIAL	THERAPEUTIC
Who	Friends, family, acquaintances	Coworkers, colleagues in community	Nurse and client
Setting	Home, away from work; any type of setting	Work, away from clients; professional community	Clinical setting; private, quiet, confidential, safe environment
Purpose	Maintain relationships; mutual sharing of information, thoughts, beliefs, ideas, feelings	Communicate to other professionals about clients, professional issues, and ideas	Promote growth and change in clients
Content	Social talk; focus on children, vacations, family, leisure, church, doing a favor, giving advice	Client's treatment plan; professional practices in work area, sharing observations, and best practices	Therapeutic talk; client expresses thoughts, beliefs, feelings, anxieties, fears, problems; client identifies needs
Characteristics	Superficial, light; not necessarily goal directed; spontaneous, enjoyable; two-way conversation, focusing on both sender and receiver, giving suggestions, advice; personal or intimate relationship occurs	Collaborative, collegial, interdisciplinary, client- or issue-focused	Learned skills; purposeful, client focused; client sets goals; planned, difficult, intense; client discloses personal information; meaningful and personal (but not intimate) relationship occurs
Skills	Uses a variety of resources during socialization	Collaborative responses, effective interactions in groups, assertive interpersonal communication skills	Uses specialized professional skills, primarily therapeutic interpersonal communication

Collegial Communication

The purpose of *collegial communication* is professional collaboration. Collegial communication occurs among colleagues in the professional work setting. In professional nursing groups within the work setting and in the community, this type of collegial communication is called *intradisciplinary*.

When psychiatric nurses interact with members of the unit's treatment team, it is called *interdisciplinary collegial communication*. The interdisciplinary team has regularly scheduled treatment team meetings designed to develop, review, and revise the client's treatment plan. It is important that all members involved in the client's treatment attend and actively participate in the meeting. Members have roles that are critical to the success of the treatment team process. Sometimes the nurse is the designated leader of the meeting and has to clearly communicate with all members of the team. Sometimes the nurse is the recorder, or the person responsible for documenting the significant information discussed in the client's treatment plan. This role requires skillful written communication techniques. Within a nursing professional group, the intent of the communication is to share knowledge, collaborate on a project, or in other ways enhance or improve the profession.

Effective cooperation has the advantage of breaking through power issues and competition that occur when teams of professionals are together. In the collaborative process, no member is more important than another member or the group as a whole. Each member's contribution is equally important to the success of the project, purpose, or goal.

The nurse therefore communicates in the collegial arena with supervisors, coworkers, physicians, consultants, members of the treatment team, and in the professional community. Simultaneously, the psychiatric nurse communicates on a therapeutic level with clients and their family members or significant others.

Therapeutic Communication

Therapeutic communication is the foundation of psychiatric nursing and *the psychiatric nurse's single most important tool*. It is an interactive process that occurs between the nurse (helper) and the client (recipient) in any health care setting. The art of interacting therapeutically is a learned skill involving both nonverbal and verbal communication. One purpose of therapeutic communication is to enhance client growth. Health-promoting interventions also occur through therapeutic communication.

Therapeutic communication is client focused, whereas social communication consists of sharing information equally between two or more individuals. Even though the nurse will engage in some social interaction with the client, such as greeting the client at the beginning of the shift, the progress toward a greater level of health occurs through the therapeutic interaction between the nurse and client.

This therapeutic interaction involves the client disclosing personal information. This sometimes includes hurtful memories and situations that bring up painful emotions. Sharing such feelings is extremely beneficial for the client because it allows him or her to identify and discuss experiences and accompanying feelings in a safe, therapeutic setting. The nurse provides a confidential and quiet setting in which the interaction takes place, encourages the client to openly discuss thoughts and feelings, and practices active listening, acceptance, and empathy.

Therapeutic communication is sometimes intimidating, not only for the client, but also for the nurse. Intense negative feelings are not easy to discuss. Many clients have not previously discussed them for fear of undesired responses such as a lack of understanding on the part of the listener, retaliation, feelings of being unworthy, and inadequacy in explaining them. The intensity of the client's feelings or verbal responses often frightens or surprises the new nurse. This is especially true when a client openly discusses such issues as wanting to die because life is not worth living. A nurse may also feel uneasy when a client discusses an emotion or feeling similar to the nurse's personal experience. If the nurse has not dealt with the personal problem effectively, this may cause anxiety.

In summary, therapeutic communication has three essential purposes: (1) to allow the client to express thoughts, feelings, behaviors, and life experiences in a meaningful way in order to promote healthy growth; (2) to understand the significance of the client's problem(s) and the role the client and the significant people in his or her life play in perpetuating those problems; and (3) to assist in the identification and resolution processes of the client's health-related behaviors. Therapeutic communication is the nurse's primary tool to help clients attain successful outcomes to the problems currently preventing them from achieving optimum health.

PRINCIPLES OF THERAPEUTIC COMMUNICATION

Personal Attributes Important for Therapeutic Communication

Nurses use their own characteristics and selves as the primary tools in psychiatric nursing, the same way singers use their voices as instruments to create music. All of the elements essential to helping another individual are within the nurse. This is both exciting and challenging.

The therapeutic use of the self begins with *knowing oneself*. You will not be able to help others unless you are first able to help yourself. Knowing yourself is a complex and lifelong learning process. It is essential to have self-knowledge before using yourself as a therapeutic tool to help others.

At the core of self-knowledge is the nurse's ability to correctly identify his or her own negative or unresolved issues. Nurses need to know what values and beliefs they hold. It is also important for them to know and understand their own family background, including dynamic cultural and social issues, values, and biases and prejudices.

Nurses need to be aware of unresolved family life issues and make every effort to resolve them as soon as they are recognized. For example, a female nurse has a long-held belief regarding women and alcohol dependency. She believes others are able to stop drinking if they really want to stop. Her belief developed because her maternal grandmother had died from alcohol-related liver disease. The nurse is perhaps unaware that she holds this belief until she has her first alcohol-dependent female client. It is only when the nurse understands and resolves her issues that she can truly succeed in the necessary separation of her own issues from those of the client.

One model of communication that can help the nurse look at self-awareness is the Johari window, developed by Joseph Luft and Harry Ingham in the 1950s (Luft and Ingham, 1955). The Johari window consists of four areas or window panes framed in a square box. The four panes—open, blind, hidden, and unknown—represent parts of the whole self (Figure 4-2).

To increase self-awareness, one must strive to increase the open area in pane 1 and decrease the blind, hidden, and unknown areas in panes 2, 3, and 4. Generally, as the nurse becomes a better communicator, pane 1, the open area, increases. As the nurse shares things about himself or herself, pane 1 grows larger and pane 3, the hidden area, decreases. In the process of asking for feedback from others, pane 2 grows smaller. As a result of the nurse becoming more self aware through interpersonal learning, pane 1, representing thoughts, feelings, and behaviors that are known to self and to others, becomes larger as the other three panes decrease in size.

Because therapeutic communication occurs for the purpose of helping others, it is vital that nurses *understand what motivates them to help others* and recognize their emotional needs so that they do not interfere with the ability to relate therapeutically to clients. Because clients do not take care of nurses' emotional needs, nurses need to meet their own emotional needs outside of work. A well-balanced, multifaceted lifestyle satisfies emotional needs. When your needs are met, you will be able to help the client through therapeutic communication.

Nurses who are *in control of their own lives and emotions* engage the client in effective communication while maintaining therapeutic control of the conversation, especially when a client is intimidating, manipulative, or threatening.

Also, nurses who are comfortable with themselves put the client's needs first by listening attentively and recognizing emotions in the client that will block a therapeutic exchange. For example, a high level of anxiety produces tunnel vision in a client, which damages communication.

Finally, *conduct a periodic self-evaluation of your responses to the client.* Questions to ask include the following (Shives, 2002):

- Am I open minded or closed minded regarding this issue?
- Am I accepting? Or am I rejecting?
- Am I being supportive? Or am I being nonsupportive?
- Am I being objective? Or am I allowing my biases to interfere with the interaction?
- Am I remaining calm and in control of my own feelings? Or am I allowing my anxiety, sympathy, or anger to surface?
- What are my true feelings? Do my nonverbal cues match my verbal communication?

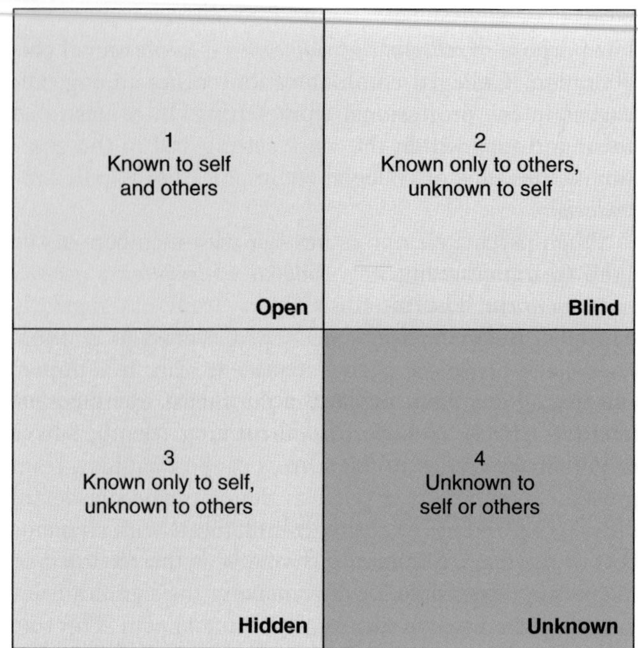

FIGURE 4-2 Johari window showing the four areas that make up the whole self.

Many employers have employee assistance programs (EAP) to help employees with personal issues that occur in the workplace that interfere with communicating effectively. Use these employee benefit services to help deal with personal issues that affect your ability to do your job well.

Roles of the Nurse in Therapeutic Communication

Nurses assume many roles during therapeutic communication with clients. One is being a professional role model. In the professional role, the nurse acts as teacher, socializer, technician, advocate, parent, counselor, and therapist. As a *role model,* the nurse is respected by staff, students, and the community. The nurse models therapeutic communication for clients, staff, and students. In the community, as well as in the health care setting, you will represent the nursing profession, and others will judge the profession based on your actions.

Clients learn about their illness and treatment methods from the nurse as a *teacher.* As a teacher, the nurse uses clear, effective communication to educate other staff and clients. The nurse as a *socializer* brings clients together for activities to prevent the social isolation of the client during hospital treatment. In the *technician* role the nurse performs a Glucometer test, administers medications, or takes vital signs. As an *advocate,* the nurse informs the client of his or her rights and responsibilities and supports the client in decision making. The advocate nurse also serves as a protector of the client by acting as a link between ethics and the law (Arnold and Boggs, 2007). The nurse in the *parent* role performs traditional nurturing tasks such as feeding, bathing, or comforting. As a *counselor*, the nurse assists the client with personal problems such as a disagreement between the client and a family member. With advanced education the nurse can also be a *therapist*, conducting individual, group, or family therapy sessions in the hospital, clinic, or community setting.

As part of the therapeutic relationship with a client, the nurse performs some or all of these roles. The number of roles the nurse assumes varies according to the type and length of the individual nurse-client relationship, as well as the setting of the interactions.

Traits of Therapeutic Communication

The following are traits of effective therapeutic communication: genuineness, positive regard or respect, empathy, trustworthiness, clarity, responsibility, and assertiveness. These characteristics allow the nurse to influence growth and change in others. They incorporate verbal and nonverbal behaviors, as well as attitudes, beliefs, and feelings behind the communication, and they are necessary for therapeutic communication to take place.

Genuineness

Genuineness is demonstrated by being consistent with both verbal and nonverbal behavior. Consistent verbal and nonverbal behavior shows that you are open, honest, and sincere. Genuineness is necessary for clients to develop trust in the nurse. You build trust when you do not appear to just be doing your job but rather when you respond with sincere interest. Genuine interaction does not mean that you have to discuss personal information or relate to the client in a social manner. It means that you remain focused on the client and respond therapeutically, using a variety of helpful responses. Do not expect a client to be open and honest if you do not display these characteristics yourself.

Positive Regard

Positive regard refers to respect and acceptance. Nurses show that they view their clients as worthy, for example, by addressing the client by the name the client prefers. Nurses accept clients for who and where they are and do not expect them to change except as it relates to their goals in treatment. Positive regard, or respect, is communicated in a variety of ways. Sitting and listening to a client, expressing concern about events affecting a client, validating the client's feelings, and effectively responding to a client's negative behavior all communicate respect. For example, a client who has just been admitted in the dayroom is found openly undressing in front of others. After assessing the situation and understanding that this activity is not harmful to others, the nurse explains to the client that undressing is for the privacy of his or her bathroom. The nurse then closes the door to allow the client to continue, but out of the view of others.

Part of positive regard is being nonjudgmental. Avoid harsh judgment of clients' behaviors and feelings because both are real and cannot be argued with, discounted, or criticized. Do not make clients feel wrong. Labeling behaviors based on your own value system is not useful. Instead, the nurse helps clients explore their behavior by discussing the thoughts and feelings that determine the behavior. When clients realize that they are not being judged, they will feel free to express their most intimate thoughts and feelings. A nonjudgmental attitude in the nurse relaxes clients by removing fears of being misunderstood or rejected. This open relationship occurs only when nurses identify their own thoughts and feelings regarding clients' behaviors.

Empathy

Empathy is the foundation of all therapeutic nurse-client relationships and is therefore an essential trait for nurses to have in order to meet their client's needs. It is difficult for clients to trust their nurse if they do not believe the nurse has an empathetic appreciation of them as individuals (McCabe, 2004; Reynolds, 2000). Empathy, or empathic understanding, is the nurse's ability to see things from the client's viewpoint and to communicate this understanding to the client. The ability to be sensitive to and communicate understanding of the client's feelings is an essential characteristic of a therapeutic relationship (May and Alligood, 2000). The nurse's ability to be fully and uniquely present with another human being is the most significant quality of a successful nurse-client relationship (Carpenito, 2000). Some research implies that empathy is a natural human trait that everyone has in varying degrees and the trait matures as we grow.

Some researchers suggest that more work is necessary in developing new ways to teach nursing students how to respond empathetically to clients (Walker and Alligood, 2001). Determining levels of empathy in students will help identify potential problematic levels that are either too low or too high. High levels of natural empathy indicate that the nurse has a tendency to overidentify and thus become too involved with clients' problems. Low levels indicate that the nurse is not able to demonstrate enough genuine concern for clients. Knowing this information will better assist the new nurse in periodic self-assessments.

Do not confuse empathy with sympathy. Sympathy is overinvolvement and sharing your own feelings after hearing about another person's similar experience. It is not objective, and its primary purpose is to decrease your own personal distress.

For example, a client tells the nurse that her father died in an automobile accident 1 month before his arrival at the hospital. The nurse responds sympathetically by saying that her own father died in an automobile accident and that it had made the nurse feel sad for a year afterward. Here the focus is on the nurse, and the client does not know how to respond. An empathic response involves an appreciation and awareness of the client's feelings and keeps the focus on the client. An empathic response is:

"I can understand how difficult that must be for you. Tell me how you are feeling now and how you have been coping with the loss." Now the focus is on the client, and the client is better able to reply.

The development of empathy poses a challenge for the psychiatric mental health nurse in the hospital setting, who typically has a brief time frame with clients and must primarily use crisis intervention principles. Lower levels of empathy from the nurse are healthier for clients in the beginning stage of the relationship. Research has shown that empathy, especially if it is expressed early in a relationship, is clearly related to positive treatment outcomes.

Empathy consists of two stages. If a client shares important and uncomfortable emotions, first be receptive to understanding the client's communication by putting yourself in the client's place. This does not mean that you need to have had the same problem or associated feeling. Then, after stepping back into the professional role, be able to communicate understanding, which demonstrates objectivity and sensitivity to the client. This understanding mirrors the client's identity and is the process the client uses to make changes to achieve positive outcomes. The following skills help nurses develop greater empathic responses:

- Attending to the client physically, by sitting in front of the client, at a slight angle, leaning slightly forward with hands and arms in an open stance
- Attending to the client emotionally by clearing your mind of other personal or work-related business and focusing your full attention on the client
- Actively listening by providing a response to each of the client's verbal and nonverbal communications
- Focusing on the client's strengths
- Expressing caring, warmth, interest, and concern through nonverbal behaviors
- Choosing the most important point of what the client is trying to say
- Demonstrating consistency between your own nonverbal and verbal communication
- Checking your empathic responses for effectiveness by looking for verbal and nonverbal clues

Active listening is closely associated with empathy because it incorporates both nonverbal and verbal behaviors necessary for therapeutic communication. Nonverbally, the nurse leans slightly forward, facing the client; uses eye contact; nods; and uses verbal phrases such as "uh huh" or "I understand." Active listening is a dynamic, interactive nonjudgmental process that requires you to listen for facts as well as the underlying meaning of the client's communication, to accurately interpret the meaning, and to provide the client with feedback regarding the nurse's understanding of the message. The end result of active listening is to fully understand the meaning of the communication (Arnold and Boggs, 2007). A nurse who listens actively is displaying interest. In one study that explored clients' experiences in communicating with nurses, clients reported that the behaviors they valued in nurses were the time the nurses gave them and the nurses' availability for them (McCabe, 2004). A client who is trying to work through problems needs to know that the nurse is there to help and wants to help.

Trustworthiness

Trustworthiness is another essential characteristic of an effective nurse. Being trustworthy means being responsible and dependable. Trustworthy nurses keep commitments and promises and are consistent in their approach and response to clients. For example, if you tell a client that you will meet him or her after lunch, then follow through with your promise, to demonstrate dependability and increase the client's trust. Clients need to know they can rely on the nurse in order to build trust. Trustworthy nurses respect the client's privacy, rights, and the need for confidentiality. Clients need to be confident that the information they share will not go beyond the health care team.

Clarity

Nurses need to communicate clearly to clients who often have difficulty processing information or thinking clearly as a result of their mental disorders. If the nurse is specific and clear, there will be less miscommunication. Clear communication means selecting simple words when speaking and asking questions to clarify meaning. Although using medical vocabulary is part of the profession, remember that clients do not always understand these complex terms. Everyday medical terms such as "taking your vital signs," "NPO after midnight," or "take these medications q.i.d.," are not common to most clients. Problems will happen if instructions and information are given in a highly technical manner. Often, clients are too embarrassed to ask for clarification. Clients appreciate nurses who not only communicate with them in an open and honest manner, but who use language that is easy to understand. The nurse therefore needs to make a conscious effort to speak at a level the client will understand. Avoid abstract, lengthy explanations. This is also true for written communication. When using written materials to educate clients, less is more. Also, make sure that all instructions are written in plain language, using the active rather than the passive voice, avoiding unclear statements, and steering clear of medical terms (American Health Consultants, 2001). Examples are as follows:

Active voice: Take your medications as directed 2 times per day (specify dosage).

Passive voice: Make sure your medication is taken as needed.

Responsibility

Responsible communication involves being accountable for the outcome of professional interactions. When communicating, you are responsible for your part in the interaction and need to make sure that your clients receive and interpret your messages correctly. Nurses who communicate responsibly, strengthen growth in others. Responsible language involves the use of "I" statements when being assertive, as described in the following section.

BOX 4-1

Behaviors of Assertive Communication

ASSERTIVE
Stands up for own rights and respects those of others. Uses expressive, directive, self-enhancing speech. Chooses appropriate words and actions.

AGGRESSIVE
Stands up for own rights but abuses those of others. Speaks in demeaning or attacking manner. Fails to monitor or control words or actions.

PASSIVE
Does not stand up for own rights and accepts the domination and bullying of others. Performs unwanted tasks and feels victimized.

EXAMPLES OF ASSERTIVE BEHAVIORS
- "I" messages (e.g., "I need," "I feel," "I will")
- Eye contact (e.g., looking directly into the eyes of the person while making or refusing a request)
- Congruent verbal and facial expressions (e.g., making certain that the facial expression matches the intent of the spoken message); a serious message accompanied by laughter negates the credibility of the message.

EXAMPLE OF ASSERTIVE PLAN FOR CHANGE
1. Target the behavior that you desire to change (e.g., how to say no and mean it).
2. List approximately 10 situations in which it is difficult to say no, and order them from least to most difficult.
3. Practice saying no, using the least threatening method first and working up to more challenging situations (e.g., imagery, tape recorder, feedback, role-playing), and practice in actual situations.
4. Say no as the first word in the practice response. This is a clear message without excuses or apologies.
5. Follow with a clear, brief, declarative statement (e.g., "I will not rearrange my schedule. I need my day off").
6. Use eye contact appropriate to the intent of the verbal message.

Assertiveness

Assertive communication is the ability to express thoughts and feelings comfortably and confidently in a positive, honest, and open manner that demonstrates respect for self while respecting others (Balzer Riley, 2004). The nurse who communicates assertively makes a conscious choice about how to communicate with others. Communicating assertively is a style choice that you can apply in any situation at any time. An assertive nurse controls negative feelings, which is important in communicating not only with clients but also with supervisors, employees, physicians, and colleagues. Box 4-1 lists behaviors of assertive communication.

You can practice some basic assertiveness techniques as a nurse. First, use responsibility language by using "I" instead of "you" (e.g., "I am responsible for the medication error" or "I feel hurt when you say that to me"). If you blame your behavior on another, you give away your power to make changes. For example, someone who states, "My mother made me angry" or "God told me to hit him," indicates that he has no power or control over his behavior and takes no responsibility for his actions. Being assertive means learning how to say no, expressing opinions and feelings, stating beliefs, and initiating conversation. Nonverbal assertive language includes using good eye contact when speaking.

Assertive messages have the same verbal and nonverbal message. Sometimes, though, clients try to cover up their true sadness by laughing or smiling while relating a painful experience when they do not know how to deal with it in another way.

Responding Techniques That Enhance Therapeutic Communication

Therapeutic responding techniques are methods that encourage clients to interact in ways that promote their growth and move them toward their treatment goals. The more skilled the nurse is in using these techniques, the better the nurse's ability to establish a trusting and collaborative nurse-client relationship that will effectively accomplish mutual goals and objectives (Schuster, 2000). These strategies create an atmosphere that promotes communication for problem solving. Table 4-3 gives examples of many of these techniques.

Silence is an important listening skill for psychiatric nurses to develop. It is not the absence of communication but rather a useful and purposeful communication tool that gives clients time to feel comfortable and respond when they are ready. It is best to use silence to serve a particular function and not to frighten or discomfort the already-anxious client. A successful interview is largely dependent on the nurse's ability to remain silent long enough to allow the client to share relevant information. Silence gives the client an opportunity to consider the communication, weigh alternatives, and formulate an answer. It also gives the nurse an opportunity to think about what she will say to the client, which will enhance the therapeutic conversation.

Active listening is vital to communicating effectively. It is not simply the act of hearing. Several techniques are incorporated into this skill such as paraphrasing the client's thoughts and feelings, understanding the meaning behind the words and phrases, and asking questions. Active listening involves focus and self-discipline and engages all of the nurse's senses.

Support and *reassurance* are provided in a genuine and honest manner. Clients need to be in an atmosphere where they are able to safely discuss sensitive information. Nurses offer both verbal and nonverbal support so that the client feels free to share thoughts and feelings, which is necessary for progress toward mental health to occur.

Sharing observations made by the nurse is important to increase the client's self-understanding. It also demonstrates to the client that the nurse is actively listening.

Acknowledging feelings is a form of client support. It is important to let the client know that his or her feelings are valid and important. There are no right or wrong answers when it comes to feelings. They cannot be taken away, argued with, or discounted.

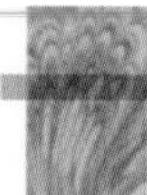

TABLE 4-3

Therapeutic Responding Techniques as Related to Steps of the Nursing Process and Phases of the Therapeutic Relationship

THERAPEUTIC RELATIONSHIP PHASE	NURSING PROCESS STEP	TECHNIQUE	EXAMPLES
Orientation	Assessment and nursing diagnosis	*Introducing self* when the client is admitted	"Hi, my name is Jennifer. I will be your nurse today."
		Offering self. The nurse demonstrates an honest, open posture, making self available to demonstrate concern and interest.	"I have some information to obtain. Let's sit here so we can begin your admission."
		Active listening. Practiced by using both verbal and nonverbal skills that show the nurse is giving full attention to the client.	The nurse faces the client and takes an open position, maintains eye contact, and uses verbal and nonverbal messages to demonstrate that the client has the nurse's full attention. "Go on. I am listening."
		Questioning. The nurse skillfully asks open-ended questions during the initial admission. Interviewing skills are necessary to avoid asking too many personal questions in one session. Direct questions are used to achieve relevance and depth. Closed questions are for gathering factual information.	"How many children do you have?" *(Closed question)* "Has this ever happened before?" *(Closed question)* "How come have you stopped taking your medication?" *(Open-ended question)* "What is that all about?" "Tell me how you feel now?" *(Open-ended question)*
		Silence. The nurse uses silence frequently so that the client has time to verbalize thoughts and feelings. It is planned and used to draw out the client. Silence should be comfortable for both client and nurse.	Sit quietly, maintain comfortable eye contact, and demonstrate interest using nonverbal nods and expressive facial movements.
		Empathizing. The nurse demonstrates warmth and acknowledges client's feelings.	"I know how hurt you must have felt. It sounds like it made you sad."
		Reality orienting/providing information. The nurse explains to the client the type of unit, gives a brief tour, and provides the client with unit information and admission paperwork.	"John, here is a copy of the unit rules. Let's go over a few important items." "You are on the locked unit now." "Today is Friday. You were admitted yesterday afternoon."
		Restating. The nurse repeats what the client says to show understanding and to review what was said.	"You say your friend's death makes you sad." "You became depressed soon after the accident?"
		Clarifying. The nurse asks specific questions to help clear up a specific point the client makes.	"Did it help when you tried any of the techniques you mentioned?" "Which technique helped the most?" "So your mother remarried soon after you were born?"
		Offering reality. The nurse presents a realistic view to the client in a reasonable manner.	"I know you think people are out to get you. I do not think that. You are safe here, and we are here to help you. This medication will help decrease those thoughts."
		Stating observations. The nurse offers a view of what is seen or heard to increase the client's verbalization.	"I see you are quite upset." "I noticed you had trouble sleeping last night."
		Fostering description of perceptions. The nurse asks the client to describe the situation.	"Help me to understand how this is affecting you right now." "What is the voice that you hear telling you?" *(To a client who is hallucinating)*
		Placing the event in time and order. The nurse asks questions to determine the relationships of events, and the nurse helps put events in perspective.	"Was the birth of your child before or after your mother died?" "Did your alcohol abuse begin immediately after your divorce?"
		Voicing doubt. The nurse discusses any uncertainty of the client's perceptions.	"I find it hard to believe that you felt no joy on hearing that she survived." "Are you sure you were in bed for one full year after that?"

TABLE 4-3

Therapeutic Responding Techniques as Related to Steps of the Nursing Process and Phases of the Therapeutic Relationship, cont'd

THERAPEUTIC RELATIONSHIP PHASE	NURSING PROCESS STEP	TECHNIQUE	EXAMPLES
Orientation, cont'd	Assessment and nursing diagnosis, cont'd	*Identifying themes.* The nurse voices issues that come up repeatedly in the course of conversation.	"It sounds like that is very important to you. You've mentioned it a few times." "When this happens over and over, how do you feel?"
		Encouraging comparisons. The nurse asks for similarities and differences among feelings, thoughts, behaviors, and various life situations.	"Was this the same way you reacted the last time it happened?"
		Summarizing. The nurse verbalizes a compilation of what has been expressed on a particular subject or event.	"Let me see if I understand your anxiety about . . ." "From what you describe, your family seems . . ."
		Focusing. Zeroes in on a subject until the important points come into clear view for both the client and the nurse.	"You talk about loss. Tell me more about the losses you've experienced." "You mentioned his drinking. Tell me more about that."
Working	Outcome identification, planning, and implementation	*Evaluating.* The nurse encourages the client to express the importance of an event.	"What does this type of behavior mean to you?" "After thinking about it, how does it affect you now?"
		Encouraging plan formulation helps the client develop steps to make changes and solve problems.	"What are the steps you'll need to take to accomplish that?"
		Assisting in goal setting encourages client to set goals during hospitalization and after hospitalization.	"I will help you set some achievable goals during your hospital stay. Do you have some ideas?"
		Providing information offers data that will help the client to set goals and develop a plan of action.	"This list and description of crisis houses will help you decide on which one will be best for you after discharge." "I have a problem-solving guide that helps people go through the necessary steps to follow in solving big problems."
		Offering alternatives fosters decision making by encouraging the client to work on arriving at healthy, growth-producing decisions.	"Looking over the pros and cons, which plan would be best for you?" "What would be your best alternative, given this situation?"
		Role-playing. The nurse plays the part of a person the client needs to say something to, in order to help the client practice what he or she wants to say.	"Let's go over what you want to say to her." "I'll play your father, and you play yourself." "Sometimes it helps to say it in the mirror a few times before the real encounter."
		Providing feedback. The nurse provides the client with supportive comments in reaction to behaviors or statements made.	"Tell me what you want to say; I'll listen and give you my feedback." "When you walked away, I felt . . ." "You will upset some people with behavior like that."
		Confronting. The nurse supports the client but directly challenges inaction on the part of the client.	"I know this is hard to do, but I believe it will help you make the right decision." "I understand your concerns; however, you have to take some steps now."
		Setting limits. The nurse provides the client with external boundaries to an expressed thought, feeling, or behavior.	"You became very angry again. To stay in the day room, you'll need to act calmer. You can walk in the hallway if you need to get up."
Termination	Evaluation	*Evaluating actions* encourages the client to look at his or her behavior and the outcomes it produces.	"When you tried to do that, how well did it work?" "When you tell her to leave, how do you think she will react?" "Was that useful for you?"

Continued

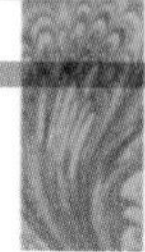

TABLE 4-3

Therapeutic Responding Techniques as Related to Steps of the Nursing Process and Phases of the Therapeutic Relationship, cont'd

THERAPEUTIC RELATIONSHIP PHASE	NURSING PROCESS STEP	TECHNIQUE	EXAMPLES
Termination, cont'd	Evaluation, cont'd	*Reinforcing healthy behaviors* offers positive responses to the client who is trying out new growth-producing behaviors and making helpful decisions.	"It sounds like you have made a healthy choice." "Standing up for yourself is new." "You've successfully tried it, so practicing it daily will be important."
		Encouraging posthospital transition helps the client see that new thoughts and actions can be accomplished after discharge.	"I know you will continue to practice being assertive." "What situations will you run into where you might try this new behavior?" "How can a relapse prevention plan assist you after you leave the hospital?" "Which coping skills will be useful to you when you return home?"

Broad, open-ended statements allow the client to assume some control over topics you will discuss. However, do not allow the client to discuss only nonrelevant topics or engage in a conversation with a superficial or social content. Ask the client questions that do not produce one-word answers. Open-ended questions result in a fuller, more revealing answer, which typically stimulates more questions.

Information giving is an ongoing process for the nurse who provides information to increase the client's knowledge about a variety of topics on his or her illness and treatment. Information decreases fears and anxiety and increases the client's fund of resources and support for his or her problem. Examples include information regarding the client's disorder, medication, aftercare support groups, structured living options, or treatment alternatives. Information is given according to the client's level of understanding and willingness to receive it.

Interpretation of what clients are sharing is useful to help them see the real meaning behind their messages. Be careful when using this technique. A client sometimes disagrees with the nurse's interpretation, which causes obstacles. Helping clients *focus* to pursue a particular topic allows them to spend their time discussing subjects of most importance. *Identification of themes* is necessary to help clients see what they repeatedly bring up in the conversation. *Placing events in order and time* is also important to help clients develop a greater perspective on events in their lives.

Clients often need encouragement to *describe their perceptions* regarding their thoughts and feelings. For example, some clients with psychiatric disorders hear imaginary voices telling them to hurt themselves or others. Ask such clients to tell the staff when this occurs so that you will be able to intervene and prevent clients' attempts to harm themselves or others. Then introduce treatment strategies to reduce this perception and minimize the clients' dysfunctional behavior. (See Chapter 12.)

To develop a sense of clients' past and current behaviors, ask clients to *compare* their present anxiety to that of their last hospitalization. Or ask clients if they have ever experienced this behavior before.

Restating what clients say lets them know that you heard and understood them. It is an active listening technique.

Reflecting is a technique used to turn around a question to obtain a response from the client. Coaching clients to answer a question helps them to accept their own ideas and feelings regarding an important event or behavior.

Clarifying is a method used to ask clients to elaborate or restate something they just said. It increases your understanding and allows clients to rethink and restate their thoughts or feelings.

Confrontation in an accepting manner is necessary for the client to be more aware of incongruent thoughts, feelings, and behaviors. This helps to bring the issue into focus, but you only use this technique after you have established a good relationship (Fortinash and Holoday Worret, 2007).

When a client is struggling to explore and solve a problem but can only see one or two solutions, *offer alternatives.* Suggesting to the client other possible solutions to the problem is not the same as giving advice. Use introductions such as "What have you thought about . . . ?," "Other clients have tried these solutions," and "Other alternatives might be . . . ." The nurse avoids phrases such as "You should," and "I think you need to solve it the way I did" (giving advice).

Voicing doubt is a technique to use when the client is having difficulty relating in a way that sounds believable. Voicing some doubt helps the client to be more realistic about perceptions and conclusions of events. Use voicing doubt cautiously, as doubt sometimes creates barriers between the client and the nurse.

Summarize the information the client provides on a regular basis. Summarizing the main points of what a client has been discussing helps focus on the most important issues related to the client's life situation. After providing the summary, the client can agree or disagree with any point, and then together the nurse and client agree on a final summary.

Role-playing provides a place for the client to act out a particular event, problem, or situation in a safe environment. The nurse can play the other part or role. The nurse also provides the client with feedback on a variety of issues within the dialog, such as voice tone, use of assertive language, identification of feelings, emotion expressed, and nonverbal behavior exhibited (Fortinash and Holoday Worret, 2007).

Special Communication Techniques

Self-Disclosure

Self-disclosure is opening up oneself to another and is an effective therapeutic skill if it is fully understood and used carefully. Experienced nurses reveal carefully selected thoughts, feelings, and life events to demonstrate to the client that they understand what the client is going through.

Disclosing your own personal beliefs, views, and life experiences occurs in social relationships on a continual basis. In intimate relationships, things that you reveal are very personal. Because a professional nurse-client therapeutic relationship exists for the purpose of helping the client, carefully think about what you will discuss before you reveal it. Because self-disclosure by the nurse is *always* for the client's benefit and *never* for the nurse's, it is important to explore the what, where, why, and when of self-disclosing to see what purpose it serves (Balzer Riley, 2004).

Make sure all self-disclosure is brief and relevant to the conversation, and do not imply that your experience is the same as the client's. Guidelines are available to help the nurse understand when to use self-disclosure. The following are acceptable purposes of self-disclosure (Deering, 1999):

- *To educate.* Will clients learn more about themselves and be able to deal better with the problems in their lives?
- *To facilitate the therapeutic relationship.* Will disclosing build rapport and help the client open up?
- *To provide concrete reflection that encourages reality testing.* Will this support the client in his or her natural feelings in response to an event?

The use of self-disclosure requires that the nurse and the client have a therapeutic relationship. The rationale for using self-disclosure comes from the belief that in doing so, the client will in turn self-disclose. Both the amount and relevance of your own self-disclosure needs to be monitored. If the self-disclosure is too lengthy, it will decrease the time the client has for disclosure and break down the interaction. If the disclosure is irrelevant to the client's problem, the client will become distracted and feel alienated from the nurse. Box 4-2 compares an example of therapeutic versus nontherapeutic self-disclosure.

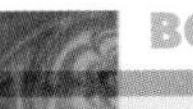

BOX 4-2

Self-Disclosure

THERAPEUTIC

Client: I'm real upset that I have to leave the hospital today.

Nurse: I have enjoyed working with you. I realize endings can be sad. It is important for you to use the tools you have learned when you go home.

The nurse is using self-disclosure in the termination phase of the relationship. She is validating the client's feelings and is also validating the relationship with the purpose of encouraging the client to transfer what they have learned in treatment to life after discharge.

NONTHERAPEUTIC

Client: That jerk of a husband had to leave me with three children to support.

Nurse: I know how you feel because my husband was just like that. He only cared about himself.

The nurse is using self-disclosure in the admission interview or beginning phase of the relationship, before there is a rapport or relationship. In addition, her comments reveal too much personal information, which she should not disclose at any time, to a client. It seems to serve the nurse's purpose, rather than the client's, to share the incident.

Both research and literature have indicated that self-disclosure is an important tool for client growth. Realize that not all self-disclosure is revealing personal information. It is sometimes as simple as sharing a feeling. Genuine, open communication can be used to create a therapeutic relationship without the use of self-disclosure. Self-disclosure enhances the relationship only when you feel comfortable using it and when it will benefit the client.

Touch

Touch, a powerful nonverbal method of communication, expresses many messages. Handshaking, holding hands, hugging, and kissing all demonstrate positive feelings for another human being. Nonessential touch is purposeful physical contact with the client other than the touch necessary for a procedure. Nonprocedural touches range from a light touch on the arm or a handshake to holding the hand or a full embrace. Touch will only communicate warmth if the nurse is comfortable with it.

Touch carries a different meaning for each person. Several variables influence the intended message of the touch, including the length of the touch, the part of the body touched, the way in which you touch the client, and the frequency of the touch.

Use caution when touching clients in a psychiatric setting. The age and gender of the client, the client's interpretation of the gesture, the client's cultural background, and the appropriateness of the touch all influence the reactions to touch.

Take potential reactions into consideration when deciding which clients to touch and what type of touch to use, if any. For example, a depressed client responds positively to touch as a gesture of concern. The nurse com-

A

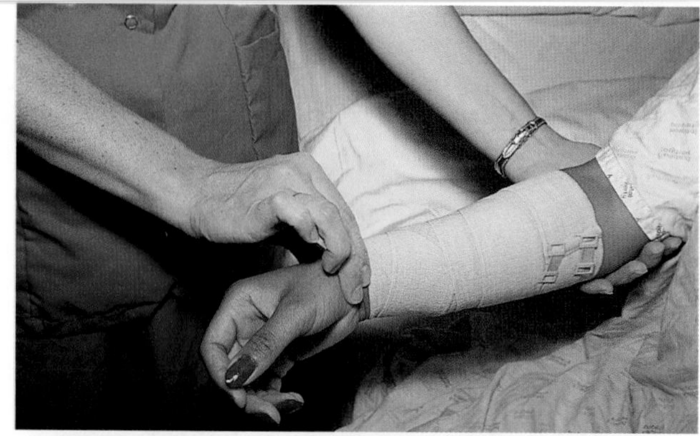

B

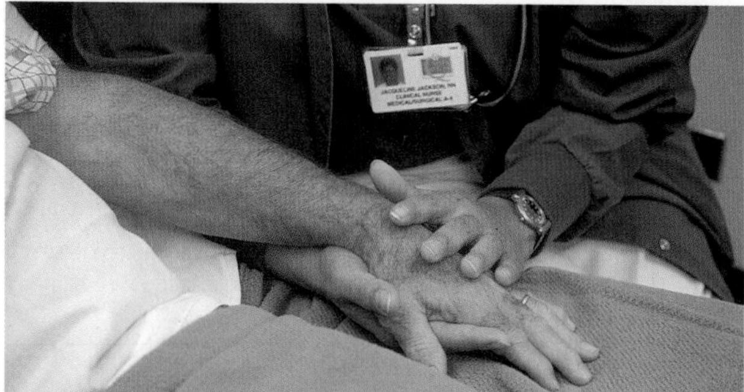

FIGURE 4-3 **A,** The nurse uses procedural touch to evaluate the client's circulation. **B,** The nurse uses nonprocedural touch to comfort the client. (From Potter PA, Perry AG: *Fundamentals of nursing*, ed 6, St Louis, 2005, Mosby.)

forts an elderly, frail client or a client who is dying, through touch. However, a paranoid, hostile client will probably think touch means confrontation and may hit the nurse. An abused client may pull away and feel frightened by a hand on the shoulder.

Procedural touch includes positioning the arm of a client when taking a blood pressure or drawing blood for laboratory work, turning a client to change a dressing or diaper, lifting or assisting a client from the bed to a wheelchair, or performing a seclusion or restraint procedure on a troubled and hostile client (Figure 4-3, *A*). *Nonprocedural touch* includes holding an older client's hand as she is expressing sadness over her husband's death, hugging an adolescent client as he leaves the hospital, shaking hands with new clients, or giving a back rub to a long-term, bedridden client (Figure 4-3, *B*).

The use of nonprocedural touch is a nurse's individual preference, as not all practitioners feel comfortable touching clients. Much depends on the nurse's comfort level, the ability to correctly interpret the situation, and the appropriate use of touch. Using touch is highly beneficial to the client's progress by enhancing the nurse-client relationship and promoting health.

Humor

Humor is a useful tool in psychiatric nursing. It is a quality that makes things seem funny, amusing, or absurd. Humor also enables us to perceive, appreciate, and express what is funny, amusing, or absurd. A sense of humor, including the ability to laugh with others and to laugh at yourself, has a positive influence on good health. Healthy humor promotes laughter between people; it encourages laughing *with* others and not *at* them. Healthy humor includes others, is appropriate to the situation, respects others, and preserves their dignity. Harmful humor excludes others. It singles out people from a group and ridicules them.

A good sense of humor is a mature coping mechanism and helps the nurse adequately handle difficult situations. It also assists in gaining a different perspective on the problem by lightening a serious mood for a few moments. Appropriate humor eases a client's concerns and communicates a sense of warmth and understanding (Bush, 2001).

Physiologically, research has linked laughter and an active sense of humor to healthy function of blood vessels. Laughter causes the endothelium, the tissue that forms the inner lining of blood vessels, to dilate which in turn increases blood flow (Goel, Plotnick, and Vogel, 2005). Laughter also reduces pain. Many theorize that laughter stimulates the brain to release the brain's natural painkillers, called endorphins, creating a natural sense of well-being and promoting the healing process. In some cases, laughing and having positive social interactions during mealtimes have aided digestion.

There are many psychologic benefits of laughter as well. Laughter functions as an immediate tension reliever and therefore decreases anxiety. It also lessens negative emotions such as anger, hostility, and resentment (Schuster, 2000).

Assess the degree to which a client has a sense of humor. In depressed clients, the outward expression of laughter and pleasure is usually missing. Clients with paranoid features are unable to laugh. In fact, they usually view others' laughter as a personal attack. This is important to remember. For example, nurses in the nursing station need to be careful not to laugh and joke behind a glass partition where paranoid clients can see them and interpret the behavior as a personal affront. On the other hand, manic clients laugh at everything, whether or not it is actually humorous. This exaggerated sense of well-being demonstrates a lack of judgment on the part of the client, and it often turns into biting sarcasm that will hurt others. Humor is nontherapeutic when a client is very ill, fearful, or anxious; is having a high level of pain; or is very depressed (Schuster, 2000).

The psychiatric mental health nurse uses humor as a therapeutic tool in a variety of ways. For example, the nurse can use it to teach the client the difference between hurtful and healthy humor, to encourage healthy humor on the unit by role modeling, and to introduce humor in formal and informal groups and individually. The use of humor will increase the flexibility of interactions and create a more relaxed environment. It enhances the client's insight and facilitates a difficult interaction for the client in a safe, low-keyed setting.

Obstacles to Therapeutic Communication

Certain obstacles occur in the client-nurse relationship that affect the nature of the communication. Some obstacles are due to the client's disorder or lack of knowledge, and some have to do with the nurse's own inability to be effective because of inexperience, lack of knowledge, or personal problems. For the relationship to grow in a healthy manner, these obstacles must be overcome.

Here are four key therapeutic obstacles for discussion: resistance, transference, countertransference, and boundary violations.

Resistance

Resistance occurs in clients who consciously or unconsciously maintain a lack of awareness of their problems in order to avoid anxiety. It takes the form of a natural and short-lived reservation about accepting a problem, or a long-term, firmly stated denial that there are problems. Resistance to change is part of human nature that both the nurse and the client need to address and manage so positive growth will occur. You can help clients overcome resistance by pointing out their progress and strengths.

For example, suppose a client resists impending discharge because of fear of failure, abandonment, or loneliness. The nurse assures the client that such fears are not uncommon at the time of termination or discharge. The nurse then reminds the client of progress made (e.g., "You've already achieved some of your goals, and have made concrete plans to continue treatment after you are discharged; these are accomplishments you didn't believe possible when you first arrived at this facility"). Such observations build the client's confidence and offer hope that will counteract resistance.

Transference

Transference is when a client unconsciously associates the nurse with someone significant in his or her life. The client transfers feelings and attitudes about the other person to the nurse. For example, a male client sees a female nurse as a mother figure because she has a mannerism that reminds him of his own mother. The client has negative feelings about his mother and, without provocation, becomes angry or bothered by the nurse's interaction with him because of this resemblance. Often, the client's intense response does not match the situation or the content of the interaction. The interaction comes to a standstill if the nurse does not address and examine the client's reasons for transference.

The nurse can deal with both resistance and transference by being prepared to hear a client's irrational and highly charged responses to the nurse. Listen to the client and then use the therapeutic techniques of clarifying and reflecting to begin problem solving. The goal is for the client to be aware and recognize the reason for the resistance.

Countertransference

Countertransference is the nurse's emotional response to a specific client. The response is irrational, inappropriate, highly charged, and generated by certain qualities of the client. It is simply the nurse's own transference. Nurses have a natural response to each client and may like or dislike some clients more than others. Countertransference occurs when the feelings are intense—either positive or negative—and are not based on reality. Because countertransference affects your ability to be an effective nurse, always observe for signs of its occurrence.

From time to time, countertransference issues will occur. Even though this is natural, it will be destructive if the nurse ignores it or treats it as insignificant. The nurse most often encounters countertransference when the client is displaying disruptive, aggressive, irritating, or resistive behaviors. If the nurse remains angry with the client as a result of these behaviors, he or she will lose the objectivity needed to promote healthy change. Nurses also find themselves attracted positively to clients in excessive ways. Recognize this and take steps to avoid countertransference.

To deal with countertransference, conduct an honest self-appraisal throughout the course of the therapeutic relationship while gaining a good understanding of the client's background and issues. If the self-appraisal reveals any problems, explore why these feelings are occurring. As soon as you recognize the problem, you need to work on it. If you are not able to handle these feelings alone, seek professional clinical help to deal with the issues.

Boundary Violations

Boundary violations occur when the nurse goes beyond the established therapeutic relationship standards and enters into a social or personal relationship with the client. Some clients also attempt to violate the boundaries of the nurse-client relationship. For example, a client asks the nurse, "How old are you?" or "Are you married?" or tries to touch the nurse inappropriately. Violations are more frequent if the nurse treats the client at odd hours or in an unusual setting, if the nurse accepts compensation or gifts for treatment, if the nurse's language or clothing is inappropriate, or if the nurse's self-disclosure or physical contact lacks therapeutic value. For example, the nurse discloses too much personal information to the client in order to benefit the nurse.

Responding Techniques That Hinder Therapeutic Communication

Earlier, this chapter presented therapeutic skills that have enhanced the communication process. There are also many responses that are counterproductive to healthy outcomes and are therefore nontherapeutic (Table 4-4).

There are several reasons why nurses fail to interact effectively. The inexperienced nurse's insecurity is one factor. A certain amount of experience and maturity greatly helps the nurse deal effectively with the difficult and complex behaviors psychiatric clients often display.

Other explanations for nontherapeutic communication are (1) the nurse has allowed necessary skills to stagnate or diminish, (2) a nurse who has worked with psychiatric clients for several years, finds he or she is on automatic pilot (repeating the same old strategies) and has lost the

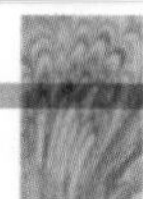

TABLE 4-4

Ineffective Responses That Hinder Therapeutic Communication

RESPONSE	DISCUSSION	NONTHERAPEUTIC RESPONSE	THERAPEUTIC RESPONSE
Offering false reassurances	The nurse, in an effort to be supportive and to make the client's pain disappear, offers reassuring clichés. This response is not based on fact. It brushes aside the client's feelings and closes off communication. Often, it is due to the nurse's inability to listen to the client's negative emotions.	"Don't worry, everything will be fine." "Every cloud has a silver lining." "Things will be better soon; you'll see."	"I know you have a lot going on right now. Let's make a list and begin to discuss them one at a time. Working toward solutions will help you to get through this."
Not listening	The nurse is preoccupied with other work that needs to be done, is distracted by noise in the area, or is thinking about personal problems.	"I'm sorry, what did you say?" "Could you start again? I was listening to another client."	"That's interesting. Please elaborate." "I really hear what you are saying . . . it must be difficult."
Offering approval	It is most important how the client feels about what he or she said or did. The client ultimately must approve of his or her own actions.	"That's good." "I agree, I think you should have told him."	"What do you think about what you said to him?" "How do you feel about it?"
Minimizing the problem	The nurse uses this response when it is difficult to hear the importance of a particular problem. This is used in an effort to make the client feel better. It cuts off communication.	"That's nothing compared to that other client's problem." "Everyone feels that way at times; it's not a big deal."	"That seems like a difficult problem for you." "That sounds pretty important for you to deal with."
Offering advice	This response undermines the client's ability to solve his or her own problems. It renders the client dependent and helpless. If the solution provided by the nurse does not work, the client will blame the outcome on the nurse. The client does not take responsibility for developing outcomes. The nurse maintains control and at the same time devalues the client.	"I think you should put your mother into a nursing home." "In my opinion, it would be wise to . . ." "Why don't you do . . ." "The best solution is . . ."	"What do *you* think you should do?" "There are several alternatives; let's talk about some. However, the final decision is yours. I will listen to your problem and help you see it clearly. We can develop a pros and cons list that will assist you in solving the problem."
Giving literal responses	The nurse feeds into the client's delusions or hallucinations and denies the client the opportunity to see reality. This does not provide a healthy response toward growth.	*Client:* "That TV is talking to me." *Nurse:* "What is it saying to you?" *Client:* "There is nuclear power coming through the air ducts." *Nurse:* "I'll turn off the air conditioner for a while."	*Nurse:* "The TV is on for everyone." *Nurse:* "There is cool air blowing from the vents. It is the air conditioning system."
Changing the subject	The nurse changes the topic at a crucial time because the discussion is too uncomfortable. It negates what the client seems interested in discussing. Communication will remain superficial.	*Client:* "My mother always puts me down." *Nurse:* "That's interesting, but let's talk about . . ."	*Nurse:* "Tell me about that."
Belittling	The nurse puts down the client's expressed feelings to avoid having to deal with painful feelings.	*Client:* "I don't want to live anymore now that my child is gone." *Nurse:* "You shouldn't feel that way."	*Nurse:* "Losing a child must be very difficult for you. Tell me more about how you are feeling."
Disagreeing	The nurse criticizes the client who is seeking support.	"I definitely do not agree with your view." "I really don't support that."	"Let's talk about the way you see that."
Judging	The nurse's responses are filled with his or her own values and judgments. This demonstrates a lack of acceptance of the client's differences. It provides a barrier to further disclosures.	"You are not married. Do you think having this baby will solve your problems?" "This is certainly not the Christian thing to do." "You are thinking about divorce when you have three children?"	"It seems hard to believe. Please explain further." "What will having this baby provide for you?" "What do you think about what you are attempting to do?" "Let's discuss this option," or "Let's discuss other options."

TABLE 4-4

Ineffective Responses That Hinder Therapeutic Communication, cont'd

RESPONSE	DISCUSSION	NONTHERAPEUTIC RESPONSE	THERAPEUTIC RESPONSE
Excessive probing	This serves to control the nature of the client's responses. The nurse asks many questions of the client before the client is ready to provide the information. This is self-protective to the nurse by avoiding the anxiety of uncomfortable silences. The client feels overwhelmed and may withdraw. The use of the "why" question places the client in a defensive position and may block further communication.	"Why do you do this?" "What do you think was the real reason?" "Why do you feel this way?" "Why do you think that way?"	"Tell me how this is upsetting to you." "Tell me what you believe to be the cause." "Tell me how you feel when that happens." "Explain your thinking on this if you can."
Challenging	This comes from the nurse's belief that if clients are challenged regarding their unrealistic thoughts, they will be coerced into seeing reality. This client will feel threatened when challenged, holding onto the beliefs even more strongly.	"You are not the Prince of Peace." "If your leg is missing, then why can you walk up and down this hall?"	"You sound like you need to feel important." "It seems to you that you are missing a leg. Tell me more about that."
Offering superficial comments	The nurse gives simple or meaningless responses to the client. It suggests a lack of understanding of the client's individuality.	"Great day, huh?" "You should be feeling good; you are being discharged today."	"What kind of day are you having?" "How are you feeling about leaving the hospital today?"
	The interactions remain superficial, maintaining distance between the nurse and client. No significant communication occurs.	"Keep the faith; your doctor should be coming anytime now."	"You look worried. Your doctor called and said he would be here within the hour."
Defending	The nurse believes that he or she must defend herself or himself, the staff, or the hospital. The nurse does not take the time to listen to the client's concerns. Effort is necessary to explore the client's thoughts and feelings.	"Your doctor is a good doctor. He would never say that." "We have an experienced staff here. They would never do that."	"What has you so upset about your doctor?" "Tell me what happened last night."
Self-focusing	The nurse shares his or her own thoughts, feelings, or problems; therefore focus is taken away from the client, who is seeking help. The nurse is more interested in what to say next than in actively listening to the client.	"That may have happened to you last year, but it happened to me twice this month, which hurt me a great deal and . . ."	"Tell me about your incident and how it relates to your sadness now."
		"Excuse me, but could you say that again? I have a response to make but I want to be sure of what you just said."	"If I heard you accurately, you said . . ."
Criticizing others	The nurse puts others down in his or her communication with the client.	*Client:* "The staff members on the evening shift let me smoke two cigarettes." *Nurse:* "The evening shift is always breaking the rules. On this shift we follow the one cigarette per break policy."	*Nurse:* "The policy is one cigarette, which we will follow."
		Client: "My daughter is hateful to me." *Nurse:* "She sounds just awful to live with."	*Nurse:* "It sounds like you are having a rough time right now with your daughter."
Interpreting or analyzing prematurely	The nurse responds before the client fully expresses thoughts and feelings about a particular problem. By rushing to a conclusion, the nurse disregards important client input and misses critical client concerns.	"I think this is what you really mean." "You think that way consciously, but unconsciously you believe . . ."	"What do you think this means?" "So you think . . .?"

6 and 10 years, because the child is accustomed to adults other than the parents, such as teachers and coaches, giving instruction and assistance. By this time the child has developed a more mature mode of communication and has a need for close relationships, both of which are helpful when interacting with the child. However, rapport and trust should be immediately established with both the child and the parent. Use concrete examples, as well as simple videotapes and books suitable for the child's age.

During preadolescence, from the ages of 10 to 12 or 13 years, when the onset of puberty begins, the preadolescent remains receptive to adults and their influence. Use some of the preadolescent's own language to communicate more effectively. Keep explanations relevant, brief, and at an appropriate level with the preteen's understanding.

The adolescent stage begins with puberty, ordinarily ages 12 or 13 years through ages 18 or 19 years. During the early adolescent years, the child is trying to form a self-identity and feel comfortable with himself or herself. The adolescent is often self-conscious, self-absorbed with his or her body image, and easily embarrassed. Respect the adolescent's privacy, as confidentiality is important in this age group. Also, you will need to relate more directly with the adolescent and less through the parents, as the adolescent is trying to separate emotionally from the parents and become independent. The early-age adolescent begins to develop abstract thinking and is usually able to understand past and present events and think about and discuss future events. Use these skills in your interactions with the early-age adolescent. As the adolescent reaches 14 or 15 years, you will find that joining an activity with the adolescent while communicating allows the adolescent to feel more comfortable with adults. Not being the adolescent's parent is an advantage and assists in the communication process. Regardless of the child's age, present a verbal and nonverbal environment in which the child or teenager feels comfortable. The degree of success that you have in communicating with a child or adolescent greatly depends on your understanding of both the developmental and chronologic age of the child. (See Chapter 5.)

Culture, Language, and Understanding

Because the United States is one of the most diverse societies in the world and part of a rapidly changing and growing multicultural world, it is imperative that you become culturally competent to deal with the diverse cultures and multicultural clients. *Cultural competence* is "a set of cultural behaviors and attitudes integrated into the practice methods of a system, agency, or its professionals that enable them to work effectively in cross cultural situations" (Sutton, 2000).

Communication is one of six areas of cultural uniqueness that you will evaluate in the initial nursing assessment because communication and culture have an impact on each other. Oral and written language, gestures, facial expressions, and body language are unique to each culture.

Cultural patterns of communication are set early in life and affect the way a person communicates ideas and feelings and makes decisions. Members within the same culture sometimes respond differently because of their own experience. Cultural competence does not suggest that the nurse needs to know everything about each culture; however, it does suggest the nurse uses communication that respects cultural differences in order to find a common communication meeting ground. Cultural competence starts with self-awareness, where the nurse reflects on his or her own values, beliefs, and attitudes, as well as knowledge of another's culture (Leininger, 2000).

Be aware of the potential *language* barriers to effective intercultural communication. A good nurse-client relationship depends on your understanding the client's point of view and frame of reference. Respecting and allowing a free exchange of the client's and family's ideas, thoughts, and feelings will promote effective intercultural communication.

For clients who are not native English speakers, the nurse's use of effective intercultural communication and learned verbal and nonverbal techniques will promote the following:

- Accurate understanding of their diagnosis, progress, and prognosis
- Assurance about what is happening and what procedures will be done
- Assurance of the expertise of the nurse and other health care providers
- Ability of clients to explain their symptoms to the nurse, to assist in their diagnosis and treatment

Nurses, therefore, need to make a special effort to provide clients with all available resources that will enhance their understanding of the situation. This includes locating an interpreter who can speak the client's language and also translate at the level required. Most hospitals have lists of local interpreters who offer their services and who will communicate technical terminology to the client. For nontechnical, uncomplicated translation, locate a hospital staff member who communicates in the client's own language. Peplau (1952, 1991) believed *understanding* is an essential component of the nurse-client relationship and as such significantly influences nurse-client interactions in the acute psychiatric setting. To manage symptoms effectively, listen and attend to clients' perceptions of their experiences (Haworth and Dluhy, 2001). Awareness of the importance of and the skills necessary to clarify individual meaning to promote understanding with clients is emphasized in cultural sensitivity and diversity training. Because each culture has varying degrees of diversity within the culture, avoid cultural stereotyping and concentrate on the uniqueness of the individual as well. It is important to note that you will not always fully understand what a client means. However, it is important not to assume to understand what a client means. Avoid "why" questions and the phrase "I completely understand." Instead, it is useful to practice learned therapeutic techniques. Here are some examples:

- Demonstrate verbal ("go on") and nonverbal (nod head) responses *to show interest and give client sufficient opportunity to respond* (active listening).
- Restate (repeat) what the client says *to ensure understanding and review what was said* (restating).
- Clarify the client's message by repeating it back in a more specific way *to further elicit the specific meaning* (clarifying).
- Ask open-ended questions ("Please explain more about..."; "Tell me more about") *to encourage the client to respond* (open-ended questions).
- Explore the client's verbal and nonverbal expressions regularly throughout the interaction *to expand understanding* (exploring).
- Summarize what the client has said at regular intervals throughout the interaction and at the end of the interaction *to confirm mutual understanding* (summarizing).

Table 4-3 describes additional examples of therapeutic techniques.

Clients experience a higher level of satisfaction and confidence with the nursing care they receive when they feel that nurses truly understand them (Shattell, 2005) (see Chapter 7).

Difficult Clients

Most nurses find it difficult to communicate with clients who are aggressive, unpopular, or distressed. Clients who exhibit *aggressive* behaviors are hostile and are often verbally or physically abusive, rejecting, and manipulative. Some have a violent past history with jail or prison time for violent offenses related to their aggressive behavior. These are unpleasant behaviors that are difficult to be around. This attacking style of behavior demonstrates a general lack of consideration and respect for others, and the natural response is to protect the self and reject the client. Even though your self-esteem and personal safety are under attack, meet the aggression assertively by setting firm limits that do not embarrass the nurse or the client. A specific behavioral treatment plan and a unified team approach are critical to treatment success. Most facilities offer assault response training and education to help staff members manage these behaviors.

Distressed clients express their physical or emotional pain both verbally and nonverbally, and sometimes continuously. Becoming too involved with a client's distress can overwhelm the nurse and interfere with effective communication. Often the nurse feels inadequate dealing with severe emotional or physical distress. It is important to remain clearheaded and to responsibly communicate understanding and concern without becoming judgmental or diminishing the client's perceptions and related feelings.

Unpopular clients have a variety of characteristics. They are unreasonably demanding, possess unacceptable personal habits, or behave in ways that are sexually inappropriate. When dealing with unpopular clients, nurses often feel frustrated, angry, or fearful. These clients are sometimes ignored or labeled as troublemakers or "problem clients." They are medicated more often, frequently admonished, and generally given less care or attention than other clients. Nurses naturally have likes and dislikes regarding client behaviors. One nurse may prefer working with a certain behavior, whereas another nurse may dislike that behavior. Some general characteristics of unpopular clients are listed in Box 4-3.

BOX 4-3

General Characteristics of Unpopular Clients

- Claim they are more ill than nurses think
- Express their dislike of the hospital
- Take up much of the nurse's time and attention
- Misuse hospitalization
- Are uncooperative and argumentative
- Are very aggressive or assaultive
- Have severe, complicated problems and a poor prognosis
- Have problems nurses think are brought on by themselves (e.g., alcohol-related disease)
- Have low morals or social stigmas
- Produce feelings of incompetence in the nurse

Difficult Co-workers

Conflicts inevitably arise in the workplace. Not only will you have to deal effectively with clients who are distressed and aggressive, but there are also times when you will deal with health care professionals who exhibit this same type of behavior. Health care is emotionally and physically demanding, which produces stress and conflict in the health care environment. There are times when colleagues become irritated, angry, argumentative, and occasionally even verbally abusive.

Conflict in health care settings has to do not only with the level of stress in the work environment, but also varying levels of responsibility, role differences, work status uncertainty, power issues, and cultural and value differences.

The best time to deal with conflict between members of the health care team is before it becomes a crisis situation. Effective communication skills are necessary to deal with a variety of conflicting professional relationships. The primary goal in dealing with workplace conflict is to find a high-quality strategy that is acceptable to all and that will result in a growth-producing outcome. The same principles of nurse-client communication, such as empathy, active listening, and respect for the dignity of others, are also necessary to have successful relationships with other health care professionals.

The skills necessary to communicate therapeutically with clients and their families are the same ones required to communicate effectively with other health care professionals. In general, it is important to consider the ego of the other person or his or her emotional vulnerability when communicating with colleagues in the work setting. Professional collegial communication also involves collaboration, coordination, networking, and sometimes negotiation and conflict resolution (Arnold and Boggs, 2007).

CHAPTER SUMMARY

- The components of communication are the stimulus (reason), the sender, the message, the medium, the receiver, and feedback.
- Environmental factors, the relationship between the sender and the receiver, the context of the communication, and the individual's attitudes and beliefs, knowledge, and perception all influence communication.
- Nonverbal communication cues involve all five senses. Ninety percent of communication is nonverbal. Verbal and nonverbal communication needs to be congruent for the communication to be effective.
- Interpersonal communication—communication between two or more people—are collegial, social, or therapeutic.
- The three purposes of therapeutic communication are to allow the client self-expression to promote healthy growth, to understand the significance of the client's problems, and to assist in the identification and resolution of the problems.
- Empathy is an important quality of therapeutic communication and is necessary to the success of the nurse-client relationship.
- Some responding techniques that enhance therapeutic communication are silence, active listening, support and reassurance, giving information, restating, reflecting, clarifying, and role-playing.
- Self-disclosure by the nurse is an effective technique when used for the right reasons, such as to benefit the client.
- Resistance, transference, countertransference, and boundary violations are obstacles to therapeutic communication.
- Certain therapeutic responding techniques correspond to specific steps of the nursing process and phases of the nurse-client relationship.
- Issues relating to the nurse's skill and self-awareness levels, the client's length of stay in treatment, the client's physical and emotional impairments, the client's age, or language and cultural differences are all challenges in effective communication.

REVIEW QUESTIONS

1 A client with paranoid schizophrenia tells the nurse, "I'm here on a secret mission for the government. Don't blow my cover." Which response by the nurse would be most therapeutic?

1. "Let's talk about something other than your mission for the government."
2. "Your admission papers do not list you as a government employee."
3. "You have lost touch with reality, which is a symptom of your illness."
4. "It sounds like you have some concerns about your privacy. You are safe here."

2 A nurse assesses a newly admitted client. Select the example of *offering self.*

1. "I've had stressful experiences in life also. Hospitalization isn't the end of the world."
2. "Tell me why you felt you had to be hospitalized for treatment of your depression."
3. "I hope you will feel better after we get your medication doses stabilized."
4. "I'd like to spend some time helping you get comfortable talking to me."

3 A military wife tearfully tells a nurse about her husband's death in a plane crash 6 months earlier. The client cries on a daily basis. She says, "I think I'm losing it. I'll never be the same." What is the nurse's best response?

1. "You will eventually get back to normal. Just start doing the things that used to be fun for you."
2. "When you find yourself starting to cry or feel sad, distract yourself by getting busy with an activity."
3. "Your husband died for our country. You should be proud of him rather than absorbed in grief."
4. "Crying and the feelings you describe are normal after such a loss. It may take a long time to grieve his death."

4 A psychiatric nurse, who works in a day program for clients with serious and persistent mental illness helps a group of clients to plan a Halloween party. One client says, "Halloween is a celebration of demons and evil." Select the nurse's most therapeutic response.

1. "Let's think of some other activities for you on the day of the party."
2. "Maybe it would be better for you to stay home on the day of the carnival."
3. "It's just a party. Your participation doesn't mean you believe in demons."
4. "The party is part of the programming. You are expected to participate."

5 A child's parent enters the nurse's station yelling, "What is wrong with you people? My daughter cut herself and you allowed it to happen. I thought my child would be safe here." Select the assertive response for the nurse.

1. "I can't respond to that. Your child is assigned to another nurse today."
2. "I can't hear you if you're screaming. Let's sit down and talk about it."
3. "Why are you always yelling when you come for visits?"
4. "I am sorry this incident happened. We are short staffed today."

*Additional self-study exercises and learning resources are available to you on the **Companion CD** at the back of the book and on the **Evolve website** at **http://evolve.elsevier.com/Fortinash/**.*

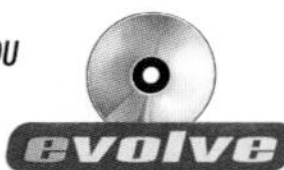

REFERENCES

American Health Consultants: Patient education management 8:9, Sep 2001.

Arnold E, Boggs K: *Interpersonal relationships: professional communication skills for nurses*, ed 5, St Louis, 2007, Saunders.

Balzer Riley J: *Communication in nursing*, ed 5, St Louis, 2004, Mosby.

Bush K: Do you really listen to patients? *Regist Nurse* 64, March 2001.

Chant S et al: Communication skills: some problems in nursing education and practice, *J Clin Nurs* 11:12-21, 2002.

Carpetino LJ: Nurses, always there for you, *Nurs Forum* 35:3-4, 2000.

Deering C: To speak or not to speak: self-disclosure with patients, *Am J Nurs* 99:34-36, 1999.

Fortinash KM, Holoday Worret PA: *Psychiatric nursing care plans*, ed 5, St Louis, 2007, Mosby.

Fox L et al: *Professional Assault Crisis Training*, Pro-ACT, San Clemente, Calif, 2004.

Haworth S, Dluhy N: Holistic symptom management: modeling the interaction phase, *J Adv Nurs* 36:302-310, 2001.

Leininger M: Founder's focus: transcultural nursing is discovery of self and the world of others, *J Transcult Nursing* 11:312-313, 2000.

Luft J, Ingham H: *The Johari window: a graphic model for interpersonal relations*, Los Angeles, 1955, University of California Western Training Laboratory.

May BA, Alligood MR: Basic empathy in older adults, *Issues Ment Health* 21:375-386, 2000.

McCabe C: Nurse-patient communication: an exploration of patients' experiences, *J Clin Nurs* 13:41-49, 2004.

O'Neill K: Kids speak: effective communication with school-aged, adolescent patient, *Pediatr Emerg Care* 18:137-140, 2002.

Peplau HE: *Interpersonal relations in nursing*, New York, 1952, Putnam.

Peplau HE: *Interpersonal relations in nursing: a conceptual frame of reference for psychodynamic nursing*, New York, 1991, Springer.

Reynolds WJ: Do nurses and other professional helpers normally display much empathy? *J Adv Nurs* 31:226-234, 2000.

Schuster PM: *Communication: the key to the therapeutic relationship*, Philadelphia, 2000, FA Davis.

Shattell M, Hogan, B: Facilitating communication: how to truly understand what patients mean, *J Psychosoc Nurs* 43:29-32, 2005.

Shives LR: *Basic concepts of psychiatric mental health nursing*, ed 5, Philadelphia, 2002, JB Lippincott.

Sutton M: Cultural competence, *Fam Pract Manag* 7:58-62, 2000.

Walker K, Alligood M: Empathy from a nursing perspective: moving beyond borrowed theory, *Arch Psychiatr Nurs* 15, 2001.

Williams K et al: Enhancing communication with older adults: overcoming elderspeak, *J Gerontol Nurs* 30:17-25, 2004.

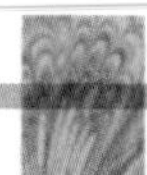

TABLE 5-3

Interpersonal Theory—Sullivan

Development results from interpersonal relationships with others in maximizing satisfaction of needs while minimizing insecurity.

ERA	AGE (YR)	BASIC CONCEPT	DEVELOPMENTAL ISSUES
Infancy	0-2	Trial-and-error learning from parental interactions of tenderness or annoyance molds development; ends with language development	Infant learns to differentiate self from others and that comfort and discomfort are connected to caregiver: parataxic mode; develops self-system: "good me" from positive paternal mood, "bad me" from negative paternal mood with mild anxiety, and "not me" from extreme parental disapproval with severe anxiety and emotional withdrawal
Childhood	2-6	Language development allows child to be educated, not trained	Language takes on symbolic function of communication; self-system continues to develop with sublimation (expression of impulses in socially acceptable ways) or develops malevolent transformation (a feeling of living among enemies)
Juvenile	6-10	Relations with peers allow children to see themselves objectively	Increased peer interactions help to give child feedback from others and widen area of interactions to include society; develops conscience; self-system develops internalized reputation and cultural stereotypes; able to distinguish fantasy and reality and develop syntaxic communication (a mature method of communicating): their own behavior is connected to others' opinions of them
Preadolescent	10-13	Develops same-sex friendships	Transition from egocentrism to love; development of friendships helps to validate personal worth through teamwork and mutual satisfaction of needs; able to work with peers toward a common goal and develop sense of oneness; all for one and one for all
Adolescent	13-17	Lust: interest in sexual activity	Sexual attractions allow adolescent to experiment with intimacy; if adults severely discourage or prevent attractions, the adolescent will feel insecure and lonely
Late adolescent	17-19	Personality integration	Able to become genuinely intimate with others by including the needs of society without excessive insecurity or anxiety; inability to achieve personality integration results in regression and egocentrism for life

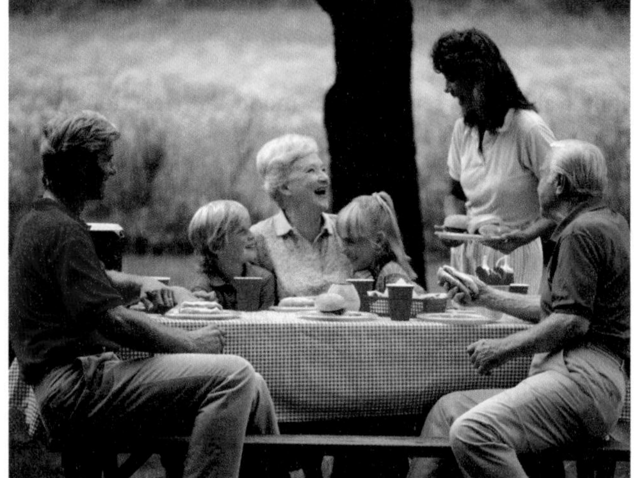

FIGURE 5-1 Healthy intergenerational involvement benefits the entire family. (©2007 JupiterImages Corporation.)

develops to cope with the high level of anxiety the child is facing in response to the parents' mood.

The *childhood era* (ages 2 to 6 years) extends from the beginning of language development to beginning social relationships with peers. Development moves from a trial-and-error system of training to actual learning through education. Children's coping mechanisms ("good me," "bad me") continue to develop from the interpersonal interactions with parents, teachers, and other caregivers. One such defense mechanism, *sublimation*, or the expression of desires in socially acceptable manners, is a positive development during this era. On the other hand, continuous punitive or extreme disapproval ("not me") will result in what Sullivan termed *malevolent transformation* (feeling that one is living among enemies). The child's anxieties will possibly develop into fears of disapproval from all authority figures and an inability to respond to positive feedback from others (Maddi, 1972). Parents who role-model malevolence educate their children to become malicious. In many cases, these children become known as the class bullies, behaving abusively to fellow students.

Ages 6 to 10 years represent the *juvenile era*, during which juveniles begin to develop friendships with peers, representing a widening of social circles. Juveniles are learning to develop elements of their conscience and personalities that will help them succeed in society. They begin to learn the importance of being members of a group, as well as gaining experience in competitive, rivalry, and compromising situations. Along with group membership, juveniles learn various ways to exclude individuals from the "in group" to the "out group," forming stereotypes about these individuals usually based on culture. Juveniles are also learning to distinguish fantasy from reality in this stage. In addition, they continue to develop aspects of their self-system in their ability to participate in a more mature form of communication, called *syntaxis*. Using this form of communication, they are able to perceive the interrelationships between their own behaviors and the reactions or responses of others. The self-system is also developing and internalizing personality patterns that Sullivan termed *supervisory patterns* that develop during the juvenile era, refine over the subsequent years, and remain with the person throughout life.

In contrast to Erikson's single stage of adolescence, Sullivan divides adolescence into three eras: preadolescence (ages 10 to 13 years), adolescence (ages 13 to 17 years), and late adolescence (ages 17 to 19 years). During *preadolescence*, friendships of same-sex friends deepen because of the need for alliances in meeting mutual needs (Maddi, 1972). Social groups continue to evolve their self-identity and become goal-focused. Preadolescents learn the importance of reciprocity (the exchange of favors or privileges) and equality in interpersonal relationships. The *adolescent era* begins at puberty with individuals experiencing sexual attraction and feelings of lust for the first time. Low self-esteem, insecurity, anxiety, and loneliness will develop if the adolescent is constantly criticized or disciplined by parents for sexual thoughts or behaviors. In the *late adolescent era*, the adolescent learns the ability to be comfortable with his or her own intimate relationships while meeting the socially acceptable expectations of society. Adolescents who have not learned to develop intimate relationships sometimes move back to the juvenile era and remain with an egocentric personality throughout life, unable to develop satisfying interpersonal relationships.

Cognitive Theory

Jean Piaget (1896-1980), a Swiss philosopher and psychologist who had his doctorate in zoology, dedicated his life work to observing and interacting with children to determine how their thinking processes differed from adults. His work established several new areas of science including cognitive theory, developmental psychology, and genetic epistemology. The application of his work on cognitive learning influenced generations of educators who applied his constructivist learning concepts to elementary level education, focusing on the child's abilities to continuously create and test new knowledge (Gallagher and Reid, 1981). This was a significant contrast to the more traditional pedagogic theory of childhood learning that viewed children as empty vessels who needed educators to fill them with knowledge.

Cognitive theory explains how thought processes are structured, how they develop, and their influence on behavior. Structuring of thought processes occurs through the development of *schema* (i.e., mental images or cognitive structures). Thought processes develop through assimilation and accommodation. When the child encounters new information that is recognized and understood within existing schema, *assimilation* of that new information occurs. If the child is not able to link the new information to existing schema, the child has to learn to develop new mental images or patterns through the process of *accommodation*. As long as the child is able to assimilate or accommodate adequately to new knowledge, the child is able to achieve *equilibrium* or mental balance. When schemas are inadequate to facilitate learning, *disequilibrium* occurs.

Piaget viewed the development of thought processes as progressing over four stages (Piaget, 1970; Piaget and Inhelder, 1969). At each stage, the development of cognitive images or structures influences the child's behavior. The child must successfully achieve goals of each stage before moving onto the next. Table 5-4 summarizes these stages. During the first stage, the *sensorimotor period* (birth to 2 years of age), the infant learns about the environment through the senses in a trial-and-error fashion that Piaget called *instrumentality*. Gradually the infant begins to recognize the difference between the self and others in the environment, or the process of *decentering*. Theorists originally believed that *object permanence*, or the ability to recognize that an object or person is in a given area or continues to exist even outside of the infant's field of vision, begins to develop toward the end of the sensorimotor period (around age 2 years). More recent research has shown that the infant gains this ability much earlier, around 6 months of age.

During the *preoperational period* (ages 2 to 7 years), the child uses of verbal and mental symbols to represent persons, objects, and actions that may or may not be present. The child also begins to exhibit pretend play, has difficulty distinguishing reality from fantasy, and focuses only on the present. Thought processes are egocentric in nature such that the child considers only his or her viewpoint, and aspects of one's self-esteem begin to show. The child's emotional state is constantly changing, and he or she is able to focus on only one emotion at a time. Later in this period, unconditional acceptance of authority begins to develop.

During the *concrete operations period* (ages 7 to 11 years), the child's thought processes are only concrete in character, which fosters the ability to sort objects and place them in some order. The child recognizes thoughts about the past and present but not thoughts about the future. The child is also able to understand conservation, or the principle that an object is able to change shape but retain the same volume. The child is also able to acknowledge the viewpoints of others and appreciate feelings such as friendship, truthfulness, and integrity.

The final period, the *formal operations period* (ages 11 to 16 years), is when the individual develops systematic ways to think about and solve problems. The individual is able to think in abstract (i.e., explaining metaphors) or hypothetical terms (i.e., "what if" statements). Thinking in terms of the future and solving or debating problems in a logical manner are also characteristic of this period.

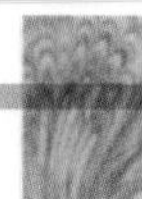

TABLE 5-4

Cognitive Development—Piaget

Development results from a tendency to organize and adapt to the environment. Intelligence development allows children to have increasingly effective and more organized interactions with the environment.

STAGE	AGE (YR)	BASIC CONCEPTS	DEVELOPMENTAL ISSUES
Sensorimotor	0-2	In-the-moment thinking: ability to differentiate self from objects	Child moves from reflexive action to instrumentability: actions lead to outcomes through trial and error; develops decentering: ability to differentiate self from objects develops object permanence: ability to hold mental representations when objects or people are out of sight
Preoperational	2-7	Here-and-now thinking: uses symbols and words to represent objects, actions, people, and places not present	Engages in pretend (symbolic) play; remains egocentric: unable to take another's point of view; cannot distinguish reality from fantasy; acquires language; only intuitively guesses about cause and effect; time is oriented in present only; can focus on only one emotion at a time; beginning development of self-system; noncontested respect for authority
Concrete operational	7-11	Past and present thinking	Able to conserve: understands that physical properties such as volume and length remain the same when there are changes in shape, group, or position; able to reverse operations; able to decenter: relates two classifications at one time; able to think about past and present events but not the future; begins to appreciate perspective of others
Formal operational	11-16	Future thinking	Able to think in abstract and hypothetical terms; able to think about possibilities rather than just what is; able to think of future events and develop strategies for solving complex problems

Cognitive development represents human's constant attempts to adapt to and make sense of their environment. Piaget's stages of cognitive development are associated with particular age spans, but they typically vary among individuals. In addition, each period is also made up of distinct structures. For example, the concrete operational period consists of more than 40 structures that deal with relationships, movements, time and space, conservation, and measurement (Brainerd, 1978). Examination of these structures has been of great value to scientists studying the development of intelligence. Educators have also applied Piaget's theory to learning activities at specific elementary school grades. Although more recent research has confirmed that Piaget probably underestimated cognitive development, particularly during the sensorimotor period, his body of work has been a major influence on those who followed in the study of human development.

Attachment Theory

John Bowlby (1908-1990) recognized the importance of maternal bonding in child development, a consistent phenomenon across all cultures. From initial animal studies, Bowlby saw bonding as a type of "protective" response by the youngster in a dangerous situation (Bowlby, 1988). Ainsworth (1989) expanded the concept of attachment to include all caregivers or "primary attachment figures" and found that infants from all cultures showed the same distress (although to different degrees) in all cultures of the world. Positive interactions with caregivers facilitate growth of secure attachments, whereas negative interactions result in insecure attachments. Bowlby viewed attachment as the core of all human development. Responses of the caregiver to the infant's distress over time result in what Bowlby called "internal working models of self and parent." These formed models influence the development of social interactions (Stroufe, Cooper, and DeHart, 1992).

According to attachment theory, children who experienced secure attachments develop into resilient, happy, and capable individuals, whereas those who faced insecure attachments tended to become antisocial, helpless, passive, or needing attention. Critics point out that this places undue emphasis on the "nurture assumption"—that is, how parents raise their children shapes their character.

Addressing these issues, Bowlby further recognized that other figures influence a child's development as their social circle expands. For example, a child experiencing helpless or passive behaviors is positively affected by a caring elementary schoolteacher who encourages, supports, and nurtures the child toward a more positive developmental process. On the other hand, a child who is greatly affected by the loss of a parent faces a more negative developmental pathway. Bowlby explained these experiences as a process of **adaptation**. Later theorists continued to build and refine on a theory of adaptation relative to human development.

Behavioral Theories

Behavioral theories, or learning theories, focus on the basic relationship between a stimulus and a response and involve the study of situations in which researchers are able to accurately predict responses. For the psychologists concerned with developing behavioral theories, it was also a way to break with the biologists and psychiatrists who believed instincts drive all human behavior and that patterns of behavior were determined at early ages. It is probably not a coincidence that the early behavioral scientists were also American, in contrast to the domination of European scientists involved in the previously discussed development theories.

Classical and Operant Conditioning

The early influences on what has come to be social learning theory were the scientific works of John B. Watson (1878-1958) and B.F. Skinner (1904-1990). Using the research techniques designed by Ivan Pavlov, Watson showed that humans learn new behaviors through the process of *classical conditioning*. He demonstrated that a conditioned stimulus paired with an unconditioned stimulus elicits a conditioned response or behavior change. When the researcher removed the unconditioned stimulus, the conditioned stimulus continued to result in the same conditioned response.

Skinner expanded on Watson's work, stating that learning does not only involve an association between a stimulus and a response. He believed that learning occurred through association of a behavior with a particular consequence. Skinner referred to this process as *operant conditioning*. He identified three basic consequences or responses to learning situations: reinforcement, extinction, and punishment. *Reinforcement* is a positive response, which then increases a particular behavior, or it is a negative response, *extinction*, which removes or eliminates the behavior. *Punishment*, or an unpleasant response, reduces the frequency of the behavior.

Social Learning Theory

Social learning theory is a general theory to explain human behavior. The term *social learning theory* first appeared in a 1941 publication by Miller and Dollard titled *Social Learning and Imitation*. They outlined the concepts that formed the foundation of several versions of social learning theory. From their early work, behaviorists were able to empirically test and validate their hypotheses.

One of the pioneers of social learning theory, Julian Rotter (1916-), questioned Freudian theory that biologic motives determined human behavior. Instead, he selected the *empiric law of effect* as the motivating factor that drives human behavior. Basically, individuals are motivated to search for positive stimulants, or *reinforcers*, and to avoid negative stimulants. He went further to say that an individual's personality is essentially linked to his or her environment. His approach to clinical psychology included study of not just one's life history, personality, and experiences, but also of one's awareness of and response to the environment. Changing either one's personality or environment affects the other. In contrast to other child development theorists, Rotter also believed that personality continues to evolve based on new life experiences or new learning opportunities, although, as one ages, the stimulants have to be more intense to effect the same degree of personality change.

Rotter's social learning theory (1982) has four main components:

1. *Behavior potential* is the degree of probability that the individual will engage in a specific behavior in a particular situation. For each specific behavior, there is a corresponding behavior potential. Rotter believed that the person seeks the behavior with the greatest potential.
2. *Expectancy* is the likelihood that a behavior will lead to a certain outcome and is based on past experiences. As the person is more likely to seek a positive outcome, or reinforcer, he or she will select the behavior with the highest expectancy of achieving a positive outcome. Expectancy is subjective, as some individuals experience unrealistic expectations that have no basis in reality (e.g., irrational expectations).
3. *Reinforcement value* is the desirability of behavior outcomes, so that those outcomes that one rates highest have the greatest reinforcement value. Again, reinforcement value is subjective, because past experiences affect it. For example, for most children, parental punishment is a negative outcome with low reinforcement value. But for some children who suffer from neglect, parental punishment has a high reinforcement value, as it is more desirable than abandonment.
4. *Psychologic situation* represents how different individuals have different explanations of the same circumstances. How individuals behave is due to their subjective analyses of the environment.

Rotter's work on social learning theory formed the basis for the well-known concept of *locus of control* (Rotter, 1992). Locus of control is an aspect of personality that deals with a person's belief of who is in control—the self or some outside force. Some have mistakenly attempted to categorize people with "internal" locus of control or "external" locus of control personalities. Rotter explained that under specific situations "internals" sometimes function more like "externals" or vice versa, based on past experiences, again reinforcing the interaction of individual and environment.

Albert Bandura's (1971) addition to social learning theory emphasized the importance of observation and *modeling* the actions, emotions, and attitudes of others. By copying the behaviors of others, individuals encode information, and this forms the basis for new behaviors. For example, children often imitate other children or adults. By role-playing and dressing up as the mother and father, children are programming their own future behaviors. Cognitive, environmental, and behavioral factors interact during observational learning processes that have four basic parts:

1. Attention to the modeled behavior
2. Retention or coding of the behavior
3. Motor reproduction of the behavior
4. Motivation and reinforcement of the reproduced behavior

Individuals are more likely to act out behaviors if they perceive that the outcomes will be valuable or result in positive reinforcement. If someone recognizes and rewards the behavior, this will further strengthen the new behavior.

Interestingly, Bandura's work with social and observational learning began from his focus on how children learn aggression (Bandura, 1986). In fact, Bandura cautioned parents and educators that television and movie violence influenced aggressive and violent behaviors in children. Although he did not claim that the media are the only source of learned aggression, he did note that they represent a key ingredient. Television network and film executives were so concerned that Bandura's warnings would result in a climate of fear among parents (and were probably more fearful of not making money) that they petitioned his removal from an expert panel to develop the 1972 Surgeon General's Report on Violence (Liebert and Sprafkin, 1988).

Bandura expanded his social learning theory to include the concept of self-reflection as a way for persons to examine their experiences, consider their own thinking processes, and adjust their thinking as a result. Self-efficacy is a form of self-reflection that affects one's behaviors; it was a central focus for Bandura's research (Bandura, 1989). Basically, individuals develop perceptions about their own effectiveness and this guides their behavior. Self-efficacy determines what individuals attempt to achieve and the amount of effort they give to achieve their goals.

Social learning theory has greatly contributed to many fields including education, health care, and behavior therapy. Most recently, researchers have applied the social learning theory to the study of how children internalize morals and values of society. Some have used the concepts of social learning theory successfully in psychomotor skill training.

Moral Development

Moral development includes moral judgment or reasoning processes and involves making decisions about right or wrong actions in a particular situation (Stroufe, Cooper, and DeHart, 1992). Piaget examined the concept of moral development and determined there were two stages of development. Before the ages of 10 or 11 years, children considered moral dilemmas differently from older children. These two different views are based on how children view "rules." For younger children, rules are absolute, coming from an authority figure. Older children learn that rules are changeable in certain situations. According to Piaget, younger children base moral judgment on consequences, while older children base judgment on motives. For example, if a child has to select which situation represents the greater wrong—the child who steals food every day to feed his poor family or the child who steals money once to buy a toy—the younger child will say the child who steals food daily is doing the greater wrong, based on the consequences or amount of harm. In contrast, the older child judges wrongness according to motives in the situation.

Lawrence Kohlberg built on Piaget's work in the area of moral development. Kohlberg (1973) completed his doctorate in psychology at University of Chicago focusing his research on moral issues faced by children and adolescents. Following Piaget's schema, Kohlberg identified six stages of moral development that are categorized into three levels (Table 5-5). Kohlberg based his model on a core sample of 72 boys, ages 10, 13, and 16 years, from lower- and middle-class families in Chicago. He asked the boys to reason out a series of moral dilemmas, and he then classified their responses according to six stages.

The first level, *preconventional morality* (about ages 4 to 10 years), consists of the following stages:

1. *Punishment and obedience orientation*, when children realize there are physical consequences in the form of punishment for bad behaviors. In this stage, children reason that authority figures lay down the rules of what is moral and children have to obey these decisions without question or punishment results.
2. *Instrumental relativist orientation*, when children focus on satisfying their own instrumental needs and occasionally the needs of others. Moral judgment is based on, "What do I get out of this decision?"

The second level, the *conventional level* (about 10 years of age through adolescence), seeks conformity and loyalty as key behaviors and consists of two stages:

1. *Interpersonal concordance* deals with the give-and-take nature of helping or good behaviors. Children receive approval by others for doing good works. Intent and character traits are also taken into account and grow in importance, such as "she means well" or "he is a loving father" in their attempts to assist others.
2. *Law-and-order orientation*, which is a stage of doing good and making moral decisions in respect of authority or because of duty to maintain social order.

The third level, the *postconventional* or *principled level* (early adulthood onward), seeks to define moral judgment and values in terms of the universal good and consists of two stages:

1. *Social-contract legalist orientation* that focuses on the legal point of view but is also open to considering what is moral and good for society.
2. *Universal ethical-principle orientation* deals with abstract and ethical moral values, rather than concrete moral rules. These include universal principles such as equality, justice, and beneficence.

Kohlberg's continued work on his stages of moral development combined the two stages of the final level. Critics of his model view his work as culturally and sexually biased. His theories are based on Western views of moral development and do not reflect other cultural views.

Carol Gilligan, an associate of Kohlberg, agreed that his premises are sometimes sexually biased. Along with his sample consisting of all males, Gilligan thought that the stages only represent masculine values that were focused

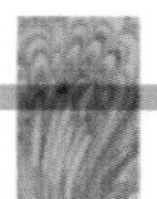

TABLE 5-5

Moral Development—Kohlberg

Moral development is influenced by the child's motivation or need, the child's opportunity to learn social roles, and the forms of justice the child encounters in the social institutions where he or she lives.

LEVEL	AGE (YR)	STAGE	DEVELOPMENTAL ISSUES
I. Preconventional (self-centered orientation)	4-10	1. Punishment-obedience orientation	Moral decisions are based on avoidance of punishment.
		2. Hedonistic and instrumental orientation	Moral decisions are motivated by desire for rewards rather than avoiding punishment, and belief that by helping others they will get help in return.
II. Conventional (able to see victim's perspective)	10-13 but can go into adolescence	3. Good boy/girl orientation	Moral decisions are based on desire for approval from others and on avoiding guilt experienced by not doing the right thing.
		4. Law-and-order orientation	Moral decisions are defined by rights, assigned duty, rules of the community, and respect for authority.
III. Postconventional (underlying ethical principles are considered that take into account societal needs)	13 to death	5. Social contract orientation	Moral decisions are based on a sense of community respect and disrespect. Rules are followed to maintain community harmony.
		6. Hierarchy of principles orientation	Moral judgments are based on principles of justice, the reciprocity and quality of human rights, and respect for the dignity of human beings as individual persons—Golden Rule: do to others as you would have them do to you.

on moral rules and responsibilities. She saw female moral values as being based in interpersonal relationships and reality situations rather than in abstract concepts. Gilligan (1982) raised another possibility to explain gender differences in forming moral values. She suggested that moral development progresses along more than one pathway: one focused on ethics, justice, and other abstract concepts and the other course focused on interpersonal relationships. At some point, each gender tends toward making one of these paths more dominant.

ADULT DEVELOPMENT

Since the time of the Chinese philosopher Confucius (511-479 BC), many viewed development on a continuum, with children and adolescents on one end and adults and old age on the other end.

There is a shortage of adult development research in comparison to studies of infancy, childhood, and adolescence. Stevens-Long (1992) attributed this lack to social, psychologic, and economic issues. Much of the emphasis on child development was in the fields of education, biology, and psychology. When education became a requirement for all children, teachers wanted to develop and test optimal teaching methodologies. Biologists and psychologists studied child development to understand human evolution.

Another reason for the lack of focus on adult development is the unsupported belief that human development plateaus at adulthood. For many years, the assumption was that adulthood was a period when external events (i.e., marriage, jobs, raising children, etc.) influenced human development rather than internal processes that were occurring during childhood. Research in adult development began evolving in the mid-1970s to include a more complex view of adulthood as a continuous and active process of growth and development. In earlier times, researchers perceived adulthood as the period of basic maintenance for the family. Little effort or time was available for creativity, self-expression, and new learning opportunities.

As human development theorists expanded in their attempts to explain concepts of personality, cognition, motivation, emotions, and intellect, it soon became apparent that values, cognitive abilities, mental and physical health, and many other factors continue to change throughout adulthood. Child and adolescent development theories with finite stages seemed inadequate to explain the dynamics of human development past 18 years of age. Many life experiences occur only during adulthood (i.e., marriage, raising children, starting or ending a career) that will significantly affect growth and development during those years. Arnold Van Gennep was one of the pioneers of adult development theory. In his book, *The Rites of Passage* (1909), he described **rites of passage** as the significant and meaningful rituals that mark and celebrate milestones and transitions in life.

Life Stage Theories

Several researchers have proposed life stage theories over the past several years. These theories divide the life span into a series of sequential transitions. Individuals who are adjusted and happy are able to achieve age-appropriate developmental tasks at each stage.

Jung's life stage theory (1971) was based on psychoanalytic theory that states that as one goes through life, one develops inner exploratory abilities that add meaning to life. He also postulated that personality differences between males and females become less distinct as people age. The final life stage deals with maintaining a balance between wisdom and senility in old age. The older person who is successful in life does not attempt to compete with youth but rather is able to deal with age changes.

Jung considered adult development on a continuum across the life cycle. He found that adults, ages 20 to 35 years, continue to develop their individuality and other personality patterns while they are establishing their families. Jung was one of the first to describe midlife transition, a period of growing awareness of masculine and feminine aspects of personality present in each individual.

Erikson was the most well known of the life stage theorists and identified eight stages of psychologic development (see Table 5-2). Each stage of development involves maintaining a balance between the *syntonic* (state of stability) and *dystonic* (state of disorder) (Erikson, Erikson, and Kiunick, 1986). A person has to adjust to move forward to the next level. The first five stages focused on children and adolescents. The remaining three stages followed adulthood from young to old age. During young adulthood, individuals struggle with *intimacy versus isolation.* They develop the abilities to have loving relationships and begin to establish long-term commitments in their relationships. Some individuals retain a sense of self-absorption and find it difficult to make and keep intimate relationships; therefore they tend to isolate themselves (Colarusso and Nemiroff, 1981).

The stage of *generativity versus stagnation* occurs during middle adulthood and is characterized by an interest of individuals in wanting to guide development of the next generation. As the children of adults grow more independent, their aging parents become more dependent. Therefore those at middle adulthood face new roles, responsibilities, and challenges. Generativity also includes the ability to evaluate and appreciate past life experiences, embrace the future, assume new relationships and responsibilities, and develop creativity. For adults who cannot achieve such outcomes and who view their lives at this point as boring or unfulfilling, their existence feels stagnate or empty.

The final stage, *ego integrity versus despair,* occurs in late life. Older adults develop a sense of acceptance of how they lived their lives and the importance of relationships they acquired throughout their lives. This stage is sometimes the climax of the previous seven stages. The individual with ego integrity is prepared to defend the dignity of one's own lifestyle and life choices. Individuals who have not successfully accomplished development tasks of earlier stages will lack ego integrity and thus feel despair about a lack of life fulfillment and death. In describing the final stage of life, Erickson stated that "the process of bringing into balance feelings of integrity and despair involves a review of and a coming to terms with the life one has lived thus far" (Erikson, Erikson, and Kivnick, 1986, p. 54).

More recently, theorists have developed a psychologic model encompassing life span development, called *selective optimization with compensation* (SOC) (Baltes, Smith, and Staudinger, 1992). This theoretic framework focuses on managing age-related gains and losses for **successful aging**. Individuals who age successfully are those who select and modify activities that enrich their lives despite energy declines. With the growth of the "old-old" population (i.e., those 85 years of age and older), theorists are applying SOC as a theoretic and practical model to understand transitions from "healthy aging" more commonly seen in older adults up to about age 80 years (termed *the Third Age*) to a nonreversible "declining aging" that seems to begin around age 85 years (termed *the Fourth Age*) (Hyer and Intrieri, 2006). Accordingly, physical and psychologic resources shift to managing losses experienced later in life. For example, an elderly individual was a professional landscaper for most of his life. Now that he is older and less mobile, he becomes *selective* in caring for a small garden *(optimization)* by setting it up in raised containers for ease of reaching *(compensation).*

Human Motivation and Development Theory

Many view Maslow's motivation and development theory (1962) as a valuable framework for understanding human needs and values from a holistic point of reference. Maslow's theoretic construct is a hierarchy of needs diagrammed in the form of a pyramid (see Figure 2-2). Maslow identifies five levels of needs, the most basic representing the base of the pyramid. From the most basic (1) to the highest (5) level, these needs include the following:

1. Biologic and physiologic
2. Safety and security
3. Affiliation or sense of belonging
4. Self-esteem
5. **Self-actualization**

Ebersole and Hess (1999) conceptualized Maslow's hierarchy of needs and applied his theory to identifying the special needs of older adults at each level. Table 5-6 identifies some of these specific needs of the older adult and potential strategies to meet those needs.

Contemporary Theorists

During adulthood, development focuses on the ability to interact with transitional aspects of the life experiences and the environment. Recognition and acceptance of the finiteness of time and the inevitability of death are essential to adult development.

Daniel Levinson, a psychosocial theorist, examined life stages from early through late adulthood (1986), broadly based on Erikson's work. In contrast to Erikson, Levinson focused less on changes within the person and more on the connection between the self and the interpersonal world. His psychosocial theory of adult development ad-

TABLE 5-6

Special Needs of Older Adults According to Maslow's Hierarchy of Needs

MASLOW'S HIERARCHY OF NEEDS	NEEDS OF OLDER ADULTS	STRATEGIES TO MEET NEEDS
Self-actualization	Finding meaning in life and death	Identify value and contributions of individual.
	Transcendence over aging process	Encourage continuity of participation in decision-making processes.
	Creativity and mastery	Reflect about past in relation to present and future.
Self-esteem	Responsible roles	Maintain aspects of roles important to individual.
	Social supports	Facilitate socialization.
	Locus of control	Promote physical appearance.
	Cognitive awareness	Facilitate decision making.
Belonging	Relationships	Identify impact of loss on individual.
	Intimacy	Support needs for intimacy and sexuality.
	Affiliations	Facilitate changes in lifestyle.
Safety and security	Sensory awareness	Obtain necessary equipment or supplies for home independence.
	Environmental safety	Assist with obtaining legal or financial help.
	Legal and economic issues	Educate older person and family regarding home safety.
Biologic integrity	Biologic needs	Provide for physical comfort.
	Comfort needs	Provide for nutritional needs.

From Ebersole P, Hess P: *Toward healthy aging: human needs and nursing responses,* ed 5, St Louis, 1998, Mosby.

dressed assessment of one's self within the world, functioning of the individual self, and relationship between the self and environment (Newton and Levinson, 1979). Psychosocial theory focuses on one's connection to the self and the environment, living life's experiences, and the creative potential of human variability.

Levinson proposed a universal life cycle consisting of specific eras sequenced from birth to old age. The *era* is the basic unit of the life cycle and lasts about 20 years (e.g., preadulthood from 0 to 20 years; early adulthood from 20 to 40 years; middle adulthood from 40 to 60 years; late adulthood from 60 to 80 years to death). A person experiences stable periods of 6 to 7 years, followed by transitional periods of 4 to 5 years. Each period consists of specific tasks for a person to encounter and achieve. From a clinical viewpoint, therapists found this framework useful in identifying transitional periods that were often times of internal conflict and thus motivation for seeking treatments (Myers, 1998). The following summarizes key events during Levinson's stages and transitions:

- Preadulthood lasts up to about age 17 years, and early adult transition occurs from ages 17 to 22 years, during which individuals begin to modify their relationships with family and friends.
- Early adulthood stage is between 17 and 45 years, characterized by periods of vitality, contradiction, and stress. Individuals face with major life tasks, including achieving goals, raising families, and establishing their position in society.
- Midlife transition is between ages 40 and 45 years. Individuals face the realization that failure to accomplish all of life's goals leads first to disappointment and then to reformulation of earlier goals.
- Middle adulthood lasts from ages 40 to 65 years. During these years adults have the greatest potential to have a positive impact on society.
- Late adult transition occurs between 60 and 65 years of age, and individuals experience some anxiety over physical decline.
- Late adulthood era occurs after 65, and individuals learn an acceptance of realities of the past, present, and future.

The Harvard Study of Adult Development, the longest and most thorough study of aging ever attempted, has followed the life course of 268 undergraduate students from 1938 to the present. The current director of the study, George Vaillant, is studying adult adaptation related to ego defense mechanisms. His book, published in 2002, *Aging Well: Surprising Guideposts to a Happier Life from the Landmark Harvard Study of Adult Development*, identifies behaviors that promote adaptation as well as maladaptation.

Using a series of interviews and questionnaires, the study followed three groups of men and women for six to eight decades. The first group consists of a sample of 268 socially advantaged Harvard graduates born about 1920. The second group is a sample of 456 socially disadvantaged urban-dwelling men born about 1930. The third group is a sample of 90 middle-class, intellectually gifted women born about 1910.

Vaillant identified six factors in middle adulthood that promote longevity:

1. Experiencing a warm, caring marriage
2. Having effective adaptive or coping strategies
3. Not smoking heavily
4. Not abusing alcohol
5. Getting adequate exercise
6. Being at recommended weight

Vaillant's study built on the intrapsychic styles of adaptation first described by Freud. The ego mechanisms of defense are the major channels toward managing instinct and affect. Ego defense mechanisms are either adaptive or pathologic in nature. Vaillant (1977) was able to develop a

BOX 5-1

Vaillant's Hierarchy of Adaptive Mechanisms

LEVEL I: PSYCHOTIC MECHANISMS (COMMON IN PSYCHOSIS, DREAMS, CHILDHOOD)
Denial (of external reality)
Distortion
Delusional projection

LEVEL II: IMMATURE MECHANISMS (COMMON IN SEVERE DEPRESSION, PERSONALITY DISORDERS, AND ADOLESCENCE)
Fantasy (schizoid withdrawal, denial through fantasy)
Projection
Hypochondriasis
Passive-aggressive behavior
Masochism, turning against the self
Acting out (compulsive delinquency, perversion)

LEVEL III: NEUROTIC MECHANISMS (COMMON IN EVERYONE)
Intellectualization (isolation, obsessive behavior, undoing, rationalization)
Repression
Reaction formation
Displacement (conversion, phobias, wit)
Dissociation (neurotic denial)

LEVEL IV: MATURE MECHANISMS (COMMON IN "HEALTHY" ADULTS)
Altruism
Suppression
Anticipation
Humor

From Vaillant GE: *Adaptation to life*, Boston, 1977, Little Brown.

theoretic hierarchy of ego defenses, grouping them according to their relative maturity and pathology (Box 5-1). As ego defense mechanisms are dynamic and mature throughout the life cycle, individuals who successfully adapt are able to select from a range of defense mechanisms to deal with problems. In healthy adults, these successful mechanisms include altruism, suppression, anticipation, and humor.

The adaptation theory as described by Vaillant (1977) is more of a conceptual model that categorizes the changes brought about by aging. Vaillant identified a series of shifts and trade-offs that occur during the aging process. The ability of the individual to let go of parts of the past while pursuing quality-of-life is critical to successful adaptation. For example, the older person often experiences sensory losses, especially in the areas of vision and hearing, and adapts to such losses by facilitating the quality of the remaining sensory perceptions. For example, the use of large-print books, direct lighting, or hearing aids enhances the older person's remaining sight and hearing. Encouraging the use of other sensory perceptual systems such as touch or taste is another way for the older individual to gather information from the environment (see the Research for Evidence-Based Practice box).

Midlife Transitions

Many young adults anxiously anticipate a midlife transition as they enter middle adulthood. As previously discussed, Levinson noted that, for many, this transition is a period of struggle or crisis (Myers, 1998). Levinson believed that up to 80% of persons experience such a period of crisis. Researchers have examined the possibility of a possible midlife crisis and whether it is universal throughout cultures and genders.

Physical changes and new responsibilities of taking care of children, grandchildren, and older parents typically characterize middle age. Also, middle-aged adults sometimes assume new work responsibilities and subsequently feel a need to reappraise their life situations and make changes while they still have the time (Huyck, 1997). The term *midlife crisis* (Jaques, 1970) described a point in time when individuals experience a life crisis as their own mortality becomes real (Shek, 1996). These realizations often result in negative outcomes such as perceptions that health is deteriorating, bad feelings about marital relations or work, inability to enjoy leisure time, and stress from caring for aging parents (Shek, 1996). The focus shifts from, "How long have I lived?" to "How many years do I have left?"

Daniel Shek examined the concept of midlife crisis among adults from Chinese descent. He found that some of the participants were unhappy with work and personal achievements, but most did not indicate dissatisfaction that was at a crisis level. Other studies (McCrae, 1984) also support the view that midlife crisis is not a universal phenomenon, nor does it cluster around any particular age-group.

The work of Arnold Kruger (1994) also focused on the presence of a midlife crisis in middle-aged adults. He concluded that the "symptoms" of a midlife crisis are in the DSM-IV criteria for adjustment disorders. Adjustment disorders are problematic responses to life events. Myers (1998) further challenged the idea of adult stages of development, noting that particular life events (working, getting married, having children, retiring) vary among cultures. For example, 40% of Jordanian women marry in their teens; that number is about 3% in Hong Kong. Regarding retirement, six times the number of men over the

RESEARCH for EVIDENCE-BASED PRACTICE

Levy B et al: Longevity increased by positive self-perceptions of aging, *Journal of Personality and Social Psychology* 83:261-270, 2002.

In this research study, 660 older adults participated in a community survey to examine the impact of positive self-perceptions of aging on longevity. These individuals had been among those who participated, in 1975, in the Ohio Longitudinal Study of Aging and Retirement (OLSAR). In the original study, subjects completed surveys about their self-perceptions of aging. Researchers also collected survival data on the original 1975 sample. Researchers found that those who held more positive self-perceptions about aging in 1975 had lived longer (an average of 7.5 years longer). The researchers controlled factors such as age, functional health, gender, and socioeconomic status. It is suggested that having a "will to live" across all life stages positively influences one's views of aging and will possibly even extend one's life.

age of 65 years in Mexico continue to work compared with men in the United States or Europe (Myers, 1998).

Role of Stress in Adult Development

The negative effects of stress on aging are well documented. A growing body of research confirms that stress plays a part in hastening cognitive and memory decline, and sometimes it even speeds aging changes in the very structure of the brain (Aldwin, 1994). The effects of stress on adult development are complex. Some researchers are examining the possibility that stress actually has a positive benefit to adult development. In many cases, individuals who have experienced a stressful life event find that they have "learned from the experience" in the long run, gaining new coping skills, increasing their self-knowledge, or enhancing social networks. These persons often feel that these stressful experiences "made them a better person." Further research is necessary in this area, as it is difficult to generalize these findings across all adult populations.

Gender Differences in Adult Development

As research in adult development has evolved, particularly in the areas of adult personality and adult learning concepts, gender differences have become apparent. Some studies have focused on a *trait approach* to adult personality that suggests personality is constant or stable over time. These studies also highlight gender differences in their approaches to adult development.

Personality is continuous for the most part, but there are some gender and age-related differences. The most stable aspects of personality include coping styles, life satisfaction factors, and goal-directed behaviors. Neugarten (1979) noted the following changes with aging:

- From ages 40 to 60 years, there is a shift from feeling in control over one's environment to perceiving the environment as more threatening, referred to as a change from *active* to *passive mastery.*
- Older adults become more *introspective and self-reflective* as they age.
- There are shifts in *sex-role expressiveness* between men and women. Men take on a more nurturing role, and women become more accepting of their aggressive tendencies.
- Older adults tend to become more *introverted.*

The longest running aging research program, the Baltimore Longitudinal Study, began in the 1950s. One aspect of the research focused on the conceptualization of personality according to the *Five-Factor Model of Personality* (McCrae, 1984). Although personality remains stable across adulthood into old age, there were gender differences in personality; for example, men became less masculine and demonstrated a lower activity level with increased age.

Life Events Framework

The life events framework proposes that major life events result in stressful circumstances that individuals respond to by changing their personalities (Miller, 1997). The model recognizes individual differences, unlike the stage theories such as Levinson's, which focus on similarities among individuals. The author noted that life events are not always age linked, particularly those that are not biologically driven such as menopause or death. Critics note that the life events framework has the following shortcomings:

- Places too great an emphasis on change
- Fails to recognize stability of personality characteristics
- Focuses to a great extent on the impact on major life events but does not recognize the impact of daily annoyances or aggravations that have additive effects

Optimum Growth

Erikson (1974a, 1974b) described what is necessary to sustain a person's opportunity and ability to grow and mature. He noted that vital individual strengths come from the stages of life. These strengths include faith, willpower, purposefulness, competence, fidelity, love, care, and wisdom. Slowly, the typical model of the elderly is changing as a result of increased longevity. Growth and maturity are now considered dynamic processes, many of which are under the control of individuals, that lead to new opportunities and rewards in later life.

Society has long focused on growth and development only during the age of youth. What if the focus moved toward adults and elders? Lillian Troll postulated this new viewpoint in writing, "To be young is to be fresh, lively, quick to learn; to be mature is to be done, complete, sedate, tired. But what if we consider a different perspective? To be young is to be unripe, unfinished, raw, awkward, unskilled, inept; to be mature is to be ready, whole, adept, wise." (Troll, 1975, p. 6).

ADULT DEVELOPMENT IN LATER LIFE

Advances in health care sciences have ensured that a larger proportion of people will be living longer with a better quality of life. More than ever as we enter the twenty-first century, aging has become an evolutionary process. Aging is a complex process involving biologic, psychologic, social, and environmental factors. How a person adapts to aging is very individualized, and no single theory adequately explains the effects of aging from a developmental perspective. New theories of aging are attempting to integrate biologic and behavioral changes to view aging as a series of life events.

The process of aging is a series of physiologic and psychosocial changes. It is important that psychiatric nurses understand normal and abnormal aging changes and their impact on such factors as activities of daily living (ADLs), mental processes, social supports, sexuality, and role development. For older adults, their physical and mental health represents the summation of health care beliefs and practices across the years. The psychiatric mental health nurse needs to consider the older person's perceptions of health and wellness as key information in the assessment and management of care.

Changing attitudes and images of aging have important implications for the psychiatric mental health nurse. Jung stated that we would not grow to be 70 or 80 years old if this longevity had no meaning for the species. Two decades ago that concept was poetically stated as follows: "The afternoon of human life must also have a significance of its own and cannot be merely a pitiful appendage to life's morning" (Campbell, 1979). This is even more significant in the new millennium. Scientists are beginning to pay attention to those words, focusing on successful aging processes as a reality rather than an ideal.

Overview of the Older Adult Population

Because those age 65 years and older use more than 70% of all health care resources, it is imperative for all health care professionals to understand basic gerontology (U.S. Census Bureau, 2000). *Gerontology* is the study of the aging process across multiple disciplines and settings. Gerontologists who receive specialized training and education in the field of aging are in many disciplines including nursing, medicine, psychiatry, social services, pharmacology, biology, and the humanities. The term *geriatrics* broadly refers to the health care and human services provided to older adults (Eliopoulos, 2001).

Demographics

Since the beginning of the twentieth century, the average growth rate of the population age 65 years and older has greatly surpassed the overall population rate according to the U.S. Census Bureau (2000). From 1900 to 2000, the older population increased more than 11 times, from 3 million to 35 million. In comparison, the total population tripled during that same period. By 2050, projections show a marked increased in the older population to more than 80 million persons. With the aging of the baby boomers, one in five individuals will be over 65 years in 2030. Older adult minority groups, including African Americans, Asians and Pacific Islanders, Native Americans, and Hispanics, will see substantial population growth into the middle of the twenty-first century.

The most rapidly growing group of the older population are those age 85 years and older, termed the *oldest old.* Currently 1.3% of the U.S. population is in this age group. By 2050, this group will grow to 19 million, or almost one fourth of the entire older population (U.S. Census Bureau, 2000). Table 5-7 presents a profile of the aging U.S. population showing several important characteristics of this growing group now and in the future.

Health Status

Overall, older adults report that their health is good to excellent (Rowe and Kahn, 1998). Socioeconomic status and availability of social support have direct effects on reports of health. Minority groups and those with low incomes consistently report poorer health, even when age is controlled. Because both males and females are living longer, a greater proportion of couples are surviving into old age. Older adults of today are more educated, with a greater portion having completed some college. More than 22% of persons age 65 years and older completed at least one year of college, compared with 12.5% in 1970. Older adults also maintain better health care practices than some younger-age groups. The most recent data from the Agency for Healthcare Research and Quality (2000) reported that older persons had better dietary habits and smoked and consumed alcohol to a lesser extent than those less than 65 years old. Only in the area of physical exercise did older adults report less activity than younger age groups.

Although a majority of older adults across all settings suffer from at least one chronic condition, illness in itself does not appear to influence individual perception of health status if functional abilities are not impaired. Functional ability is categorized as ADLs and instrumental ADLs (IADLs). Nurses include physical and psychosocial functions in a functional assessment. This chapter discusses assessing the functional abilities of older adults later.

A Life Span Perspective of Aging

Gerontologists in a variety of scientific fields have attempted to explain the developmental processes of aging from biologic and behavioral perspectives. A variety of theories on aging exist because scientists do not agree on a single definition of aging. The literature has described chronologic, biologic, psychologic, and social definitions of aging extensively, but they do not adequately describe the process of aging. Therefore, scientists and philosophers have developed theories to explain the meaning, causes, and factors related to the aging process.

Biologic Theories of Aging

Biologic theories of aging are classified into various categories based on causative factors. Most biologic theories view the process of aging as either a normal, gradual wearing down of all systems or an abnormal series of cellular damage or mutations eventually leading to the body's inability to make repairs (Schneider and Rowe, 1990).

One method of classifying biologic theories of aging relates to categorizing predisposing factors as intrinsic or extrinsic to the organism. Intrinsic, or genetic, theories focus on the process of aging as internal to the organism. Researchers estimate that genetic factors account for about 30% of variance in life expectancy with lifestyle and environmental influences having more profound effects on aging than they previously thought (Lao et al., 2005). Certain genetic diseases, including several types of cancers and high cholesterol syndromes that lead to heart disease, have a negative impact on life expectancy (Rowe and Kahn, 1998).

Extrinsic or nongenetic theories propose that aging occurs as a result of environmental factors acting on the organism, such as radiation, ozone, drugs, and toxic substances, which, researchers have theorized, damage cellular structures, leading to aging and death.

Researchers have not agreed on any single biologic theory to explain the aging process. A combination of

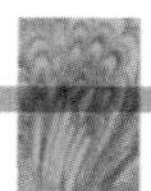

TABLE 5-7

Profile of the Older US Population: 2000 and 2050 Comparisons

ETHNIC GROUP	OLDER POPULATION IN 2000 (%)	OLDER POPULATION IN 2050 (%)
Caucasian	69.4	50.1
African American	12.7	14.6
Asian, Pacific Islander	3.8	8.0
Other Races	2.6	3.3
Hispanic	12.6	24.4

OTHER FACTS

Sex ratios will continue to decline (number of males per 100 females) as age increases:
- Ratio of 82 for males 65-69 years old
- Ratio of 44 for males 85-89 years old
- Ratio of 26 for males 95-99 years old

Eight states will double their older population by 2020: Nevada, Arizona, Georgia, Washington, Alaska, Utah, Colorado, and California.

Increasing numbers of older women live in poverty compared with older men:
- Currently 16% of older women are at or below poverty level, compared with 9% of men.
- 2 million of the 2.3 million older poor living alone are women.
- Poverty rates are higher for older minorities.

Modified from US Bureau of the Census: US interim projections by age, sex, race, and Hispanic origin, Washington, DC, 2004; www.census.gov/ipc/www/usinterimproj; and US Bureau of the Census: Sixty-five plus in the United States. In *Current Population Reports*, P23-190, No. 178RV, special studies, Washington, DC, 1996, US Department of Commerce, Economics and Statistics Administration.

genetic and environmental factors best explains why individuals age differently. Four biologic theories of aging most examined by researchers follow.

Genetic Theory. The genetic theory of aging represents a group of basic aging theories, all of which focus on an internal genetic code that drives the aging process. The basis of the theory is that genes are categorized as juvenescent or senescent. *Juvenescent* genes promote and maintain growth and vigor through the adult years, whereas *senescent* genes become active in middle adult and later years and initiate a process of decline and deterioration. However, this theory lacks empirical evidence to support that there is an "aging" gene.

Another popular genetic theory is the *biologic clock theory* (Schneider and Rowe, 1990), which suggests that a programmed internal genetic clock regulates an organism's development and subsequent decline. This internal clock runs down over a predetermined length of time. Supporters of this theory point to certain normal physiologic changes in humans that happen with time, such as hair graying and menopause.

Although the biologic clock theory gives dramatic evidence for boundaries of the human life span, there are limitations to this theory. One limitation is the inability to generalize in vitro studies to in vivo studies. Second, the theory does not explain what factor triggers the end of cellular replication and the beginning of cellular degeneration. Finally, the theory does not explain extreme cases of longevity.

Researchers have a suggested a final genetic theory, *error theory*, to explain the development of harmful genes that interfere with biologic processes such as protein synthesis (Hayflick, 1985). Damage to biologic synthesis results in the development of damaged cells that interfere with normal biologic functions. The proliferation of cancerous cells is an example of a process in which normal cells become unusual through some error process.

Immunologic Theory. Most biologists agree that changes in the immunologic system after puberty influence the process of aging. Antibody production declines, and autoimmune responses change in response to the decline. The result is that the body's ability to differentiate normal and abnormal or foreign substances fails. This response occurs sometimes in cases of tissue rejection in organ transplantation.

Immune function significantly declines with aging. By age 85 years, an individual's immune system functions at 5% to 10% of the system's level at puberty. Rheumatoid arthritis and mature-onset diabetes are two diseases commonly experienced in older age that caused by alterations to the immune system. Although no one knows exactly how or why the immune system exhibits a functional decline with aging, the appearance of autoantibodies in the serum of older persons is common. Autoantibodies are antibodies particular to an individual's own normal serum or tissue. Researchers hypothesize that their appearance signals declines in immune system function (Navratil, Sabatine, and Ahearn, 2004).

Cross-Linkage Theory. Collagen tissue, an important component of connective tissue that maintains the structure of cells, tissues, and organs, changes with aging. Collagen provides the elasticity necessary in many types of tissue such as cardiac and muscle. With age the combination of chemical changes and external stimuli causes the formation of molecular bonds in collagen, or cross-links that tend to stabilize the collagen fibers, resulting in rigid, fragile tissue. Scientists do not understand the mechanism that triggers the formation of cross-links, but they believe that the most active period of cross-link development is between age 30 and 50 years.

Cross-links also form in elastin in connective tissue. Elastin is similar to collagen in that it maintains tissue flexibility and permeability. The effects of cross-linking in elastin fibers are most pronounced in the changes in facial skin with aging. Skin becomes brittle, dry, saggy, and appears translucent (see-through). The formation of cross-links is probably not the only cause of aging, but collagen alterations at the cellular level affect structural and functional changes associated with aging.

Free Radical Theory. Biologists theorize that some environmental stimuli, such as radiation, ozone, and certain chemicals, interfere with cellular activity, resulting in the production of free radicals, which are compounds the body produces in cells as a result of environmental stimuli. They sometimes interact with various cellular structures, causing damage to normal cellular function. Free radicals are also formed during the normal process of cellular oxygenation when the cell removes waste products. Although the cell is capable of neutralizing and removing such by-products, researchers theorize that over time the cell loses its capacity to eliminate waste and repair itself. Researchers are continuing to study the potential effectiveness of antioxidants such as vitamins A, C, and E in protecting cellular structures.

Sociologic Theories of Aging

Sociologists have observed that an individual's role, relationships, and social experiences change as he or she ages. Sociologic theories of aging attempt to explain the social aspects of the aging process. Sociologists developed three of the earliest theories in the 1960s. These three theories—*disengagement*, *continuity*, and *activity*—all take a different approach to the social aspects of aging. Common to the three theories is the focus on action and adaptation by the individual (i.e., the aging person needs to change or adjust to new situations). Relocation to a nursing home is often traumatic for the older person who is not able to adjust to the highly structured institutional routines. Social theories that focus more on the interaction between the aging individual and the environment have evolved.

Disengagement Theory. The **disengagement theory** was the first sociologic aging theory developed by social gerontologists. In 1961, Cumming and Henry published the results of their exploratory study of 275 healthy, financially stable persons, ages 50 to 95 years, who lived in Kansas City. They theorized that a process of mutual withdrawal naturally occurs between the aging individual and society that is inevitable and universal in its occurrence. The retirement process is an example of this disengagement. Society clearly identifies the age of 65 years as the time for retirement. Identifying a retirement marker, or target, is also a mechanism for society to open the opportunity for a young person to enter the workforce. According to Cumming and Henry (1961), if the older person is prepared for retirement, he or she will have an easier time "disengaging" from society. The older person's social ties continue to shrink, causing the individual's further withdrawal into self.

The disengagement theory has been the most controversial of the social aging theories. Most of the criticism focuses on its presumed universality and on the fact that it does not allow for biologic or personality differences between individuals. In addition, it presumes that the individual will see disengagement as an obligation to society. How ready and accepting older persons are to change roles determines their ability to adjust and, subsequently, their life satisfaction.

Havighurst, Neugarten, and Tobin (1968) reexamined the original data used to formulate the disengagement theory and arrived at different conclusions in support of disengagement. For example, they found that individual personality traits and past experiences influence how an individual in society adapts to aging. A person who is withdrawn early in life will probably continue to withdraw and adapt if his or her social ties also support withdrawal behaviors. Society today is less insistent that older adults completely disengage. For example, some industries are hiring retired persons on a part-time or per diem basis or using them as expert consultants. It is a combination of one's personal preferences and the needs of society, rather than personal preference or societal needs alone, that determines the degree and pattern of disengagement.

Continuity Theory. Theorists developed the **continuity theory** out of Havighurst, Neugarten, and Tobin's reformulation of the disengagement theory (1968). The basis of the continuity theory is that people adapt best when they are allowed to be who they are. With aging, people become "more like themselves" (i.e., as an individual ages, he or she attempts to maintain continuity and consistency of habits, beliefs, norms, values, and other aspects of the personality). If a person is having difficulties adjusting to changes such as retirement or relocation, the continuity theory says that it is not the process of aging that interferes with adaptation but rather personality factors or the individual's social environment that influences adaptation. The continuity theory allows for individual differences in the aging process and theorizes that each individual's personality contains a self-maintaining component, meaning that the individual's long-standing behavior patterns enhance coping and adjustments to new situations across the life span (Atchley, 1989).

Activity Theory. Those who support the **activity theory** believe that maintaining an active lifestyle and social roles offsets the negative effects of aging (Figure 5-2). Activity theorists postulated that by retaining a high level of participation in his or her socioenvironment, the older individual will report a higher level of overall life satisfaction and a more positive self-concept. Four propositions were initially identified in the conceptualization of the activity theory (Lemon, Bengston, and Peterson, 1972):

1. The greater the loss in social roles (both formal and informal), the less the activity participation.

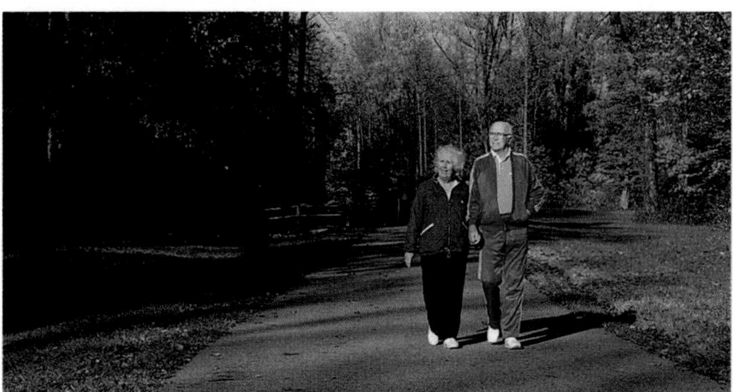

FIGURE 5-2 Continuing interest and activity in a favorite hobby helps to preserve cognitive and physical function. (From Sorrentino SA: *Mosby's textbook for nursing assistants,* ed 4, St. Louis, 1996, Mosby.)

2. The more activity maintained, the greater the social role support for the older person.
3. Maintaining stability of social roles supports a person's positive self-concept.
4. The more positive a person's self-concept, the greater the degree of life satisfaction experienced.

Many have not accepted this activity theory because of the lack of empiric evidence to support these postulates. The importance, type, and availability of a particular activity as perceived by the older person is an essential consideration affecting self-concept and life satisfaction. It is possible that the activity theory only applies to older persons who are able to participate in meaningful activities and social interactions.

Psychologic Theories of Aging

Studying human behavior and attempting to explain why persons act the way they do have been the focus of developmental psychologists since Freud, the founder of psychoanalysis. Because in many cases older adults do not exhibit the same patterns of behavior as their younger counterparts, theorists developed psychologic theories and models of aging. Whereas sociologic theories of aging focus more on the interaction between the aging individual and his or her socioenvironment within an age *cohort* (group with one or more factors in common) or a culture, developmental psychologists examine human development from an *intrapsychic* or mental viewpoint. Few of the human development theories address characteristics of developmental change in older adults. Most of the developmental theories focus on a single area of one's *psyche*, or the center of thought processes, emotions, and behavior. For example, Freud's theory and practice focused on sexual aspects across the human life span. A focus on cycles or stages during which the individual performs key developmental tasks or events is apparent in most of the developmental theories.

New Theories and Emerging Models of Aging

In the field of theory, aging theories are in their infancy. This is especially true with psychologic theories, most of which theorists developed after World War II. New theories of aging include behavioral genetics, gerotranscendence, and gerodynamics theories. Emerging models of aging focus on successful aging and explore the complexities of health and aging from the perspective of older adults.

Behavioral genetics theory examines the relevant impact of genetic and environmental factors on biologic and behavioral differences among individuals across the life span (DeFries et al., 2000). *Gerotranscendence theory* looks at aging from three levels: cosmic, the self, and social relations. The theory implies that aging brings on changes such as (1) changes in time perception, (2) acceptance of the mysteries of life and death, (3) altruistic behavior, and (4) an increased need for solitude and reflection (Tornstam, 1997). *Gerodynamics theory* is based on several physics theories, including general systems theory and chaos theory. Gerodynamics postulates that individuals pass through a series of transformations, or life events, and are thereby changed in some way (Schroots, 1995). Individuals respond differently to these events, which either weaken or strengthen the individual. Those who age successfully have the ability to cope with traumatic events and maintain healthy lifestyles. As yet, these theories need additional testing to support the concepts.

Models of healthy aging are beginning to come from explorations of reports by older adults of their perceptions regarding attributes of successful aging. Later in this chapter, what researchers are learning about healthy aging is discussed in terms of how this knowledge will restructure views about developmental aging. New models of healthy aging go beyond what is typically considered the dimensions of health (i.e., physical, functional, psychologic, and social) and attempt to understand how older adults interpret their health and well-being (see the Research for Evidence-Based Practice box).

RESEARCH for EVIDENCE-BASED PRACTICE

Bryant L, Corbett K, Kutner J: In their own words: a model of healthy aging, *Social Science and Medicine* 53:927-941, 2001.

In this qualitative research study, 22 older adults participated in semistructured interviews to identify what factors distinguish healthy from less healthy aging. A model of healthy aging became apparent from analysis of the interviews. Participants described health as "going and doing," a perspective they viewed as being important to their well-being. Whereas some of the less healthy elders focused on the physical aspects of health, the majority of participants viewed healthy aging as the presence of the following components: (1) having something worthwhile and meaningful to do, (2) retaining the necessary abilities to meet potential challenges, (3) getting the needed resources to perform activities, and (4) having the will to go and do.

Process of Aging

The process of aging incorporates physiologic and psychosocial changes within the individual. As described in several of the biologic and psychosocial theories of aging, external or environmental factors affect aging in many ways. The physiologic changes that come with aging are universal. Because the changes that characterize normal physiologic aging reflect pathologic changes, health care providers often confuse normal and abnormal aging processes. Although aging is ultimately irreversible, people are still able to significantly delay disease and disability even into very old age (Rowe and Kahn, 1998).

Psychosocial changes during aging in the areas of cognition, personality, social interactions, sexuality, and roles are even less distinct. Personality and socioenvironmental factors play a huge role in determining psychosocial aging changes. Particular aspects of such processes as cognition and memory decline with aging, whereas other aspects remain the same or are even enhanced with advanced age.

Physiologic Aging

The physiologic aging changes considered part of normal aging affect all body systems, but not necessarily at the same rates. It is important to have an understanding of the common physiologic aging changes, as some of these changes indicate the development of pathologic conditions. Many of these changes begin as early as the fourth and fifth decades of life. There are also individual differences in the rates of aging of some biologic systems because of factors such as heredity, environment, lifestyle, and nutrition (Kane, Ouslander, and Abrass, 2003). In keeping with the focus of this textbook, the following section discusses the physiologic changes of the nervous system.

Nervous System. Unlike cells of other body systems, the cells of the nervous system do not reproduce. There is a loss of nerve cells with normal aging, but the degree of loss differs, depending on the structure of the nervous system. The aging pigment, lipofuscin, is deposited in nerve cells, and neurofibrillary plaques and tangles form in the aging brain. These plaques and tangles sometimes indicate Alzheimer's disease but are also apparent in normal aging brains in the absence of dementia (see Chapter 15).

The amount of neurotransmitters also decreases with normal aging. A decrease in acetylcholine and epinephrine sometimes causes changes in cognitive functioning such as memory storage. Because of the redundancy of nerve cells, it is impossible to generalize that all older persons have diminished memory or cognitive abilities. Decreases in another neurotransmitter, serotonin, is also part of normal aging. Serotonin is important in the regulation of activities such as sleeping, drinking, and breathing. Serotonin also affects temperature regulation, heart rate, and affect. Reductions in the amount of serotonin result in the older person's inability to respond to physical and psychologic stressors in an appropriate manner (see Chapters 6, 11, and 24).

The normal aging process influences the sleep cycle as well. Older adults usually complain of frequent periods of restlessness or insomnia. Some go to the bathroom often during the night and, as a result, they nap during the day to make up for the loss of night sleep. Periods of rapid eye movement (REM) sleep also decrease with aging.

CLINICAL ALERT

Because many drugs are excreted through the kidneys, it is important to test creatinine clearance, which is an indicator of the proportion of muscle mass. Reduced creatinine clearance indicates a decrease in muscle mass, so dosages of medication that the kidneys absorb will sometimes need to be reduced for older clients.

CLINICAL ALERT

It is important for psychiatric–mental health nurses to recognize that many mental health problems develop or are identified at certain ages. For instance, schizophrenia is most often diagnosed in late adolescence or early adulthood but is uncommon after age 50 years. Certain forms of dementia are also more commonly identified at particular ages. For example, symptoms of Pick's disease are often evident by middle age, but symptoms of Alzheimer's disease are typically observed by age 75 years.

Functional Assessment. In view of all of the physiologic changes older adults experience throughout the life span, most individuals are able to cope with the minor aches and pains attributed to normal aging. Coping mechanisms usually fail when the older person is unable to function and carry out ADLs independently. Most situations that bring the older person to the primary care practitioner involve an inability to carry out specific functional tasks. Therefore, it is important to assess the older person's functional status and its effect on the person's daily life.

Functional assessment usually consists of evaluating two areas. The first area, ADLs, includes categories of personal care such as bathing, grooming, toileting, and transferring. The second area, IADLs, addresses activities important for the individual to function in the community. IADLs include shopping, preparing meals, and getting around. Box 5-2 shows the major categories of ADL and IADL assessment.

Activities of Daily Living. ADLs focus on the physical skills necessary to function from day to day. Nearly 31% of adults age 65 years or older reported some degree of activity limitations caused by physical, mental, or emotional problems (Centers for Disease Control and Prevention, 2004). Older African Americans and Hispanics tended to have more difficulties with ADLs (Federal Interagency Forum on Aging Related Statistics, 2004). Older adults reported having the greatest amount of difficulty bathing, walking, and transferring between the bed and the chair.

Instrumental Activities of Daily Living. The ability of the individual to function in the community is an important aspect of the functional assessment. Approximately 17.5% of older adults report difficulty with at least one IADL. Performing heavy housework was a problem by over 31% of older adults, followed by problems shopping (17%), doing light housework (12%), and managing money (11%) (National Centers for Health Statistics, 2002).

BOX 5-2

ADL and IADL Functional Assessment Categories

ADL CATEGORIES	IADL CATEGORIES
Bathing	Shopping
Dressing	Meal preparation
Hair care	Transportation
Mouth care	Use of telephone
Nutrition/assist with feeding	Medication usage
Ambulation/mobility	Housekeeping
Mental status	Laundry
Elimination	Financial management

There is a subjective, as well as objective, component of IADLs. Assessing the ability of the older person to perform daily skills needed to function in the community is important. In addition, the nurse needs to assess the meaning of the activity to the individual. For example, taking care of shopping needs is not as important to some individuals as housekeeping or meal preparation. An older individual who fears going out into the community because of safety issues will essentially become isolated. Another older person may have difficulty chewing and swallowing, so meal preparation seems like a difficult task.

Both aspects of the functional assessment, ADLs and IADLs, are relevant indicators for identifying outcomes of illness, both physical and mental. Often changes in ADLs and IADLs are the indication of a new illness. Individuals respond differently to physical aging changes, so the ability to function independently is more predictive of outcomes of aging than physical aging changes alone.

Psychosocial Aging

Psychosocial aging changes typically focus on an individual's responses to particular events across the life span. Past coping mechanisms are not always effective in adjusting to stressful events in later life. Because the life events of old age differ from those of younger ages, adaptation is sometimes more difficult for older adults. Miller (1990) distinguished the life events of older adults as follows:

- They are viewed as losses, rather than gains.
- They are most likely to occur close together with less time to adjust to each event.
- They are more intense and demand greater energy than is available for the coping process.
- They are longer lasting and often become chronic problems.
- They are inevitable and bring a feeling of powerlessness.

Preparing for some life events will facilitate adjustment in old age. For instance, some employers offer preretirement counseling for older employees in preparation for retirement. Psychosocial aging changes are reflected in several areas, including cognition and memory, personality, social support, sexuality, and role status. From a developmental perspective, the meaningfulness of life events is important in determining patterns of psychosocial aging in these particular areas. A great deal of research is necessary before researchers are able to draw any conclusion regarding normal versus abnormal psychosocial aging. The following section explores the current state of knowledge on psychosocial aging from a developmental perspective.

Cognition and Memory. Probably no other area of aging research has been studied to such an extent as cognition, especially in the areas of intelligence and memory. Evidence on the development of cognitive functions into old age is becoming clearer with studies that have followed older subjects over time. It is now apparent that cognitive functioning shows as much variability in aging as do physiologic indicators (MacDonald, Hultsch, and Dixon, 2003).

Several factors contribute to the variability in cognitive functioning observed in older adults. These factors include health status, genetic profile, socioeconomic status, education, and lifestyle behaviors (Herzog and Wallace, 1997). In turn, cognitive losses often result in functional impairment and physical disabilities, causing a spiraling decline for the older person.

Cognitive behaviors are divided into several interrelated processes including intelligence, memory, attention, reaction time, and problem solving. These divisions are random and researchers base them on how they typically study cognitive behaviors.

Studies of intelligence during the 1940s reported that older adults experience declines in all aspects of intelligence including knowledge acquisition, calculating, vocabulary, and abstract thought. The problem with these early studies was that researchers used the cross-sectional method to collect the data, comparing younger-age groups with older adult groups. The younger-age groups consistently had higher intelligence scores on the various tests, prompting researchers to conclude that intelligence declines with aging (Woodruff, 1983). Later longitudinal studies, which followed the same older subjects over a period of time, found that intelligence showed little or no decline in healthy aging persons. Declines that occurred were in the oldest age-group (Schaie and Willis, 1991).

Horn and Cattell (1967) theorized that age-related differences in intelligence are possibly due to distinctions between two types of intelligence that seem to develop from birth. *Crystallized intelligence* develops from knowledge gained through the accumulation of experience and education. Crystallized intelligence declines slightly, remains the same, or even increases with aging, depending on one's life experiences. On the other hand, neurophysiologic processes across the life span affect *fluid intelligence*. Declines in the nervous system with aging that affect one's attention span or reaction time reflect a loss of fluid intelligence. Instruments that measure intelligence using performance standards show declines in intelligence with aging (Birren and Schaie, 1985), and even some gerontologists have questioned these conclusions. Some older adults have shown an increased time in completing intelligence performance tests because they are more cautious and take additional time to make correct choices.

Much aging research is devoted to the study of memory processes during aging. It is unfortunate that society equates aging with memory loss. Older persons are often portrayed on television or in movies as forgetful. A common joke is, "There are three telltale signs you are getting old. The first is loss of memory, and the other two . . . I forget." There is much that we still do not know about the process of memory perception, storage, and retrieval.

Most of the early theories of memory focused on the three components of memory (i.e., perception or encoding, storage, and retrieval). Memory was categorized as short or long term, or as primary, secondary, or tertiary. These categorizations were based on the length of storage time and the process of retrieval.

Other memory theories focused on the encoding processes, which gave different types of information in various ways. For instance, information that the brain processes in a more complex manner, such as algebraic equations, is stored in a deeper area of memory and will last longer. Information that the brain easily recognizes requires less attention. For example, tasks such as starting a car are almost automatic. Researchers believe that automatic processing of information does not change with aging (Friedman, 2000). Offering cues to older adults will help them recall information stored in deeper areas of memory.

Theorists developed the contextual theory of memory from the information-processing model. This theory expands the information-processing model by including individual factors that sometimes impact memory, such as learning behaviors, past experiences, personality, degree of motivation, physical health, and socioeconomic status (Perlmutter et al., 1987).

Certain types of memory decline as a part of normal aging. *Explicit memory*, the ability to recall a specific name or place, tends to decline in aging (Rowe and Kahn, 1998). *Working memory*, the type of memory needed to perform daily activities, does not show an aging decline. Because older adults often take longer to process information (also normal to aging) and have some specific recall problems, they often fear that this is an indicator of Alzheimer's disease. It is important to explain that this is not true and to encourage older adults to seek ways to improve cognitive functioning through training and practice.

Self-perception of memory changes and self-efficacy also influence memory performance (Ryan, 1992; Ryan and See, 1993). The concept of *metamemory* refers to one's self-perceptions of memory changes and their effect on memory processes (Hertzog, Dixon, and Hultsch, 1990). For example, an older person falsely believes that memory loss is part of aging and perceive that forgetfulness indicates the start of memory decline. In reality, forgetting information is also due to a lack of attention to detail in a particular situation. Further study is necessary to determine whether an individual is able to mentally control or influence the development of memory across the life span.

Attention span refers to the ability to concentrate throughout the performance of some task. With aging, the ability to maintain the attention span through completion of complex tasks diminishes because complex tasks require dividing one's attention among several tasks at the same time. Some misinterpret these normal aging changes with the attention span as dementia. Two other segments of attention also show some decrements in aging. *Vigilance*, or the ability to sustain attention over longer periods of time, and *selective attention*, or the ability to discriminate and focus on relevant information, are less acute in older adults.

Increased reaction time/decreased speed of performance on intelligence tests is one of the most obvious changes in normal aging, but researchers still do not fully understand how this happens. Unfamiliarity with performance tests or increased cautiousness caused by fear of failure and resulting in test anxiety sometimes affect reaction time in older adults.

Problem-solving ability is a higher cognitive function. The complexity of the problem, past experiences, the amount of information that is irrelevant to a situation, and the individual's level of education are factors that influence problem solving. There is little knowledge about normal changes in higher cognitive functioning during aging. Most older persons are able to live and function effectively in the community.

Personality. Personality traits develop over the life span, influenced by internal and external environmental factors. An individual's ability to cope with stress and adapt to change molds an individual's personality. How individuals perceive themselves, *self-concept*, reflects their personality. In general, most personality traits remain stable during the aging process. Personality influences how an individual interacts and reacts within the socioenvironment (see Chapter 13).

Personality theorists have attempted to identify specific traits that predict successful aging. Individuals described as introverted are more self-centered and internalize behaviors and responses. Extroverted personalities focus more on the outside world and are described as outgoing. Certain personality traits assist individuals in adapting to aging better than others. The individual's ability to adapt to change determines successful aging more than a particular category of personality traits.

Some traits intensify with aging, such as that of cautiousness, which is often an effective safety mechanism for older adults. For example, the older person tends to drive a car with more caution, drive only in daylight hours, or avoid high speeds. In unfamiliar situations or when several choices are available, older adults tend to act more cautiously. They also tend to prefer familiar tasks, places, or situations.

Locus of control is another aspect of personality that remains stable over time (Reid, Haas, and Hawkings, 1977). Individuals with an *internal locus of control* perceive that they actively control their own destiny. On the other hand, individuals with an *external locus of control* believe they have no control over their destiny and think that their behaviors have no effect on any outcomes. Another phenomenon, the *secondary locus of control*, describes individuals with an external locus of control who learn to adapt to their beliefs. This has also been termed *learned helplessness*. These individuals learn dependency and prefer others to decide for them.

Social Support and Interactions. In an extensive review of the literature, Broadhead et al. (1983) presented Kahn and Antonucci's comprehensive definition of social support as interpersonal transactions that include one or more of the following behaviors: (1) expressing positive affect between individuals, (2) affirming or approving of another person's behaviors, and (3) providing direct aid or assistance to another. Different individuals within one's social network provide different types of support.

Hyde (1988) suggested that the quality, rather than the quantity, of social relationships is significantly related to life satisfaction among older adults. The quality of social support is a key area for interventions in the training of health care providers. Social support is part of a communication process in which facilitation of communication skills improves the quality of support (Albrecht and Adelman, 1984).

Social networks are generally the web of social ties that surround a person and include several characteristics important in the study of the health and well-being of older adults. These include the following:

- Size of the social network
- Frequency of social contacts
- Quality of the interactions
- Intimacy or closeness among members
- Strength of the relationships
- Geographic location of members
- Reciprocity (sharing) of assistance

Social networks and social supports are different concepts. Considering the network as the web or structure, social support refers to the emotional or tangible assistance obtained from the social resource network. Not all social ties are supportive, and not all social supports come from the closest social network such as a son or daughter living near older parents. Oxman and Berkman (1990) proposed a three-component model of social relationships that included the quantitative and qualitative nature of social relationships. Because many have associated social relationships with subsequent physical and mental illness in older adults, an assessment tool that addresses the multidimensional aspects of social relationships is important. Table 5-8 presents an example of some of the assessment questions (Oxman and Berkman, 1990).

Sexuality and Intimacy. Physical aging changes related to the reproductive system occur in men and women. Several factors influence psychologic aspects of sexuality and intimacy in older adults, including past experiences, attitudes toward intimacy, societal views about sexuality in older adults, and functional status.

Many older adults feel a newfound freedom in their sexual behaviors because they no longer need to focus on concerns regarding pregnancy. The unavailability of an acceptable partner, stereotypes that older adults are asexual, or fears of inability to initiate and maintain sexual performance frustrate some of these feelings. Older women probably experience the greatest effects because many become widowed or suffer from the effects of longstanding values about sexual taboos.

Only in recent years have older persons, especially those over 80 years, been subjects of studies of sexuality. Bretschneider and McCoy (1988) reviewed the available studies of psychosocial aspects of sexuality and aging. The following summarizes some of their findings:

- The frequency of sexual activity decreases with aging, but the interest and ability in sexual function do not necessarily decline with aging.

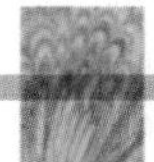

TABLE 5-8

Social Relationship Components and Characteristics

COMPONENTS	CHARACTERISTICS	SAMPLE QUESTIONS
Social network	Marital status/confidant	Are you married? Is there any one special person that you feel very close and intimate with?
Structure and composition	Number, kinship	How many children/close family members do you have?
	Proximity	How many live within an hour's drive?
	Frequency and type of contact	How many do you have phone or letter contact with at least once per month?
Type and amount of social support and function	Emotional	How frequently did someone try to make you feel better about your illness in the past month?
	Tangible aid	How frequently did someone help you get your medication in the past month?
	Guidance	How frequently did someone suggest that you call the doctor in the past month?
Perceived adequacy of social support	General	In the past year, did you need more help with daily tasks than you received?
	Specific	How helpful was it for your children to try to make you feel better about your illness?

From Oxman T, Berkman L: Assessment of social relationships in elderly patients, *Int J Psychiatr Med* 20:65, 1990.

- Older individuals who are in normal health and functioning have the ability to maintain sexual activity.
- Declines in sexual activity are mostly related to lack of a partner, especially for women.
- Psychosocial factors that prevent sexual activity by older adults include stereotypic beliefs, attitudes, and personality factors.
- Sexual behaviors and beliefs generally remain stable across the life span.
- Men remain more sexually active than women across the life span.

Role Transitions. Older persons also experience role changes along with the other changes of aging. Some of these role changes are more obvious than others, and individuals adapt to role changes in different ways. How important the role is to an individual influences how well the older person is able to cope with a role transition. From a developmental perspective, roles contain various tasks a person has to perform in life. Each role has different life tasks. Some tasks are new to the person if the role is a completely new one, and other tasks are similar to ones performed early in life, as in role reversals.

Retirement. Retirement implies a major role transition for many individuals. Because individuals live longer and retire earlier, the retirement period may last for 30 to 40 years. Only recently have researchers begun to explore gender differences in adaptation to retirement. Life events surrounding retirement affect adaptation more than the retirement process itself (Jonsson, Josephsson and Kielhofner, 2000). Particular life events even cause retirement. For instance, a middle-aged woman takes an early retirement because she needs to care for her older mother at home who has Alzheimer's disease. This individual's adjustment to retirement is negative because of a conflict between the woman's role in the workforce and her caregiver role.

Loss of a Spouse. A major role transition occurs after loss of one's spouse, when adaptation requires the survivor to perform tasks the partner previously performed. Couples who have shared responsibilities across the life span have less difficulty with the role changes. Personality traits seem to influence adjustment to widowhood. For example, a widow who let her husband take care of finances finds herself overwhelmed by the new responsibility, or the husband who lost his wife never learned how to cook or clean and is also overwhelmed. If the surviving spouse adapts to change, he or she will rapidly adjust and learn these tasks. The widower sometimes finds himself the center of attention by family members who want to assist him, as well as by widows looking for male companionship.

Grandparent Role. The role of the grandparent is another transition. The grandparent who adjusts successfully provides grandchildren with a viewpoint that often differs from that of the parents but is equally positive. Many grandparents take on the role of full- or part-time surrogate parents.

Role Reversal. When physical or mental deterioration is present, this often reverses the roles of the parent and child. Most often the oldest female child, on reaching middle age, provides care for the incapacitated older parent. This is an especially difficult transition for the female middle-aged child who has just completed raising her own children and who was planning her own retirement in a few years. If the caregiver is a middle-aged man, it is often an awkward situation because his wife has to adapt to a role for which she sometimes has no emotional connection (i.e., caring for the older parent-in-law). Supporting the caregiver is as important as supporting the care receiver under these circumstances.

Table 5-9 summarizes some normal aging changes discussed in this section and areas for functional assessment.

Mental Assessment. Gerontologists are attempting to develop adequate standardized tests designed specifically for older adults to assess their mental status and cognitive functioning. Designing reliable instruments for older adults continues to be a challenge because of the interrelationships among several factors including health status, physical/mental aging changes, socioenvironmental variables, and life events. Thus, the context of what many consider normal development for an older individual is the focus of any mental status assessment.

Several mental status assessment instruments are available to evaluate mental and cognitive functions. Most instruments examine mental status in view of the individual's ability to function in daily living activities. However, the mental status assessment is not sufficient to provide a diagnosis of a disorder. Other sources of information, such as the health history, physical examination, diagnostic/laboratory tests, and psychosocial factors, are necessary for diagnosis.

The mental status assessment of older adults includes the following areas: appearance, mood, communication, thought processes, perceptual and motor abilities, attention, memory, consciousness, and orientation. Appearance, behaviors, and responses of the older client are areas for attention by the health care provider performing the assessment. For instance, the older person states that he or she has no suicidal ideations, but appearance indicates self-neglect and behaviors include withdrawing from social networks and accumulating drugs. It is important to identify such inconsistencies.

Several screening instruments are available for the health care provider to give a quick assessment of mental status. Each instrument addresses different areas of the mental status examination. Often these brief instruments provide an initial baseline of cognitive functioning for use in further in-depth assessment and screening for diagnosis and subsequent interventions.

The Mini-Mental State Examination (MMSE) is one of the most commonly used instruments to screen for cognitive disorders in older adults (Folstein, Folstein, and McHugh, 1975). It assesses several dimensions of cognitive function, including orientation, memory, attention, and speech. Out of a total score of 30, normal persons score 25 and above, whereas individuals diagnosed with dementia score lower than 20 points.

TABLE 5-9

Functional Assessment of Common Psychosocial Aging Changes

AREA	NORMAL AGING CHANGES	AREAS FOR FUNCTIONAL ASSESSMENT
Cognition and memory	Normal crystallized intelligence ↓ Fluid intelligence (slight, gradual) ↑ Reaction time ↓ Divided attention ↓ Vigilance ↓ Selected attention ↑ Information-processing time ↑ Cautiousness	Degree of external stimulation Environmental distraction Assess barriers to learning (e.g., sensory impairments, relevancy/level of information, learning environment) Assess factors influencing memory process (e.g., education level, learning style, past experiences, physical/mental health, motivation)
Personality	Stability of most personality traits ↑ Cautiousness ↑ Rigidity (slight)	Adaptive coping strategies Decision-making processes Adjustment to change (e.g., retirement, change in housing, loss)
Social support and interactions	Perceived social support affected by several factors (personality, health status, past experiences, coping style) Changes in social network (size, intimacy, geographic location, reciprocity of assistance) Changes in source of social support with aging	Attitude/perception of social support Past experience with social support Social network Types of social support needed Sources of social support
Sexuality and intimacy	Sexual behaviors/interests maintained across life span in absence of physical/mental disorders ↓ Sexual activity in males ↓ Intensity of sexual responses Lack of partner is greatest factor affecting sexual activity	Attitudes toward expressions of sexuality and intimacy Means to maintain sexual behaviors/interests Availability of privacy in environment Risk factors blocking sexual behaviors
Role transitions	Retirement Widowhood Grandparenting	Importance of past roles/tasks Responses to retirement Effects of retirement on spouses Impact of loss of spouse Ability to take on new tasks in ADLs/IADLs Social supports/network Relationships with children/grandchildren Parenting role

ADLs, activities of daily living; *IADLs,* instrumental activities of daily living.

Another commonly used instrument is the Short Portable Mental Status Questionnaire (SPMSQ) (Pfeiffer, 1975). Although it is not adequate to provide a diagnosis of dementia, many frequently use this tool to screen cognitive abilities in older adults, including orientation, immediate and remote memory, thought processes, and concentration (Box 5-3). The SPMSQ scoring is particularly sensitive to population differences in cognitive abilities related to education or ethnic background, which impact cognitive functioning (Fillenbaum et al., 2001).

Human Development in the Twenty-First Century

Something historic will occur on January 1, 2011: the date that the first baby boomer will turn 65 years old. Society's entire perception of aging will continue to evolve over the following 20 to 30 years as the older adult population experiences unprecedented growth during that time frame. Images of aging and attitudes toward older persons are gradually changing for the better. As the aging population grows more ethnically and racially diverse, a reexamination of cultural values about aging is necessary. In fact, the entire body of knowledge on human development will probably need revising, as research in aging has begun to refocus efforts to understand successful aging. In particular, scientists are examining health, learning, and creativity as areas to promote quality of life for older adults.

Images of Aging

Images of aging and attitudes of society toward older adults have been changing over the plast several years. Unfortunately, society has usually focused on the negative aspects of aging. The term **ageism** has been used to describe the stereotypic views of older adults (Butler, 1987). The myth of the "burden of the elderly" has been gradually rejected with the growing body of scientific evidence disproving the notion that to be old is to be sick (Rowe and Kahn, 1998).

In 1995, the American Association of Retired Persons (AARP) published a study titled *Images of Aging in America* (Speas and Obenshain, 1995). The purpose of this report was to examine knowledge, perceptions, and attitudes about aging. One's personal experience with older adults was the strongest predictor of perceptions and attitudes toward aging. Most Americans had misconceptions about older adults, reflecting a lack of knowledge about aging.

BOX 5-3

Short Portable Mental Status Questionnaire

INSTRUCTIONS

Ask questions 1 to 10 in this list and record all answers. Ask question 4a only if the patient does not have a telephone. Record the total number of errors based on 10 questions.

1. What is the date today? (month, day, year)
2. What day of the week is it?
3. What is the name of this place?
4. What is your telephone number?

4a. What is your street address? *(Ask only if patient does not have a telephone.)*

5. How old are you?
6. When were you born? (month, day, year)
7. Who is the president of the United States now? (last name)
8. Who was the President just before him? (last name)
9. What was your mother's maiden name?
10. Subtract 3 from 20 and keep subtracting 3 from each new number, all the way down.

SCORING

For white subjects with at least some high school education, but not more than high school education, research has established the following criteria:

0-2 errors	Intact intellectual functioning
3-4 errors	Mild intellectual impairment
5-7 errors	Moderate intellectual impairment
8-10 errors	Severe intellectual impairment

Allow one more error if subject has only grade school education.
Allow one more error for African-American subjects, using identical educational criteria.
Allow one less error if subject has education beyond high school.

From Pfeiffer E: A short portable mental status questionnaire for the assessment of organic brain deficit in elderly patients, *J Am Geriatr Soc* 23:433, 1975.

On a positive note, many subjects showed a lack of stereotypes and myths about aging. These findings have important implications for health care professionals who work with older adults.

In 2004, researchers repeated this study with noticeably similar results. Many people continued to have false impressions about aging and older adults. Adults with fewer economic resources and significant health issues expressed the greatest anxiety about getting older. Similar to the 1990s study, the current study found little evidence of intergenerational conflict (Abramson and Silverstein, 2004).

Cultural Impact

Cultural beliefs also influence one's attitudes toward older adults. Culture influences the responses of older adults to health, illness, and treatment. Some cultures subscribe to health care practices or home remedies that are in direct opposition to modern health care practices. The health care professional needs to examine his or her own feelings toward differing cultural beliefs and health care practices of older clients. The incorporation of some home remedies into the older client's care plan sometimes increases compliance, but only if these remedies do not conflict with treatment.

Various cultures hold different views regarding aging. Since ancient times, the contributions of older adults to a society affect the status of older adults within a particular cultural group. For example, Far Eastern cultures value the wisdom of their elders and thus hold the older population in high respect. In contrast, some primitive cultures have considered older adults a burden, unable to hunt and provide for the tribe. Such cultures have sometimes sent older adults away from the tribe.

In the current Western culture, there is greater support for views of successful aging. The focus on age has presented the public with issues relating to functional, economic, and political aspects of aging that future older persons will experience. The situation of today's older population is possibly the most optimistic in terms of the availability of social and economic resources, but future generations of older persons face difficult resource issues (Conrad, 1992). The costs may outweigh the contributions by future older persons in society, and cultural values toward older adults may change.

Refocusing on Healthy Aging

Perceptions of health and wellness develop across the life span and affect attitudes and behaviors related to health care practices. For older adults, their physical and mental health represents the result of health care beliefs and practices across the years. In 2002, 73% of older adults rated their health as good to excellent, similar to results from a decade earlier. In 2002, the percentage of older adults reporting poor or fair health was 27% (29% in 1991). As older adults age, the percentage reporting good to excellent health declines regardless of gender or race. The greatest differences are among Caucasian men. Of those Caucasian men ages 65 to 74 years, 79% report good health or better, whereas 65% of them ages 85 and older report good to excellent health. Regardless of age group or gender, Caucasians overall report good to excellent health as compared to other ethnic groups (Federal Interagency Forum on Aging-Related Statistics, 2004).

Perceived health affects disease and disability among older adults. Rogers (1995) found that in older persons suffering from multiple chronic conditions and disability, those who perceived their overall health as very good to excellent lived longer than persons who considered themselves to be in poor health.

The MacArthur Foundation Study (Rowe and Kahn, 1998) has brought together 10 years of scientific knowledge and expertise related to aging. They identify three components necessary for successful aging:

1. Avoidance of disease and risk factors
2. Maintaining high cognitive and physical abilities
3. Engagement with life through productive relationships and behaviors

The early identification of risk factors and disease prevention/health promotion behaviors has a significant impact on the development and progress of several chronic diseases. For example, exercise is beneficial for helping older adults to prevent heart disease, hypertension, and diabetes. A regular, moderate program of aerobic and strength training for older adults is both safe and effective in improving function.

Challenging the mind as well as the body is important to maintain mental capabilities. Not all cognitive processes decline in aging, and most of these changes occur very late in life. Older persons who maintain a high level of self-efficacy, a measure of one's self-esteem, appear to manage well both mentally and physically.

Maintaining social relationships and continuing some sort of meaningful activities contribute positively to aging. Social networks often shrink for older adults who outlive their peers and relatives. Older persons find support in caring relationships with friends or family members. Grandparents find joy in having their grandchildren visit for extended periods, offering a break to the parents. In terms of productive activities, many older retirees remark that they are much busier after retirement, with new projects and volunteer work. With the aging of the baby boomers, the focus on successful aging is more of a reality than an ideal.

Refocusing on Learning and Aging

A large body of literature has focused on adult learning theory. In contrast to children, adults prefer self-directed learning and incorporate past experiences in new opportunities. Adults also prefer to learn about things that have application to their daily lives. Older adults continue to learn well into their 70s or 80s. Physical limitations affect speed of learning, so teaching methods need to be adapted for older learners. Older adults also need to have a choice as to how they best learn materials (i.e., auditory, visual, or tactile).

When teaching older adults, nurses need to link their lesson to experiences or activities older adults are familiar with or have enjoyed, especially social activities. For example, encourage older adults who enjoyed the years raising their own children to join a foster grandparent program or a senior volunteer program where they develop new relationships and learn about new resources. Intergenerational programs are also growing in popularity. Elementary and high schools are joining with senior communities to share learning experiences. Retired persons teach young people about skills such as woodcrafting. In turn, young people give in return and teach the older persons about computers and the Internet.

Refocusing on Creativity and Aging

In his book, *The Creative Age: Awakening Human Potential in the Second Half of Life* (2000), Gene D. Cohen provided evidence that the human potential for creativity continues well into old age. He found that although information processing slows down as one ages, older persons are able to go on to learn new information by modifying how they process this information through slowly digesting bits of data or thoughtfully asking questions to clarify key points. Studies on computer training of persons over the age of 65 years reported that practicing increased both the speed and accuracy of their computing.

In another example, older persons tend to have difficulty bringing up certain words. In contrast, persons in their 80s who keep on challenging themselves reading, writing, or doing crossword and word game puzzles have continued to grow their vocabularies. Research has even demonstrated links between creative activities and the consequential positive feelings with increased production of protective immune cells. Creativity is also possibly linked to delaying the onset of Alzheimer's disease. Continually challenging oneself mentally is a way to build up reserves of neurologic structures and connections.

CHAPTER SUMMARY

- Whatever the directions and results of future studies on aging and human development, it is clear that human development does not occur in isolation. The constant influence of biologic, psychosocial, and environmental factors creates a dynamic system in which human development occurs across the life span.
- Human development also begins at a much earlier age than previously believed, and it continues into much later years than researchers ever anticipated.
- It is important for the psychiatric mental health nurse to consider that development is a continuous process. Although there are common markers of human development at particular ages, there is a great degree of human variation.
- External factors such as culture or traditions also have a significant influence on human development, so the nurse needs be aware of these factors and take them into account when caring for clients.
- Understanding that many aspects of human development continue to grow and change well into old age provides the nurse additional opportunities to promote and stimulate successful aging.

REVIEW QUESTIONS

1 To assess that a 4-year-old child is in the initiative versus guilt developmental stage according to Erikson, the nurse asks the parent,

1. "Can your child put on socks without help?"
2. "What activities does your child participate in with other children?"
3. "Does your child get upset when you leave the room?"
4. "Does your child do chores to help you out at home, such as picking up toys?"

2 A 10-year-old child has this nursing diagnosis: *Delayed growth and development related to insufficient opportunities to interact with other children as evidenced by inability to engage in group play.* Select the best outcome for this child's plan of care. Within 2 months, the child will:

1. Voluntarily join a team sport.
2. Find useful ways to engage in solitary play.
3. Attend three sessions with a certified child psychologist.
4. Have an improved sense of self and peers.

3 A nurse cares for a 77-year-old retired physician hospitalized with pneumonia. Which form of address would be most appropriate to use with this client?
1. The client's first name
2. Mr. or Ms., followed by the client's surname
3. Doctor, followed by the client's surname
4. An endearing term, such as "Honey" or "Sweetie"

4 Which change(s) in neurotransmitters are expected in the normal aging process? You may select more than one answer.
1. Decreased serotonin
2. Increased glutamate
3. Decreased acetylcholine
4. Decreased epinephrine
5. Decreased lipofuscin

5 A nurse offers an educational presentation in a senior citizens center. Which activity/activities might the nurse suggest to promote healthy, successful aging? You may select more than one answer.
1. A swim aerobics class
2. Woodworking
3. Watching television
4. Crossword puzzles
5. Drinking four to six glasses of wine daily

Additional self-study exercises and learning resources are available to you on the ***Companion CD*** *at the back of the book and on the* ***Evolve website*** *at* ***http://evolve.elsevier.com/Fortinash/.***

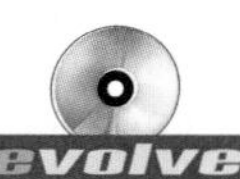

REFERENCES

Abramson A, Silverstien M: *Images of aging in American 2004: selected findings*, American Association of Retired Persons, 2004; www.aarp.org/research/reference/agingtrends/aresearch-import-926.html.

Agency for Healthcare Research and Quality: *Medical expenditure panel survey*, Rockville, Md, 2000, Agency for Healthcare Research and Quality.

Ainsworth M: Attachments beyond infancy, *Am Psychol* 44:709, 1989.

Albrecht T, Adelman M: Social support and life stress: new directions for communication research, *Hum Communication Res* 11:3, 1984.

Aldwin C: *Stress, coping, and development: an integrative approach*, New York, 1994, Guilford.

Atchley R: A continuity theory of normal aging, *Gerontologist* 29:183, 1989.

Baltes P, Smith J, Staudinger U: Life-span developmental psychology, *Annu Rev Psychol* 23:65, 1992.

Bandura A: *Social learning theory*, New York, 1971, General Learning Press.

Bandura A: *Social foundations of thought and action: a social cognitive theory*, Englewood Cliffs, NJ, 1986, Prentice-Hall.

Bandura A: Human agency in social cognitive theory, *Am Psychol* 44:1175, 1989.

Beers M, Berkow R: *Merck manual of geriatrics*, ed 3, New York, 2000, John Wiley and Sons.

Birren J, Schaie K: *Handbook of the psychology of aging*, ed 2, New York, 1985, Van Nostrand Reinhold.

Bowlby J: *A secure base: clinical applications of attachment theory*, London, 1988, Routledge.

Brainerd, C: *Piaget's theory of intelligence*, Englewood Cliffs, NJ. 1978, Prentice-Hall.

Bretschneider J, McCoy N: Sexual interest and behavior in healthy 80 to 102 year olds, *Arch Sex Behav* 17:109, 1988.

Broadhead W et al: The epidemiologic evidence for a relationship between social support and health, *Am J Epidemiol* 117:521, 1983.

Butler R: Ageism. In Maddox G, editor: *The encyclopedia of aging*, New York, 1987, Springer.

Campbell J: *The portable Jung*, New York, 1979, Penguin Books.

Cohen G: *The creative age: awakening human potential in the second half of life*, New York, 2000, Avon Books.

Colarusso CA, Nemiroff RA: *Adult development*, New York, 1981, Plenum Press.

Conrad C: Old age in the modern and postmodern western world. In Cole T, Van Tassel D, Kastenbaum R, editors: *Handbook of the humanities and aging*, New York, 1992, Springer.

Cumming E, Henry W: *Growing old: the process of disengagement*, New York, 1961, Basic Books.

DeFries J et al: *Behavioral genetics*, New York, 2000, Worth.

Ebersole P, Hess P: *Toward healthy aging: human needs and nursing responses*, ed 5, St Louis, 1999, Mosby.

Eliopoulos C: *Gerontological nursing*, ed 5, Philadelphia, 2001, JB Lippincott.

Erikson EH: *Eight stages of man in childhood and society*, New York, 1963, WW Norton.

Erikson EH: *Childhood and society*, ed 2, New York, 1974a, WW Norton.

Erikson EH: *Dimensions of a new identity: Jefferson lectures*, New York, 1974b, WW Norton.

Erikson EH: *The life cycle completed*, New York, 1982, WW Norton.

Erikson EH, Erikson J, Kivnick H: *Vital involvement in old age: the experience of old age in our time*, New York, 1986, WW Norton.

Federal Interagency Forum on Aging Related Statistics: *Older Americans 2004: key indicators of well-being;* www.agingstats.gov, 2004.

Fillenbaum G et al: Impact of estrogen use on decline in cognitive function in a representative sample of older community-resident women, *Am J Epidemiol* 153:137, 2001.

Folstein M, Folstein S, McHugh P: "Mini-mental state": a practical method of grading the cognitive state of patients for the clinician, *J Psychiatr Res* 12:189, 1975.

Friedman D: Event-related brain potential investigations of memory and aging, *Biol Psychol* 54: 175, 2000.

Freud S: *The ego and the id*, New York, 1923, WW Norton.

Gallagher J, Reid D: *The learning theory of Piaget and Inhelder*, Monterey, Calif, 1981, Brooks/Cole.

Gilligan C: *In a different voice*, Cambridge, Mass, 1982, Harvard University Press.

Havighurst R, Neugarten B, Tobin S: Disengagement and patterns of aging. In Neugarten B, editor: *Middle age and aging*, Chicago, 1968, University of Chicago Press.

Hayflick L: Theories of biological aging. In Andres R, Bierman E, Hazzard W, editors: *Principles of geriatric medicine*, New York, 1985, McGraw-Hill.

Herzog A, Wallace R: Measures of cognitive functioning in the AHEAD study, *J Gerontol* 52B:37, 1997.

Hertzog C, Dixon R, Hultsch D: Relationships between metamemory, memory predictions, and memory task performance in adults, *Psychol Aging* 5:215, 1990.

Horn J, Cattell R: Age differences in fluid and crystallized intelligence, *Acta Psychol* 26:107, 1967.

Huyck M: Middle age, *Acad Am Encyclopedia* 13:390, 1997.

Hyde R: Facilitative communication skills training: social support for elderly people, *Gerontologist* 28:418, 1988.

Hyer L, Intrieri R: *Geropsychological interventions in long-term care*, New York, 2006, Springer.

Jaques E: Death and the mid-life crisis. In Jaques E: *Work, creativity, and social justice*, London, 1970, Heinemann.

Jonsson H, Josephsson S, Kielhofner G: Evolving narratives in the course of retirement: a longitudinal study, *Am J Occupational Ther* 54:463, 2000.

Jung C: The stages of life. In Campbell J, editor: *The portable Jung*, New York, 1971, Viking Press.

Kane R, Ouslander J, Abrass I: *Essentials of clinical geriatrics*, New York, 2003, McGraw-Hill.

Kohlberg L: Stages and aging in moral development: some speculations, *Gerontologist* 13:497, 1973.

Kohlberg L: The development of children's orientations toward a moral order. In Damon W, editor: *Social and personality development essays on the growth of the child*, New York, 1983, WW Norton.

Kruger A: The mid-life transition, crisis or chimera? *Psychol Rep* 75:1299, 1994.

Lao J et al: Genetic contribution to aging: deleterious and helpful genes define life expectancy, *Ann N Y Acad Sci* 1057:50, 2005.

Lemon B, Bengston V, Peterson J: An exploration of the activity theory of aging: activity types and life satisfaction among inmovers to a retirement community, *J Gerontol* 27:511, 1972.

Levinson DJ et al: *The seasons of a man's life*, New York, 1986, Ballantine Books.

Liebert RM, Sprafkin J: *The early window: effects of television on children and youth*, ed 3, New York, 1988, Pergamon.

MacDonald S, Hultsch D, Dixon R: Performance variability is related to change in cognition: evidence from the Victoria Longitudinal Study, *Psychol Aging* 18: 510, 2003.

Maddi S: *Personality theories: a comparative analysis*, Homewood, Ill, 1972, Dorsey Press.

Maslow A: *Toward a psychology of being*, New York, 1962, Van Nostrand.

McCrae R: Situational determinants of coping responses: loss, threat, and challenge, *J Pers Soc Psychol* 46:919, 1984.

Merck Institute for Aging and Health: *The state of aging and health in America 2004*, Washington, DC, 2004, Merck Company Foundation.

Miller C: *Nursing care of older adults: theory and practice*, Glenview, Ill, 1990, Scott, Foresman.

Miller M: Life changes scaling for the 1990s, *J Psychosom Res* 43:279, 1997.

Miller N, Dollard J: *Social learning and imitation*, New Haven, Conn, 1941, Yale University Press.

Myers D: Adulthood's ages and stages, *Psychology* 5:196, 1998.

National Centers for Health Statistics: *Limitation of activity: difficulty performing instrumental activities of daily living*, National Centers for Health Statistics, 2002; www.cdc.gov/nchs.

Navratil JS, Sabatine JM, Ahearn JM: Apoptosis and immune responses to self, *Rheum Dis Clin North Am* 30:193, 2004.

Neugarten BL: Time, age, and the life cycle, *Am J Psychiatry* 136:887, 1979.

Newton PM, Levinson DJ: Crisis in adult development. In Lazare A, editor: *Outpatient psychiatry: diagnosis and treatment*, Baltimore, 1979, Williams & Wilkins.

Oxman T, Berkman L: Assessment of social relationships in elderly patients, *Int J Psychiatr Med* 20:65, 1990.

Pennebaker J: The effects of traumatic disclosure on physical and mental health: the values of writing and talking about upsetting events, *Int J Emerg Ment Health* 1:9, 1999.

Perlmutter M et al: Aging and memory, *Annu Rev Gerontol Geriatr* 7:57, 1987.

Pfeiffer E: A short portable mental status questionnaire for the assessment of organic brain deficit in elderly patients, *J Am Geriatr Soc* 23:433, 1975.

Piaget J: *The science of education and the psychology of the child*, New York, 1970, Grossman.

Piaget J, Inhelder B: *The psychology of the child*, New York, 1969, Basic Books.

Reid D, Haas G, Hawkings D: Locus of desired control and positive self-concept of the elderly, *J Gerontol* 32:441, 1977.

Rogers R: Sociodemographic characteristics of long-lived and healthy individuals, *Popul Dev Rev* 21:33, 1995.

Rotter J: *The development and application of social learning theory*, New York, 1982, Praegor.

Rotter J: Cognates of personal control: locus of control, self-efficacy, and explanatory style: comment, *Appl Prevent Psychol* 1:127, 1992.

Rowe J, Kahn R: *Successful aging: the MacArthur Foundation study*, New York, 1998, Pantheon Books.

Ryan E: Beliefs about memory changes across the adult life span, *J Gerontol* 47:41, 1992.

Ryan E, See S: Age-based beliefs about memory changes for self and others across adulthood, *J Gerontol* 48:199, 1993.

Schaie K, Willis S: *Adult development and aging*, Boston, 1991, Little Brown.

Schneider E, Rowe J: *Handbook of the biology of aging*, ed 3, San Diego, 1990, Academic Press.

Schroots J: Gerodynamics: toward a branching theory of aging, *Can J Aging* 14:74, 1995.

Shek D: Mid-life crisis in Chinese men and women, *J Psychol* 130:109, 1996.

Speas K, Obenshain B: *Images of aging in America: final report*, American Association of Retired Persons, Chapel Hill, NC, 1995, FGI Integrated Marketing.

Stevens-Long J: *Adult life: developmental processes*, ed 4, Palo Alto, Calif, 1992, Mayfield.

Stroufe A, Cooper R, DeHart G: *Child development: its nature and course*, New York, 1992, McGraw-Hill.

Sullivan H: *The interpersonal theory of psychiatry*, New York, 1953, WW Norton.

Tornstam H: Gero-transcendence: the contemplative dimension of aging, *J Aging Stud* 11:143, 1997.

Troll L: *Early and middle adulthood*, Monterey, Calif, 1975, Brooks, Cole, p. 6.

US Census Bureau: *Census of population: general population characteristics (2000)*, Washington, DC, 2000, US Department of Commerce, Economics and Statistics Administration.

Vaillant G: *Adaptation to life*, Boston, 1977, Little, Brown.

Vaillant G: *Aging well: surprising guideposts to a happier life from the landmark Harvard study of adult development*, New York, 2002, Little Brown.

Van Gennep A: *The rites of passage*, Chicago, 1909, University of Chicago Press.

Woodruff D: A review of aging and cognitive processes, *Res Aging* 5:139, 1983.

Chapter 6

Neurobiology in Mental Health and Disorder

CANDICE A. FRANCIS

Between stimulus and response there is space. In that space is our power to choose our response. In our response lies our growth and our freedom.

VIKTOR FRANKL

OBJECTIVES

1 Identify the basic anatomic structures of the central nervous system.
2 Describe the physiologic functions of the central nervous system.
3 Describe the normal functioning of neurons.
4 Discuss the role of common neurotransmitters in the functioning of the central nervous system.
5 Describe the electrochemical mechanism of the central nervous system.
6 Identify criteria for client care related to neuroimaging testing.
7 Identify emerging technologies with a significant impact on the future of psychiatric nursing.
8 State uses for current neurobiologic findings in planning care for clients with a psychiatric disorder.
9 Identify potential areas for further nursing research related to neurobiology.

KEY TERMS

action potential, p. 118
alexia, p. 116
amygdala, p. 116
aphasia, p. 115
autonomic nervous system, p. 113
axon, p. 117
basal nuclei , p. 116
Broca's area, p. 115
central nervous system, p. 113
cerebral cortex, p. 114
cerebrum, p. 113
corpus callosum, p. 114
cortex, p. 113
dendrites, p. 117
fissures, p. 114
frontal lobe, p. 114
gray matter, p. 113
gyri, p. 114
hippocampus, p. 117
hypothalamus, p. 117
limbic system, p. 116
neuroglia, p. 113
neuron, p. 113
neuroplasticity, p. 126
neurotransmitter, p. 119
occipital lobe, p. 115
parietal lobe, p. 116
peripheral nervous system, p. 113
premotor cortex, p. 115
primary motor cortex, p. 114
somatic association cortex, p. 115
stem cells, p. 123
sulci, p. 114
synapse, p. 117
temporal lobe, p. 115
thalamus, p. 116
Wernicke's area, p. 115
white matter, p.113

Visit the *Neurology Review* section of your **Companion CD** when you see this icon to view an animation illustrating the concept described in the text.

Neuroscientific discovery and developments continue to advance at a remarkable pace and contribute to the evolving understanding of brain function. This research provides new strategies for clinicians, clients, and families addressing mental disorders. Many now recognize mental disorders as brain-based illnesses. Although some still misunderstand mental disorders and stigmatize those clients, research on brain biology has helped reshape perceptions of mental illness. To understand treatment approaches to psychiatric illness, the psychiatric mental health nurse requires a firm foundation in the fundamentals of neurobiology, physiology and genetics, and how these affect treatment of psychiatric disorders. Increased knowledge in this area has changed the way mental health care providers perceive and treat mental disorders. This chapter reviews the fundamentals of neurobiology and examines concepts and clinical approaches to the treatment of mental illness with regard to our growing knowledge of neuroscience.

UNDERSTANDING NEUROBIOLOGIC FUNCTIONS

The biologic model of psychiatric illness is not a new phenomenon, but the availability of new tools makes it increasingly more sophisticated. Science has advanced beyond merely making educated guesses about how the brain works and has developed scientific models that allow for testing brain-based interventions and developing new effective treatments (Gur, 2002). The best psychiatric mental health care begins with an understanding that the symptoms associated with psychiatric disorders are usually manifested behaviorally. Clients with psychiatric disorders frequently behave in ways society considers "not normal." They often express their disorders through responses such as hearing voices, considering suicide, or wearing a winter coat on a hot summer day. These abnormal perceptions, thoughts, and behaviors usually have a neurobiologic basis. Knowledge of normal brain structure and function helps mental health care providers to offer an optimal level of treatment to people with brain-based illnesses. Understanding the structural or neurochemical defects that affect clients with psychiatric disorders helps psychiatric nurses to more effectively assess clients' responses and plan interventions.

NEUROANATOMY AND NEUROPHYSIOLOGY OF THE HUMAN NERVOUS SYSTEM

Human thoughts, feelings, and actions begin in the central nervous system. The brain acts as the primary mediator-organ, controlling and determining how people interact with the world. All human responses are the result of the complex interaction between underlying neuroanatomy and neurophysiology, as well as the genetic, environmental, and developmental factors that influence those systems.

Neuroanatomy

The brain is one of the most important structures in the human body. Although it weighs only 3 to 5 pounds, the brain contains approximately 140 billion cells, making it the most complex and vital of human organs (Gribbin, 2002). The human nervous system is composed of two separate but interconnected anatomic divisions. The first division, the **central nervous system** (CNS), is composed of the spinal cord and brain. The second division, the **peripheral nervous system** (PNS), contains peripheral nerves, 12 pairs of cranial nerves that originate just outside of the brain stem, and 31 pairs of spinal nerves arising from the spinal cord. These peripheral nerves transmit sensory (incoming) information toward the CNS and motor (outgoing) information away from the CNS to muscles and glands that are controlled by the CNS.

Although the PNS and certain interactions with the **autonomic nervous system** (ANS) are of critical importance to human functioning, the understanding of psychiatric disorders depends on in-depth understanding of the structure and function of the CNS. For that reason, this chapter focuses on the CNS and how the nurse will use that knowledge to provide care to individuals who have psychiatric and neurologic disorders.

Brain cells are categorized as either neurons or neuroglia. **Neurons** generate and conduct electrical signals. **Neuroglia** provide the mechanical and physiologic support for neurons. **White matter** is composed of the axons of neurons that are insulated by myelin. White matter makes up the core of major brain structures such as the cerebrum and cerebellum. The **gray matter**, or **cortex**, typically covers the surface of these organs. The cortex is the functional area of the brain where neurons communicate with each other and where neurotransmitters are concentrated.

Cerebrum

The **cerebrum** is the largest part of the brain and it is divided into two halves called cerebral hemispheres. The cerebral hemispheres contain important functional areas such as the cerebral cortex, basal nuclei, and limbic system.

The cerebral hemispheres account for more than 70% of the neurons in the CNS and are responsible for functions such as hearing, vision, language, cognitive functions, control of muscles, and sensory interpretation. The left hemisphere is dominant in almost 95% of people and mainly controls motor and sensory functions on the right side of the body. The right hemisphere controls functions on the left side of the body. Most right-handed people, and half of left-handed people, have a dominant left hemisphere. In rare cases, some people have mixed dominance, with one side dominant for language expression and the other for motor functions such as handwriting.

Effective coordinated human activity requires a complex interrelationship and communication within and between the two hemispheres. A large bundle of white matter called the **corpus callosum** connects the two hemispheres. Sensorimotor information constantly flows between the two hemispheres via nerve pathways in the corpus callosum. The corpus callosum has to be intact for full, smooth, and coordinated communication between the hemispheres.

The outermost surface of the **cerebral cortex** contains corrugated wrinkles with many grooves and indentations. Shallow grooves are called **sulci**, and the deeper grooves extending deep into the brain are called **fissures**. The raised areas are called **gyri**. The sulci and gyri dramatically increase the overall surface area of the cerebrum. The cerebral cortex is typically composed of only six layers of cells, but it covers an area that, if spread out, equals almost 2.5 square feet. In contrast, the cortex of a chimpanzee would cover only a single sheet of paper, while a rat's cortex occupies an area roughly equal to the size of a postage stamp (Gribbin, 2002). Most discussions on cerebral functions focus on the outer layer, the cerebral cortex.

The cerebrum is divided by the major fissures into four distinct functional regions called lobes. These are the frontal, temporal, occipital, and parietal lobes (Figure 6-1). Although these lobes often work together, each has distinct functions. The normal functions of each lobe, along with typical symptoms of disturbances in each cerebral cortical region of the brain, are described in Table 6-1. Many symptoms exhibited by clients with neurologic disorders and mental disorders are a disturbance in the normal functioning of one or more these cerebral lobes.

The **frontal lobe** is the largest lobe, and human beings as a species have the best-developed frontal lobes of all animals. Much of what makes human behavior unique is due to the functioning of the frontal lobe. The frontal lobe contains several important structures. The **primary motor cortex** lies in front of the large central sulcus and is also called the precentral gyrus. As a primary cortex, it is responsible for directly controlling voluntary motor activity of specific muscles. Neurons originating from the primary motor cortex are directly traced to peripheral nerves that innervate the muscles of the body. As they exit the brain, they form a pyramid-shaped bulge called the corticospinal nerve tract. Because of its unique shape, this system of nerves is also called the pyramidal tract. The pyramidal tract passes through the intersection of the medulla and spinal cord. It is at this point that the nerve tracts cross over, or decussate, to the opposite side of the body. This helps to explain why the right motor cortex actually controls voluntary motor activity on the left side

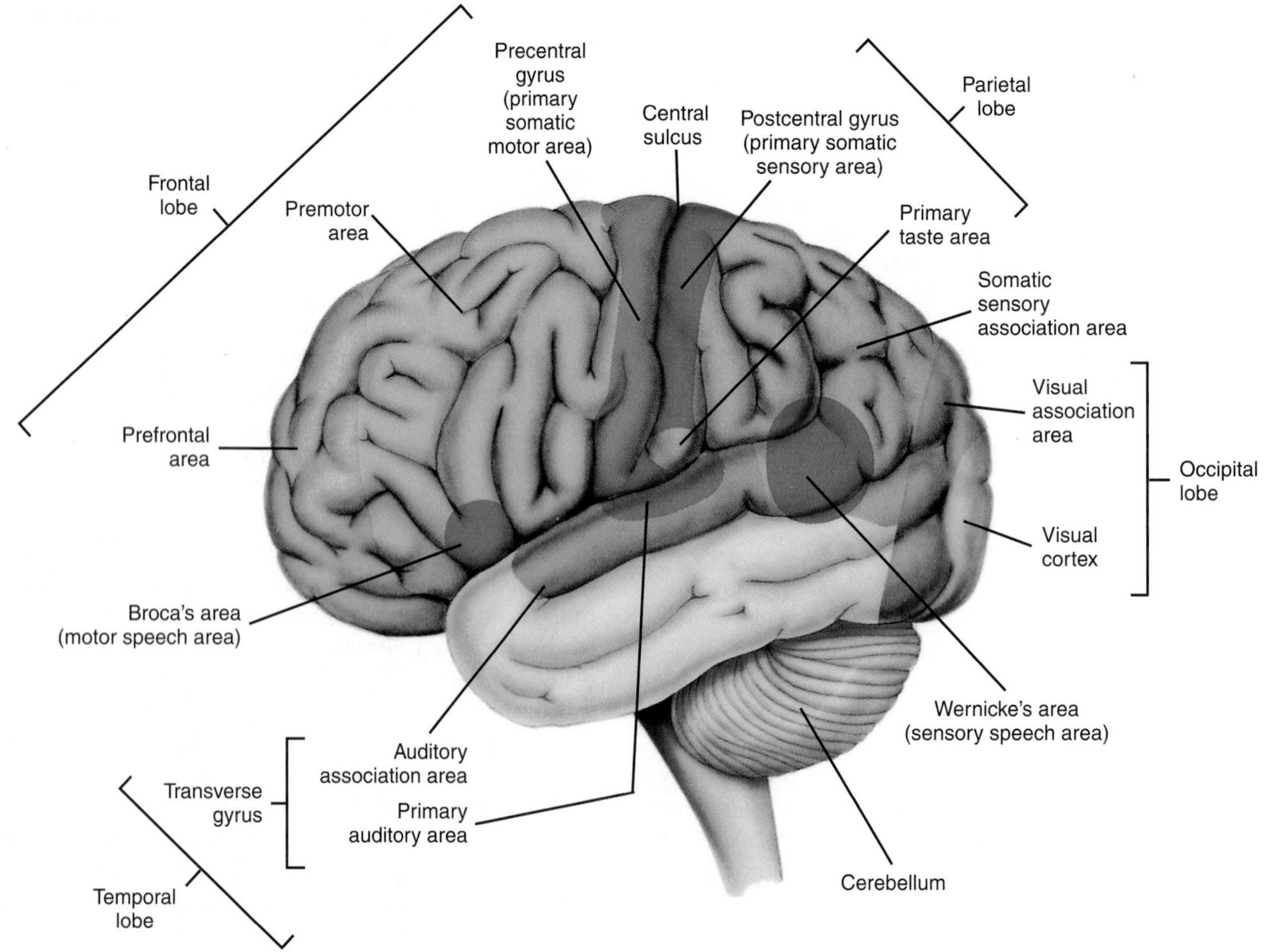

FIGURE 6-1 Functional areas of the cerebral cortex. (From Thibodeau GA, Patton KT: *Anatomy & physiology,* ed 6, St Louis, 2007, Mosby.)

of the body and the left motor cortex controls motor activity on the right side of the body.

The frontal lobe also contains two other important structures. The **premotor cortex** is responsible for the coordinated movement of multiple muscles, and the **somatic association cortex** integrates motor commands. Researchers have identified a number of brain regions as association regions. In fact, some estimate that 70% to 75% of all cortical regions are association regions that integrate functions in the primary region. The primary regions are generally involved in analysis, initiation, interpretation, and integrative activities. In the case of the frontal lobe, the somatic association cortex is the area of the brain responsible for coordinating learned motor skills. Cognition, memory, and analytic functions are largely functions of a third region of the frontal lobe known as the prefrontal cortex. Damage to this area of the frontal lobe causes changes in personality. Other functions of the prefrontal cortex, sometimes described as executive functions, include reasoning, planning, prioritizing, sequencing behavior, insight, flexibility, and judgment (Young and Pigott, 1999). Normal frontal cortical functions help suppress and moderate more primitive impulses and actions. The frontal cortex also allows a person to appropriately process incoming sensory stimuli, reason, focus on tasks, and respond to social cues. Difficulty in performing these activities often manifests as symptoms of psychiatric disorders. Two key functions, working memory and behavioral inhibition, have increasingly become targets of research interest as scientists explore the neurobiology of psychiatric disorders (Dubin, 2002). Another important area usually localized only in the left frontal lobe is **Broca's area**, which controls the muscles necessary to speak. Damage to Broca's area from causes such as accidents or stroke results in the inability to speak (motor aphasia). Speech is a vital part of communication and appropriate social interaction.

The **temporal lobe** is responsible for some functions of language, memory, and emotion. **Wernicke's area** is a specialized area of the temporal lobe responsible for organizing words so they will be recognized and express the correct emotional content. Written speech, verbal speech, and the visual recognition that is critical to communication are all functions of the temporal lobe. Language is one example where two distinct regions, Broca's area in the frontal lobe and Wernicke's area in the temporal lobe, work together to facilitate normal communication. **Aphasia**, a communication disorder, sometimes has several origins within the brain, most notably Wernicke's area of the temporal lobe and Broca's area in the frontal lobe. The auditory association area of the temporal lobe is involved with memory, especially those connected to visual and auditory cues.

The **occipital lobe** contains the primary visual cortex and is most responsible for visual functioning. Color recognition, the ability to recognize and name objects, and the ability to track moving objects are functions of the occipital lobe. The occipital lobe is sensitive to hypoxia, and trauma to this region of the brain sometimes results in blindness, even if the optic nerves and eyes remain in-

TABLE 6-1

Normal Functions and Symptoms of Dysfunction of the Cerebrum

LOBE	LOCATION	NORMAL FUNCTION	SYMPTOMS OF ALTERATIONS IN BRAIN FUNCTIONING
Frontal	Anterior, or front area, of brain	Programming and execution of motor functions Higher thought processes such as planning, ability to abstract, trial-and-error learning, and decision making Intellectual insight, judgment Expression of emotion	Changes in affect such as flattening Alteration in language production Alteration in motor functioning Impulsive behavior Impaired decision making Concrete thinking
Parietal	Posterior to central sulcus	Sensory perception: taking in information from environment, organizing it, and communicating this information to rest of brain Association areas that allow for such things as accurately following directions on a map, reading a clock, building a birdhouse, or dressing oneself	Altered sensory perceptions such as decreased consciousness of pain sensation Difficulty with time concepts such as inability to keep appointment times Alteration in personal hygiene Alteration in ability to calculate numbers Inability to adequately perform common motor actions of writing Mixing up right and left Poor attention span
Temporal	Lies beneath skull on both sides; commonly called the temple	Primarily responsible for hearing and receiving information via ears	Auditory hallucinations Increased sexual focus Decreased motivation Alterations in memory Altered emotional responses Sensory aphasia
Occipital	Most posterior of brain lobes—back of head	Primarily responsible for seeing and receiving information via eyes	Visual hallucinations

tact. Lesions of the occipital lobe can cause visual hallucinations and other abnormalities of visual functioning, such as **alexia**, or the inability to read.

The **parietal lobe** of the brain functions as the primary sensory processing center. The postcentral sensory gyrus area of the parietal lobe, or the somesthetic cortex, interprets sensory information. This includes visual, tactile, and auditory information. Posterior to the somesthetic cortex is the somesthetic association area. Again, as an association area, it is responsible for organizing, integrating, and analyzing sensory information that the primary sensory cortex in the postcentral gyrus will interpret more specifically.

Basal Nuclei. The **basal nuclei**, also known as basal ganglia, are concentrations of cell bodies closely involved with motor functions and association. Basal nuclei are concentrations of gray matter located within the white matter of the cerebrum and midbrain. They have many connections to both the superficial cortex above and the deep midbrain structures below. Among the most well known basal nuclei are the caudate lobe, putamen, globus pallidus, and substantia nigra. These basal nuclei translate movements such as walking while it is happening, and they also modulate and correct muscle functioning that allows movements to occur in a coordinated manner. The basal nuclei aid in the learning and programming of motor behavior. Activities that are well learned and rehearsed over the course of a person's life often become automatic. Complex motor skills involved in walking, eating, or driving become so natural that a person does not have to think consciously to perform them. This helps to explain why some people with dementia retain some of these complex behaviors long after a severe memory or language loss.

Conditions such as Huntington's disease and Parkinson's disease are associated with basal nuclear dysfunction and their inability to effectively communicate with the cerebral cortex (Montoya, 2006). Some medications used to treat psychiatric disorders alter the basal nuclei (Box 6-1). For example, chlorpromazine (Thorazine) and haloperidol (Haldol) are two older neuroleptic antipsychotic medications that sometimes cause hypertonicity, or dystonia, a condition marked by excessive muscle tone.

Limbic System. Instincts, primitive drives, sexual arousal, fear, aggression, and other emotions are part of the functions of the structures deep within the brain called the **limbic system** or limbic lobe. It is often called a *system* because researchers believe its functions are a result of the interrelated, closely coordinated actions of its various structures. Table 6-2 and Figure 6-2 identify some of the structural components of the limbic system. Part of the limbic system, the **amygdala**, is instrumental in emotional functioning and in regulating affective responses to events. The amygdala modulates common emotional states such as feelings of anger and aggression, love, and comfort in social settings. The limbic system's function of emotional regulation is linked with the olfactory pathways that connect to the amygdala. Some suggest that this explains why certain smells evoke strong emotional responses and memories in some individuals The limbic system holds increasing interest for researchers trying to identify the biologic etiology of bipolar disorder. Some researchers have hypothesized that the rapid misfiring of neurons in the amygdala is instrumental in the development of the typical symptoms of bipolar disorder. Researchers are also studying the amygdala in an attempt to better understand abnormal fear reactions such as panic and violent-rage behaviors (Carlson, 2001).

The **thalamus**, a part of the brain collectively referred to as the diencephalon, is another part of the limbic sys-

BOX 6-1

Extrapyramidal Symptoms: Adverse Effects From Antipsychotic Medications

- ***Acute dystonia.*** Marked by prolonged, often painful, muscle contractions that often occur in the eye (oculogyral crisis), tongue (glossospasm), neck (torticollis), and back (retrocollis). The nurse assesses a client who complains of a stiff neck, backache or other muscle aches, and pains after receiving antipsychotic medication to either rule out or treat this extrapyramidal symptom. Treatment includes antiparkinson medication.
- ***Akathisia.*** Possibly a result of the blockade effect of these drugs on the neurotransmitter dopamine. Signs include motor restlessness, a subjective sense of anxiety, and an inability to lie down or sit still.
- ***Pseudoparkinsonian symptoms.*** Marked by decreased motor movements, muscle rigidity, drooling, masklike facies (blunted or flat facial expression), and shuffling gait (walk). Treatment includes antiparkinson medication.
- ***Tardive dyskinesia.*** A significant adverse effect of antipsychotic drug therapy. Usually an irreversible and late-onset complication, it is characterized by the presence of abnormal, stereotyped, rhythmic movements of the limbs and torso; tongue protrusion; and chewing movements. Will affect any muscle in the body, including the diaphragm; usually occurs after abrupt termination of the drug, after reduction in dosage, or after long-term, high-dose therapy. Nurses minimize incidence with careful dose management, drug holidays, and administration of antiparkinson drugs.

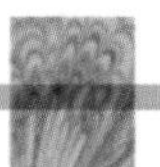

TABLE 6-2

Structures of the Limbic System

STRUCTURE	FUNCTION
Amygdala	Modulates emotional states Regulates affective responses to events
Thalamus	Relays all sensory information, except smell Filters incoming information regarding emotions, mood, and memory to prevent cortex from becoming overloaded
Hypothalamus	Regulates basic human functions such as sleep-rest patterns, body temperature, and physical drives of hunger and sex
Hippocampus	Controls learning and recall of an event with its associated memory

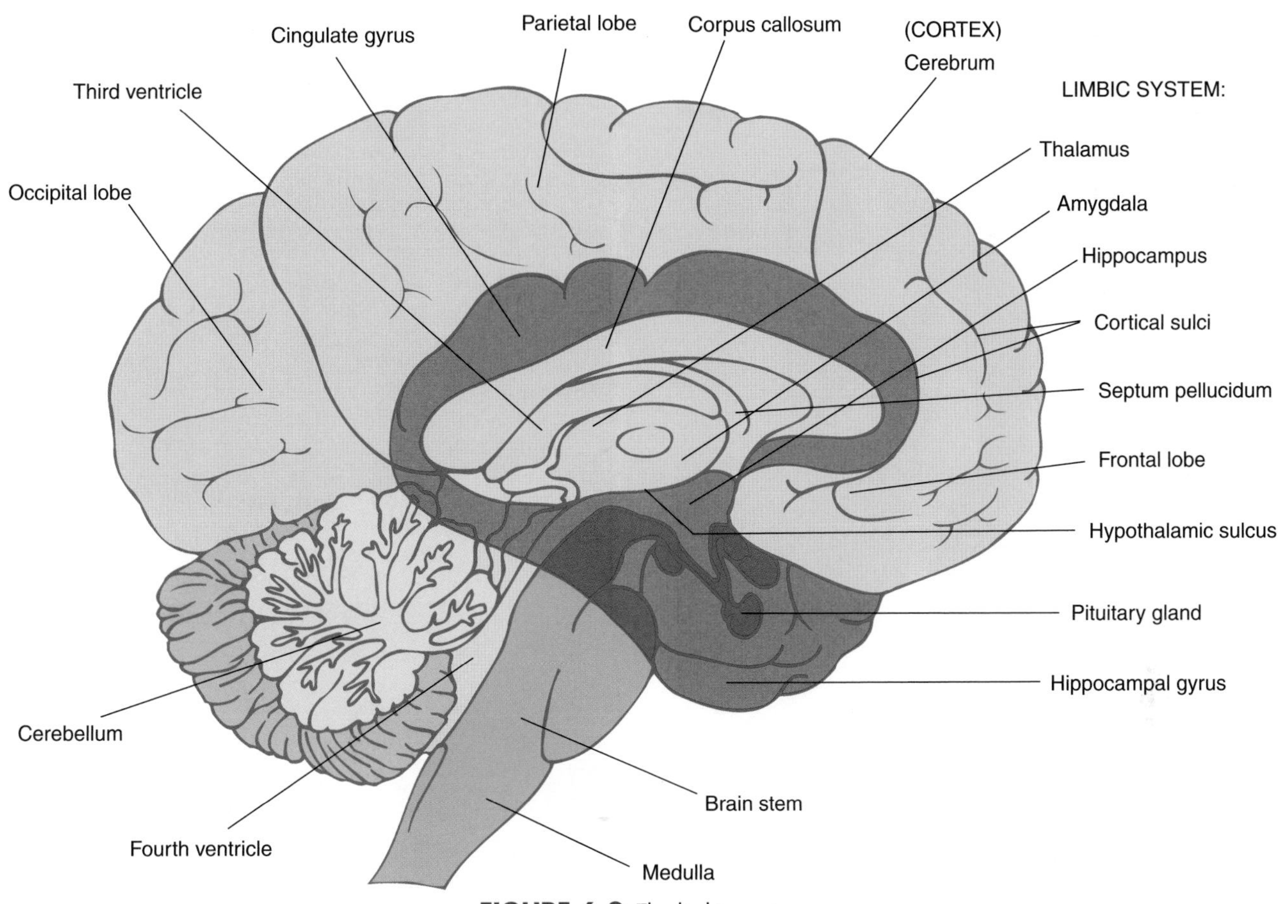

FIGURE 6-2 The limbic system.

tem. It is primarily a structure that acts as gateway directing sensory information to the cerebral cortex. All sensory information, except smell, comes from the PNS to the cerebral cortex of the CNS via the thalamus. This critical structure helps to filter incoming sensory information and to direct it to specific regions of the cortex where it can be interpreted and evaluated more fully. This includes sensory information that influences emotions, mood, and memory.

The **hypothalamus** is another functional part of the limbic system that rests deep within the brain and helps regulate some of the most basic human functions including sleep-rest patterns, body temperature, thirst, and physical drives of hunger and sex. Research indicates that some symptomatic behaviors, such as appetite and sleep problems in the depressed client, the seasonal mood changes of seasonal affective disorder (SAD), and temperature regulation problems in clients with schizophrenia (e.g., wearing winter coats in the summer) are a hypothalamic dysregulation. Because of the close physical and physiologic association with the pituitary, hypothalamic activity influences hormonal regulatory events attributed to the pituitary as well.

The **hippocampus** is located deep within the temporal lobe below the thalamus (see Figure 6-2). It has direct connections with the hypothalamus and the amygdala, and it plays a major role in the encoding, consolidation, and retrieval of memories. Clients with Alzheimer's disease have damage to the hippocampus, resulting in difficulties with short-term memory and learning ability.

Neurophysiology

Among the billions of cells that make up the human brain, approximately 10% are neurons. The neurons are directly responsible for impulse conduction that allows the brain to initiate signals and process information. Each neuron has thousands, if not hundreds of thousands, of connections to other neurons. The connections, called **synapses**, allow various areas of the brain to communicate with each other, to interpret sensory information, and to initiate stimuli to activate muscles. This constant brain nerve cell (neuronal) activity accounts for the complex perceptions and behaviors that make us human. The vast numbers of synaptic interconnections makes the brain far more complex and sophisticated than any computer.

There are several types of neurons in the brain. Nuclei and other major organelles are typically in a region of the cell known as the cell body or cyton. Two kinds of processes originate from the cell body region. **Dendrites** carry electrical impulses toward the cell body, while the **axon** carries impulses away from the cell body. Axons end at small presynaptic axon terminals. Figure 6-3 illustrates one common type of neuron, called a motor neuron, that stimulates glands and muscle cells.

FIGURE 6-3 Structural features of neurons: dendrites, cell body, and axon. (From Lewis SM et al: *Medical-surgical nursing: assessment and management of clinical problems,* ed 7, St Louis, 2007, Mosby.)

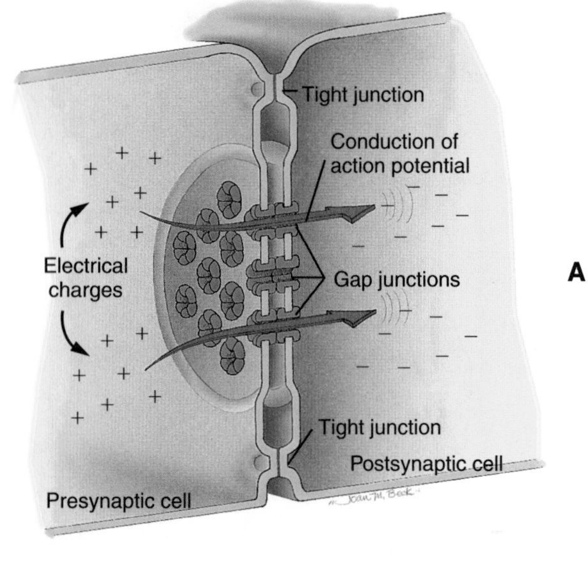

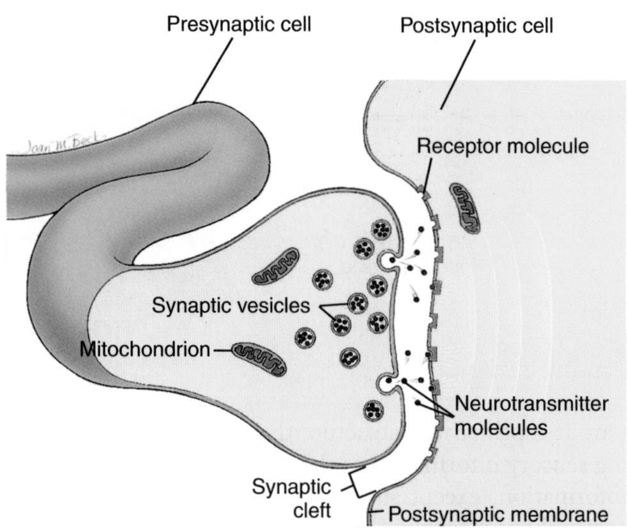

FIGURE 6-4 Electrical and chemical synapses. **A,** Electrical synapses involve gap junctions that allow action potentials to move from cell to cell directly by allowing electrical current to flow between cells. **B,** Chemical synapses involve transmitter chemicals (neurotransmitters) that signal postsynaptic cells, possibly inducing an action potential. (From Thibodeau GA, Patton KT: *Anatomy & physiology,* ed 6, St Louis, 2007, Mosby.)

Nerve Cell Electrical Function: Action Potential

All neurons are capable of detecting, processing, and conducting electrical signals known as **action potential**. Neurons in the CNS are also capable of generating their own electrical impulses. Cells conduct electricity by concentrations of ions such as sodium, potassium, and chloride. These ions differ inside and outside of the cell. Because these ions carry an electrical charge, the difference in the distribution of electrically charged ions on the two sides of the membrane creates an electrical potential, or ability to conduct an electrical current. The neuronal membranes allow selective movement of these ions across the membrane. An action potential occurs as a result of the movement of ions across the cell membrane, temporarily shifting the electrical charge on each side of the nerve cell membrane.

Many kinds of events initiate action potentials given sufficient stimulus strength. Typically, when an action potential reaches the synaptic terminal, it causes a change in the permeability of the membrane, allowing chemical neurotransmitter substances to be released into the gap or synaptic cleft between adjacent, or neighboring, neurons. Figure 6-4 illustrates a typical synaptic structure. The

TABLE 6-3

Common CNS Neurotransmitters

MOLECULAR CLASS	NAME OF NEUROTRANSMITTER	ACTIVITY	DISTRIBUTION
Biogenic amine (catecholamine)	Acetylcholine (ACh)	Excitatory	Motor neurons, pons, forebrain
Amino acids	Aspartate	Excitatory	CNS
	Glutamate	Excitatory	Primary exciter in CNS
	γ-Aminobutyric acid (GABA)	Inhibitory	Primary inhibitor in CNS
	Glycine	Inhibitory	Spinal cord
Monoamines	Dopamine	Excitatory	Basal nuclei, limbic system
	Serotonin (5-HT, 5 hydroxytryptamine)	Excitatory	Brain stem, pons, medulla
	Norepinephrine	Excitatory	Pons, medulla
Neuropeptides	Many	Excitatory	CNS, PNS
Gases	Nitrous oxide (NO)	Uncertain	Brain, blood vessels
	Carbon monoxide (CO)		

movement of neurotransmitters across cell membranes plays a large role in mental health and mental disorders.

Nerve Cell Chemical Function: Neurotransmitters

As the depolarization of neurons reaches the synapse, the action potential is no longer effective in communicating directly with the next neuron in sequence. The space between the two cell membranes in most synapses is about 20 to 30 nanometers (nm). Although this is small, it is too large for most action potentials to cross directly. So communication between one neuron and another depends on the release of chemicals known as **neurotransmitters** by the presynaptic cell and their reception on the postsynaptic membrane. Neurotransmitter movement, while much slower than action potentials, is effective in sending and regulating signals from one neuron to the next. It is the specificity of neurotransmitter receptor sites on the postsynaptic membrane that forms the basis of chemical control of all neurologic functions.

Neurotransmitters are categorized several ways. For our purposes, we will classify them according to their chemical structure. Additionally, they are also identified as either *excitatory* or *inhibitory* in nature when reaching the postsynaptic membrane. Considerable available research identifies brain regions with the highest concentrations of various transmitter substances and associates various brain functions and malfunctions with specific neurotransmitters. Although more than 100 substances are identified as neurotransmitters or probable neurotransmitters, Table 6-3 summarizes the most widely recognized neurotransmitter substances of the CNS. For a substance to qualify as a neurotransmitter, it will display the criteria described in Box 6-2.

Many synthetic and naturally occurring toxins, street drugs, anesthetics, and medications used to treat psychiatric disorders function at the level of the synapse where cell sites have specific receptors. Similarly, an increasing number of neurologic dysfunctions are attributed to abnormalities associated with neurochemical transmitter substances.

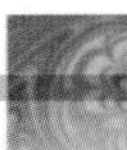

BOX 6-2

Criteria for a Substance To Be Labeled a Neurotransmitter

- The chemical is synthesized in the neuron.
- The chemical is present in the presynaptic terminal and released in amounts sufficient to exert a specific effect on a receptor neuron.
- When applied exogenously (as per drug) in a reasonable concentration, the drug mimics the action of the endogenously released neurotransmitter.
- A specific mechanism exists for removing it from its site of action, the synaptic cleft.

Once a neurotransmitter is attracted to the postsynaptic membrane, typically at receptor sites that are specific to the particular neurotransmitter, it is deactivated. Deactivation happens by one of three primary means:

1. The neurotransmitter leaves the area through natural diffusion of a substance from an area of high concentration to one of low concentration.
2. The neurotransmitter is broken down by enzymatic degradation.
3. The neurotransmitter undergoes reuptake and is transported back into storage in the presynaptic neuron.

Specific Neurotransmitters. Specific neurotransmitters are located in different regions and areas of the brain, allowing for highly differentiated regional functions of the brain. The intricate interaction of nerve cells and distribution of various neurotransmitters in different areas of the brain form the basis for all complex activities of the CNS.

Acetylcholine (ACh) was the first substance discovered to be a neurotransmitter. It is almost everywhere in the brain, but particularly high concentrations occur in the basal nuclei and motor cortex of the brain. Neurons using ACh as a neurotransmitter are often called cholinergic. There are two types of acetylcholine receptors:

muscarinic and nicotinic. Many drugs, such the older neuroleptic antipsychotics, interact with ACh and its receptor sites to produce anticholinergic side effects, which occur when muscarinic acetylcholine receptors are blocked. Side effects include dry mouth, blurred vision, constipation, and urinary retention. These side effects are troubling to clients and are a common reason why clients stop using their medications and fail to comply with the treatment regimen. In severe cases, muscarinic receptor blockade produces confusion and delirium in clients, especially in older clients. Nicotinic receptors respond positively to nicotine and are common in neuromuscular synapses as well as in some CNS and PNS regions. Nicotine, found in tobacco, binds with the nicotinic receptor sites and is able to mimic the effects of ACh released in some centers of the brain that are associated with pleasure, making nicotine highly addictive. Exposure to excessive levels of nicotine will sometimes cause paralysis. Nicotine is also an effective insecticide and a common cause of poisoning in children. Good client teaching and nursing care designed to manage the side effects and adverse effects of drugs are significant aspects of psychiatric mental health nursing.

Glutamate (glutamic acid) is an amino acid and the most widely distributed excitatory neurotransmitter in the brain. Some theorize that excessive glutamate activity is a part of the neurodegenerative process seen in such illnesses as schizophrenia and Alzheimer's disorder (Alexander et al., 2002; Goff and Coyle, 2001; Stahl, 2000). γ-Aminobutyric acid (GABA), chemically derived from glutamate, is the brain's principal inhibitory neurotransmitter. Nerve cells stimulated by inhibitory neurotransmitters such as GABA will be turned off, which slows or stops actions completely in postsynaptic neurons.

Dopamine is a neurotransmitter well localized in the CNS. Dopaminergic neurons occur in several brain regions including the substantia nigra, midbrain, and hypothalamus. Dopamine-containing cells in the midbrain project to the limbic cortex. Researchers think that these areas are the parts of the brain that malfunction in schizophrenia.

Norepinephrine or noradrenaline is concentrated in a small area of the brain known as the locus ceruleus. Many studies now indicate that clients suffering from mood disorders, particularly major depression, suffer from a deficit of norepinephrine. Sympathetic nerves that innervate smooth muscles in blood vessels have a heavy concentration of norepinephrine, which helps to explain its role in elevating blood pressure in the fight-or-flight response. When released directly into the bloodstream, norepinephrine acts as a hormone that enhances the effect of locally released norepinephrine at neuromuscular junctions. Both norepinephrine and its chemical relative, epinephrine, are synthesized from the amino acid tyrosine. Norepinephrine, epinephrine, dopamine, serotonin, and histamine belong to the class of neurotransmitters known as monoamines. Norepinephrine-producing neurons are sometimes referred to as adrenergic.

Serotonin has a pattern of action similar to norepinephrine and is made from tryptophan, another amino acid. Serotonin production occurs in the brain stem and is also widely dispersed throughout the cerebral cortex and the spinal cord. Serotonin helps to regulate a constant internal environment. Maintaining a normal body temperature, normal eating and sleep-rest patterns, and normal moods is dependent on adequate levels of serotonin. Clinically significant problems occur when clients have low levels of serotonin, and many behavioral symptoms common to depression occur when available serotonin is depleted.

Researchers suspect that two other gases—*carbon monoxide* (CO) and *nitric oxide* (NO)—function as neurotransmitter-like substances. NO and CO are both poisonous, unstable gases found in automobile emissions. Nitric oxide shares few of the characteristics of other neurotransmitters. It is not stored in synaptic vesicles. NO actually works in the opposite direction and feeds back toward the presynaptic neurons, and has no known specific receptor sites. Yet it functions as a chemical messenger in the brain and in peripheral blood vessels. It is involved in blood vessel contraction in the clitoris and penis during sexual arousal. Research suggests that nitric oxide plays a role in the brain's memory function and is possibly part of the complex illness of major depression (McLeod, Lopez-Figueroa, and Lopez-Figueroa, 2001). Research indicates that carbon monoxide acts in similar ways.

Other larger neuropeptide molecules such as *cholecystokinin* and *endorphins*, whose functions are still being researched, occur at multiple sites in the brain. Researchers think these molecules play a role in the complex functioning of the brain.

Clinical Significance of Neurotransmitters. Extensive research has been directed toward developing new drugs that operate at the synaptic level within the brain. Any chemical that mimics, competes, destroys, or prevents a neurotransmitter from binding on specific receptor sites on the postsynaptic membrane alters the effectiveness of communication between neurons. Researchers have made countless advances in the treatment of psychiatric disorders. This is due to an increased understanding of neurotransmitters as well as an understanding of the way neurotransmitters are synthesized and deactivated. A brief discussion of some of the more common brain-related illnesses linked to neurotransmitter dysfunctions follows. Table 6-4 summarizes specific disorders and related neurotransmitters.

Depression. Serotonin and its close chemical relatives, dopamine and norepinephrine, are the neurotransmitters most widely involved in various forms of depression. The two major classes of antidepressants—tricyclic and selective serotonin reuptake inhibitors (SSRI) agents—differ primarily in their effects on either norepinephrine or serotonin levels. This explains why certain drugs, such as fluoxetine or paroxetine, that specifically target serotonin may not be effective for some clients but work well for others (see the Case Study presented later in the chapter). The selective serotonin reuptake inhibitor (SSRI) class of

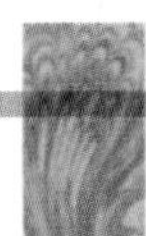

TABLE 6-4

Relationship of Neurotransmitter Dysfunction to Mental Disorders

NEUROTRANSMITTER	DYSFUNCTION	MENTAL DISORDER
Dopamine	Increase	Schizophrenia
Serotonin	Decrease	Depression
Norepinephrine	Decrease	Depression
γ-Aminobutyric acid (GABA)	Decrease	Anxiety disorders
Acetylcholine	Decrease	Alzheimer's disease

antidepressants inhibits the reuptake of serotonin by the presynaptic secreting cells. This reduces the availability of serotonin for subsequent release. Other antidepressants function as monoamine oxidase inhibitors (MAOIs). Monoamine oxidase (MO) is an enzyme that typically deactivates serotonin and dopamine. Deactivating this enzyme leaves the system unable to turn off the effects of these transmitter substances on postsynaptic neurons. Conversely, an enzyme or drug that acts opposite to MO or is an MAOI reduces the transmission of signals between neurons. Catechol *O*-methyl transferase (COMT), an enzyme normally responsible for deactivating norepinephrine, is sometimes present in excess in certain synapses. Too much of this enzyme prevents adrenergic neurons from effectively communicating with one another. Antidepressants that inhibit or reduce COMT levels restore neuronal communication ability. Because norepinephrine is also important in regulating activities such as heart rate and blood pressure, antidepressants operating on the norepinephrine system may have adverse side effects on these functions.

Anxiety. A number of conditions related to anxiety such as panic disorders and extreme phobias are triggered by an overproduction of some excitatory neurotransmitters causing a hyperexcitability of the postsynaptic membrane. GABA, one of the key inhibitory neurotransmitters in the CNS, normally counteracts the effect of these transmitters. Many antianxiety medications such as diazepam (Valium) or alprazolam (Xanax) act by stimulating GABA synthesis, which then modulates the effect of excitatory neurotransmitters. This produces a calming effect in clients experiencing anxiety.

Schizophrenia. A complex disorder such as schizophrenia most likely has multiple contributing factors including genetic predisposition, prenatal development, and the environment. The direct cause of symptoms manifested in schizophrenia is probably a disruption of normal neurotransmitter activity, particularly dopamine. One plausible explanation for schizophrenia is the dopaminergic theory, which hypothesizes that the dopamine levels in people with schizophrenia are elevated. Some maintain that at least six other neurotransmitters—glutamate, serotonin, norepinephrine, acetylcholine, GABA, and cholecystokinin—are also involved in schizophrenia. The most commonly prescribed antipsychotic drugs suppress dopamine and similar transmitter substances. Current treatment continues to focus primarily on the dopaminergic theory.

Parkinsonism. Most researchers agree that the immediate cause of parkinsonism is a deficiency of dopamine, particularly in the basal nuclei involved in motor coordination. Characteristically, patients suffering from Parkinson's disease display tremors, a shuffling gait, and a progressive lack of motor control. Clients sometimes have a loss of facial motor control, slurring speech, and make facial expressions that are flat or masklike. Public figures such as the late Pope John Paul II, boxer Muhammad Ali, and actor Michael J. Fox displayed several of these symptoms, raising public awareness of the condition. The causes of dopamine deficiency in Parkinson's patients appear to be both genetic and environmental. Currently, parkinsonism is treated with L-dopa, a dopamine precursor capable of crossing the blood-brain barrier of the brain. According to the theory, brain cells containing the appropriate enzymes will convert the L-dopa into dopamine.

Alzheimer's Disease. Alzheimer's disease is among the leading causes of disability and death of older adults in the United States, and the number of affected persons increases each year. Acetylcholine is the neurotransmitter primarily involved in Alzheimer's disease. Decreased levels of ACh produce many of the behavioral manifestations of the disease, such as memory loss and disorientation. This helps to explain why drugs such as donepezil (Aricept) are useful in the treatment of Alzheimer's disease. Aricept and other similar drugs inhibit the cholinesterase enzyme that breaks down ACh thus increasing the amount of available acetylcholine, therefore prolonging the onset of symptoms of Alzheimer's disease (Stahl, 2000).

Both Parkinson's and Alzheimer's diseases are examples of recognized organic brain disorders. They are included in this discussion because of their relationship to specific transmitter substances and because the devastating effects of these degenerative conditions are clearly linked to mood disorders and dementia that psychiatric mental health nurses encounter. The Case Study is an example of a neurodegenerative disorder, multiple sclerosis, that frequently has associated symptoms of a mental disorder.

CASE STUDY Shawn, a 43-year-old woman, was diagnosed with multiple sclerosis 5 years ago. She was taking gabapentin (Neurontin) and paroxetine (Paxil), and muscle pains and migraine headaches made it difficult for her to sleep. She also complained of feeling depressed and hopeless as a result of the recent exacerbation of debilitating MS symptoms. Shawn reported a 10-pound weight loss in the past 2 months.

CRITICAL THINKING

1 What questions will the nurse ask at this time?

2 What changes will the nurse suggest to improve Shawn's insomnia?

INTERRELATED SYSTEMS

Evidence is now clear that the CNS operates in delicate balance with other body systems. Research demonstrates that the CNS both affects and is affected by the immune system, the endocrine system, and the body's natural biologic rhythms, as well as other systems. The following are some examples of the interactions between body systems and how the disruption of these systems sometimes results in mental, emotional, and behavioral dysfunction and disorder.

Psychoneuroimmunology

Psychoneuroimmunology (PNI) studies the relationship between the neurologic, endocrine, and immune systems and behaviors associated with these systems. Cytokines, chemical messengers between immune cells, signal the brain to produce changes of activity in the endocrine system as well as the immune system. Research studies focus on the relationship of cytokines and the pathophysiology of medical diseases such as cancer, allergies, and autoimmune diseases. More recent studies focus on psychiatric disorders such as major depression, schizophrenia, and Alzheimer's disease (Kronfol and Remick, 2000).

Brain receptor sites for neuropeptides produced by the immune system are associated with changes in emotions and behaviors. Stress causes the discharge of corticotropin-releasing factors that suppress the immune system. Studies indicate that negative emotions, anxiety, and psychiatric disorders such as schizophrenia and mood disorders are sometimes associated with a decreased functioning of the immune system. Posttraumatic stress syndrome is associated with long-term immunosuppression (Kawamura, Kim, and Asukai, 2001).

Neuroendocrinology

Neuroendocrinology studies the relationship between the nervous system and the endocrine system. A number of hormones, including epinephrine, actually function as neurotransmitter-like substances. This affects chemical communication between many cells, even ones that are distant from the source of the hormone. Several hormonally based disorders result in medical conditions that produce psychiatric symptoms, as described next.

Research studies correlate hypothyroidism with depressive symptoms and Addison's disease with depression and fatigue. Other endocrine disorders are linked to autoimmune conditions such as Graves' disease, which causes excessive thyroid secretion. This sometimes follows an acute infection suggesting an immunologic origin for Graves' disease. People who suffer from Graves' disease commonly report symptoms of emotional stress, nervousness, fatigue, weight loss, heat intolerance, and gastrointestinal symptoms. Also, because schizophrenia and other psychiatric disorders occur more frequently during the reproductive period of life when sex hormones are most active, this suggests an endocrine-related origin.

Chronobiology

Chronobiology is the study of the biologic rhythms of the body, such as the circadian rhythms. These rhythms manifest in metabolic rate, sleep-wakefulness cycles, blood pressure, hormone levels, and body temperature. Researchers think the brain controls these rhythms and their interactions with various endocrine organs. Many psychiatric and medical disorders occur more frequently when sleep patterns and biologic rhythms are disrupted.

Many hypothesize that dreams result from the activation of electrical activity in brain regions that recall recent memories and reinforce long-term memories. One theory maintains that mental disorders are the result of brain circuits that are not activating competently because of abnormal brain wave patterns. When incompetent brain circuits are activated while the individual is awake, clients often report hallucinations and illusions. While sleeping, these incompetent brain circuits appear to produce bizarre or illusory dreams (Kavanau, 2000). Psychoactive drugs modify brain waves in psychotic clients, which temporarily restore more normal brain circuits. Antidepressants increase brain waves and suppress or reduce rapid eye movement (REM) sleep. Electroconvulsive therapy suppresses abnormal brain waves, allowing more normal slow waves to dominate. Additional information on sleep disorders is in Chapter 18.

Sundowning, or *Sundowner's syndrome*, is the exacerbation, or worsening, of psychotic or depressive symptoms during the afternoon or evening resulting in confusion and disorientation. Some studies connect sundowning with a disturbance of circadian rhythms. Psychiatric and medical conditions such as Alzheimer's disease also disrupt the client's circadian rhythm (Volicer et al., 2001). Decreased exposure to light during the winter months has also shown to produce depressive symptoms in clients suffering from seasonal affective disorder (SAD). PMH nurses need to be aware of these examples of chronobiologic disruptions that produce symptoms of mental illnesses.

EMERGING CONCEPTS IN PSYCHOBIOLOGY

Genetic Research

Genetics is the study of genes and the role they play in the functioning of living organisms. The Human Genome Project that began in 1990 resulted in the identification of all of the genes contained on the 23 pairs of human chromosomes. The knowledge of precise locations of genes responsible for every human biologic characteristic, as well as their biochemical structure, has opened up endless possibilities for research into the genetic causes of nearly every human disease or condition. This includes psychiatric disorders. However, recognizing that genes only determine the potential to develop any normal or abnormal condition significantly complicates the problem of identifying genetic causes of specific psychiatric disorders. Excellent evidence attributes disorders such as Huntington's disease and Parkinsonism to specific genes. For example, both diseases are located on chromosome number 4, but evidence for genetic causes of some other specific neurologic disorders is not so clear.

Because there appear to be familial tendencies in some disorders, researchers are attempting to specify schizophrenia genes. According to the most current literature, there are as many as 150 genes on nearly a dozen different chromosomes that contribute to the causes of schizophrenia, making the situation more complex (Lewis et al., 2003; Badner and Gershon, 2002). Research indicates that schizophrenia results from the interaction of multiple genes rather than a single gene. In theory, defective genes code for incorrect synthesis of neurotransmitters, or their deactivating enzymes, or other factors interfere with the proper transmission of vital chemical agents.

Research has also identified genes that are linked to bipolar disorder and substance dependence (Schindler et al., 2001). This helps to explain why certain psychiatric disorders recur in families and why first-degree relatives of individuals with psychiatric disorders have increased risk for developing the same or similar disorders. The genetic origins of other psychiatric dysfunction and disorders, namely attention deficit hyperactivity disorder, antisocial personality disorder, and violent behaviors, are being explored (Doyle, Roe, and Faraone, 2001; Raine et al., 2000).

Although few researchers believe that a single gene causes a psychiatric illness, genetics clearly plays a significant role in influencing mental health and disorder. The interaction of genes is highly complex, and the link of genes to behavior remains controversial. It appears that many genes influence psychiatric illness and the dysfunctional behaviors that are symptomatic of those illnesses (Petronis et al., 2003). There is also increased evidence that environmental and developmental conditions in utero contribute to the expression of these genes that subsequently manifest as abnormal behavior.

Stem Cell Technology

Stem cell technology is perhaps the most controversial and promising technique that will lead to treatments and cures for neurobiologic disease and injury. **Stem cells** are cells that have the complete genome intact and have not yet differentiated, or developed, into a specific cell type. A fertilized egg is *totipotent*, or has total potential to develop into an entire human being. As embryonic cells replicate, some become specialized genes while others are turned off. Adult stem cells have already differentiated, or begun to develop to a certain degree. For example, some adult stem cells have already developed into epithelia rather than connective tissue cells or muscle or nervous tissues. Although there are adult stem cells in a variety of tissues including bone marrow, some connective tissues, and even brain tissue, the ability to successfully culture them and use them for therapeutic purposes is currently limited.

The reason why stem cell technology is so promising is because undifferentiated stem cells from embryos have the potential to develop into any type of cell, so researchers are able to control gene expression deliberately. Specialized stem cells can be developed into organs for transplants and have fewer complications from tissue rejection. The controversy surrounding stem cell research is an ethical issue, primarily regarding the source of embryos that provide undifferentiated stem cells. Many public figures have taken seemingly rational and passionate but opposing points of view increasing the intensity of the debate. These points of view will shape public policy and the direction of stem cell research, which will determine matters of life and death. Debate continues for or against the use of embryos or amniotic fluid as researchers seek cures and treatments for conditions and diseases and remedies that stem cells might provide.

Regardless of the source of stem cells, adult or embryonic, numerous technical challenges remain, but the potential therapeutic applications for this research seem unlimited at the moment. Active research continues on numerous neurobiologic conditions including brain and spinal cord injury, neurogenetic disorders affecting brain development, and degenerative conditions such as amyotropic lateral sclerosis (ALS), Parkinson's disease and Alzheimer's disease, among others (Shihabuddin et al., 1999). The implications of stem cell research for the future of psychiatric nursing are promising as is the potential of stem cell therapy itself.

DIAGNOSTIC AND EVALUATION PROCEDURES

Neuroimaging

Before modern neuroimaging techniques were available, clinicians had few noninvasive tools to examine the human brain, with the exception of the x-ray. The brain remained a mystery. The development of imaging techniques since the early 1980s has dramatically changed the understanding of brain structure and function. Brain anatomy and physiology has now been mapped in exquisite detail, providing valuable information using a variety of techniques. Useful neuroimaging techniques available today include ultrasonography (US), computed tomography (CT), magnetic resonance imaging (MRI), functional magnetic resonance imaging (fMRI), positron emission tomography (PET), and single photon emission computed tomography (SPECT) (Figure 6-5). Unlike older x-ray technology that uses film, these techniques use computers to generate images. Table 6-5 identifies common nursing considerations for clients undergoing neuroimaging tests.

Ultrasonography

Ultrasonography, also known as echoencephalography, uses high-frequency sound waves to form images of brain spaces and masses. Because ultrasonography does not use

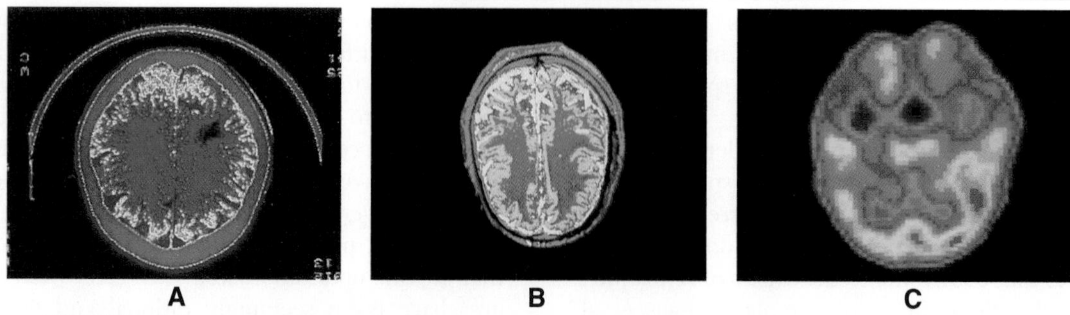

FIGURE 6-5 Neuroimaging techniques. **A,** Computed tomography scan. **B,** Magnetic resonance imaging scan. **C,** Positron emission tomography scan. (From Thibodeau GA, Patton KT: *Anatomy & physiology,* ed 6, St Louis, 2007, Mosby.)

harmful radiation, many prefer this technique to examine developing brains. It was developed for medical purposes following World War II and has been widely used to create images of developing fetuses as well as various organs within the body, including the brain.

Computed Tomography

Following the development of sonography, a new neuroimaging technique based on x-rays was developed in 1972. Scientists conducted research to develop this technology at Electronic Music Industry, a branch of Capitol Records. Money from the sale of Beatles records partly funded the research. This technique used to be called computerized axial tomography (CAT). A CT scan of the brain provides a three-dimensional view of brain structures by imaging serial thin sections through the brain or other anatomic structure. These multiple sections help differentiate fine densities, unlike a normal x-ray film. Anatomic abnormalities in the brain as revealed in CT scans are not specific to any type of psychiatric disorder and do not serve as a specific test for disorders. However, they do provide suggestive evidence of brain-based problems. Clients with schizophrenia, bipolar disorder, other mood disorders, alcoholism, multi-infarct dementia, and Alzheimer's disease have shown nonspecific brain abnormalities in CT scans. Many use the CT scan because it is available and cost effective. Disadvantages include lack of screening sensitivity, underestimation of brain atrophy, and inability to image in the sagittal and coronal views.

Magnetic Resonance Imaging

Formerly known as nuclear magnetic resonance (NMR), MRI has become an excellent tool and a substitute for actual exploratory surgery. It is also advantageous because it uses radio waves instead of harmful radiation and provides images that are sharper than CTs. MRI is unaffected by bone, and, unlike CT, it is able to view brain structures close to the skull. It also differentiates between white matter and gray matter tissue.

MRI is not appropriate for all clients because of several contraindications to its use. Box 6-3 indicates the client groups who must avoid MRIs. Clients with claustrophobia are often unable to complete the study because the MRI machine is enclosed and clients are required to remain motionless. Because of the confining environment and excessive noise of the equipment, nurses need to focus on client teaching before the test and closely monitor the client's anxiety levels during testing. Newer open-structured MRI equipment has made MRI testing easier for clients. MRIs show neuroanatomic changes in clients with schizophrenia that include increased size of ventricles, temporal lobe reductions, hippocampal reductions, and cortical atrophy as evidenced in Figure 12-1.

Functional MRI. fMRI is a modification of the basic MRI and detects brain activity by measuring oxygen consumption and metabolic differences in various parts of the brain. fMRI reveals that clients with Alzheimer's disease often have lower glucose metabolism in the cortical regions (Alexander et al., 2002). fMRI is an effective tool for identifying specific functional areas of the brain associated with behaviors. The science of neuroinformatics, which includes techniques such as fMRI, has become the equivalent of the Human Genome Project of the twenty-first century by helping to map the human brain.

Positron Emission Tomography and Single Photon Emission Computed Tomography

Positron emission tomography (PET) is based on the basic principles of CT scanning. PET scanning remains at the forefront in neuroimaging procedures because of the information it provides regarding brain function in addition to structure. Patients undergoing a PET scan have radioactive substances such as glucose introduced into the blood supply of the brain. When positron-emitting radionuclei interact with electrons, an image is produced. Both particles cease to exist and are converted into two photons that travel in opposite directions and are detected as color variations indicated on a screen. The machine and procedure require a support team of physicists, chemists, and computer experts and are expensive.

SPECT and PET are also called radionucleide scanning techniques, because both involve the introduction of radioactive substances into the blood supply of the brain. SPECT is particularly useful in visualizing vascular struc-

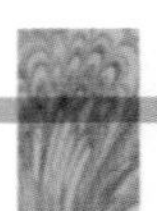

TABLE 6-5

Nursing Considerations with Neuroimaging Procedures

TEST	GENERAL CONSIDERATIONS	COMMON NURSING CARE	COMMON CONTRAINDICATIONS
ANATOMIC IMAGING			
Computed tomography (CT)	Three-dimensional view of brain structures Differentiate fine-density structures, unlike normal x-ray film Examination time: 15-30 min Clear fluids meal before test	Explain purpose of test and all procedures. Reassure client that test is safe and that radiation exposure is not a concern. Assess client's anxiety level and monitor for symptoms of claustrophobia. Reassure client that hearing monotonous noise is common. Instruct client to lie still to ensure good imaging. If using contrast iodine, monitor for gastrointestinal upset, flushing, and perceptions of excess warmth.	Allergy to iodine (not all CT requires iodine) Inability to lie completely still Claustrophobia
Magnetic resonance imaging (MRI)	Separates view of white matter from gray matter tissue Examination time: 15-60 min	Explain purpose of test and all procedures. Reassure client that test uses magnets, not radiation; radiation exposure is not a concern. Assess client's anxiety level and monitor for symptoms of claustrophobia. Instruct client to lie still to ensure good imaging. Instruct client that a clear plastic helmet with antenna will be put over head. Reassure client that hearing monotonous noise is common.	Inability to lie completely still Claustrophobia Pacemakers Metallic implants, plates, or screws Life support equipment needed for client Infusion pumps Generally not used when client is pregnant
FUNCTIONAL IMAGING			
Positron emission tomography (PET)	Two-dimensional view of brain structures Measures physiologic and chemical functioning such as glucose uptake by cells in brain, as well as information on anatomic structures Short half-life isotopes used	Explain purpose of test and all procedures. Inform client that isotopes are radioactive and discuss concerns. Assess client's anxiety level and monitor for symptoms of claustrophobia. Explain that there will be time interval of about 45 min between injection of isotope and scanning procedure. Explain that client may be blindfolded and have earplugs to decrease environmental stimulus during testing. Instruct client to lie still to ensure good imaging. Make sure client does not fall asleep during procedure—this will affect test results.	Inability to lie completely still Claustrophobia Severe anxiety level Recent use of sedating/tranquilizing medication because these medications alter cellular glucose use patterns Breast-feeding Requires expensive cyclotron
Single photon emission computed tomography (SPECT)	Two-dimensional view of brain structures Measures physiologic and chemical functioning such as glucose uptake by cells in brain, as well as information on anatomic structures Long half-life isotopes used No onsite cyclotron required	As for PET above.	Breast-feeding Inability to lie completely still Claustrophobia

tures in the brain and in diagnosing disorders such as cerebrovascular accidents (CVAs).

These techniques are particularly useful for demonstrating variable levels of brain activity and associated blood flow within the brain. SPECT scans have detected abnormalities in the frontal cortex, occipital, and temporal lobes, and parahippocampal gyrus in clients with panic disorders.

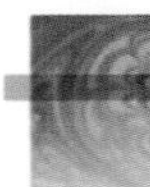

BOX 6-3

Client Group Contraindications for MRI

- Individuals with pacemakers
- Individuals with metallic objects such as screws, prostheses, and orthopedic devices
- Clients on life-support systems

CLIENT and FAMILY TEACHING GUIDELINES

BIOLOGIC BASIS OF PSYCHIATRIC DISORDERS

- Determine a mutually acceptable time and location for the teaching session.
- Select an environment that is favorable for learning.
- Identify the client's readiness for learning.
- Identify the client's motivation for learning.
- Identify the client's knowledge about the topic and accuracy of that knowledge.
- Identify with the client the specific content that is requested and required.
- Define a measurable outcome with the client to determine that learning has occurred.
- Define the evaluation method used to determine the effectiveness of teaching.
- Use multiple teaching-learning approaches, such as visual and auditory, based on client's needs.
- Monitor the client's anxiety level during the teaching session, as increased anxiety will decrease information processing.
- Identify alternative resources available to the client to increase learning potential.
- Identify the process that the client will follow to access support persons if the client requires more reinforcement.

NEUROBIOLOGY AND PSYCHIATRIC NURSING

Psychiatric mental health nursing provides care to clients with brain-based illnesses. Increasingly, a strong background in neurobiology is part of the standards of practice for psychiatric mental health nursing (American Nurses Association, 2006). By synthesizing the findings of the nursing assessment discussed in Chapter 3 and the nurse's understanding of psychobiologic issues, effective nursing care will assist clients in achieving wellness.

As we are learning, each structure and each neurochemical produced and used by the brain has a specific function. The brain is a dynamic, continually changing environment, and researchers are discovering more of the complexities of the brain. In adults, the brain seems less able to repair itself after injury or replace degenerative cells when compared with other parts of the body. This **neuroplasticity**, or the ability of the brain to change its structure and function, is providing insights into the role of certain brain areas in the development of illness (Mohr and Mohr, 2001). New understanding and application of concepts such as the neuroplastic nature of brain tissue are also leading to new approaches for treating disorders. Until now, many believed that the capacity of the brain to repair itself after injury or to replace degenerative cells was minimal, particularly in adults, but current research reveals brain cell regeneration in several conditions.

Genetics and stem cell research are just two emerging technologies that are opening the door to potential treatments for psychiatric illnesses. Much of the stigma attached to psychiatric illness was due to a lack of understanding regarding the biologic basis of these disorders. Therefore, effective client and family teaching is an important function of the role of the psychiatric mental health nurse as researchers discover new information regarding the structures and functioning of the CNS. The Client and Family Teaching Guidelines box displays the highlights of effective client teaching regarding the biologic basis of psychiatric disorders. Psychiatric mental health nurses will continue to play an important part by directly assisting clients with brain-based disorders and by teaching and informing clients, families, and the general public about advances in neurobiology.

New research findings continue to change the way people with psychiatric disorders are cared for and treated. The Research for Evidence-Based Practice box highlights the importance of critical thinking as psychiatric mental health nurses approach and plan modifications of care based on new research findings.

Knowledge of the neurobiologic basis of psychiatric disorders is essential in effective psychiatric mental health nursing practice. Nurses need to include biologic principles in all aspects of nursing care, from assessment to evaluation, to ensure comprehensive and quality nursing. More and more information will be available regarding structure and functioning of the brain, and because of this, the role and function of the psychiatric mental health nurse will continue to change. Staying current with dynamic development in the field will continue to stimulate and positively challenge the truly professional psychiatric mental health nurse.

RESEARCH for EVIDENCE-BASED PRACTICE

Gross-Isseroff R et al: The suicide brain: a review of postmortem receptor transporter binding studies, *Neuroscience and Biobehavior Review* 22:653, 1998.

Some research has reported that the brains of individuals who commit suicide are different from the brains of individuals who have died of natural causes. Postmortem examination of the receptor/transport binding sites of the brain tissue of suicide victims and of individuals who have died of natural causes show that the brains of suicide victims have unique, specific neurochemical characteristics that make "suicide brains" different from the brains of individuals who have died of natural causes. Scientists are using such studies to formulate a hypothesis of molecular markers that will possibly help define and identify individuals at risk for suicidal behavior. Researchers are developing tests to measure identified markers. When these markers are specifically identified and prove to be reliable in their ability to predict suicidal behavior, the test will likely become a routine aspect of mental health evaluation.

CHAPTER SUMMARY

- Current knowledge about the brain and its functions is continually changing.
- The brain is the most complex and one of the most important organs in the human body because of its multiple functions.

- Psychiatric disorders are brain-based illnesses with anatomic or physiologic components.
- It is imperative for nurses to understand the anatomy and physiology of the brain and other systems that interact with the nervous system. Nurses also will become familiar with psychobiologic approaches to treat psychiatric disorders.
- One key to understanding treatment strategies for psychiatric disorders is to recognize the role that neurotransmitter substances play in neural communication.
- Nurses will become familiar with psychobiologic approaches to treat psychiatric disorders.
- Modern neuroimaging techniques help explain structure and function and their relation to brain differences and psychiatric illnesses.
- Emerging fields in neuroscience such as genetics and stem cell research will continue to bring advanced technologies that lead to improved care for patients suffering from neurobiologic disorders.

REVIEW QUESTIONS

1 Which statement by a family member of a person with schizophrenia demonstrates effective learning about the disease?

1. "The disease was probably caused by problems with several genes. These genes cause changes in how certain brain chemicals work."
2. "The disease could be cured if our politicians and laws allowed for more stem cell research. Adult stem cells hold so much promise."
3. "The disease probably resulted from the mother's smoking during pregnancy. Nicotine is actually a neurotransmitter."
4. "If our family had more money, we could afford the promising psychoneuroimmunologic treatments available in other countries."

2 Which assessment finding best indicates release of norepinephrine?

1. Pulse rate changes from 70 to 62.
2. Pupil size changes from 8 mm to 3 mm.
3. Client begins complaining of "intestinal cramping."
4. Blood pressure changes from 126/70 to 158/84.

3 These clients are scheduled to have magnetic resonance imaging (MRI). For which client(s) should additional assessment information be gathered before the diagnostic procedure? You may select more than one answer. A client with:

1. A history of wounds from exploding shrapnel during military service
2. A co-occuring diagnosis of bleeding peptic ulcers for the past 3 years
3. Current complaints of extreme sensitivity to loud noises
4. Reports of allergies to iodine, eggs, and shellfish
5. A 3-year history of Parkinson's disease

4 An adult has panic attacks. Which neurotransmitter is most implicated in this problem?

1. Norepinephrine
2. Acetylcholine
3. Serotonin
4. γ-aminobutyric acid (GABA)

5 A nurse plans the care for an adult with a tumor in the brain's frontal lobes. Initial interventions should focus on the client's anticipated problems with:

1. Motor function and judgment
2. Sensory and calculation abilities
3. Interpretation of visual stimuli
4. Hearing and hygiene

*Additional self-study exercises and learning resources are available to you on the **Companion CD** at the back of the book and on the **Evolve website** at **http://evolve.elsevier.com/Fortinash/**.*

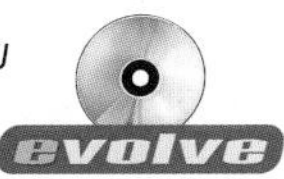

ONLINE RESOURCES

American Academy of Sleep Medicine: **www.aasmnet.org**

American Society of Neuroimaging: **www.asnweb.org**

Center for Sleep and Circadian Biology: **www.northwestern.edu/cscb**

Encyclopedia of Psychology: Psychobiology: **www.psychology.org/links/Publications/Psychobiology**

International Society of Developmental Psychobiology: **www.oswego.edu/isdp**

National Institute of Mental Health: The Human Brain Project: **www.nimh.nih.gov/neuroinformatics/**

National Sleep Foundation: **www.sleepfoundation.org**

Society for Light Treatment and Biological Rhythms: **www.sltbr.org**

REFERENCES

Alexander GE et al: Longitudinal PET evaluation of cerebral metabolic decline in dementia: a potential outcome measure in Alzheimer's disease treatment studies, *Am J Psychiatry* 159:238-245, 2002.

Amen DG: Brain SPECT imaging in psychiatry, *Prim Psychiatry* 5:83-87, 1998.

American Nurses Association: *Scope and standards of psychiatric mental health practice*, Washington, DC, 2006, American Nurses Publishing.

Badner JA, Gershon ES: Meta-analysis of whole-genome linkage scans of bipolar disorder and schizophrenia, *Mol Psychiatry* 7:405-411, 2002.

Carlson NR: *Physiology of behavior*, ed 7, Boston, 2001, Allyn & Bacon.

Doyle AE, Roe CM, Faraone SV: The genetics of attention deficit hyperactivity disorder, *Prim Psychiatry* 8:65-71, 2001.

Dubin MW: *How the brain works*, Williston, Vt, 2002, Blackwell Science.

Goff D, Coyle J: The emerging role of glutamate in the pathophysiology and treatment of schizophrenia, *Am J Psychiatry* 158:1367-1377, 2001.

Gribbin J: *How the brain works: a beginner's guide to the mind and consciousness*, New York, 2002, Doring Kindersley.

Gross-Isseroff R et al: The suicide brain: a review of postmortem receptor transporter binding studies, *Neurosci Biobehav Rev* 22:653, 1998.

Gur R: Functional imaging is fulfilling some promises, *Am J Psychiatry* 159:693-694, 2002.

Kavanau J: Sleep, memory, maintenance and mental disorders, *J Neuropsychiatry* 12:199-208, 2000.

Kawamura N, Kim Y, Asukai N: Suppression of cellular immunity in men with a past history of posttraumatic stress disorder, *Am J Psychiatry* 158:484-486, 2001.

Kronfol Z, Remick, D: Cytokines and the brain implications for clinical psychiatry, *Am J Psychiatry* 157:683-694, 2000.

Lewis CM et al: Genome scan meta-analysis of schizophrenia and bipolar disorder, part II, *Am J Human Genetics* 73:34-48, 2003.

McLeod TM, Lopez-Figueroa A, Lopez-Figueroa MO: Nitric oxide, stress and depression, *Psychopharmacol Bull* 35:24-41, 2001.

Mohr WK, Mohr B: Brain, behavior, connections, and implications: psychodynamics no more, *Arch Psychiatr Nurs* 15:171-181, 2001.

Montoya A et al: Brain mapping and cognitive dysfunction in Huntington's disease, *J Psychiatr Neuroscience* 31:21-29, 2006.

Petronis A et al: Monozygotic twins exhibit numerous epigenetic differences: clues to twin discordance? *Schizophrenia Bull* 29:169-178, 2003.

Raine A et al: Reduced gray matter volume and reduced autonomic activity in antisocial personality disorder, *Arch Gen Psychiatry* 57:119-129, 2000.

Rapoport JL: The neurodevelopmental model of schizophrenia: update 2005, *Mol Psychiatry* 10:614, 2005.

Schindler KM et al: Candidate genes for schizophrenia: further evaluation of KCNN3, *Prim Psychiatry* 8:51-53, 2001.

Shihabuddin LS et al: Stem cell technology for basic science and clinical applications, *Arch Neurol* 6:29-32, 1999.

Stahl SM: *Essential psychopharmacology: neuroscientific basis and practical applications*, ed 2, New York, 2000, Cambridge University Press.

Thibodeau G, Patton K: *Anatomy and physiology*, ed 6, St Louis, 2007, Mosby.

Volicer L et al: Sundowning and circadian rhythms in Alzheimer's disease, *Am J Psychiatry* 158:704-711, 2001.

Young GB, Pigott SE: Neurobiological basis of consciousness, *Arch Neurol* 56:153-157, 1999.

Chapter 7 Cultural, Ethnic, and Spiritual Considerations

RUTH N. GRENDELL

Culture is the widening of the mind and of the spirit.
JAWAHARLAL NEHRU

OBJECTIVES

1. Differentiate the concepts of culture, race, and ethnicity.
2. Discuss characteristics that are common to all cultures.
3. Discuss the need for a nurse's self-evaluation in order to provide competent cultural care to persons from other socio-cultural backgrounds.
4. Analyze selected socialization issues—acculturation, assimilation, ethnocentrism, and xenophobia—as they relate to cultural heritage, mental health beliefs, and practices.
5. Perform a cultural assessment using the Heritage Assessment Tool.
6. Formulate potential nursing diagnoses related to a client's cultural or ethnic orientation.
7. Discuss adaptive methods to use in planning and implementing therapeutic nursing interventions for a client's cultural or ethnic orientation.
8. Conduct a self-assessment of spiritual beliefs.
9. Develop a spiritual assessment to use when pastoral care is not available.
10. Describe a therapeutic plan of care for a person in spiritual distress.

KEY TERMS

acculturation, p. 132
ageism, p. 132
assimilation, p. 132
cultural awareness, p. 134
cultural competence, p. 134
cultural heritage, p. 130
culture, p. 130
culture of poverty, p. 130
culture shock, p. 132
ethnicity, p. 130
ethnocentrism, p. 132
faith, p. 137
heritage consistency, p. 131
heterosexism, p. 132
racism, p. 132
religion, p. 137
sexism, p. 132
spirituality, p. 137
xenophobia, p. 132

CULTURE AND ETHNICITY

The book *The Spirit Catches You and You Fall Down* by Anne Fadiman (1997) is required reading in many colleges and universities across the United States to introduce students and faculty to concepts related to cultural awareness. It is a fascinating true account of conflicts and misunderstandings between cultures. The story describes how a Hmong refugee family from Laos interacted with the culture of the Western (allopathic) health care system in the treatment for Lia, a young child who had been diagnosed with epilepsy. Lia's parents believed she was ill because she lost one of her three souls and it was replaced by a spirit. They recognized her seizures as "the spirit catches you and you fall down." Her illness was a great concern for them, but they felt that she had been chosen for a special purpose because persons with epilepsy often become shamans or healers in the Hmong culture. To them, Lia was a special child who would someday have power to envision things that others could not and have empathy for those who become ill.

As Lia's seizures increased in number and severity, and there was no traditional healer to help them, they frequented the local American hospital emergency services for help. Here they encountered health care personnel who did not speak their language, who knew nothing about their belief system, and who repeatedly misdiagnosed Lia's complicated health problems. To the parents, some of the health care procedures such as blood draws and other invasive procedures were more harmful than the illness itself. They did not understand the instructions that health care providers gave, and no translators were available. The health care personnel complained that the family did not adhere to the prescribed medical plan. The parents and the health care providers all wanted a healthy life for Lia. However, because of the different cultural beliefs and language problems, the result was tragic.

Unfortunately, this is not an isolated incident. As nations become multicultural, conflicts are inevitable. Conflicts between cultures are most commonly due to ineffective intercultural verbal and nonverbal communication, prejudices, and lack of understanding or acceptance of each other's values and beliefs. Individuals construct their worldviews through their own socialized cultural lenses. Until individuals view the world through the lenses of persons of another culture—*or walk in their moccasins*—they cannot understand how prejudgments and fears affect perceptions and interactions with each other.

Defining Culture

The term **culture** is usually associated with ethnicity and race and is the defining boundary that makes one culture different than another. However, culture is more than just a boundary. It is the structural background that shapes a person's worldview and all the lived experiences and heritage. Culture actually has many definitions. "It is a set of values, beliefs and behaviors that influence the way that members of the group express themselves" (Catalano, 2000, p. 321). Culture is the integrated pattern of human behavior of members of a racial, religious, or social group passed on to future generations and results in the development of a **cultural heritage**.

The cultural background is a core component of **ethnicity**, which is a race or group of people who have common traits and customs. An example of ethnicity is the more than 200 American Native Indian groups. These groups share many common cultural values but have different life patterns. The groups have their individual languages, traditions, values, and symbols. Each group belongs to the Native American culture, but each subculture perceives itself as distinctive. Ethnic pride sometimes leads to conflicts between the subcultures (Spector, 2003).

Subcultures

There are subcultures within each major culture. Subcultures develop when members of the group develop new values that they honor more than the values of their dominant culture (Catalano, 2000). Although these groups accept many of the traditional values of the main culture, they modify or abandon some values because of influences within or outside the different subculture groups. Sometimes individuals actually belong to several subcultures related to age, gender, occupation, social/economic status, geographic location, family style, alternative lifestyles, and ethnicity. Teenagers, young adults, and older adults are representatives of subcultures. Some individuals also belong to several *subsets* within a subculture. For example, some students in a high school belong to clubs (sports, music, drama), use a special language (slang), wear a particular clothing style, develop specific habits and lifestyles, or have friendships and values that differ from the other subset groups. The differences sometimes lead to intrapersonal and interpersonal conflicts.

Many studies have been published about the generation gap between the age-groups within a culture, particularly in the Western world. Each generation has its separate group awareness, a particular lifestyle, and a belief system and worldview that define the social norms. Each generation has a particular impact on society and has its own mental and physical health problems. Table 7-1 outlines the current generations in the United States. Consider how the social and physical environments, the advances in science and technology, and the specific mental and physical health care needs have influenced each generation. Members of the G.I. Generation are currently the "old" frail elderly; and 95% of the members of the Silent Generation have entered retirement. The eldest members of the baby boomer generation are entering senior age status (see Table 7-1).

A subculture that is important to include in this discussion is the **culture of poverty**. *Poverty* is not being able to obtain what is necessary to adequately live in a particular cultural context (Revision notes UK, 2005) (Figure 7-1). Poverty has become a global social and economic burden because of the increased numbers of people entering and remaining in poverty over the past several decades. The characteristics, special needs, and issues

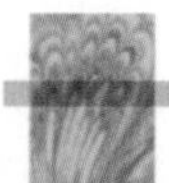

TABLE 7-1

Current U.S. Generation Subcultures

GENERATION	BIRTH YEARS
G.I., World War II, or Greatest Generation	1900-1924
Silent Generation (includes Korean War veterans)	1925-1945
Baby boomers	1946-1964
Baby busters	1958-1968
Generation X	1965-1981
Generation Y	1984-2004
Generation Z (the Millennials)	2005-2025

related to living in poverty are diverse, complex, and include several subsets of individuals with mental illnesses (the different age groups that range from teenaged runaways, to families, to the poor elderly; individuals addicted to drugs or alcohol; and those who suffer from posttraumatic stress disorders such as war veterans, refugees, and legal or illegal immigrants). Many of the homeless population are repeatedly jailed for vagrancy, stealing, or for committing violent acts and are sent back into the homeless environment after serving the required sentence. During imprisonment, any public assistance is withdrawn, often taking several months to be reestablished, and the cycle of poverty continues.

A subset in the culture of poverty is the working poor, or people who receive the minimum wage and exist on housing and food allowances through public assistance or pensions. The working poor also includes people who receive survivor benefits, persons with mental or physical disabilities, children of incarcerated parents, and single-parent families and large families with children under 18 ("Putting a Face on Poverty," 2005; U.S. Department of Health and Human Services, 2006).

All of these individuals experience discrimination and live under the stigma associated with poverty. Many live for the moment and cannot plan for the future. Access to health care is minimal and it is most often received for emergency circumstances. They are frequently unable to see the importance of prescribed therapy or are unable to self-manage the treatment requirements.

Many of the poor population are illiterate or do not have the education or the necessary skills to obtain higher-paying jobs. A report of interviews with poor young single mothers, 18 to 23 years of age, indicated that they feel isolated from their peers, have lost family support, and are struggling to care for their children. However, they recognize the need for education and are motivated to prepare themselves for higher paying jobs and to support themselves. They do not want to depend on public assistance for an extended period of time and are hoping to continue their education somehow. Without financial and other forms of assistance, this is difficult to accomplish (Jennings, 2005).

Cultural Heritage

Heritage consistency is how closely a person's lifestyle matches, or reflects, the typical lifestyle of one's own culture. Common themes and roles all cultures address include the family, marriage, parenting roles, education, health, work, and methods of education. A major component of heritage consistency is a cultural, ethnic, or national religion, or a belief in a divine or superhuman power or powers. The religion consists of a system of

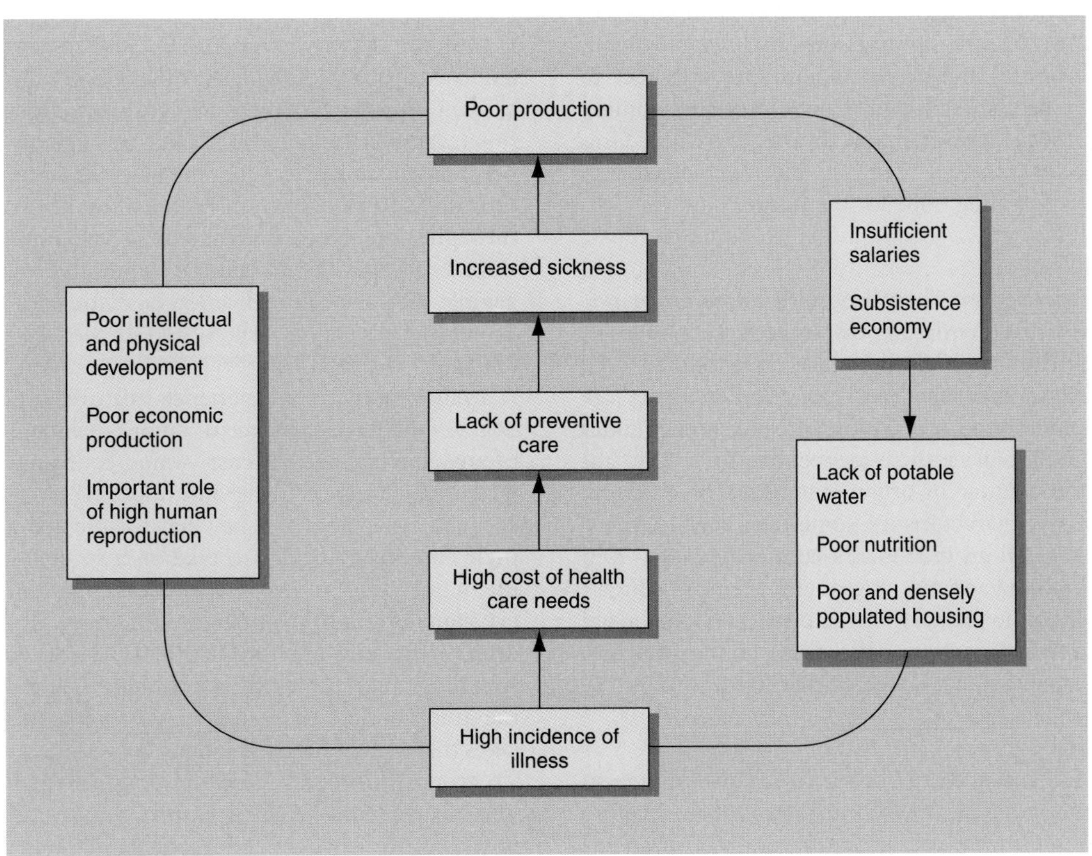

FIGURE 7-1 The cycle of poverty (From Spector RE: *Cultural diversity in health and illness*, ed 6, Upper Saddle River, NJ, 2004, Pearson.)

beliefs, practices, and ethical values (Spector, 2003). Many cultures view physical and mental illnesses as a spiritual problem or as punishment for behaviors that are opposite of the religious codes and morals of the cultural group. Some cultures believe traditional healers, rituals, talismans, and folk (generic) medicines and practices will restore health.

Individuals also express cultural heritage through language; works of art, music, and dance, ethnic clothing; customs and traditions; holiday celebrations; diet; and expressions of spirituality. Culture includes the behavioral responses and decisions regarding significant life experiences such as birth, rights-of-passage ceremonies, illness, pain, death, and mourning practices. Culture is a learned process or socialization that begins at birth and continues throughout the person's life span. Individuals rarely consider the influence of culture unless the individual purposely studies one's own culturally determined behavior (Clark, 2002). In other words, cultural values are powerful forces that affect all aspects of a person's life, both consciously and unconsciously.

An illustration of strong cultural heritage is Mardi Gras, an important celebration for residents of New Orleans, Louisiana. In spite of the tragedies caused by Hurricane Katrina in August 2005, the people of New Orleans decided they had to demonstrate their spirit of survival and celebrate this special event. Displaced residents returned to share in the celebration. Many of those who remained struggle with posttraumatic stress disorders and the exacerbation of mental and physical illnesses, unemployment, and loss of housing, and they are waiting for assistance to clean up the debris. Although many worry that coming hurricane seasons may bring more disaster, the Mardi Gras celebration is a treasured tradition, and they believe it is important for instilling hope for the future.

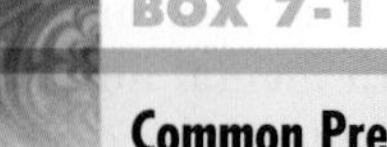

BOX 7-1

Common Prejudices or Biases

- **Racism**. The belief that members of one race are superior to those of other races.
- **Sexism**. The belief that members of one sex are superior to the other sex.
- **Heterosexism**. The belief that everyone is or should be heterosexual and that heterosexuality is best, normal, and superior.
- **Ageism**. The belief that members of one age group are superior to those of other ages.
- **Ethnocentrism**. The belief that one's own cultural, ethnic, or professional group is superior to that of others. One judges others by his or her own yardstick and is unable or unwilling to see what the other group is really about.
- **Xenophobia**. The morbid fear of strangers and those who are not of one's own ethnic group.

From American Nurses Association: *Multicultural issues in the nursing workforce*, Washington, DC, 1993, The Association.

Cultural Diversity

Different characteristics between cultures are either *primary characteristics* or *secondary characteristics*. Examples of primary characteristics are nationality, race, color, gender, age, and religious beliefs. Secondary characteristics are social economic status, occupation and education, gender issues, geographic place of residence, length of time absent from the country of origin, and sexual orientation. The secondary characteristics sometimes have a more powerful effect on an individual's cultural identity, even though these characteristics are sometimes more difficult to identify than the primary characteristics. Nurses avoid generalization or stereotyping based on minimal information about the individual or the culture (Box 7-1).

Changing Trends

Since the mid-1960s, there has been a massive migration of immigrants and refugees from many countries into the United States, Canada, Britain, and several European nations; they are seeking political and religious freedom and economic opportunities. The *melting pot* theory, a common belief that **acculturation**, the acceptance of the values and traditions of the host country, takes place as the immigrants adjust to their new environment, is no longer true. Acculturation is sometimes referred to as **assimilation**, which is the gradual process of developing a new cultural identity. The process is complete when the individual becomes fully merged into the dominant cultural group.

Examples of *cultural assimilation* include developing the ability to speak fluently in the host country's language, assuming a new name, and moving to a nonethnic neighborhood. *Marital assimilation* occurs through intermarriage between members of different cultures, thus forming a new subculture. *Structural assimilation* occurs primarily through social interactions and the development of friendships between different cultural groups. This includes engaging in personal and social activities in impersonal groups such as church, school, and the workplace (Spector, 2003).

Many immigrants experience **culture shock**—a sudden or violent disturbance of emotions including a sense of anxiety, fear, and distrust—when confronted with different standards of living and opposing worldviews and societal expectations. They have difficulty abandoning their cultural traditions to take on a strange new way of life. They prefer to live in their own communities for social support and to maintain their cultural heritage. Children and young adults usually adapt to their new surroundings more quickly even though they are subject to the traditions of the older family members. It usually takes three generations or longer for members of a minority group to integrate into the dominant culture of the new environment. Therefore, the United States and other host countries have actually become multicultural nations, now referred to as salad bowls rather than melting pots (Catalano, 2000).

CLINICAL ALERT

Authorities believe that an increase in group **suicide pacts** among Japanese teenagers and young adults is due to Internet chat rooms that offer specific strategies to end life. Individuals agree to meet and carry out the plan together. Many of the individuals were depressed, had been subjected to bullying, experienced broken relationships, were in abusive situations, or were disconnected from their families (Tabuchi, 2006). School nurses and other health care providers and teachers need to be aware of the potential problems young immigrant students encounter in the unfamiliar environment, especially in the early weeks and months. Cultural awareness programs need to be encouraged throughout the school system.

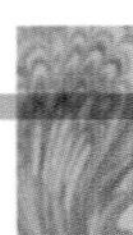

TABLE 7-2

Estimates of Population Groups in the United States: 2003

	POPULATION (%)*	
ORIGIN		
Latin America	53.3	
Asia	25	
Europe	13.7	
Other world regions	8	
IMMIGRATION RATES		
Since 2000	13.6	
1990s	36.6	
1980s	24	
1970s	13	
	FOREIGN BORN (%)	**NATIVE BORN (%)**
GEOGRAPHIC DISTRIBUTION		
Northeast	22.2	18.5
South	29.2	36.5
Midwest	11.3	24.1
West†	37.3	21
AGE CATEGORIES		
<18	8.9	27.8
18-24	80.1	60
25-44	45.1	21
45-64	24.7	23.5

From the U.S. Census Bureau: Current population survey, 2003 annual social and economic supplement. In Larsen, LJ: *The foreign-born population in the United States 2003,* Current Population Reports, P20-551, Washington, DC, 2004, U.S. Census Bureau.
*33.5 million foreign born (11.7% of the total U.S. population).
†52.7% of immigrants from Central America reside in the West.

Environmental Mixture of Cultures

A current estimate from the U.S. Census Bureau indicates that 33.5 million foreign-born individuals represent 11.7% of the nation's population. These percentages are rapidly changing because of the increase in the number of immigrants each year (Table 7-2). The foreign-born category includes naturalized citizens, lawful permanent residents (immigrants), temporary migrants (foreign students), refugees (humanitarian migrants), and people who are living in the United States illegally. Persons born in the United States and its islands such as Puerto Rico or persons born abroad of U.S. parents are considered to be "native born." Many immigrants obtain U.S. citizenship following the 5-year residency requirement; however, fewer foreign-born persons under 25 years of age have graduated from high school. They usually marry at an early age and have larger families than the comparative native-born group. Approximately 16.6% live below the poverty level compared with 11.5% of the native born. Many of the individuals of immigrant parents under 18 years of age were born in the United States (U.S. Census Bureau, 2003).

The U.S. population reached the 300 million mark in 2006. Most of the growth is due to natural causes—more births than deaths. However, 42% of the current population increase is due to the arrival of immigrants. Many of the immigrants are young and in their prime child-bearing years (Kim, 2006). Consider the contributions and the challenges that they bring.

Western Health Care System as Culture

At the beginning of this chapter, the Western (or allopathic) health care system was referred to as a culture. Consider how the defining characteristics apply. Health care providers in this system are socialized into their various specialty areas through education, internalized beliefs and values, traditions and clothing, habits, standards, and language transmitted to them by the previous generation. Scientific evidence is the only acceptable method for establishing truth and gaining new knowledge. Members believe the Western system of health care delivery is superior to any other method. They are privileged to know specific items of information related to health and illness and perceive themselves as the experts in stating what health care should be.

The beliefs of the Western health care system consist of standard definitions of health and illness, the necessity for routine physical examinations and diagnostic procedures, compliance with prescribed treatment regimens, and the advantages of technology. The known causes of disease are bacteria, viruses, chemical carcinogens, environmental pollutants, and lifestyles, among other factors. For centuries, allopathic medicine followed a philosophy of dualism, the separation of the body, mind, and spirit, and therefore treatment was directed primarily toward physiologic issues. Health care providers viewed pain as a cultural phenomenon, and responses to pain varied according to the person's cultural background. Health care providers stereotyped individuals from different cultures according to their emotional and behavioral pain responses. We are currently aware that pain is simply what the person says it is and exists when the person says it does (McCaffrey and Pasero, 2004). Pain, along with its physiologic and emotional effects, is currently considered as the fifth vital sign included in the routine client assessment.

The public's increased interest and use of alternative therapies challenges the Western health care culture. Immigrants from all of the cultures have also introduced their traditional methods, and many clients, fearing criticism, do not share their information with health care providers. Until recently, many health care providers have not included inquiry about the client's self-care practices or were unaware of the many types of alternative therapy that clients use. Within the past several years, health care providers have become more aware of alternative therapies and have included some into the plan of care as complementary measures. Some of these include biofeedback and meditation. Most of the alternative and complimentary therapies from China and other Far Eastern countries are now widely accepted.

Cultural Awareness

Cultural awareness is the initial step toward effective interaction among individuals from different cultures. This awareness develops through understanding and valuing all aspects of another person's culture. It also involves an awareness of one's own culture, including the overt and covert prejudices and biases toward other cultures.

Cultural awareness enables the person to do the following (Leonard and Plotnikoff, 2000):

- See the world through multiple perspectives
- Enhance communication and interpersonal skills
- Model open-mindedness
- Explore one's personal cultural identity and values
- Reflect on how identity and values impact the view of the world

Various self-assessment tools are available. These tools have you listen to comments from individuals from a different culture and reflect on how your culture affects them. They also help you recognize behaviors that may offend people from another culture. Examples of items on an assessment tool include reflecting on one's personal prejudices and biases, one's ability to "think in" and speak a second language, the degree of knowledge one has about the history and traditions of different cultures, one's personal interest in understanding more about other cultures, and whether one has had any meaningful interactions with people of another culture (San Diego State University, 2005).

The self-assessment tool in Box 7-2 allows one to calculate the points from the responses that indicate a high, average, or low degree of cultural awareness. Several resources and classes are available to help individuals to develop cultural awareness. Not all self-assessment tools are accurate. However, the tools help people to gain insight and understanding of the important factors in developing cultural awareness. It is important to realize that cultural values are neither right nor wrong. Many groups established certain values for survival purposes, but in another culture's view these values are harmful (Catalano, 2000). This is especially true when dealing with health care issues.

Culturally Competent Health Care

Cultural competence requires respect for diversity and an understanding of the attitudes, beliefs, behaviors, practices, and communication patterns of multiple cultures and their languages (Medrano, Setzer, Enders et al., 2005). Culturally competent health care requires the development of interpersonal skills, communication skills, and awareness and sensitivity to the uniqueness of individuals. It is also an ongoing process as each new encounter presents the opportunity to gain additional knowledge and skills. Establishing trust is an important aspect in developing an effective relationship between the client and the care provider. Nurses need to use a gradual approach to complete an accurate assessment that includes initially asking general questions to ease a client's anxiety and to demonstrate interest in that person as an individual before he or she will reveal personal information.

Transcultural Communication

Effective communication is necessary for culturally competent care. Clear and effective communication is important in any exchange between individuals, and it is especially important when there are cultural and language differences. Learning to listen is fundamental to the communication process, which is extremely complex and involves multiple verbal and nonverbal components. The nurse and other health care providers need to be aware of the meaning of gestures, body positions, facial expressions, eye movements, and the tone of voice during all communication with individuals from various cultures (Catalano, 2000). Sometimes health care professionals speak authoritatively and use too many medical terms.

Some groups, including Native Americans, use a soft tone of voice. Members of Arab groups sometimes use dramatic emotional communication styles that seem hostile. Other groups, such as Asian-Pacific people, nod their heads and smile to show respect, but health care providers from another culture often interpret these behaviors as understanding and agreement when they actually are neither.

High-Context and Low-Context Cultures. One set of factors that dramatically influence communication and understanding between people of different cultures is the values of each culture regarding the decision-making process. A model taken from anthropology, sociology, and psychology defines behaviors and communication styles of cultural societies as *low context* (individualistic) or *high context* (collectivistic). The model suggests that an individualistic, or low-context, society is one in which people care for themselves and their immediate family. Low-context societies emphasize thinking and values that are centered on the individual: autonomy, individual initiative, the right to privacy, emotional independence, and universalism (arriving at rules of conduct that are applied to everyone). Although there are wide variations among persons in any culture, these qualities are generally char-

BOX 7-2

Self-Assessment of Cultural Awareness

I understand that the term *culture* implies an integrated pattern of human thoughts, communication methods, actions, customs, beliefs, values and institutions of racial, ethnic, religious, or social group. I also understand that *competence* implies a capacity to function effectively. Therefore, within this perspective I will use this self-assessment tool to determine my ability to provide culturally competent care to individuals who belong to various cultural groups.

Responses: A = strongly agree, B = agree, C = disagree, D = I don't know

____ 1. I acknowledge cultural differences and similarities that exist, and I refuse to label one culture superior or inferior to another.
____ 2. I understand that the therapeutic relationship is based on respect for the client and adherence to acceptable social and cultural communication patterns.
____ 3. I understand the features of a culture to take into consideration when planning and implementing culturally competent care.
____ 4. I am aware that I have subconscious biases and prejudices that affect my ability to adequately assess the needs of individuals from another culture.
____ 5. I always try to determine the norms for nonverbal communication within a culture and family that affect my interactions with people from that culture.
____ 6. I use various resources to determine the diseases/disorders that are endemic (common) to a culture.
____ 7. I respect the uniqueness of individuals from different cultures and avoid stereotyping.
____ 8. I look for educational information that reflects different cultures.

When interacting with individuals and families who have limited English proficiency, I always keep the following in mind:

____ 9. A person's limitation for communicating in English is not a reflection of intelligence.
____10. I am willing to work with the individual and family and others to find effective methods of communication.
____11. During an interview, I ask about the individual's beliefs and practices.
____12. I inquire about the individual's and the culture's customs/beliefs related to major life events.
____13. I provide written instructions and alternative illustrations as often as possible to accompany any verbal communication and make sure the client understands the content.
____14. I am comfortable in working with an interpreter, and I take time to clarify of the content the interpreter presents to the client.
____15. I am aware of the resources available to me at my institution and on the Internet that will assist me in developing educational materials for clients from different cultures.
____16. I inquire about family colloquialism (dialect, expressions) that affects communication.
____17. I am able to intervene when I observe others being insensitive toward clients from a different culture.
____18. I avoid imposing my values on people from a different culture.
____19. I accept and am considerate that male/female roles vary significantly among different cultural and ethnic groups and the client's reluctance to discuss certain matters or to receive care provided by me.
____20. I accept that religion and other beliefs influence how individuals and families respond to illnesses, disease, and death.
____21. I stay informed on the major health concerns and issues for ethnically and racially diverse client populations residing in the local area.
____22. I have taken professional development and training to enhance my knowledge and skills in the provision of services and supports to culturally, ethnically, racially, and linguistically diverse groups.
____23. I am actively involved in developing education materials that account for average literacy and that are culturally appropriate for individuals and families who receive care at my facility.

Modified from Giger J, Davidhizar R: *Transcultural nursing,* ed 4, St Louis, 1999, Mosby.

acteristic of persons who function in a democratic environment in which most members of the society have a legal voice and advocate for themselves. These cultures emphasize individual thinking and an analytic style of approaching a situation without considering the context or social situation in which the individual is acting. In general, this kind of thinking is typically American and is found in other Western cultures. Successful communication in this type of culture includes being assertive (including making direct eye contact), advocating for oneself, thinking through problems independently, and arguing for a point of view. It is typical for Americans to use this style of interaction as a standard. However, the rest of the world does not always function with these understandings.

In contrast, a high-context society is one in which people are included in strong groups throughout their lifetimes. These persons stress a "we" consciousness, collective identity, group solidarity, sharing, group decision making, collective duties and obligations, emotional dependence, and particularism or arriving at rules of conduct that are applied to persons depending on their particular role in society (Ito, 2005; Autgis and Raneer, 2004; Xue and Zhou, 2003).

Several high-context cultural cues are present and noticeable to the observer. For example, those from a high-context culture tend to use communication that is more global and based on standards external to the person, such as social position. Successful communication in this culture depends on the physical context and the cultural information internalized in the communicators. More of the message comes from nonverbal symbolization and cultural roles in the society.

Many Asian and some South American, French, Hispanic, African-American, and Native-American cultures share high-context culture characteristics. This cultural environment supports the development of persons who base their decisions on group input. Sometimes people from these cultures do not want to argue in public, use indirect language to communicate, and are also hesitant to make direct eye contact. Roles of women and men in some cultures determine appropriate interaction with professional persons or those outside the family (Harris, 2003). An example of communication conflict between members of high- and low-context cultures follows (Her and Culhane-Pera, 2004):

> A primary physician conducted a thorough examination of an elderly Asian non–English-speaking gentleman who was very ill. The physician informed the son about a plan of therapy that included additional diagnostic procedures, possible surgery or the use of long-term medication therapy, and monitoring. The son stated that he understood and thanked the physician for his help, and they would let him know their decision when his uncle arrived from Laos "sometime this year." The physician was shocked and questioned himself about what he had done incorrectly and what more he could have done to emphasize the severity of the father's condition.

The globalization effects created by social, political, educational, and economic interchanges have resulted in more acceptance of values held by Westernized low-context cultures by some of the high-context societies. Remember, however, that wide individual variations exist within any culture, and knowing that a client is from a particular culture is just a starting point.

Guidelines for Communicating With Non–English-Speaking Clients. Consider the following when interacting with clients (Box 7-3).

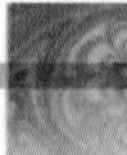

BOX 7-3

Guidelines for Communicating With Non–English-Speaking Clients

- Use interpreters rather than translators. Translators just restate the words from one language to another. An interpreter decodes the words and provides the meaning behind the message.
- Use dialect-specific interpreters whenever possible.
- Use interpreters trained in the health care field.
- Give the interpreter time alone with the client.
- Provide time for translation and interpretation.
- Be aware that interpreter's affect the reporting of symptoms, insert their own ideas, or omit information.
- Avoid the use of relatives, who sometimes distort information or are not objective.
- Avoid using children as interpreters, especially with sensitive topics.
- Use same-age and same-gender interpreters whenever possible.
- Maintain eye contact with both the client and the interpreter to elicit feedback and read nonverbal cues. (NOTE: Some cultures interpret constant eye contact as disrespectful or aggressive.)
- Remember that clients usually understand more than they express; thus, they need time to think in their own language. They are alert to the health care provider's body language, and they sometimes forget some or all of their English in times of stress.
- Speak slowly without exaggerated mouthing, allow time for translation, use the active rather than the passive tense, wait for feedback, and restate the message. Do not rush; do not speak loudly. Use a reference book with common phrases, such as *Roget's International Thesaurus* or *Taber's Cyclopedic Medical Dictionary.*
- Use as many words as possible in the client's language, and use nonverbal communication when you and the client are unable to understand each other's language.
- If an interpreter is unavailable, the use of a translator is acceptable. Be alert that translation sometimes leaves out parts of the message, distorts the message, sends information not given by the speaker, and sometimes the client does not fully understand the messages.

From Purnell LD, Paulanka BJ: *Transcultural health care,* Philadelphia, 1998, F.A. Davis, as cited in Catalano J: *Nursing Now! Today's issues, tomorrow's trends,* ed 2, Philadelphia, 2000, F. A. Davis. NOTE: Social class differences between the interpreter and the client sometimes results in the interpreter's not reporting information that he or she perceives as superstitious or unimportant.

Personal Space. Personal space, or territory, is an important consideration when interacting with individuals from various cultures. The space may be perceived as violated when the distance between two individuals is too close or too far away. In some cultures, such as the Jewish, Arab, Turkish, and Middle-Eastern, people are comfortable with standing closely when speaking to each other. These individuals may interpret an American health care provider as cold and distant (Catalano, 2000).

Touch. Touch also has different cultural meanings, ranging from implying a person's power or authority, anger, or sexual arousal, to expressing empathy and friendliness. Some consider touching inappropriate, and it is sometimes a cause of miscommunication. In some Arab cultures, men and women do not display affection or touch each other when in public. Some Native-American cultures interpret eye contact as "stealing the soul from the body." Mexican-American and other South American groups believe eye contact invokes the *mal de ojo*, or the evil eye. In some cultures, individuals embrace and kiss each other on both cheeks when greeting and again when departing. It is important to know the appropriate methods for greeting people, when touching such as a handshake is acceptable, or whether physical contact is forbidden. Some people perceive physical contact as inappropriate when a person from a different culture or gender performs a physical examination, takes a pulse, provides personal care, or performs a procedure. It is necessary to explain what is happening and the purpose before performing the physical contact. Some cultures, including some African and Arab groups, require that a hospitalized female client have a female companion present and be treated by only female health care providers (Catalano, 2000; personal experience).

Time Orientation. Time orientation is also a factor in communication with clients. In some cultures, time is of little importance and people from these cultures give little attention to the exact time of an appointment. Living in the present is the norm. In Western cultures, people are more future oriented and prefer designing plans, making schedules, and organizing activities. Differences in time orientation interfere with adherence to medication schedules and the treatment regimen, and may result in failure to meet the intended outcomes of long-term health care plans. Some health care providers are frustrated by this discrepancy and avoid talking with the client. When a breakdown in communication occurs, the client sometimes feels isolated, distrusts the provider, withdraws or becomes angry, and eventually abandons the health care system.

Biologic Characteristics. The assessment also considers biologic characteristics related to susceptibility to certain diseases, variability of skin and body structure, metabolism of medications, enzyme deficiencies, and high-risk behaviors such as smoking and substance addiction (Catalano, 2000). Later, the chapter will discuss assessing a person's spirituality beliefs.

Translation Services. Guidelines for obtaining translation services are important. Communicating an important and often complex health care matter is difficult without the use of the client's specific language. Nurses often use translation services, so a good interview question before accepting a position in a particular health care facility is whether professional translation services are available. It is important to acquire accurate translation, using an educated, credentialed, or certified translator if possible. Using a family member or additional hospital staff is often convenient but not recommended, because the client often wishes to avoid embarrassing the translator or revealing information that is culturally inappropriate. Many factors affect the accuracy of the translation, so the translator needs to take care to avoid bias. It is a good idea to use standard communication techniques when asking questions through an interpreter, beginning with general information and asking sensitive questions after establishing communication. Some communication patterns in low-context cultures use fewer words and more nonverbal communication. Therefore, it may seem as though the translator is not asking the questions posed by the interviewer. It is important to consider the communication context and preference of the client and translator. The care team needs to incorporate a plan of adequate translator involvement for sufficient ongoing assessment of the client's status. Important cultural needs also include dietary needs. In addition, reading materials, especially client education materials, need to be in the client's language.

SPIRITUALITY

It is often difficult to separate religious and spiritual values from ethnic and cultural beliefs. People often use the terms *religion* and *spirituality* synonymously. However, the nature of spirituality is broad and involves the search for answers to questions, such as the following:

- Why are we here?
- What am I supposed to be doing with my life?
- How am I to make meaning out of my suffering?
- What really happens to the soul after death?
- Why did this happen to me?
- Why is God punishing me?

Advances in technology, the global disasters, wars, threats of nuclear destruction, and the genome mapping project have created additional questions that are often disturbing to the integrity of the self and the meaning of life.

Spirituality is (1) an integrative energy that produces inner harmony or wholeness, (2) a sense of coherence, (3) the driving force that permeates all aspects that give meaning to life, (4) a sense of transcendence over reality—"drawing strength from inner resources, living fully for the present, a sense of inner knowing" (Catalano, 2000, p. 350). Spirituality provides a set of self-determined values that are the basis for living. Hope is a central concept of spirituality, and the faith factor helps provide coping skills. Religion is a personal set or institutionalized system of shared religious attitudes, beliefs, and practices (Koenig, 2004).

Faith is the belief and trust in God, or a supreme being. It is also the ability to draw on spiritual resources without having physical and empiric proof. It is an internal certainty that comes from one's own experience with the divine. Faith, although only a part of spirituality, is an essential component. It is through one's experience of faith that a deep individual spirituality assists one in the challenges and celebrations of life. The goals are as follows:

- Provide an image of the divine
- Provide an image of humanity
- Provide an understanding of the relationship between the divine and humanity
- Help to examine thoughts of divine punishment, reward, or neutrality
- Help to give belief and meaning to life
- Help to find a sense of duty, vocation, calling, or moral obligation
- Help to examine one's experience of the divine and sacred
- Help to cope with situations and conflict with spiritual understanding
- Provide a format for spiritual rituals and practices
- Provide a faith community
- Provide authority and guidance for one's system of belief, meaning, and ritual

Religion usually includes a set of beliefs that aid in explaining the meaning of life, suffering, health, and illness. A *religious perspective* of spirituality views the soul as a means of relating to a supreme being and to others. Some call the supreme being the divine creator of the universe, God, a divine mystery, or use other similar names. Religious practices nurture the soul. Religion determines the important rituals that are meaningful during transitions in life, the type of foods to eat, times for fasting, and services to attend. Examples of rituals surrounding the birth process include baptism of the infant at a specific time, circumcision, postpartum practices for the new mother, and a specific burial site for the placenta. Certain traditional rites of passage into adulthood are honored, as well as the rituals surrounding death.

Some express spirituality by participating in an organized religious community and by adhering to a set of rules of behavior. Traditional spiritual healing practices include the use of prayer, meditation, fasting, belonging to religious support groups, reading scriptures and religious literature, and listening to inspiring music. One study revealed that 63% of the individuals who responded indicated they wanted their spiritual needs considered in the plan of care (Myerstein, 2004).

A *secular perspective* of spirituality is made up of a set of positive values—such as love, honesty, truth, optimism, and others—that the person chooses as a standard or purpose to live by. The person renews spirituality through loving relationships; through experiencing the beauty of nature, art, music, poetry, and literature; and other activities that assist in fulfilling life goals. The soul does not need to be a religious concept. The soul is an image of the person that extends beyond the physical self such as an energy field or aura that is characterized by a color and movement. The soul is often considered as a life force, referred to as *chi* in the Chinese culture, as *ki* in the Japanese culture, and as *prana* in Indian faith systems. Reiki, shiatsu, and therapeutic touch are practices that renew or balance the energy force. Some believe the use of herbs, aroma therapy, and others provides a balance between all living things, the earth, and the universe (Catalano, 2000).

Some major spiritual considerations include the fear of death and loss, both of self and others. Spirituality allows one to cope with these feelings by providing a sense of hope and meaning to experiences that would otherwise be crippling. Having a spiritual understanding that one's connection with creation is more than merely a physical existence helps to ease the fear and pain of loss. Feeling connected to the divine eases feelings of abandonment, grief, and alienation and promotes self-acceptance. Spirituality is often a key component in the healing process and an integral part of the client's treatment plan.

Significant spiritual questions tend to remain constant, regardless of the health care need. Issues such as loss, fear, death, abandonment, and feelings of alienation are sometimes present in clients who have both physical and psychiatric illnesses. Responses to these feelings range from finding new meanings and strength, to acceptance, to grief, to a sense of hopelessness. An objective in a spiritual intervention is to first acknowledge and validate these feelings and then help the client consider ways to rewrite his or her life story in a way that includes these experiences. One's spirituality can be a significant help during these times.

A spiritual crisis may occur when religious or spiritual beliefs conflict with a necessary procedure or a treatment protocol, such as agreeing to a therapeutic abortion, permitting a blood transfusion, or making end-of-life decisions. Situational spiritual distress is sometimes related to the death or illness of a significant other person, beliefs that the family, peers, or health care providers oppose, or to other separations such as divorce. Spiritual distress also occurs when a person is separated from spiritual or cultural support systems and when personal beliefs and values are challenged. In some cases, spiritual beliefs and practices are harmful to a person's mental and physical health (Meyerstein, 2004; Carpenito, 2002).

Spiritual Support

Before caregivers provide effective spiritual interventions, it is critical to identify people who are at significant spiritual risk. *Spiritual distress* is a nursing diagnosis that is defined as "the state in which the individual or group experiences a disturbance in the belief or value system that provides strength, hope, and meaning to life" (Carpenito, 2002, p. 897). Individuals at spiritual risk are those who have a high spiritual need, coupled with low spiritual resources to meet that need. These individuals have more risk for poor outcomes and are the primary focus for outcome-based spiritual care (Koenig, 2004).

The traditional definitions of mental health and illness differ among cultures and individuals. However, many cultural beliefs do not separate illnesses of the body from illnesses of the mind. Ancient beliefs attributed illnesses of the body or mind to the work of evil spirits outside the body, such as witchcraft and voodoo curses, or through evil spirits that entered the body or mind. Some societies believed that evil was caused by someone within the community who was "different." That person was punished or removed from the community, and then a cure could be found. Special healers used their skills to remove the power of the spirits. Healing methods included, among others, the use of purgatives, bloodletting, the application of leeches, and herbal mixtures. Sometimes groups have said special prayers and incantations and made sacrifices on the ill person's behalf. Modern societies consider these practices primitive. However, some people consider these traditions sacred and continue using the cultural practices. Today, some religious faiths promote praying to saints, lighting candles, making pilgrimages to shrines, and anointing with oil. Faith healers and practitioners of therapeutic touch often perform the "laying on of hands" as a healing practice.

Culturally competent care includes providing spiritual support and pastoral counseling to clients in the psychiatric setting. The provision of these services and assurance of access for all clients is a standard set forth by credentialing organizations. In general, one of the pastoral services offered by institutions or within communities is to contact appropriate representatives of the client's faith tradition. Having these services available is often of great comfort to the mentally ill. Certified pastoral counselors (CPCs) are skilled in communicating with mentally ill persons. The nurse's role is to find out if clients wish to make use of these persons by visitation, prayer, or other faith tradition. Part of the typical psychiatric intake assessment includes determining whether there are any spiritual or religious concerns. Usually the nurse will contact a representative of the client's faith tradition to meet with the client or the health care team to discuss the client's preferences and concerns and make plans to meet the individual's needs.

Visits from a religious practitioner often comforts clients with depression or who are in crisis. Frequently, representatives of faith traditions such as elders, rabbis, priests, ministers, imams (for followers of the Islam [Moslem] faith), and other spiritual leaders come to psychiatric units to visit people from their communities. Occasionally, individuals with serious mental disorders experience delusions that are spiritual or religious. As explained in Chapter 12, challenging or debating the truth of a person's delusions is not therapeutic, and spiritual delusions are no exception. The nurse does not agree with the client's delusions but avoids arguing or debating the specifics of a delusion and focuses on decreasing the person's anxiety or agitation.

Nurses need to be consciously aware of their own personal beliefs or lack of beliefs about spirituality and religion and not impose them on clients. Nurses remain neutral and unbiased. For example, advising the client that a particular spiritual practice will cure a mental illness is inappropriate, even if the nurse believes this is true. Engaging in spiritual or religious practice with individuals on a psychiatric unit is also inappropriate. The nurse elicits information about what is causing the person distress without discussing specific spiritual or religious content. CPCs are skilled in counseling clients and consulting with staff about these problems and assist the health care team in ways to address particular concerns of individual clients. Many times, an individual will make a decision that is difficult for the health care provider to accept. In some settings, the CPC will meet with the staff to assist them in understanding and accepting what they believe are controversial decisions made by the clients and their families (Catalano, 2000).

Intervention Tools

There are a variety of spiritual interventions for use that range from formal to informal rituals and practices. For example, formal Christian rituals include sacraments, such as baptism, communion, and anointing. Additional formal practices include worship or memorial services, as well as formal confession and absolution. On many of these occasions, a chaplain involves members of a local faith community, either in a leadership or a support role. Often the agency chaplain is in contact with local worship communities to provide appropriate information for formal prayer services at a local church or synagogue when requested by a client.

Informal rituals and practices include pastoral counseling, the use of individual or group prayer at the hospital, the reading of scripture, and the distribution of devotional books, cards, and other related materials. The use of rosaries or prayer beads, the playing of music, and the use of icons or pictures often allow clients to express the more experiential, noncognitive side of their spirituality. Some individuals use visual imagery, such as in the telling of sacred stories from various traditions. Access to audiotapes and videotapes of the client's own religious community worship services or activities can be especially helpful.

Religious practices often are beneficial for clients, but for those who do not have a formal religion, other spiritual interventions are useful. Group therapies that encourage clients to extend themselves and to find meaning in life are helpful. In addition, several other creative forms of expression such as art, music, and dance therapy often address clients' spiritual needs.

Spiritual Assessment

Assessing an individual's spiritual need and determining interventions that will be helpful and appropriate in addressing that need is an essential component of a chaplain's role in a health care system. Discovering the client's perception of his or her spirituality requires the ability to acknowledge your own biases and a willingness to put them aside during the interaction.

A pastor or chaplain usually addresses spirituality. If there is no pastoral care department in the facility, and if the client has no specific faith community, these spiritual issues may not be addressed. Even in cases where the client has a faith community, some are reluctant to examine areas of spirituality that deal with mental illness. Therefore, nursing interventions that address spirituality are important. Box 7-4 provides a spiritual assessment tool.

Other helpful assessments focus on the items listed here. The core factors underlying this assessment model are *belief* and *meaning*. An individual views life in terms of what he or she perceives is important and gives meaning to life. Some areas the interviewer will consider are as follows:

- What beliefs does the person have that give meaning and purpose to life?
- What are the important symbols that reflect these beliefs?
- How does the person's life story reflect or demonstrate these underlying themes?
- Do any areas of the person's life story come into conflict with these underlying, foundational beliefs?
- Do any current situations or problems come into direct conflict with these beliefs?
- Is the person able to consciously communicate these beliefs?
- In what ways are these beliefs an unconscious part of the person's worldview?

Vocation and Obligation

Out of one's perception of belief and meaning comes a sense of how to live life. The following axis is closely linked to the one presented earlier and demonstrates that people usually do what they consider important. If a task, action, or thought has no meaning, the person is much less likely to do that action or to follow through on

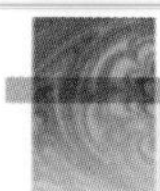

BOX 7-4

Spiritual Assessment Tool

The following reflective questions may assist you in assessing, evaluating, and increasing awareness of spirituality in yourself and others.

MEANING AND PURPOSE

These questions assess a person's ability to seek meaning and fulfillment in life, manifest hope, and accept ambiguity and uncertainty:
What gives your life meaning?
Do you have a sense of purpose in life?
Does your illness interfere with your life goals?
Why do you want to get well?
How hopeful are you about obtaining a better degree of health?
Do you feel that you have a responsibility in maintaining your health?
Will you be able to make changes in your life to maintain your health?
Are you motivated to get well?
What is the most important or powerful thing in your life?

INNER STRENGTHS

These questions assess a person's ability to manifest joy and recognize strengths, choices, goals, and faith:
What brings you joy and peace in your life?
What can you do to feel alive and full of spirit?
What traits do you like in yourself?
What are your personal strengths?
What choices are available to you to enhance your healing?
What life goals have you set for yourself?
Do you think that stress in any way caused your illness?
How aware were you of your body before you became sick?
What do you believe in?
Is faith important in your life?
How has your illness influenced your faith?
Does faith play a role in your health?

INTERCONNECTIONS

These questions assess a person's positive self-concept, self-esteem, and sense of self; sense of belonging in the world with others; capacity to pursue personal interests; and ability to demonstrate love of self and self-forgiveness:
How do you feel about yourself right now?
How do you feel when you have a true sense of yourself?
Do you pursue things of personal interest?
What do you do to show love for yourself?
Can you forgive yourself?
What do you do to heal your spirit?

These questions assess a person's ability to connect in life-giving ways with family, friends, and social groups and to forgive others:
Who are the significant people in your life?
Do you have friends or family in town who are available to help you?
Who are the people to whom you are closest?
Do you belong to any groups?
Can you ask people for help when you need it?
Can you share your feelings with others?
What are some of the most loving things that others have done for you?
What are the loving things that you do for other people?
Are you able to forgive others?

These questions assess a person's capacity for finding meaning in worship or religious activities and a connectedness with a divinity:
Is worship important to you?
What do you consider the most significant act of worship in your life?
Do you participate in any religious activities?
Do you believe in God or a higher power?
Do you think that prayer is powerful?
Have you ever tried to empty your mind of all thoughts to see what the experience might be?
Do you use relaxation or imagery skills?
Do you meditate?
Do you pray?
What is your prayer?
How are your prayers answered?
Do you have a sense of belonging in this world?

These questions assess a person's ability to experience a connection with life and nature, an awareness of the effects of the environment on life and well-being, and a capacity for concern for the health of the environment:
Do you feel a connection with the world or universe?
Are you concerned about the survival of the planet?
How does your environment impact your state of well-being?
What are your environmental stressors at work and at home?
What strategies reduce your environmental stressors?
Do you have any concerns for the state of your immediate environment?
Are you involved with environmental issues such as recycling environmental resources at home, work, or in your community?

From Dossey BM: Holistic modalities and healing moments, *Am J Nurs* 6:44, 1998. SOURCES: Burkhardt MA: Spirituality: an analysis of the concept, *Holist Nurs Pract* 3:69, 1989; Dossey BM et al, editors: *Holistic nursing: a handbook for practice*, ed 2, Gaithersburg, Md, 1995, Aspen.

thoughts about that task. When life circumstances place the person in a position where actions come into conflict with core beliefs and meaning systems, crisis and significant stress may result. The following questions are included in this axis:

- What sense of duty, vocation, calling, or moral obligation does this person have?
- How actively has this client been able to express these in the past?
- What impact does the client's current situation/illness have on these perceptions?

Experience

The person examines both hopeful and worrisome questions that surround the emotional experiences of a person of faith. Questions to examine in this axis include the following:

- What experience of the divine or sacred has this person had?
- What emotions or moods are associated with these contacts?
- How does the client's current situation relate to these experiences?

Courage and Growth

This axis examines how the person adapts to situations that confront and conflict with the client's core beliefs and meanings. Questions in this axis examine how a client may deal with extremely stressful and challenging issues and include the following:

- How spiritually adaptable is the client?
- How has the client coped in the past with situations that were in conflict with his or her current spiritual understanding?
- Must new experiences fit into existing belief systems, or can the person's beliefs adapt with new experiences?
- How concrete is the person's spirituality?
- How adaptable is the person currently?

Ritual and Practice

- What are the spiritual rituals and practices of this individual?
- Are they formal or informal?
- Does the individual experience them on a regular basis?
- How do they support the individual?
- How do the client's current circumstances affect these rituals?

Community

- *Family of origin.* How did the client's family of origin share spiritual experiences?
- *Current family structure.* How does the client's current family share spiritual experiences? How does the client view participation in a faith community?
- *Faith community of origin.* How formal was the client's faith community of origin? How informal? How active or inactive was the client?
- *Current faith community.* How formal is the client's current faith community? How informal? How active or inactive is the client?

Authority and Guidance

- What is the source of this client's system of belief, meaning, and ritual?
- When faced with problems, tragedy, or doubt, where does the client look for guidance?
- Does the client look for answers from internal or external sources?
- Is this source fixed, or is it flexible? (Fitchett, 1997)

Stages of Faith

A key concept in understanding spiritual development is that a person's faith tends to become internalized as one develops. During development, one's sense of faith, meaning, moral values, and judgment moves from an external locus of control to an internal locus of control. In determining how best to assist a client in using his or her spirituality to address mental illness, it is essential to determine the client's stage of spiritual development. This is important for determining what interventions, if any, are appropriate. Several significant models of both faith development and moral/spiritual development will help inform a chaplain of the client's spiritual needs.

The first model is James Fowler's (1981) stages of religious development theory (Box 7-5). In this theory, Fowler states that an individual passes through various stages in a linear fashion, based on age. This theory is much like many of the other individual development theories.

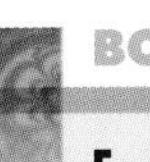

BOX 7-5

Fowler's Stages of Religious Development

STAGE 1: INTUITIVE-PROJECTIVE FAITH
A developmental stage that begins in early childhood
Intuitive images of good and evil
Fantasy and reality are the same

STAGE 2: MYTHICAL-LYRICAL FAITH
A developmental stage that can begin in middle to late childhood
More logical, concrete thought
Literal interpretation of religious stories
God is like a parent figure

STAGE 3: SYNTHETIC-CONVENTIONAL FAITH
A developmental stage that can begin in early adolescence
More abstract thought
Conformity to the religious beliefs of others

STAGE 4: INDIVIDUATING-REFLEXIVE FAITH
A developmental stage that can begin in late adolescence to early adulthood
Individuals begin to take full responsibility for their religious beliefs
In-depth exploration of one's values and religious beliefs

STAGE 5: CONJUNCTIVE FAITH
A developmental stage that can begin in middle adulthood
Individuals become more open to paradox and opposing viewpoints
Stems from awareness of one's finiteness and limitations

STAGE 6: UNIVERSALIZING FAITH
A developmental stage that can begin in late adulthood
Individuals transcend belief systems to achieve a sense of oneness with all beings
Conflict events are no longer viewed as paradoxes

Stages of Moral Development

A second important model that helps assess a client's spirituality and how illness or the current situation has challenged the client's spirituality is Kohlberg's six stages of moral development theory. Kohlberg theorized that individuals move, in a linear fashion with age, through key areas of faith and spiritual reasoning. The theory indicates that individuals all move through one or more of the following stages:

Preconventional	I. Avoids breaking rules to avoid punishment
	II. Bases moral action on satisfying needs
Conventional	I. Pleases others and does what is expected
	II. Maintains order and follows the law

Postconventional	I. Determines moral actions based on individual rights and community standards
	II. Believes in universal ethical principles that can guide actions

Based on the work of Kohlberg and Fowler, the following model looks at four areas of spirituality, each having implications for effective pastoral interventions.

Impartial Spirituality

- They believe individuals are amoral.
- They tend to do things in their own interest. ("What's in it for me?")
- They are generally individuals who are not involved in faith communities.
- Some have a casual, cultural acquaintance with a formal faith community.
- They represent a significant minority of the population.

Institutional Spirituality

- These individuals are regular church attendees.
- They follow institutional rules.
- They do things because they are told to do them.
- They follow a good person/bad person concept.
- They probably make up the largest percentage of the population.

Individual Spirituality

- These individuals are seekers who have left a formal religious community.
- They often challenge the beliefs of formal religious communities.
- They seek new answers or personal answers to questions, problems, or crises.
- They appear on the surface to be in the impartial stage of faith.
- They represent a smaller minority of the population.

Integrated Spirituality

- These individuals have internalized their faith.
- These people obey rules because they fully accept them and feel that they are just and right.
- They may or may not belong to formal faith communities.
- They are seen as teachers or mystics.
- They make up a very small percentage of the population.

An accurate assessment of the client's stage of faith is important. It helps determine the type of interventions a nurse will use. As always, these models also have their limitations, and individuals tend to move along a continuum of spirituality and faith rather than being locked into a particular stage. In some instances, a crisis is the initiator of a person's movement, in either direction along the continuum. An individual in the first stage might likely be operating out of a "bargaining" position when dealing with a spiritual crisis that questions a core meaning held by the individual. An intervention that helped that individual become connected with a faith group, perhaps a return to a youthful experience of faith, provides some additional spiritual tools that were not otherwise available to the person. It is probably less effective to attempt to use interventions that encouraged and supported challenges to existing spiritual norms for a person in either the first or second stage, but it is an effective intervention to use when dealing with an individual in the third stage. For individuals who are in the fourth stage, who are often older adults, the best possible pastoral intervention is in learning from them and accepting their unique spiritual legacy.

Selected Cases of Clinical Spiritual Interventions

Pain

Kathleen, a client with depression and anxiety, also had a serious case of pancreatitis, which required an inpatient stay of about 30 days. A few weeks after her discharge, she returned to talk. As she talked, she confessed that the experience had made a significant impact on her faith and spiritual viewpoint. When faced with agonizing pain for the first time in her life, this middle-aged woman confided that the physical agony she felt connected her emotionally for the first time with the concept of "torment and damnation." Although her existing spiritual beliefs helped her to cope with the symptoms of her illnesses, the experience of excruciating pain caused her to question some of the fundamental spiritual principles that had guided her up to that point. Especially challenged during this illness was her understanding of the relationship between the divine and humanity, and her concept of ultimate punishment and reward.

Spiritual Torment

Steven, a devout Mormon in his mid-50s, was in spiritual torment. His permanent developmental delay, coupled with his bipolar illness, had prevented him from marrying. His own understanding of his religious principles, whether or not they were completely accurate according to that faith tradition, led him to believe that he would never "be able to enter heaven." He usually made this statement as part of a tearful, tormented lament. His own strong faith was "punishing" him. An appropriate intervention in this case was to listen to and acknowledge Steven's pain and help connect him with responsible members of his faith community with whom he could discuss his concerns.

Punishment

Mary, a woman in her mid-50s, was a devout Catholic. She believed that her lifelong bouts of major depression were an appropriate "punishment" for the sexual abuse she had experienced as a child. She clung to the belief that she was responsible for the abuse and that the attention she received and the enjoyment she felt at the time only confirmed her worthlessness and lack of capacity to be loved as an adult. In this case, where Mary deeply believed in her denominational faith system, religious authority figures spoke with much more authority than either physicians or other health care team members. Mary was introduced to an empathetic priest who was also a trained psychotherapist. The interventions all centered on Mary's own belief system and included helping Mary to see herself as a survivor of abuse rather than as the responsible party. A sacramental ritual particular to her denomination was also included to eliminate Mary's deeply held "need" to be punished.

Voices

Fred, a patient with schizophrenia and a member of a charismatic Protestant group, stated that he had the "gift of wisdom." Fred's schizophrenic symptoms included auditory hallucinations. On further discussion, Fred revealed that during worship services it was quite common for him and others to rise and to "speak in tongues," a regular occurrence within his denomination. He also revealed that the voices he heard were negative and frequently told him to harm himself. In Fred's case, the hospital chaplain provided the interventions. Without challenging the faith experience that Fred described having during worship services, the chaplain was able to help Fred see a difference between the negative voices that told him to harm himself and any prophetic experience that Fred had within the understanding of his own religious concepts. From this distinction, Fred's reluctance to maintain his antipsychotic medication regimen diminished. This improved medication maintenance gave Fred a better quality of life and fewer hospitalizations.

Guilt

Terry, a woman in her mid-40s with bipolar disorder, felt guilty because of how she behaved during previous manic phases of her illness. These actions included both risky sexual behaviors and irresponsibility with her finances. Terry came from a mainstream, liturgical Protestant tradition whose culture had emphasized both "personal responsibility" and "spiritual consequences" for one's own actions. Terry believed that she was "condemned" and that there was nothing she could do to change that. In ongoing discussions, the nurse educated Terry about her illness and instructed her on how to manage her symptoms more effectively by correctly using and monitoring her medications. Terry was eventually able to view her illness in the same way she viewed a chronic physical illness, such as diabetes. This decreased her feelings of guilt. To help maintain her medication compliance, Terry also began to incorporate part of her faith tradition in her ongoing care by using the daily prayer rituals of her faith to help her take her medication.

Hyperreligiosity

Hank, a religiously preoccupied individual with schizoaffective disorder, often lectured others when anyone engaged him in conversation. Any attempt to relate to Hank using the more traditional religious language of his own faith background caused him to begin a long, rambling, confused, and pressured ranting about his "special connection" to God "as a prophet." To engage Hank in spiritual discussions for either assessment or intervention purposes, it was necessary to use language that he did not identify as religious. By engaging Hank in discussions about meaningful areas of spirituality in ordinary language rather than spiritual language, the staff avoided the words that usually triggered Hank's tangential responses. He then had more meaningful conversations with staff.

SELECTED TRADITIONAL AND CULTURAL MENTAL HEALTH BELIEFS

In some cultures there is no distinction between physical or mental illness. Symptoms are somaticized by complaints of fatigue, dizziness, weight loss, nausea, headache, chest pain, or insomnia. Some African Americans consider stress as source of physical problems. Latinos often view the person with mental illness as a victim of circumstances with no responsibility for the illness, such as a blow on the head, a sudden fright, anxiety, or witchcraft. People from some cultures believe alcohol or drug addiction is due to a moral weakness. Puerto Ricans perceive evil spirits as the cause of mental illness. Mental illness is a cause of shame for Chinese and Japanese families. In some cultures, people seek help only when psychosomatic symptoms appear.

An overview of mental health beliefs and practices from different selected cultures follows. This information is not intended to stereotype any group, but merely to describe the known traditional means that some members or families of a given group use to cope with a mental health problem.

American Indian Communities

The traditional belief equates health with living in total harmony with nature and possessing the ability to survive under exceedingly difficult circumstances. Evil spirits and witchcraft are sometimes the causes of illness. The medicine man or woman may chew on the root of jimson weed that induces a trancelike state and a vision to identify the specific evil cause of the person's illness. In some tribes, the healer builds a sand painting or sprinkles pollen around the sick person and then sits in meditation about the possible causes of the illness. Personal observation of the traditional Navajo squaw dance ceremonies or the Hopi butterfly dance demonstrates the importance of these rituals. The government hospitals on Navajo reservations include a Hogan for the medicine man to use when treating clients.

Remedies include purification ceremonies, immersion in water, and the use of sweat lodges, herbal medicines, and special rituals. Singers chant to ease the spirit of the sick person. Purification "awakens the body and the senses and prepares a person for meditation" (Spector, 2003, p. 181).

Mental illness includes "ghost sickness," a preoccupation with death and the deceased person that is thought to be due to witchcraft. Alcohol addiction, suicide, and domestic violence are major mental health problems.

Asian/Pacific Islander Communities

The Asian/Pacific Islander populations are a diverse mixture of people from many cultures who speak multiple languages. In addition several dialects are often spoken within cultures, further limiting communication between groups. The nations of origin include China, Japan, Hawaii, the Philippines, Vietnam, Asian India, Korea,

Samoa, Guam, and the remaining Asian/Pacific islands. Health is a state of spiritual and physical well-being—a harmony with nature, a balance of the forces of yin (the inner body, or viscera, or the front of the body) and yang (the outer surface of body or the back part of the body). Yin restores life strength, and yang protects the body from outside forces. The person lives in peaceful interaction between mind and body when the forces are in balance. The universe is indivisible, and each person has a function within it. Health care practices are based on the ancient philosophies of Buddha, Confucius, and Tao; most of the people use versions of Chinese medicine such as acupuncture, acupressure, massage, moxibustion (application of heat), cupping, bleeding using leeches, herbal remedies, and consultation with traditional healers (see Chapter 25).

Mental illness creates stigma and shame for the family, and the family often cares for the client in private. Individuals often seek health care much later in the course of the disease with a feeling of hopelessness. Mental illnesses are often identified in somatic terms. The illnesses include the *anger syndrome* caused by the suppression of anger, anxiety, paranoia symptoms, compulsive neuroses, depression, and fear that body or its functions will be offensive to others (Spector, 2003).

Black American (African-American) Communities

Members of the black American communities in the United States have their origins in Africa and a cultural heritage that is a mixture of the Caribbean, Native American, and northern European cultures. In 2000, there were 34,659,190 African Americans in the United States, or 12.3% of the total population, and approximately one-third were reported as living in poverty (U.S. Census Bureau, 1999).

In this culture, health means a harmony with nature. The body, mind, and spirit are one entity. Illness is due to demons or spirits or by actions of the person's own accord. The family often has a matriarchal structure, and there are strong, large, extended family networks. There is a continuation of tradition and a strong religious connection within the community. Prayer and the laying on of hands are common methods for treating illness. Many black Americans tend to use traditional medicines and healers to treat physical and mental illnesses when they are knowledgeable in this area and have access to this resource. Several diagnostic techniques include the use of biblical phrases and material from folk medicine books, observation, and entering the spirit of the client. Some black Americans stay away from health clinics because they do not trust the system, feel discriminated, or lack funds.

Individuals who follow the Muslim faith believe that foods affect thoughts and behaviors; therefore, they eat kosher foods to protect from illnesses. Fasting is a part of traditional celebrations such as Ramadan.

Voodoo is a traditional practice of white magic (harmless magic) and black magic (dangerous magic). Slaves from the West Indies brought voodoo to the United States in the late 1700s and early 1800s. Some integrated the rituals and practices into Christian rituals used by some black communities today. Some black people attribute their illness to a "fix" or a "hex" put on them by a person who is angry with them. Bad voodoo is greatly feared. A voodoo priest or elderly woman healer sometimes uses herbal remedies to treat mental illnesses.

Hispanic Communities

Hispanic communities include Mexico, Puerto Rico, Cuba, Central and South America, and Spain as their countries of origin. These groups of people are the fastest growing group in the United States. The term *Chicano* is used as a universal identifier of all Americans of Mexican descent. Their belief is that the natural world is not separated from the supernatural world. The traditional definition of health is related to good luck, a reward for good behavior, or a gift from God. To maintain health, individuals wear religious medals or amulets, have relics in the home, and attend religious services and prayer. Herbs and spices help to prevent illness, which is an imbalance in the body or a punishment for wrongdoing. Meals consist of a combination of hot (spicy) and cold (nonspicy) foods to maintain a balance.

There are subtle differences among the Spanish groups regarding the classification of illness, its causes, and treatment. Illness is caused by an imbalance of hot and cold or wet and dry substances. Other causes are external magic or supernatural forces, such as casting the "mal ojo," the "evil eye"; development of a strong emotional state from fright, and soul loss or envy and bad luck. Some people believe that evil spirits or forces cause mental illness. Folk healers, or *curanderos*, are well known within their communities for their holistic services with roots in Aztec, Spanish, spiritualistic, homoeopathic, and scientific elements. The *curandero* may be born with the gift of healing, learns by apprenticeship especially in the use of herbs, or receives a calling to be a healer. The *Santeria* or *Santero*, folk healer for Puerto Ricans, use storytelling to help people cope with daily difficulties.

Religious rituals are common healing practices. The types of practices include making promises, visiting shrines, and offering candles, medals, flowers and prayers to saints. Altars, shrines, and pictures of saints are placed in many homes.

Mental illnesses are thought to be hereditary; others occur because of a hex, worry, fright, or injury. Emotional illnesses are believed to be due to jealousy or rage. Drug addiction is a vice or a moral illness and others will judge the person for immoral behaviors (Spector, 2003).

Communities of European Origin

Members of this community have origins throughout Europe and in 2003 made up 15% of the foreign-born population of the United States (www.census.gov). The 2000 census counted 211,460,626 people who indicated their heritage as European, or 75.1% of the total U.S.

population. Those noting two races (Caucasian was one) constituted 77.1% of the population. In general, this population expresses a low-context cultural heritage and speaks a variety of languages. They typically value individual strengths and independence and do not emphasize community identification as much as some of the other groups. Traditional religious practice is common, and many nationalities are represented in this group. Careful assessment, as in all the other groups, is key to understanding the individual. Individuals in this population often seek traditional medical care; many use alternative health care before seeking allopathic treatment. This culture is beginning to have a clearer understanding of mental illness, but many still view it as a moral failing.

The Jewish population is a subculture of the European population even though many of the Jews emigrated from countries from all over the world. There is an emphasis on community and multigenerational continuity. Most Jews celebrate the important religious holidays. The religious beliefs range from completely secular to the orthodox traditions. Some of the aging survivors of the Holocaust experience *survivor guilt* and present symptoms of chronic posttraumatic stress disorder. In biblical times, they perceived mental illness as demon possession; visions were proof of contact with the divine. Currently, some still view mental illness as punishment for disobedience, creating a social stigma; however, there is more acceptance of therapeutic measures. The most common mental symptoms include paranoia and neuroses. The patterns of illness are related to religious and cultural experiences. Certain holidays, such as days of mourning, are triggers for dysfunctional mental symptoms including suicidal thoughts.

Healing practices include prayer, reading Psalms and religious texts, participating in religious rituals, and activities that provide a distance and the opportunity to reflect and find new options (Myerstein, 2004).

THE ROLE OF THE NURSE

Nursing traditionally maintains a holistic view when caring for clients and their families and has incorporated cultural and spiritual content within the academic context and in all levels of actual client care, including all phases of the nursing process and discharge planning. Psychiatry also now recognizes the necessity for inclusion of cultural and spiritual content. The *Diagnostic and Statistical Manual of Mental Disorders* (DSM-IV-TR) includes several problems that may cause noncompliance with treatment. Among those are client's personal cultural or religious beliefs, values, and judgments concerning the advantages and disadvantages of accepting a treatment regimen (APA, 2000). In the first report on mental health by the United States surgeon general, multiple entries appear that emphasize the influence of culture and spirituality in the role of mental wellness and illness (U.S. Department of Health and Human Services, 1999). The report covers many aspects of mental health and mental illness that the American Psychiatric Association will address in upcoming decades.

Definitions of mental health and illness, as well as entire concepts of mental health and illness, are different within different societal structures. The DSM-IV-TR (APA, 2000) provides information about syndromes that occur in particular cultures (culture-bound syndromes) (Table 7-3).

The purpose of cultural competence is to ensure that the nurse gives clients of all cultures every opportunity to

Text continued on p. 148

TABLE 7-3

Culture-Bound Syndromes

CULTURE	IDIOM	BEHAVIOR	POTENTIAL RELATIONSHIP WITH DSM-IV-TR AXIS CLASSIFICATION
Malaysia Polynesia Puerto Rico Navajo Indian	*Amok* *Cafard* or *cathard* *Mal de pelea* *Iich'aa*	Brooding, episodes of intrusive thoughts, violent outbursts, aggressive behavior followed by exhaustion, amnesia	Occurs at onset or exacerbation of a chronic psychotic process or during a brief psychotic episode
Latino (especially women from the Caribbean and Latin Mediterranean people)	*Atique de nervios*	Uncontrollable screaming, crying, trembling May exhibit aggressive behavior Fainting and seizures sometimes occur Suicide intent Behaviors frequently occur after stressful event related to the person's family	Anxiety, mood, dissociation, or somatoform disorders Distinguished from panic attack classification by no expressions of fear or apprehension
Latino	*Bilis, colerea, muina*	Perceived cause is inner core imbalance (of hot/cold or material/spiritual) caused by suppression of anger or rage Symptoms: headache, nervous tension, trembling, screaming, gastric upset; possible loss of consciousness Chronic fatigue after acute episode	

Data from American Psychological Association: *Diagnostic and statistical manual of mental disorders*, ed 4, Washington, DC, 2000, American Psychological Association; US Department of Health and Human Services and SAMSHA: web resources 2006; www.mentalhealth.samhsa.gov.

Continued

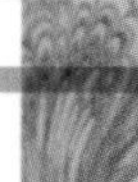

TABLE 7-3

Culture-Bound Syndromes, cont'd

CULTURE	IDIOM	BEHAVIOR	POTENTIAL RELATIONSHIP WITH DSM-IV-TR AXIS CLASSIFICATION
West Africa, Haiti	*Boufee delirante*	Sudden outburst of agitation, aggressive behavior, confusion, jerky movements May have hallucinations (visual and auditory) and paranoid behavior	Resembles brief psychotic disorder episode
West Africa	*Brain fag, brain tiredness*	Difficulty concentrating or remembering; feeling that brain is "fatigued" Other somatic symptoms include pain, pressure in head/neck, blurred vision, heat or burning Often expressed by high school or university students	Resembles symptoms of anxiety, depressive, and somatoform disorders
Far East, India, Sri Lanka, China	Folk term *Dhat* (or *jiryan*) *Sukrapraena* *Shen-k uei*	Severe anxiety associated with weakness, exhaustion and discharge of semen, white discoloration of urine	
Southern United States and Caribbean groups	Falling out Blacking out	Sudden collapse (usually preceded by dizziness or "swimming in the head") Temporary loss of vision Feels paralyzed	Compared to conversion disorder or dissociation disorder
Several American Indian tribes	Ghost sickness	Preoccupation with death or deceased Fear of danger Anxiety, hallucinations, confusion, anorexia, fainting, dizziness	
Korean folk syndrome	*Hwa-byung (wool-hwa-byung)* English term: anger syndrome	Caused by suppression of anger Insomnia, panic, fear of impending death, palpitations, dyspnea, chest pressure, indigestion, generalized aches and pain	
Malaysia China Assam Thailand	*Koro* (and other local terms) *Shuk yang, shook yong* *Jinjinia bemar* *Rok-joo*	Sudden severe anxiety that penis (vulva and nipples in female) will recede into body and be possible cause of death	Symptoms meet criteria for a DSM-IV-TR mood or anxiety disorder Diagnosis included in *Chinese Classification of Mental Disorders* (CCMD-2)
Malaysia, Indonesia Siberian groups Thailand Ainu, Sakhalin, Japan Philippines	*Latah* *Amurakh, irkunii, ikota, olan, myriachit, menkeiti* *Bah tschi, bah-tsi, baah-ji* *Imu* *Mali-mali, silok*	Syndrome seen in many parts of the world More prevalent in middle-aged females in Malaysia Dissociation/trancelike behavior Echolalia (parrot-like repetitions); echopraxia (imitation of actions of others)	Dissociation disorder
Latino (United States and Latin America)	*Locura*	Severe form of psychosis Possibly caused by inherited or vulnerability to many life difficulties Poor social skills Auditory and visual hallucinations, unpredictable behavior Some exhibit violent behavior	
Mediterranean cultures and other parts of the world	*Mal de ojo* (evil eye)	Children are especially vulnerable; also seen in women Sleep disturbances; crying, diarrhea, vomiting, fever in child or infant	

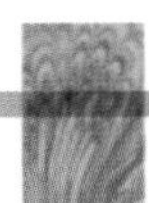

TABLE 7-3

Culture-Bound Syndromes, cont'd

CULTURE	IDIOM	BEHAVIOR	POTENTIAL RELATIONSHIP WITH DSM-IV-TR AXIS CLASSIFICATION
Latino (United States and Latin America) Greeks in North America	*Nervios* *Nevra*	Broad term to describe vulnerability to stressful life experiences Headache (brain aches), irritability, gastrointestinal disturbances, sleep disturbances, dizziness *(mareos)*	
Arctic and subarctic Eskimo communities	*Pibloktoq* (term may vary by region)	Sudden dissociation event; convulsive seizures and sometimes coma follows Before the episode, the person is withdrawn, irritable, or exhibits bizarre behavior	
Chinese	*Qi-gong psychotic reaction*	Acute dissociation episode; paranoia Can occur following practice of qi-chong, a health-enhancing exercise Vulnerability increases with overinvolvement with exercise	Included in the *Chinese Classification of Mental Disorders* (CCMD-2)
Southern United States (among African American, European Americans and Caribbean societies) Latino societies	*Rootwork* *Mal puesto* *Brujeria*	Anxiety, gastrointestinal disturbances, fear of being poisoned/killed ("voodoo death") Attributed to hexes, spells, roots; "root doctor" (a traditional healer) is able to remedy this situation	
Portuguese Cape Verde Islanders and immigrants to the United States	*Sangue dormido "sleeping blood"*	Pain, numbness, tremor convulsions, paralysis, blindness, heart attack, infection, miscarriage	
China	*Shenjing shairuo "neurasthenia"*	Fatigue Multiple symptoms including headaches, pains, difficulty concentrating, sleep disturbances, and so on	Symptoms meet criteria for a mood or anxiety disorder Diagnosis included in the *Chinese Classification of Mental Disorders* (CCMD-2)
Taiwan China	*Shen-k'uei* *Shenkui*	Severe anxiety/panic symptoms, numerous somatic complaints, and sexual dysfunction Often considered life threatening	
Korea	*Shin-byung*	Anxiety with numerous somatic complaints Sometimes develops into dissociation Thought to be caused by possession of ancestral spirits	
African and European Americans from the Southern United States	*Spell*	Trance state with ability to "communicate" with the deceased or spirits Folk tradition does not consider these episodes as medical problems; often misinterpreted in clinical settings	
Latino (Mexico, Central America, South America); similar syndromes and beliefs are found throughout the world	*Susto ("soul loss");* also referred to *asespanto, pasmo, tripa ida, perdida del alm, chibih*	Presumed cause is a frightening event Multiple somatic symptoms occur shortly after the fright or a long time later Considered life threatening and ritual healings are used	Related to posttraumatic stress disorder and somatoform disorder
Japan	*Taijin kyofusho*	Phobia: a fear that own body parts and functions are offensive to others	Resembles social phobia Syndrome is in the official Japanese diagnostic system for mental disorders

Continued

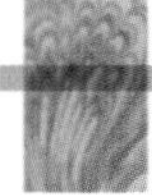

TABLE 7-3

Culture-Bound Syndromes, cont'd

CULTURE	IDIOM	BEHAVIOR	POTENTIAL RELATIONSHIP WITH DSM-IV-TR AXIS CLASSIFICATION
Ethiopia, Somalia, Egypt, Sudan, Iran and other North African and Middle Eastern societies	*Zar*	Possession of a spirit Episodes of dissociation, bizarre behavior and sudden verbal outbursts Withdrawal from social group and has a "relationship" with the spirit Not considered as an illness by the community	

Data from American Psychological Association: *Diagnostic and statistical manual of mental disorders,* ed 4, Washington, DC, 2000, American Psychological Association; US Department of Health and Human Services and SAMSHA: web resources 2006; www.mentalhealth.samhsa.gov.

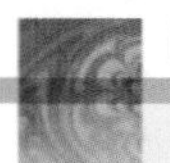

BOX 7-6

LEARN Model for Cross-Cultural Health Care

*L*isten to the patient and family's concepts of the illness, reactions to the Western health care system approaches, and their desires for therapy.

*E*xplain your assessment, using drawings, videotapes, and test results.

*A*cknowledge differences and similarities between the person from a different culture and the health care system perspectives; emphasize similarities.

*R*ecommend the diagnostic and therapeutic approaches and *listen* to the patient and family's responses.

*N*egotiate all areas of care, accommodating the patient and family's cultural beliefs and practices.

Modified from Her C, Culhane-Pera K: Culturally responsive care for Hmong patients, *Postgraduate Medicine* 116:39-46, 2004.

RESEARCH for EVIDENCE-BASED PRACTICE

Her C, Culhane-Pera K: Culturally responsive care for Hmong patients, *Postgraduate Medicine* 116:39-46, 2004.

Approximately 187,000 Hmong live throughout the United States, primarily in Minnesota, California, Wisconsin, and South Carolina. The traditional concepts of illness and traditional methods including interventions through shamans and use of herbal remedies for healing remain very important. Health is viewed as a balance of the social, natural, and supernatural realms. Treatment involves realigning these forces into harmony. The transparent spirit world surrounds daily reality. The people resist many of the healing methods used by the Western health care system. The Hmong brought many physiologic conditions and mental disorders related to posttraumatic stress and severe or chronic recurrent major depression. A series of case histories provided an overview of the cultural beliefs and practices surrounding physiologic and psychologic illnesses of Hmong refugees. Several themes were discovered: (1) apprehension about the effects of invasive procedures, surgical procedures, and the potential for impaired spiritual health; (2) concern about the effects of long-term medications, particularly if the condition does not necessarily cause a person to feel ill (imbalanced); (3) expectations for a quick recovery; (4) a belief that activities, food, temperature, and weather influence the hot-cold balance. The patriarchal structure values family-based decision making, and the family relied on their leaders if a disease was serious and the family perceived the treatment plan as dangerous. The use of a culturally sensitive approach demonstrates respect for the patient's cultural beliefs.

receive information about treatment in ways that they understand, considering their education, acculturation, and language (Box 7-6). The Research for Evidence-Based Practice box describes how learning about the traditions and beliefs of a culture will lead to culturally responsive care.

As mentioned previously, it is necessary to use a gradual approach for obtaining information from an individual from another culture. Because most clients with mental health problems do not react well to pencil-and-paper questionnaires, it is helpful to be knowledgeable of the scope and nature of these questions in order to gather the information effectively. In some mental care institutions, clients respond to a crisis questionnaire and a recovery questionnaire. The questions ask what the client believes the crisis event is and how the health care providers can assist in meeting a positive recovery outcome (Huggins, 2006).

The nurse and other health care providers are important advocates in helping clients and families understand various treatment methods in our multilingual and ethnically diverse environments. This is particularly important in the area of mental health, given the complex terminology and multiple behaviors and symptoms that require accurate interpretation by a culturally aware staff. Interpreters need to be able to attach accurate meaning and purpose to a client's language so that the client will clearly understand nursing implications for effective treatment. Cultural diversity helps nurses and professionals in other health care disciplines recognize that people are more alike than different and that everyone deserves the best possible physical and psychologic treatment regardless of language, culture, and ethnicity.

Several theories are proposed for incorporating cultural content while using the nursing process. Madeleine Leininger's *Culture Care Diversity and Universality: A Theory of Nursing* (1991) is the only nursing theory that specifically addresses the client's holistic cultural needs. Leininger noted that there are common or similar patterns, values, and meanings related to health and illness manifested by many cultures, and the differences are based on the worldview and the spiritual, social, and environmental context of a particular culture. Her sunrise enabler model is a tool that examines the influences of the multiple factors involved in designing efficient culture care. Watson's theory of human caring and Neuman's systems model are other nursing models used frequently in designing and implementing culturally congruent health care plans (Fawcett, 2000).

CLINICAL ALERT

Mrs. Williams is a 50-year-old woman whose husband died about 14 months earlier of a myocardial infarction. She came to the family practice clinic because she began to have chest pain and wondered if she also had cardiac problems. While obtaining a history, the practitioner noticed that Mrs. Williams was still dressed in black and added the diagnosis of "delayed bereavement" to the history. The practitioner failed to assess Mrs. Williams in terms of her cultural expression of grief. Mrs. Williams is Hispanic, and it is customary for people of many Hispanic cultures to wear black for a year or longer. It would be socially unacceptable for Mrs. Williams to do otherwise. Nurses need to avoid making assumptions.

The Nursing Process

The principal nursing tool in mental health is the *therapeutic use of self*. Often in the nurse-client relationship, sensitive cultural issues manifest themselves and impact client care. Therefore, understanding the significance of culture and its influence on clients' mental and physical health is important for nurses in all settings of health care delivery. This understanding will affect every step of the nursing process as well as the client's interpretation of life events.

ASSESSMENT

The assessment process is the foundation for all other steps of the nursing process. During assessment, the nurse formulates a perspective of the client's needs and problems. The nurse's personal biases, assumptions, cultural meanings, and nursing experience all influence the process.

Using the Heritage Assessment Tool (Box 7-7) when assessing clients is an entry point for gathering culture-specific data. In some instances, a more comprehensive assessment is necessary. Some assessment tools include additional information related to interpretation of time, attitudes related to personal space or territory, the format for names, social greetings and departures, family roles, expected and taboo behaviors; nutrition and deficiencies; pregnancy and childbearing practices, rituals related to illness and death, and the use of folklore practices (Catalano, 2000).

NURSING DIAGNOSIS

The nurse needs to be as specific as possible when conducting an assessment to determine the client needs and problems and identify specific nursing diagnoses. Nursing diagnoses are the same for clients from diverse cultural backgrounds, with a few exceptions. Actual culture-related nursing diagnoses include those related to communication barriers, sociocultural conflict, language barriers, and differences in health and illness beliefs and practices.

The process of making a nursing diagnosis is important because these diagnostic categories often help other staff members to frame a client's health concerns and potential outcomes. Accurate nursing diagnoses reflect the client's unique cultural perspective. If assessment is inaccurate, the nursing diagnosis will be incorrect. The nurse, viewing client behavior through an ethnocentric lens, interprets the client's behavior as dysfunctional. Box 7-8 describes common mistakes nurses make as a result of culture-related misunderstandings when making nursing diagnoses.

OUTCOME IDENTIFICATION

The nurse's understanding of cultural issues is crucial to ensure that the outcomes involve client participation. This also ensures that the outcomes fit the clients' needs and wishes. Often clients fail to achieve desired outcomes because those outcomes are inconsistent with their cultural worldview. Many clients will agree with the nurse, whom they see as the expert. In reality, however, the clients do not plan or are unable to follow through with the client educational and discharge planning because, from their perspective, it makes no sense to them and is not relevant to their problems. This leads to further misdiagnosis, especially the diagnosis of *noncompliance*. This happens most often when a client wants to use a traditional healing method or another culture-specific approach and sees the allopathic-oriented nursing intervention as conflicting with the traditional ways of achieving health.

PLANNING

Nurses are more likely to include a client's beliefs in the mental health care plan when the nurse considers the meaning of the client's behavior and communication in the context of his or her culture and traditions. When establishing goals of care and planning nursing interventions, the nurse considers each client's particular situation and challenges. Ideally, the family and the client's community are partners in developing and implementing the client's treatment plan.

IMPLEMENTATION

Holistic and culturally sensitive care plans that fit with the client's culture and needs evolve over time. The care plan is a living document, and the nurse adjusts the plans as goals are met and other goals are identified. For example, if the client is using ethno-medications, the nurse determines what type and how they react with conventional medications. Also, it is important to maintain effective verbal and nonverbal communication between the

BOX 7-7

Heritage Assessment Tool

1. Where was your mother born?
2. Where was your father born?
3. Where were your grandparents born?
   a. Your mother's mother?
   b. Your mother's father?
   c. Your father's mother?
   d. Your father's father?
4. How many brothers and sisters do you have?
5. What setting did you grow up in?
   a. Urban
   b. Rural
   c. Suburban
6. What country did your parents grow up in?
   a. Father
   b. Mother
7. How old were you when you came to the United States?
8. How old were your parents when they came to the United States?
   a. Mother
   b. Father
9. When you were growing up, who lived with you? (ask this way)
   a. Nuclear family
   b. Extended family
   c. Single-parent family
   d. Other
10. Have you maintained contact with any of the following:
    a. Aunts, uncles, cousins? (1) Yes (2) No
    b. Brothers and sisters? (1) Yes (2) No
    c. Parents? (1) Yes (2) No
    d. Your own children? (1) Yes (2) No
11. Did most of your aunts, uncles, and cousins live near to your home when you were growing up?
    a. Yes
    b. No
12. Approximately how often did you visit your family members who lived outside of your home when you were young?
    a. Daily
    b. Weekly
    c. Monthly
    d. Once a year or less
    e. Never
13. Was your original family name changed?
    a. Yes
    b. No
14. Do you have a religious preference?
    a. Yes (if yes, please specify)
    b. No (1 point for yes, but 0 for no)
15. Is your spouse the same religion as you?
    a. Yes
    b. No
16. Is your spouse the same ethnic background as you?
    a. Yes
    b. No
17. What kind of school did you go to?
    a. Public (0)
    b. Private
    c. Parochial
18. As an adult, do you live in a neighborhood where the neighbors have the same religion or ethnic background as you do?
    a. Religion (1) Yes (2) No
    b. Ethnicity (1) Yes (2) No
19. Do you belong to a religious institution?
    a. Yes
    b. No
20. Would you describe yourself as an active member?
    a. Yes
    b. No
21. How often do you attend your religious institution?
    a. More than once a week
    b. Weekly
    c. Monthly (0)
    d. Special holidays only (0)
    e. Never
22. Do you practice your religion in your home?
    a. Yes (please specify, 1 point for each example)
    b. Praying
    c. Bible reading
    d. Diet
    e. Celebrating religious holidays
    f. No
23. Do you prepare foods of your ethnic background?
    a. Yes
    b. No
24. Do you participate in ethnic activities?
    a. Yes (please specify, 1 point for each example)
    b. Singing
    c. Holiday celebrations
    d. Dancing
    e. Festivals
    f. Costumes
    g. Other
    h. No
25. Are your friends from the same religious background as you?
    a. Yes
    b. No
26. Are your friends from the same ethnic background as you?
    a. Yes
    b. No
27. What is your native language (the language your parents may have spoken other than English)?
28. Do you speak this language?
    a. Prefer
    b. Occasionally (0)
    c. Rarely (0)
29. Do you read this language?
    a. Yes
    b. No

The greater the number of *yes* answers, the more likely the client is to strongly identify with a traditional heritage. (The one *no* answer that indicates heritage identity is "Was your name changed?") This assessment may be scored 1 point for each yes from question 10, except where noted (0), and 2 points for no if the person's family name was not Americanized. Again, a high score, usually greater than 15 points, indicates identification with a traditional background.

From Spector RE: *Cultural diversity in health and illness*, ed 6, Upper Saddle River, NJ, 2004, Pearson.

BOX 7-8

Commonly Misapplied Nursing Diagnoses

Common NANDA nursing diagnoses frequently misapplied because of a lack of understanding of cultural issues include:

- **Defensive coping and noncompliance**. Clients from minority cultures that have experienced discrimination, bias, and stereotyping are often resistant to appropriate nursing interventions, especially in the area of teaching and discharge planning. Suspicion and mistrust cause the nurse to misunderstand a client's behaviors and mislabel them.
- **Ineffective role performance and impaired parenting**. Use of these diagnoses requires an understanding of the client's culture-specific roles and parenting activities. They are often different from those of the nurse and the majority culture.
- **Impaired social interaction and impaired verbal communication**. Misunderstanding occurs when the nurse fails to take into account culture-specific interaction patterns. Silence, infrequent eye contact, shame, fear, and language barriers all affect clients' ability to interact. The gender of the nurse and the gender of the client also influence communication because many cultures have specific gender-role behavioral codes.
- **Disturbed thought processes**. Thought patterns and processes that appear distorted are sometimes related to culture-specific expressions of anxiety and fear. Careful assessment will enable the nurse to accurately diagnose anxiety or fear in many clients rather than assume that underlying thought processes are altered.

client and the caregivers and obtain an interpreter if necessary. Promoting the client's understanding of the allopathic system and the rationale for the care often increases compliance.

Clients who are members of cultural communities often mistrust the system in general and the nurse in particular, especially if the nurse comes from a different cultural background. Trust issues are important in mental health nursing care and, because of the nurse's professional role, responsibility for the therapeutic relationship rests primarily on the nurse. For example, researchers have noted that race is a powerful issue in treatment. In particular, it affects how medication is administered, the level and frequency of interventions, and the outcome of intervention. Symptom presentation and prevalence of disorder also differ across cultural groups.

Faison and Mintzer (2005) reported that the elderly population is growing in size and in racial and ethnic diversity worldwide. Growing public health concerns are depression and suicide in the elderly, and different cultural communities have not always understood access to mental health service. There is a great need for care providers and the public to understand mental health issues in the diverse aging population and to develop strategies to meet their needs. Cohen et al. (2005) noted that United States–born blacks and African Caribbeans from the English-speaking and French-speaking islands were more likely to seek services and be treated. A majority of participants in the treatment group in this study were diagnosed with depression, were younger, experienced impaired ability for daily functions, and had a family history of mental illness and minimal social or religious supports. The use of social support systems in the intervention process is crucial in effectively caring for these older clients (Kim, 2002). Involving family members and other members of the client's cultural group in the assessment, planning, and intervention process facilitates nursing care and ensures more effective client outcomes.

EVALUATION

The nurse evaluates whether the client has been able to maintain his or her cultural beliefs regarding mental health and illness. In doing this, the nurse evaluates mental health care from a multicultural nursing perspective to determine if the client outcomes have been achieved. The nurse respects the client's needs and beliefs and remains open to communicate. The discharge plan needs to be realistic and culturally congruent. If the client does not feel invested in the treatment choices, he or she is less likely to be effective after discharge. Thus, evaluation of nursing interventions is based on culturally sensitive and realistic client outcomes. The Case Study on p. 152 demonstrates the use of the assessment and intervention tools.

CHAPTER SUMMARY

- Cultural awareness is the initial step toward effective interaction among individuals from different cultures and involves an awareness of one's own culture, including the prejudices and biases toward other cultures.
- Cultural competence requires a respect for diversity and the understanding of the attitudes, beliefs, behaviors, practices, and communication patterns of multiple cultures and their languages.
- Culture is a set of values, beliefs, and behaviors that influence the way that members of the group express themselves; it is also the integrated pattern of human behavior for members of a racial, religious, or social group that is transmitted to succeeding generations as a cultural heritage.
- The communication aspects of language, space, and time orientation have various practices among different cultures.
- Secondary characteristics of cultural diversity (social economic status, occupation and education, gender issues, geographic place of residence, length of time absent from the country of origin, and sexual orientation) have a powerful effect on an individual's cultural identity even though these characteristics are not as easy to identify as the primary characteristics.
- Heritage consistency is the concept that describes how much a person identifies with his or her cultural background.
- The nurse and other health care providers need to be aware of the meaning of gestures, body positions, facial expressions, and eye movements, and the tone of voice during all communications with individuals from various cultures.

Continued on p. 153

CASE STUDY

This case illustrates the use of the assessment and intervention tools referred to in this chapter. It also reflects some of the significant aspects of spiritual care as they apply to both clients and nurses. It also demonstrates the value of spiritual care as perceived by a client and physician.

HOLISTIC ASSESSMENT

The client is a 66-year-old woman who has been hospitalized for an extensive period (approximately 6 weeks). The initial problems were major depression, anxiety, and a degenerative spinal condition that required several surgeries. The spinal condition is treatable, but the process will leave her with some permanent restrictions in movement and some possible residual pain. The client currently has significant chronic leg and lower back spasms and states that medication gives her little relief. Both the pain and the restrictions resulting from surgery have exacerbated her depression and anxiety.

The client has been divorced for almost 40 years. Immediately after her divorce, she and her four children moved 1500 miles away from her family and friends so that she could seek employment in a manufacturing environment. Although two of her children live close by, only one child is in regular contact with the client. The client has a Lutheran background, but she has no local connection to a congregation and has not attended church regularly since leaving her hometown. Both the client and her physician are extremely interested in her having regular visits for spiritual care, and both have stated that the visits provide the client with significant help and support.

THE CLIENT'S BELIEF AND MEANING

Being independent, strong, and self-sufficient are important goals in life, which are to be valued and pursued.

THE CLIENT'S VOCATIONS AND OBLIGATIONS

The client's goal was to support, raise, and care for herself and her children without being dependent on others. She still seeks to care for her adult daughter—asking the spiritual caregiver to meet with her daughter to talk about performing a marriage ceremony.

THE CLIENT'S EXPERIENCE AND EMOTION

The client has had a life of struggle, which has been balanced against the rewards of accomplishing her goal to be independent and her pride in being self-sufficient.

THE CLIENT'S COURAGE AND GROWTH

The client is now struggling to find some meaning in her pain and suffering.

THE CLIENT'S RITUAL AND PRACTICE

The client has a strong, dependent need to have the poem "Footprints," the Twenty-Third Psalm, and the Lord's Prayer read to her; she requests few other institutional rituals.

THE CLIENT'S COMMUNITY

The client's community is small, consisting of her children, their spouses, and several grandchildren, mostly living some distance from the client.

THE CLIENT'S SOURCE OF AUTHORITY AND GUIDANCE

The client's source of authority and guidance is largely external and comes from her early Midwestern social norms and experiences with institutional religion. She grants pastors a great deal of power, authority, and control; the client also believes that common religious articles such as the Bible and prayer cards have an almost magical authority and power.

THE CLIENT'S STAGE OF FAITH DEVELOPMENT

The client is basically in stage 1, the impartial stage of faith, and is now possibly seeking to move into the early phase of stage 2, the institutional religion stage.

LEVEL OF SPIRITUAL RISK

This client is at significant spiritual risk. She has an extremely high need for spiritual care and has very limited to nonexistent resources with which to meet this need. In making a triage assessment of how to assign scarce pastoral care resources, this client's particular situation calls for a significant amount of qualified pastoral care.

SPIRITUAL CARE PLAN

Using the assessment tools as previously described, the spiritual pastoral care plan was to see the patient often—daily if possible. During these visits the spiritual intervention tools of prayer, presence, and short scripture readings were used to help bolster the client's sense of God's care for her and to support her in the healing process. Another intervention strategy was to help the patient explore her stated desire to be connected to a local Lutheran church and to help identify ways in which to do this. In addition, the spiritual caregiver helped the client explore, to the extent of her desire and capability, what meaning there is for her in this illness and in her future physical limitations. The intent of this goal was to help the client find possible new meanings in her life as a result of this illness.

The benefit to the client in pursuing these spiritual care plan goals was the provision of help, support, and comfort. This spiritual support helped ease her sense of torment and pain, resulting in a reduced experience of suffering. The benefit to the hospital in pursuing these spiritual care plan goals was greater client satisfaction. As the client experienced significant relief in the periods after her spiritual care, her requests for nursing interventions decreased. The client was also more satisfied with her overall care and was less anxious about her prognosis. The client's physician reported that she was quite satisfied with the hospital's ability to address the client's spiritual needs and that in doing so the hospital helped the client to experience less pain and discomfort.

CRITICAL THINKING

1. Assess and prioritize the client's psychiatric, physical, and spiritual areas of concern, ensuring that all areas are addressed.
2. Describe the benefits of collaborating with the hospital chaplain in addressing the client's spiritual needs as part of a holistic assessment.
3. Given your knowledge of the stages of faith and the client's spiritual and religious background, which stage of faith best fits this client? What is the rationale for your choice?
4. How can your assessment of this client's family history of struggle, pride, and pain be used to guide you in your spiritual assessment? Consider the stages of the spiritual dimension as a guide.

- Religious beliefs are a part of cultural heritage and have a strong influence on lifestyle, ethics, health care, and life decisions.
- Religion is a personal set or institutionalized system of religious attitudes, beliefs and practices.
- Spirituality is (1) an integrative energy that can produce inner harmony or wholeness; (2) a sense of coherence; (3) the driving force that permeates all aspects that give meaning to life; (4) a sense of transcendence over reality.
- Faith is the belief and trust in God (or supreme being), and the ability to draw on spiritual resources without having physical and empiric proof. It is an internal certainty that comes from one's own experience with the divine.
- Health is three-dimensional, encompassing the body, mind, and spirit.
- Belief and meaning make up the central core principles underlying an individual's spiritual dimension, and culture as well as life experiences influence it.
- Spirituality is an essential human dimension that helps connect people to each other, the community, and the world, and clients express their spirituality in a variety of ways.
- There is a growing belief that a quality spiritual assessment is significantly beneficial in reducing a client's feelings of powerlessness and despair.
- For some individuals a chaplain represents the ultimate authority for one's spiritual health, just as the nurse or physician often is the authority for one's physical or mental health.
- Research on spirituality and healing has grown, but there needs to be greater focus on mental health and spirituality.

REVIEW QUESTIONS

1 A family immigrates to the United States from Honduras. Which member(s) of the family are most likely to experience culture shock? You may select more than one answer.
1. Father
2. Mother
3. Teenage daughter
4. 8-year-old son
5. 3-year-old son

2 A nurse assesses an adult client with a foot ulcer that will not heal. The client is of Cuban heritage, has been in the United States for 2 years, and is fluent in English. Which question should the nurse include in the assessment?
1. "Do you believe evil spirits caused your problem?"
2. "What are your main cultural values and beliefs?"
3. "Have you used any folk medicine treatments on your foot?"
4. "How have you been treating your foot sore at home?"

3 An adult client recently diagnosed with cancer states, "I've lived my life according to the Bible. I don't understand why God has forsaken me." Which nursing diagnosis applies?
1. Spiritual dysfunction
2. Disturbed thought processes
3. Hopelessness
4. Spiritual distress

4 A nurse provides discharge instructions to a client of Vietnamese heritage who immigrated to this country 1 year ago. Which strategy would be important to assure the client's understanding of the instructions?
1. Use a professional interpreter.
2. Handwrite the instructions.
3. Show the client a video.
4. Contact a bilingual translator.

5 A Native American adult is hospitalized. The emergency department assessment indicates auditory and visual hallucinations. The client states, "My dead father told me to kill myself to save me from the bad spirits." What would be an appropriate nursing intervention for the nursing care plan?
1. Consult the family, with the client's consent, for a spiritual healer from the client's tribe.
2. Initiate a consultation between the hospital chaplain and the client.
3. Assign only Native American staff members to provide this client's care.
4. Provide the client with frequent periods alone for meditation and prayer.

Additional self-study exercises and learning resources are available to you on the ***Companion CD*** *at the back of the book and on the* ***Evolve website*** *at* ***http://evolve.elsevier.com/Fortinash/.***

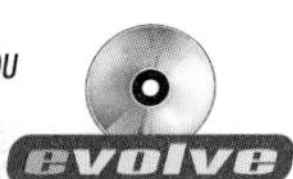

ONLINE RESOURCES

Cultural Awareness Assessment, San Diego State University: www.sa.sdsu.edu/forstudents/cultural3.html

National Consumer Supporter Technical Assistance Center: Cultural Competency Initiative Toolkit: **www.ncstac.org/content/culturalcompetency/index.htm**

Transcultural Nursing: **www.madeleine-leininger.com**

REFERENCES

American Psychiatric Association: *Diagnostic and statistical manual of mental disorders*, Fourth Edition, Text Revision. Washington, DC, American Psychiatric Association, 2000.

American Nurses Association: *Discrimination and racism policy statement* (to be reviewed and updated 2006), Washington, DC, 1998, American Nurses Association.

Autgis T, Raneer A: Personalization of conflict across cultures: a comparison among the U.S., New Zealand and Australia, *J Intercultural Commun Res* 33:109-119, 2004.

Carlson B et al: Oregon hospice chaplains: experiences with patients requesting physician-assisted suicide, *J Palliative Med* 8:1160-1167, 2005.

Carpenito L: *Nursing diagnosis: application to clinical practice*, ed 9, Philadelphia, 2002, Lippincott.

Catalano JT: *Nursing now! Today's issues, tomorrow's trends*, ed 2, Philadelphia, 2000, F.A. Davis.

Cohen C et al: Comparison of users and non-users of mental health serves among depressed older urban African Americans, *Am J Geriatr Psychiatry* 13:545-553, 2005.

Fadiman A: *The spirit catches you and you fall down*, New York, 1997, Farrar, Straus & Giroux.

Faison W, Mintzer M: The growing ethnically diverse aging population: is our field advancing with it? *Am J Geriatr Psychiatry* 13:541-544, 2005.

Fawcett J: Leininger's theory of culture care diversity and universality. In *Analysis and evaluation of contemporary nursing knowledge*, Philadelphia, 2000, F.A. Davis.

Fitchett G: *Developing outcome-focused spiritual care: facing the challenge of filling a new wineskin*, unpublished monograph presented to the national meeting of the College of Chaplains, 1997.

Fowler JW: *Stages of faith*, San Francisco, 1981, Harper.

Harris J: Learning to listen across cultural divides, *Listening Professional* 2:4, 20-21, 2003.

Her C, Culhane-Pera K: Culturally responsive care for Hmong patients, *Postgrad Med* 116:39-46, 2004.

Ito K: A history of Manga in the context of Japanese culture and society, *J Pop Cult* 38:456-475, 2005.

Jennings P: What mothers want: welfare reform and maternal desire, *J Sociol Soc Welf* 31:113-200, 2005.

Kim G: U.S. Population is nudging toward the 300 million mark, *San Diego Union Tribune*, p A-3, Jan 20, 2006.

Kim M et al: Primary health care for Korean immigrants: sustaining a culturally sensitive model, *Public Health Nurs* 19: 191-200, 2002.

Koenig H: Religion, spirituality and medicine: research findings and implications for clinical practice, *South Med J* 97: 1194-1205, 2004.

Leininger MM: *Culture care diversity and universality: a theory of nursing*, New York, 1991, National League for Nursing Press.

Leonard B, Plotnikoff G: Awareness: the heart of cultural competence. *AACN Clin Issues Adv Pract in Acute Clin Care* 11:51-59.

McCaffery M, Pasero C: *Pain: clinical manual*, ed 2, St Louis, 2004, Mosby.

Meadows M: *Moving toward consensus on cultural competency in health care: closing the gap*, Office of Minority Health, Jan 2000; www.omhre.gov.

Medrano M, Setzer J, Enger S, Costello R, Benaventa V: Self-assessment of cultural of cultural and linguistic competence in an ambulatory health system, *J Health Care Manage* 50: 371-385.

Myerstein I: Psychopathology and psychotherapy: a clinician's view, *J Relig Health* 43:329-341, 2004.

Putting a face on poverty, *Canada & World Backgrounder* 70:8-12, 2005.

Revision notes UK, 2005; www.revision-notes.co.uk/revision/623.html.

San Diego State University: Cultural awareness assessment, 2006; retrieved Mar 2, 2006, from www.sa.sdsu.edu/forstudents/cultural13.html.

Spector R: *Cultural diversity in health and illness*, ed 6, Upper Saddle River, NJ, 2003, Prentice Hall Health.

Tabuchi H: Concern rises over suicides in Japan, *San Diego Union-Tribune*, p A-3 (Associated Press), Mar 11, 2006.

US Census Bureau: 1999; retrieved Feb 25, 2006, from www.census.gov.

US Census Bureau: 2003; www.census.gov/prod/2004/pubs/p20-s51/pdf.

US Department of Health and Human Services: Poverty thresholds and poverty guidelines, 2006; retrieved Feb 25, 2006, from http:/aspe.hhs.gov/poverty/06poverty.shtml.

Xue F, Zhou S, Zhou P: Visual strategies in United States and Chinese television ads, conference papers, International Communication Association annual meeting, San Diego, Calif, 2003; retrieved Feb 28, 2006, from EbschoHost, www.ebscohost.com.

Chapter 8

Legal and Ethical Aspects in Clinical Practice

ROBERT L. ERB, JR.

The law is reason, free from passion.
ARISTOTLE

OBJECTIVES

1 Review key events in the history of mental illness and its legal treatment.
2 Describe and discuss the various forms of admissions to mental health facilities.
3 Explain the difference between confidentiality and privileged communication.
4 State the impact of federal legislation on patient privacy.
5 Identify situations in which the duty to warn is applicable.
6 List the rights of mental health clients and identify how these rights apply in practice.
7 Distinguish between the concepts of competency to stand trial and the insanity defense.
8 Apply the elements of malpractice to a current practice situation.
9 Describe the purpose and implementation of psychiatric advance directives.

KEY TERMS

breach of duty, p. 165
clear and convincing evidence, p. 157
commitment, p. 156
competency to stand trial, p. 164
duty to warn, p. 159
expert witness, p. 165
forensic psychiatric nurses, p. 165
least restrictive alternative, p. 156
legal duty, p. 165
mandatory outpatient treatment, p. 157
privileged communication, p. 158
psychiatric advance directives, p. 157

HISTORICAL REVIEW

According to Sales and Shuman (1994), law and mental health have been linked for many years. Even in ancient Rome, the law was concerned about the legal status of the mentally disabled. Should the individual have a guardian? Could the individual enter into a contract? According to Roman law, the person with a mental disability could not form a marriage contract, and if the law made a person a ward (dependent), the person did not have any legal rights (Brakel, Parry, and Weiner, 1985).

During the Middle Ages, people believed that the mentally ill were possessed by demons. The king could hold custody of property of the mentally ill. Profits were applied to the maintenance of the individuals and their households. When a person was thought to be incompetent because of mental illness, a jury of 12 men decided whether or not to commit the individual to the care of a friend, who received an allowance for taking care of the individual (Brakel, Parry, and Weiner, 1985).

In the American colonies of the seventeenth century, the lack of facilities meant that families had to care for people with mental illnesses. If a person had no family or friends, the individual wandered from town to town—in some instances in the company of transient groups. There was no distinguishing between a homeless person and a person with a mental illness; therefore, all were treated as itinerant, poor persons. As early as 1676, the state of

Massachusetts passed a law to manage people who had mental illnesses and were dangerous. The individual could be detained, but generally there were no procedures for commitment of a person with a mental illness at this time (Brakel, Parry, and Weiner, 1985).

It was not until 1752 that Pennsylvania Hospital in Philadelphia opened to treat people with mental illnesses (Laben and MacLean, 1989). In Williamsburg, Virginia, in 1773, the state opened a facility, specifically for treatment of people with mental illnesses. The next state institution built was in Lexington, Kentucky, in 1824 (Brakel, Parry, and Weiner, 1985).

In 1841, Dorothea Dix, American educator, began her crusade for placing individuals with mental illnesses in specially built hospitals rather than placing them in poorhouses and jails. During the following years, Dix traveled throughout the United States, pressing for moral and humane treatment of people with mental illnesses (Laben and MacLean, 1989).

During the late nineteenth and early twentieth centuries, various states passed laws on civil commitment procedures for people with mental illnesses. From 1900 to 1955, the population in mental institutions grew from 150,000 to 819,000 inpatients in state and county mental hospitals (LaFond, 1994). Passage of the Community Mental Health Centers Act of 1963 authorized funds to build community treatment centers. Shortly thereafter, civil rights lawyers began to challenge the treatment of people with mental illnesses. During the Vietnam War era, a distrust of government appeared. Activism began with concern about the treatment of people with mental illnesses and their rights. Society gave more consideration to individual rights; especially questioning the long-standing practice of hospitalizing individuals for many years, in some instances without much treatment (LaFond, 1994).

Large numbers of individuals were released into the community, raising concerns that there were not appropriate facilities and services to adequately care for them within the community. Because of the increasing number of people with mental illnesses in the community and the appointment of more conservative judges who were reluctant to become involved in the administration of hospitals, recommendations for expanding the mental health commitment laws began. In California, state legislation (Lanterman-Petris-Short Act of 1969) passed an act that allowed psychiatrists and other designated professionals to hold individuals for an evaluation period of 72 hours. The individuals, *on the basis of a mental disorder*, had to be a danger to self, danger to others, or "gravely disabled" (i.e., unable to provide or use food, clothing, or shelter for themselves).

In an extensive review of the literature, Lamb and Weinberger (1998) described a variety of factors limiting adequate access to mental health services: closure of long-term treatment facilities (state hospitals), lack of developed treatment resources in the community, lack of understanding by police officers and the general population, and the creation of strict civil commitment standards. As a result, a large number of mentally ill individuals are now in jails and prisons; surveys estimate that up to 15% of inmates have severe mental illness.

The impact of managed behavioral health organizations on hospitals, clinics, and clients themselves is a growing concern with ethical and legal consequences. In an effort to control the rising costs associated with psychiatric treatment, many insurance plans carve out the management of mental health benefits to managed behavioral health organizations. Authorization for access to treatment and ongoing use of mental health benefits is often a complicated maze for clients and clinicians alike. Insurance mental health benefits (if they are offered at all) have historically had many more restrictions on their use or are paid at significantly lower rates than health benefits for other chronic medical illnesses such as diabetes and heart disease. This is largely due to the stigma still associated with mental illness.

Nurses and physicians need to consider their legal and ethical responsibilities when managed care organizations pressure to limit or deny client access to treatment or payment for services. Pressure to prematurely discharge clients from inpatient facilities is increasing (Simon, 1998). The advocacy role of nurses to help clients to obtain, maintain, and fully utilize mental health benefits is critical. Although managed care organizations will deny authorization or stop paying for mental health services, the potential liability for denying services remains with the physician, nurse, and hospital (Simon, 2001).

COMMITMENT

Commitment is a term referring to the various ways that an individual enters mental health treatment. States have varying terms and mechanisms associated with commitment, but in general there are three common types: voluntary commitment, emergency commitment, and longer term judicial or civil commitment.

An important concept related to the location and nature of mental health treatment is the concept of **least restrictive alternative**. Least restrictive alternative means providing mental health treatment in the least restrictive environment, using the least restrictive treatment. In the mid-1960s, an elderly woman who was hospitalized at St. Elizabeth's in Washington, D.C., filed a writ of habeas corpus so that she could be released into the community. At that time, there were few alternatives to hospitals for treatment. The court ruled that there needed to be alternatives to inpatient facilities, including halfway houses, nursing homes, and day treatment programs (*Lake v. Cameron*, 1966).

Developing a treatment plan involves consideration of all alternatives, including such options as inpatient treatment, partial hospitalization or intensive outpatient treatment, home health services, and foster and respite care. An individual residing in a community that has developed many care options is the least likely to be hospitalized. The cost of health care services is also an important factor. The nurse needs to select the least restrictive, most clinically appropriate, and most cost-effective intervention to assist the client.

Voluntary Commitment

Nurses are the most familiar with clients who access treatment voluntarily by consenting to be admitted and treated. Nurses treat clients whose clinical conditions vary widely in their psychiatric severity on a voluntary basis. However, voluntary clients who are seeking a discharge from the hospital but who are an immediate danger to themselves or others may be placed on an emergency commitment status pending further evaluation and treatment.

Emergency Commitment

Severe mental illness sometimes affects a client's cognitive functions so that he or she refuses treatment for a variety of reasons. Some individuals with psychosis, paranoia, delusions, or hallucinations reject psychiatric treatment for fear of being harmed or on the basis of some strange rationale that only they understand. Persons suffering from severe mood disturbances who are depressed and suicidal sometimes refuse to enter treatment because of a sense of hopelessness and a wish to die. When the effects of the client's mental illness result in an immediate risk of self-harm or harm to others, an emergency commitment is appropriate. In some states, if the effect of the mental illness is such that the client is unable to provide food, clothing, or shelter for himself or herself (i.e., "gravely disabled"), an emergency commitment is also appropriate. (See Chapter 29.)

Emergency commitment differs from a judicial or indefinite commitment. Emergency commitment is for a shorter period and generally has more restrictive criteria for admission. Usually a state requires that a mental health official, such as a physician, psychologist, social worker, or advanced practice nurse, see the individual. Some states require a licensed physician. Once the individual is brought to the inpatient unit, a second mental health professional, usually a physician, has to make an examination. This procedure protects the rights of the individuals. Usually within a short period (5 days or less, excluding weekends and holidays) a probable cause hearing has to take place to continue the person's hospitalization.

Taking away an individual's freedom through a commitment procedure is a serious matter. The U.S. Supreme Court has established the standard of **clear and convincing evidence** as the standard of proof that must be met for commitment. The criminal standard of "beyond a reasonable doubt" is not used.

Civil or Judicial Commitment

A judicial or civil commitment is for a longer time than an emergency commitment. The legal basis for extended detention of an individual for treatment lies in the *parens patriae* power of the state to protect and care for individuals with disabilities and the police power of the state to protect the community from persons who are a threat. For a judicial commitment, the individual has to be given time to prepare a defense that states why hospitalization is not necessary. The client has the right to have his or her attorney cross-examine the mental health professionals regarding the necessity for continued inpatient treatment.

Although many usually use judicial or civil commitment for longer term inpatient or residential treatment, at least 35 states have passed legislation for **mandatory outpatient treatment** (Torrey and Kaplan, 1995). In California, A.B. 1421 Court-Ordered Outpatient Treatment was effective January 1, 2003, but was applicable only in those counties adopting a resolution authorizing its application. The purpose of mandating outpatient mental health treatment is to break the cyclical pattern of clients who, when discharged from an inpatient treatment facility, discontinue medication, deteriorate, exhibit dangerous behavior, and subsequently require readmission to the acute psychiatric care setting. Nurses need to acknowledge their advocate role and yet balance clients' need for progressive mental health treatment. This includes activating clients' participation in outpatient treatment programs that address the recurring nature of chronic mental illness.

PSYCHIATRIC ADVANCE DIRECTIVES

Virtually all states have developed statutes governing the use of advanced directives, focused on anticipatory planning regarding general medical and psychiatric care (Appelbaum, 2004). Some states have special provisions and have made psychiatric models that allow a competent person to describe warning signs of declining mental health and consent or refuse a treatment method These models also allow a competent person to agree to commitment in a psychiatric care facility for a determined period of time and to appoint a surrogate (substitute) decision maker (Backlar et al., 2001).

Following the principle of medical advance directives for health care, **psychiatric advance directives** (PADs) are legal documents utilized when a patient is unable to participate in the decision-making process (O'Connell and Stein, 2005). Implementation of PADs reduces the average hospital length of stay, impacts the burden on the mental health legal system, and significantly decreases involuntary commitments (Sherman, 1998; Backlar and Macfarland, 1996).

CONFIDENTIALITY

The Health Insurance Portability and Accountability Act (HIPAA) of 1996 now regulates the protection and privacy of health information. This law guarantees the security and privacy of health information and outlines standards for enforcement. The final HIPAA Privacy Rule went into effect April 14, 2003, for all health care providers (individuals or organizations who send bills or are paid for health care). The Privacy Rule defines protected health information (PHI) as any individually identifiable health information that an organization keeps, files, uses, or shares in an oral, electronic, or written form (Sharp

LEGAL CASE REPORT: Clinical Case Implications

Sexually Violent Predator: Commitment Standard • *Kansas v. Hendricks* (1997)

In a controversial 5-to-4 decision, the U.S. Supreme Court upheld a statute enacted by the state of Kansas. Leroy Hendricks had been convicted of sexual offenses against children. He had a 40-year history of sexual involvement with children, and he had been convicted on several occasions. Before his release, the state of Kansas petitioned to have Hendricks civilly committed under the state's Sexually Violent Predator Act. When he was stressed or pressured, he was unable to control his impulses. A jury in a lower state court found him to be a sexually violent predator, and the court civilly committed him. The court defined his pedophilia as a mental abnormality, but on appeal to the Kansas State Supreme Court, the commitment was overturned because a mental abnormality did not meet the commitment standard, which was based on mental illness.

On appeal to the U.S. Supreme Court, the justices commented that "states have, over the years, developed numerous specialized terms to define mental health concepts. Often these definitions do not fit precisely with the definitions employed by the medical community." The Court maintained that the person must have an inability to control behavior and can be held until he or she is no longer dangerous to others. Hendricks had admitted at the jury trial that he could not control his behavior. "This admitted lack of volitional control, coupled with a prediction of future dangerousness, adequately distinguishes Hendricks from other dangerous persons who are perhaps more properly dealt with exclusively through criminal proceedings. Hendricks' diagnosis as a pedophile, which qualifies as a 'mental abnormality' under the Act, thus plainly suffices for due process purposes."

Because no effective treatment was being offered at this point, treatment was "nonexistent." The Court asserted, "We have never held that the constitution prevents a state from civilly detaining those for whom no treatment is available, but nevertheless pose a danger to others." Treatment is not required for those who are dangerously mentally ill. There are built-in safeguards to ensure against an indefinite duration. The commitment is reviewed annually, and if the person can demonstrate in the future that there is no longer dangerous behavior, release can be granted.

The dissenting opinion focused on several issues; the act was meant to segregate violent sexual offenders and be a meaningful attempt to provide treatment. This had not been accomplished. "As of the time of Hendricks' commitment, the state had not funded treatment, it had not entered into treatment contracts, and it had little, if any, qualified staff." Offenders were not committed until sentences were near completion, there were no less restrictive alternatives, and any treatment available was not offered until the sentence had been completed.

Since this ruling, some states have moved toward enacting laws that would place sexual offenders who have completed their sentences in mental health facilities. This action places a responsibility on mental health professionals to develop programs of intervention that will lead to reducing the symptoms of these sexual offenders.

HealthCare Medication Guidelines, 2002). Both civil and criminal penalties of fines or prison sentences were established under HIPAA for the knowing violation of patient privacy. Mental health records, including psychotherapy and drug and alcohol treatment, have special additional privacy protection under the regulation.

Nursing Implications

Nurses need to be knowledgeable about federal and state privacy regulations and understand their relevance to information management in the nurse's practice area. The American Nurses Association code of ethics (ANA, 1982) also defines the importance of keeping a client's information confidential. At the time of admission to a mental health facility, admission often requests that clients sign a release of information document. The release of information usually includes the following:

- The information that will be released
- The persons or parties the information will be shared with, such as other health care providers and insurance providers
- The purpose for releasing the information
- The period of time the information will be released

The release of confidential client information even for the best-intended purposes is risky. Even when presented with a subpoena for the release of PHI, consulting with an attorney from the nurse's place of employment before releasing any information is advisable.

The confidentiality of the client's information and the necessity for having a signed release from the client before releasing information, even to family members who are closely involved with the client's daily care, present challenges for the nurse. For instance, a paranoid client who refuses to sign a release of information for his parents who are the caregivers will result in the nurse having to tell the parents when they telephone, "I'm sorry, but I'm not able to give you any information at this time." However, it is possible to also say, "but if you have information that you think would be important for me to know, I can listen to you." In this way, the family is able to communicate important medical or behavioral history to the treatment facility without the nurse releasing any information about the client without his or her permission.

PRIVILEGED COMMUNICATION

Privileged communication is different from confidentiality. It is enacted by statute to designated professionals such as the clergy, attorneys, psychologists, or physicians. Reflecting a major change in direction, several states are now including nurses and other health care professionals under these conditions. The provisions of these statutes allow certain information given to the professionals by clients to remain secret during any litigation. The privilege belongs to the client, and only the client can assert or waive this privilege. These statutes

LEGAL CASE REPORT: Clinical Case Implications

Privileged Communication • *Jaffee v. Redmond* (1996)

In a U.S. Supreme Court decision, the justices ruled that a social worker, according to Illinois law and the Federal Rule of Evidence 501, did have privileged communication and that her client could use privilege in keeping communications between them confidential. The client, Mary Lu Redmond, a police officer, had in the process of her duties shot and killed Ricky Allen. In a wrongful death lawsuit filed by Allen's estate after his death, the social worker and Redmond declined to answer questions concerning what took place in the therapeutic sessions. The judge directed the jury that the notes concerning the sessions must be negative in relation to the defendant. The jury sent back a verdict of $545,000 against the defendant, Redmond, on state and federal claims. Even though the therapist was not an advanced practice nurse, if a state has a nurse therapist-client privilege, it seems likely that federal courts, on the basis of this decision, would recognize the privilege. Nurses need to be aware of the privileged communication in the state where they are practicing.

exclude the mandatory reporting of child, elder, impaired adult, and (in some instances) domestic violence; some communicable diseases relating to public safety; and information that will prevent a felony, such as murder, from occurring.

DUTY TO WARN AND PROTECTION: TARASOFF

In the mid-1970s, a landmark case changed the manner in which mental health professionals dealt with warning their clients' intended victims. That case, *Tarasoff v. Regents of the University of California* (1976) was about a young University of California student from India, Prosenjit Poddar. He had a relationship with Tatiana Tarasoff and had misinterpreted a New Year's Eve kiss as a serious romantic gesture. After several months had passed, she told him that she wished to date other men and that she did not view their relationship as serious. He subsequently became depressed and sought mental health counseling. He communicated to his therapist that he would harm Tarasoff, who at that time was in South America. One day he ran out of the therapist's office and was detained by the campus police and released. After Tarasoff's return, he went to her home and fatally wounded her with a knife. The family of the victim brought suit against the University of California, and after the case reached the Supreme Court of California, the justices ruled "protective privilege ends where the public peril begins." This ruling, **duty to warn**, established the responsibility of a treating mental health professional to notify an intended, identifiable victim. Other states have enacted similar statutes since *Tarasoff v. Regents of the University of California* (1976) to ensure that mental health professionals warn potential identifiable victims.

Nursing Implications

Nurses need to be aware of any case law related to duty to warn/Tarasoff within their jurisdiction. Nurses, especially advanced practice nurses, should know when to refer a client for commitment and when to warn their client's potential intended victims. Many mental health treatment facilities have duty to warn/Tarasoff policies and procedures in place that will guide nurses and other clinicians in the notification and documentation process.

RIGHTS OF CLIENTS

Up until the last quarter of the twentieth century, few gave any attention to the rights of individuals in mental health facilities; mental health laws protecting client rights are therefore relatively new (Wexler and Winick, 1992). These days, when individuals enter a mental health facility, they usually retain their civil rights, unless clearly restricted by using due process to certify that an individual lacks the capacity or competence. These individuals retain the right to vote, to manage financial matters, to enter into contractual relationships, and to assert the constitutional right to seek the advice of an attorney. Other basic rights usually include the right to send and to receive unopened mail, to wear one's own clothes, to receive visitors, to keep and use personal possessions, and to have access to a telephone.

Clients also have a right to be informed regarding potential risks, benefits, and reasonable alternatives before giving consent for any specific therapy, surgery, or treatments, including medication. Nurses need to disclose serious side effects that will be uncomfortable or irreversible to the client. Clients are able to give informed consent unless there has been a judicial ruling to the contrary. In documented emergency or endangering situations, however, nurses are able to administer medications and treatment without the client's consent.

Many states require that all clients receive a written summary of their rights in their own language on admission to an inpatient facility. In California, a list of client rights (including the name and telephone number of the Office of Patient Advocacy) is required to be publicly posted in every mental health treatment facility. For non–English-speaking clients, it is important that the client rights are in their own language or presented via a qualified interpreting service. Treatment facilities are expected to know the dominant languages of the clients that they serve and to make provisions to have client rights available in those languages.

Nursing Implications

The education of clients regarding their rights is an ongoing advocacy process and a major focus for nurses. Clients' diminished mental status and cognitive function at the time of admission when client rights are reviewed often means that nurses have to use a variety of educational methods and repeat the material as a part of the treatment plan.

SECLUSION AND RESTRAINTS

Since the Middle Ages, mental health facilities have used seclusion and restraints (S/R) to control the behavior of persons with mental disorders. In October 1998, the *Hartford Courant* published a five-part investigative series of articles on "Deadly Restraints." It included a national survey that documented 142 deaths over the most recent decade that were directly related to the use of S/R. Congressional hearings followed, and federal reforms were proposed and implemented shortly thereafter (see the Research for Evidence-Based Practice box).

Effective August 2, 1999, the Health Care Financing Administration (HCFA), now called the U.S. Centers for Medicare and Medicaid Services (CMS), introduced new standards for the use of S/R for all Medicare and Medicaid participating hospitals. CMS declared that "the patient's right to be free of restraints is paramount" (Pennsylvania Department of Public Welfare, 2000). The new rules stated that health care professionals were to use S/R only when less restrictive alternatives to ensure client safety had failed, such as talking to the client. Coercion, discipline, punishment, or staff convenience were unacceptable reasons for placing a person in seclusion or restraints. However, the most notable change was the implementation of the "1-hour rule," which requires a face-to-face evaluation by a licensed independent practitioner (LIP) within 1 hour of the initiation of restraints used for behavioral management. The face-to-face assessment is required even if the client has been released from restraints before the arrival of the LIP. The definition of the LIP varies by state. In addition to physicians, psychologists and advanced practice nurses are sometimes able to order restraints, depending on the individual's license.

RESEARCH for EVIDENCE-BASED PRACTICE

Johnson ME: Being restrained: a study of power and powerlessness, *Issues in Mental Health Nursing* 19:191, 1998.

Researchers conducted a phenomenologic study with 10 adult participants—5 men and 5 women—relating to their experiences of being restrained. Interviews were transcribed in their entirety. All participants had been controlled with leather restraints on a psychiatric unit. Generally, the attitude of psychiatric nurses had been that assisting clients with external limits helped them to feel safe and protected. Usually the restraint resulted from failure to conform to unit rules or from a feeling on the part of the staff that the behavior of these clients was escalating and out of control. Results of the study indicated that the participants felt coerced, vulnerable, helpless, and dehumanized. Johnson commented that "We need to use restraints as a last resort." This study supports the need to use least restrictive interventions to help clients regain control, such as talking to clients, presenting anxiety-reducing strategies, or offering medications, before using physical restraint, whenever possible.

The second major reform came from the Joint Commission on Accreditation of Healthcare Organizations (JCAHO), now known as The Joint Commission (TJC). TJC issued new Restraint and Seclusion Standards for Behavioral Health effective January 1, 2001 (Restraint and Seclusion Standards, November 2000). The new TJC standards concurred with CMS's "1-hour rule" and, in addition, added a new requirement that the client's family and legal representatives be notified when restraints are used and the LIP is to engage the clinical staff in reviewing alternative interventions. The staff is also now required to perform continuous in-person observation of any client in restraints for the duration of the restraint procedure. Clients who are in seclusion only are to be monitored in person for the first hour. After that, the staff is able to use audio and video equipment.

The third set of reforms were in the Children's Health Act of 2000, which included national standards restricting the use of seclusion and restraints in psychiatric facilities and in nonmedical community children's programs previously not covered by CMS and TJC standards.

The health care community has dramatically reduced the use of S/R, partly as a result of the new standards, but also because of a new commitment on the part of mental health professionals to change S/R practice. From 1997 to 2000, Pennsylvania successfully reduced the incidence of restraint and seclusion in its nine state hospitals by 74%, with no increase in staff injuries and without any additional funds. The state hospitals implemented key concepts, including identifying the use of seclusion/restraints as a treatment failure, restriction of the use of S/R to emergency situations only, having adequate numbers of staff, and providing staff training in crisis prevention and intervention.

Nursing Implications

In inpatient settings nurses play a primary role in maintaining or changing unit culture with regard to the use of S/R. The leadership role of nurses in staff training, treatment planning, and performance improvement activities related to decreasing S/R is critical. "Never underestimate the difference one person can make" (Sharp HealthCare Medication Guidelines, 2002).

RIGHT TO TREATMENT

In the 1980s a movement began in Alabama for the right to treatment for people with mental illnesses. With financial limitations within the mental health system, employees at Bryce Hospital were laid off because of a budget shortfall. As a result of this situation, a class action suit on behalf of the employees and clients was filed, alleging that with fewer employees the clients could not receive the proper treatment. The case was settled by consent decree in 1986. Many jurisdictions continue to follow some of the standards and guidelines specified, including the right to privacy and dignity, the right to the least restrictive treatment, and individual treatment plans. These plans included a statement of problems and intermediate and long-range treatment goals (with a timetable for attainment with rationale for the specified treatment) (Laben and MacLean, 1989; *Wyatt v. Stickney*, 1972).

The U.S. Supreme Court ruled that health care professionals cannot keep an individual in a mental hospital without treatment if he or she is nondangerous and capable of defining and carrying out a plan of self-care in the community. Mr. Donaldson had been hospitalized in Florida for more than 14 years and wanted to be released. Because of his religion, he declined to take medication or other treatment. He was denied the privilege of going out on the grounds. He had a friend who was willing to assist him on discharge from the hospital. The ruling was limited, but it did set the standard that the state cannot detain individuals who are nondangerous without providing some mode of treatment (*O'Connor v. Donaldson*, 1975).

In the later decision *Youngberg v. Romeo* (1982), the U.S. Supreme Court ruled that a young man with profound retardation was entitled to "minimally adequate training" to provide him with safe conditions. The court stated that a qualified professional's judgment about this matter is "presumptively valid." There was great concern at the time that the right-to-treatment movement was over, but that is not entirely true: courts have upheld the concept of providing adequate treatment (Appelbaum, 1987; *Woe v. Cuomo*, 1986). However, Stefan (1993) reported that "conditions and treatment in many state institutions are still so appalling that plaintiffs still can establish a departure from professional judgment in a well-litigated case." Therefore, the new generation of mental health nurses has a professional obligation to help patients seek out and engage treatment for mental illness at the least restrictive level. This will provide the greatly needed protective care regarding health care discrimination for this underserved health care population (Mental Health Equitable Treatment Act of 2001).

RIGHT TO REFUSE TREATMENT

In the late 1970s and early 1980s, two well-known cases were litigated in the states of Massachusetts and New Jersey, based on the right to refuse psychotropic medication. In the New Jersey case, Mr. Rennie was diagnosed with a psychotic disorder (schizophrenia) at one point and manic depression (bipolar disorder) at another time. There was no agreement about the appropriate medication to be administered. He was given the antipsychotics fluphenazine (Prolixin) and chlorpromazine (Thorazine) at different times. He suffered from documented side effects such as akathisia (a restlessness manifested by the inability to lie down or sit still) and wormlike movements of the tongue (symptoms indicative of tardive dyskinesia, a serious side effect). He refused to take his medication. Rennie filed suit to prevent the involuntary administration of medications. After the courts heard the suit on four different occasions, they decided that voluntary and involuntary clients had the right to refuse medication.

During emergency situations, if there is potential danger, clients can be forcibly medicated. In the case of an involuntary client, as long as nurses follow due process guidelines as established and the administration complies with accepted professional judgment, medication can be given (*Rennie v. Klein*, 1979, 1981). The administrative procedure includes the physician communicating with the client about his or her mental health condition and outlining the plan of care with the client when possible. If the client refuses, the medical director of the facility reviews the treatment recommendations and is authorized to call in an outside psychiatrist for consultation (Weiner and Wettstein, 1993).

Rogers v. Okin was originally filed in 1975 (Rogers, 1979, 1980) as a class action suit to direct a state hospital from certain seclusion practices and forcibly medicating clients. In this case, the courts reached a different conclusion. Instead of deferring to administrative procedures that rely on professional judgment, the right to refuse treatment is upheld if the client is involuntary and competent. If the person is ruled incompetent, the judge uses the substituted judgment standard to determine administration of medication. The judge looks at whether the client, if competent, would have chosen medication administration. In this decision the court ruled that only a judicial authority, and not the decision of the physician or the guardian, was vital (Weiner and Wettstein, 1993).

Nursing Implications

Nurses practicing in mental health facilities need to be aware of the state and case laws and policies and procedures for that jurisdiction regarding the administration of medication to voluntary and involuntary competent clients. Frequent nursing assessment for side effects and careful documentation of clients' complaints related to side effects are essential for adjustment or discontinuance of medication. Nurses need to carefully analyze and questions the reason for the refusal of medication: Is it because of the client's denial of the illness or symptomatology of the condition, or is it because of side effects or displeasure with the treatment staff? Client and family medication education by nurses, along with physicians and pharmacists, and a reassuring therapeutic relationship will greatly assist in medication adherence and will minimize refusal (Sharp HealthCare Medication Guidelines, 2002; Laben and MacLean, 1989) (see Chapter 24).

ELECTROCONVULSIVE THERAPY

The administration of electroconvulsive therapy (ECT) is still controversial, resulting in part from its portrayal in movies as a traumatic procedure. However, in many instances it is an effective treatment for life-threatening depression. The client needs to give informed consent for the procedure, which includes being knowledgeable about the risks and benefits. A potential side effect is memory loss that is usually temporary but is sometimes irreversible.

The question of who can give informed consent is an issue. Previously, the American Psychiatric Association (1978) advised that if an incompetent client could not give informed consent, then a relative of the client is sufficient. Later, Parry (1985) stated that if there is a question of

LEGAL CASE REPORT: Clinical Case Implications

Involuntary Commitment • In the Interest of R.A.J. (1996)

In a recent case a son petitioned for involuntary commitment of his 62-year-old father, R.A.J. The court found probable cause at a preliminary hearing to commit R.A.J. for no more than 14 days to the state hospital. At the hospital he was diagnosed with bipolar disorder and alcohol abuse. At a later hearing, it was not concluded that he had a chemical dependency, but a judgment was issued that he was mentally ill, had impairment, and could be hospitalized for up to an additional 90 days. Because he was refusing to take medication, the court ordered that this intervention was the least restrictive and that he could be involuntarily medicated with haloperidol (Haldol) and carbamazepine (Tegretol), or with risperidone (Risperdal) and carbamazepine, for 90 days. R.A.J. then appealed the decision related to the forced medication order. R.A.J. contended that he had agreed to take the risperidone but not the other medication. The hospital argued that if one medication was refused, the client had "effectively refused necessary treatment." The court noted that it must find by clear and convincing evidence that the treatment was necessary, that the client refused it, that medication was the least restrictive alternative, and that the benefits outweighed the risks. The following items were also taken into consideration:

- The danger that the client represented to himself or others
- The client's current condition
- The client's past treatment history
- The results of previous medication trials
- The efficacy of current or past treatment modalities concerning the client
- The client's prognosis
- The effect of the client's mental condition on his capacity to consent

The court ruled that refusal to take one medication instead of the two prescribed amounted to refusal of treatment for the "purposes of the forced medication statute." The medication haloperidol could be given in injectable form if R.A.J. refused the oral risperidone. The benefits outweighed the risks, and medication was the least restrictive form of treatment.

competence, legal consultation or court guidance takes place. California recognizes that both voluntary and involuntary clients are sometimes capable or incapable of giving informed consent. A court hearing is held for incapable clients to determine whether the ECT treatment will be administered.

In the state of Washington, a client has the right to refuse ECT unless there is clear and convincing evidence that it is necessary. The state must have compelling evidence that ECT is necessary and would be effective, and that other forms of treatment have not been beneficial or are not available (Washington Antipsychotic Medication: ECT, 1993). Some states, such as Tennessee, have regulations related to administration of ECT to minors (Tenn. Code Ann. §33-3-105). Other states limit the number of treatments that a health care provider is able to give to an individual within a certain time frame (Weiner and Wettstein, 1993). California limits the duration of the validity of the client's informed consent to 30 days, during which a maximum of 15 treatments may be administered. In addition, an oversight ECT committee consisting of three ECT qualified psychiatrists have to review each series of ECT treatments to determine the appropriateness and efficacy of that treatment (California Health & Safety Code, Title 9). Health care facilities have to report data on a quarterly basis to the state Department of Health. Data include the number of ECT treatments administered by age group and any serious medical complications. (See Chapter 23 for more information on ECT including nursing implications.)

RESEARCH

The federal government has established guidelines that apply to research on human subjects. The major objective is to provide informed consent to the person who has agreed to participate in research projects. Some of the guidelines include a clear statement of the following:

- Purpose of the research
- Risks and possible discomforts to the subject
- Possible benefits to the individual or to others
- Alternative treatment procedures
- Confidentiality of records
- Sources for further information
- Availability of compensation if injury occurs.

It is most important to note that the research is voluntary and clearly reflects autonomy on the participants' part (45 CFR §46.116) (Box 8-1).

Alzheimer's disease and other dementias will increase in numbers as the population ages. Because there are no animal models of this degenerative process, human experimentation is necessary (Dukoff and Sunderland, 1997). The National Institutes of Health has discovered that clients in the early stages of dementia are able to select health care proxies (substitutes) despite some "minimal memory problems and word-finding difficulties"; in the early stages they continue to "possess the capacity to make independent decisions." As a safeguard to this process, a biochemist assesses all clients. In this manner, as the disease progresses and the research participants are no longer capable of giving informed consent, clients will have a health care proxy to speak for them.

Nursing Implications

Nurses need to be aware of research guidelines in their particular area of practice, especially when they are involved with research projects to fulfill educational or clinical requirements. Many health care facilities are encouraging staff nurses to participate in research, and a thorough awareness of guidelines, including legal and regulatory implications, is imperative.

BOX 8-1

Experimental Subject's Bill of Rights

1. A statement that the procedure or treatment involves research, an explanation of the purposes of the research, the expected length of the subject's participation, an estimate of the subject's expected recovery time after the experiment, and identification of any procedures that are experimental.
2. An explanation of the procedures the subject will follow and any drug or device to be used, including the purposes of such procedures, drugs, or devices. If researchers are giving a placebo to a portion of the subjects involved in a medical experiment, all subjects need to be informed of this fact; however, they need not be informed as to whether they will actually receive a placebo.
3. A description of any reasonably foreseeable or expected risks or discomforts to the subjects.
4. A description of any benefits to the subject or to others that may reasonably be expected from the research.
5. A disclosure of appropriate alternative procedures or courses of treatment, if any, that will possibly be advantageous to the subject and their relative risks and benefits.
6. A statement describing how the researchers will maintain the confidentiality of records that identify the subject. For research subject to the Food and Drug Administration (FDA) regulations, this statement also has to specify that the FDA has the right to inspect the records of subjects participating in studies involving a drug or device subject to FDA regulation.
7. For research involving more than minimal risk, an explanation as to whether any compensation or medical treatments are available if injury occurs. This includes a description of the compensation and where a subject can obtain further information.
8. A statement that participation is voluntary, refusal to participate will involve no penalty or loss of benefits to the subject, and the subject has the right to end participation at any time without penalty or loss of benefits.
9. The name, institutional membership, if any, and address of the person or persons actually performing and primarily responsible for conducting the experiment.
10. The name of the sponsor or funding source, if any, or manufacturer if the experiment involves a drug or device, and the organization, if any, under whose general authority the experiment is being conducted.
11. The name, address, and telephone number of an impartial third party not associated with the experiment for the subject to address complaints about the experiment.
12. An offer to answer any questions concerning the experiment or procedures involved, a person to contact for answers to relevant questions about the research and the research subject's rights, and the person to contact in the event of a research-related injury.

From California Health and Safety Code Section 24172.

THE AMERICANS WITH DISABILITIES ACT

The Americans with Disabilities Act (42 USC §12101) is a substantial breakthrough in discrimination against people with mental illnesses; however, there are specific exclusions. The definition includes mental barriers that limit the ability of the individual in one or more major activities. Enforcement of the statute depends on the person's limitations. Courts have ruled that if a person's mental condition is stabilized, there is no disability (*Mackie v. Runyon*, 1992). However, such people are protected if the fact that they once had a mental disability (such as depression) is used against them in the employment situation. Some exclusions include persons who use controlled substances for unlawful purposes and individuals who take prescribed drugs without the supervision of a health care professional (Parry, 1985). In addition, people who are a direct threat to others are excluded. However, it is important to recognize that this must be based on actual behavior of the individual and not on the mental disability itself.

An employer cannot ask a person about prior history of mental health treatment as part of an application process for employment. The employer can evaluate the individual as to the ability to perform the job functions. Questions about prior use of health care insurance coverage are also not permissible (Weiner and Wettstein, 1993).

ADVOCACY

The term *advocacy* refers to speaking in favor of or arguing for a cause. As a result of the mental health movement begun in the 1970s, states developed advocacy programs for clients. Many states initiated internal grievance procedures allowing clients to express views on their treatment. Under the Protection and Advocacy for Mentally Ill Individuals Act of 1986, all states were required to designate an agency that is responsible for maintaining the rights of people with mental illnesses. The names vary from state to state. For example, in Tennessee, Tennessee Protection and Advocacy, Inc. (TPA), is the organization responsible for implementation of this Act. There has been some controversy in regard to this movement; some mental health professionals say that advocacy sets up adversarial (opposing) relationships. Advocates need to have some understanding of the nature of mental illness and how the mental health system works (Laben and MacLean, 1989).

Nursing Implications

With the increasing prevalence of managed care, patient or client advocacy has become a major part of the nurse's responsibility, especially in the case of nurse psychotherapists and psychiatric case managers who are seeking appropriate care for their clients from third-party payers. Simon (1998) has written that psychiatrists have to advocate with managed care organizations for the care they consider necessary. This strategy incorporates nurses calling managed care companies to obtain authorization for client care. Nurses need to be well informed about the client's right to appeal denial of services that a mental health provider believes is a "medical necessity." Nurses need to help clients strongly pursue appeals particularly in a case where the client is living in the community and the mental health provider believes there is a potential for dangerousness to self and others. Documentation that the client has been clearly informed of these rights is also advisable. In addition to the responsibility to pursue appeals, the nurse is often responsible for providing adequate data so a utilization reviewer is able to make an informed decision.

It is critical that nurses have a keen understanding of each client's rights and report to the health care provider and administration when those rights are violated. Nurses have a long history of being in the best position to serve as outspoken advocates for the client; to continue in this role, they need to be aware of the changing laws and guidelines relative to mental health treatment.

FORENSIC EVALUATIONS

Individuals who have mental health problems and who are charged with or convicted of crimes fall within the category of forensic mental health services. In the 1960s and 1970s, there were many exposés in the professional journals and newspapers of treatment of these individuals. In many instances, persons were sent to institutions for evaluation and remained there for years without resolution of criminal charges. Procedural due process for many was nonexistent. Many forensic units were isolated and provided inadequate treatment. These conditions began to change in 1972 with the landmark decision *Jackson v. Indiana*. Jackson was mentally challenged and hearing and speech impaired. He was found incompetent to stand trial. Because of his disabilities, he probably would never become competent to stand trial. At that time Indiana required hospitalization in a mental hospital until return to competency. Jackson was not going to become competent, so hospitalization would literally sentence him to a form of detention for life. His criminal charge was robbery for a total of $9.

The U.S. Supreme Court ruled that an individual could be hospitalized only for a reasonable length of time (not defined) and that the 3½ years that Jackson had been detained was too long. If the state wanted to hospitalize him longer, he had to be civilly committed, meeting commitment standards. Otherwise he had to be released. Because of this ruling, in the state of Tennessee, the population of the forensic unit went from 185 to 50 within 2 years (Laben and Spencer, 1976).

Competency to Stand Trial

Competency to stand trial is a narrow concept. Criteria include the following: Does the individual charged with the crime understand the criminal charges? Is there an understanding of the legal process and the consequences of the charges? Can the individual advise an attorney and defend the charges? Essentially it is the person's awareness of the legal process that the mental health professional has to evaluate (see the Research for Evidence-Based Practice box).

If the judge, prosecuting attorney, or defense attorney believes that competency is an issue, a request by the attorney results in a *court ordered evaluation* (COE) asking for the evaluation of the person's competency to stand trial. Many states recognize not only the psychiatrist as the competent evaluator on this issue but also psychologists, social workers, and advanced practice psychiatric nurses who have been educated and trained in this evaluation process. Many now perform evaluations on an outpatient basis, resulting in return to the courts and a more timely resolution of the charges (Laben and MacLean, 1989).

> **RESEARCH for EVIDENCE-BASED PRACTICE**
>
> Applebaum KL, Fisher WH: Judges' assumptions about the appropriateness of civil and forensic commitment, *Psychiatric Services* 48:710, 1997.
>
> Researchers completed a survey of Massachusetts district court judges related to forensic evaluations; 58 of 160 responded. The judges were asked, when civil commitment was available and the charge was a minor offense, why were individuals committed for a 20-day forensic evaluation for competency to stand trial? An overwhelming majority (93.1%) admitted concerns about the treatment of individuals in a civil commitment to a mental health facility. Some of the reasons for this strategy included that the defendant did not meet commitment standards and that on some occasions psychiatric hospitals deny admission to offenders who meet commitment criteria unless the court orders the admission. A forensic commitment does not allow for early discharge; the defendant must remain for 20 days and must appear in court before discharge. "This study confirms suspicions that judges order pretrial evaluations to fill perceived gaps in the civil system."

Criminal Responsibility (Insanity Defense)

Competency to stand trial relates to the present mental condition of the defendants and their current ability to make a defense in court. The insanity defense relates to the state of mind at the time of the offense. This concept comes from the legal doctrine of *mens rea*. For a person to be found guilty, the individual must be able to form intent. If, because of mental illness, intent cannot be formed and the person is possibly responding to hallucinatory voices, there is no guilt involved (Shah, 1986).

The first well-known case came from England where the M'Naghten Rule was declared. The set of circumstances involved Daniel M'Naghten, who shot and mistakenly murdered the secretary to the prime minister instead of his intended victim, Sir Robert Peel. M'Naghten intended to kill Peel because he had an irrational belief that Peel was plotting against him. He was found not guilty by reason of insanity, which caused great anxiety in that country. Subsequently, a panel of 15 judges met and defined what has become known as the M'Naghten Rule. An accused will not be held responsible if at the time of the commission of the act, he was "laboring under such a defect of reason, from disease of the mind, as to not know the nature and quality of the act he was doing, or if he did know it, that he did not know he was doing what was wrong" (Shah, 1986).

Much criticism of this doctrine emerged in the 1960s and 1970s, and some states subsequently adopted a modern interpretation of the insanity defense, which states that a person is not responsible for criminal conduct if at the time of such conduct, as a result of mental disease or defect, the person lacks substantial capacity either to appreciate the criminality (wrongfulness) of the conduct or to conform his or her conduct to the requirements of the law (*Graham v. State of Tennessee*, 1977). This definition is derived from the Model Penal Code.

After a person is found not guilty by reason of insanity, he or she is usually hospitalized and sent to a psychiatric unit for evaluation of commitability. Many states have stricter release standards for individuals found not guilty by reason of insanity because, although they have been found not guilty, they have committed a criminal act (Laben and MacLean, 1989).

Guilty but Mentally Ill

Several states have adopted a new plea of guilty but mentally ill (GBMI). The individual is found guilty, but because of the plea that mental illness caused the person to commit the crime, the person is sent to prison and treated for the mental illness. Many thought that fewer people would adopt an insanity defense with the GBMI plea. This has not always proved to be the case; in Michigan the numbers of those pleading this form of the insanity defense increased, although in Georgia the numbers have decreased (Callahan et al., 1992).

Nursing Responsibilities in the Criminal Justice System

In at least one state, advanced practice nurses can testify to the issue of competency to stand trial. Nurses should not take this lightly and should seek special education before testifying on this issue. In most states, psychologists with doctoral degrees and psychiatrists testify concerning the insanity defense. Many states have highly specialized psychiatric units staffed with **forensic psychiatric nurses** trained in clinical observation and treatment of violent offenders.

MALPRACTICE

Because of the irreversible side effects of some medications given to individuals with mental health problems and the trend of short-term hospitalizations, nurses working in psychiatric settings need to be aware of situations that will potentially lead to a malpractice lawsuit. *Negligence*, the primary basis for malpractice lawsuits, is a civil dispute between two or more citizens or a health care facility. A person alleges that a professional ignored or committed an act that a reasonably prudent professional would not do. The action of the professional causes injury resulting in measurable damages.

Elements of a Malpractice Suit Based on Negligence

To bring a suit, the plaintiff must establish that a nurse had a **legal duty** or relationship to that person to provide a certain standard of care. The second aspect to establish in that relationship is a **breach of duty**. The care is then measured by the reasonably prudent nurse standard: What would another nurse working in a mental health facility have done in the same situation? Usually **expert witnesses** testify regarding adherence or departure from the standard of care. Some jurisdictions look to a reasonably prudent nurse standard; however, with the development of standards of care by the American Nurses Association and American Psychiatric Nurses Association in relationship to psychiatric nursing practice, these guidelines could be applied in a lawsuit (Statement on Psychiatric Mental Health Nursing Practice, 1994). A poor outcome does not necessarily mean that an act of negligence has occurred. The next element that a court explores is whether the injury *(damages)* was predictable based on the nurse's actions and the set of circumstances that followed. The court explores whether the nurse was the causal link in the injury that occurred. This is defined by establishing the connection between the nurses acts of negligence and the alleged damages using two tests that are accepted throughout the United States: (1) *but for test*—the alleged damages would not have occurred but for the act of negligence, and (2) *substantial factor test*—the negligence was a substantial factor in causing the alleged damages. For example, did the nurse give the wrong medication, or did the nurse not know about drug interactions with certain medications that led to the injury? The last element that a court has to determine is whether there is a proven injury because of the nurse's behavior. The most damaging and reckless behavior a nurse could be associated with would involve *gross negligence*, defined as acting with willful and conscious disregard of the rights and safety of others.

Documentation

The state or the mental health facility where the nurse is practicing often regulates the information that needs to be documented in a mental health record. Although many mental health professionals view comprehensive charting as a challenge, reflected clinical information is not just a record of the care of the client; it is also a legal document that is valuable in any litigation that takes place.

Adequate legible documentation is the best means of defense against a lawsuit and the best way to validate that the nurse and other health care professionals adhered to their scope of practice and a safe standard of care. It is important to be specific and to document symptoms by

LEGAL CASE REPORT: Clinical Case Implications

Nurse's Responsibility • *Hatley v. Kassen* (1992)

Pennie Johnson had been mentally ill for 10 years. She had been an outpatient in a forensic unit, because long-term inpatient treatment was considered nontherapeutic. Because of her long-term history, a difficult client file had been established to assist treating physicians. In February 1988, a state trooper picked her up on a toll road, at which time she threatened suicide. She was taken to a county hospital. In the nursing assessment, Johnson stated that she was feeling increasingly depressed and had ingested medication that exceeded the prescribed dosage. She continued to take this medication in front of the hospital staff, at which time it was removed from her.

She was examined by Dr. Kalra, who decided to discharge her because he thought her condition had not changed. Johnson asked both the nurse who assessed her and the nursing supervisor, Ms. Kassen, RN, to return her medication. She announced that if they did not return the medication, she would throw herself in front of a car. Kassen told Johnson that, if she would return home in a taxicab paid for by the hospital, Kassen would return the medication. Johnson declined the offer. A security officer was instructed to escort her out of the hospital. There was disputed testimony as to whether the physician knew of her threats. Thirty minutes after leaving the hospital, Johnson stepped in front of a truck and was killed.

Johnson's parents brought an action for damages against Kassen. In the lower court decision, a summary judgment (granted when no genuine issue of material fact is presented) was awarded to the physician and the hospital, and a directed verdict was entered in favor of Kassen (a decision that is directed to the jury by the judge because the opposing party has not sufficiently presented its case) (Weiner and Wettstein, 1993). The Court of Appeals of Texas reversed the decision and sent the case back to the lower court for further litigation, stating that the doctor and the nurse were not entitled to official immunity because they were employed at a government hospital.

The court, in its decision, did note the testimony of three expert witnesses regarding Kassen's nursing care. Two nurse experts testified that Kassen's actions were substandard once she knew that Johnson had communicated suicidal intentions with a specific plan. A psychiatric expert in the field of suicidology testified that Kassen should have sought the advice of the physician or supervisor before releasing Johnson after the suicidal threats.

One judge wrote a dissenting opinion. This justice believed that Johnson had threatened for 10 years to commit suicide and had never done so; therefore it was not foreseeable that Johnson would follow through with her threat, and therefore it was not negligence on Kassen's part. "I would hold that threats of suicide cannot enslave the intended victim to either submission or damages—especially threats that have been 'empty' for years."

This case was sent for retrial, so the final results are unknown. However, elements of the case are useful for analytic purposes. The nurses and doctor had a duty to a client who was brought to the emergency department. Several experts testified that once a client has a suicide plan, some form of hospitalization should be instituted or—at the least—a supervisor notified or another discussion held with the physician. On the basis of this testimony, it might be concluded that the nurse's action fell below the standard of care. Because the nurse permitted the client to leave the hospital, she could be targeted as a causal agent in the resulting death. Damages could be awarded for the incident (Weiner and Wettstein, 1993).

writing in quotes what the client expresses to you, such as "I am hearing voices that say I am a bad person." Recording the actual words of the client is more definitive than simply noting, "The client is hallucinating," especially if the words are destructive to the client or others. Nurses need to chart in a timely and legible manner. Recording at the time something happens is more adequate than block charting, which is usually briefer and not as definitive (*Nurse's Handbook of Law and Ethics*, 1992). A client's record is a sequential document; thus, it does not save space for late entries. Nurses need to label late entries as such and initial them.

In a mental health record, it is especially important to document when the person has achieved the goals outlined in the treatment plan. If the individual has an exacerbation of the illness, the treatment plan needs to reflect the change. Informed consent concerning the giving of psychiatric medications is an important aspect of the chart, especially medications such as some neuroleptics, which cause irreversible side effects or provide chemical restraint.

Records are an excellent source for communicating with other mental health professionals on the staff, as well as other agencies. Records are also used to validate reimbursement for care that the agency gave the client. Because managed care is becoming more common, nurses need to carefully record a clear outline of all of the client's symptoms to document a necessity for continued, decreased/increased level of care (e.g., controlled structured environment, increased observation, medication stabilization, and continued hospitalization). For example, if routine hospitalization is for 5 days but the client continues daily to verbalize suicidal thoughts, recording this information is critical for extended permission to continue the hospitalization.

Do not use improper abbreviations that the agency does not authorize. Nurses need to obtain records from other facilities or other treating professionals to provide an accurate long-term picture of how the client was treated on prior occasions.

Nurses need to document in writing all client education, aftercare plans, participation in a treatment team, or referral to other agencies for care as well. Accurate recording of vital signs is essential, especially when clients are taking psychotropic medications. Nurses will need to define and communicate their observations on the efficacy of prescribed medication in the chart and to the physician. Clearly document all notifications and order clarifications. Nurses also need to complete any nursing assessments that the organization requires. Careful documenting also means spelling words correctly and making sure sentences are grammatically correct. If a nurse makes an error in documentation, she or he needs to place a single

LEGAL CASE REPORT: Clinical Case Implications

Responsibilities of Treating Therapists • *Estates of Morgan v. Fairfield Family Counseling Center* (1997)

Matt Morgan was playing a card game with his parents and sister when he left the room, returned with a gun, and shot and killed his parents. His sister was injured but survived. Matt had problems in his senior year in high school and after graduation had difficulty retaining employment. He was "verbally abusive" to his parents, and they had become afraid of him. In January 1990, police removed him from his home as he was attempting to fight with his father.

After a period of wandering, Matt eventually presented to the emergency department at a hospital in Philadelphia. He was diagnosed with schizophreniform disorder and transferred to a mental health facility. He had delusions that the government was affecting his body and the airwaves so that he was unable to watch television or listen to tapes or radio, and he had delusions of persecution, ideas of reference, and thought broadcasting. He was given thiothixene (Navane) and was admitted to a respite unit.

During the 12-week stay at the respite unit, Matt continued to receive thiothixene and intensive therapy. He had paranoia concerning his family, but this decreased, and he was able to admit that the medication helped him to manage his symptoms. He acknowledged that his conflicts with his family, especially his relationship with his father, could be attributed to his mental illness. The treating physician thought it was in Matt's best interest to return to his home and be followed at the Fairfield Family Counseling Center (FFCC). His parents came to get him at the end of June 1990, and he was first seen in the FFCC on July 16, 1990.

A psychotherapist initially saw Matt, and then he was referred to Dr. Brown, a contract psychiatrist for medication evaluation, on July 19, 1990. Dr. Brown reported that Matt had been in a mental health unit "of some sort" in Philadelphia and that he was out of medication. He wrote, "He comes to the mental health clinic for his medication, continued care, and help in completing a Social Security Disability form." Dr. Brown concluded that Matt had some form of atypical psychosis and did not appear to have a thought disorder or schizophrenia. Dr. Brown also noted that he thought Matt might be malingering in an attempt to obtain disability. Dr. Brown wrote that it was "wise to defer diagnosis, continue the medication, obtain Matt's records from Philadelphia, and schedule another appointment for a month later." When Matt returned for his appointment, the records from the mental health unit in Philadelphia were available, but the court reported that it was clear from Dr. Brown's testimony that he never read them or attempted to contact the treating physician.

Dr. Brown reduced the dosage of thiothixene and wrote again about the possibility of malingering. Dr. Brown saw Matt on October 11, 1990, for the last time; he prescribed a tapering and discontinuation of the thiothixene. He stated that Matt would continue in psychotherapy. Matt was referred to a vocational counselor to assist him in finding employment. Between October and January 1991, Matt remained in psychotherapy and vocational counseling. However, his mother reported that Matt's condition was deteriorating. He was pacing and showed a quiet demeanor, withdrawal, and irritability. She said that Matt had given a deposit toward the purchase of a gun and asked that he be placed back on medication. The vocational counselor thought that the mother was overprotective. When Matt failed to keep his appointment with the psychotherapist in January of 1991, it was decided that the only person who should see him was the vocational counselor. Matt's condition continued to worsen, his parents became afraid of him, and he once again developed symptoms of paranoia. During of May 1991, Matt's mother continued to report Matt's deterioration. An appointment was scheduled with Dr. Brown, but Matt did not keep it. Matt's employer also reported that he was "too weak to push a lawnmower, was on the verge of passing out, and did not seem to be totally in touch with reality." On June 14, 1991, Matt's mother wrote a letter to FFCC seeking help for her son. She explained her concerns about his potential violence. The vocational counselor and a licensed social worker conducted an assessment. FFCC had an unwritten policy that no involuntary commitment would be initiated without family involvement; but when the family attempted such course of action, the probate court informed them that it would need the vocational counselor's approval.

On July 20, 1991, Matt's parents sent a letter to a psychologist employed at FFCC who reviewed the record, talked with the vocational counselor and social worker, and determined that Matt could not be given medication against his will and could not be hospitalized. Another social worker commented on July 25, 1991, that Matt was losing weight and deteriorating. That evening Matt shot his family.

In an action for negligence brought by the parents' estate, expert witnesses for the plaintiffs, the Morgan estates, testified that Dr. Brown's treatment of Matt was negligent for failure to read the prior treatment reports, for failure to diagnose, for discontinuing needed medication, and for failure to closely monitor Matt after discontinuation of the medication. The fact that a vocational therapist was making commitment decisions was of particular concern. One expert testified that it was foreseeable that without medication, this created a potential for violent behavior; the expert added, "The only reason Matt killed his parents is because he was taken off medication and didn't receive good care."

The expert witnesses testified that at the point Matt refused medication because of his deteriorating condition, the action should have included "strong family involvement, making Matt's participation in vocational therapy contingent upon continued treatment, and telling Matt that he faced involuntary hospitalization unless he resumed taking his medication."

The court in its ruling stated that "a relationship between the psychotherapist and the patient in the outpatient setting constitutes a special relationship justifying the imposition of a duty upon the psychotherapist to protect against the patient's violent propensities. The outpatient setting embodies sufficient elements of control to warrant the imposition of such a duty, and such a duty would serve the public's interest in protection from the violently inclined mental patient in a manner that is consistent with Ohio law."

The trial court had dismissed this action, and the court of appeals affirmed in part and reversed in part. The Supreme Court held that the psychotherapist had a duty to protect against the client's potentially violent behavior. The case was returned to the trial court to settle the issues of whether the defendants were negligent and whether a summary judgment in the defendant's favor was warranted.

What nurses need to learn from this case is that any treating therapist needs to be aware of the duty to hospitalize and protect families and the public when appropriate. Consultation by nurse clinicians with mental health professionals who have legal authority to commit is essential.

line through the words without making them illegible and then initial the error.

Sexual Misconduct

In studies that have been conducted with social workers, psychiatrists, and psychologists, researchers estimate that up to 14% of these professionals have had a sexual relationship with a client (Weiner and Wettstein, 1993). There has not been a study of nurses; however, cases for removal of a nursing license for such activity are on record (*Heinecke v. Department of Commerce*, 1991). All mental health professions consider such behavior unethical, and in many states this behavior is criminal, especially if it is within a few months of the therapeutic relationship. Some states have mandatory reporting laws for a second therapist who becomes knowledgeable about such behavior (Strasburger, Jorgenson, and Randles, 1991).

Many of the cases are settled out of court (*Hall v. Schulte*, 1992). When information about the relationship is presented to a jury, members tend to be sympathetic to the client, except when a client appears to have encouraged the relationship. Because the client comes to a therapist with a problem, the issue of the transference phenomenon becomes pronounced, resulting in true lack of consent to become involved with the therapist (Weiner and Wettstein, 1993).

Suicide and Homicide

Malpractice suits and wrongful death actions for homicidal clients' injury to a third party and death from suicide have become more common. Some states have ruled that individuals working in government agencies have sovereign immunity and are protected from liability in malpractice situations (*Poss v. Department of Human Resources*, 1992; *Smith v. King*, 1993). When conducting nursing assessments that include a suicidal component, use extreme caution. For example, when an individual threatens *intent* of suicide with a defined plan and demonstrates *lethality* and access to the *means* to commit suicide, nurses must communicate this information, in a timely manner, to a mental health provider. Then health care providers must follow the appropriate steps to provide client safety, including involuntary commitment, to escape liability. If there is a question, the nurse should seek legal consultation. However, "clinicians are not liable for errors of clinical judgment; they are liable only for departures from the relevant standard of care, given the clinical situation" (Weiner and Wettstein, 1993, p. 119).

Because of the previously described decision regarding *Tarasoff v. Regents of the University of California*, it is important to communicate with the mental health treatment team when a client threatens to harm someone. Many states require that health care providers notify a potential victim or police of this occurrence. Some states have limited the warning to include only identifiable victims (*Leonard v. Iowa*, 1992; Rudegair and Appelbaum, 1992). Failure to comply with the required notification will lead to exposure and major liability.

ETHICAL ISSUES

Ethical issues are connected to legal implications for nursing care. *Ethics* is that body of knowledge that explores the moral problems about specific issues. In nursing practice, look at the rules, principles, and ethical guidelines that the nursing profession has developed to guide conduct (Davis and Aroskar, 1991). Laws reflect the moral character of a society and are developed (it is hoped) with an ethical basis; therefore, consider ethical principles when evaluating a dilemma or problematic situation. Many ethical problems occur in the arena of mental health law when statutes conflict with a nurse's personal beliefs.

Autonomy

The term *autonomy* refers to having respect for an individual's decision or self-determination about health care issues. This point is especially important with problems such as the right to die and, in mental health, treatment in the least restrictive alternative. When involuntary commitment is necessary, it is difficult for mental health providers to have to follow the law rather than do what the client currently desires. The caregiver will want to allow the client to make decisions, but if the individual is demonstrating intent by threatening suicide with an active plan, proceeding against the wishes of the person is necessary for safety and compliance with the law. This kind of decision in ethical terms is called a *paternalistic decision*, or *parentalism* (Purtilo, 1993). This often causes a great deal of anxiety for the new health care professional.

In addition, it is sometimes difficult for families when the member who is mentally ill and refusing treatment has to be involuntarily hospitalized. Educating the family about the illness, being supportive, and allowing all of the family to express their frustration, anxieties, and (perhaps) anger will be helpful for the family.

Olsen (1998) has raised an interesting question about autonomy and privacy in relation to video monitoring of psychiatric clients who are placed in seclusion. One loses autonomy when secluded or restrained, and compounding this situation with video monitoring is threatening to a client. To justify the use of such strategies, Olsen has recommended that health care providers keep a record that a monitor is being used and the therapeutic reason for such use. The client needs to be informed of the monitoring, perhaps by placing a sign in the seclusion room. Olsen contends that only staff with clinical responsibility for care of the client should have access to the monitor, that only clinically competent staff should monitor clients, and that the nurse should perform personal visualization and assessment of the client. "Ethical treatment means balancing the good of a safer environment with the potential of harm from a loss of privacy."

Beneficence

Individuals who work in the health care field have a special duty and responsibility to act in a manner that is going to benefit and not harm clients. The term *beneficence* refers to bringing about good (Purtilo, 1993). The goal in mental health treatment is to assist individuals in returning to a mentally healthy way of life.

The moral rule of *primum no nocere* ("first do no harm") is vital in clinical interventions with persons with mental illnesses. Situations in which this issue will possibly occur include giving neuroleptic medications when certain side effects are irreversible. Another instance is the consideration of giving ECT to a client who has failed to respond to antidepressive medication and continues to be suicidal. It is known that memory loss is sometimes a side effect. Do the beneficial aspects of the treatment outweigh the possible side effects? This dilemma causes anxiety for the client, family, and mental health professional in the decision-making process.

Certainly, when a mental health professional considers a sexual relationship with a client, preventing harm is the major consideration. According to the literature, the professional who becomes involved with a client uses denial and rationalization that the client desires the relationship, that the therapeutic relationship has ended, or that it took place outside of the therapeutic time (Russell, 1993). Russell writes that it is important for students to become aware of their own sexual feelings and possible attraction to a client, and that this is an important part of the mental health curriculum, especially for students who later hope to specialize in this area.

Distributive Justice

According to Purtilo (1993, p. 84), *distributive justice* refers to the "comparative treatment of individuals in the allotment of benefits and burdens." "The principle of justice holds that a person should be treated according to what is fair, given what is due or owed" (Chally and Loriz, 1998, p. 17). During times of health care cost constraints, who is going to get treatment and the cost of the treatment are frequent topics of debate. In managed care, mental health care is not always treated equally as physical health; the mental health needs of clients are often compromised. Many nurses working in a mental health setting find that, to access mental health care, it is necessary to become an active advocate for the client with the primary care provider. When there is an annual cap (limit) on the amount of money that a managed care organization is allowing for each individual in a health care plan, resistance to treating a person with a serious and persistent mental illness will occur, especially when this person needs a variety of services over a long time.

A major question is the treatment site for individuals with medical and mental health problems. It is not uncommon for a mental health unit to not want to admit a person with serious physical health problems, and a medical unit may not want to admit someone with severe mental health problems who also has a physical problem. These issues are going to become more widespread as the nation moves more toward managed care to control health care costs. How is the United States going to divide the health care dollar, and where will individuals with mental illnesses fit into the picture (Lazarus, 1994)?

An editorial in the *American Journal of Psychiatry* reported that "under managed care, the actual dollar amounts spent on all mental illness treatment have decreased" (Leslie and Rosenheck, 1999, p. 1250) There is growing concern that because people with the diagnosis of major depression have high rates of health care utilization, the managed care organizations will "dump" them or fail to provide adequate care, resulting in longer illnesses.

Mental health parity (equality) bills have been introduced and passed in some states. In addition, some states have passed their own statutes giving clients a bill of rights in relation to reimbursement for mental health care. Maryland has a law that requires coverage for mental health and substance abuse care (Goldstein, 1998).

CHAPTER SUMMARY

- Balancing the rights of the mentally ill versus the community has been and continues to be a struggle.
- Alternatives to inpatient mental health treatment need to consider the least restrictive environment using the least restrictive treatment.
- There are three types of commitments for a client with a mental illness: an emergency commitment, a voluntary commitment, and an involuntary indefinite commitment.
- Clients need to be informed about treatment, including risks and alternatives, on admission.
- A civil or judicial commitment of a client is legally based in *parens patriae,* the power of the state to protect and care for disabled individuals, and the police power of the state to protect the community from persons who are a threat.
- Half of the states in the United States have enacted preventive or mandatory outpatient treatment, in which clients can be returned to the hospital if they discontinue treatment medication, deteriorate, or exhibit dangerous behavior after discharge.
- Clients with mental illnesses retain their civil rights on entering a mental hospital or other inpatient treatment center. Clients need to receive a summary of their rights on admission.
- Restrain clients only to prevent physical injury to the clients themselves or to others, and only a psychiatrist or licensed physician is able to order nonemergency seclusion or restraint.
- Clients who are ruled competent and are voluntarily or involuntarily committed have a right to refuse treatment and medication.
- The U.S. Supreme Court ruled that individuals charged with or convicted of a crime could only be hospitalized for a reasonable length of time. To be committed longer requires a person to be civilly committed or released.
- Competency to stand trial is based on a person's current awareness of the legal process as evaluated by a mental health professional.
- The insanity defense comes from the concept that for a person to be found guilty, the person must be able to form intent and relate to his or her state of mind at the time of the offense.

- Several states have adopted a new plea, guilty but mentally ill (GBMI). Because of the plea that states mental illness caused the commission of the crime, the person is sent to prison and treated for mental illness.
- Nurses working in psychiatric settings need to be aware of situations that will possibly lead to malpractice lawsuits.

REVIEW QUESTIONS

1 An individual is found not guilty by reason of insanity after planting explosive devices in a local church. What would be the nurse's expectation regarding this person?

1. The individual will be treated for mental illness in a prison or other forensic setting.
2. The individual will be unable to provide useful assistance to the defense attorney.
3. The individual will have a new trial after psychiatric stability has been attained.
4. The individual will be unable to act with intent at the time of the offense because of mental illness.

2 An adult client assaulted another client in an acute psychiatric unit and was unable to be managed through less restrictive means. The client was restrained at 1345. By what time must the client have a face-to-face assessment by the physician?

1. 1445
2. 1545
3. 1745
4. 1345 on the following day

3 Which individual with a mental illness may need emergency or involuntary hospitalization for mental illness?

1. The individual who sees visions of angels dancing on the television screen.
2. The individual who throws a lamp at the owner of a local department store.
3. The individual who resumes using cocaine after 1 year of being clean.
4. The individual who stops taking prescribed antipsychotic medications.

4 A nurse at a local mental health clinic prepares to give a client with schizophrenia a regularly scheduled monthly antipsychotic medication injection. Just before the nurse gives the injection, the client says, "Wait! I've changed my mind. I don't want to take that medicine anymore." Which initial action by the nurse would be legally and ethically appropriate?

1. Say, "You have a right not to take it, but let's talk about how that could affect your illness."
2. Remind the client that this medication has been used for months with no adverse effects.
3. Assess the client for evidence of dangerousness to self or others.
4. Call for assistance to restrain the client and proceed with the scheduled injection.

5 A nurse's neighbor asks, "Why aren't people with mental illnesses kept in state institutions anymore?" Select the nurse's accurate response(s). You may select more than one answer.

1. "Better drugs for mental illness now make it possible for many people to live in their communities."
2. "There are less restrictive settings available now to care for individuals with mental illness."
3. "Our nation has fewer people with mental illness; therefore, fewer hospital beds are needed."
4. "Psychiatric institutions are no longer popular as a consequence of negative stories in the press."
5. "Funding for treatment of mental illness has shifted to community rather than institutional settings."

6 Benjamin Franklin invented the lightning rod, a device that saved lives and property in early American history. He refused to patent the invention because he wanted it widely shared for the well being of humankind. Franklin's action can best be correlated to which ethical principle in health care?

1. Autonomy
2. Beneficence
3. Distributive justice
4. Parity

*Additional self-study exercises and learning resources are available to you on the **Companion CD** at the back of the book and on the **Evolve website** at **http://evolve.elsevier.com/Fortinash/.***

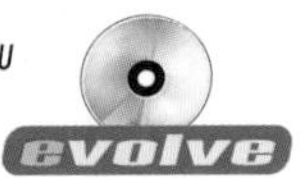

REFERENCES

American Nurses Association: *Code for nurses,* Kansas City, Mo, 1982, American Nurses Association.

American Psychiatric Association: *Electroconvulsive therapy: task force report 14,* Washington, DC, 1978, The Association.

Americans with Disabilities Act (42 USC §12101).

Appelbaum P: Resurrecting the right to treatment, *Hosp Community Psychiatry* 38:703, 1987.

Appelbaum P: Law & psychiatry: psychiatric advance directives and the treatment of committed patients, *Psychiatr Serv* 55:751, 2004.

Backler P, Macfarland BH: A survey on use of advanced directives for mental health treatment in Oregon, *Psychiatr Serv* 47, 1387, 1996.

Backlar P et al: Consumer, provider, and informal caregiver opinions on psychiatric advanced directives, *Adm Policy Ment Health* 28:427, 2001.

Brakel SJ, Parry J, Weiner BA: *The mentally disabled and the law,* ed 3, Chicago, 1985, American Bar Foundation.

California Health & Safety Code 24172, Experimental subject's bill of rights, California Welfare & Institutions Code, Title 9.

Callahan LA et al: Measuring the effects of the guilty but mentally ill (GBMI) verdict, *Law Hum Behav* 16:441, 1992.

Chally PS, Loriz L: Ethics in the trenches: decision making in practice, *Am J Nurs* 98:17, 1998.

Davis AJ, Aroskar MA: *Ethical dilemmas and nursing practice,* ed 3, Norwalk, Conn, 1991, Appleton & Lange.

Dukoff R, Sunderland T: Durable power of attorney and informed consent with Alzheimer's disease patients: a clinical study, *Am J Psychiatry* 154:1070, 1997.

45 CFR §46.116.

Goldstein A: Ahead of the fed: how some states are already regulating managed care, *Time,* p 30, July 13, 1998.

Graham v. State of Tennessee, 541 SW2d 531 (Tenn 1977).
Hall v. Schulte, 836kP2d 989 (Ariz Or of App 1992).
Health Insurance Portability and Accountability Act of 1996.
Heinecke v. Department of Commerce, 810 P2d 459 (Utah App 1991).
Jackson v. Indiana, 406 US 715 (1972).
Laben JK, MacLean CP: *Legal issues and guidelines for nurses who care for the mentally ill*, Owings Mills, Md, 1989, National Health Publishing.
Laben JK, Spencer LD: Decentralization of forensic services, *Community Ment Health J* 12:405, 1976.
LaFond JQ: Law and the delivery of involuntary mental health services, *Am J Orthopsychiatry* 64:409, 1994.
Lake v. Cameron, 364 F2d 657 (DC Cir 1966 *en banc*).
Lamb HR, Weinberger LE: Persons with severe mental illness in jails and prisons: a review, *Psychiatr Serv* 49:483, 1998.
Lanterman-Petris-Short Act of 1969.
Lazarus A: Disputes over payment for hospitalization under mental health "carve-out" programs, *Hosp Community Psychiatry* 45:115, 1994.
Leonard v. Iowa, 491 NW2d 508 (Iowa Sup Ct 1992).
Leslie DL, Rosenheck R: Shifting care to outpatient mental health care: use and cost under private insurance, *Am J Psychiatry* 156:1250, 1999.
Mackie v. Runyon, 804 F Supp 1508 (1992).
Mental Health Equitable Treatment Act of 2001.
Nurse's handbook of law and ethics, Springhouse, Pa, 1992, Springhouse.
O'Connell M, Stein C: Psychiatric advance directives: perspectives of community stakeholders, *Adm Policy Ment Health* 32: 241-265, 2005.
O'Connor v. Donaldson, 422 U5 563 (1975).
Olsen DP: Ethical consideration of video monitoring psychiatric patients in seclusion and restraint, *Arch Psychiatr Nurs* 12:90, 1998.
Parry J: Mental disabilities under the APA: a difficult path to follow, *Ment Phys Disabil Law Rep* 17:100, 1985.
Pennsylvania Department of Public Welfare, Office of Mental Health and Substance Abuse Services: *Leading the way toward a seclusion and restraint-free environment—Pennsylvania's seclusion and restraint reduction initiative*, Harrisburg, Pa, 2000, Office of Mental Health and Substance Abuse Services.
Poss v. Department of Human Resources, 426 SE2d 635 (Go Or App 1992).
Purtilo R: *Ethical dimensions in the health professions*, ed 2, Philadelphia, 1993, WB Saunders.
Rennie v. Klein 416 F Supp 1294 (1979); 653 F2d 836 (3rd Cir 1981); 454 US 1978 (1982).
Restraint and Seclusion Standards for Behavioral Health effective January 1, 2001, Joint Commission for the Accreditation of Healthcare Organizations website, November 2000.
Rogers v. Okin, Right to Refuse Treatment for a Mental Illness, 478 F Supp. 1342 (Mass, 1979); F .2d 1 (1st Cir, 1980).
b. 45CFR 46.116 Code of Federal Regulations, Title 45, Public Welfare, 45 CFR section 46.116, General Requirements for Informed consent, Department of Health and Human Services, National Institutes of Health, Office for Protection of Research Risks, 1991.
Rudegair TS, Applebaum PS: On the duty to protect: an evolutionary perspective, *Bull Am Acad Psychiatry Law* 20:419, 1992.
Russell J: *Out of bounds sexual exploitation in counseling and therapy*, London, 1993, Sage.
Sales BD, Shuman DW: Mental health law and mental health care: introduction, *Am J Orthopsychiatry* 64:172, 1994.
Shah S: *Criminal responsibility in forensic psychiatry and psychology*, Philadelphia, 1986, FA Davis.
Sharp HealthCare Medication Guidelines, San Diego, California, 2002.
Sherman PS: Computer-assisted creation of psychiatric advance directives, *Commun Ment Health J* 34:351, 1998.
Simon RI: Psychiatrists' duties in discharging sicker and potentially violent inpatients in the managed care era, *Psychiatr Serv* 49:62, 1998.
Simon RI: *Psychiatry and law for clinicians*, ed 3, Washington, DC, 2001, American Psychiatric Publishing.
Smith v. King, 615 So2s 69 (Ala Sup Ct 1993).
Statement on psychiatric mental health nursing practice and standards of psychiatric mental health clinical nursing practice, Washington, DC, 1994, American Nurses Publishing.
Stefan S: What constitutes departure from professional judgment? *Ment Phys Disabil Law Rep* 17:207, 1993.
Strasburger L, Jorgenson L, Randles R: Criminalization of psychotherapist-patient sex, *Am J Psychiatry* 148:859, 1991.
Studer Q: Sharp HealthCare Leadership Development session, November 2002.
Tarasoff v. Regents of the University of California, 529 P2d 553 (Cal 1974) and 551 P2d 334 (Cal 1976).
Tenn Code Ann §33-6-201, 33-10-103, 33-3-105.
Torrey EF, Kaplan RS: A national survey of the use of outpatient commitment, *Psychiatr Serv* 46:778, 1995.
Washington Antipsychotic Medication: ECT: legislative and regulatory developments, *Ment Phys Disabil Law Rep* 17:206, 1993.
Weiner BA, Wettstein RM: *Legal issues in mental health care*, New York, 1993, Plenum Press.
Wexler DB, Winick BJ: Therapeutic jurisprudence and criminal justice mental health issues, *Ment Phys Disabil Law Rep* 16:225, 1992.
Woe v. Cuomo 638 F Supp 1506 (ED NY 1986).
Wyatt v. Stickney 344 F Supp 373 (1972).
Youngberg v. Romeo 461 US 308 (1982).

PSYCHIATRIC DISORDERS

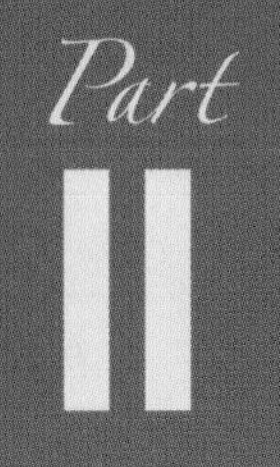

Chapter 9 Anxiety and Anxiety Disorders

PAMELA E. MARCUS

Worry is a thin stream of fear trickling through the mind. If encouraged, it cuts a channel into which all other thoughts are drained.

ARTHUR SOMERS ROCHE

OBJECTIVES

1. Discuss the four stages of anxiety and their manifestations.
2. Explain how the body adapts to stress according to Selye's general adaptation syndrome.
3. Describe the various defense mechanisms an individual uses when feeling anxious.
4. Identify the defining characteristics of anxiety in the NANDA classification.
5. Describe the coping mechanisms of trauma victims that assist the nurse in evaluating the risk for posttraumatic stress disorder.
6. Explain the advantages of the humanistic nursing model in providing care to clients experiencing varying levels of anxiety.
7. Apply the nursing process to provide comprehensive nursing care to clients with anxiety disorders.
8. Relate the biologic model to target symptoms and therapeutic agents for psychopharmacologic intervention in anxiety and related disorders.
9. Design a teaching plan for family members of clients with obsessive-compulsive disorder.
10. Discuss the usefulness of clinical rating scales in evaluating treatment outcomes of clients with anxiety disorders.

KEY TERMS

agoraphobia, p. 183
anxiety, p. 173
anxiolytic, p. 190
compulsions, p. 185
defense mechanisms, p. 174
dissociation, p. 184
humanistic nursing, p. 178
obsessions, p. 185
panic anxiety, p. 182
panic attacks, p. 182
phobias, p. 183
repression, p. 184
stress, p. 179

Anxiety is an integral part of the universal human experience. For most people, it is a vague, subjective feeling of uneasiness with no identifiable object, resulting from an external threat to one's integrity. The function of **anxiety** is to warn the individual of impending threat, conflict, or danger. Anxiety is also a state of tension, dread, or impending doom, coming from external influences that threaten to overwhelm the individual. When a person receives a signal of approaching danger, this motivates the individual to act, whether it means fleeing the threatening situation or controlling dangerous impulses. Some even freeze or do not act.

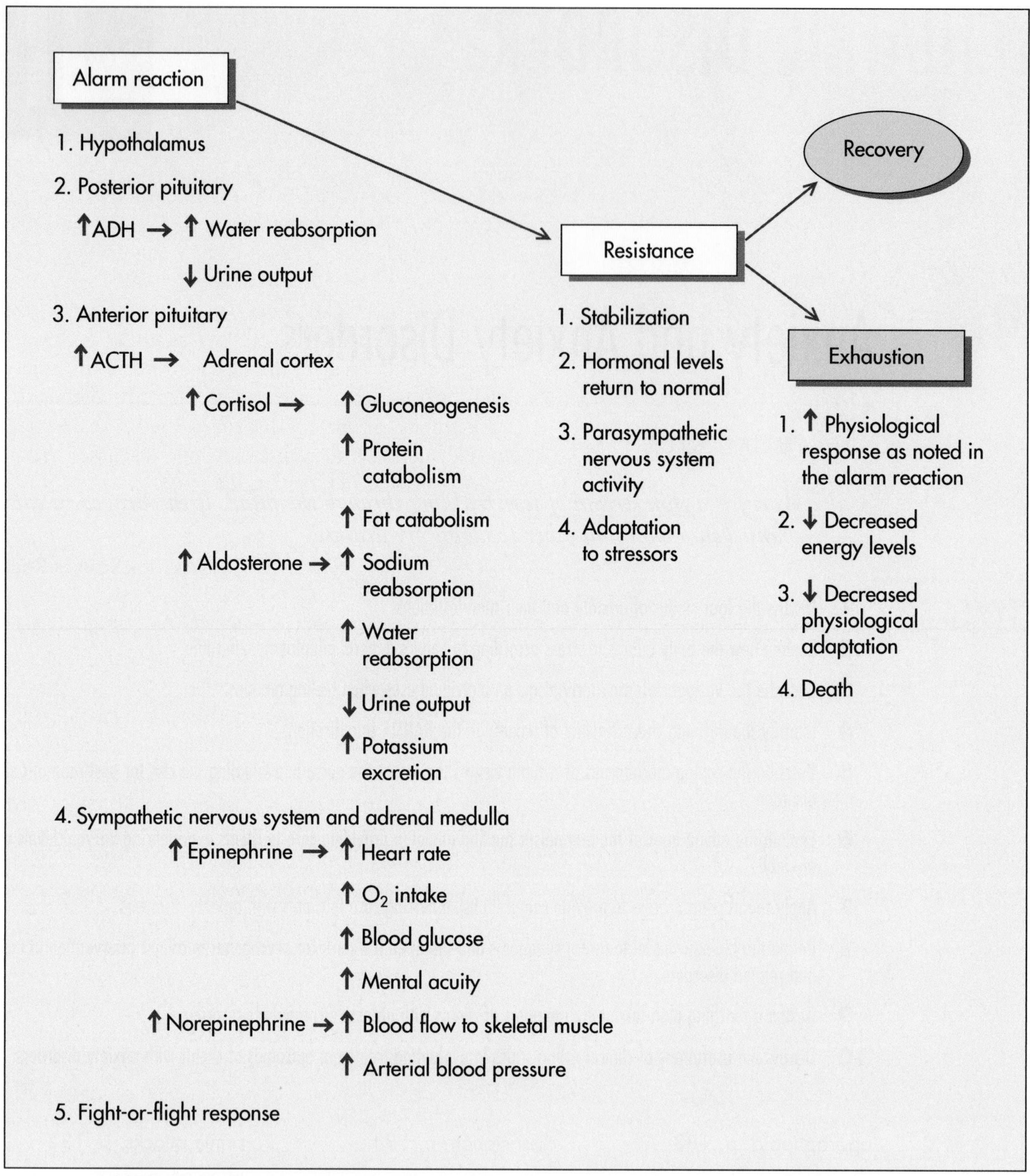

FIGURE 9-1 General adaptation syndrome (GAS). (From Potter PA, Perry AG: *Fundamentals of nursing*, ed 6, St Louis, 2005, Mosby.)

A helpful way to conceptualize the physiologic and behavioral changes that occur during stress is by understanding the general adaptation syndrome (GAS) identified by Hans Selye (1907-1982), a pioneer in stress research (Figure 9-1). The GAS occurs in three stages (Potter and Perry, 2004):

1. In the *alarm stage* (fight-or-flight), the adrenal glands release stress hormones that prepare the body to deal physically with the stressful event the individual is confronting. The rising hormone levels activate the autonomic nervous system, which increases blood volume, blood glucose, blood oxygen level, and an enhanced arousal level. Pupils dilate, muscles tense, and the body is ready for flight or fight (Figure 9-2).
2. In the *resistance/recovery stage*, the body maintains its protective responses to the stressor and stabilizes/recovers its normal physical state as the threatening situation eases.
3. In the *exhaustion stage*, the body is no longer able to function in an activated state without an assault to the immune system. Exhaustion occurs when the stress level persists and the body's defense mechanisms weaken. Some extreme cases result in death.

Defense mechanisms are the primary methods the ego (self) uses to control or manage anxiety (Table 9-1). Defense mechanisms protect us from threats to the physical,

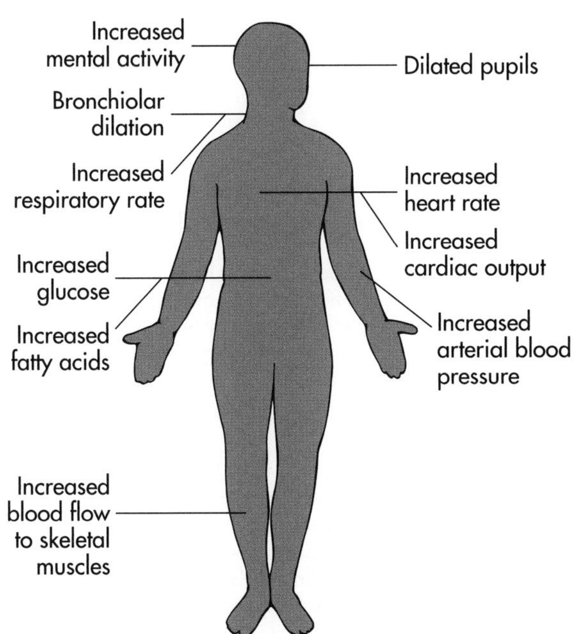

FIGURE 9-2 Fight-or-flight response. (From Potter PA, Perry AG: *Fundamentals of nursing*, ed 6, St Louis, 2005, Mosby.)

mental, and social aspects of ourselves. We all use defense mechanisms in various stages of life. For example, a person with a history of being abused as a child uses the repression defense mechanism to control the anxiety related to the trauma. Repressing the painful event enables the individual to engage in normal activities, such as school, sports, making friends, and even marriage and parenthood. The pain of the trauma eventually becomes too difficult to repress, so the person uses dysfunctional methods to manage anxiety, which disrupts the person's life. Therapy helps these individuals confront the traumatic event, and their level of functioning increases as they learn to manage anxiety in a healthier way.

An example of a commonly used defense mechanism—identification—is seen in the teenager who dresses and grooms like the most popular girls in school. She is using the defense mechanism to identify with the peers she admires to diffuse her own identity with theirs and thus be accepted as one of the group. Being different carries the threat of rejection, which creates overwhelming anxiety in most teens. Eventually, many young people grow into confident adults who find their own identities. All defense mechanisms reduce anxiety, and most people use a variety of them occasionally to get through a difficult time or to meet the challenges of a developmental milestone. Individuals who use defense mechanisms rigidly or consistently will not grow and develop emotionally as healthy, responsible beings. This is often noted in individuals diagnosed with personality disorders. For example, a person with an antisocial personality disorder often relies on the defense mechanism projection to control anxiety by projecting his own inadequacies onto another person or situation. In one sense, projection effectively reduces anxiety, yet by constantly using projection, the individual fails to confront and deal with his vulnerabilities and ceases to grow (see Chapter 13).

Psychoanalytic theory says that at an unconscious level, the consequence of ignoring anxiety signals is the threat of being "destroyed" or of no longer existing. Anxiety responses exist on a continuum (Table 9-2), and individuals are more or less successful at using various defense mechanisms to control their own anxiety experiences. Those who are less successful at using these mechanisms, or who rely primarily on less adaptive defense mechanisms, sometimes develop the symptoms of anxiety disorders because they have not successfully managed anxiety. Treatment for anxiety disorders, therefore, includes functional methods to reduce anxiety, discussed later in this chapter (also see Chapters 13 and 23).

HISTORIC AND THEORETIC PERSPECTIVES

In *Interpersonal Relations in Nursing*, Hildegard Peplau (1952), a pioneer of psychiatric mental health nursing, identified stages of anxiety on a continuum. Her work illustrates the view of anxiety and tension developed by Harry Stack Sullivan (1882-1949), a prominent American-born psychiatrist and expert in developmental theory. Nurses further began to explore these stages while providing care using the clinical practice guidelines. Figure 9-3 describes anxiety's continuum as mild, moderate, severe, and panic. Optimally functioning people generally operate in the mild range of anxiety. The mild stage of anxiety facilitates learning, creativity, and personal growth. Nursing students and other learners often experience mild anxiety as they strive to excel in their work. Occasional movement to the moderate stage is an adaptive mechanism to cope with pleasant or unpleasant situations. For example, a nursing student who is giving an important oral presentation or who is anticipating a difficult test experiences moderate anxiety. When the student manages the stressor, he or she will then move back along the continuum to mild anxiety. Moderate and severe anxiety is either acute or chronic. In severe anxiety, the person focuses energy primarily on reducing the pain and discomfort of anxiety, rather than on coping with the environment. Consequently, this impairs the individual's level of functioning, and the person often requires help to reverse the situation. In panic anxiety, the individual is disorganized, with increased motor activity, a distorted visual-perceptual field, loss of rational thought, and decreased ability to relate to others. Table 9-2 fully explains the responses to the stages of anxiety.

In addition to describing anxiety by degree, there are also different types of anxiety. Signal anxiety is the type of anxiety experienced when a person identifies a precipitant. It is important to note that although signal anxiety is learned, it results from situations that have

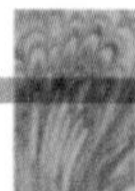

TABLE 9-1

Defense Mechanisms

DEFENSE MECHANISM*	DEFINITION	EXAMPLE
HIGH ADAPTIVE LEVEL		
Humor	The use of humor assists the person to manage everyday stressors	The comedian talks about his substance abuse and current recovery with humorous stories that the audience can identify with
Sublimation	Channeling maladaptive thoughts and feelings such as aggression into socially acceptable behaviors	A young man experienced being bullied as a child and becomes a policeman; he channeled his feelings of anger and inability to deal directly with the bully into observing law and order and protecting others
Suppression	Avoiding thinking about problem areas intentionally, unlike repression which is unintentionally put into play	The student nurse focuses all his energy on his school assignments to avoid several problems happening at home
MENTAL INHIBITIONS: COMPROMISE FORMATION LEVEL		
Displacement	Transferring a feeling or response toward one person onto another less threatening person or object	A mother was angry with her teenage daughter for doing poorly in school and disobeying, so she goes to the gym and has a rigorous game of racquetball
Dissociation	An alteration in an awake state where the person feels detached from his or her surroundings	The client describes feeling detached from his body, looking down at his body from the corner of the room
Repression	Unintentionally pushing back disturbing thoughts, desires, or experiences from the conscious mind; more intense than suppression, which is intentional	When describing her childhood that included sexual abuse, the client is unable to recall a lot of her early experiences and appears detached from them
MINOR IMAGE DISTORTING LEVEL		
Devaluation	Attributing negative qualities to self or others	The client finds fault in every aspect of the hospitalization experience
DISAVOWAL LEVEL		
Denial	An unconscious refusal to acknowledge some painful reality or subjective experience that others identify	The client consumes a six-pack of beer every day; he does not identify a problem with alcohol consumption
Projection	Attributing strong conflicting feelings or faults to another person	The client is angry at the nurse for setting limits but accuses the nurse of being angry with him
MAJOR IMAGE DISTORTING LEVEL		
Splitting of self-image or image of others	Inability to integrate positive and negative aspects of self or others or integrate own strengths and weaknesses; viewing self, others, and situations as being either all good or all bad	The client cannot identify anything about self or others that is positive and only identifies the negative characteristics; views things only in black and white and cannot see shades of gray

*From American Psychiatric Association: *Diagnostic and statistical manual of mental disorders*, ed 4, text revision, Washington, DC, 2000, APA.

been successfully repressed, or coped with, by using another defense mechanism. Consequently, the precipitant is successfully excluded from one's consciousness. Signal anxiety is the predominant etiologic factor in phobic disorders. A cue in the environment causes anxiety, which becomes severe in nature, resulting in a panic attack. The individual is unaware of the cue initially; the original experience involving the cue is repressed. For example, Sherry is shopping at a grocery store, and she becomes severely anxious when passing an individual who smells of alcohol. Sherry had an uncle who drank alcohol heavily and was abusive when intoxicated. When she passed this person who had similar characteristics of her uncle, it reminded her of the fear she experienced when her uncle visited her family after drinking.

Trait anxiety is a function of personality structure. As a part of the developmental processes or events, some individuals have more traumatic experiences or have less success in coping with these events, resulting in unresolved conflict or confusion. These individuals have an anxiety diathesis, or predisposition to anxiety when stressed. They have a higher probability of worrying than someone who does not have a trait anxiety as part of his or her personality structure. Situations that re-create or represent the original conflict or experience evoke a more severe anxiety response in persons with a higher level of trait anxiety. For example, a woman worries excessively about her own children being injured or catching colds because her mother was chronically ill for much of her childhood. As a result, she limits their activity and is anx-

TABLE 9-2

Responses to Anxiety

ANXIETY LEVEL	PHYSIOLOGIC	COGNITIVE/PERCEPTUAL	EMOTIONAL/BEHAVIORAL
Mild	Vital signs normal; minimal muscle tension; pupils normal, constricted	Perceptual field is broad; awareness of multiple environmental and internal stimuli; thoughts are often random but controlled	Feelings of relative comfort and safety; relaxed, calm appearance and voice; performance automatic; habitual behaviors occur
Moderate	Vital signs normal or slightly elevated; tension experienced; client is uncomfortable or experiences pleasure (labeled as "tense" or "excited")	Alert; perception narrowed, focused; optimum state for problem solving and learning; attentive	Feelings of readiness and challenge, energized; engages in competitive activity and learns new skills; voice, facial expression interested or concerned
Severe	Fight-or-flight response; autonomic nervous system excessively stimulated (vital signs increased, diaphoresis increased, urinary urgency and frequency increased, diarrhea, dry mouth, appetite decreased, pupils dilated); muscles rigid, tense; senses affected; hearing decreased; pain sensation decreased	Perceptual field greatly narrowed; problem solving difficult; selective attention (focuses on one detail); selective inattention (blocks out threatening stimuli); distortion of time (things seem faster or slower than actual); dissociative tendencies; detachment; vigilambulism (automatic behavior)	Feels threatened, startles with new stimuli; feels on "overload"; activity increases or decreases (may pace, run away, wring hands, moan, shake, stutter, become very disorganized or withdrawn, freeze in position/be unable to move); appears and feels depressed; demonstrates denial; complains of aches or pains; is agitated or irritable; need for space increases; eyes move around room, or gaze is fixed; some close eyes to shut out environment
Panic	Above symptoms increase until sympathetic nervous system release occurs; person becomes pale; blood pressure decreases; hypotension; muscle coordination poor; pain, hearing sensations minimal	Perception totally scattered or closed; unable to take in stimuli; problem solving and logical thinking highly improbable; perception or unreality about self, environment, or event; dissociation often occurs	Feels helpless with total loss of control; client is angry, terrified; becomes combative or totally withdrawn, cries, or runs away; completely disorganized; behavior is usually extremely active or inactive

From Green E, Katz J, Marcus, P: Practice guideline for management of anxiety. In Green E, Katz J, editors: *Clinical practice guidelines for the adult patient,* St Louis, 1995, Mosby.

ious and overprotective. These anxious behaviors can be passed on to her children and continue to affect future generations.

State anxiety develops in situations identified as conflictual or stressful and in which the individual experiences limited control. This is often perceived as anxiety that has occurred before. The "butterflies" in the stomach feeling that some students experience before an important examination is an example of mild state anxiety. A person who was bitten by a dog in the past and who experiences an increased heart rate when seeing a large dog walking down the street is displaying a more moderate form of state anxiety. A woman with a strong family history of cancer who delays making an appointment with her primary health care provider after noticing a lump in her breast demonstrates severe and maladaptive state anxiety. Free-floating anxiety is a pervasive sense of dread or doom unattached to any idea or event. This type of anxiety often results in a panic state if stressors exceed the person's ability to cope.

State and trait anxiety are important concepts for nurses because nurses use a rating scale known as the State-Trait Anxiety Inventory to differentiate and estimate between the types of anxiety. Individuals with high levels of trait anxiety are likely to experience higher levels of state anxiety when confronted with significant stressors. Nurses who are able to estimate their clients' levels of trait anxiety during the assessment process are better able to select interventions directed at helping clients cope with high state anxiety responses to identified stressors.

Anxiety in the Context of Psychiatric Mental Health Nursing

Many people use the term *anxiety* in a variety of contexts. However, it is important to be precise when using it. Inherent in all nurse-client relationships is the nurse's goal in making the relationship meaningful and moving it forward. Another important nursing goal is to facilitate choices through the relationship. Although all relationships are not nursing, the basis for all nursing is a relationship. A nursing relationship does not imply equal participation or responsibility on the part of the nurse and the client, but rather the nurse's intention to establish a connection. Caring for an unconscious anesthetized client or for an individual experiencing psychosis or dementia es-

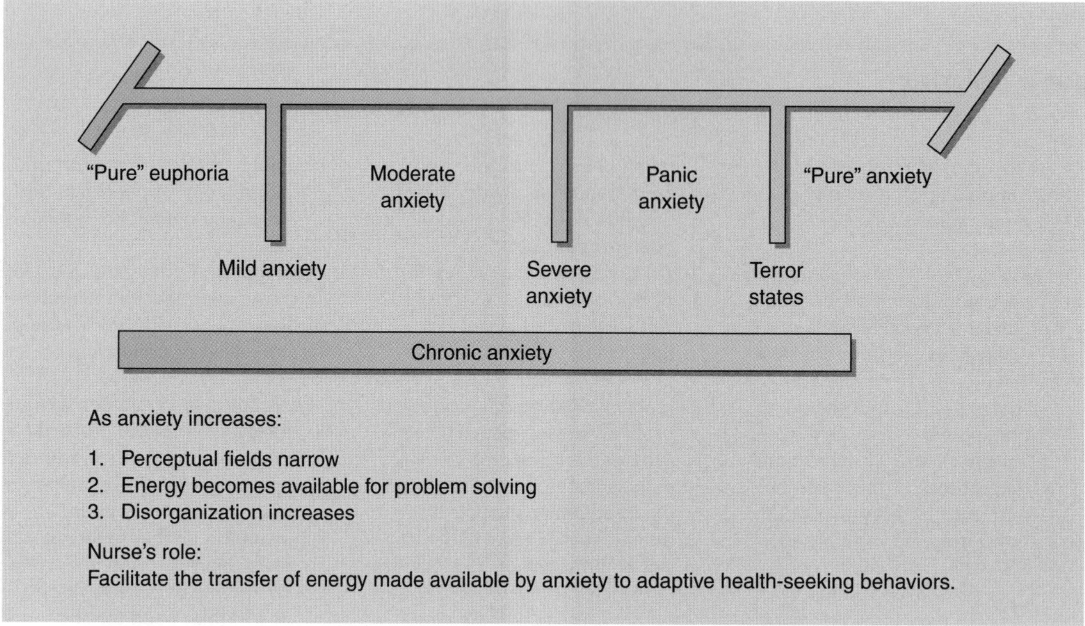

FIGURE 9-3 Hildegard Peplau's construction of the anxiety continuum. (From Peplau H: *Interpersonal relations in nursing: a conceptual frame of reference for psychodynamic nursing,* New York, 1991, Springer.)

tablishes a connection; therefore, it is a relationship. For psychiatric mental health nurses, the primary goal of the nurse-client relationship is to become available to the individual. Through establishing a relationship, both the client and the nurse have the opportunity to develop their potentials as human beings, with the understanding that the focus of therapy is the client. Recognizing and managing anxiety and making appropriate choices are critical for both the client and the nurse in the relationship.

Influence of Hildegard Peplau

In the 1950s, Peplau described the nurse as a person who relates *to* the client rather than *with* the client. She presented the phases of the nurse-client relationship in a social learning model that today appears maternalistic but was nonetheless consistent with the meaning of developmental theory and mental health nursing practice at the time. In fact, both seasoned and novice colleagues consider Peplau the matriarch of psychiatric mental health nursing.

According to Peplau, it is critical that nurses recognize the choices or potentials that exist in the emerging relationship between the client and the nurse. In *Interpersonal Relations in Nursing,* Peplau (1952) addressed the term *unexplained discomfort,* which includes the needs, frustrations, and conflicts that occur within the relationship. She considers them experiences that influence behavior by providing energy to the relationship. According to Peplau, nurses need to examine anxiety as it occurs in nurses and clients and in the communication of the interpersonal relationship.

Peplau also presented a method for the nurse to examine the relationship between the nurse and the client. This method is process recording. Process recording helps nurses develop self-awareness about the way they relate to clients and emphasizes the value of the nurse-client relationship (see Chapter 4). The defining purpose of process recording is to provide a practical vehicle for nurses to reflect on the content of the interaction in a safe, effective manner. As nurses review their responses to clients or "the nursed," Peplau's position is that nurses will develop a growing awareness of their responses. This is a critical factor in helping clients to achieve their goals and to function optimally. Peplau's anxiety continuum is a theory that many use in the treatment of anxiety disorders.

Humanistic Nursing Theory

Humanistic nursing theory is also applicable in treating anxiety and anxiety disorders. Patterson and Zderad (1976) developed a theory of **humanistic nursing** based on existential theory and the phenomenologic method. The cornerstone of their theory is an interactive process that occurs between two persons: one needing help and one willing to give help. Nurses and clients interact; the client calls, and the nurse responds. Humanistic nursing differs from Peplau's interpersonal nursing in that in humanistic theory the nurse is a participant in the process. The nurse tries to be fully present in the process and is in relationship *with* the client, rather than *to* the client, as defined in Peplau's theory. In humanistic theory the nurse's availability to the client is critical to the process of nursing.

Anxiety in Psychiatric Practice

Descriptions of anxiety as a phenomenon of concern in mental health are relatively recent. Psychiatry as a medical specialty had its origins in France in the late eighteenth century. Before that time, care for the insane (lunatics) fell to the law or to the church. Foucault (1988) has asserted that "madness" replaced death as a major theme in human experience. During the Age of Reason and into the nineteenth century, early psychiatric practitioners concerned themselves with the psychoses, those mental disorders believed to pose the greatest risk to society. However, in the second half of the nineteenth century, as the roots of psychoanalytic theory developed, anxiety (or "neuroses") emerged as a source of a variety of emotional and behavioral disturbances.

ETIOLOGY

Biologic Model

Roots of the biologic model for anxiety disorders date back to the nineteenth-century writings of Charles Darwin. Darwin postulated that emotional expression and anatomic structures both changed in the course of evolution to enable the species to adapt to its environment. Darwin further identified certain emotions as being universally demonstrated through expression, using motor and postural changes. In the early part of the twentieth century, investigators linked the endocrine system with emotions, first through establishing the relationship of the adrenal medulla in the production of epinephrine, resulting in the fight-or-flight response.

Selye (1956) built on this work after World War II, using observations of stress and anxiety demonstrated by soldiers who served in combat. A new conceptualization of **stress** replaced the former "psychic trauma." Selye expanded on the notion that the endocrine system and the central nervous system, particularly the hypothalamus and pituitary gland, have a reciprocal relationship. At the same time, researchers conducted important investigations regarding the effects of neuropharmacology on the autonomic nervous system (ANS) in regulating cardiovascular, gastrointestinal, and motor responses. The ANS, particularly the sympathetic nervous system, was responsive to environmental stimuli, including emotional states. A comprehensive discussion of Selye's theory appears in Chapter 27.

As the ability to understand the physiologic state by observing the living brain in imaging techniques such as positron emission tomography (PET) and the functional magnetic resonance imaging (fMRI), the role of stress and the brain functioning has become more apparent. The amygdala is particularly important to understand as it relates to fear responses, particularly in posttraumatic stress disorder (PTSD). The amygdala is involved in the fight-or-flight response. Some have hypothesized that the different anxiety disorders affect different parts of the amygdala (National Institute of Mental Health [NIMH], 2002). The medial prefrontal cortex organizes the response to a traumatic episode, and the hippocampus has the spatial and contextual memory of the trauma. Chronic stress possibly causes changes in the hippocampus (Korn, 2002; NIMH, 2002).

Genetic considerations are important when assessing individuals with anxiety disorders. When performing a functional magnetic resonance imaging (fMRI), researchers found that some of the research subjects had one or two copies of a short variate of the human serotonin transporter gene as opposed to the long variate of this same gene. The transporter gene helps to code protein in the neuronal area that recycles secreted serotonin from the synapse. In the study done by Hariri and Weinberger (2002), they found that individuals with the shorter transporter gene had more amygdala activation when matching angry or fearful faces while having a fMRI. Further study is necessary in this area. In one genetic study of panic disorder, Heun and Maier (1995) showed an 8% to 17% risk in first-degree relatives. NIMH is studying the genetic impact on most major psychiatric disorders in the NIMH Human Genetics Initiative (NIMH, 2002). By studying and understanding brain functioning and genetics, researchers will make new advances in the use of pharmaceutical agents to assist patients with anxiety-related disorders (see Chapter 24).

Psychodynamic Model

In psychoanalytic terms, anxiety is a warning to the ego that it is in danger from either an internal or an external threat. Anxiety is involved in the development of personality and personality functioning and in the development and treatment of neuroses and psychoses. Freud's work is the basis for anxiety neurosis existing as a separate classification.

Three types of anxiety are identified in psychoanalytic theory: reality anxiety, moral anxiety, and neurotic anxiety. Reality anxiety is a painful emotional experience resulting from the perception of danger in the external world, such as the fear of the possibility of a terrorist attack. Fear is the response to external danger, and consequently anxiety parallels fear. Moral anxiety is the ego's experience of guilt or shame. An example of moral anxiety is experiencing guilt for expressing anger at a family member. Neurotic anxiety is the perception of a threat according to one's instincts. According to Freud's theory of "signal anxiety," anxiety is a signal of impending emergence of threatening, unconscious mental content. Neurotic symptoms develop in an attempt to defend against anxiety—including somatic symptoms, obsessions, compulsions, and phobias (described fully in this chapter and in Chapter 10).

Interpersonal Model

Both the interpersonal and the social psychiatry models view anxiety as a response to the individual's external environment rather than the relatively simple psychoanalytic view of a response to instinctual drives. Interpersonal theorists, particularly Sullivan, regarded symptom formation as a result of expectations, insecurities, frustrations, and conflicts between individuals and primary groups. Primary groups include families, work colleagues, and friends.

Like psychoanalytic theorists, interpersonal theorists place a great deal of emphasis on early development and experiences in relation to future mental health. According to Sullivan, the individual's first experience of anxiety is the infant's perception of the anxiety of the mothering person. The self-system develops in the context of approval or disapproval from significant others. Disapproval results in a threat to the self-system, a fear of rejection—in other words, anxiety.

Interpersonal theorists define anxiety broadly. According to Sullivan, anxiety is the first great educative experience in living. Also according to Sullivan, one of the great tasks of psychology is to discover the basic vulnerabilities to anxiety in interpersonal relations rather than to try to deal with the symptoms of anxiety.

Environmental Model: Social Psychiatry

Social theorists emphasize the role of social conditions in deviant behavior and assert that symptoms, including anxiety and its manifestations, result from the dynamic relationship between individuals and their environment. Social psychiatry evolved after World War II when researchers began using a large number of community and epidemiologic surveys to develop a model for understanding the role of vulnerability, predisposition, and stressors in symptom formation. Social psychiatry views factors such as socioeconomic status, racial inequalities, and fear of a terrorist attack as stressors equivalent to combat in the military. Individuals respond to the environment on a continuum, either adaptively or with symptom formation—mental illness or physical illness. The mediating factor in this response is the individual's ability to manage anxiety. Social psychiatric influences, particularly with respect to sampling methodology and the use of standardized questionnaires and scales, have contributed significantly to the current research base for the anxiety disorders.

Behavioral Model

Clinicians who believed the psychoanalytic model and methods were lacking, designed behavioral models in psychiatry and psychology. They identified experimental psychology as a resource for ideas from which to develop new treatments. In behavioral models, based on learning theory, the etiology of anxiety symptoms is a generalization from an earlier traumatic experience to a benign setting or object. An example is an awkward child whose parents ridiculed him while bowling. As a result, he associates embarrassment and shame with sports events in indoor facilities and develops panic attacks during basketball games. The same kinds of cognitive operations that link embarrassment with sporting events link cognitions of the expectation of embarrassment with the idea of a sporting event, and the individual begins to experience panic attacks while reading the sports page. Consequently, in this model, anxiety occurs when an individual encounters a signal that *predicts* a painful or feared event.

Early behavioral therapists directed their efforts at the anxiety disorders. In 1958, Wolpe, a physician working with soldiers experiencing symptoms of posttraumatic stress disorder (PTSD), reported success using systematic desensitization applied to simple phobias (Wolpe, 1973). Systematic desensitization is a method that comes from the learning theory. The therapist exposes a deeply relaxed client to a graded hierarchy of phobic stimuli. Others have redefined this method further into *in vivo desensitization*, whereby the therapist exposes the individual progressively to more anxiety-provoking situations. These live exposure treatments take a variety of forms, including graded practice, participant modeling, and prolonged or brief duration. In 1981, behaviorists demonstrated that 60% to 79% of patients with agoraphobia experienced clinically significant improvement by using the methods of systematic desensitization.

Table 9-3 demonstrates the clinical manifestations of anxiety, which take into account the biologic, cognitive,

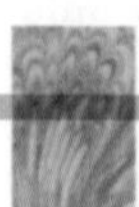

TABLE 9-3

Clinical Manifestations of Anxiety: Symptoms and Responses

MANIFESTATION	SYMPTOM/RESPONSE
Physiologic	
Cardiovascular system	Palpitations, racing heart, increased blood pressure, fainting, decreased blood pressure
Respiratory system	Rapid, shallow breathing, pressure in chest, shortness of breath, gasping, lump in throat
Gastrointestinal system	Loss of appetite or increased appetite, abdominal discomfort or feeling of fullness, nausea, heartburn, diarrhea
Neuromuscular system	Hyperreflexia, insomnia, tremors, pacing, clumsiness, restlessness, flushing, sweating, muscle tension
Genitourinary system	Decreased libido, frequency or urgency of urination
Cognitive	Decreased attention, inability to concentrate, forgetfulness, impaired judgment, thought blocking, fear of injury or death
Behavioral	Rapid speech, muscle tension, fine hand tremors, restlessness, pacing, hyperventilation
Affective	Irritability, impatience, nervousness, fear, uneasiness

behavioral, and affective patterns of behavior. This table is a good tool to help nurses recognize the manifestation anxiety has on the body systems, as well as on thought patterns and behavior.

EPIDEMIOLOGY

A 12-month study conducted to determine the extent of anxiety disorders in the population showed that 20% of individuals in the United States have a type of anxiety disorder (Kessler et al., 1994). The NIMH research on anxiety disorders reports that more than 19 million adult Americans have anxiety disorders. A number of anxiety disorders, such as obsessive-compulsive disorder (OCD), social phobia, and body dysmorphic disorder, begin in childhood and continue into adulthood.

Researchers conducted a study to examine the prevalence of mood and anxiety disorders. The statistics gathered demonstrated that 9.21% of individuals in the United States have reported symptoms of mood disorders, and 11.08% of the reported population had anxiety disorders. In this same population, 9.35% reported having substance abuse. The associations between substance use, mood disorders, and anxiety disorders are significant, according to a CDC study (2004).

Almost all clients presenting with agoraphobia in clinical samples have a current diagnosis or history of panic disorder. In contrast, epidemiologic samples identify more clients with agoraphobia without a history of panic disorder. Agoraphobia is more common in women than in men.

Simple phobia is common in the general population, with reported lifetime prevalence rates of 10% to 12% (American Psychiatric Association [APA], 2000). Overall, the prevalence of simple phobia is higher for women than for men. However, there is a higher prevalence of fear of heights and blood injection injury among men—30% to 45%, as compared with 10% to 25% in other categories.

In contrast to other anxiety disorders, in clinical samples equal numbers of men and women seek treatment for social phobia. In community-based samples, however, social phobia is more common among women. Lifetime prevalence rates vary from 3% to 13% (APA, 2000). In outpatient treatment settings, rates of social phobia range from 10% to 20% of persons seeking treatment for anxiety disorders. Similarly, OCD is equally common in men and women; researchers estimate the lifetime prevalence at 2.5% (APA, 2000).

Estimates for the prevalence of PTSD range from 3% to 58% of at-risk individuals. This wide variability is due to both sampling methods and the population assessed. Community-based samples for prevalence range from 1% to 14% (APA, 2000).

Age of Onset

In general, anxiety disorders develop during adolescence and early adulthood. The typical age of onset for panic disorder varies from late adolescence to the mid-30s. Rare cases have an onset in childhood, and a small number develop symptoms after age 45 years. Acute and posttraumatic stress disorders develop at any age.

There are two ages of onset for specific phobias, situational type. There is a peak of onset in childhood and another peak in early adulthood. Other types of phobias usually have an onset in childhood.

Cultural Variance

Most research supporting the development of the DSM-IV-TR classification occurred in the United States; consequently, symptoms defining disorders are representative of that culture. However, take care to establish cultural norms when evaluating clients for anxiety and related disorders. For example, some cultures restrict women's participation in public activities; thus, agoraphobia is less commonly diagnosed. Fears of magic or spirits are present in many cultures and are pathologic only when the fear is excessive in the context of that culture. Many cultures have rituals to mark important events in people's lives. The observation of these rituals is not indicative of OCD unless it exceeds norms for that culture, is exhibited at times or places inappropriate for that culture, or interferes with social functioning.

It seems that with the exception of OCD and social phobia, anxiety and related disorders exhibit a higher prevalence among women than among men. This observation possibly represents a cultural variation. Overall, women are more likely than men to present for treatment or come in contact with health care providers. Leskin and Sheikh (2004) evaluated gender differences in panic attacks in a study. The results of the study found that women demonstrated more severe symptoms of panic attacks, particularly in the area of respiratory symptoms such as difficulty breathing or feeling as though they would faint or be smothered. The researchers decided to examine the role premenstrual hormones played in the severity of symptoms. They did a review of the literature and concluded that women often have more respiratory symptoms because of the influence of the dysregulation of GABA/benzodiazepine receptor complex when the women had premenstrual dysphoric disorder. Further research in this area is necessary.

Comorbidity (Co-occurrence)

Anxiety disorders do not exist in a clinical vacuum. Understanding the co-occurrence of different anxiety disorders with other Axis I disorders is helpful in providing comprehensive treatment. There is a high comorbid rate of anxiety and depression. Often patients with these disorders are at a 15-fold increased risk of suicidal ideation than patients who have neither disorder (Goodwin et al., 2001). Clients with major depression often had an 18.8% increased risk of panic and a 15.3% increased risk of agoraphobia. There is substantial co-occurrence between substance abuse disorders and anxiety disorders.

OCD exists with other anxiety disorders, as well as substance abuse, major depression, and eating disorders. In Tourette's syndrome, 30% to 50% of clients also have

OCD; however, the rate of Tourette's syndrome among OCD clients is lower, with estimates ranging from 5% to 7%.

Acute and posttraumatic stress disorders are associated with increased risk for major depression, other anxiety disorders, somatization disorder, and substance abuse disorders. Because of the nature of the disorder and its presentation after a significant event, it is difficult to determine whether the co-occurring condition developed before the stress disorder or as a consequence of it.

CLINICAL DESCRIPTION

Panic

In the nineteenth century, clinical syndromes similar to panic disorder and agoraphobia began to appear in the literature. In 1871, an American physician, Da Costa, described panic attacks occurring in soldiers who served in the Civil War. Around the same time, Westphal, a German physician, presented clinical data on four patients with classic agoraphobic syndromes. Freud first named panic attacks as occurring when "the connection between anxiety and threatened danger is entirely lost from view . . . spontaneous attacks . . . represented by intensely developed symptoms . . . tremor, vertigo, palpitations of the heart" (Freud, 1963). Freud also noted the co-occurrence of the anxiety disorders and depression.

World Wars I and II contributed to the development of the knowledge base of the anxiety disorders, as did the work of the noted cardiologist Paul Dudley White. He and his colleagues collected data on a number of patients who did not have organic heart disease. They named the clinical syndrome *neurocirculatory asthenia*. In the same institution, neuropsychiatrists identified a similar symptom complex and named it *anxiety neurosis*. Both the cardiologists and the neuropsychiatrists were describing what today we call *panic disorder*.

Panic anxiety refers to anxiety symptoms that occur during panic attacks. Panic anxiety is differentiated from generalized anxiety by the sudden onset of distressing physical symptoms combined with thoughts of dread, impending doom, death, and fear of being trapped.

Panic Attack

It is important to note panic attacks are not in the DSM-IV-TR classification as psychiatric illnesses. Rather, **panic attacks** are symptoms, potentially meeting some of the defining characteristics of many of the disorders described in this chapter. Panic attacks are sudden, spontaneous episodes accompanied by symptoms such as a racing heart or palpitations, dizziness, dyspnea, and a feeling that death is imminent.

Panic attacks occur in a variety of anxiety disorders, including panic disorder, social phobia, simple phobia, and PTSD. Panic attacks occur in specific, cued situations (as with simple phobias) or are unexpected (uncued) (APA, 2000). The DSM-IV-TR Criteria box lists the symptoms of a panic attack.

DSM-IV-TR CRITERIA

Panic Attack

A distinct period of intense fear or discomfort in which four or more of the following symptoms develop abruptly and reach a peak within 10 minutes:

1 Palpitations, pounding heart, accelerated heart rate
2 Sweating
3 Trembling or shaking
4 Sensations of shortness of breath or smothering
5 Feeling of choking
6 Chest pain or discomfort
7 Nausea or abdominal distress
8 Feeling dizzy, unsteady, lightheaded, or faint
9 Derealization (feelings of unreality) or depersonalization (being detached from oneself)
10 Fear of losing control or going crazy
11 Fear of dying
12 Paresthesias (numbness or tingling sensations)
13 Chills or hot flushes

From American Psychiatric Association: *Diagnostic and statistical manual of mental disorders*, ed 4, text revision, Washington, DC, 2000, American Psychiatric Association.

Panic Disorder

An individual is diagnosed with panic disorder if the following two criteria are met: (1) recent and unexpected panic attacks are present, and (2) at least one of the attacks has been followed for 1 or more months by (a) persistent concern about having additional attacks, (b) worry about the implications of the attack or its consequences (e.g., losing control, having a heart attack, "going crazy"), or (c) a significant change in behavior related to the attacks.

In panic disorder without agoraphobia, the individual is free from agoraphobic symptoms, the panic attacks are not related to direct effects of a substance (illicit drugs, medication), and the attacks are not due to a physiologic condition (e.g., hyperthyroidism). In addition, the anxiety is not better explained by another mental disorder, such as OCD (for example, a fear of contamination) or PTSD (e.g., in response to stimuli associated with a severe stressor).

To be diagnosed with panic disorder with agoraphobia, the individual must meet the criteria for panic disorder, as well as experience debilitating agoraphobic symptoms. These agoraphobic symptoms are feeling anxiety about being in areas where it is difficult to escape or where no assistance is available, such as being in a crowd, being on a bridge, or traveling in a subway train. The individual with agoraphobia avoids these situations or stays home if the agoraphobia involves fear of being outside the house alone.

Panic disorder is primarily seen in ambulatory settings. Nurses are among the first health care providers that clients with new-onset panic disorder come in contact with, either in a clinic or physician's office or, more typically, in a hospital emergency department. The sudden onset of physical symptoms and the pervasive feelings of impending doom are frightening, and the client often responds by seeking reassurance from a caregiver. However, it is not uncommon for clients with panic disorder to have been ill for 8 to 10 years before presenting for treatment and to have experienced one or two attacks per week. In addition, clients have learned to avoid those situations that trigger attacks. Some attacks begin with a feeling of general unease, followed quickly (in a few seconds to minutes) by the onset of physical symptoms.

Phobias

The prominent features of phobic disorders, or **phobias**, are that the client experiences panic attacks in response to particular situations or learns to avoid the situations that cause panic attacks.

Agoraphobia

To meet the first DSM-IV-TR criterion for panic disorder with agoraphobia, the person must experience recurrent, unexpected panic attacks, with at least one attack followed by one of the following for a month: (1) persistent concern about having additional attacks, (2) worry about the implications or its consequences, or (3) a significant change in behavior related to the attacks. The second criterion is that the individual experiences **agoraphobia** (i.e., anxiety about being in places or situations from which escape is difficult [or embarrassing] or in which help is not readily available in the event of an unexpected or situationally predisposed panic attack). Agoraphobic fears typically involve characteristic clusters of situations that include being outside the home alone, being in a crowd or standing in line, being on a bridge, and traveling in a bus, train, or car. The third criterion is that the person avoids agoraphobic situations or has stress or anxiety about having a panic attack, or the individual requires the presence of a companion. The fourth criterion stipulates that panic attacks are not due to the direct effects of a substance or a general medical condition. Finally, the anxiety or phobic avoidance is not better explained by another mental disorder, as described in the panic disorder section (APA, 2000).

Agoraphobia exists apart from panic disorder according to DSM-IV-TR criteria. The individual with agoraphobia without a history of panic disorder meets the criteria for agoraphobia as just described but has no history of panic attacks. The description of agoraphobia includes "in the event of suddenly developing panic-like symptoms that the individual fears could be incapacitating or extremely embarrassing, for example, fear of going outside because of fear of having a sudden episode of dizziness or a sudden attack of diarrhea." If the individual has a co-occurring medical condition, the fear described is clearly in excess of the fear usually associated with that disorder.

Specific Phobias

The DSM-IV-TR criteria define a specific phobia as a marked and persistent fear that is excessive or unreasonable, cued by the presence or anticipation of a specific object or situation, such as animals, insects, heights, flying, or seeing blood. Exposure to the phobic stimulus invariably provokes an anxiety response, which takes the form of a cued panic attack (i.e., the individual experiences symptoms listed in the DSM-IV-TR Criteria box). Children with a specific phobia express their anxiety by crying, throwing tantrums, freezing, or clinging. Persons with a simple phobia (except children) recognize that their fear is excessive or unreasonable. Persons avoid phobic situations or endure them with distress. The avoidance, anticipatory anxiety, or distress interferes significantly with the person's routine, occupational, or social functioning, or there is marked distress about having the phobia. It is important to consider if another Axis I mental disorder is causing the phobias (APA, 2000).

Social Phobia

Social phobia, or social anxiety disorder, is a marked and persistent fear of one or more social or performance situations in which the person is exposed to unfamiliar people or to possible criticism by others. The individual fears that he or she will act in a way (or show anxiety symptoms) that will be humiliating or embarrassing. To make this diagnosis in a child, the child must demonstrate the capacity for social relationships with familiar people, and the anxiety must occur in interactions with peers. In addition, exposure to the feared social situation almost invariably provokes anxiety, which often takes the form of a situationally bound panic attack. Children express their fear by crying or exhibiting tantrum-like behavior. Adults acknowledge that their fear is excessive or unreasonable. Individuals with social phobia avoid social or performance situations or endure them with intense anxiety and distress (APA, 2000).

Individuals with social phobia are unable to work well in a group. If an individual is in the psychiatric hospital for a co-occurring disorder, such as substance abuse, using the group format causes undo anxiety and is not therapeutic. The individual is able to work on problem areas with individual attention and medication such as the selective serotonin reuptake inhibitor (SSRI) antidepressant paroxetine (Paxil) (see Case Study, p. 184).

Posttraumatic Stress Disorder

PTSD was first defined as a diagnostic category in DSM-III. Before that time, the pattern of responses after traumatic events was most common in soldiers and the syndrome was called *shell shock* or *combat fatigue.*

PTSD is a model diagnostic category for psychiatric disorders from a theoretic perspective: the causal factors are identifiable. PTSD describes an individual's reaction to traumatic events in human experience beyond combat, including the experiences of adult and child survivors of sexual abuse, physical abuse, disasters, and the grieving process. Cases of PTSD are expected to rise as a result of disasters such as occurred on September 11, 2001, Hurricane Katrina, and the Iraq War, which will have an im-

CASE STUDY Ken is a 19-year-old freshman at a local college. His friends brought him to the emergency department from a fraternity party one Saturday night with acute alcohol intoxication. He is referred to the college health service.

During his initial evaluation, the nurse asks Ken about his patterns of drinking. He reports that he began drinking at age 14 when one of his friends suggested having a beer or two before attending a school dance. He reported that ever since he started school, he has been unable to participate in the easy conversation or social chitchat common among fellow students. However, he did not have the same experience with family members. He was afraid that he wouldn't have anything to contribute to the conversation. He began to worry about his appearance and his tendency to trip over his own feet.

When Ken reached high school, he found that this uneasiness was beginning to isolate him from others in his age-group. At home, his parents usually began dinner parties with a glass of wine or a cocktail, so when his friend suggested a beer before the dance, Ken eagerly accepted. To his surprise, he found that once he arrived at the dance, he was relaxed and able to interact. He was even able to ask two girls to dance!

He continued to drink before arriving at parties, dances, football games, and just about any other social activity. He was worried that he was an alcoholic. The clinical specialist at the health service talked with Ken at length about social phobia and prescribed the antidepressant paroxetine (Paxil). Ken also began attending a group focused on behavioral strategies to cope with anxiety (see Chapter 23).

CRITICAL THINKING

1. What cues does Ken offer that will lead to the most appropriate nursing diagnoses for him?
2. What are two beliefs Ken formed that led to his experience at the fraternity party?
3. Using information in this chapter and information in Chapter 14, what would be the prognosis for Ken?
4. What is an alternative pharmacologic choice for Ken? (See Chapter 24.)
5. How would you describe the advantages of group therapy to Ken?

pact on the health care system for years to come. Controversy still exists in refining the level of intensity required of an event or an experience to meet the definition of trauma and in separating PTSD symptoms from other co-occurring disorders, including substance abuse, depression, and anxiety.

To be diagnosed with PTSD, the individual must have experienced a traumatic event before the onset of symptoms. The individual must have experienced, witnessed, or been confronted with an event that involved actual or threatened death or serious injury, or a threat to the physical integrity of self or others. The individual's response must have involved intense fear, helplessness, or horror. Children express their response with agitated or disorganized behavior.

The second group of defining criteria for PTSD involves various mechanisms of reexperiencing the traumatic event. One of the following must be present: recurrent and intrusive disturbing recollections of the occurrence, including thoughts, images, or perceptions. The person sometimes experiences recurrent dreams of the incident, acting or feeling as though the event was recurring, and feeling the experience of psychologic distress when internal or external cues resemble the trauma. This includes physiologic reactions after exposure to internal or external cues that resemble the incident.

The person with PTSD avoids stimuli associated with the trauma and experiences a numbing of general responsiveness if reminded via cues of the incident. Numbing and avoidance are evident by at least three of the following:

- Efforts to avoid thoughts, feelings, or conversations about the trauma
- Efforts to avoid persons or places that evoke memories of the trauma
- Inability to remember an important aspect of the trauma (**repression**)
- Diminished interest or participation in significant activities
- A feeling of estrangement or detachment from others
- Restricted range of affect
- A sense of impending doom (no expectation of a career or normal life span)

The fourth criterion describes symptoms of increased arousal that were not present before the trauma. Two of the following must be present: sleep disturbances, irritability or angry outbursts, difficulty concentrating, hypervigilance, and exaggerated startle response. Symptoms must persist for more than 1 month and cause significant impairment in social or occupational or other significant areas of functioning.

PTSD is also acute if symptoms have occurred for 1 to 3 months or as chronic if the symptoms have persisted for at least 3 months. When the onset of symptoms is more than 6 months after the traumatic event, there is a specific definition of delayed onset (APA, 2000).

Acute Stress Disorder

Acute stress disorder differs from PTSD in three ways: the individual experiences at least three symptoms indicating dissociation, the time frame of development and duration of symptoms is shorter, and the dissociative symptoms prevent the individual from adaptively coping with the trauma. Three of the following indications of **dissociation** must be present: subjective sense of numbing or detachment, reduced awareness of surroundings (being in a daze), derealization (unreal feeling), depersonalization (feeling alienated), and dissociative amnesia. In terms of time, the symptoms last from 2 days to a month. The onset of the dissociative experience occurs during the traumatic experience or develops immediately afterward. The defining characteristic is that the symptoms cause significant distress or impairment in social and occupational functioning. For example, the individual is unable to perform some necessary task, such as obtaining necessary medical or legal assistance or mobilizing personal resources.

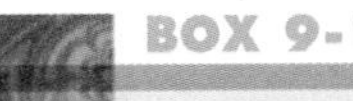

BOX 9-1

Generalized Anxiety Disorder Self-Test

The following questions will help you determine if you are experiencing symptoms of generalized anxiety disorder (GAD). Simply answer yes or no, then take this to your health care professional to see if further evaluation and treatment are necessary.

Yes or No?	Are you troubled by the following:
Y N	Excessive worry, occurring more days than not, for at least 6 months?
Y N	Unreasonable worry about a number of different situations, such as work, school, or health?
Y N	Your inability to "shut off" your worry?

Yes or No?	Are you bothered by at least three of the following:
Y N	Restlessness, feeling keyed up or on edge?
Y N	Being easily tired?
Y N	Concentration problems?
Y N	Irritability?
Y N	Muscle tension?
Y N	Trouble falling asleep, trouble staying asleep, or restless/unsatisfying sleep?
Y N	Anxiety that interferes with your daily life?

Having more than one illness at the same time makes it difficult to diagnose and treat the different conditions. Conditions that sometimes complicate anxiety disorders include depression and substance abuse, among others. The following information will help your health care professional to evaluate you for GAD.

Yes or No?	In the last year, have you experienced the following:
Y N	Changes in sleeping or eating habits?
Y N	Feeling sad or depressed more days than not?
Y N	A disinterest in life more days than not?
Y N	A feeling of worthlessness or guilt more days than not?
Y N	An inability to fulfill responsibilities at work/school or home because of alcohol or drug use?
Y N	Being arrested because of alcohol or drugs?
Y N	The need to continue using alcohol or drugs even though doing so is causing problems for you or your loved ones?

Modified from the Anxiety Disorders Association of America, www.adaa.org.

Generalized Anxiety Disorder

Excessive anxiety and worry (apprehensive expectation) that occurs more days than not for at least 6 months characterizes generalized anxiety disorder (GAD). This anxiety involves concerns about a number of events and activities. The person finds it difficult to control the worry. Three of the following six symptoms must be present to some degree for at least 6 months: restlessness or feeling on edge, being easily fatigued, difficulties with concentration, irritability, muscle tension, and sleep disturbance. The focus of the anxiety and worry is not due to features of another Axis I disorder (worry about having a panic attack, as in panic disorder, or fear of contamination, as in OCD) and is not a part of PTSD. The anxiety or worry interferes with normal social or occupational functioning and is not due to the direct effects of a substance or a general medical condition, and it does not occur exclusively in the presence of another Axis I disorder (mood disorder, psychotic disorder, or pervasive developmental disorder). Box 9-1 offers a self-test for GAD.

CASE STUDY

Phillip is a 31-year-old accountant who has been disabled from his job with a national firm for 8 months. He reports that he has been hospitalized for treatment of depression, which he has experienced since college. Despite his depression, he graduated with honors, was certified as a public accountant, and finished graduate school.

Phillip first was treated for OCD 2 years after graduate school when he began experiencing trouble with his supervisor. A number of the firm's clients had complained that he was unable to either give them completed tax forms or file for the necessary extensions in a timely manner.

Treatment with paroxetine relieved Phillip from his counting and checking behaviors, but he presently spends his time preoccupied with thoughts about killing himself. He is unable to decide on a method of suicide that will not endanger his family's entitlement to his accidental death insurance policies. However, he has plans to have a fatal automobile accident. After relating this lethal suicidal plan to his nurse psychotherapist, Phillip is admitted to an inpatient facility to prevent a suicidal gesture and to stabilize the medication regimen.

CRITICAL THINKING

1 What type of treatment plan is indicated for Phillip, using safety as a priority?
2 What three collaborative treatment approaches are important in Phillip's long-term therapy?
3 Which methods can be used to measure the outcomes Phillip achieves as a result of his treatment?

Obsessive-Compulsive Disorder

OCD is the presence of either obsessions or compulsions. DSM-IV-TR defines **obsessions** as recurrent and persistent thoughts, impulses, or images that a person experiences at some time during the disturbance as intrusive and inappropriate and cause marked anxiety or distress. These thoughts, impulses, and images are not simply excessive worry about real problems. The individual attempts to suppress or ignore these thoughts and impulses or to neutralize them with some other thought or action. Persons with OCD recognize that the obsessional thoughts are part of their own thoughts as opposed to coming from somewhere else, as in thought insertion, which may be present with schizophrenia (see Chapter 12).

Compulsions are repetitive behaviors that the person feels driven to perform in response to an obsession. Some examples include repeated hand washing and checking many times to ensure that appliances are unplugged before leaving the house (see Case Study above). The behaviors or thoughts are an attempt to prevent or reduce the distress invoked by the obsession or to prevent some dreaded threatening situation (such as a fire in the example of checking appliances). However, these behaviors or mental processes are either not connected in a realistic way with what they intend to prevent or are clearly excessive.

CLIENT and FAMILY TEACHING GUIDELINES

OBSESSIVE-COMPULSIVE DISORDER

TEACH THE CLIENT'S FAMILY

- Obsessive-compulsive disorder is a chronic anxiety disorder that responds to different treatment strategies.
- The client experiences recurrent thoughts that interrupt his or her day-to-day functioning. To decrease the overwhelming anxiety felt as a result of the thought pattern, the client manifests compulsions or behavior patterns. Some of the thoughts are counting, checking (to see if the stove is off or the door is locked), and concern about germs.
- Thoughts, impulses, and images are involuntary and worsen with stress.
- Books and Internet resources can be helpful (e.g., *Loving Someone with OCD* by K.J. Landsman or the website of the Obsessive-Compulsive Foundation: www.ocfoundation.org).

TEACH THE CLIENT

- It is important to apply behavioral and cognitive strategies to manage the anxiety and reduce the symptoms of the disorder by attending to them when the thought patterns are more pervasive and the compulsions most disruptive.
- Medication management is an effective treatment modality and usually involves treatment with a drug in the antidepressant category.
- Different classes of drugs have different side effect profiles; recognizing and reporting side effects are important for managing the client's drug therapy.
- Achieving symptom control through pharmacotherapy takes months.
- Obtaining information via self-help books or online can be helpful.

Except in children, individuals recognize that the obsessions or compulsions are excessive or unreasonable at some point in the disorder. The obsessions or compulsions cause marked distress, are time consuming, or significantly interfere with the person's normal routine or occupational functioning. If another Axis I disorder is present, the content of obsessions or compulsions is not restricted to it (e.g., food rituals in anorexia, hair pulling in trichotillomania) (see Client and Family Teaching Guidelines box).

Many have investigated the etiology of OCD. Researchers believe it results from a trauma to the basal ganglia or cortical connections (Blackman, 1997). There is possibly a genetic predisposition that is triggered by an infection or environment stressors (Blackman, 1997). In 1989, PET scan studies demonstrated differences in functioning of the caudate nucleus of the basal ganglia and parts of the frontal lobe. This finding has implication for treatment, including identifying the most effective medication, as well as cognitive behavioral psychotherapy (CBT). The SSRI medications of fluoxetine (Prozac), fluvoxamine (Luvox), paroxetine (Paxil), and sertraline (Zoloft) are indicated (Fredman and Korn, 2002). Developing a nursing care plan with the aim of understanding the symptoms and the difficulty they impose on the client is important.

PROGNOSIS

The prognosis for anxiety disorders is related to factors specific to the disorder, the client, and the clinician. Clients treated for panic disorder with or without agoraphobia follow a typically chronic course. Follow-up studies indicate that 6 to 10 years after treatment, 30% of clients are well, 40% to 50% are improved but still symptomatic, and 20% to 30% are the same or slightly worse (APA, 2000).

Specific phobias that persist into adulthood generally do not end. The course of social phobia is often continuous, with onset or reemergence after stressful or humiliating experiences. The prognosis for OCD is similar to that for other anxiety disorders, with increasing and decreasing symptoms related to stressors. However, 15% of clients demonstrate a chronically deteriorating course with progressive compromise of social and occupational functioning.

For acute and posttraumatic stress disorders, the prognosis is closely related to an individual's exposure to the stressful event, as well as to one's premorbid functioning (client's functioning just before onset of illness) and support systems. Persons with acute stress disorder by definition either recover in 4 weeks or are diagnosed with PTSD. Approximately half of those diagnosed with PTSD recover in 3 months; half continue to experience symptoms persisting for longer than a year after the trauma. A positive outcome is more likely if there are few competing stressors at the time that symptoms develop, if the client seeks early treatment and follows it, and if the client has above average intelligence.

DISCHARGE CRITERIA

Client will:

- Identify situations and events that trigger anxiety and select ways to prevent or manage them.
- Describe anxiety symptoms and levels of anxiety.
- Discuss the connection between anxiety-provoking situations or events and anxiety symptoms.
- Explain relief behaviors openly.
- Identify adaptive, positive techniques and strategies that relieve anxiety.
- Demonstrate behaviors that represent reduced anxiety symptoms.
- Use learned anxiety-reducing strategies.
- Demonstrate ability to problem-solve, concentrate, and make decisions.
- Verbalize feeling relaxed.
- Sleep through the night.
- Use appropriate supports from the nursing and medical community, family, and friends.
- Acknowledge the inevitability of occurrence of anxiety.
- Discuss ability to tolerate manageable levels of anxiety.
- Seek help from appropriate sources when anxiety is not manageable, including websites such as Obsessive-Compulsive Anonymous (OCA) (www.members.aol.com/west24th/index.html).

- List the medication used to control the symptoms as well as the appropriate dosage and scheduled times.
- Continue postdischarge anxiety management including medication and therapy.

The Nursing Process

ASSESSMENT

Assessment of anxiety disorders is conducted in a variety of settings. New treatment modalities have improved the quality of life and level of participation in activities for people with anxiety disorders. Nurses no longer expect to encounter clients with psychiatric disorders only in traditional psychiatric settings. It is important for all nurses to identify dysfunctional manifestations of anxiety in order to implement treatment promptly.

Nurses primarily see panic disorders in ambulatory settings. Nurses are among the first health care providers to come in contact with clients who are experiencing their first symptoms of panic disorder, either in a clinic or a physician's office or, more typically, in a hospital emergency department. The sudden onset of physical symptoms and the pervasive feelings of impending doom are frightening, and the client often responds by seeking reassurance from a caregiver. It is these physical symptoms that bring clients to the emergency department with the concern that they are experiencing a heart attack and impending death.

The client with agoraphobia sometimes comes to the attention of a nurse when preparing a client for diagnostic testing that includes a computed tomography (CT) scan or magnetic resonance imaging (MRI). The client who is agoraphobic may become visibly anxious at the prospect of entering a confined space when the nurse describes the procedure and the equipment.

Most often clients with anxiety symptoms do not present with anxiety as their reason for seeking treatment. Anxiety by definition is a vague, nonspecific feeling of discomfort. Nurses who use an assessment tool that addresses each identified human response pattern will obtain cues from the client experiencing anxiety that indicate further assessment. The guidelines for a comprehensive nursing assessment, listed in Box 9-2, are adaptable for any practice setting. When thought of as a list of questions, an admission interview becomes a task for nurses and consequently an ordeal for clients. As the nurse becomes more experienced, she or he will integrate assessment into the continuing nursing process, and inquiring about human response patterns evolves into a less threatening interaction between client and nurse.

NURSING DIAGNOSIS

To determine which nursing diagnoses will most effectively guide treatment for clients with anxiety and related disorders, the nurse relies on information obtained in the assessment process. The nurse identifies defining characteristics for the target diagnoses from the client, and the nurse and client jointly identify etiologic factors or risk factors.

Etiologic factors influence the selection of the intervention. It is impossible to anticipate each potential diagnosis for all of the disorders discussed in this chapter. Diagnoses are prioritized according to clients' needs. Typical diagnoses for clients with anxiety disorders include the following:

- Risk for suicide
- Anxiety
- Death anxiety
- Stress overload
- Self-mutilation
- Hopelessness
- Powerlessness
- Social isolation
- Disturbed sensory perception
- Disturbed thought processes
- Insomnia
- Impaired memory
- Deficient knowledge
- Fear
- Fatigue
- Chronic low self-esteem
- Disturbed body image
- Risk-prone health behavior
- Ineffective role performance
- Ineffective coping
- Defensive coping
- Ineffective denial
- Impaired social interaction
- Compromised family coping
- Interrupted family processes
- Spiritual distress
- Decisional conflict
- Noncompliance
- Posttrauma syndrome
- Risk for posttrauma syndrome

OUTCOME IDENTIFICATION

Outcome criteria differ according to the characteristics of each client's nursing diagnoses and associated (DSM-IV-TR) diagnoses. Determining outcomes before implementing the plan will guide both nursing interventions and evaluation. Nursing diagnoses are associated with outcomes (goals) to serve as a guide in outcome development. In practice, nurses generally determine outcomes by the patient's presentation of clinical manifestations.

Generalized Anxiety Disorder

Client will:

- Demonstrate significant decrease in physiologic, cognitive, behavioral, and emotional symptoms of anxiety.
- Demonstrate effective coping skills.
- Exhibit enhanced ability to make decisions and problem solve.
- Demonstrate ability to function adaptively in mild anxiety states.
- Discuss the medication regimen and take the medications as prescribed.

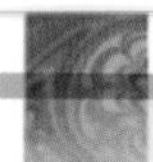

BOX 9-2

Nursing Assessment Guidelines According to Human Response Patterns

EXCHANGING: A PATTERN INVOLVING MUTUAL GIVING AND RECEIVING
Assess eating and elimination patterns. Clients with anxiety disorders and somatization disorders have frequent appetite disturbances and such gastrointestinal complaints as gas, constipation, and diarrhea. Urinary frequency is another associated symptom.

COMMUNICATING: A PATTERN INVOLVING SENDING MESSAGES
Observe for tics, stuttering, or other unusual speech patterns. Note whether the client maintains eye contact throughout the interview, and whether there are any instances of blushing. There is co-occurrence between Tourette's syndrome and obsessive-compulsive disorder; blushing and difficulty communicating with authority figures are common in social phobia.

RELATING: A PATTERN INVOLVING ESTABLISHED BOND
In taking a social history, be particularly attentive to the client's affect in describing roles and role-related problems including occupational function, financial issues, and role in the home. Ask about the client's role satisfaction and what contributes to it. Note whether the client presented alone for the appointment with the provider. If the client came with someone, what is the client's relationship to the individual? Clients with multiple roles are at risk for role strain, characterized by anxiety symptoms. Alternatively, if the individual describes an isolated existence, search tactfully for contributing factors to this isolation. Clients with severe obsessive-compulsive disorder are isolated in part because their degree of involvement with rituals is a competing demand on their time available for social and occupational functioning.

VALUING: A PATTERN INVOLVING THE ASSIGNING OF RELATIVE WORTH
Inquire about cultural background and values. Be particularly attentive when assessing a client with a cultural experience different from your own. In addition to various culture-bound syndromes that are related to anxiety, some clients exhibit behaviors and cognitive patterns that are adaptive and syntonic in one culture yet are labeled pathologic in another.

CHOOSING: A PATTERN INVOLVING THE SELECTION OF ALTERNATIVES
Assess the client's usual methods of coping with stressors. What aspects of the client's life are stressful? If the individual is part of a family unit, how does the family cope with change? Does the individual use alcohol to cope with stressful situations or public appearances? Social phobia is often diagnosed only after a maladaptive substance use disorder is identified. What is the client's usual method of decision making? Does the individual usually follow recommendations? What strategies does the person use to enhance success? Clients with obsessive-compulsive disorder most often experience a disturbance in this pattern. Clients develop obsessional thinking and ritualistic behaviors to cope with perceived threats (which range from intrusive thoughts to adaptive motor responses that become overgeneralized). Nurses who suspect symptoms of obsessive-compulsive disorder should ask the client quite frankly if the individual has any particular ways that he or she needs to perform tasks and if interruptions during the performance of these are stressful. Clients with other anxiety disorders, particularly generalized anxiety disorder, often express difficulties coping and making choices, fearing they will make the wrong decision.

MOVING: A PATTERN INVOLVING ACTIVITY
In inquiring about an individual's history of physical disability, remember to ask about any episodes of motor dysfunction that may indicate conversion symptoms. If the client indicates past traumatic injury, ask about the circumstances. *Although posttraumatic stress disorder develops after combat situations, sexual abuse, and disasters, it also follows less dramatic events, such as automobile accidents, and is sometimes related to grief or bereavement as well.* Questions about traveling, sports activities, and hobbies will yield content suggesting agoraphobic symptoms.

PERCEIVING: A PATTERN INVOLVING THE RECEPTION OF INFORMATION; AND KNOWING: A PATTERN INVOLVING THE MEANING ASSOCIATED WITH INFORMATION
These two patterns together compose the traditional mental status examination. Orientation and memory questions are key to identifying anxiety disorders. *Look for signs of hesitation or pressured speech and thought pattern in answering questions about an individual's history that indicate periods of intense anxiety. Listen carefully, as the client describes past medical treatment, for clusters of illnesses that suggest an increase of anxiety exhibited by somatic concerns.*

FEELING: A PATTERN INVOLVING THE SUBJECTIVE AWARENESS OF INFORMATION
Ask directly about experience of pain and fears. Anxiety symptoms are easier to identify if the nurse prompts the client for actual incidents (e.g., "Are your muscles tight from time to time, is your mouth dry, do you perspire a lot—particularly when you're expecting something unpleasant?" "Have you had more difficulty concentrating lately?" "Have you ever had these feelings come out of nowhere?") *Endorsement of several of the defining characteristics of panic attack warrants a more thorough evaluation for panic disorder and agoraphobia.* Explore the client's experiences of guilt and shame for signs of social phobia.

- Identify when to call the therapist for more visits when a crisis occurs.
- Demonstrate the use of mindful meditation when experiencing symptoms of heightened anxiety.

Obsessive-Compulsive Disorder

Client will:

- Participate actively in learned strategies to manage anxiety and decrease obsessive-compulsive behaviors, such as using mindful meditation.
- Describe increasing sense of control over intrusive thoughts and ritualistic behaviors.
- Demonstrate ability to cope effectively when thoughts or rituals are interrupted.
- Spend less time involved in anxiety-binding activities and instead use time gained to complete activities of daily living and participate in social/recreational activities.
- Successfully manage times of increased stress by integrating knowledge that thoughts, impulses, and images are involuntary, thus reducing sense of responsibility and consequent anxiety.
- Discuss the medication regimen and take the medications as prescribed.

- Identify when to call the therapist for more visits when a crisis occurs.

Posttraumatic Stress Disorder

Client will:

- Demonstrate concern for personal safety by beginning to verbalize worries.
- Participate actively in support group.
- Identify and involve significant support system.
- Assume decision-making role for own health care needs.
- Acquire and practice strategies for coping with anxiety symptoms such as breathing techniques; progressive relaxation exercises; thought, image, and memory substitution; and assertive behaviors (see Chapter 23).
- Discuss the medication regimen and take the medications as prescribed.
- Identify when to utilize a PRN medication to decrease the heightened anxiety response to a cue in the environment.
- Contact the therapist for immediate help when a crisis occurs.
- Identify the need to call the therapist for more visits when symptoms increase.

PLANNING

Treatment planning for the client with anxiety disorders in the current health care environment is complex and varied. Clients with severe OCD were formerly hospitalized for structured behavioral programs.

Today, both clinicians and administrators in inpatient facilities are struggling to balance effective treatment with the high costs associated with these specialty units. Increasingly, inpatient hospitalization is available only for short periods of time for clients at risk to themselves or others. Rather than assuming their traditional roles of providing direct care to clients in inpatient facilities, nurses are becoming case managers. As case managers, nurses provide information on treatment alternatives to clients and families.

IMPLEMENTATION

The role of a nurse in the implementation of a care plan for clients with anxiety and related disorders depends on the setting. The following interventions are useful for clients with anxiety symptoms, regardless of diagnosis or treatment setting.

Nursing Interventions

1. Maintain safety for the client and the environment. *A client's anxiety can escalate to a panic state, which can frighten and harm the client and others. The nurse's first priority is to protect the client and the environment.*
2. Assess own level of anxiety and make a conscious effort to remain calm. *Anxiety is readily transferable from one person to another.*
3. Recognize the client's use of relief behaviors (pacing, wringing of hands) as indicators of anxiety. *Early interventions help to manage anxiety before symptoms escalate to more serious levels.*
4. Inform the client of the importance of limiting caffeine, nicotine, and other central nervous system stimulants. *Limiting these substances prevents/minimizes physical symptoms of anxiety, such as rapid heart rate and jitteriness.*
5. Teach the client to distinguish between anxiety that is connected to identifiable objects or sources (illness, prognosis, hospitalization, known stressors) and anxiety for which there is no immediate identifiable object or source. *Knowledge of anxiety and its related components increases the client's control over the disorder.*
6. Instruct the client in the following anxiety-reducing strategies. *These help lessen anxiety in a variety of ways and distract the client from focusing on the anxiety* (see Chapter 23):
   a. Progressive relaxation technique
   b. Mindful meditation (Box 9-3)
   c. Slow deep-breathing exercises
   d. Focusing on a single object in the room
   e. Listening to soothing music or relaxation tapes
   f. Visual imagery or nature related DVD productions
7. Help the client build on coping methods that the client used to manage anxiety in the past. *Coping methods that were previously successful will generally be effective in subsequent situations.*
8. Activate the client to identify support persons who will help the client perform personal tasks and activities that current circumstances make difficult (such as a partial hospitalization program or a short stay hospitalization). *A strong support system will help the client avoid anxiety-provoking situations/activities.*
9. Assist the client in gaining control of overwhelming feelings and impulses through brief, direct verbal interactions. *Individual interactions executed at appropriate intervals will reduce/manage client's anxious feelings/impulses.*

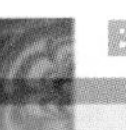

BOX 9-3

Mindful Meditation

- The individual learns meditation to reduce stress by concentrating on her or his body.
- The individual pays attention to the act of breathing to enhance concentration.
- The individual observes the act of breathing, attending to the intake and exhale of each breath.
- Meditation discourages intrusive thoughts; the client agrees to deal with the subject of the intrusive thought at a later time.
- The individual benefits by feeling in control of his or her body. There is a reduction of pain and anxiety, and the individual feels hopeful.

From Ott, MJ: Mindfulness meditation: A path of transformation and healing. *J Psychosoc Nurs Ment Health Serv,* 42(7):22-29, 2004.

10. Help the client structure the environment so that it is less noisy. *A less stimulating environment creates a calming, stress-free atmosphere that reduces anxiety.*
11. Assess the presence and degree of depression and suicidal ideation in all clients with anxiety and related disorders. *A thorough assessment results in early intervention that will possibly prevent self-harm.*
12. Administer **anxiolytic** (antianxiety) medication as a least restrictive measure. *Medication is often the first appropriate method to reduce debilitating anxiety.*
13. Help the client to understand the importance of the medication regimen and to take it as prescribed. *Medication is an effective addition to other psychosocial therapeutic interventions when necessary.*

Additional Treatment Modalities

Biologic Interventions

Pharmacologic Interventions. Pharmacologic interventions alone or in combination with cognitive behavioral interventions are among the most successful treatments for anxiety and related disorders. Since the early 1960s, benzodiazepines have been used widely in the treatment of anxiety disorders. They are relatively safe and effective for short-term use in controlling debilitating symptoms of anxiety. Longer term treatment of these drugs raises issues of tolerance, abuse, and dependence.

SSRIs, antidepressants now widely used to treat anxiety disorders, are particularly effective in treating OCD and panic disorders. Fluoxetine and fluvoxamine are for OCD, paroxetine is for GAD, OCD, panic disorder, PTSD, and social phobia. Sertraline is for OCD, panic disorder, and PTSD; and venlafaxine is for GAD (Fredman and Korn, 2002).

Pharmacologic treatment for PTSD is largely symptomatic. Varying combinations of antidepressants, antipsychotics, and, to a lesser extent, benzodiazepines are used (see Chapter 24).

Electroconvulsive Therapy. The primary indication for electroconvulsive therapy (ECT) is depression. However, ECT is sometimes a treatment for anxiety disorders when other treatments are too high a risk or have failed. For example, in clients with OCD who have only a partial response to clomipramine and who are suicidal, ECT is a reasonable treatment alternative. No one fully knows how ECT operates, but many think it is related to improving transmission of dopamine, norepinephrine, and serotonin and release of hypothalamic and pituitary hormones (Keltner and Folks, 2005) (see Chapter 23).

Psychotherapy

Psychotherapeutic intervention takes place in group or individual settings. One advantage of group therapy is the opportunity for the client to learn from the successes and failures of others with similar symptoms. Behavioral and cognitive behavioral therapies have been widely effective in treating a variety of anxiety disorders (see Chapter 23).

Behavioral Therapy. Behavioral treatments, including systematic desensitization, are among the most effective treatments for panic disorder with agoraphobia. First, the therapist and client define the phobic stimulus. Together they define a hierarchy for the phobic stimulus. The client and therapist then expose the client to events on the hierarchy that increase the client's degree of anxiety. As the client and therapist move through the hierarchy, the client progressively masters increasing levels of anxiety until she or he encounters the phobic stimulus (see Chapter 23).

Cognitive Behavioral Therapy. Cognitive behavioral therapy is widely used in the treatment of anxiety disorders. The success of this approach centers on the client's understanding that symptoms are a learned response to thoughts or feelings about behaviors that occur in daily life. The client and therapist identify the target symptoms and then examine circumstances associated with the symptoms. Together they plan strategies to change either the cognitions or the behaviors. Cognitive behavioral therapy is short term and demands active participation on the part of both the client and the therapist (see Chapter 23).

Psychologic First Aid. Psychologic first aid is currently recommended as an initial response if a person or groups of individuals encounter a traumatic event or loss. This involves protecting individuals who have experienced or witnessed the trauma from any further injury or harm by reducing their psychologic arousal. Support for individuals who are demonstrating distress is obtained by

MEDICATION KEY FACTS Anxiety Disorders

Pharmacologic treatment includes benzodiazepines (alprazolam [Xanax], clonazepam [Klonopin], diazepam [Valium], lorazepam [Ativan]), and nonbenzodiazepines (buspirone [Buspar]). Other medications include antidepressants and pregabalin (Lyrica).

BENZODIAZEPINE

- May cause physical and psychologic dependence.
- Alcohol and other central nervous system depressants may potentiate action, especially in elderly patients.
- Blood dyscrasias (fever, sore throat, bruising, rash, and jaundice) are rare.
- *Herbal considerations:* Kava kava and St. John's wort may potentiate action.
- *Dietary considerations:* Grapefruit juice may increase blood concentration and risk of toxicity.

NONBENZODIAZEPINE (BUSPIRONE)

- MAOIs may increase BP; *do not use together.*
- Lower potential for abuse, addiction, or tolerance.

ADDITIONAL TREATMENT MODALITIES

Anxiety Disorders

- Biologic
  - Pharmacologic
    - Benzodiazepines
    - Selective serotonin reuptake inhibitors
    - Tricyclic antidepressants
    - Monoamine oxidase inhibitors
  - Electroconvulsive therapy
- Psychotherapy
  - Behavioral therapy
  - Cognitive behavioral therapy
  - Psychologic first aid

keeping families together so that there is support among family members. Information about stress reduction and common side effects of trauma must be given to individuals who have been involved with the trauma in order to help them return to their pre-event psychologic state. It is important to provide information on where they can receive further assistance for their psychologic need. The research suggests that brief cognitive behavioral therapy may be the intervention of choice to prevent further trauma related maladaptive responses (Gray, Litz, Papa, 2006). Research utilizing critical incident stress debriefing (CISD) has been inconclusive for preventing individuals from developing acute stress disorder or PTSD after a traumatic incident.

Additional treatment modalities and collaborative interventions include consultation with occupational therapists, vocational rehabilitation counselors, and psychologists, depending on the particular treatment needs of a client. A summary of additional treatment modalities appears in the Additional Treatment Modalities box and in Chapter 23.

EVALUATION

A number of valid, time-tested tools are available that yield reliable information for anxiety disorders. Although these are not for nurses specifically, clinical rating scales offer a method to track changes in symptoms over time with a numeric value. These changes are correlated with discrete interventions (such as instituting a behavioral program or a change in medication). Two rating scales commonly used with clients exhibiting anxiety disorders are the Yale-Brown Obsessive-Compulsive Scale (Y-BOCS) and the Hamilton Anxiety (HAM-A) Scale.

Ideally, the nurse evaluates client progress toward the identified outcomes at every interaction with the client. If the client does not make satisfactory progress, the nurse modifies either the expected outcomes or the interventions. The nurse examines all factors that relate to the outcomes, including what occurred in the previous phases of the nursing process, the role of the nurse in setting client and clinician expectations, the clarity of communicating client goals with the client, and other intervening events that have occurred since the outcomes were set.

NURSING CARE PLAN

Susan, a 47-year-old woman, presented to the employee health department of a teaching hospital after walking there from her office. She was complaining of chest pain and shortness of breath. The staff instituted the standard cardiac workup for clients with new-onset chest pain. Susan's medical history included psoriasis. Her vital signs were remarkable for a pulse of 116; her electrocardiogram and laboratory work were within normal limits.

Susan mentioned to the staff that her son had died 3 months ago. She was referred to a research team conducting a study on panic disorder and saw a clinical specialist in psychiatric mental health nursing. Susan participated in the research protocol after giving informed consent. During the course of the interview, she revealed that her deceased son, an only child, had been an alcoholic whose death was a suicide. She was presently considering separating from her husband of 27 years who was involved in a long-term extramarital affair. Her screening was positive for limited-symptom panic attacks that were increasing in frequency. She agreed to an extended evaluation after her initial interview.

During her evaluation, Susan and the nurse explored her symptoms of anxiety and depression, the exacerbation of her psoriasis, and her chronic headaches, which had become worse since her son's death.

On moving back from the West Coast, Susan had obtained her first job in 24 years. In addition to concern about financial matters and her son's alcoholism, she now worried frequently about her performance at work. She revealed that her husband's extramarital affair had been occurring for several years and related his behavior to their sexual difficulties. The nurse recommended a medication trial. Susan refused medication because of her fears of addiction and loss of control.

DSM-IV-TR DIAGNOSES

Axis I	Generalized anxiety disorder (with limited-symptom panic attacks)
	Bereavement
	Partner relational problem
Axis II	Deferred
Axis III	Psoriasis
	Headaches
Axis IV	Problems with primary support system
Axis V	GAF = 60 (current); GAF = 75 (past year)

Nursing Diagnosis *Anxiety related to change in role functioning, recent loss of son (complicated grieving), threat to socioeconomic status, and stressors exceeding ability to cope, as evidenced by uncertainty, intermittent sympathetic nervous system stimulation, restlessness, and exacerbation of medical condition (psoriasis)*

NOC Anxiety Self-Control, Symptom Control, Psychosocial Adjustment: Life Change, Neurologic Status: Autonomic, Coping

NIC Anxiety Reduction, Anticipatory Guidance, Teaching: Individual, Counseling, Coping Enhancement

Continued

NURSING CARE PLAN—cont'd

CLIENT OUTCOMES	NURSING INTERVENTIONS	EVALUATION
Susan will identify common situations that provoke anxiety.	Assign "homework" to client (e.g., keeping a panic attack and headache diary). *Documenting anxiety responses helps client link symptoms with precipitating events.* During weekly sessions, review with Susan, her log of panic symptoms. *Discussing the linking of events/situations with anxiety symptoms teaches Susan which stressor events provoke anxiety so she will learn to manage/avoid them.*	Susan identifies returning home after work as a critical time for symptoms to develop. She reports that she visits her mother or does errands daily.
Susan will describe early warning symptoms of anxiety.	Assist Susan in associating her panic attack symptoms with thoughts about separation from her husband. *This will help illustrate to Susan specific situations in her life that result in panic anxiety.*	Susan reports that she does not experience headaches when her husband is traveling.
Susan will report willingness to tolerate mild to moderate levels of anxiety.	In weekly sessions, explore with Susan the advantages and disadvantages of separation and divorce. *These discussions will help Susan problem-solve options that offer some control over her anxiety.*	Susan reveals unwillingness to live alone.
Susan will demonstrate adaptive coping mechanisms.	During weekly sessions, discuss options that will allow Susan maximum control over her choices. *Increased choices over life situations tend to minimize anxiety responses to some degree.*	Susan informs her husband that she wants a trial separation. Her husband moves into their son's former room.

Nursing Diagnosis *Complicated grieving related to ineffective coping response to son's death, as evidenced by anxiety on returning home; disturbed sleep pattern; expression of guilt, sadness, and crying; and difficulty with concentration*

NOC Grief Resolution, Psychosocial Adjustment: Life Change, Role Performance, Sleep, Coping, Family Coping

NIC Grief Work Facilitation, Guilt Work Facilitation, Emotional Support, Family Support, Family Integrity Promotion, Coping Enhancement

CLIENT OUTCOMES	NURSING INTERVENTIONS	EVALUATION
Susan will return to her home directly after work, without going immediately to bed.	Explore with Susan her usual patterns of behavior before her son's death. Identify possible modifications of those behaviors. *These discussions will help Susan to focus on alternative activities/behaviors that minimize complicated grieving patterns and increase coping skills.*	Susan describes cooking dinner for her son. She identifies other constructive activities to perform to modify that routine.
Susan will be able to talk with family and significant others about her son's death.	Promote recognition that others also experience the loss of Susan's son. *This will help Susan recognize that others share her grief, which is comforting during critical times.*	Susan is able to visit with her mother and talk about her son without experiencing panic symptoms.
Susan will be able to use her son's former bedroom as a functional part of the house.	Initiate discussion of ways Susan and her husband can plan for disposal of some of their son's possessions without feeling disloyal to his memory. *Discussing difficult topics at appropriate times with a trusted nurse helps feelings emerge and helps client continue in the grieving process.*	As part of their trial separation agreement, Susan's husband moves into their son's room.

Nursing Diagnosis *Decisional conflict related to uncertainty surrounding personal values and beliefs, as evidenced by delayed decision making and physical signs of distress when faced with decisions, specifically her relationship with her husband*

NOC Information Processing, Decision Making, Personal Autonomy, Family Social Climate, Family Functioning, Family Coping

NIC Self-Awareness Enhancement, Values Clarification, Decision-Making Support, Mutual Goal Setting, Support System Enhancement

CLIENT OUTCOMES	NURSING INTERVENTIONS	EVALUATION
Susan will make an informed decision about her relationship with her husband.	During weekly sessions, explore with Susan her expectations of marriage, how her relationship with her husband has changed over the course of their marriage, and what part she played in the changes. *This type of exploration will help Susan to clarify values and expectations about her role in the marriage, which will assist her in making critical life choices.*	Susan describes increasing involvement with her son as his substance abuse worsened and the consequent problems in an already strained marriage. She reports frequent conflict with her husband over his own drinking.

CLIENT OUTCOMES	NURSING INTERVENTIONS	EVALUATION
Susan will identify potential outcomes of separation and divorce and prioritize them according to social, financial, and interpersonal values.	Review with Susan some of the important relationships in her life. Support her considerations in the values clarification process. *It is critical that the nurse be aware of his or her own values and choices and maintain clear distinctions between his or her worldview and that of the client.*	Susan describes her parental relationships as conflict ridden, with her father frequently abusing alcohol. She is critical of her mother's domination of her father. She acknowledges long-standing differences with her husband over sexual issues and feelings of disgust toward her husband when he smells of beer.

Nursing Diagnosis *Chronic low self-esteem related to unresolved developmental issues, as evidenced by self-negating verbalizations, evaluation of self as unable to deal with decisions, and passive dependence on marital partner*

NOC Self-Esteem, Role Performance, Social Interaction Skills, Stress Level, Personal Autonomy

NIC Self-Esteem Enhancement, Role Enhancement, Counseling, Emotional Support, Socialization Enhancement, Coping Enhancement

CLIENT OUTCOMES	NURSING INTERVENTIONS	EVALUATION
Susan will identify specific interactions with her husband that result in physical and psychologic anxiety symptoms and threaten her self-esteem.	Teach Susan to use a diary to put her interactions with her husband and her responses in writing. *Putting things in writing will help Susan to record interactions with her husband that result in anxiety symptoms and low self-esteem.*	Susan effectively identifies interactions with her husband that promote physical and psychologic symptoms of anxiety such as headaches and limited-symptom panic attacks. She admits these negative interactions make her "feel bad" about herself and she wants to change course.
Susan will develop a more positive self-evaluation through role-play sessions with the clinical nurse specialist.	During weekly sessions, the nurse and Susan will role-play responses that seem more satisfactory to Susan. *This will help Susan to distinguish anxiety-producing interactions and modify her responses through role-playing and other teaching strategies, which will increase her self-esteem.*	Susan reports fewer episodes of headaches and limited-symptom panic attacks. Susan frequently describes reinitiating discussions with her husband that she previously identified as being unsatisfactory. She says she feel "better" about herself as a person.
Susan will demonstrate assertive behaviors and more positive interpersonal relationships.	Provide Susan with feedback about behaviors observed. *This will give Susan information about her responses/behaviors so she will begin to modify/manage them.*	Susan initiates the subject of marital therapy with the nurse. Susan requests that her husband join her in weekly sessions to deal with issues involving the husband's use of alcohol, his extramarital affair, and their sexual difficulties.
Susan will admit feeling angry when she was unable to assert herself and will be able to describe her feelings and the reasons for them more accurately.	Help Susan identify and label angry feelings. *This will help Susan to begin processing her feelings more accurately and not misinterpret feelings or their meaning.*	Susan says she is able to openly assert herself and name her feelings about her husband and their marriage difficulties.

Nursing Diagnosis *Sexual dysfunction related to values regarding sexual intimacy conflict, as evidenced by ineffective role performance with husband and inability to achieve desired satisfaction*

NOC Sexual Functioning, Role Performance, Self-Esteem, Social Interaction Skills

NIC Sexual Counseling, Role Enhancement, Self-Esteem Enhancement, Anxiety Reduction

CLIENT OUTCOMES	NURSING INTERVENTIONS	EVALUATION
Susan will demonstrate ability to achieve an ongoing intimate relationship with her husband.	Provide an open, neutral atmosphere where Susan and her husband are able to discuss their differences regarding the level of interest in intimate relations and achievement of satisfaction. *This will encourage positive discussions about sexuality in a nonthreatening environment.*	Susan and her husband report increased mutually satisfying sexual intimacy.

CHAPTER SUMMARY

- Anxiety disorders encompass a wide variety of illnesses that share the common symptoms of anxiety.
- Etiologic models for anxiety include biologic, psychosocial, psychodynamic, and social theories.
- Anxiety disorders have high co-occurrence with depression and substance abuse.
- Anxiety disorders are more common among women, although obsessive-compulsive disorder is equally common in both men and women.
- Treatment of anxiety disorders is multidisciplinary and usually involves more than one treatment modality.
- Inpatient treatment of anxiety disorders is increasingly rare and is generally confined to managing acute exacerbations if the person becomes a danger to self or others or if the symptoms are so severe that they greatly reduce self-care functions.
- The nursing role in the treatment of clients with anxiety symptoms varies. Nurses in all treatment settings will assist the client and family with education about the disorders and their treatment.
- Nursing care plans for clients with symptoms of anxiety reflect the understanding that managing anxiety effectively is part of daily living.
- Nurses actively participate in behavioral interventions structured to decrease phobic responses.
- Rating scales are an effective means for nurses to measure the success of strategies implemented to reduce anxiety.

REVIEW QUESTIONS

1 A client with generalized anxiety disorder receives a new prescription for amitriptyline (Elavil) 50-mg qHS. The client finds information on the Internet that states the drug is an antidepressant. The client calls the nurse saying, "The doctor gave me the wrong drug. I have anxiety, not depression." Select the nurse's best response.

1. "It's not a mistake. Some antidepressant medications also work well for managing anxiety."
2. "Thank you for phoning about this error. I'll confer with the physician and call you back."
3. "You misinterpreted the information. Amitriptyline is a benzodiazepine, not an antidepressant."
4. "The Internet is not always a reliable source for medication information."

2 A woman gets a report of abnormal cells from a Pap smear. She calls her attorney to prepare a will and tells her family, "I won't be around much longer." Which nursing diagnosis and etiology best apply to this situation?

1. Deficient knowledge related to reasons for pap smears
2. Fear related to misinterpretation and misinformation about Pap tests
3. Disturbed thought processes related to malignant cancer
4. Risk-prone health behavior related to a negative vision for the future

3 An adult invites eight people to dinner. This person has never given a dinner party and wants to prepare every menu item. On the morning of the party, the adult multitasks and makes progress preparing each food. As the time approaches for the guests to arrive, which change indicates an increased anxiety level?

1. Blood pressure and pulse rates increase slightly. The person notices feelings of mild muscle tension.
2. Muscles become tense. The person must stop cooking to use the bathroom every 10 to 15 minutes.
3. Fond memories of family reunions, and the good foods that were served, drift in and out of the person's thoughts.
4. The person notices there are cobwebs in the corner of the dining room and removes them before the guests arrive.

4 Place the following behaviors resulting from anxiety in order from most to least adaptive.

1. An adult describes the aftermath of being in a serious automobile accident saying, "I felt like I was floating above the car instead of being in it."
2. After a pregnancy, a woman continues to gain weight until she is more than 80 pounds overweight. She says, "There's no reason for me to diet or exercise. I'm just a huge blimp."
3. A nursing student fails a major exam and states, "If the instructor had known how to teach the subject, I would have made an A."
4. A man gets a chocolate stain on his necktie while eating a cookie and chuckles, "Oh well, I guess that's the way the cookie crumbles."

5 After 3 weeks of hemoptysis (coughing blood), a person finally seeks treatment. A chest x-ray film is taken and the person waits for the results. When the physician explains the report, the person complains, "I can't understand what you're saying. You're talking so fast. All I hear is a loud clicking on my watch." The client is wet with perspiration. Which level of anxiety is evident?

1. Mild
2. Moderate
3. Severe
4. Panic

*Additional self-study exercises and learning resources are available to you on the **Companion CD** at the back of the book and on the **Evolve website** at **http://evolve.elsevier.com/Fortinash/**.*

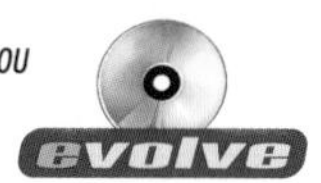

ONLINE RESOURCES

Anxiety Disorders Association of America: **www.adaa.org**

National Center for Post-Traumatic Stress Disorder: **www.ncptsd.va.gov**

National Alliance on Mental Illness: **www.nami.org**

National Institute of Mental Health: **www.nimh.nih.gov**

National Mental Health Association: **www.nmha.org**

Obsessive-Compulsive Foundation: **www.ocfoundation.org**

Posttraumatic Stress Disorder Alliance: **www.ptsdalliance.org**

REFERENCES

American Psychiatric Association: *Diagnostic and statistical manual of mental disorders*, ed 4, text revision, Washington, DC, American Psychiatric Association, 2000.

American Psychiatric Association: *Clinical practice guidelines: acute stress disorder and post traumatic stress disorder*, Washington, DC, American Psychiatric Association, 2004.

American Psychiatric Association: *Clinical practice guidelines: panic disorder*, Washington, DC, American Psychiatric Association, 2006, www.psych.org/psych_pract/treatg/pg/pg/panic.

Anxiety Disorder Research at the National Institute of Mental Health: *Fact sheet*, June 27, 2002, www.nimh.nih.gov/publicat/anxresfact.cfm.

Blackman S: OCD: past, present and future, *Psychiatric Times* XIV:5-14, 1997.

Fortinash KM, Holoday Worret PA: *Psychiatric nursing care plans*, ed 4, St Louis, 2007, Mosby.

Foucault M: *Madness and civilization*, New York, 1988, Vantage.

Fredman S, Korn, ML: Anxiety disorders and related conditions, *Medscape*, June 20, 2002, www.medscape.com/viewprogram/1917-pnt.

Freud S: Introductory lectures on psychoanalysis. In *The standard edition of the complete psychological works*, London, 1963, Hogarth Press (originally published in 1917). (classic)

Freud S: *The standard edition of the complete psychological works*, London, 1963, Hogarth Press. (classic)

Goodwin R et al: Panic and suicidal ideation in primary care, *Depress Anxiety* 14:244-246, 2001.

Gray MJ et al: Crisis debriefing: what helps, and what might not, *Curr Psychiatry* 5:17-26, 2006.

Hall CS: *A primer of Freudian psychology*, Cleveland, 1954, World (classic).

Hariri AR: The amygdala response to emotional stimuli: a comparison of faces and scenes. *NeuroImage* 17:317-323, 2002.

Heun R, Maier W: Relation of schizophrenia and panic disorder: evidence from a controlled family study, *Am J Med Genet* 60:127-132, 1995.

Hollander E et al: Clomipramine vs desipramine crossover trail in body dysmorphic disorder, *Arch Gen Psychiatry* 56:1033-1044, 1999.

Keltner NL, Folks DG: *Psychotropic drugs*, ed 4, St Louis, 2005, Mosby.

Kessler RC et al: Lifetime and 12 month prevalence of DSM III-R psychiatric disorders in the United States: results from the National Comorbidity Survey, *Arch Gen Psychiatry* 51:8-19, 1994.

Korn M: Recent developments in the science and treatment of PTSD, *Medscape*, June 20, 2002, www.medscape.com/viewprogram/1917-pnt.

Landsman KJ et al: *Loving someone with OCD: help for you and your family*, Oakland, Calif: New Harbinger, 2005.

Leskin GA, Sheikh JI: Gender differences in panic disorder, *Psychiatric Times* XXI:1-7, 2004.

Medical Letter on the CDC and FDA: Mental health epidemiology: substance use and mood and anxiety disorders common in the U.S. Atlanta, Aug 29, 2004, News Rx, p 84.

NANDA International: *NANDA nursing diagnoses: definitions and classifications 2007-2008*, Philadelphia, 2007, NANDA.

National Institutes of Mental Health (NIMH): *Effects of chronic stress on the hippocampus*, Bethesda, Md, 2002, Korn.

National Institutes of Mental Health (NIMH): Gene may bias amygdala response to frightful faces, *NIMH News Release*, www.nimh.nih.gov/events/pramygdala.cfm, retrieved Dec 23, 2003.

Ott, MJ: Mindfulness meditation: a path of transformation and healing, *J Psychosoc Nurs Ment Health Serv*, 42:22-29, 2004.

Patterson JG, Zderad LT: *Humanistic nursing*, New York, 1976, Wiley.

Peplau H: *Interpersonal relations in nursing*, New York, 1952, Putnam (classic).

Peplau H: *Interpersonal relations in nursing: a conceptual frame of reference for psychodynamic nursing*, New York, 1991, Springer.

Potter PA, Perry AG: *Fundamentals of nursing*, ed 6, St Louis, 2004, Elsevier.

Selye H: *The stress of life*, New York, 1956, McGraw-Hill (classic).

Wolpe J: *The practice of behavior therapy*, ed 2, New York, 1973, Pergamon Press (classic).

Chapter 10 Somatoform, Factitious, and Dissociative Disorders

PAMELA E. MARCUS

Your pain is the breaking of the shell that encases your understanding.

KAHLIL GIBRAN

OBJECTIVES

1. Name four physical symptoms reported by clients with somatization disorder.
2. Discuss two treatment strategies that reduce the symptoms of somatization disorder.
3. Apply the nursing process for managing clients with somatization disorder.
4. List two symptoms of pain disorder and interventions useful in reducing symptoms.
5. Describe a major symptom of conversion disorder and an effective nursing response.
6. Identify two symptoms of hypochondriasis and two nursing interventions.
7. Describe the symptoms of body dysmorphic disorder.
8. Formulate three nursing assessment questions to ask an individual with suspected body dysmorphic disorder.
9. Describe the symptoms of factitious disorder.
10. Identify two nursing interventions helpful in reducing symptoms of factitious disorder.
11. Relate the biologic patterns to target symptoms and therapeutic agents for psychopharmacologic intervention in somatization disorder and body dysmorphic disorder.

KEY TERMS

body dysmorphic disorder, p. 199
conversion disorder, p. 198
dissociation, p. 201
factitious disorder, p. 200
hypochondriasis, p. 199
la belle indifference, p. 199
pain disorder, p. 198
somatization disorder, p. 197

HISTORIC AND THEORETIC PERSPECTIVES

Somatoform disorders include a group of disorders that convert anxiety into physical symptoms for which there is no identifiable physical diagnosis. Theorists believe the physical symptoms are linked to psychobiologic factors, which are not intentional or under the conscious control of the client (unlike malingering). *Soma* is the Greek word for body, and somatization is the expression of psychologic stress through physical symptoms. The etiology of somatoform disorders and other disorders that express anxiety through physical symptoms can be traced to the work of Briquet, for whom somatization disorder was originally named (*Briquet's syndrome* or *hysteria*). In 1859, Briquet wrote about somatization in his book *Treatise on Hysteria*. For longer than 10 years, he followed 430 patients who had a diagnosis of hysteria or a focus on bodily concerns and sensations; he intended to dispute the belief that hysteria did not have any etiology in the female reproductive system or what he termed a "wandering uterus." His hypothesis was that hysteria was caused by an impact on the nervous system as a result of life stressors, such as marital conflict, child abuse, and family losses.

The results of Briquet's study found that 14% of his patients demonstrated symptoms after a psychologic trauma, such as a rape, witnessing a fire, or witnessing a sibling jump from a high window. He described other stressors that were related to conflict in the individual or the family, such as unplanned pregnancy, conflict in the marriage, or issues related to in-laws' input into their adult children's marital dynamics.

Briquet's research subjects were 87 individuals who were under the age of 12 and had been abused or neglected. He described these children as being held constantly in fear. Briquet also studied nuns, household servants, and prostitutes. The results of his research demonstrated that hysteria was rarely found in nuns. There were 197 prostitutes in his research population. Of these prostitutes, 104 had hysteria. An additional 29 prostitutes had intense nervous reactions, which were similar to mild forms of hysteria (Briquet, 1859; Loewenstein, 1990).

ETIOLOGY

Somatoform disorders reflect complex interactions between the mind and the body with serious impairment in the person's social and occupational functioning. Psychoanalytic theory suggests that psychogenic complaints of pain, disease, or loss of functioning are generally related to repressed aggression or sexuality. In conversion disorder, for example, the individual may be expressing a forbidden thought or wish by converting it into physical symptoms that are more appropriate and acceptable, and which also provide sympathy, care, and attention from others. Some theorists see hypochondriasis as an acceptable way to express anger or hostility resulting from past losses or disappointments. The physical symptoms supply the person with the help and concern needed to make up for his or her troubled past. Others see hypochondriasis as a defense against guilt or a low self-concept. In this case, the physical symptoms may be a well-deserved punishment. In pain disorder, the pain may be the person's way of gaining the love and care of others or a reprimand for actual or perceived wrongful acts. In body dysmorphic disorder, some theorists believe that the person gives a special meaning to the body or body part that is related to an event that occurred early in psychosexual development. The body or body part is the symbol of the earlier event that is repressed. Examples of body dysmorphic disorder may be seen in people who undergo extensive, painful cosmetic surgeries that seem distorting and disfiguring to others.

Biologic Theory

In biologic terms, changes in structure and function of the brain because of prolonged stress or trauma can result in somatoform disorders by altering the individual's perceptions and interpretations of bodily functions. It is puzzling why some persons develop an anxiety disorder, whereas others develop a somatoform disorder and many clients experience both. Neurotransmitters such as serotonin and norepinephrine are closely involved with depression and anxiety, but they are also known to modulate pain. Individuals experiencing severe pain generally have abnormal levels of neurotransmitters (Gallagher & Cariati, 2002).

Behavioral Theory

Behaviorists believe that some individuals learn to use somatic symptoms to communicate helplessness and manipulate others. Attention from others tends to exacerbate somatic symptoms in these individuals. Nurses and doctors in the United States are trained to respond to clients who report pain. Pain is considered the fifth vital sign in this country and must be addressed on admission and throughout the client's hospital stay (Sharp HealthCare, 2006). Somatic symptoms are also reinforced by having clients' avoid activities they find boring or unhelpful to their perceived pain.

Cognitive Theory

Cognitive theorists believe that clients with somatic symptoms misinterpret the meaning of body functions and sensations and become overly alarmed by them. Cognitive theorists advocate cognitive therapy to help clients reinterpret the meaning of body sensations (discussed later in this chapter and in Chapter 23).

EPIDEMIOLOGY

The epidemiologic data of this group of disorders differ in incidence and prevalence (Box 10-1). In regard to these disorders, it is interesting to note that some believe that an increase in diagnoses may be caused by a greater awareness of the disorder, whereas others think the increase is the result of overdiagnosis of the disorder in highly suggestible individuals.

CLINICAL DESCRIPTION

Somatoform Disorders

Somatization Disorder

Somatization disorder was formerly called hysteria and Briquet's syndrome (Briquet, 1859). Briquet developed a checklist of somatic concerns commonly voiced by the population as a whole. If a client had reported concerns in 13 out of 35 items, the individual had Briquet's syndrome. The checklist was shortened for DSM-IV-TR and is outlined here. The characteristic pattern of clients presenting with somatization disorder is one of frequently seeking and obtaining medical treatment for multiple, clinically significant somatic complaints. To meet DSM-IV-TR criteria, the symptoms must begin before age 30 years and are not adequately explained by any general medical disorder or the direct effects of a substance. For example, patients with multiple sclerosis, systemic lupus erythematosus, or other chronic debilitating diseases who have an onset in early adulthood frequently present with multisystem complaints, but do not have somatization disorder because a general medical condition better explains their symptom complex.

Distribution of symptoms in somatization disorder requires that symptoms have a distinct pattern that differs from general medical conditions if the following three criteria are met: (1) there is involvement of multiple organ

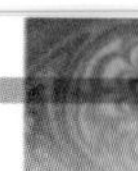

BOX 10-1

Epidemiology of Somatoform, Factitious, and Dissociative Disorders

SOMATOFORM DISORDERS

Somatization Disorder

Widely variable lifetime prevalence from 0.2% to 2% among women and less than 0.2% in men
Occurs in all cultures; most prevalent in South America (Gureje et al., 1997)
60% to 80% of the population may have somatic symptoms without known organic cause

Conversion Disorder

Widely varied reported cases from 11/100,000 to 500/100,000 in the general population
Reported in up to 3% of outpatient referrals to mental health clinics
Conversion symptoms identified in between 1% and 14% of general medical-surgical patients

Pain Disorder

Prevalence unknown
Association with both psychologic issues and general medical condition seems fairly common
Association with only psychologic factors appears much less common

Hypochondriasis

1% to 5% in general population
2% to 7% among primary care outpatients

Body Dysmorphic Disorder

Prevalence unknown
5% to 40% in mental health settings with co-occurring anxiety or depressive disorders
6% to 15% in cosmetic surgery and dermatology settings

FACTITIOUS DISORDER

Limited information on prevalence as this disorder generally involves deception, which is difficult to recognize
More common in females than in males; Munchausen is the most chronic and severe form, in which a person feigns illness or injures self to gain sympathy, more common in males
Higher prevalence in specialized treatment settings

DISSOCIATIVE DISORDERS

Dissociative Amnesia

Recent increase in reported cases involving previously forgotten early childhood memories

Dissociative Fugue

0.2% in general population
Prevalence may increase during times of extraordinary stressful events

Dissociative Identity Disorder

Recent increase in reported cases

Depersonalization Disorder

Lifetime prevalence in community and clinical settings unknown
Half of all adults may experience a single brief episode in lifetime, usually stress-induced

Data from American Psychiatric Association: *Diagnostic and statistical manual of mental disorders*, ed 4, text revision, Washington, DC, 2000, American Psychiatric Association.

systems (gastrointestinal, sexual/reproductive, and/or neurologic), (2) the symptoms exhibit an early onset and chronic course without development of physical signs or structural abnormalities (e.g., degenerative changes in bones and joints associated with complaints of pain), and (3) clinical laboratory abnormalities commonly associated with general medical conditions are absent. The specific diagnostic criteria are listed in the DSM-IV-TR Criteria box. Nurses in a general hospital or clinical practice setting are more likely to encounter clients with somatization disorder than those working in inpatient psychiatric units.

Pain Disorder

The predominant focus of the clinical presentation in **pain disorder** is pain in one or more anatomic sites. The severity of the pain calls for clinical attention and causes clinically significant impairment in one or more areas of functioning. Psychologic factors have an important role in the onset, severity, exacerbation, or maintenance of the pain. This experience of pain is not due to a mood, anxiety, or psychotic disorder and does not meet the criteria for dyspareunia (painful coitus or intercourse). This disorder is a pain disorder associated with psychologic factors if an associated medical condition does not play a major role in the onset, severity, and maintenance of symptoms. If a general medical condition plays a major role in the maintenance of the syndrome, the disorder is *pain disorder associated with both psychologic factors and a general medical condition*. Both disorders are either acute (if the duration is less than 6 months) or chronic (the pain is extended beyond 6 months).

Conversion Disorder

Clients who present with conversion symptoms exhibit one or more symptoms or deficits that affect voluntary motor or sensory function. These appear to be related to a neurologic or general medical condition. These symptoms or deficits are not caused by a general medical condition, the direct effects of a substance, or as a culturally sanctioned behavior or experience. The symptom is not intentionally produced and is not limited to pain or sexual dysfunction; nor does it occur exclusively in the context of somatization disorder. The conversion symptoms cause clinically significant distress or impairment in social, occupational, or other important areas of functioning. Common symptoms are blindness, paralysis, deafness, seizures, anesthesia, or abnormal motor movements (American Psychiatric Association [APA], 2000) (see Case Study).

The critical defining characteristics of **conversion disorder** are as follows: (1) psychologic factors are identi-

DSM-IV-TR CRITERIA

Somatization Disorder

A A history of many physical complaints beginning before age 30 that occur over several years and result in treatment being sought or significant impairment in social, occupational, or other important areas of functioning.

B Each of the following criteria must have been met, with individual symptoms occurring at any time during the course of the disturbance:

1 *Four pain symptoms:* a history of pain related to at least four different sites or functions (e.g., head, abdomen, back, joints, extremities, chest, rectum, during menstruation, during sexual intercourse, or during urination)

2 *Two gastrointestinal symptoms:* a history of at least two gastrointestinal symptoms other than pain (e.g., nausea, bloating, vomiting other than during pregnancy, diarrhea, or intolerance of several different foods)

3 *One sexual symptom:* a history of at least one sexual or reproductive symptom other than pain (e.g., sexual indifference, erectile or ejaculatory dysfunction, irregular menses, excessive menstrual bleeding, vomiting throughout pregnancy)

4 *One pseudoneurologic symptom:* a history of at least one symptom or deficit suggesting a neurologic condition not limited to pain (conversion symptoms such as impaired coordination or balance, paralysis, or localized weakness; difficulty swallowing or lump in throat; aphonia (loss of voice); urinary retention; hallucinations; loss of touch or pain sensation; double vision; blindness; deafness; seizures; dissociative symptoms such as amnesia; or loss of consciousness other than fainting)

C Either 1 or 2:

1 After appropriate investigation, each of the symptoms in criterion B cannot be fully explained by a known general medical condition or the direct effects of a substance (e.g., a drug of abuse or a medication).

2 When there is a related general medical condition, the physical complaints or resulting social or occupational impairment is in excess of what would be expected from the history, physical examination, or laboratory findings.

D The symptoms are not intentionally produced (as in factitious disorder or malingering).

From American Psychiatric Association: *Diagnostic and statistical manual of mental disorders,* ed 4, text revision, Washington DC, 2000, American Psychiatric Association.

fied as being related to the onset or exacerbation of the symptom; (2) specific, identifiable conflicts or stressors precede the development of the conversion symptoms; and (3) the person demonstrates an obvious lack of concern about the seriousness of the symptoms, which is inconsistent with the problem. This lack of concern is the **la belle indifference,** or "beautiful indifference," a hallmark symptom of conversion disorder.

Hypochondriasis

"Don't be such a hypochondriac!" is a common theme in American culture and perhaps other cultures as well. Parents say it to children who complain of stomachaches before school on the day of an important test. Sometimes even nursing students say it to each other as they worry about potential signs and symptoms while learning and acquiring knowledge related to medical, surgical, or psychiatric mental health nursing. Such instances, however, probably do not reflect true **hypochondriasis** as defined in the DSM-IV-TR.

Six major criteria are associated with this diagnosis. First, the individual focuses on fears of having—or the idea of having—a serious medical disorder based on the individual's misinterpretation of bodily symptoms. Second, this misinterpretation of symptoms persists despite appropriate medical evaluation and reassurance. Third, the individual's preoccupation with symptoms is not as intense or distorted as it would be in a delusional disorder, nor is it as restricted as in body dysmorphic disorder. The fourth criterion states that the preoccupation causes clinically significant distress or impairment in social, occupational, or other major areas of functioning. To meet the fifth criterion, the duration of the disturbance must be at least 6 months. Hypochondriasis is not due to another anxiety disorder, somatoform disorder, or major depressive episode.

Body Dysmorphic Disorder

Body dysmorphic disorder (BDD) is when a client has a preoccupation with an imagined defect in appearance. If the individual has a slight physical anomaly, the person's concern is markedly excessive. This preoccupation causes

CASE STUDY

Juan is a 34-year-old client on a neurologic unit in a Department of Veterans Administration medical center. He has been treated on the psychiatric service in this facility for a number of years and was diagnosed with schizophrenia, based primarily on his prominent and constant visual and auditory hallucinations involving his drill sergeant. In the past he has taken the antipsychotic medication haloperidol (Haldol).

Juan was born in Puerto Rico and joined the Marines in San Juan when he turned 18. He was unable to complete basic training because he experienced a psychotic episode during which he assaulted his drill sergeant. Juan was admitted to the neurology department when one morning he told his family he was unable to walk. Juan had no recent falls or other injuries. Providers did not find any abnormalities on his physical examination or computerized tomography (CT) scan. During a mental status examination, Juan reported that he no longer heard any voices. Nursing assessment also revealed Juan's lack of concern about a seemingly serious problem like paralysis. The psychiatric mental health nurse specialist learned from Juan's family that about a month before his admission, Juan's appeal for a service-related disability was turned down. His family was depending on that financial supplement to help them obtain better housing, a goal they had voiced on many occasions.

CRITICAL THINKING

1 What are two symptoms that indicate Juan is experiencing a conversion disorder?

2 How does the recent behavior of Juan's family play a role in his current symptomatology?

3 Which of Juan's symptoms might be labeled *la belle indifference* (beautiful indifference)?

4 How does Juan's assaultive behavior during his psychotic episode influence his perceived paralysis?

5 What are two behavioral outcomes that would indicate Juan's ability to better cope with his disorder?

clinically significant distress or impairment in social or occupational functioning. This preoccupation is not the result of another mental disorder.

Body dysmorphic disorder usually begins in adolescence, but sometimes may begin in childhood. Diagnosis may take years because clients can hide their symptoms. Onset can be gradual or abrupt (APA, 2000). Depending on how the client experiences the severity of the symptoms or the extent the client focuses on the perceived deficit, behavior patterns sometimes cause difficulties at school or at work. Examples of symptoms include excessive grooming, checking in the mirror, and skin picking. Often, the client reports poor grades as a result of this preoccupation of the body imperfection. For example, a client uses a mirror to check her or his hair multiple times a day, if the hair is a focus symptom for the client. Other clients stop participating in sports, have numerous school absences, and if the symptoms are severe, the person quits school. When experiencing severe symptoms, the client often becomes hesitant to leave the home. Some become violent and angry when frustrated about the perceived deficit. For example, a person who is preoccupied with a perceived problem with his hair breaks the mirror by throwing the brush against the bathroom mirror in a fit of anger (see Case Study).

There is a high risk of completed suicide in clients with body dysmorphic disorder. In their study population of 185 subjects followed for 4 years, Phillips and Menard (2006) found out that 2 individuals completed suicide during this study period (see Research for Evidence-Based Practice box).

When assessing the individual with body dysmorphic disorder, it is important to ask if the patient has any worries about his or her body appearance. This includes hair, facial features, hips, fingers, and any other body area that the client identifies as concerning. Ask directly about the concern and how the person perceives the deficit. Determine the amount of time the client spends thinking about the imagined defect. What actions has the person taken to hide or get rid of the deficit, such as makeup, surgery, or baggy clothes? How has the concern about the deficit affected the person's ability to function at school, work, socially, and within the family. Understanding the client's subjective experience will assist the nurse in planning care that considers the individual's needs (Phillips, 2006; Slaughter and Sun, 1999).

Factitious Disorder

Individuals with **factitious disorder** intentionally produce physical or psychologic signs and symptoms to assume the sick role. The individual does this behavior for economic gain, avoiding school or legal responsibility, or to improve physical well-being. Both men and women have symptoms of factitious disorder. Peebles et al. (2005) described six cases in girls ranging in age from 9 to 15. Two of these girls were avoiding attendance at school; the other four had unresolved psychologic conflicts. This illness is often unreported. Some adults demonstrate factitious disorder in prison, the military, and groups that are controversial. Some individuals develop factitious disor-

CASE STUDY

Crystal is a 23-year-old executive secretary. She was referred to a mental health practice group by the fourth plastic surgeon with whom she had consulted regarding dermabrasion surgery to remove three 2-centimeter (cm) flat scars from her right upper arm. Although she lives in a coastal Florida city, Crystal wears only long-sleeved jackets, blouses, and dresses. The garments are always loosely fitted. Crystal is certain that people notice her "lumpy" arm and make comments about it; therefore, she goes to extreme lengths to prevent this embarrassment and suffers the consequences of an extremely hot climate. She refuses to go to the beach with friends or swim in front of anyone because of the preoccupation with her scars.

CRITICAL THINKING

1 What intervention would help Crystal become aware of her preoccupation?
2 What three outcome strategies can Crystal perform that would reduce her exaggerated perceptions?
3 What are two verbal outcome statements that would illustrate Crystal's progress in managing her problem?
4 How can Crystal be educated to understand the role medication plays in decreasing her symptoms?
5 What are two behavioral outcomes that would indicate Crystal's ability to better cope with her disorder?

RESEARCH for EVIDENCE-BASED PRACTICE

Phillips KA, Menard W: Body dysmorphic disorder: a prospective study, *American Journal of Psychiatry* 163:1280-1283, 2006.

The authors enrolled 200 subjects to study the course of body dysmorphic disorder (BDD) over a 4-year period. The study included individuals who had the delusional variant of BDD. Fifty-two percent of the subjects in this study came self-referred, and 48% were referred by professionals. Researchers first interviewed the subjects in person and assessed them weekly for severity of symptoms and for on going psychiatric treatment. They evaluated suicidal ideation and severity of suicidal symptoms as well. The researchers in this study were not applying any therapeutic interventions for the study participants. The subjects were receiving care by other practitioners.

On intake, 147 of 185 subjects reported a history of suicidal ideation; 51 had a history of a suicidal attempt. The research subjects identified the focus of the BDD symptoms as the precipitating cause of the suicidal attempt. On conclusion of the study, two male subjects who were receiving psychiatric care completed suicide. Nine subjects attempted suicide during the study period, with a total of 30 suicidal attempts between them. Of the 185 individuals in the total study group, 167 received psychiatric care during the course of the study.

The study concludes that individuals with BDD have a high risk of suicidal completion. They present risk factors other than the symptoms of BDD, such as multiple psychiatric hospitalizations, are often single or divorced and have poor social supports, poor self-esteem, a high anxiety level, depression, and hostility.

It is important for the nursing staff to thoroughly assess the client with BDD for suicidal ideation and level of risk. It is important for the staff to monitor their own reaction to an individual with BDD, because if a staff member does not share the same perception of the body deformity as the client, then she or he may not understand the level of stress the client is experiencing.

der after an actual physical illness. Some clients also have symptoms of depression, hypochondriasis, anxiety, borderline personality disorder, conduct disorder, and antisocial disorder. The adult clients are often knowledgeable in medical terminology, and many work in health care systems. Providers often make the diagnosis of factitious disorder based on inexplicable laboratory results (Krahn et al., 2003).

Often, health care providers are reluctant to make this diagnosis. Clients undergo expensive procedures, which often endanger their lives. Countertransference causes the staff to be abrupt and inappropriately confront the client. This damages the therapeutic relationship and does not provide the client with appropriate care. Evidence that indicates the best method of intervention is still in need of research. Confrontation can be ineffective as a means of intervention. Another intervention that is helpful is a supportive empathetic relationship that helps the client to change the maladaptive behaviors. The practitioners works with these clients as a multidisciplinary team to provide consistent comprehensive care. This team consists of medical practitioners as well as psychiatric practitioners. Note that malingering differs from factitious disorder in that individuals who malinger have external incentives, such as relief from work, and no intrapsychic need to maintain the sick role.

Dissociative Disorders

Dissociative Amnesia

In persons with dissociative amnesia, the defining symptom is one or more episodes of inability to recall important personal information, usually of a traumatic or stressful nature, that is too extensive for ordinary forgetting to explain (**dissociation**). The disturbance does not occur exclusively during the course of dissociative identity disorder and does not result from the effects of a substance (blackouts during ethyl alcohol intoxication) or a general medical condition (amnesia after head trauma).

Dissociative Fugue

Dissociative fugue is a sudden, unexpected travel away from home or one's customary place of work, with an inability to recall one's past (or where one has been). The individual demonstrates confusion about personal identity or assumes a new identity, which is sometimes partial ("filling in the blanks"). As in dissociative amnesia, the disturbance does not occur in the context of a dissociative identity disorder and is not due to the effects of a substance or to a general medical condition.

Dissociative Identity Disorder

No other disorder in current psychiatric nosology (classification) has aroused as much controversy as dissociative identity disorder (DID). DSM-IV-TR criteria for DID are straightforward. The first criterion is that the individual must demonstrate two or more distinct identities or personality states, each with its own relatively enduring pattern of perceiving, relating to, and thinking about the environment and self. Second, at least two of these personality states recurrently take control of the person's behavior. The individual is unable to recall important personal information that is too extensive for ordinary forgetting to explain. These behavior patterns and thoughts do not result from the effects of a substance (e.g., blackouts or chaotic behavior during alcohol intoxication) or a general medical condition (complex partial seizures). In children the symptoms are not due to imaginary playmates or other fantasy play.

Depersonalization Disorder

Essential features are persistent or recurrent episodes of feelings of detachment or estrangement from one's self. Sensations of being outside of one's body or mental processes or an observer of one's body often occur. Various types of sensory anesthesia, lack of affective response, and a sense of lacking control of one's actions or speech are often present. The individual has intact reality testing (e.g., awareness of the situation). Depersonalization is a common experience, and the diagnosis is made only if symptoms are severe enough to cause marked distress or impaired functioning. A separate diagnosis is not made if the experience occurs exclusively during the course of another mental disorder such as schizophrenia, panic disorder, acute stress disorder, or another dissociative disorder or is not caused by the physiologic effects of a substance or general medical condition.

PROGNOSIS

The somatoform disorders, with the exception of conversion disorder, are chronic and fluctuating and rarely remit fully. The prognosis for persons with somatization disorder is related to factors specific to the disorder, the client, and the clinician. One follow-up study on body dysmorphic disorder indicates that in 1 year, full remission was 0.09% and partial remission was 0.21%.

In this study, 84.2% of the subjects were receiving mental health treatment. The authors concluded that the probability of relapse was 0.15% in clients whose symptoms were partially or fully remitted (Phillips et al., 2006). Conversion disorders usually remit within 2 weeks; however, there is recurrence in 20% to 25% of cases. A single recurrence of symptoms is predictive of future episodes. Factors that have been identified with a good prognosis are identifiable stressors at the time that symptoms develop, early treatment, and above-average intelligence. The dissociative disorders have varying prognosis ranging from a rapid, complete recovery (fugue) to both episodic and continuous chronic courses (dissociative identity disorder). Dissociative identity disorder frequently reemerges during periods of stress or relapse of substance abuse (APA, 2000).

DISCHARGE CRITERIA

Client will:

- Identify situations and events that trigger somatic concerns or dissociative states and select adaptive ways to prevent or manage them.

- Describe somatic symptoms and thoughts or stressors that may have increased the client's level of anxiety.
- Discuss the connection between anxiety-provoking situations or events and somatic symptoms or dissociation.
- Explain relief behaviors openly.
- Identify adaptive, positive techniques and strategies that relieve anxiety and decrease the focus on somatic concerns.
- Demonstrate behaviors that represent reduced somatic focus or dissociation states.
- Use learned stress-reducing strategies, such as mindful meditation.
- Demonstrate an ability to problem-solve, concentrate, and make decisions.
- Sleep through the night.
- Use appropriate supports from the nursing and medical community, family, and friends.
- Determine the difference between somatic concerns and an illness state with laboratory and other objective test confirmation of pathology.
- Discuss the ability to tolerate manageable levels of stress and emotionality.
- List the medication used to control the symptoms as well as the appropriate dosage and scheduled times.

The Nursing Process

ASSESSMENT

It is important for the nurse to thoroughly assess each client without judging the possibility that the client is feigning the physical symptoms. Obtaining history, collaborative history with family members and collaborating with other treating practitioners, will assist staff in providing the client with comprehensive care. Understanding the possible anxiety precipitants of the somatic concerns will help the client to reduce his or her focus on the physical sensations or concerns.

NURSING DIAGNOSIS

To determine which nursing diagnoses will most effectively guide treatment for clients with somatoform disorders, factitious disorders, and dissociative disorders, the nurse relies on information obtained in the assessment process. The nurse identifies defining characteristics for the target diagnoses from the client, and the nurse and client jointly identify etiologic factors. Etiologic factors influence the selection of intervention. Nursing diagnoses are prioritized according to clients' needs. Typical diagnoses for clients with somatoform disorders, factitious disorders, and dissociative disorders include the following:

- Risk for suicide
- Risk for self-directed violence
- Risk for other-directed violence
- Self-mutilation
- Risk for self-mutilation
- Anxiety
- Death anxiety
- Hopelessness
- Powerlessness
- Insomnia
- Chronic pain
- Fatigue
- Fear
- Health-seeking behaviors
- Disturbed body image
- Chronic low self-esteem
- Ineffective coping
- Defensive coping
- Social isolation
- Risk for loneliness
- Risk-prone health behavior
- Ineffective role performance
- Noncompliance
- Impaired social interaction
- Ineffective denial
- Impaired memory
- Disturbed sensory perception
- Disturbed thought processes
- Deficient knowledge
- Imbalanced nutrition: less than body requirements
- Imbalanced nutrition: more than body requirements
- Activity intolerance
- Impaired physical mobility
- Spiritual distress
- Sexual dysfunction
- Interrupted family processes
- Compromised family coping
- Decisional conflict
- Relocation stress syndrome

OUTCOME IDENTIFICATION

Outcome criteria differ according to the characteristics of each client's nursing diagnoses and collaborative (DSM-IV-TR) diagnoses. Determining outcomes before implementating the plan will guide both nursing interventions and evaluation. Nursing diagnoses are associated with outcomes (goals) and serve as guides in outcome development. In practice, nurses generally determine outcomes by the patient's presentation of clinical manifestations.

General Outcome Expectations

Client will:

- Contact the nursing staff if thoughts are suicidal or harmful toward others.
- Identify situations and events that trigger somatic concerns or dissociative episodes and select ways to prevent or manage them.
- Describe somatic symptoms that occur with the increase in levels of anxiety.
- Discuss the connection between anxiety-provoking situations or events and somatic symptoms or dissociative states.
- Explain relief behaviors and thoughts openly.

- Identify adaptive, positive techniques and strategies that relieve anxiety and decrease somatic focus or the dissociative episodes.
- Demonstrate behaviors that represent reduced somatic symptoms or provide the client with a means of reassociation when experiencing a dissociative state.
- Use learned anxiety-reducing strategies such as mindful meditation (see Box 9-3).
- Demonstrate the ability to problem solve, concentrate, and make decisions.
- Verbalize the feeling of being relaxed and less concerned about somatic sensations or disorders.
- Sleep through the night for 6 to 8 hours.
- Use appropriate supports from the nursing and medical community, family, and friends.
- Learn to manage anxiety at tolerable levels without dissociating or focusing on somatic sensations.
- Seek help from appropriate sources when there is an awareness of new somatic concerns.
- List the medication used to control the symptoms as well as the appropriate dosage and scheduled times.
- Continue postdischarge symptom management including medication and other therapies.

Somatization Disorder

Client will:

- Construct an exercise program that includes anxiety-reducing techniques.
- Address two positive somatic responses (e.g., massage therapy, the satisfied feeling after a successful exercise session).
- Keep an intake log to document somatic preoccupation and stressors (including intrusive thoughts or concerns).
- Help the therapist to coordinate the information from the primary care provider and any other involved specialists.
- Take the medication as prescribed and be able to identify the rationale for the medication.
- Contact the therapist for more frequent visits if somatization increases.

Dissociative Identity Disorder

Client will:

- Alert the therapist or use a hotline such as 1-800-SUICIDE or 1-800-273-TALK when feeling suicidal.
- Respond to his or her name when addressed by a member of the treatment team.
- Refer to self in the first-person pronoun form: "*I* think."
- Identify periods of increasing anxiety.
- Inform others of dissatisfaction in a nonthreatening manner.
- Use assertive-response behaviors to meet needs (see Chapters 4 and 23).
- Keep a written journal to identify stressors and when the dissociation occurs.
- Take medications as prescribed.
- Identify when to utilize a prn medication to decrease the heightened anxiety response to a cue in the environment.
- Contact the therapist if symptoms increase.

PLANNING

Treatment planning for the client with anxiety and related disorders in the current health care environment is complex and varied. Clients with severe body dysmorphic disorder (BDD) often need hospitalization to prevent a suicidal occurrence. In the past, treatment for dissociative identity disorder also occurred in special units with a prolonged hospitalization.

Today both clinicians and administrators in inpatient facilities are struggling to balance effective treatment with the high costs associated with these specialty units. Increasingly, inpatient hospitalization is available only for short periods of time for clients at imminent risk to themselves or others. Rather than assuming their traditional roles of providing direct care to clients in inpatient facilities, nurses are increasingly involved as case managers. As case managers, nurses provide clients and families with information on treatment alternatives.

IMPLEMENTATION

The role of a nurse in the implementation of a care plan for clients with somatization disorders depends on the setting. The following interventions are useful for clients with somatic symptoms, regardless of the diagnosis or treatment setting.

Nursing Interventions

1. Identify the degree of suicidal ideation and depression in clients with all types of anxiety and associated disorders. *A thorough evaluation of clients with anxiety disorders and associated disorders will help to prevent suicide and other destructive behaviors early in the intervention process.*
2. Monitor one's own level of anxiety and make a conscious effort to remain calm. *Anxiety is readily transferable from one person to another. Individuals with somatoform illness have a risk of an increase of symptoms during times of increased anxiety.*
3. Recognize that the client's use of relief behaviors focuses on somatic sensations as indicators of anxiety. *Early interventions help to manage anxiety before symptoms escalate to more serious levels.*
4. Educate the client about the importance of limiting caffeine, nicotine, and other central nervous system stimulants. *Limiting these substances prevents or minimizes physical symptoms of anxiety, such as rapid heart rate and jitteriness, which may cue other somatic concerns.*
5. Teach the client to distinguish between somatic sensations that are connected to identifiable objects or sources (such as a cold, pain from a fall) and somatic concerns for which there is no immediate identifiable object or source but are a reaction to an increase in

MEDICATION KEY FACTS Somatoform, Factitious, and Dissociative Disorders

Pharmacologic interventions are symptom-oriented. Medications include the following:
- Anxiolytics for associated anxiety
- Antidepressants for associated depression
- Antipsychotics for any underlying psychosis

Patients diagnosed with dissociative disorder are usually not good candidates for psychopharmacotherapy and seldom derive more than limited symptomatic benefits.

anxiety. *Knowledge of anxiety and its related components increases the client's control over the disorder.*

6. Instruct the client to perform the following strategies *to reduce anxiety and distract the focus on somatic concerns* (see Chapter 23):
   a. Progressive relaxation technique
   b. Slow deep-breathing exercises
   c. Focusing on a single object in the room
   d. Soothing music or relaxation tapes
   e. Visual imagery (guided imagery)
7. Help the client build on coping methods that helped to manage anxiety in the past. *Coping methods that were previously successful will generally be effective in subsequent situations.*
8. Activate the client to contact support persons who will increase socialization and provide emotional support as the client attends work or school, even when client is feeling poorly. *A strong support system helps the client avoid anxiety-provoking situations or activities.*
9. Help the client gain control of overwhelming feelings and impulses through brief, direct verbal interactions. *Individual interactions at appropriate intervals help reduce or manage a client's anxious feelings or impulses.*
10. Help the client to understand the importance of the medication regimen and the need to take medications as prescribed. *Medication is an effective adjunct to other psychosocial therapeutic interventions when necessary.*

Additional Treatment Modalities

Biologic Interventions

Pharmacologic Interventions. Pharmacologic interventions alone or in combination with cognitive behavioral interventions are among the most successful treatments for somatoform disorders. Selective serotonin reuptake inhibitors (SSRIs), antidepressants now widely used to treat somatoform disorders, have been particularly effective in treating body dysmorphic disorder (BDD). Pharmacologic treatment of dissociative identify disorder (DID) is largely symptomatic. Varying combinations of antidepressants, antipsychotics, and, to a lesser extent, benzodiazepines are used. Researchers are currently studying the best medication regimen for individuals with somatoform disorders. For example, they recently studied clomipramine (Anafranil) versus desipramine (Norpramin) for individuals with body dysmorphic disorder. Clomipramine was more effective for individuals with this disorder than desipramine. Clomipramine improved the individual's ability to function, including the clients who have delusions accompanying the body dysmorphic disorder (Hollander et al., 1999). (For more specific information about dosages and side effect profiles, see Chapter 24.)

Psychotherapy

Psychotherapeutic intervention takes place in group or individual settings. One advantage of group therapy is the opportunity for the client to learn from the successes and failures of others with similar symptoms. Behavioral and cognitive behavioral therapies have been widely effective in treating a variety of anxiety disorders (see Chapter 23).

Cognitive Behavioral Therapy. Many therapists use cognitive behavioral therapy to treat clients with somatoform disorders and dissociative disorders. The success of this approach centers on the client's understanding that symptoms are a learned response to thoughts or feelings about behaviors that occur in daily life. The client and therapist identify the target symptoms and then examine circumstances associated with the symptoms. Together they plan strategies to change either the cognitions (thoughts) or the behaviors. Cognitive behavioral therapy is short term and demands active participation on the part of both client and therapist (see Chapter 23).

EVALUATION

Ideally the nurse and the client together evaluate the client's progress toward the identified outcomes at every interaction. If the client does not make satisfactory progress, the nurse modifies either the expected outcomes or the interventions. The nurse examines all factors that relate to the outcomes, including what occurred in the previous phases of the nursing process, the role of the nurse in setting client and clinician expectations, the clarity of communicating client goals with the client, and other intervening events that have occurred since the outcomes were set. It is important for the nurse to remember that the somatoform disorders and the dissociative disorders are chronic and enduring. It takes patience and support for the client to determine the pattern of his or her behavior and to incorporate methods to initiate change.

NURSING CARE PLAN

Mary is a 40-year-old woman who has seen four primary practitioners in the last 2 weeks. A nurse is currently evaluating her for chronic constipation and intolerance of several different foods. At her gynecologic appointment last week, she had concerns about having excessive menstrual bleeding and cramps. Mary went to the chiropractor in the early part of this week with vague back pain. She reports several concerns about her ability to walk, as sometimes she has a weakness in her knees and overall she feels tired and weak. She has been having arguments with her boyfriend and has been concerned that he will end the relationship because of her significant complaints about her body. Mary has been having some stress at work. She has been calling in sick frequently, and her employer is requesting a note from her practitioner each time she calls in. Mary is afraid that her supervisor will reprimand her for absenteeism.

The nurse practitioner performed a thorough physical examination, which was negative. Mary's recent laboratory values were within normal limits. The nurse practitioner obtained Mary's past medical records with the client's permission and noticed a pattern of multiple physician visits with similar complaints assessed in the past 2 weeks. The nurse practitioner made the diagnosis of somatization disorder.

DSM-IV-TR Diagnoses

Axis I	Somatization disorder
Axis II	Deferred
Axis III	History of gastroesophageal reflux disease (GERD), chronic constipation, intolerance of several different foods
	Headaches, back pain
	Sexual dysfunction (inability to lubricate), excessive menstrual bleeding, cramps
	Weakness in knees resulting in concerns about ambulating
	Reports of feeling tired and weak
Axis IV	Problems with primary support system
	Occupational concerns
Axis V	GAF = 60 (current); GAF = 75 (past year)

Nursing Diagnosis *Disturbed sensory perception related to subjective experience of feelings of pain, weakness, gastrointestinal and genitourinary symptoms, as evidenced by chronic constipation and intolerance of several different foods, excessive menstrual bleeding and cramps, and vague back pain*

NOC Stress Level, Distorted Thought Self-Control, Cognitive Orientation, Neurological Status: Spinal Sensory/Motor Function

NIC Anxiety Reduction, Cognitive Restructuring, Neurologic Monitoring, Surveillance: Safety, Self-Esteem Enhancement, Environmental Management

CLIENT OUTCOMES	NURSING INTERVENTIONS	EVALUATION
Mary will identify common situations that provoke anxiety and somatic concerns.	Assign "homework" to client (e.g., keeping a body concern diary). *Documenting somatic responses helps client link symptoms with precipitating events.* During weekly sessions, review Mary's diary of somatic symptoms. *Discussing the linking of events/situations with the somatic symptoms teaches Mary which stressor events provoke anxiety so she will learn to manage them.*	Mary identifies early morning, before preparing for work, as a critical time for symptoms to develop. She reports that her feelings of dread surrounding the volume of work her supervisor expects her to complete occur frequently when she prepares for work in the morning.
Mary will describe early warning symptoms of anxiety.	Assist Mary in associating her somatic symptoms with thoughts about her workload. *This will illustrate to Mary specific situations in her life that result in somatic sensations and concerns.*	Mary reports that she does not experience gastrointestinal or other painful symptoms when her supervisor is out of the office.
Mary will report willingness to tolerate mild to moderate levels of somatic concerns without calling in ill or seeking medical attention.	In weekly sessions, explore with Mary her concerns about her job and her relationship with her boyfriend. *These discussions will help Mary problem solve options that offer some control over her anxiety and her somatic concerns.*	Mary is able to talk to her boyfriend about her willingness to seek some professional help to decrease her body's response to anxiety and alleviate her multiple somatic concerns.
Mary will demonstrate mindful meditation to reduce her anxiety and somatic concerns. (See Box 9-3.)	During weekly sessions, demonstrate relaxation exercises, such as mindful meditation to assist Mary in reducing her anxiety level and somatic discomfort. *Relaxation exercises help an individual to reduce the somatic anxiety responses.*	Mary reports enjoying using mindful meditation twice a day: once in the morning before preparing for work and once before leaving work for home. She feels this intervention has helped her to feel calmer.

Nursing Diagnosis *Impaired social interaction related to multiple somatic concerns restricting the client's ability to socialize, as evidenced by boyfriend voicing frustration with client's somatic concerns; also the client's girlfriends have stopped asking the client to join them on outings because of her frequent somatic concerns*

NOC Stress Level, Fear Level, Social Involvement, Self-Esteem, Social Interaction Skills, Role Performance

NIC Anxiety Reduction, Coping Enhancement, Socialization Enhancement, Self-Esteem Enhancement, Support System Enhancement

Continued

NURSING CARE PLAN—cont'd

CLIENT OUTCOMES	NURSING INTERVENTIONS	EVALUATION
Mary will be able to go shopping with her girlfriends without discussing a somatic concern.	Explore with Mary her usual patterns of behavior when asked to go out with her friends. Identify possible modifications of those behaviors. *These discussions will help Mary to focus on alternative activities/behaviors that minimize dysfunctional behavioral patterns and increase coping skills.*	Mary describes telling her girlfriend details of each one of her physical concerns. She acknowledges her girlfriend's frustration when Mary continued relating her fatigue. Mary was able to identify why her friend was reluctant to ask her to join her in a social situation.
Mary will utilize yoga and mindful meditation to decrease her somatic concerns.	Encourage Mary to utilize an exercise program such as yoga and a relaxation program such as mindful meditation to reduce her somatic concerns. *Exercise and relaxation exercises reduce anxiety and somatization.*	Mary purchased and used a yoga tape to begin the yoga program. She expressed enjoying mindful meditation.

Nursing Diagnosis *Health-seeking behaviors related to multiple somatic concerns as evidenced by going to four practitioners in a 2-week period to report many health concerns*

NOC Health Beliefs, Knowledge: Health Promotion, Participation in Health Care Decisions, Personal Health Status, Personal Well-Being

NIC Health Education, Self-Modification Assistance, Coping Enhancement, Teaching: Individual, Decision-Making Support, Mutual Goal Setting

CLIENT OUTCOMES	NURSING INTERVENTIONS	EVALUATION
Mary will agree to choose one health care practitioner to coordinate all of her health care needs.	The nurse practitioner encourages Mary to choose one practitioner to coordinate her health care needs. *This prevents multiple expensive and unnecessary medical tests. This also allows the practitioner to monitor Mary for somatic concerns on a continuing basis.*	Mary agrees with the nurse practitioner and requests that she become her primary provider along with the nurse's supervising medical doctor.
Mary will reduce her somatic concerns when her health care needs are met on a regular basis.	The nurse practitioner sets up a regular schedule for Mary's evaluations. The nurse practitioner plans to see Mary every month for half an hour to evaluate somatic concerns. *A structured schedule will ensure Mary that her health care needs are being met and will reduce her somatization.*	Mary agrees to attend monthly sessions to present her health care concerns.

CHAPTER SUMMARY

- Treatment of somatoform disorders and dissociative disorders is multidisciplinary and usually involves more than one treatment modality.
- Inpatient treatment of somatoform disorders is usually the result of suicidal risk and the failure of treatment in an outpatient setting.
- The nursing role in the treatment of clients with somatoform disorders and dissociative disorders varies. Common to all treatment settings is the nurse's role in client and family education about the disorders and their treatment.
- Nursing care plans for clients with symptoms of somatoform disorders reflect the understanding that managing anxiety effectively is part of daily living.
- Nurses actively participate in behavioral interventions structured to decrease the somatic responses.

REVIEW QUESTIONS

1 A nurse assesses a client suspected to have somatization disorder. Which findings support the diagnosis? You may select more than one answer. The client:

1. Is currently 46 years old.
2. Reports headaches, burning urination, knee problems, and hemorrhoids.
3. Is also diagnosed with Graves' disease.
4. Names six current physicians providing care.
5. Complains of skimpy, irregular menstruation.
6. Complains of frequent episodes of double vision.

2 A nurse interviews a client diagnosed with conversion disorder. Which comment is most likely from this client?

1. "Since getting a divorce, I've had crushing chest pain, but I don't think it really means anything."
2. "I have daily problems with nausea and vomiting. I think I'm getting seriously dehydrated."
3. "Sexual intercourse is so painful that I avoid it. I'm afraid that's going to destroy my marriage."
4. "I get big lumps in my throat and can't swallow when I eat. I'm afraid I might have cancer."

3 A client reports fears of having breast cancer and says to the nurse, "I've missed so much work having three mammograms in the past 6 months. No problems showed up, but I'm sure that's because the radiologic technicians were not qualified to correctly perform mammograms." Which disorder would the nurse suspect?
1. Dissociative fugue
2. Factitious disorder
3. Hypochondriasis
4. Pain disorder

4 A nurse counsels a client diagnosed with body dysmorphic disorder. Which nursing diagnosis would be a priority for the plan of care?
1. Ineffective role performance
2. Anxiety
3. Disturbed body image
4. Risk for self-directed violence

5 A client with dissociative identity disorder is hospitalized for the fourth time after overdosing. The client does not remember overdosing. Select the best initial nursing outcome for this situation. Client will:
1. Inform staff when feeling the urge to harm self.
2. Not switch personalities for the next 7 days.
3. Discuss childhood issues that relate to anxiety.
4. Assume a decision-making role for his or her own health care needs.

Additional self-study exercises and learning resources are available to you on the ***Companion CD*** *at the back of the book and on the* ***Evolve website*** *at* ***http://evolve.elsevier.com/Fortinash/.***

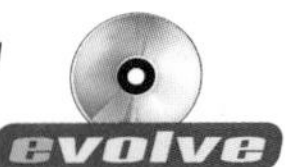

Online Resources

National Alliance on Mental Illness: **www.nami.org**

National Institute of Mental Health: **www.nimh.nih.gov**

Mental Health America: **www.nmha.org**

REFERENCES

American Psychiatric Association: *Diagnostic and statistical manual of mental disorders*, ed 4, text revision, Washington, DC, American Psychiatric Association, 2000.

Briquet P: *Traits de l'hysterie*, Paris, 1859, J Bailliere.

Gallagher RM, Cariati S: Clinical update: the pain-depression conundrum: bridging the body and mind, Oct 2, 2002; retrieved Jan 4, 2005, from Medscape website: www.medscape.com/viewprogram/2030.

Gureje O et al: Somatization in cross-cultural perspective: a World Health Organization study in primary care, *Am J Psychiatry* 154:989-995, 1997.

Hollander E et al: Clomipramine vs desipramine crossover trial in body dysmorphic disorder, *Arch Gen Psychiatry* 56:1033-1044, 1999.

Krahn LE et al: Patients who strive to be ill: factitious disorder with physical symptoms, *Am J Psychiatry* 160:1163-1169, 2003.

Loewenstein RJ: Somatoform disorders in victims of incest and child abuse. In Kluft RP, editor: *Incest-related syndrome of adult psychopathology*, pp 75-107, Washington, DC, 1990, American Psychiatric Press.

Peebles R et al: Factitious disorder and malingering in adolescent girls: case series and literature review, *Clin Pediatr* 44:237-244, 2005.

Phillips KA, Menard W: Suicidality in body dysmorphic disorder: a prospective study, *Am J Psychiatry* 163:1280-1283, 2006.

Phillips KA et al: A 12- month follow-up study of the course of body dysmorphic disorder, *Am J Psychiatry* 163:907-913, 2006.

Sharp HealthCare Pain Program: Sharp Memorial Hospital and Sharp Mesa Vista Hospital, San Diego, Calif, 2006.

Slaughter JR, Sun AM: In pursuit of perfection: a primary care physician's guide to body dysmorphic disorder, *Am Fam Physician* 60:1738-1745, 1999.

Chapter 11

Mood Disorders and Adjustment Disorders

BONNIE M. HAGERTY and KATHLEEN L. PATUSKY

When sorrows come, they come not single spies, but in battalions.
WILLIAM SHAKESPEARE

OBJECTIVES

1. Describe theories for the etiology of mood disorders including neurobiologic, ethologic, and psychosocial theories.
2. Discuss the etiology for adjustment disorders.
3. Compare and contrast the DSM-IV-TR classifications of depressive, bipolar, and adjustment disorders.
4. Discuss the epidemiology and course of depressive, bipolar, and adjustment disorders.
5. Apply the nursing process for clients with mood and adjustment disorders.
6. Describe independent and collaborative interventions nurses and other mental health care providers use with clients who have mood and adjustment disorders.
7. Examine personal feelings, thoughts, and reactions to clients with mood disorders that affect the therapeutic relationship and management of client care.

KEY TERMS

adjustment disorders, p. 215
affect, p. 227
anhedonia, p. 218
atypical depression, p. 225
bipolar disorder, p. 220
dysthymia, p. 219
euthymia, p. 226
flight of ideas, p. 220
hypomania, p. 222
kindling, p. 210
learned helplessness, p. 214
melancholic depression, p. 224
mood, p. 227
neuroplasticity, p. 210
neurotransmission, p. 209
nihilism, p. 219
postpartum mood disorder, p. 225
psychomotor agitation, p. 219
psychomotor retardation, p. 219
schemata, p. 214
seasonal affective disorder, p. 225
selective gene expression, p. 212
temperament, p. 227
unipolar depression, p. 218

MOOD DISORDERS

Mood disorders, sometimes known as affective disorders, are a major public health problem in the United States. Data indicate that mood disorders are a leading cause of disease burden, morbidity, and mortality worldwide (Murray and Lopez, 1997). Dysregulation of mood or affect characterizes mood disorders; however, these illnesses involve changes in all areas including physiology, cognition, and behavior. In addition to the effects of mood disorders have on individual and family suffering, interpersonal relationships, career and work productivity, and societal and health system costs, these illnesses are also sometimes fatal: 15% of those afflicted commit suicide. Depression is also linked to morbidity and mortality when it is associated with other illnesses such as cardiovascular disease. As a result of these serious consequences, there has been ongoing research about the etiology, clinical course, outcomes, and treatment modalities for mood disorders.

Mood disorders involve dysfunctional mood expression that includes deep, incapacitating depression; irritability and intense elation; or joy. This differs from depression and elation that are normal responses to life events. For example, a person who has suffered a loss will feel grief and sadness and will sometimes even experience physical symptoms and problems with thinking. Success or exciting life events generate mood elevation, elation, and euphoria. Most people experience mood swings associated with loss or success. The mood changes in mood disorders, however, are more pronounced and are characterized by their pattern over time, which includes frequency of occurrence, duration, and intensity. Additional symptom clusters that occur with mood disturbance include changes in sleep, appetite, thinking, activity, self-worth, and suicidal thinking. Thus, these illnesses affect the total person, not just mood.

HISTORIC AND THEORETIC PERSPECTIVES

Over the centuries, many have recognized disturbances in mood. Hippocrates described changes in temperament. Kraepelin (1921) distinguished between dementia praecox, the chronic progressive deterioration of cognition and functioning, and the cyclic recurrence of abnormal mood. Freud (1957) differentiated between maladaptive depression and grief in his famous article "Mourning and Melancholia," which described the psychodynamic genesis of depression. Leonhard (1974), a German psychiatrist, proposed the separation of manic-depressive illness into two types: bipolar (history of depression and mania) and unipolar (history of depression only). This differentiation is the basis for the current clinical depiction of bipolar disorder and unipolar disorders.

Mental health professionals currently recognize various forms of unipolar and bipolar disorders that include a broad spectrum of mood disorders with varied features and clinical characteristics. Mood disorders have commanded more public attention as a result of their pervasiveness and recognition of their serious, damaging consequences. New treatments, including the use of medications such as fluoxetine (Prozac) and treatments such as electroconvulsive therapy, have created social controversy. Famous people with high media profiles have publicly acknowledged their struggles with mood disorders. Historians are now presenting information that many prominent people, including Abraham Lincoln, Winston Churchill, Vincent Van Gogh, Ernest Hemingway, Sylvia Plath, and Herman Melville, experienced a serious mood disorder.

ETIOLOGY

In spite of continuing investigation, there is no single explanation for the cause of mood disorders. Many researchers and clinicians support the hypothesis that mood disorders have neurobiologic, ethologic, psychosocial, and cognitive factors that contribute to the development of depression and mania. Some types of mood disorders are more related to certain specific etiologic factors. For example, research findings suggest that depression includes several distinct syndromes that health care providers can differentiate clinically over time (Kendler et al., 1996). Each theoretic perspective helps to explain some aspect of mood disorders, but none fully accounts for their development. In general, these etiologic factors are primarily neurobiologic, ethologic, or psychosocial and are summarized in Box 11-1.

BOX 11-1

Etiologic Factors Related to Mood Disorders

NEUROBIOLOGIC FACTORS
Altered neurotransmission
Neuroendocrine dysregulation
Genetic transmission

ETHOLOGIC FACTORS
Evolutionary psychology/biology

PSYCHOSOCIAL FACTORS

Psychoanalytic Theory
Depression is a result of loss.
Mania is a defense against depression.

Cognitive Theory
Depression is a result of negative processing of thoughts.

Learned Helplessness
Depression is a result of a perceived lack of control over events.

Life Events and Stress Theory
Significant life events cause stress, neurobiologic changes that result in depression or mania.

Neurobiologic Factors

Since the mid-1990s, research on the etiology of mood disorders has focused on the biologic mechanisms that are related to their onset and clinical course. Although this research has shown a link between physiology, genetics, and mood disorders, none has established direct cause-and-effect relationships. The more common biologic theories include those related to altered neurotransmission and neuroendocrine dysregulation.

Neurotransmission

Research on the biology of mood disorders has emphasized neurotransmitter disturbances. Researchers initially became interested in **neurotransmission** after investigating the action of antidepressant drugs. In 1954, scientists discovered that clients treated with reserpine for hypertension developed depression. Several years later, they found that isoniazid had an antidepressant effect on persons being treated for tuberculosis. Researchers introduced imipramine as an antidepressant in 1958, and research began on the mechanisms of action in the brain. Results from this line of research became the basis for discovering the important role that neurotransmitter play in psychiatric disorders. Brain neurotransmitters functioning affects mood regulation and, in the case of mood disorders, dysregulation of mood. Neurotransmitter activity also controls a wide range of behavior and functions, including appetite, arousal, sleep, cognition, and movement.

Many believe that monoamine neurotransmitter systems, especially those of norepinephrine and serotonin, their metabolites, and their receptors, are somehow altered during episodes of depression and mania. Neurotransmitter availability and receptor change theories state that there is less than normal neurotransmission activity in depression and more than normal neurotransmission activity in mania.

Researchers now consider neurotransmitter theories of mood disorders simplistic and incomplete. More recent research focuses on changes in receptors, ion channel processes, and neurotropic growth factors, such as brain derived neurotropic factor (BDNF), that nourish the cells (Eisch et al., 2003). These neurotrophins that nourish the brain cells atrophy or fail to regenerate under stressful conditions. This deprives the neurons of adequate nutrition. These complex physiologic mechanisms are consistent with theories that propose long-term changes in the brain, such as kindling, that occur with mood disorders.

Post (1992) has described a phenomenon called **kindling** in which stress initially alters neurotransmission mechanisms, resulting in a first episode of depression. This initial episode creates an electrophysiologic sensitivity to future stress, which means that it will take less stress to trigger another depressive or manic episode. In essence, kindling creates new hardwiring of the brain or long-lasting alterations of neuronal functioning that influence many cellular processes and structures, including changes in cell dendrites, and changes in cellular metabolism. This process is based on **neuroplasticity**, or the ability of neurons to regenerate or restructure. The kindling model is consistent with the cyclic and progressive nature of mood disorders and suggests that health care providers treat clients early for their mood episodes and keep clients on medication for extended periods to avoid physiologic alterations and deterioration over time.

Technologic advances in studying the brain provide additional support for the theory of disturbances in brain functioning during depression. Positron emission tomography (PET) enables researchers to examine brain physiology of depressed persons as compared with normal control subjects PET allows researchers to examine metabolism of glucose and oxygen and to compare brain functioning in individuals both during their depressive episode and after their recovery. Figure 11-1 depicts the differences that are apparent using PET scanning of depressed, recovered, and normal control brains. Figure 11-2 indicates alterations in blood flow in brains of depressed persons. PET scanning has shown that the prefrontal cerebral cortex and the limbic system (including the amygdala) appear to have physiologic disruptions in the brains of persons experiencing depression. Researchers also use magnetic resonance imaging (MRI) and single photon emission computed tomography (SPECT) to produce images of the functioning of the brain.

Although research continues on the specific mechanisms of these biochemical processes, the complexity of the biologic structural and physiologic changes that occur with mood disorders continues to pose challenges for investigation. Inconsistent definitions and criteria for depression and mania also make research more difficult. In addition, neurotransmission is a complex activity that includes multiple processes, such as neurotransmitter synthesis and release, receptor site function and change, interactions among the various neurotransmitters and hormones, and the action of these transmitters and hormones on genetic material.

Neuroendocrine Dysregulation

The involvement of the neuroendocrine system is another area of research on the biologic factors of mood disorders. Studies have associated the dysregulation of the limbic hypothalamic-pituitary-adrenal (HPA) axis with depression. The hypothalamus, pituitary, adrenal glands, and hippocampus make up the HPA axis, which controls physiologic responses to stress. The hypothalamus regulates endocrine functions and the autonomic nervous system. It is also involved in behaviors such as those related to fight, flight, feeding, sleep, and sex. The hypothalamus manufactures serotonin, a major neurotransmitter responsible for mood disorders. In response to stress, the hypothalamus releases corticotropin-releasing hormone (CRH), which stimulates the anterior pituitary to secrete adrenal corticotropic hormone (ACTH). In turn, ACTH triggers the release of cortisol into the blood from the adrenal cortex. Serum cortisol is elevated during stress and is associated with stimulation of the autonomic nervous system, increasing levels of epinephrine and norepinephrine. Through an elaborate feedback mechanism, levels of cortisol signal the hypothalamus via the hippocampus to increase or decrease CRH production. Researchers do not yet fully understand the specific physiologic mechanisms through which stress signals this process to begin. Stress-input signals possibly come from the amygdala, autonomic nervous system, or cerebral cortex (Young et al., 2004).

The HPA axis is often hyperactive in clients with depression. As many as 50% of clients with moderate to severe depression exhibit elevated serum cortisol levels. Over time, high levels of cortisol damage the hippocampus. There is evidence associating decreased hippocampal volume with recurrent and chronic depression. Serious consequences include cognitive impairment, particularly memory difficulties (Sapolsky, 2000).

The functioning of the HPA axis is related to the 24-hour cycle of circadian rhythms that control physiologic processes. Clients with mood disorders have disrupted or irregular cyclic patterns. Blood cortisol is normally low in the early morning and highest in late afternoon, although constant increases are often apparent in depression. Clients with mood disorders also have disrupted sleep-wake cycles. Persons with mania have a decreased need for sleep, whereas many with depression experience hypersomnial (excessive sleep). During depression, clients experience decreased rapid eye movement (REM) latency and decreased shallow, slow delta wave sleep, thus fragmenting

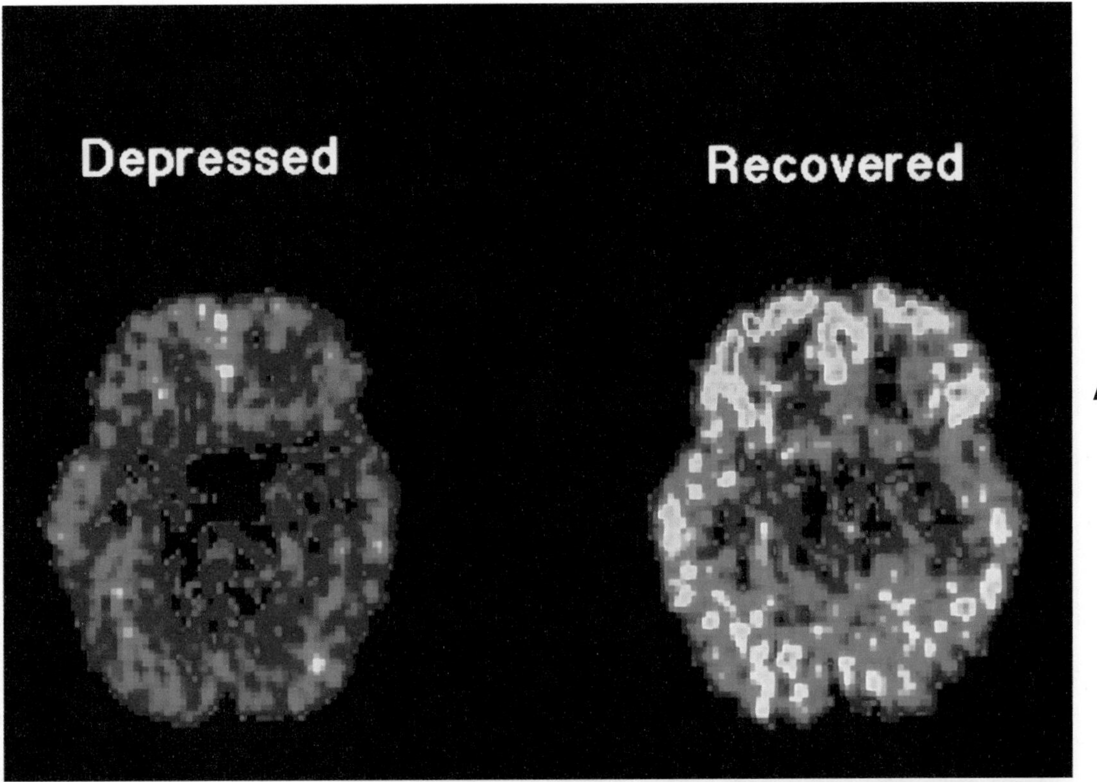

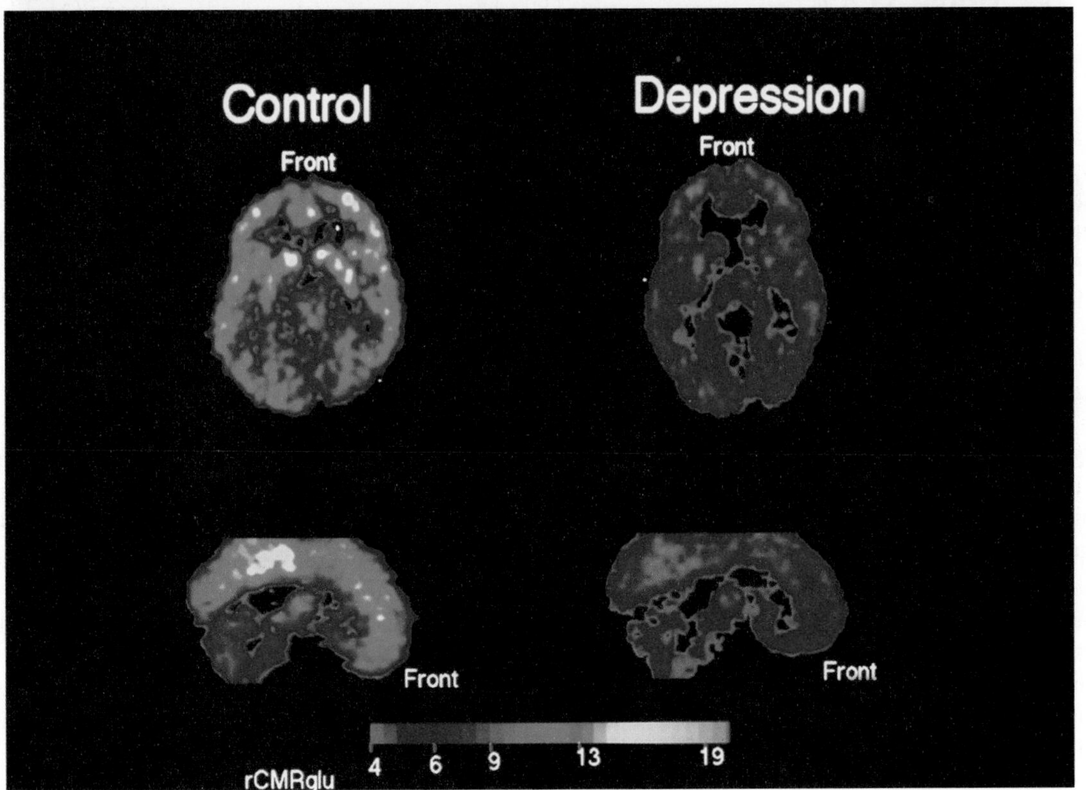

FIGURE 11-1 **A,** Positron emission tomography (PET) scans of the brain in the same individual during depression *(left)* and after recovery through treatment with medication *(right)*. Several brain areas, particularly the prefrontal cortex *(at top)*, show diminished activity *(darker colors)* during depression. **B,** PET scans of a normal subject *(left)* and a depressed subject *(right)* reveal reduced brain activity *(darker colors)* during depression, especially in the prefrontal cortex. A form of radioactively tagged glucose was used as a tracer to visualize levels of brain activity. (Courtesy Mark George, MD, National Institute of Mental Health Biological Psychiatry Branch, U.S. Department of Health and Human Services.)

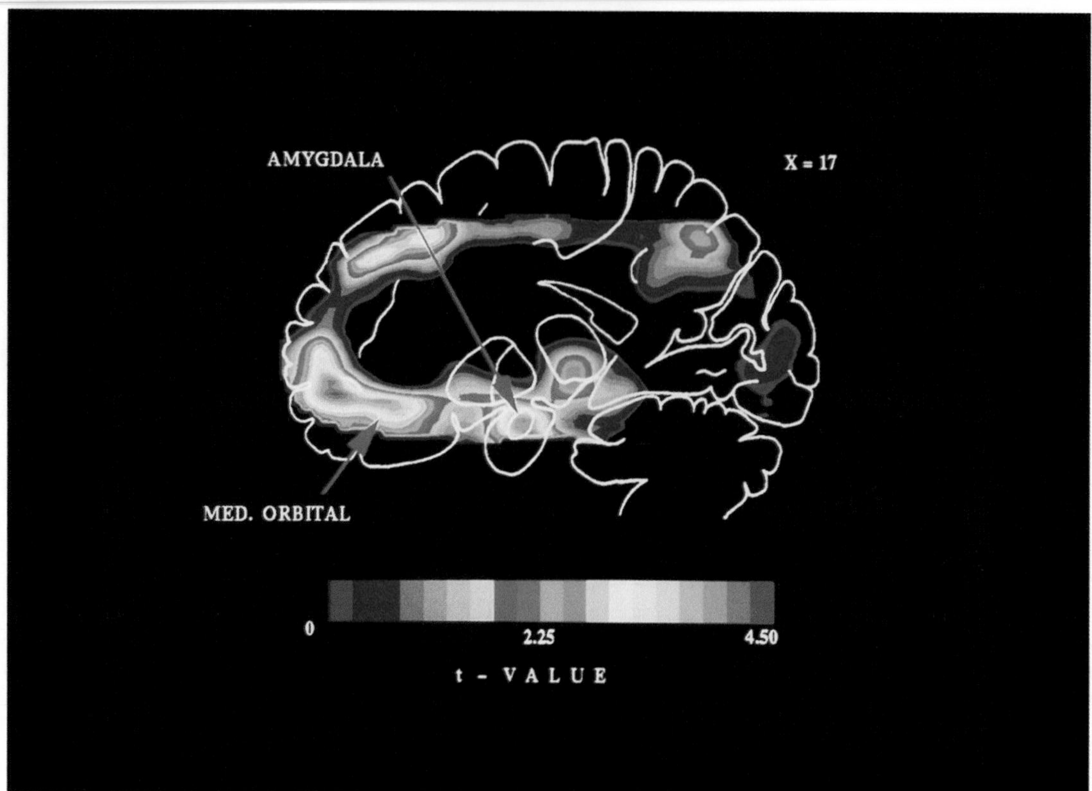

FIGURE 11-2 PET scan indicates increased blood flow in the amygdala and prefrontal cortex in persons with major depression of the familial pure depressive disease subtype. The scan is a composite of images of 13 individuals. (Courtesy Wayne C. Drevets, MD, Department of Psychiatry, Washington University School of Medicine, St Louis.)

the sleep-wake cycle. Even seasonal patterns appear to have some relationship to mood disorders, with episodes of depression often occurring during periods of decreased light. Thus, many alterations are evident in chronobiology.

Genetic Transmission

Mood disorders tend to occur in certain families, and many believe that genetics are responsible for their manifestation (Kendler et al., 2006). Studies on families, twins, adoption, and molecular genetics provide data on the heritability of mood disorders.

In family studies, researchers select families who exhibit mood disorders and then examine the morbid risk relatives have for developing these disorders. Researchers then compare this with the general population. Results of these studies demonstrate consistently that first-degree relatives of persons with bipolar disorder and unipolar depression have a greater risk for developing a mood disorder. This risk is particularly high for relatives of persons with bipolar disorder, possibly indicating that genetics plays a greater role in bipolar disorders than in unipolar depression.

Researchers have based twin studies on the assumption that monozygotic twins share the same genes and that dizygotic twins have about 50% of their genes in common. Results of twin research provide additional evidence for the genetic transmission of mood disorders. If one monozygotic twin suffers from bipolar disorder, there is a high rate that the other twin will have a disorder as well. In some studies, up to 100% of other the twins developed a mood disorder, usually bipolar illness. Although there are high rates of concordance for dizygotic twins, they tend to be less than those for monozygotic twins. For unipolar disorders the concordance rates continue to be higher for monozygotic twins, and both twin types have a higher concordance than the general population (Kendler, 2001).

Using adoption studies, researchers examine the contributions of both the environment and genetic transmission. In general, adoption studies also show that genetic factors play a role in mood disorders. Most studies have focused specifically on bipolar disorder and have found that the biologic parents of adult adoptees who were diagnosed with bipolar disorder have a much higher incidence of the disorder than parents of adoptees with no mood disorder.

Although all of the preceding information indicates that genetics is partly responsible for the development of mood disorders, the research has not revealed specific genes or genetic mechanisms. Advancing research in molecular genetics and genetic analysis are promising. The search for the specific genetic basis of mood disorders continues, with special emphasis on genetic location and genetic processes, including the role of **selective gene expression** (Barondes, 1998). The interaction between genes and the environment further complicates genetic research, though many think this is an important component of the genetics of mood disorders (Hamet and Tremblay, 2005). Many researchers agree that genetic expressions and genetic transmission of mood disorders hold the key to future major advances in understanding, diagnosing, and treating depression and bipolar disorders (Van den Bree and Owen, 2003).

Ethologic Factors

Ethologic theories of human development rely on evolutionary concepts as explanations of mood disorders. Human behavior serves the survival of the species and helps individuals adapt to their environments. Psychiatrist John Bowlby (1969), for example, concluded that bonding and attachment between mothers and their infants evolved because helpless infants needed adequate protection for continued development. Ethologic approaches to development and biology have existed since the time of Charles Darwin, but renewed interest in the field has extended these approaches to offer a different perspective on the occurrence of mood disorders.

Evolutionary Psychology/Biology

Evolutionary psychology is a way of thinking about any topic within psychology. The basic idea is that natural selection designed the human mind to solve problems of adaptation. All human minds develop reasoning and regulatory mechanisms that organize the interpretation of experiences, account for recurrent concepts and motivations, and provide universal meaning structures that help us understand the behavior of others. Evolutionary biology is a related field that examines the selective advantage of human traits and biology (Nesse, 2002). Both areas explore how human beings have adapted and are still adapting to changes in the environment. They also try to identify defenses that seem like diseases but are actually evolved protective mechanisms. In exploring mood disorders, the focus is on proximate explanations such as brain chemistry, past experiences, or personality. From an evolutionary perspective, the focus is on the purpose of a mood disorder and why it persists in the present.

Researchers have not examined the evolutionary function of bipolar disorder, but many considered the function of depression. On the surface, depression and its main symptoms (lack of energy, fearfulness, loss of interest, sleep and eating disorders) do not seem to promote survival; however, some suggested a number of possible functions (Watson and Andrews, 2002). Depression possibly serves as a cry for help, or sometimes it forces the loser of a social conflict to accept defeat, stopping the winner's oppressive behavior. Depression also possibly forces a partner to have greater involvement. Depression may serve a social rumination function—that is, the symptoms permit the individual to focus on and analyze social problems. Depression may have a social motivation function in that the severity of symptoms may influence reluctant social partners to provide help or withdraw demands. Nesse (2002) also suggested that depression prevents wasted effort by allowing the individual to disengage from unreachable goals.

One ethologic perspective suggests a number of treatment approaches. During assessment, nurses need to consider social factors that are limiting the individual's ability to function in all areas of life. The social system is an important element in ethology; therefore group and family therapies are encouraged, as well as multidisciplinary teamwork. The ethologic perspective questions the use of antidepressant medications, as they interfere with the client's ability to address issues within the social environment. If medications are used, they do not replace work on the social problems. In the ethologic view, medications are not for removing the very suffering that provides motivation for life change in an adaptive depressive episode (Watson and Andrews, 2002).

Psychosocial Factors

Psychosocial explanations for the development of mood disorders represent a range of theoretic perspectives, including psychoanalytic theory, learned helplessness, cognitive theory, life events and stress theory, and personality theory.

Psychoanalytic Theory

The basic premise of psychoanalytic theory is that unconscious processes result in expression of symptoms, including depression and mania. Freud (1957) distinguished between depression and normal grief, citing both as a response to real or symbolic loss. According to Freud, loss generates intense, hostile feelings toward the lost object. The person then turns these feelings inward onto the self (anger turned inward), creating guilt and loss of self-esteem. Thus, depression is linked with loss and aggression.

Psychodynamically, mania is a defense against depression. The client denies feelings of anger, low self-esteem, and worthlessness and reverses the affect so that there is a triumphant feeling of self-confidence. Mania represents a conquered superego with little inclination to control id impulses. Yet over time, this distorted view of reality waivers, and the client demonstrates outward hostility toward others, often focusing on the weaknesses of others that are similar to the internal weaknesses they are avoiding.

Few data support the psychodynamic theories of depression and mania, but there is some evidence that clients with depression have experienced more early childhood loss and deprivation than persons without depression (Brown and Harris, 1978; Bowlby, 1969). Clinicians also note that anger is often associated with depression, although the relationship between anger and depression remains obscure. Many people who experience early childhood loss and anger never experience depression, whereas many who do not experience a visible or acknowledged loss do experience depression. The psychoanalytic theory is only one of many explanations that attempt to explain the intrapsychic dynamics of depression and mania. The relevance of this theoretic perspective is in its references to the early childhood environment in which loss, disruption, or chaos triggers stress that in turn triggers the physiologic mechanisms described previously.

Cognitive Theory

The cognitive model of depression points to errors of logical thinking as causative factors for depression. It assumes that underlying cognitive structures, some of which are not fully conscious, influence mood. These cognitive structures, or schema, are shaped by early life experiences and are predisposed to negative processing of information. In a diatheses-stress model, when persons predisposed to depression with negative schemata encounter stress, the negative processing is activated, resulting in depressive thinking (Beck, 1967).

Beck (1967) differentiated among levels of cognition that influence depression: automatic thoughts, schemata or assumptions, and cognitive distortions. *Automatic thoughts* are thoughts a person is aware of, although they appear briefly and a person usually does not recognize them. They form the person's perception of a situation, and it is this perception, rather than the objective facts about the situation, that results in emotional and behavioral responses. If the perceptions are distorted, inferences and responses will be maladaptive. For example, a shy college graduate was unable to find a teaching position and took a job as a secretary in a law office. Other staff did not invite her to lunch with them. She viewed this as rejection and decided that no one liked her. She later discovered that no one on the staff had attended college and they had interpreted her shyness as dislike because she was working at a job that was beneath her.

Schemata are internal representations of the self and the world. They facilitate information processing because the mind uses them to understand, code, and recall information. Beck (1967) proposed a triad of thinking (schemata) that gives rise to the development of depression:

1. Negative, self-deprecating views of self
2. Pessimistic views of the world, so that life experiences are interpreted in a negative way
3. The belief that negativity will continue into the future, promoting a negative view of future events

These mind-sets result in the misinterpretation of events and situations so that the client's cognitive schema of self as worthless and the world and future appear hopeless. This faulty cognitive processing leads to assumptions and continued errors of logic that result in depressive symptoms and an ongoing negative view of life. This is exemplified when people state that they know that they will never make it through college. *Cognitive distortions* link schemata and automatic thoughts. Faulty information processing includes cognitive distortions, such as *overgeneralization* (drawing general conclusions based on isolated incidents), *dichotomous thinking* (perceiving events and experiences in only one of two opposite categories), and *magnification* (placing a distorted emphasis on a single event or error). The following example illustrates each of these types of distortion. A 23-year-old beauty pageant contestant was not selected as a finalist. She concluded that the judges hated everything about her (overgeneralization). She was convinced that the other contestants were either beautiful and smart or unattractive and dull (dichotomous thinking). She was convinced that the judges were trying to tell her not to compete (magnification).

Hopelessness/Learned Helplessness Theory

Cognitive theory states that depression results from altered cognition. One such altered cognition is **learned helplessness**, demonstrated by the development of helplessness, apathy, powerlessness, and depression. According to the original theory as proposed by Seligman (1975), uncontrollable, stressful events that a person experiences result in the lack of motivation to act in response to the environment.

Learned helplessness theory was modified to specify that, in the face of current events and past experiences, persons have the expectation (cognition) that external events are uncontrollable (Abramson et al., 1978). This in turn results in helplessness, passivity, and sadness, which lead to other symptoms of depression, such as decreased appetite and low self-esteem.

Further revision of the theory resulted in the *hopelessness theory of depression*. In this theory revision hopelessness is a sufficient cause of depression. The individual's inferred negative outcomes and negativity about the self are key elements of depression. Helplessness is only a part of hopelessness. With the occurrence of an unpleasant event, persons at risk for depression and having negative expectations attribute instability, globalization, and excessive importance to those events. For example, a client perceives that she is not able to recover from divorce (instability), that her entire life is ruined (globalization), and that her former marriage is the only focus of her life (importance).

More recently, researchers have postulated that cognitive vulnerability, or a person's negative cognitive style, in the presence of negative life events leads to hopelessness, which results in the valid and distinct subtype of *hopelessness depression*. Symptoms of this type of depression include apathy, lack of energy, slow initiation of voluntary behavior, and psychomotor retardation. Studies provide some support for hopelessness depression, but additional testing with more general client populations is necessary.

A lack of social support during times of negative life events often leads to increased hopelessness and helplessness and depression. Research with human immunodeficiency virus (HIV) clients has supported this model, with hopelessness rather than low social support as the key contributor to depression. The influence of low social support on hopelessness was necessary to account for depression (Johnson et al., 2001). More research is necessary to identify other mechanisms that lead to the specific symptom pattern of hopelessness depression.

Life Events and Stress Theory

The relationship of life events and stress to mood disorders is widely acknowledged. In studying depression, researchers have been interested in the quantity and nature of life events and in the size and perceived support from the client's social network. Brown and Harris (1978) reported that stressful social factors (e.g., lack of an intimate, confiding relationship with a significant other; having three or more children at home; being unemployed; and loss of one's mother before age 11 years) contributed significantly to vulnerability for depression. Holmes and Rahe (1967) indicated that all life events, even pleasant ones, are capable of causing various degrees of stress. Thus, even a vacation or a joyous wedding may generate high levels of stress. The person's perception or appraisal of an event is as important as the change in daily life caused by the event. Factors such as social support and the person's perception of that support as wanted or unwanted, sufficient or insufficient, also influence the effect of an event. Life events most likely influence the development and recurrence of depression through the psychologic and, ultimately, biologic experiences of stress.

Ravindran et al. (2002) associated depressive illness with increased stress perception, reduced perception of positive events, reliance on coping styles that use emotion rather than rational thought, and quality of life.

Early life stress, including child abuse and loss, influences the development of depression probably by disrupting HPA axis functioning. Chronic hypersecretion of CRF and cortisol and autonomic nervous system (ANS) activation during neurologically vulnerable times of development sensitize physiologic stress responses and even generate brain changes (Gillepsie and Nemeroff, 2005). Thus, individuals who experience early life stress become vulnerable in how their stress response influences the onset and course of depression.

Researchers have examined the occurrence of stressful life events and depression with regard to gender differences. Stressful life events triggered episodes of depression in women, mediated by genetic risk factors (Kendler et al., 1999). Whereas women reported more interpersonal stressors, men reported more legal and work-related stressful life events. At the same time, most life events influenced the risk for depression in men and women in similar ways. Researchers concluded that the greater prevalence of depression in women versus men was not due to differences in the rate of reported stressful life events or to a greater sensitivity of women to the harmful influences of stressful life events (Kendler et al., 2001). Marital status has been a risk factor for higher severity of depressive symptoms in women than in men. Greater role demands and more chronic family stress among women, as well as higher education and the presence of children in the household, may explain the difference (Barnow et al., 2002). There have been less data about the relationship between stressful life events and bipolar disorder, although studies have suggested a role of disrupted social routines or circadian rhythms. Malkoff-Schwartz et al. (2000) studied the influence of social rhythm disruption as a stressful life event on clients with pure mania, pure depression, cycling episodes, and recurrent unipolar depression. The researchers found that stressful life events, especially social rhythm disruption, influenced the onset of manic episodes. The authors suggested that interventions to minimize stress and social rhythm disruption in clients with a history of mania will help prevent the onset of manic episodes.

Life stressors sometimes can lead to **adjustment disorders**, which are different from major depression. The main distinction between an adjustment disorder and major depression is that a specific psychosocial stressor can be identified for the adjustment disorder. In acute cases, the adjustment disorder occurs within 3 months of a stressor. In chronic cases, symptoms last longer than 6 months after the occurrence of the stressor. During this time, the individuals have difficulty functioning in their roles or interpersonal relationships. Symptoms usually decrease once the stressor is removed. In some cases, symptoms disappear outside of the setting linked with the stressor, especially when the stressor is location specific (e.g., the work setting). Adjustment disorders, or adjustment reactions, can occur in response to any type of stressor, including but not limited to loss, change in life style, maturational crisis, or even success or gain.

An adjustment disorder can occur in anyone, regardless of age, gender, or socioeconomic status, when a single stressor or multiple stressors overwhelm a person's coping skills. There is often no preexisting mental disorder, and the symptoms of adjustment disorder are time limited. The stress response is highly individualized and what one person experiences as highly stressful is sometimes an irritant or a challenge to another person. Loss and change frequently characterize the identified stressors.

EPIDEMIOLOGY

Mood disorders, particularly depression, are common. Data from the National Comorbidity Survey Replication suggest that the lifetime prevalence of developing major depressive disorder is 16.2%, with twice as many women developing the disorder (Kessler et al., 2003). The lifetime prevalence of bipolar disorder is about equal for men and women, 1.4% and 1.3%, respectively. Women have a lifetime prevalence of 21.3% for major depression and 8.0% for dysthymia, whereas men have a lifetime prevalence of only 12.7% for major depression and 4.8% for dysthymia. These differences begin to occur around age 13 (Hankin and Abramson, 2001). Researchers have proposed a number of theories to account for gender differences in the rates of depression, including hormonal or biologic differences, social roles, and cognitive processing. However, no one has adequately explained these gender differences for depression, and additional research is necessary to determine why women are at higher risk for depression (Kuehner, 2003).

The first episode of a mood disorder seems to be occurring at younger ages. The average age for onset of bipolar illness is the mid to late twenties although children and teenagers are now being diagnosed. Although the average age of onset for unipolar depression has been the middle 30s, there is some evidence that onset is occurring in younger individuals (Lewinsohn et al., 1993). Although the most frequent age of onset for depression is the 25- to 44-year age-group, people in younger age-groups have an ever-increasing risk of developing depression. Data indicate that when the onset of depression is at an early age (teens or early 20s) or at age 55 years or over, it is usually more prolonged and chronic (Greden, 2001). Persons presenting with depression that is diagnosed in their 20s or 30s often report not having depression in their early years. Rates of depression do not significantly increase during menopause. The risk of developing depression and mania increases if there is a positive family history for mood disorders (Perlis et al., 2006).

Sociocultural factors are sometimes related to the onset of depression and mania. Depression seems to occur less frequently in African Americans than in either white or Hispanic groups in the United States. It also appears that depression is more frequent in lower socioeconomic groups, whereas bipolar disorders are more frequent in higher socioeconomic groups. Although depression and mania occur throughout the world, ethnicity and culture influence the expression of symptoms. For example, Asians describe more somatic symptoms of depression, whereas people from Western cultures describe more mood and cognitive changes.

In an increasingly stressful society characterized by mobility, family disruptions, and economic stressors, women and younger persons are manifesting depression more than in previous generations. Persons with depression often seek help from their primary care providers for physical symptoms such as fatigue, insomnia, headache, and loss of appetite. Research indicates that primary care providers do not always correctly diagnose depression or treat it appropriately (Solberg et al., 2005). Box 11-2 summarizes epidemiology data for mood disorders.

The adjustment disorders have received little research attention, despite recognition of their frequent occurrence. These disorders have occurred in 5% to 21% of adults in outpatient psychiatric settings, 7.1% of adults in psychiatric inpatient settings, and 13.7% of medical inpatients (Jones et al., 2002). Reliable data are not available for children or adolescents, although adjustment disorders are common in these age-groups.

BOX 11-2

Epidemiology of Mood and Adjustment Disorders

- 16.2% of the general population develop a mood disorder.
- 21.3% of women and 12.7% of men develop major depression.
- Average age of onset for bipolar illness is mid- to late-20s or earlier.
- Average age of onset of depression is mid-20s to 30s, although probably earlier.
- Depression occurs more frequently in whites and Hispanics than in African Americans.
- Depression occurs more frequently in lower socioeconomic groups.
- Bipolar disorders occur more frequently in higher socioeconomic groups.
- Adjustment disorders occur in 5% to 21% of adults in psychiatric outpatient settings.

Nurses need to anticipate the frequent diagnosis of adjustment disorders in children and adolescents. Children and adolescents are in the developmental process of acquiring coping skills. The occurrences of stressors, particularly those that appear suddenly, involve loss, or disrupt a sense of family security, overwhelm coping skills. Stressors include a death in the family, disruption of the family because of a natural disaster, divorce, or diagnosis of a physical illness. The potential for suicidal ideation and behavior, especially among adolescents, necessitates immediate treatment. A comparison of nonsuicidal with suicidal adjustment disordered adolescents revealed that the suicidal patients were more likely to have received previous psychiatric treatment, demonstrate poor psychologic functioning, report the recent suicide of a significant other, report dysphoric mood, or display psychomotor restlessness (Pelkonen et al., 2005).

Adjustment disorders present most frequently in primary care and medical settings. When researchers studied medical inpatients to compare characteristics of adjustment disorder with major depression, the patients with adjustment disorder were more likely to be older, widowed, and living alone with less severe symptoms (Casey, 2001).

Mood Disorders Across the Life Span

Most information about mood disorders presented in textbooks and literature addresses the average adult, generally covering ages between 18 and 65 years. There is growing concern, however, with the increase in mood disorders among children and adolescents. At the same time, there are changes in the way mood disorders are perceived with older adults. It is important to recognize that there will be new variables when mood disorders, particularly depression, present at either end of the life span.

Mood Disorders in the Young

Mood disorders presenting in childhood or adolescence are significant for three reasons: (1) they generate extraordinary pain and distress for young individuals who are not prepared to understand or deal with the resulting emotions and behaviors, (2) they initiate major difficulties during a period of time essential to development and therefore influence the rest of the life span, and (3) they produce tremendous stress and concern for the entire family unit. Assessment of children and adolescents needs to address not only symptomatology of the current illness episode but also the influence a mood disorder is having on normal development and social learning, as well as the impact of the disorder on family dynamics and coping status.

Concerns with childhood psychiatric disorders begin during infancy, addressed by the specialty of *infant mental health*. The focus within this specialty is generally on the influence of parenting and parent-infant relationships. Research on the emergence of mood disorders in children places greater emphasis on inborn and environmental issues. Temperament is one such inborn factor. In one study of young children, the temperamental trait of behavioral disinhibition was associated with higher rates of mood disorders (Hirshfeld-Becker et al., 2002). Familial relationships are an environmental factor that researchers have explored at length. For example, attachment relationships are associated with depression from infancy through adolescence. Most recently the diagnosis of early-onset bipolar disorder (EOBD) has gained acceptance. Bipolar disorder was once thought to emerge by early adulthood, but the diagnosis has been made as early as age 5 years. The symptom profile of EOBD overlaps with that of other childhood psychiatric disorders, some of which may be comorbid. The main differential characteristic seems to be that EOBD symptoms show a cyclical pattern not evident in other disorders.

Mood disorders in adolescents have received much attention. Depression often appears as irritable hostility and is often comorbid with anxiety and personality disorders, as well as drug use. A longitudinal study of more than 900 children revealed that 13% of the group developed depression between ages 14 and 16 years. At age 21, the depressed individuals were three times more likely than nondepressed adolescents to have a subsequent depression and twice as likely to have an anxiety disorder (Fergusson and Woodward, 2002). A randomized treatment trial with depressed adolescents showed that interpersonal psychotherapy offered at school-based health clinics provided effective treatment (Mufson et al., 2004). Bipolar disorder in adolescents sometimes presents initially as recurrent depressive episodes, developing into bipolar I disorder in 10% to 15% of cases. When manic episodes occur during adolescence, they are associated with psychotic symptoms, school truancy, antisocial behavior, or substance abuse (American Psychiatric Association [APA], 2000).

Mood Disorders in the Elderly

Just as the picture of mood disorders has changed for children and adolescents, new information has emerged for mood disorders in older adults. Researchers have categorized late-life depression into three subtypes: (1) early-onset depression with lifelong vulnerability, (2) late-onset depression in reaction to severe life stress, and (3) late-onset depression with vascular risk factors. Vascular depression has been associated with physical findings of white matter hyperintensities apparent during MRI. The presence of this physical finding has been connected with poor treatment results (van den Berg et al., 2001).

Estimates of late-life depression have ranged from 3% to 57%. One study of a rural Greek population showed a prevalence of mild to moderate depression of 27% and a prevalence of moderate to severe depression of 12%. Cognitive impairment was a strong risk factor, with unmarried status and particular medical conditions more common among depressed individuals (Papadopoulos et al., 2005). The recognition of late-life depression has increased with the understanding that depressed older adults are less likely to report depressed mood and more likely to report somatic symptoms, including apathy, fatigue, difficulty sleeping, and loss of interest in usual activities. About 25% of subsyndromal or minor depression in older adults met the criteria for major depression within 2 years (Alexopoulos et al., 2002a). However, both major and minor depressions respond well to treatment, especially when pharmacotherapy and psychotherapy are combined.

Nurses need to consider social differences in the treatment plans for older adults with depression. Often there is no available support system. Getting a family's help is sometimes difficult and sometimes even adds to the older adults' stress level, depending on the relationship. Some family members view depressive symptoms as a part of normal aging and need instruction on the nature, treatment, and positive prognosis of depression. Furthermore, the values and attitudes of the older adult will influence treatment participation. Generational differences in the acceptance of psychiatric treatment lead the older adult to refuse care or deny the need for care. When asked if they are depressed, some older adults say they are not. However, asking about the somatic and activity changes (e.g., What activities do you enjoy these days? Are you participating in the same activities you did a few months ago?) will provide a clearer picture of depressive symptoms.

Apart from direct effects of depression in older adults, findings that depression has a relationship with cognitive disorders are of particular concern. It is possible that depression is an early sign of dementia, a risk factor of dementia, or that depression initiates a physiologic effect that results in damage to the hippocampus and dementia. Researchers offered provisional criteria to identify depression in patients with Alzheimer's disease, and current studies seek to validate this. These criteria include requiring three (instead of five) depressive symptoms from the DSM-IV list; expansion of the symptom list to include irritability and social isolation or withdrawal; assessing for decreased positive affect rather than loss of interest; and no longer requiring that symptoms occur nearly every day, although they represent a change from previous behavior (Alexopoulos et al., 2002b).

Ultimately depression is of particular concern with older adults because the symptoms often result in life-threatening situations within a rather short time. For example, vegetative symptoms lead to dehydration and electrolyte imbalance, and they compromise any existing medical conditions. Higher mortality in older adults with depression is due to suicide, comorbid medical illness, and impairment of physical functioning. In one study, late-onset depression was associated with mortality for both men and women. With men mortality was also associated with severity of depression; with women mortality was associated with self-rated vascular and cardiac conditions. Researchers concluded that older women with depression require closer follow-up monitoring of vascular conditions (Steffens et al., 2002).

Mood disorders at either end of the life span are just as responsive to treatment as mood disorders during midlife. The important idea to keep in mind is that the features and considerations are somewhat different. Research is providing new knowledge on child, adolescent, and older adult mood disorders. The challenge is to keep up with changes in the characterizations of illness and the progress in available treatments.

CLINICAL DESCRIPTION

Mood disorders are primarily changes in mood; however, cognitive, physiologic, and behavioral changes are also evident. They are defined by a pattern of episodes over time and by a pattern of symptoms in each episode. Mood disorders are classified in the DSM-IV-TR as depressive disorders (unipolar) or bipolar disorders or other mood disorders. The following sections describe the signs and symptoms of mood disorders.

Types of Mood Disorders

Depressive Disorders

Persons diagnosed with a depressive disorder (unipolar depression) have experienced only episodes of depression with no manic or hypomanic episodes. This is also referred to as **unipolar depression**. The DSM-IV-TR Criteria box lists criteria for a major depressive episode. The clinical symptoms of depressive disorders are listed in the Clinical Symptoms box.

Major Depressive Episode, Single or Recurrent. An episode of major depression is indicative of a first episode or of a recurrent episode of major depression. Symptoms occur as a result of the disorder and not from the effects of a substance, medical condition, or loss of a loved one within the previous 2 months.

Emotional Symptoms. Two primary symptoms of major depression are depressed mood and **anhedonia**, or loss of interest and pleasure in activities. For clients to be diagnosed with major depression, one of these symptoms must be present most of the day, nearly every day, for at least 2 weeks. Clients describe their mood as depressed, sad, empty, or numb. They report difficulty experiencing pleasure or satisfaction from their usual activities, including eating, sex, or going out with friends. Although clients describe feelings of sadness or frequent crying, some persons with depression are unable to describe feelings and report disinterest, disconnection, or an inability to feel emotion. Anxiety, irritability, or anger is also sometimes present. Clients also report feelings of loneliness, helplessness, or hopelessness. The affect of a person with depression is flat and constricted, with minimal expression, or appears rather normal as the person attempts to disguise his or her inner struggles.

Cognitive Symptoms. Criteria for major depression involving cognition include a diminished ability to think, concentrate, or make decisions; recurrent thoughts of death; and an excessive focus on self-worthlessness and guilt. Many clients describe difficulty concentrating on a task or conversation. Reading a newspaper or following the train of thought in a lecture may be overwhelming. Clients are sometimes unable to make decisions about routine concerns, such as what clothing to put on in the morning or what to buy at the grocery store. They have problems at their job, including problems with executive functions originating in the frontal lobe of the brain, resulting in an inability to organize, begin, and complete their work. Recurrent thoughts of death are often evident, including thoughts of suicide, death from natural

DSM-IV-TR CRITERIA

Major Depressive Episode

A Five (or more) of the following symptoms have been present during the same 2-week period and represent a change from previous functioning; at least one of the symptoms is either (1) depressed mood or (2) loss of interest or pleasure. NOTE: Do not include symptoms that are clearly due to a general medical condition or mood-incongruent delusions or hallucinations.

1 Depressed mood most of the day, nearly every day, as indicated by either subjective report (e.g., feels sad or empty) or observation made by others (e.g., appears tearful). NOTE: In children and adolescents, it can be irritable mood.
2 Markedly diminished interest or pleasure in all, or almost all, activities most of the day, nearly every day (as indicated by either subjective account or observation made by others).
3 Significant weight loss when not dieting or weight gain (e.g., a change of more than 5% of body weight in month) or decrease or increase in appetite nearly every day. NOTE: In children, consider failure to make expected weight gains.
4 Insomnia or hypersomnia nearly every day.
5 Psychomotor agitation or retardation nearly every day (observable by others, not merely subjective feelings of restlessness or being slowed down).
6 Fatigue or loss of energy nearly every day.
7 Feelings of worthlessness or excessive or inappropriate guilt (which may be delusional) nearly every day (not merely self-reproach or guilt about being sick).
8 Diminished ability to think or concentrate, or indecisiveness, nearly every day (either by subjective account or as observed by others).
9 Recurrent thoughts of death (not just fear of dying), recurrent suicidal ideation without a specific plan, or a suicide attempt or a specific plan for committing suicide.

B The symptoms do not meet criteria for a mixed episode.
C The symptoms cause clinically significant distress or impairment in social, occupational, or other important areas of functioning.
D The symptoms are not due to the direct physiologic effects of a substance (e.g., a drug of abuse, a medication) or a general medical condition (e.g., hypothyroidism).
E The symptoms are not better accounted for by bereavement (i.e., after the loss of a loved one, the symptoms persist for longer than 2 months or are characterized by marked functional impairment, morbid preoccupation with self-worthlessness, suicidal ideation, psychotic symptoms, or psychomotor retardation).

From American Psychiatric Association: *Diagnostic and statistical manual of mental disorders,* ed 4, text revision, Washington, DC, 2000, American Psychiatric Association.

CLINICAL SYMPTOMS

Depressive Disorders

MAJOR DEPRESSION

Emotional
Anhedonia
Depressed mood, sadness
Irritability

Cognitive
Diminished ability to think, concentrate, or make decisions
Recurrent thoughts of death
Excessive focus on self-worthlessness and guilt

Behavioral
Significant weight loss or gain, change in appetite
Insomnia or hypersomnia
Psychomotor agitation or retardation
Fatigue
Sleep disturbances

Social
Withdrawal from family and social interactions
Problems at work from inability to organize, initiate, or complete work
Financial problems

DYSTHYMIC DISORDER

Emotional
Depressed mood
Anhedonia
Irritability or angry mood

Cognitive
Feelings of low self-esteem and inadequacy
Feelings of guilt and brooding about the past
Difficulty with concentration, memory, and decision making
Attitudes of pessimism, despair, and hopelessness

Behavioral
Chronic fatigue

Social
Social withdrawal

CLINICAL ALERT

Be alert to **suicidal ideation and intent** with clients with depression and clients with mania who are cycling into depression or whose insight and judgment are impaired. A particularly high-risk time is 1 to 6 weeks after the initiation of antidepressant therapy, before it reaches its full therapeutic effect.

causes, or existential thoughts about dying. At times, these thoughts occupy a large portion of the client's waking hours. Negative thinking is often apparent, with feelings of worthlessness and excessive guilt. Clients think about past deeds and their negative view of themselves and the world. Clients with severe depression sometimes become delusional with fixed beliefs that cannot be changed by logic; delusions focus on persecution, punishment, **nihilism** (belief of nonexistence or nothingness), or somatic concerns.

Behavioral Symptoms. Behavioral symptoms that are criteria for major depression are significant weight loss or gain or change in appetite, insomnia or hypersomnia, psychomotor agitation or psychomotor retardation, and fatigue. Weight gain or weight loss is significant when it represents a 5% change in body weight in 1 month. Sometimes the weight change is not apparent, but the client reports a major change in appetite. Sleep disturbances are common, and clients report not being able to sleep (insomnia) or sleeping too much (hypersomnia). **Psychomotor agitation** is evident when the client appears to be restless, paces, fidgets, or is irritable. With **psychomotor retardation** the client appears slowed down in movement and in speech. Their entire body is slowed resulting in symptoms such as constipation and difficulty digesting food. Persons with depression appear listless and disheveled. They sometimes do not carefully attend to their dress, appearance, or hygiene. They exhibit a stooped posture and make little eye contact. Many clients report feelings of fatigue and loss of energy, citing an inability to accomplish tasks and an increased need for naps. They often appear very tired. Fatigue causes many clients to visit their family physician or nurse practitioner, believing that the fatigue is indicative of a physical problem. Thus, depression is often initially diagnosed during a visit to the primary care provider.

Social Symptoms. For major depression to be diagnosed, the symptoms must cause personal distress and significant impairment in social and occupational functioning. Some clients withdraw from family and social interactions. Although some people are able to function at work with relatively little impairment, this often comes at great personal and family expense as their energy for social interaction is exhausted. When the person is unable to work, financial problems often jeopardize the family. Family members begin to feel confused, angry, guilty, abandoned, and sad.

Marital distress is often a cited stressor at least 6 months before the onset of a depressive episode (Schmaling and Becker, 1991). During an episode the client's erratic behavior, mood, and cognition alienate a loved one, who becomes frustrated with how to help the partner. Unfortunately, it appears as though marital distress continues even after the acute episode subsides. Continued marital strain has been cited as a factor in episode recurrence (Schmaling and Becker, 1991).

Dysthymic Disorder. **Dysthymia** differs from major depression in that it is a chronic, low-level depression. To receive this diagnosis, the client must have had depressed mood and at least three of the following symptoms for most of the day, nearly every day, for at least 2 years (1 year for children and adolescents): poor appetite or overeating, insomnia or hypersomnia, low energy, low self-esteem, poor concentration or difficulty making decisions, and feelings of hopelessness. There cannot have been a manic or hypomanic episode. The client may have experienced an episode of major depression before the onset of dysthymia, provided there were at least 6 months with no signs or symptoms of depression. After 2 years of dysthymia, some clients are diagnosed with major depression superimposed on dysthymia if symptoms increase in severity. The dysthymic disorder is not due to the effects of a substance or medical condition. Psychotic features are usually not present in this disorder.

Emotional Symptoms. The predominant symptom that must be present for the diagnosis of dysthymia is depressed mood. Clients report feeling chronically "down, gloomy, sad." Many are unable to remember a time when they felt good or their usual self. Another symptom indicative of dysthymia is a generalized loss of interest or pleasure in activities, but unlike major depression, anhedonia is not a primary emotional symptom. Another symptom is irritability or angry mood. Some clients find themselves feeling impatient with family members or coworkers and have angry outbursts. Many feel bad about their irritable state but are unable to control it.

Cognitive Symptoms. Cognitive symptoms of dysthymia include low self-esteem and inadequacy; guilt and brooding about the past; difficulty with concentration, memory, and decision making; and negative thinking evidenced by pessimism, despair, and hopelessness. Clients with dysthymia often have little regard for themselves and are overwhelmed by a sense of inadequacy and a lack of self-confidence. They reflect on past actions and attribute personal guilt to their circumstances. Negativity is pervasive in what they do and say; life seems hopeless, and situations are full of pessimism and despair. Clients often report poor memory and decreased concentration on tasks and have problems making decisions, but the impairment is usually not as severe as impaired cognition during major depression.

Behavioral Symptoms. Clients with dysthymia commonly complain of chronic fatigue. They are exhausted from usual activities and often believe that they have a physical illness or chronic fatigue syndrome. Clients make repeated visits to their health care provider, hoping to determine the cause of their fatigue. Along with the fatigue, clients display decreased activity and productivity. Everything becomes a chore, and it often becomes difficult to complete tasks in the usual amount of time.

Social Symptoms. Social withdrawal is common with dysthymia. Clients are tired, irritable, and depressed and no longer get satisfaction from outings or activities with family and friends. Clients' mood states and negativity prevent people from wanting to be with them, increasing their isolation from others.

Depressive Disorders Not Otherwise Specified. There are types of depression that do not meet the criteria for the depressive disorders presented thus far or that will be disorders in their own right. Some of these include premenstrual dysphoric disorder, minor depressive disorder, recurrent brief depressive disorder, and the postpsychotic depression of schizophrenia. *Dysphoria* refers to a depressed, sad mood. The reader is referred to the DSM-IV-TR classification for more extensive descriptions of these diagnoses.

Bipolar Disorders

A **bipolar disorder** occurs when the client experiences both episodes of depression and episodes of mania or hypomania over time. Bipolar disorders are the pattern of manic, hypomanic, and depressed episodes over time. The depressed and manic episodes are not due to the effects of a substance, including antidepressant medication, electroconvulsive therapy, or light therapy. Clients may be diagnosed with a bipolar I or a bipolar II disorder (see the DSM-IV-TR Criteria box). Although the public continues to refer to bipolar disorders as manic depression, that is a term for a single, polarized disorder. A bipolar disorder encompasses the range (spectrum) of possible disturbances in mood. The clinical symptoms of bipolar disorders are in the Clinical Symptoms box.

Manic Episode. *Manic episodes* occur when there is an abnormally and persistently elevated, expansive, or irritable mood for at least 1 week. At least three of the following symptoms must also be present: inflated self-esteem, decreased need for sleep, more than usual talkativeness, racing thoughts, distractibility, increase in goal-directed activity, and excessive involvement in pleasurable activities (see the DSM-IV-TR Criteria box on p. 222). *Mixed episodes* occur when both manic and major depressive criteria are met nearly every day for 1 week (see the DSM-IV-TR Criteria box on p. 222).

Emotional Symptoms. To be diagnosed as having a manic episode, the client must exhibit an abnormally and persistently elevated, expansive, or irritable mood for at least 1 week. The client appears euphoric, with periods punctuated by irritability and anger. Some clients report minimal euphoria but describe irritability as their primary mood. Emotional lability, where mood and affect fluctuate between euphoria and anger, is common.

Cognitive Symptoms. Inflated self-esteem and grandiosity are common symptoms of mania. Clients report that they are confident, capable, and can do things better than others. As the mania becomes more intense, clients describe themselves in glowing terms and may believe that they are capable of amazing feats and achievements. Delusions of grandeur are sometimes evident during severe episodes of mania as clients believe that they possess extraordinary gifts and talents, are famous, or personally know someone famous. These delusions of inflated self-worth and ability represent mood-congruent psychotic features of mania. Cognitively, clients with mania also experience thought-flow disturbance with racing thoughts and flight of ideas. **Flight of ideas** is a type of thought disorder in which somewhat connected thoughts occur quickly, resulting in little elaboration and rapid changing of subjects. It becomes difficult to block out incoming stimuli, and the client becomes distractible, responding to irrelevant stimuli. Clients with mania often deny the seri-

DSM-IV-TR CRITERIA

Bipolar I and Bipolar II Disorders

TYPE	CHARACTERISTICS
Bipolar I Disorder	
Single manic episode	Only one manic episode No past major depressive episodes
Most recent episode: hypomanic	Current hypomania At least one previous manic episode
Most recent episode: manic	Current mania At least one previous depressive, manic, or mixed episode
Most recent episode: mixed	Meets criteria for both manic and depressive current episode At least one past major depressive or mixed episode
Most recent episode: depressed	Current depressive episode At least one past manic or mixed episode
Bipolar II Disorder	No previous full manic episode At least one past major depressive episode and past or current hypomanic episode

Modified from American Psychiatric Association: *Diagnostic and statistical manual of mental disorders*, ed 4, text revision, Washington, DC, 2000, American Psychiatric Association.

ousness of their status and lack judgment regarding personal, social, and occupational needs and activities.

Behavioral Symptoms. Increased talkativeness, increased goal-directed behavior or agitation, and excessive involvement in pleasurable activities are notable symptoms of mania. As the mania progresses, clients become more talkative and their speech is pressured (delivered with urgency). The rate of speech often increases and becomes rapid. There is a decreased need for sleep and, clients do not feel tired. Some clients exhibit extremes in appearance, wearing bright colors, unusual dress, and heavy makeup. Clients begin and engage in more activities, taking on additional tasks and initiating new projects. Productivity appears to increase as the client begins more tasks, but as the mania becomes more intense, actual productivity decreases as clients become more distractible, disorganized, and agitated. They begin to physically move faster—pacing, fidgeting, rarely letting their body stay still. It becomes more difficult for the client to eat and drink because of excessive movement and activity and decreased appetite. As insight and judgment become more impaired, clients become involved in activities that they perceive as pleasurable but that carry a high risk for harm or negative consequences. Clients often report engaging in extramarital affairs, promiscuity, spending sprees, gambling, wild driving, and unwise business deals. These behaviors often have serious health, financial, legal, and interpersonal consequences.

Social Symptoms. At first, mania seems to promote sociability, and clients become more outgoing and active; however, before long, insight and judgment fail, and these same clients become intrusive—interrupting others' conversations and activities, changing from euphoria to anger, and disrupting social interactions. Clients with mania find it difficult to set both physical and emotional boundaries, interfering in the physical space and personal issues of others. The funny, witty client becomes angry and isolated as the mood escalates and intensifies.

Perceptual Symptoms. One symptom of mania is distractibility, in which attention is easily and frequently drawn to irrelevant external stimuli. Clients appear unable to screen out secondary stimuli (e.g., noises, other voices, and visual attractions) that are not necessary or relevant to the task at hand. Distractibility interferes with attention, concentration, and memory. Perceptual disturbances also occur in the form of hallucinations. Manic hallucinations occur in any sensory mode but are usually auditory, with themes that pertain to grandiosity, power, and, occasionally, paranoia. These indicate manic psychosis.

CLINICAL SYMPTOMS

Bipolar Disorders

MANIC EPISODE

Emotional

Abnormally and persistently elevated, expansive, or irritable mood

Cognitive

Thoughts of inflated self-esteem and grandiosity
Thought-flow disturbance with racing thoughts and flight of ideas

Behavioral

Increased talkativeness
Decreased need for sleep
Increased goal-directed behavior or agitation
Excessive involvement in activities thought to be pleasurable

Social

Increased sociability
Intrusive, interruptive, and disruptive during conversations or activities
Fluctuations between euphoria and anger

Perceptual

Distractibility
Hallucinations

CYCLOTHYMIC DISORDER

Behavioral

Periods of hypomania
Periods of depressed mood and anhedonia
Irritability or angry mood
Chronic fatigue

Cognitive

Feelings of low self-esteem and inadequacy
Feelings of guilt and brooding about the past
Difficulty with concentration, memory, and decision making
Attitudes of pessimism, despair, and hopelessness

Social

Social withdrawal

Hypomanic Episode. Manic and hypomanic episodes share symptom criteria, and they differ primarily

DSM-IV-TR CRITERIA

Manic, Mixed, and Hypomanic Episodes

MANIC EPISODE

A A distinct period of abnormally and persistently elevated, expansive, or irritable mood, lasting at least 1 week (or any duration if hospitalization is necessary).

B During the period of mood disturbance, three (or more) of the following symptoms have persisted (four if the mood is only irritable) and have been present to a significant degree:

1. Inflated self-esteem or grandiosity
2. Decreased need for sleep (e.g., feels rested after only 3 hours of sleep)
3. More talkative than usual or pressure to keep talking
4. Flight of ideas or subjective experience that thoughts are racing
5. Distractibility (i.e., attention too easily drawn to unimportant or irrelevant external stimuli)
6. Increase in goal-directed activity (either socially, at work or school, or sexually) or psychomotor agitation
7. Excessive involvement in pleasurable activities that have a high potential for painful consequences (e.g., engaging in unrestrained buying sprees, sexual indiscretions, or foolish business investments)

C The symptoms do not meet criteria for a mixed episode.

D The mood disturbance is sufficiently severe to cause marked impairment in occupational functioning or in usual social activities or relationships with others, or to necessitate hospitalization to prevent harm to self or others, or there are psychotic features.

E The symptoms are not due to the direct physiologic effects of a substance (e.g., a drug of abuse, a medication, or other treatment) or a general medical condition (e.g., hyperthyroidism).

NOTE: Manic-like episodes that are clearly caused by somatic antidepressant treatment (e.g., medication, electroconvulsive therapy, light therapy) should not count toward a diagnosis of bipolar I disorder.

MIXED EPISODE

A The criteria are met both for a manic episode and for a major depressive episode (except for duration) nearly every day during at least a 1-week period.

B The mood disturbance is sufficiently severe to cause marked impairment in occupational functioning or in usual social activities or relationships with others, or to necessitate hospitalization to prevent harm to self or others, or there are psychotic features.

C The symptoms are not due to the direct physiologic effects of a substance (e.g., a drug of abuse, a medication, or other treatment) or a general medical condition (e.g., hyperthyroidism).

NOTE: Manic-like episodes that are clearly caused by somatic antidepressant treatment (e.g., medication, electroconvulsive therapy, light therapy) should not count toward a diagnosis of bipolar I disorder.

HYPOMANIC EPISODE

A A distinct period of abnormally and persistently elevated, expansive, or irritable mood, lasting throughout at least 4 days, that is clearly different from the usual nondepressed mood.

B During the period of mood disturbance, three (or more) of the following symptoms have persisted (four if the mood is only irritable) and have been present to a significant degree:

1. Inflated self-esteem or grandiosity
2. Decreased need for sleep (e.g., feels rested after only 3 hours of sleep)
3. More talkative than usual or pressure to keep talking
4. Flight of ideas or subjective experience that thoughts are racing
5. Distractibility (i.e., attention too easily drawn to unimportant or irrelevant external stimuli)
6. Increase in goal-directed activity (either socially, at work or school, or sexually) or psychomotor agitation
7. Excessive involvement in pleasurable activities that have a high potential for painful consequences (e.g., engaging in unrestrained buying sprees, sexual indiscretions, or foolish business investments)

C The episode is associated with an unequivocal change in functioning that is uncharacteristic of the person when not symptomatic.

D The disturbance in mood and the change in functioning are observable by others.

E The episode is not severe enough to cause marked impairment in social or occupational functioning or to necessitate hospitalization, and there are no psychotic features.

F The symptoms are not due to the direct physiologic effects of a substance (e.g., a drug of abuse, a medication, or other treatment) or a general medical condition (e.g., hyperthyroidism).

NOTE: Hypomanic-like episodes that are clearly caused by somatic antidepressant treatment (e.g., medication, electroconvulsive therapy, light therapy) should not count toward a diagnosis of bipolar II disorder.

From American Psychiatric Association: *Diagnostic and statistical manual of mental disorders,* ed 4, text revision, Washington, DC, 2000, American Psychiatric Association.

in their severity and duration. *Hypomanic episodes* are not severe enough to cause significant impairment in social and occupational functioning or to require hospitalization. However, for diagnosis, it must be evident that the mood and behavioral disturbances of **hypomania** represent a definite change in the person's usual functioning for at least 4 days. During a hypomanic phase, clients appear extremely happy and agreeable, at ease with social conversation, and humorous. Although the moments of elevated mood seem desirable, they represent dysfunctional affective states during which the client is not fully in control of moods and accompanying behavior. Many clients often report that they like the experience of hypomania. They perceive that during these episodes they are productive, creative, and function at a higher level. Yet this is a dangerous time because hypomania can escalate to mania. As judgment declines, clients sometimes fail to recognize the consequences of their actions. Some clients report going off their medication in order to experience hypomanic episodes. The criteria for hypomanic episodes are presented in the DSM-IV-TR Criteria box.

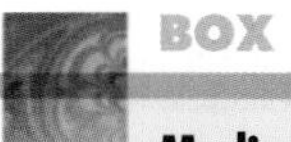

BOX 11-3

Medical Conditions and Substances Associated With Mood Disorders

MEDICAL CONDITIONS	SUBSTANCES
Hypothyroidism/ hyperthyroidism	Digitalis
Mononucleosis	Thiazide diuretics
Diabetes mellitus	Reserpine
Cushing's disease	Propranolol
Pernicious anemia	Anabolic steroids
Pancreatitis	Oral contraceptives
Hepatitis	Disulfiram
Human immunodeficiency virus	Sulfonamides
Multiple sclerosis	Alcohol and other substances of dependence
	Marijuana

Cyclothymic Disorder. Cyclothymic disorder is a chronic mood disturbance of at least 2 years' duration (1 year for children and adolescents), with many periods of hypomanic symptoms, depressed mood, and anhedonia. Clients with cyclothymic disorder have not been without the symptoms for more than 2 months over a period of 2 or more years; however, these symptoms are less severe or intense than those in major depressive or manic episodes.

Additonal Types of Mood Disorders

The DSM-IV-TR also provides diagnostic criteria for mood disorders resulting from general medical conditions and from substance use. In these instances, the depressed or elevated mood and accompanying symptoms are due to some general medical condition or to the ingestion of or withdrawal from medications or other substances. Box 11-3 lists examples of the types of medical conditions and substances commonly associated with the development of mood disorders.

Medical Conditions and Mood Disorders

When mood disorders and medical conditions are concurrent, the presentation, treatment, and prognosis of both are often complicated and compromised. Comorbidity (co-occurrence) is identified in several ways:

- A medical client develops a mood disorder as a stress response to a serious medical condition.
- A medical client develops a mood disorder as a physiologic response to either medical pathology or medications.
- A psychiatric client with a persistent mood disorder develops common medical disorders.
- A psychiatric client with a persistent mood disorder has an exacerbation of symptoms as a result of medical pathology or treatment.
- Health care providers identify previously unrecognized relationships between mood and medical disorders.

Medical conditions are often stressful and frightening, and some result in a depressive reaction to the situation or a major depression. A variety of medical disorders are associated with depression. In one study of 176 consecutive clients between ages 20 and 60 years admitted to medical units, 32% met criteria for a major depression. Most episodes were mild to moderate rather than severe, and researchers included all types of medical problems apart from malignancies or neurologic illnesses. The rates of depression were similar for acute and chronic illnesses (Sharma et al., 2002). Another study of more than 2500 community residents concluded that the prevalence of major depression was elevated in individuals who reported one or more chronic medical conditions (Gagnon and Patten, 2002). Medical illnesses introduce insecurity and powerlessness into the lives of individuals who are already physically vulnerable. For example, the uncertainty of organ transplant has been associated with depression and other coping problems. After heart transplant surgery, the lack of a sense of personal control has been associated with depression (Bohachick et al., 2002).

The pathophysiology of a medical condition, or a response to the medications given for a medical condition, sometimes results in a mood disorder. Research has implicated disorders of nearly every body system with co-occurring mood disorders. *Cardiovascular disorders* have been linked with major depression to a great extent. Major depression and depressive symptomatology are common in clients with coronary artery disease and significantly increase risk and complicate recovery from a range of cardiac events. Depression after myocardial infarction (MI) increases mortality, especially during the first 18 months after the MI (Strik et al., 2001). More recently, the association of cardiac events with vessel inflammation has resulted in the description of a possible causal pathway. One theory is that the inflammatory process of cardiac disease results in lower tryptophan levels. Because tryptophan is associated with serotonin availability, the decrease in both levels puts clients at risk for mood disturbances and depression (Murr et al., 2002).

Neurologic disorders are closely linked with depression. Depression after stroke is particularly common. Estimates suggest that an average 20% of poststroke clients have major depression, and another 21% meet criteria for minor depression. When onset of major depression occurred shortly after a stroke, vegetative symptoms were more frequent than if the onset appeared later (12 to 24 months poststroke). Late-onset depression was more frequently associated with poor social functioning. Both early- and late-onset depression were attributed to etiology provoked by brain injury (Tateno et al. 2002). Researchers have suggested that early treatment of poststroke depression has a significant influence on the rehabilitation and recovery of activities of daily living (ADLs) function of stroke clients (Chemerinski et al., 2001). Depression is a significant symptom in Parkinson's disease (PD). Clinical manifestations included apathy, psychomotor retardation, memory impairment, pessimism, irrationality, and suicidal ideation without suicidal behavior. In one study, 52.5% of clients with PD were severely depressed, and

37.5% were mildly to moderately depressed. The depression was associated with stage of disease and functional capacity, with significantly higher depression among clients in the severe stage of PD (Gupta and Bhatia, 2000).

Endocrine disorders are also involved in the emergence of psychiatric disorders. In one study, researchers suggested that there is a relationship between type 2 diabetes mellitus and bipolar I disorder, separate and apart from effects of age, race, gender, medication, and body mass (Regenold et al., 2002).

Additional disorders that result in mood disturbances are also the focus of much research. For example, scientists have long studied cancer and thyroid disease with regard to mood disorders. Alternatively, a number of medical conditions mimic psychiatric illness. The problem lies in determining the root cause of symptoms, whether they are the result of medical, psychiatric, or psychologic pathology. In the process of treatment, nurses must take care to ensure that medication administration does not further complicate illnesses. Many medical drugs are associated with the emergence of mood disorders. At the same time, many side effects of psychotropic drugs are initially assessed as medical in nature (e.g., cardiac or blood pressure changes seen with certain antidepressant drugs). Ultimately the assessment of medical clients must include the psychiatric component.

Psychiatric clients are at least as likely as individuals without psychiatric disorders to develop medical problems ranging from the common cold to serious medical disorders. This is particularly problematic because psychiatric clients have not always received timely or adequate medical care. Consequently, psychiatric clients tend to present at more advanced stages of illness, with more complicated psychosocial factors influencing care. Clients with a preexisting psychiatric disorder will present for treatment on any hospital inpatient unit. Unless the treatment plan considers the psychiatric disorder along with the medical illness, problems often occur with medication compatibility, accurate interpretation by staff of client behavior, client cooperation with and involvement in care, or client ability to follow treatment instructions after hospitalization. For example, major depression and bipolar disorder increase the risk for HIV, increasing the morbidity of HIV-related illnesses by blocking treatment. Many clients with untreated mental illnesses do not follow antiretroviral therapies, whereas treatment of mood disorders has improved adherence to treatment and clinical outcomes of HIV infection (Angelino and Treisman, 2001).

Among psychiatric clients the pathophysiology of, or treatment received for, a medical disorder promotes the return of psychiatric symptoms or the emergence of a new disorder. For example, when clients are admitted to the hospital, a complete history of previous medications is not always available. If the client does not continue psychotropic medications, the symptoms of a preexisting mood disorder will return, or the client will experience a withdrawal response from medications.

CLINICAL ALERT

Rapid discontinuation of some antidepressants results in withdrawal symptoms. **Tricyclic antidepressant discontinuation syndrome** sometimes results in gastrointestinal symptoms (nausea, vomiting, abdominal cramps, diarrhea), general distress (headaches, lethargy, sweating), sleep disturbances (insomnia, excessive dreaming, nightmares), affective symptoms (anxiety, agitation, low mood, mania, hypomania), movement disorders, or cardiac arrhythmias. **SSRI discontinuation syndrome** sometimes manifests as gastrointestinal (GI) symptoms (nausea, GI distress), general distress (flulike symptoms, lethargy, sweating), sleep disturbance, affective symptoms (anxiety, irritability, crying spells, agitation, confusion), problems with balance (dizziness, light-headedness, vertigo, ataxia), or sensory abnormalities (paresthesias, numbness, tremor). SSRI discontinuation syndrome is especially likely with the shorter-lasting SSRIs and is most problematic with fluvoxamine (Luvox), nefazodone (Serzone), paroxetine (Paxil), and venlafaxine (Effexor). The nurse needs to instruct patients to avoid missing doses of antidepressants, reassure patients that withdrawal symptoms are usually mild and short lived, and anticipate that most antidepressants will need to be tapered gradually.

Comorbidity (Co-occurrence)

Current research is expanding our awareness of medical and psychiatric comorbidity, with new knowledge and new questions available every day. There is high co-occurrence of mood disorders with other major mental illnesses (Rush et al., 2005), especially substance abuse and dependence. Psychiatric clients are living longer than they did in previous generations. Consequently, clinics are seeing an increase in clients with comorbid (co-occurring) medical and psychiatric disorders who are also showing signs of dementia. Epidemiologic data indicate that from 30% to 50% of clients with Alzheimer's disease (AD) have significant depressive symptoms. As a result, researchers are trying to develop criteria that will define the course of depression in AD. Others are making an effort to identify criteria for vascular depression, a subtype occurring within acute and chronic cerebrovascular pathology. Thus, two new diagnostic categories will become available, separate from existing depressive disorders. Ultimately, nurses need to be aware of the comorbidity of mood and medical disorders in all treatment settings.

Additional Symptom Features of Mood Disorders

The DSM-IV-TR recognizes that there are features of mood disorders that indicate various subtypes of unipolar and bipolar disorders. Persons experiencing an episode of major depression, whether it is part of a unipolar or bipolar pattern, sometimes demonstrate melancholic, atypical, or seasonal features. Postpartum onset represents another type of mood disorder.

Features of **melancholic depression** include anhedonia and a lack of reactivity to any pleasurable stimulus, a distinct quality of mood in which the client perceives the depression as different from the feeling after the death of a loved one, depression that is worse in the morning (diurnal variation), sleep disturbance of early morning awak-

CLINICAL SYMPTOMS

Additional Mood Disorders

MELANCHOLIC DEPRESSION

Emotional

Anhedonia
Increased depression in the morning

Cognitive

Excessive feelings of guilt

Behavioral

Waking at least 2 hours before normal and being unable to fall back to sleep
Psychomotor retardation or agitation
Significant weight loss

ATYPICAL DEPRESSION

Emotional

Mood reactivity
Ability to react to positive stimuli

Cognitive

Sensitivity to interpersonal rejection

Behavioral

Significant weight gain or increase in appetite
Hypersomnia
Leaden paralysis

SEASONAL AFFECTIVE DISORDER

Emotional

Depression between October/November and March/April

POSTPARTUM DEPRESSION

Behavioral

Difficulty caring for child

ening at least 2 hours before the usual time, marked psychomotor retardation or agitation, significant weight loss or loss of appetite, and excessive guilt.

Features of **atypical depression** include mood reactivity, loss of the ability to react to positive stimuli, significant weight gain or increase in appetite, hypersomnia, leaden paralysis or a heavy feeling in the arms and legs, and a long-standing pattern of being sensitive to interpersonal rejection.

A seasonal pattern occurs when there is a regular, temporal relationship between the onset and the remission of an episode of major depression (unipolar or bipolar) at a particular time of the year. This pattern must be evident for 2 consecutive years with no intervening, nonseasonal episodes. Seasonal episodes of altered mood must outnumber any nonseasonal episodes over a lifetime. This pattern is commonly called **seasonal affective disorder** (SAD). Clients with SAD often develop depression during October or November and find it diminishing in March or April. Atypical features are also associated with SAD. A seasonal pattern also occurs with bipolar disorder, particularly bipolar II disorder, in which increased light triggers manic or hypomanic episodes.

Some women will experience a **postpartum mood disorder,** including depression or mania, after the birth of a child. About 10% to 15% of new mothers have postpartum depression (Righetti-Veltema et al., 2002). This usually occurs within 4 weeks of the birth and consists of symptoms of depression or mania described earlier. In its severe form, new mothers become psychotic, hearing voices and experiencing delusions. Some new mothers who are clinically depressed have a great deal of difficulty providing childcare; in fact, the child is sometimes at risk for neglect or injury. Many women describe transient mood changes after delivery are less severe and end within a few weeks.

A summary of clinical symptoms of these additional types of mood disorders is in the Clinical Symptoms box.

ADJUSTMENT DISORDERS

Adjustment disorders manifest with a variety of symptoms, most of which are similar to other psychiatric disorders, particularly mood disorders. Sadness or mood disturbances, withdrawal, and preoccupation with the stressors lead the clinician to conclude that the person is experiencing major depression. Adjustment disorders, however, are generally of a briefer duration. The nervousness and distress of adjustment disorders sometimes mimics a generalized anxiety disorder, but the criteria symptoms for generalized anxiety disorder are not met for the required time frame. Although acute stress disorder and posttraumatic stress disorder are also responses to a stressor, the nature of the stressor with these disorders is much more severe and perceived as life threatening (Casey, 2001).

The diagnostic criteria for adjustment disorders are in the DSM-IV-TR Criteria box on p. 226. There is clinical significance when the level of distress exceeds usual expectations or when social, occupational, or school functioning is impaired. For example, a conflict with a coworker results in prolonged sleep disturbance and depressed mood or a pattern of calling in sick to work. Adjustment disorder is often diagnosed if a stressor is identified and the patient's symptoms are not severe enough to meet criteria for a more severe disorder.

The diagnostic category of adjustment disorders has been controversial for many reasons. The criteria are seen as overlapping with depressive and anxiety disorders, so many have questioned its validity. Reactions to stress are highly individualized, both in perception and in expression, so specific symptoms are difficult to identify. The absence of biologic markers, the close link with environmental factors, and the lack of clear measurable criteria are problematic. Some have questioned how adjustment disorders differ from normal adaptive reactions, with a concern that current diagnostic and treatment practices overmedicalize a process that is not truly pathologic. Critics have noted that in primary care settings, clinicians categorize psychiatric disorders as distress requiring no specific intervention, distress requiring intervention, or psychiatric disorder. These critics suggest that assessing patients with adjustment disorder along

DSM-IV-TR CRITERIA

Adjustment Disorders

A The development of emotional or behavioral symptoms in response to an identifiable stressor(s) occurring within 3 months of the onset of the stressor(s).

B These symptoms or behaviors are clinically significant as evidenced by either of the following:

1 Marked distress that is in excess of what would be expected from exposure to the stressor

2 Significant impairment in social or occupational (academic) functioning

C The stress-related disturbance does not meet criteria for another specific Axis I disorder and is not merely an exacerbation of a preexisting Axis I or Axis II disorder.

D The symptoms do not represent bereavement.

E Once the stressor (or its consequences) has terminated, the symptoms do not persist for more than an additional 6 months.

Specify if:

Acute: if the disturbance lasts less than 6 months

Chronic: if the disturbance lasts for 6 months or longer

Adjustment disorders are coded based on the subtype, which is selected according to the predominant symptoms. The specific stressor(s) can be specified on Axis IV.

With depressed mood

With disturbance of conduct

With anxiety

With mixed disturbance of emotions and conduct

With mixed anxiety and depressed mood

Unspecified

From American Psychiatric Association: *Diagnostic and statistical manual of mental disorders,* ed 4, text revision, Washington, DC, 2000, American Psychiatric Association.

these guidelines will permit spontaneous resolution where possible and prevent unnecessary expensive treatment (Casey et al., 2001).

PROGNOSIS

Scientists are now giving more attention to understanding the life course of persons with mood disorders. The bipolar disorders have historically been perceived as recurrent, with cycles of mania and depression interspersed with periods of **euthymia**. The pattern of cycles varies from person to person, with episodes of depression, mania, and euthymia varying widely in duration. Some individuals experience rapid shifts in mood, known as *rapid cycling.* It is often more difficult to treat persons who exhibit this pattern. The bipolar disorders have a high rate of recurrence and relapse. Factors that contribute to relapse include the number of and recovery from previous episodes, a family history of bipolar disorder, functional incapacity associated with episodes, past psychotic episodes, and past suicide attempts (Consensus Development Panel, 1985). However, many recurrences are controllable with proper treatment and monitoring.

There is evidence of differences between the depression period of bipolar disorder and the depression of major depressive disorder including family history of bipolar disorder, earlier age of onset, more depressive episodes, and individual symptom differences. Symptom differences include more sadness, insomnia, cognitive difficulties, and somatic complaints in bipolar disorder (Perlis et al., 2006).

Major depression is a serious, recurrent disorder for the majority of persons with the disorder (Greden, 2001). Research indicates that 50% to 85% of clients with unipolar depression experience a subsequent episode and that recurrent episodes tend to be increasingly intense with shorter time periods between episodes (Greden, 2001). The mean duration of an episode is 16 weeks (Kessler et al., 2003). Data suggest that nearly two thirds of people who experience major depression will suffer at least one recurrence within 10 years. Negative long-term effects impair self-care, productivity, social functioning, occupational functioning, and physical health (Greden, 2001). Fifteen percent of people with depression eventually commit suicide (Hirschfeld et al., 1997).

These data show the need for education, lifetime monitoring, and maintenance treatment for many persons with depression. The prognosis for major depressive disorder is good because with adequate treatment, it is controllable with medications, psychotherapy, and self-help strategies. However, clients need to be aware of the recurrent nature of their disorder and educated about the importance of recognizing symptoms and seeking help early when depression begins. Unfortunately, many persons do not recognize the onset of their recurrences (Hagerty et al., 1997), and less than a third of the people who experience depression seek help, putting them at risk for future, more severe depression.

Dysthymia often continues for years before individuals seek assistance for their symptoms. Many people are unaware that the chronic, low-level depression that is draining their energy is a form of depression that is treatable. Unfortunately, more than 50% of persons with dysthymia go on to develop major depression (Horwath et al., 1992).

With proper treatment the prognosis for maintaining individual functioning with a mood disorder is favorable. Inevitably, failure to seek help, lack of education regarding the disorder, lack of proper diagnosis and appropriate treatment, not following a treatment plan, or resistance of the symptoms to usual interventions mean that some persons will become so impaired that their daily functioning will diminish for long periods.

DISCHARGE CRITERIA

Most clients with a mood disorder are not hospitalized. They generally receive outpatient treatment. Because of insurance constraints and availability of services, both settings have become increasingly limited in the amount of time available to clients for treatment. Inpatient stays range from 4 to 7 days unless symptoms are severe. Outpatient visits are usually limited to 20 per year, unless the client pays privately for care. Consequently, the goals of treatment are quite different for hospital versus outpatient treatment, and realistic outcomes within the available time frame are sometimes different from ideal expectations. When clients are discharged from the hospital, the expectation is for clients to have outpatient treatment so that progress will continue. Clients require attention to ensure that they meet the following realistic criteria for each setting before discharge, whereas continued improvements in delivery of care aim for the ideal criteria.

Hospital Discharge Criteria

Realistic

Client will:

- Verbalize plans for the future, including absence of imminent suicidal intent or behavior.
- Verbalize plan for seeking help (a contract) if suicidal thoughts become intensified or if thoughts progress to plans.
- Demonstrate ability to manage basic self-care needs, such as personal hygiene, or verbalize strategies to acquire assistance.
- Identify psychosocial or physical stressors that have negative influences on mood and thinking.
- State positive and helpful strategies to cope with threats, concerns, and stressors.
- Identify signs and symptoms of the mood disorder, including prodromal (early) signs that indicate the need to seek help.
- Describe how to contact appropriate sources for validation or intervention when necessary.
- Verbalize knowledge about medication treatment and necessary self-care strategies.

Ideal

Client will:

- Describe mood state and demonstrate ability to identify changes from euthymic mood.
- Verbalize realistic perceptions of self and abilities that are positive and hopeful.
- Verbalize realistic expectations for self and others.
- Use learned techniques and strategies to prevent or minimize symptoms.
- Engage family or significant other as a source of support.
- Structure life to include appropriate activities that promote social support, minimize stress, and facilitate healthy living (e.g., diet, exercise).

Outpatient Discharge Criteria

Realistic

Client will:

- Verbalize plans for the future, including absence of imminent suicidal intent or behavior.
- Verbalize plan for seeking help (a contract) if suicidal thoughts become intensified or if thoughts progress to plans.
- Demonstrate an ability to manage basic self-care needs, such as personal hygiene, or verbalize strategies to acquire assistance.
- Describe mood state and demonstrate ability to identify changes from euthymic mood.
- Identify psychosocial or physical stressors that have negative influences on mood and thinking.
- State positive and helpful strategies to cope with threats, concerns, and stressors.
- Identify signs and symptoms of the mood disorder, including prodromal (early) signs indicating the need to seek help.
- Describe how to contact appropriate sources for validation or intervention when necessary.
- Use learned techniques and strategies to prevent or minimize symptoms.
- Verbalize knowledge about medication treatment and necessary self-care strategies.

Ideal

Client will:

- Verbalize realistic perceptions of self and abilities that are positive and hopeful.
- Verbalize realistic expectations for self and others.
- Engage family or significant other as a source of support.
- Structure life to include appropriate activities that promote social support, minimize stress, and facilitate healthy living (e.g., diet, exercise).

The Nursing Process

ASSESSMENT

Mood is the key variant in mood disorders. In the performance of a mental status examination by the nurse, consideration of related phenomena enhances the assessment of mood. **Mood** is a feeling state reported by the client that often varies with external and internal changes. This implies that the state is prolonged over a course of time, and the identification of a specific cause is often difficult. **Affect** is the expression of a client's feeling state that is observable by others. The expression of affect is highly changeable. **Temperament** is observable differences in the strength and duration of a client's tendency to respond to circumstances and degree of emotionalism expressed. Many consider this a product of a person's biologic constitution. The term is generally applied when speaking of infants or children, but nurses need to remember that temperament patterns influence a variety of phenomena that extend into adulthood, including impulse control and attachment. *Emotion* is the client's experience of a feeling state, and clients are often able to identify previous experiences that are highly intense and variable. *Emotional or affective reactivity* is the degree to which a client tends to respond to external and internal changes with feeling states. This is evident in how the client responds to questions. *Emotional regulation* refers to the client's ability to control or modify the occurrence and intensity of feeling states. *Range of affect* is the span of emotional expression the client shows. Limitations of range are described as restricted, blunted, or flat (Box 11-4).

The prevalence and incidence of mood disorders demand that nurses be alert for symptoms of depression and

BOX 11-4

Mental Status Criteria

- **Mood:** The internal manifestation of subjective feeling state
- **Affect:** The external expression—manifestation of a feeling state
- **Temperament:** Observable differences in the intensity and duration of arousal and emotionality
- **Emotion:** The experience of a feeling state
- **Emotional reactivity:** The tendency to respond to internal or external events with emotion
- **Emotional regulation:** The ability to control or modify the occurrence and intensity of feelings
- **Range of affect:** The span of emotional expression experienced and displayed

mania. Most persons experiencing a mood disorder, particularly depression, never seek psychiatric care. More often, these individuals visit family practitioners, clinics, or emergency departments reporting symptoms of fatigue, lack of activity, or vague physical complaints. Many do not realize that they are experiencing a mood disorder. They are treated for a medical problem such as an acute cardiac event, cancer, or stroke but have an underlying mood disorder that increases their risk for morbidity and mortality.

Clients with mood disorders pose a challenge because their primary symptom is one of depression or emotional elation. Their affective dysregulation often evokes emotional responses in nurses who find themselves feeling depressed, anxious or angry while caring for the individual. The negativity of depression or the expansive euphoria, hyperactivity, and grandiosity of mania may also promote fatigue, irritability, and negativity in the nurse. Therefore when caring for clients with mood disorders, nurses must maintain awareness of their own personal reactions to the client and the ways in which these reactions affect the nurse-client relationship and subsequent care.

Clients experiencing mood disorders are in emotional pain and are suffering. They are unable to change their emotional state at will. Yet many have heard people close to them, including health professionals, make comments such as, "Pull yourself together," or "Get a hold of yourself." These clients need validation that their emotional state is not their fault, that they are experiencing a psychiatric disorder. Clients need acceptance and respect.

It is important that nurses appear confident, straightforward, and hopeful. Reassuring comments such as "I know you'll feel better soon" are not helpful, because they are false reassurance. It is appropriate to express hope with comments such as "I've known many clients with depression, and they have felt better within several weeks of starting on their medications."

Communication with the person with depression depends on the severity of the depression. Clients with severe depression are sometimes physically and cognitively slowed down and have problems with attention, concentration, and decision making. Simple, clear communication is most helpful in this situation. The nurse needs to be more directive if the person is having a difficult time making decisions and functioning (e.g., "It's time for lunch. I'll go with you," rather than, "Would you like to go to lunch?"). As clients' conditions improve, they cognitively process more complex information, concentrate better, and make decisions more easily.

Communication with clients experiencing mania is also difficult. Their hyperactivity, expansive or irritable mood, and inability to filter stimuli are barriers to effective communication. Nurses need to be simple, clear, direct, and firm. Clients need to know that the nurse cares about them and is concerned about their behavior. Acute episodes of mania are not appropriate times for the nurse to examine the client's feelings and motives. Interactions need to be brief and direct, minimizing unnecessary stimuli. It is also important not to threaten or challenge a client during a manic episode, because in some situations the client will escalate, responding with anger or rage.

Information from the client experiencing a mood disorder is sometimes minimal or inaccurate because of the client's cognitive impairment, altered mood, or behavioral disturbances. A family member or significant other is an important source of information when the client is not reliable. Interviews need to be short and more directive if the client is having behavioral or cognitive difficulty.

Assessment of the client with depression or mania includes information about his or her presenting problem and mental status, past psychiatric history, social and developmental history, family history, and physical health history. Assessment instruments assist with the specificity of data collection. For assessing depression, these instruments include the Beck Depression Inventory (BDI), Carroll Rating Scale for Depression (CRSD), and Zung Self-Rating Depression Scale. One scale used to assess mania is the Manic State Rating Scale. Nurses will ask clients to assess their own level of depression or mania by having them rate it on a 10-point scale (e.g., "If zero represents feeling fine and 10 represents the worst depression you have ever experienced, how would you rate your depression now?"). This allows for daily comparisons of mood using specific empirical data.

Physiologic Disturbances

Body physiology changes during episodes of depression and mania. During moderate or severe depression, body processes frequently slow down. The client with depression reports and exhibits neurovegetative signs of depression, which include psychomotor retardation, fatigue, constipation, anorexia (loss of appetite), weight loss, decreased libido (sex drive), and sleep disturbances. These symptoms relate to changes in body processes that cause disruption and slowing of normal physiology. Some clients also describe vague physical symptoms such as headache, backache, gastrointestinal pain, and nausea. Sleep disturbance is a common problem. Clients describe ini-

CASE STUDY Robert, age 36, arrives at his primary care clinic for a physical exam because of extreme fatigue, loss of energy, hypersomnia, muscle aches, loss of 21 pounds, and headaches. These symptoms have made it difficult for him to function at his job as a store manager and enjoy activites with his friends. He is convinced that he has mononucleosis or Lyme's disease. You are assessing Robert before the nurse practitioner enters the examination room.

CRITICAL THINKING

1. What are important questions for the nurse to ask Robert at this time?
2. What laboratory tests might be appropriate?
3. What specific signs and symptoms suggest that Robert might be depressed?
4. Why is it important for Robert to get help immediately for his depression?

CASE STUDY Allison, age 28, a divorced mother of two children, arrives at the hospital emergency department accompanied by her mother. She has been unable to sleep for several weeks, cries easily, paces around the house, is irritable, has gained 18 pounds in 2 months, and no longer calls her friends. Her mother has been staying with her to take care of Allison's children. Although her mother has been concerned about Allison's behavior for the past several months, she decided to bring her to the hospital when Allison began talking about death and guns. Allison blames her behavior on her frustration with her asthma; she is wheezing.

CRITICAL THINKING

1. What information suggests that Allison may be experiencing atypical depression?
2. What additional information would be helpful for the nurse to know about Allison to develop nursing diagnoses and goals?
3. What are the care priorities for Allison at this point?
4. Which nursing diagnoses would be relevant for this client?
5. What long- and short-term outcomes, based on the nursing diagnoses, might be established with Allison?

tial insomnia (the inability to fall asleep after going to bed), middle insomnia (waking up in the middle of the night and being unable to return to sleep easily), and terminal or late insomnia (waking up in the early hours of the morning and being unable to return to sleep). Hypersomnia occurs when the client sleeps excessively but never feels rested. Clients with depression have a decreased or increased appetite with corresponding changes in weight. Clients often describe food as tasteless (see the Case Study above, left).

The client experiencing mania also has difficulty sleeping. Not feeling the need for sleep, the client sleeps only a few hours a night or not at all, but feels rested. Hyperactive behavior and the inability to attend to tasks often prevent the client from eating properly, resulting in dehydration and inadequate nutrition. As the client becomes increasingly stimulated, metabolic activity increases, and vital signs become elevated. Without proper intervention, clients with mania are at physical risk for dehydration, malnutrition, hypertension, fever, and cardiac arrest, which may lead to death.

NURSING DIAGNOSIS

The nurse uses objective and subjective data obtained during the assessment of clients with mood disorders and adjustment disorders to arrive at relevant nursing diagnoses. Data from all sources, including the client, significant others, and other professionals, are organized into a pattern of relationships that reflect the client's major areas of health care needs (see the Case Study above, right and the Nursing Assessment Questions box). Box 11-5 lists nursing diagnoses relevant to clients experiencing a mood or adjustment disorder. Nurses will prioritize diagnoses according to client needs and problems.

OUTCOME IDENTIFICATION

Outcome criteria for clients with mood disorders include short- and long-term client behaviors and responses that indicate improved functioning. These criteria are based on nursing diagnoses and are achieved through implementation of planned nursing care. Outcomes are established for phases of treatment including the acute phase of the illness, continuation of treatment to prevent relapse, and long-term maintenance. Outcome criteria provide the nurse with direction for evaluating client response to treatment and ongoing maintenance of health. Outcomes for clients with adjustment disorder will be related to the nature of the stressor and strategies for managing it, as well as current symptomatology, such as sleeping problems, that need focused interventions.

Client will:

- Remain safe and free from harm.
- Verbalize suicidal ideations and contract not to harm self or others.
- Verbalize absence of suicidal or homicidal intent or plans.
- Express desire to live and not harm others.
- Make plans for self for the future, verbalizing feelings of hopefulness.
- Engage in self-care activities in accordance with ability, health status, and developmental stage.
- Develop a plan to manage inadequate sleep.
- Develop a plan to achieve and maintain adequate nutrition.
- Establish a pattern of rest/activity that enables fulfillment of role and self-care demands.
- Make decisions based on examination of options and problem solving.
- Report absence of hallucinations/delusions.
- Initiate satisfying social interactions with and assistance from significant others or peers.
- Demonstrate participation in milieu, group, and community activities.
- Report increased communication and problem solving among family members regarding issues related to the disorder.

NURSING ASSESSMENT QUESTIONS

Mood Disorders

1 How would you describe your mood? *To assess client's insight into feeling state*
2 Have you noticed a change in your behavior within the past month? *To determine client's awareness of behavioral changes*
3 Do you feel that people are noticing a change in your behavior, such as irritability or hyperactivity? *To determine client's sensitivity to others' observations of behavioral changes*
4 What activities have you found enjoyable over the past month? Did you enjoy them as much as you previously did? Can you imagine an event or situation that would give you pleasure? Have you been able to enjoy food or sex over the past month? *To determine client's current quality of life*
5 When did you first begin to feel depressed or elated? Did others comment that your mood seemed more depressed (or higher) than usual? Have you ever felt this way before? When? What was it like? *To establish behavioral patterns*
6 How has your sleep been? Are you able to fall asleep at night? Stay asleep? Do you find yourself waking up early and being unable to return to sleep? Are you sleeping more than usual in a 24-hour period? How much? Are you sleeping less than usual? How much? *To determine sleep patterns*
7 How has your appetite been in the past month? How much weight have you lost or gained in the past month? *To determine nutritional/metabolic status*
8 How has your energy level been? Do you feel tired every day? Do you ever feel as though your limbs are heavy? Do you have more energy than usual? *To assess fatigability*
9 How has your concentration been? Are you able to attend to things such as reading the newspaper? Can you concentrate on projects or activities to finish them? What has your decision making been like? Have you had racing thoughts? *To evaluate cognitive abilities*
10 How have you felt about yourself lately? Have you felt guilty more than usual about things you have done? *To determine client's level of self-worth/self-esteem*
11 Have you felt particularly slowed down, or have others told you that you seemed to move or speak more slowly than usual? *To determine presence of sensorimotor retardation*
12 Have you felt particularly "speeded up" to the point where you noticed it or someone told you this? *To evaluate presence of mania/hypomania*
13 Have you had thoughts of death or suicide? How often? What specifically have you thought about doing to harm yourself? What prevented you from committing suicide? Have you had thoughts of harming or killing someone else? How often? What specifically have you thought about doing to harm someone else? *To determine suicidal/homicidal intent/plans*
14 What have you been doing lately to manage your feelings? Has it helped? *To assess for effective coping mechanisms/strategies*
15 How has your mood affected your job? Your family? Your social life? Your interpersonal relationships? *To assess pervasiveness of client's present mood state*
16 Have your received treatment from a mental health professional in the past? What kind of treatment? Did it help? *To determine presence and effectiveness of any past treatment*

- Describe alternative coping strategies for responses to stressors, strengths, and limitations.
- Report increased feelings of self-worth and confidence.
- Engage in activities and behaviors that promote confidence, belonging, and acceptance.
- Describe information about the disorder, including the course of illness and personal symptom patterns, as well as available, ongoing resources.
- Identify medications, including action, dosage, side effects, therapeutic effects, and self-care issues.
- In conjunction with a mental health provider, practice self-management of the illness, including monitoring and identifying prodromal (early) symptoms of recurrence and initiating strategies to deal with recurrent symptoms.
- Follow prescribed professional and self-care treatment strategies.

PLANNING

Recent information about the epidemiology and recurrent course of depression and mania provides the basis for caring for clients with mood disorders in the hospital and in the community. Nursing care not only addresses the acute episodes of the disorder but the client's ongoing risk for recurrent episodes. Interventions during the acute depressive or manic episodes are effective, but too often the client is left with little understanding of the clinical course of the illness and the importance of long-term management and self-care strategies. Nurses need to plan interventions for each client based on his or her particular behaviors, needs, and concerns. When planning client care, the nurse purposefully involves and includes the client, the client's significant others, and additional health care providers. Using prioritized nursing diagnoses derived from assessment data, interventions are selected and planned to facilitate achievement of desired client outcomes.

IMPLEMENTATION

The plan of action for clients with mood disorders varies depending on whether the client' mood is depressed or manic. In the short term, nursing and collaborative interventions are available that are effective in reducing the acuity of the episode and promoting more optimal functioning. With the current trend of short-term hospitalizations, nurses in the hospital setting do not have the opportunity to observe the client's recovery from the episode. Nurses document and communicate projected treatment responses to the client and to other nurses, mental health professionals, and significant others who will care for the client in the community. Nurses who work with clients in the community are able to

BOX 11-5

NANDA Nursing Diagnoses for Depression and Mania

DEPRESSION	MANIA
Activity intolerance	Risk-prone health behavior
Adult failure to thrive	Caregiver role strain
Anxiety	Impaired verbal communication
Constipation	Compromised family coping
Ineffective coping	Defensive coping
Death anxiety	Ineffective coping
Deficient diversional activity	Ineffective denial
Disturbed energy field	Disturbed energy field
Fatigue	Impaired environmental interpretation syndrome
Complicated grieving	Interrupted family processes
Delayed growth and development	Risk for deficient fluid volume
Ineffective health maintenance	Delayed growth and development
Hopelessness	Ineffective health maintenance
Insomnia	Insomnia
Deficient knowledge	Deficient knowledge
Risk for loneliness	Risk for loneliness
Noncompliance	Noncompliance
Imbalanced nutrition: less than body requirements	Imbalanced nutrition: less than body requirements
Imbalanced nutrition: more than body requirements	Imbalanced nutrition: more than body requirements
Risk for impaired parenting	Risk for impaired parenting
Powerlessness	Ineffective role performance
Ineffective role performance	Self-care deficit: bathing/hygiene; dressing/grooming; feeding
Readiness for enhanced self-care	Disturbed sensory perception
Self-care deficit: bathing/hygiene; dressing/grooming; feeding	Sexual dysfunction
Chronic low self-esteem	Sleep deprivation
Sexual dysfunction	Impaired social interaction
Impaired social interaction	Spiritual distress
Social isolation	Risk for suicide
Chronic sorrow	Ineffective therapeutic regimen management
Spiritual distress	Ineffective family therapeutic regimen management
Risk for suicide	Disturbed thought processes
Ineffective therapeutic regimen management	Risk for other-directed violence
Risk for self-directed violence	Risk for self-directed violence
Readiness for enhanced hope/power	

From NANDA International: *NANDA nursing diagnoses: definitions and classification 2007-2008,* Philadelphia, 2007, NANDA International.

see treatment responses over time. Initial treatment responses help to dictate continued care and prevention of recurrences over time. Interventions for clients with adjustment disorders will consider the nature of the stressor as well as the client's immediate symptoms to address.

Mood disorders, although primarily disturbances in mood regulation, affect the whole person—physically, cognitively, socially, and spiritually. Short-term interventions in the hospital or community address priority issues such as preventing self-harm, promoting physical health (e.g., adequate nutrition, bathing, grooming, sleep), monitoring effects of medications, and assisting with altered thought flow and impaired communication. Other concerns to address include promoting social interaction; improving self-esteem; understanding the mood disorder and its treatment; the need to follow the treatment plan; and the plan for discharge and continuation of services. One goal is to help clients improve their quality of life. Because episodes of depression and mania affect the entire family, involving the client's significant others provides an opportunity for them to understand the disorder and to support clients in their recovery. Figures 11-3 and 11-4 depict clinical pathways, which specify collaborative interventions relevant to mood disorders.

Nursing interventions for clients with mood disorders cover a wide range of biopsychosocial areas, with consideration of the effects of depression and mania on the physiologic, cognitive, psychologic, behavioral, and social areas. Intervention for clients experiencing depression and mania requires that nurses maintain self-awareness and boundaries regarding their own reactions to clients, because client depression, irritability, anger, negativity, euphoria, and hyperactivity can readily influence nursing responses. It is potentially difficult and exhausting to interact with clients who provoke personal feelings and reactions during highly emotional encounters. Nurses accomplish initiating and maintaining a therapeutic connection with clients by being consistent, caring, concerned, empathetic, and genuine. Clients with mood disorders often have a difficult time developing a therapeutic alliance and typically avoid interpersonal connection with others. A knowledgeable, nondemanding, and matter-of-fact approach is reassuring to clients and promotes their confidence in the nurse.

Nursing Interventions

1. Conduct a suicide assessment as necessary *to ensure the client's safety and prevent harm to self or others.*
2. Maintain a safe, harm-free environment through close and frequent observations *to minimize the risk of self-harm or violence.*
3. Establish rapport and demonstrate respect for the client *to facilitate the client's willingness to communicate thoughts and feelings.*
4. Assist the client in verbalizing feelings *to promote a healthy, expressive form of communication.*
5. Identify the client's social support system and encourage the client to use it *to minimize isolation and loneliness and provide assistance with monitoring the illness and treatment.*
6. Praise the client for attempts at alternate activities and interactions with others *to encourage socialization and promote self-esteem.*
7. Gently refuse to be part of secrecy agreements with the client; instead encourage the client to share important and relevant information with staff *to promote the client's participation in care and responsibility for own actions.*
8. Monitor and implement strategies to ensure adequate fluid intake and output, food intake, and weight *to ensure adequate nutrition and hydration and adequate weight for body size and metabolic needs.*

Text continued on p. 235

ST. JOSEPH HOSPITAL

DRG Number : ______
Primary Physician : ______
Physician(s) in Consult : ______
Anticipated Discharge Date : ______
Actual Discharge Date : ______
Financial : ______

MAJOR DEPRESSION CLINICAL PATHWAY©

CARE NEEDS	DAY OF ADMIT	LEVEL 1	LEVEL 2	LEVEL 3	LEVEL 4	LEVEL 5
CONSULTS/ ASSESSMENTS:	MD. CM. SW. RN. OT. Consults? Medical? Other?	Psy eval? Fam mtg? Complete all assess.	Complete family mtg. Complete psy testing if ordered.	SW/CM process family mtg w/pt. Complete psy consult if ordered.	OT reassess? Transfer summaries.	Send results of assess to out-pt Tx.
HEALTH MAINTENANCE Sleep Disturbance. ADL's. Diet. Med Dx ______ ______ ______	Chem 19. CBC. UA. Tox? T_3T_2Tsh? Pg? TCA/Li/Other? Sleep? ADL? Medical (below)? Nutri? VS ______ Ortho? - - - - - - >	Lab results? Nutri? Sleep? ADL? Review prot? Medical? VS ______ - - - - - - - - - - >	Nutri? Sleep? ADL? Review prot? Medical? VS ______ - - - - - - - - - - >	Nutri? Sleep? ADL? Review prot? Medical? VS ______ - - - - - - - - - - >	Nutri? Sleep? ADL? Review prot? Medical? Med refer to med f/u. VS ______ - - - - - - - - - - >	VS ______
PROGRAM: Target Sx ______ ______ ______ Meds. Teaching needs. Stressors. Compliancy. Tx	Orientation Prot. Rest 24"? Sx? Groups? Med orders? Consent form? Teaching needs? Stressors? Tx compliancy?	Shift Assess Prot. Multidis Tx plan mtg. Assess need for alt pathway. Groups per prot. Comm mtg: ______ ______ Meds/SE? Chart to target Sx. Tx compliancy?	Shift Assess Prot. Groups per prot. ______ ______ ______ Tx compliancy? Med/SE? Chart to target Sx. Prov med sheets.	Shift Assess Prot. Groups per prot. ______ Med group. D/C planning ______ Tx compliancy? Med/SE? Chart to target Sx. 1 unit resp.	Shift Assess Prot. Multidis Tx plan? Groups per prot. ______ ______ ______ Chart to target Sx. Med/SE? Tx compl?	Daily Assess Prot. D/C Prot.
SAFETY - Harm to self, others, and destruction of property. Elopement. Potential for falls. Sexually acting out.	Suicide Prot.? Safety Prot.? SFC? Verbal contract? Mental status? E?	Suicide Prot.? Mental status? Safety Prot.? SFC? E? OW Prot.? ______	Suicide Prot.? Mental status? Safety Prot.? SFC? E? OW Prot.? ______	Suicide Prot.? Mental status? Safety Prot.? SFC? E? OW Prot.? ______	Suicide Prot.? Mental status? Safety Prot.? SFC? E? SI review opt if ret. OW Prot.? ______	Review opt if SI reoccurs. Use of support systems.
DISCHARGE PLANNING: Compliancy. F/u. Teaching. MHC Financial	CM/SW 1 data - family? placement? F/up? Release of info. LOS expectation. DSHS form? Insurance?	Housing? LOS. F/up resources? Support system? Contact fam. Assign fam. grp. Contact MHC/out-pt Tx.	Placement?. MHC call liaison? Formulate f/up plan. Fam. attend sup/ed group. LOS.	Finalize f/up plan. LOS. Arrange for trans on day of D/C. Assess for therapeutic pass.	Liaison from MHC to see. Review Sx & cues to reoccurrence. Consider long-term care. Resources for meds. Coord D/C w/fam.	Check transportation & meds by 8 am for D/C by 11 am.

MAJORDEP.PIH 2/28/92

Axis I ______ Axis II ______ Axis III ______ Axis IV ______ Axis V ______

PERMANENT PART OF THE PATIENT RECORD

NOTE: This is not a Physician Order

FIGURE 11-3 Clinical pathway: major depression. (Coyright 1991, St. Joseph Hospital, Tacoma, Wash.)

Barnes and Jewish Hospitals
Department of Nursing
Patient Clinical Management Path

Admission ______________________
D/C Date ______________________
Estimated LOS ______________________
Case Manager ______________________

Case Type & Number **(DRG – 430) Bipolar Affective Disorder**

	Day 1/Adm. Loc ( )	Var. n/a m u	Day 2 – 3 Loc ( )	Var. n/a m u	Day 4 – 6 Loc ( )	Var. n/a m u	Day 7 – 9 Loc ( )	Var. n/a m u
Date								
Procedure/Test	Organic Workup (MD), EEG (MD), CT (MD), MRI (MD), EKG (MD), CXR (MD), Electrolytes (MD), Lithium Level (MD), Drug Screen (MD), Thyroid Studies (MD), Routine Labs (MD), Other ________ (MD)		Lab Results (ID abnormals)		-----> Psych Testing complete		Labs ________ Tests ________ Med. Blood Levels ________	
Consults	Medical (MD) Behavior Med. (MD) Psych Testing (MD) Other ________ (MD)		ID additional consults		----->		----->	
Meds/Tx	Meds ordered per MD including PRN to control behavior. ECT (MD) – permits (Nsg) – teaching (Nsg) – team notified (Nsg)		Monitor antidepressant, lithium, tegretol, valproic acid, PRN Meds. Other anti-psychotic meds; if mania DC antidepressant ----->		-----> ----->		-----> ----->	
Activity	Voluntary/Involuntary SP/EP (MD, Nsg) Fall precautions (MS, Nsg)		Assess ADL's -----> -----> Integrate into milieu Participate in groups Individual therapy		-----> Assess precautions -----> -----> ----->		-----> -----> -----> -----> ----->	
Nutrition	Assess appetite (MD, Nsg) Assess elimination patterns (MD, Nsg)		-----> -----> Teaching diet		-----> -----> ----->		-----> -----> ----->	
Discharge Planning	Legal Guardian ID (Nsg) Assess support system (Nsg, MD, SW, AT) Initial Plan (MD/Nsg)		SW Acknowl. note Placement issues MTP signed (MD/Nsg/SW)		Family Mtg		Plans discussed with patient (MD) -----> Weekly Progress Note (MD, SW, Nsg, TR) Completes SW assess Referrals Resources MTP developed	
INTERVENTIONS: Assessment Functional Assessment	H+P & Psych orders (MD) Nsg Assessment and ADB SW notified – pt/family Proper envir. assessed Mini Mental (Nsg) Assess LOF (Nsg, SW, AT) Assess methods to control behavior (Nsg) Remove ext. stimuli (Nsg)		Ongoing assess & treatment (MD, Nsg, SW, TR) BM initial Assess. Assess for dystonia If ADL assess needed OT referral		-----> Assess: – thought patterns – orientation – cog. skills – task completion		-----> Assess task completion Encourage incr. LOF -----> Assess lifestyle changes ----->	
Patient Teaching	Orient pt/family to unit (Nsg) Bill of Rights Given (Nsg)		Ed. Pt/family to various therapies MED Educ. Primary Nurse (Nsg)		-----> ----->		-----> ----->	

Signature & Initials

Refer to Nurses Notes for documentation regarding variances.

FIGURE 11-4 Clinical pathway: bipolar affective disorder. (Copyright 1994, Gina Bufe.)

Continued

	Day 10 – 12 Loc ( )	Var. n/a m u	Day 13 – 14 Loc ( )	Var. n/a m u	Day 15 Loc ( )	Var. n/a m u	Discharge Expected Outcome
Date							
Procedure/Test	Labs ________ Tests ________ Med. Blood Levels ________		Labs ________ Tests ________ Chart copied if appropriate		DC Orders Written		
Consults	----->		F/u appts made		----->		
Meds/Tx	-----> -----> Begin ECT outpt. arrangements		-----> -----> ----->		Perscriptions written		Pt will verbalize/ demonstrate imp. of medication +/or other therapies in maintaining optimal level of fcn after DC as evidenced by ________
Activity	-----> -----> -----> -----> ----->		Do teaching r/t follow up therapy		Plans finalized r/t outpt therapy		
Nutrition	-----> -----> ----->		DC teaching r/t nutrition		----->		
Discharge Planning			DC teaching w/family Weekly progress notes (MD, SW, TR, Nsg) DC teaching on utilization of skills learned while in hosp and how to integrate to home. Written information r/t resource given.		MTP closed or remains ongoing Final DC instructions given to pt/family F/U appt finalized		Pt will return to least restrictive/most supportive environment after DC with improved coping skills and identified resources as demonstrated by ________ ________.
INTERVENTIONS: Assessment	-----> ----->		-----> ----->		Final assessments & DC summary written.		
Functional Assessment	MMSE (Neg) -----> -----> -----> ----->		----->		----->		
Patient Teaching	-----> ----->		-----> -----> DC teaching		Final DC teaching to patient. Patient's responses to teaching documented		

*SW works M – F

Addressograph:

Teaching (initial and date when complete)

1. Medication Education ________
2. Education on illness ________
3. Social Skills ________
4. Coping Skills ________
5. ADL's ________
6. Self-Esteem ________
7. Dealing with Anger ________
8. Communication Skills ________
9. Dealing with Sadness ________
10. Decision Making ________
11. Other ________

*Document patient response in progress notes

FIGURE 11-4, cont'd Clinical pathway: bipolar affective disorder. (Copyright 1994, Gina Bufe.)

9. Promote self-care activities, such as bathing, dressing, feeding, and grooming, *to establish the client's level of functioning and increase self-esteem.*
10. Assist the client in establishing daily goals and expectations *to promote structure and direction and minimize cognitive difficulties.*
11. Plan self-care activities around those times when the client has more energy *to increase activity tolerance and minimize fatigue.*
12. Reduce choices of clothing, activities, and tasks and increase choices as the client improves cognitively *to make decision making easier and minimize stress.*
13. Assess the client's cognitive/perceptual process *to ascertain the existence of hallucinations/delusions that are troubling or harmful for the client.*
14. Assist the client in identifying negative, self-defeating thoughts and modifying them with realistic thoughts *to promote more accurate, positive thoughts about self, others.*
15. Encourage the client to attend therapeutic groups that provide feedback regarding thinking *to reframe thinking with the support of others* (see Chapter 23).
16. Provide simple, clear directives/communication in a low-stimulus environment *to assist with focus, attention, and concentration with minimal distractions.*
17. Teach the client and significant others about the disorder and treatment when the client is able to learn *to increase knowledge, promote adherence to treatment, and minimize guilt about the disorder.*
18. Gradually increase levels of activity and exercise *to minimize fatigue and increase activity tolerance.*
19. Identify sources of external stress and assist the client in coping with them in a more effective manner *to minimize stressors and promote adaptive coping mechanisms.*
20. Establish limits with clients with mania in a firm, consistent, and caring way *to provide acceptable boundaries for behavior.*
21. Teach the client and significant others how to self-manage their illness at home, including identifying prodromal (early) symptoms, seeking help, and implementing appropriate strategies *to prevent or minimize recurrent episodes.*

Additional Treatment Modalities

Psychopharmacology

Although there is no "cure," since the 1950s there have been major advances in the use of medications to treat the symptoms of mood disorders. Investigation of the neurobiology of depression and mania has provided directions for development of these new medications. In addition to a focus on the effects of antidepressants on neurotransmitters, research suggests that these medications produce changes in gene expression and neuroplasticity (Yamada et al., 2005). Because there are multiple types of medications that seem to work with various individuals and their types of depression and mania, selecting the drug and the dosage that is effective for any individual is often a difficult process. Nurses need to explain to clients that some individuals do not respond to the first or even second medication prescribed but that most people do find a medication that works well for them.

MEDICATION KEY FACTS
Adjustment Disorders

Pharmacologic interventions for adjustment disorders are symptom oriented to treat symptoms that may cause clinically significant functional impairment. Medications prescribed include antianxiety drugs, antidepressants, and occasionally antipsychotics.

There are various types of antidepressant medications used to treat persons with episodes of major depression and some persons with dysthymia. These include tricyclics, heterocyclics, MAOIs, SSRIs, and most recently joint serotonin and norepinephrine reuptake inhibitors (NSRIs). These medications have powerful effects not only on mood but also on the entire syndrome of depression symptoms, including the neurovegetative symptoms. Not surprisingly, medications also cause side effects that create discomfort and even danger. Taken in large quantities, many are toxic or even lethal. In addition, these medications usually have a lag period of 1 to 6 weeks for initiation of therapeutic effects, during which time the side effects are often the most pronounced. As the medication begins to exert its therapeutic effect, the side effects often diminish. The nurse needs to be aware that a time for higher suicide risk is within several weeks after the client has started an antidepressant. In view of data regarding the recurrent nature of depression and how it impairs functioning over time, many clients are now taking these medications for years, or for an entire lifetime. Debate continues about the safety, benefits, and problems associated with taking antidepressants during pregnancy.

Mood stabilizers are effective in treating mania in clients with bipolar disorders. The primary, most widely used mood stabilizer is lithium. Lithium acts as a salt within the body, and its blood levels are closely linked to the client's hydration and sodium intake. Side effects of lithium include neuromuscular and central nervous system effects (tremor, forgetfulness, slowed cognition), gastrointestinal effects (nausea, diarrhea), weight gain and hypothyroidism, and renal effects (polyuria). Nurses monitor blood levels to ensure an adequate, but not toxic, level. Usually, blood levels of 0.6 to 1 mEq/L are appropriate for maintenance therapy, whereas in the treatment of acute mania, levels of up to 1.5 mEq/L are necessary. The therapeutic-range blood level for lithium is narrow; toxicity can occur quickly and is evidenced by vomiting, oversedation, ataxia, and, finally, seizures. Lithium blood levels over 1.5 mEq/L are toxic. Lithium is excreted through the kidneys, so nurses need to use caution with clients with renal disease. Warn clients taking lithium to use diuretics only with extreme caution and under close supervision, because diuretics elevate lithium blood levels quickly. Changes in hydration through perspiration, vomiting, and restricted fluid intake promote elevated lithium levels and toxicity.

MEDICATION KEY FACTS Depressive Disorders

CYCLIC ANTIDEPRESSANT

Selective Serotonin Reuptake Inhibitors (SSRIs)

Citalopram (Celexa), fluoxetine (Prozac), paroxetine (Paxil), sertraline (Zoloft), venlafaxine (Effexor)

- First-line antidepressant therapy.
- May cause fatal reaction with MAOIs causing serotonin syndrome, hypertensive crisis, rigidity, and neuroleptic malignant syndrome (NMS).
- A life-threatening condition called *serotonin syndrome* can occur when medicine used to treat migraine headaches (5-hydroxytryptamine receptor agonists [triptans]) and medicines used to treat depression (SSRIs and SNRIs) are used together.
- Episodes of self-harm and potential suicidal behavior reported higher in patients under age 18.
- *Herbal considerations:* St. John's wort and SAM-e may cause serotonin syndrome.

Atypical New-Generation Antidepressant

- May cause fatal reaction with MAOIs causing NMS, serotonin syndrome, autonomic instability.
- Elderly are more sensitive to the drug's anticholinergic, cardiovascular, and sedative effects.
- *Herbal considerations:* St. John's wort and SAM-e may increase risk for serotonin syndrome.

SPECIFIC ATYPICAL NEW GENERATION ANTIDEPRESSANTS

Selective Serotonin Norepinephrine Reuptake Inhibitors (SNRIs)

Venlafaxine (Effexor), duloxetine (Cymbalta)

- Indicated for social anxiety disorder and general anxiety disorder.
- Venlafaxine is not approved for indications in children and adolescents because of the lack of efficacy and concerns about increased hostility and suicide ideation.

Norepineprine Dopamine Reuptake Inhibitors (NDRIs)

Bupropion (Wellbutrin)

- Second-line agent in cases of SSRI or SNRI treatment resistant depression (bupropion).
- Wellbutrin-SR and Zyban indicated for smoking cessation.
- *Herbal considerations:* Ephedra may cause hypertensive crisis.

Serotonin-2 Antagonist/Reuptake Inhibitors (SARIs)

Trazodone (Desyrel)

- May increases risk for hypertensive crisis with MAOIs.

Noradrenergic/Specific Serotonergic Antidepressants (NaSSAs)

Mirtazapine (Remeron)

- Poses a higher risk of seizures than tricyclic antidepressants (mirtazapine).
- MAOIs may increase the risk of hyperpyretic crisis, hypertensive episodes, and severe seizures.
- Episodes of self-harm and potential suicidal behaviors reported in patients under age 18.

NONSELECTIVE CYCLIC AGENTS

Tricyclic Antidepressants (TCAs)

Amitriptyline (Elavil), clomipramine (Anafranil), imipramine (Tofranil), desipramine (Norpramin), doxepin (Sinequan), nortriptyline (Aventyl)

- MAOIs may increase the risk of NMS, seizures, hypertensive crisis, and hyperpyresis.
- *Herbal considerations:* St. John's wort and SAM-e may increase risk for serotonin syndrome.

Monoamine Oxidase Inhibitor Agents (MAOI)

Phenelzine (Nardil), tranylcypromine (Parnate), selegiline transdermal patch (Emsam)

- MAOIs are prescribed as third-line agents after SSRI or TCAs have been tried.
- Signs of toxicity include increased headache and palpitations.
- MAOIs should not be used within 14 days of taking SSRIs.
- Avoid anticholinergics, anesthetics, amphetamines, appetite suppressants, nasal decongestants, antihypertensives, CNS depressants, sympathomimetics, cyclic and newer antidepressants as it may increase hyperpyretic crisis, seizures, hypertensive episode, or serotonin syndrome. Some over-the-counter cough and cold medications contain sympathomimetics; it is prudent to consult the pharmacist when purchasing over-the-counter medicines.
- *Herbal considerations:* Parsley and St. John's wort pose risk for serotonin syndrome.
- *Dietary considerations:* Avoid caffeine, chocolate, and all tyramine-containing foods (such as aged cheese), within several hours of ingestion as it may cause sudden, severe hypertension or hypertensive crisis.

NEW AGENT: SELEGILINE TRANSDERMAL SYSTEM (EMSAM)

- A patch version of a monoamine oxidase inhibitor for adults with major depression.
- *Dietary considerations:* No tyramine dietary modifications needed at 6 mg per 24 hours as monoamine oxidase activity in the digestive system is not affected. Higher doses increase risk for hypertensive crisis, and tyramine-containing foods and beverages should be restricted.

Anticonvulsants are now often being prescribed for mood stabilization. These medications, including carbamazepine, valproate, gabapentin, and lamotrigine, are used when the client is unable or unwilling to take lithium or when other medications have been ineffective. In many settings, anticonvulsants are the drugs of choice for mood stabilization. Lamotrigine is especially promising because research indicates that it is useful as a mood stabilizer, particularly with clients experiencing bipolar depression that has been difficult to treat.

Other medications prescribed for clients during episodes of depression or mania include benzodiazepines, on a time-limited basis for associated anxiety symptoms, sedative-hypnotics or trazodone for sleep regulation, and antipsychotics for relief from hallucinations, delusions, and extremely agitated behavior. Although antidepressants and mood stabilizers assist with minimizing and regulating symptoms related to anxiety and sleep, their therapeutic effects take longer to occur than the other medications mentioned here.

Although physicians or advanced practice nurses prescribe medications, the nursing care related to administration of psychopharmacologic agents is extensive. The nurse needs to understand the mechanisms of action, dosages (therapeutic), side effects, and self-care considerations of each medication. This enables the nurse to explain the

MEDICATION KEY FACTS Bipolar Disorders

MOOD STABILIZERS

- Pharmacologic treatment for acute mania in bipolar disorder to include lithium, carbamazepine, divalproex, and lamotrigine.
- Second-generation (atypical) antipsychotics are approved for treatment of acute bipolar mania and olanzapine indicated to treat acute bipolar depression (see Chapter 12 for Medication Key Facts related to antipsychotics).
- Antidepressants are typically used only in combination with other medications because of the risk for switching into mania or accelerating the rate of mood cycling.
- Antidepressants (citalopram, fluoxetine, paroxetine, bupropion, venlafaxine) are also indicated to treat acute bipolar depression. Clonazepam (benzodiazepine) is used for treatment or adjunct therapy for treatment of acute mania (see Chapter 9 for Medication Key Facts related to benzodiazepines).

Lithium Salts

Lithium carbonate (Lithotabs, Eskalith, Lithobid)

- Require therapeutic drug monitoring to prevent toxicity. Therapeutic serum level is 0.6-1.2 mEq/L; toxic serum level is greater than 1.5 mEq/L.
- A lithium serum concentration of 1.5-2.0 mEq/L may produce vomiting, diarrhea, drowsiness, confusion, incoordination, coarse hand tremor, muscle twitching, and T-wave depression on ECG.
- Acute toxicity may be characterized by seizures, oliguria, circulatory failure, coma, and death.
- *Herbal considerations:* Dandelion, goldenrod, juniper, and parsley increase lithium effects and toxicity.
- *Dietary considerations:* Monitor sodium intake as significant changes will alter lithium excretion. Black/green tea, coffee, cola nut, guarana, plantain, yerba maté may decrease lithium levels.

ANTICONVULSANTS

Divided into three classes (first, second, and third generation) and indicated for manic symptoms.

First-Generation Anticonvulsants

Klonopin (Clonazepam) (see Chapter 9 for Medication Alerts related to benzodiazepines)

Second-Generation Anticonvulsants

Carbamazepine (Tegretol), valproic acid (Depakene), divalproex sodium (Depakote)

- Require therapeutic serum level (50-100 mcg/ml; toxic serum level is >100 mcg/ml).
- Toxic reactions include blood dyscrasias.
- Do not use together with MAOIs; may cause fatal reactions (seizures and hypertensive crisis).
- *Herbal considerations:* Gingko and quinine increases anticonvulsant action.
- *Dietary considerations:* Grapefruit and grapefruit juice may increase the absorption and blood concentration of carbamazepine.

Third-Generation Anticonvulsants

Gabapentin (Neurontin), topiramate (Topamax), lamotrigine (Lamictal), oxcarbazepine (Trileptal)

- Gabapentin (Neurontin) has been found to be ineffective for treatment of bipolar disorders.
- Abrupt withdrawal of these drugs may increase seizure frequency.
- Use caution with lamotrigine, especially in children for potentially life-threatening rash (Stevens-Johnson syndrome); slow titration of dosage is warranted.
- *Herbal considerations:* Ginkgo increases anticonvulsant effect, and ginseng and santonica decrease effects.

medication to clients and observe for intended and unintended effects. Through teaching clients more about their medications, the nurse promotes and encourages adherence to the treatment plan and the minimization of negative effects. Clients are able to discuss their concerns and to make informed decisions about their treatments.

Many of these medications require special considerations that clients need to understand to ensure efficacy and safety. Because many clients discontinue their antidepressants and mood stabilizers too early or do not take them as prescribed, nurses need to emphasize the importance of staying on the medication to prevent relapse, recurrence, and continuation of changes in the brain. Nurses teach clients specific self-care activities associated with medication, such as the required dietary restrictions for MAOIs, precautions regarding hydration and salt intake for lithium, and management of anticholinergic effects of the tricyclics. The Client and Family Teaching Guidelines boxes on p. 238 present teaching plans for clients taking SSRIs and lithium, respectively.

Biologic Intervention

Electroconvulsive Therapy. Electroconvulsive therapy (ECT) involves the use of electrically induced seizures to treat severe depression or, less frequently, intense mania

CLINICAL ALERT

Serotonin syndrome is an idiosyncratic medication reaction with a fairly rapid onset that occurs with excessive accumulation of serotonin (5HT1A). In depressed clients, serotonin syndrome results from high doses or concurrent use of such medications as serotonin reuptake inhibitors (including tricyclic antidepressants), serotonin precursors (e.g., L-tryptophan), serotonin agonists (e.g., buspirone), MAOIs, or other medications that influence serotonin levels (e.g., cold or allergy preparations, cocaine, lithium, ginseng, or St. John's wort). Risk factors include genetic predisposition (MAO activity), acquired disorders (liver, pulmonary, or cardiovascular disease), or iatrogenic situation (medications). At least three of the following symptoms contribute to the diagnosis: mental status changes, agitation, myoclonus, hyperreflexia, fever, diaphoresis, ataxia, or diarrhea. Symptoms also include abdominal pain, elevated blood pressure, tachycardia, irritability, hostility, increased motor activity, or mood change. Severe reactions manifest as high fever, cardiovascular shock, or death. Early identification is important. The nurse will obtain a full history of all medications being taken (including over the counter); instruct patients and families to report immediately any subtle changes of confusion, unusual behavior, or agitation; and monitor vital signs carefully. If a nurse suspects serotonin syndrome, the nurse will discontinue the medications and notify the physician.

CLINICAL ALERT

Clients need to avoid *foods* containing tyramine while taking MAOI antidepressants *to prevent* **hypertensive crisis.** These include avocados; yogurt; aged cheese; smoked or pickled fish, meat, or poultry; processed meats; yeast; overripe fruit; chicken or beef liver pate; red wine; beer; liqueurs; and fava beans. Foods to use in moderation include caffeine beverages, cottage and cream cheese, soy sauce, chocolate, and sour cream. *Medications* to avoid include over-the-counter cough and cold medicines, appetite suppressants, muscle relaxants, allergy remedies, hay fever remedies, narcotics, analgesics, and several prescription medications. The nurse needs to ask the client to contact the physician or nurse *before* taking any over-the-counter medication. Tell client to avoid common cold remedies and diet medications.

CLIENT and FAMILY TEACHING GUIDELINES

Serotonin Selective Reuptake Inhibitors

TEACH THE CLIENT

- The purpose of SSRIs is to treat depression. The medication alters brain nerve cells, thus increasing the availability of serotonin. A deficiency of serotonin in the brain is possibly related to the onset of depression.
- It is important to take the medication as prescribed; changing the dosage or missing a dose will prevent it from helping the depression.
- Common side effects of SSRIs include nausea, increased anxiety, and insomnia. These side effects often diminish once the medication begins to exert its therapeutic effect.
- Sexual side effects, including delayed ejaculation, impotence, or anorgasmia, are not uncommon. Discuss any such difficulties with your health care provider before making any medication changes on your own.
- The medication usually does not immediately improve symptoms of depression. It usually takes 1 to 6 weeks before you feel the effects of the medication. At first, you will still feel depressed but will have more energy and look less depressed. These medications often work from the outside inward.
- The medication needs to be taken as prescribed, even after you feel better. It needs time to have positive effects on the brain that will minimize the chances for future episodes of depression.

CLIENT and FAMILY TEACHING GUIDELINES

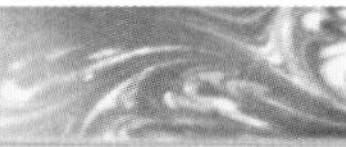

Lithium

TEACH THE CLIENT

- Lithium is a mood stabilizer for persons with mania and depression.
- Lithium alters brain neurotransmission, changes cell membrane function, and inhibits release of thyroid hormone. It is not clear how lithium specifically stabilizes mood.
- Before starting lithium, health care providers will perform laboratory tests to ensure adequate functioning of the heart, kidneys, thyroid gland, and electrolytes.
- It is important to take lithium daily as prescribed to maintain a steady blood level of the medication. Do not take extra doses to make up for missed doses.
- Lithium sometimes takes a week to begin working and to develop a steady blood level. Your health care provider will have you get your blood drawn to check lithium blood levels. Blood for the lithium level must be drawn about 12 hours after the last dose of lithium (e.g., if you take your dose at 8 PM, your blood level must be drawn at 8 AM).
- Common side effects of lithium include increased urine output, increased thirst, fine tremors, muscle weakness, nausea, weight gain, and diarrhea.
- Lithium levels can be increased rapidly, leading to toxicity. Signs of toxicity include nausea and vomiting, marked tremors, muscle weakness, muscle twitching, lack of coordination, sluggishness and drowsiness, confusion, seizures, and coma. Toxicity can occur as blood levels rise above 1.5 mEq/L.
- It is important to maintain a stable blood level of lithium. Do not change the amount of sodium (salt) in your diet, because decreasing salt will increase the amount of lithium in the blood.
- Any activity or situation that affects your fluid and salt intake or output will change the level of lithium in your blood. Exercise, sunbathing, and vomiting are examples of situations in which you lose salt and fluid, increasing your lithium level. It is important to contact your health care provider if you believe that your lithium level changed or if you experience any side effects or early toxic signs.
- Other drugs can affect your lithium level. Medications (e.g., diuretics, ibuprofen, verapamil) can raise lithium levels. Be sure to check with your health care provider before taking any new prescribed or over-the-counter medications.
- Lithium causes birth defects if taken during the first trimester of pregnancy. Tell your health care provider if you intend to become pregnant or are pregnant.

not controlled with lithium or antipsychotics. Although scientists introduced ECT in the 1930s, its use decreased after the discovery of antidepressants and lithium. Procedures have been developed for ECT that make it a safe and effective treatment for many individuals who have not achieved a treatment response with medication or other types of treatment. Researchers do not know how ECT alleviates depression and mania, but they believe it is related to the alteration of neurotransmission. A more complete discussion of ECT is presented in Chapter 23.

Transcranial Magnetic Stimulation. Transcranial magnetic stimulation is an intervention currently being investigated for its antidepressant effects. It is a noninvasive procedure in which an electromagnet is placed on the scalp. Electrical current is generated by rapid pulsing in the magnetic field, causing the cortical neurons to depolarize. Although the specific mechanisms involved in its antidepressant effect remain unclear, this intervention increases monoamine concentrations in the brain when used repetitively. Initial research has been encouraging with respect to its effects with unipolar depression (Fitzgerald et al., 2006; George et al., 1999).

Vagal Nerve Stimulation. Vagal nerve stimulation is one development for the treatment of depression. A device called the vagal nerve stimulator device is implanted in the left chest wall under the collarbone and electrically stimulates the vagus nerve. Research is trying to determine the effectiveness of this treatment for major depressive disorder, although early findings are promising (George et al., 2006; Hammerly, 2001).

Deep Brain Stimulation. In this treatment, an electrode is inserted deep into the brain and an electrical current stimulates the brain. The application of this treatment to mood disorders is recent and current research examines its use with clients with treatment-resistant depression (George et al., 2006).

Phototherapy. Seasonal affective disorder (SAD) is a type of mood disorder, and its features are in the DSM-IV-TR classification. Phototherapy is one type of treatment that has effectively lessened symptoms of this recurrent, seasonal disorder. The exact mechanism of action remains unclear, although researchers believe that exposure to morning light causes a circadian rhythm shift (phase advance) that regulates the normal relationships between sleep and circadian rhythms and ultimately affects mood regulation.

Clients are referred for phototherapy after a careful and complete psychiatric history that documents the occurrence of SAD. Phototherapy consisting of a minimum of 2500 lux is usually administered on waking in the morning. Clients sit or lie in front of the light box for 30 minutes to several hours, depending on the strength of the light source. An antidepressant effect usually occurs within 2 to 4 days and is complete after 2 weeks. Maintenance therapy consists of sitting in front of the lights for about 30 minutes each day. Side effects are rare, although some clients do report irritability, headaches, or insomnia. Phototherapy is not effective for everyone with a diagnosis of SAD; some fail to respond, and others experience only a partial response. Because phototherapy requires a large amount of time each day, research is in progress that examines alternative methods to acquire the additional light, including the use of light visors and lights that shine onto the bed in early morning before awakening (Hammerly, 2001).

Alternative and Complementary Therapies

Natural and alternative remedies for illness have become popular. Nurses need to be knowledgeable about approaches such as exercise, homeopathy, and massage (Zahourek, 2000). Persons frequently turn to health food stores for vitamins and other supplements, yet there is minimal evidence about the effects of these products on depression and mania. Some have claimed that St. John's wort, believed to change serotonin levels, has antidepressant effects. Research has not consistently supported this result. In fact, St. John's wort is not recommended for severe depression or bipolar disorder and sometimes causes serotonin syndrome when taken with other medications that increase serotonin levels (Hammerly, 2001). SAMe (S-adenosylmethionine) is also possibly a natural antidepressant, making brain cells more responsive to neurotransmitters and showing clinical effectiveness in alleviating postpartum depression. However, SAMe triggers manic episodes in some individuals with bipolar disorder (Hammerly, 2001; Murray, 2002). Fish oils, also known as omega-3 fatty acids, do appear to affect health, including alleviating depressive symptoms and promoting cardiovascular health (Murray et al., 2002). More research is necessary on the effectiveness, long-term effects, and drug interactions of these natural supplements. Because these substances are available over the counter as food products rather than as medications, concern also exists about quality control in their preparation, purity, and dosing accuracy. As more people seek alterative and complementary approaches to their health care, it is important that nurses ask clients about their use of such products, as natural supplements interact with prescribed medications and influence medication response. Also see Chapter 25 for additional information.

Family Intervention

Mood disorders affect the entire family, not just the client who is experiencing the depression or mania. Most often the family or significant others become known to the nurse during the client's acute episode of depression or mania. Conflicts and communication problems, which existed in the family network before the onset of the episode, intensify, and the usual role functioning is disrupted.

Nurses in both the hospital and community interact with the client's family, who often appreciate the opportunity to vent feelings of confusion, anger, concern, or frustration. Teaching family members about the client's disorder, especially the biologic nature of the disorder, allows them to rethink the situation and minimize blame on the client. Many are relieved to hear that their loved one's behavior can be explained and is manageable. They also find it helpful to know that the client's behavior (e.g., irritability, inability to accept love, and negativity) is not a personal offence to other family members but is part of the symptomatology of depression or mania. Nurses run family education groups in the hospital and in the community, inviting family and clients to learn more about the disorder and its impact on the family.

Nurses also work together with other mental health professionals, including advanced practice nurses, regarding assessing the need for family therapy. Nurses observe client-family interactions, listen to their concerns, and identify potential problem areas. Nurses make referrals for marital therapy or family therapy.

Interventions that include preparing the family for a client's discharge from the hospital facilitate the client's return to functioning in the community. Data suggest that even after symptoms stop, the client who has experienced affective episodes continues to have difficulty in his or her interpersonal and occupational functioning (Greden, 2001; Klerman and Weissman, 1992).

Group Intervention

Group intervention provides multiple benefits to clients with mood disorders, including socialization, education about their disorder and more useful coping mechanisms, the opportunity to vent feelings, the establishment of personal goals, and the realization that others have similar problems. These benefits help reduce isolation and hopelessness. Nurses assess clients' ability to participate in groups based on their behavior, mental status, psychologic readiness in view of the nature of the particular group, and physiologic status. For example, clients with mania who are hyperactive and extremely agitated are not able to focus on the group discussion and become overstimulated and disruptive in the group. Some clients with severe depression with psychomotor retardation and cognitive impairment have a difficult time and become overwhelmed by a formal group. Certain types of groups (e.g., a unit community meeting or activities groups) are less structured and less imposing to clients than formal group therapy.

In addition to assessing clients' readiness for groups, nurses encourage their attendance at the appropriate functions. Some clients need to be directed with statements such as "It's time for group now. I'll walk there with you." Others require only encouragement or reminders.

Nurses who are qualified conduct groups along with other nurses or therapists. Nurses initiate and lead groups such as social skills training and educational groups. Clients often need to discuss their experiences and reactions after the completion of a group. Nurses listen, allow clients to ventilate feelings, and reinforce the new insights or perceptions that clients experience.

Psychotherapeutic Intervention

Although the effectiveness of antidepressant and mood-stabilizing medications is undisputed, psychotherapeutic interventions are also important in the treatment of mood disorders. Psychopharmacologic agents pose a number of problems for many clients. These medications often have major side effects that create discomfort, interfere with usual functioning, and promote noncompliance. Alternative treatment is necessary for the 20% to 30% of persons with mood disorders who do not respond to medications. Also, although mood disorders represent alterations in neurobiologic functioning, numerous psychologic, social, and interpersonal issues that require psychotherapeutic intervention are associated with episodes of depression and mania.

Types of psychotherapy that have been used to treat mood disorders and associated psychosocial issues include cognitive therapy, behavioral therapy, interpersonal relationship therapy, and psychodynamic therapy. Although each of these differs with respect to the underlying theoretic framework, goals, and approach, there are some commonalities. Therapeutic success is related to several factors: the nature of the relationship between the therapist and client; the provision of understanding, support, help, and hope; the establishment of a framework for understanding and interpreting clients' problems; and the provision of an opportunity to explore and try out new coping strategies.

Cognitive Therapy. Cognitive therapy, as outlined by Beck (1967), addresses systematic errors in the client's thinking that maintain negative cognitive processing. The goal of the therapy is to identify underlying cognitive schemata and specific cognitive distortions. Schemata are internal models of the self and the world that individuals use to perceive, code, and recall information. Nurses ask clients to identify their automatic thoughts, silent assumptions, and random inferences so that they are able to examine negative thoughts and assumptions logically. This helps the client challenge these thoughts against realistic attributes and subsequently validate or refute them.

Cognitive therapy has been effective in treating outpatients with unipolar mild to moderate depression. In studies that have investigated the effectiveness of medication versus cognitive therapy, findings indicate that both appear to be equally effective for outpatients with depression and often provide some modest gain when used in combination (Scott, 1996). In addition, the use of cognitive therapy also increases the rate of symptom improvement in depression, although longer term follow-up studies fail to find differences over time. Researchers have not completely explored the use of cognitive therapy with inpatients experiencing severe depression, although there are indications that it is useful for symptom reduction (Hollon et al., 2002).

Behavioral Therapy. Behavioral therapy, often used in conjunction with cognitive therapy for treating mild to moderately depressed outpatients, is an effective treatment for depression, comparing favorably with medication and cognitive therapy. There is less information about its usefulness with persons experiencing mania.

The behavioral approach is based on learning theory. Abnormal behaviors such as the symptoms of depression and mania represent behaviors acquired as a result of aversive (negative) environmental events. Positive environmental responses to the maladaptive behaviors or avoidance of negative consequences reinforce these. The behavioral therapist works with clients to determine specific behaviors to modify and to identify the factors that evoke and reinforce these behaviors. Using role modeling, role playing, and situational analysis, nurses assist clients in learning and practicing different adaptive behaviors that bring positive environmental reinforcement. The therapy is not concerned with understanding underlying issues or pathopsychology; it is concerned only with those behaviors that are changeable. Behavioral therapy has several advantages (e.g., shorter treatment duration than other types of therapy, focus on specific behaviors to modify) and is applicable to various types of clients.

Interpersonal Therapy. The therapist using interpersonal therapy views depression as developing from pathologic, early interpersonal relationship patterns that continue to be repeated in adulthood. The emphasis is on social functioning and interpersonal relationships, with particular emphasis on the milieu, or the environment. Life events, including change, loss, and relationship conflict, trigger earlier relationship patterns, and the client experiences a sense of failure, decreased importance, and loss. The goal of the therapy is to understand the social context of current problems based on earlier relationships and to provide symptomatic relief by solving or managing current interpersonal problems. The client and therapist select one or two current interpersonal problems and examine new communication and interpersonal strategies for managing relationships more effectively.

Interpersonal therapy is often effective for clients with mild to moderate depression, although there is no indication that it is more effective than other types of psychotherapy. Some research suggests that when used in combination with medications, interpersonal therapy helps clients stick to medication treatment and lengthens the time between the recovery period and recurrence of a major depression episode (Klerman, 1992; Frank et al., 1991).

Psychodynamic Therapy. Psychodynamic therapy comes from Freud's psychoanalytic model (see Chapter 23). Depression is a result of early childhood loss of a love object and ambivalence about the object; projection of anger onto the ego, resulting in blockage of the libido (sex drive); and unresolved intrapsychic conflict during the oral or anal stage of psychosexual development. Thus, these damage self-esteem, and the person repeats the primary loss pattern throughout life. Through the relationship with the therapist, the client uncovers repressed past experiences, experiences a catharsis or a release of feelings, confronts defenses, interprets current behavior, and works through early loss and cravings for love.

Scientists have not fully researched the effect of psychodynamic psychotherapy on depression or mania. Many have modified techniques used in this therapy over time, and there have been problems with standardizing the approach for research purposes. For some clients, psychodynamic psychotherapy assists in developing insights that promote behavioral change. Many clients, including those with severe depression, however, are unable or unmotivated to participate in this type of therapy and, for some, problems such as self-care deficits, psychomotor retardation, and fatigue take priority.

Self-Management Intervention

In the current health care environment with fewer financial resources and difficulty with access to health care, more and more clients have to self-manage their chronic illnesses. Self-management type approaches for chronic illnesses such as asthma and cardiac disease have reduced health care costs and improved longer term health outcomes (Clark et al., 2001). There is little documentation of specific interventions to teach and help clients and their families to better manage their mood disorder on an ongoing, daily basis. Related research has shown that depression management and relapse prevention strategies, including extra visits with a depression specialist and telephone follow-up calls, result in greater adherence to antidepressant medication regimens and fewer depressive symptoms (Katon et al., 2001). Pollack (1996) described the ways in which persons with bipolar disorder self-manage their illness and noted that professionals need to better understand these strategies to assist clients in using them and preventing relapse.

Nurses have a major role in educating clients with mood disorders about their illness and helping them to develop strategies for ongoing management of the disorder and its impact on their lives. Nurses are able to teach clients self-management strategies such as identifying early symptoms of recurrence (see the Research for Evidence-Based Practice box), problem solving about potential options for intervention, and building a collection of self-management strategies for times of increased stress and potential recurrence.

The keys to treatment of adjustment disorders are support and normalization. Patterns of treatment often follow the guidelines available for use with crisis intervention (see Chapter 20). Patients need to feel that support is

RESEARCH for EVIDENCE-BASED PRACTICE

Hagerty BM, Williams RA, Liken M: Prodromal symptoms of recurrent major depressive episodes: a qualitative analysis, *American Journal of Orthopsychiatry* 67:308, 1997.

Hagerty, Williams, and Liken (1997) conducted a qualitative study to determine clients' experiences with onset of symptoms in recurrent depression. They conducted four focus groups with 16 persons who had at least three well-documented episodes of major depression. The focus groups were audiotaped and videotaped, and results were transcribed for analysis. Using phenomenologic analysis, the researchers identified themes in the focus group content. Results showed that participants experienced distinct phases as they were entering a recurrent episode of depression. These phases were termed, "Something's not right," "Something's really wrong," "the Crash," and "Connection." Participants reported that sometimes these phases occurred over a short period of time (days), whereas sometimes they were more insidious. Participants agreed that once they experienced "the crash," descending into the acute depressive episode, it was too late to initiate activities to prevent the episode. All participants reported occurrence of a "prodromal" phase of symptom onset in which specific signs and symptoms in patterns unique to them. Many of these early signs and symptoms were different than those listed as DSM criteria for diagnosing depression. Based on study results, the researchers theorized that persons with recurrent depression often did have a prodromal phase in which early signs and symptoms were identifiable; clients learned to monitor for and recognize these early signs, make judgments about their depression, and initiate strategies to prevent or minimize the oncoming episodes.

available to help sort out their feelings, options, and resources. At the same time, they need to learn that it is normal for people to have difficulty dealing with stressful situations and that they have the capacity to learn new ways of coping more effectively.

In a randomized controlled study of individuals on a first-time sick leave for adjustment disorder, researchers tested a three-stage intervention model (van der Klink et al., 2003). The first stage consisted of psychoeducation, helping patients to understand the source of their stress and loss of control. Nondemanding daily activities were encouraged. In the second stage, patients drew up a list of stressors and developed problem solving responses to each. In the third stage, patients practiced their problem-solving strategies and initiated more demanding activities. Throughout the intervention, the patients' personal responsibility in recovery was emphasized. As compared with a control group who received "usual" care, significantly more of the intervention group had returned to work after 3 months. Sick leave was shorter for the intervention group, and the incidence of recurrence was lower. Both the control and intervention groups experienced a similar decrease of symptoms. Van der Klink and van Dijk (2003) concluded that treatment of adjustment disorders needs to include stress inoculation training (using the stages described identified here), relaxation training, cognitive restructuring, and a gradual resumption of activities within specific time frames.

The treatment of adjustment disorders for children and adolescents includes additional methods. Family therapy addresses tension between family members. Some parents need assistance to understand the child's view of the stressor. Individual therapy helps to identify the meaning of the stressor for the child or adolescent. Brief, focused, and time-limited therapy concentrates on teaching relaxation techniques and cognitive problem solving. Group or classroom interventions are also helpful. The purpose of treatment for children and adolescents is to support existing coping strategies and teach new ones appropriate to the developmental stage of the patient.

The use of medications for the treatment of adjustment disorders is also controversial. Many clinicians believe that adjustment disorders will remit on their own or with only supportive brief psychotherapy. Some maintain that medicating the problem deprives people of the opportunity to learn how to cope with stressful situations. The exception is the adjustment disorder with depressed mood. One retrospective study compared the response to antidepressants (SSRIs) of patients with major depression and patients with adjustment disorder in the primary care setting. Both groups achieved a similar clinical response, but patients with adjustment disorder had twice the response rate of patients with major depression (Hameed et al., 2005). The researchers concluded that antidepressant therapy provides an effective treatment for adjustment disorder with depressed mood. Initially, limited use of antianxiety medications may be necessary.

Although adjustments disorders are time limited and transient, hospitalization is sometimes necessary if a patient reports suicidal ideation or behavior. Estimates of suicidality are varied and contradictory. By one report, the rate of suicidal behavior was around 4%, less than for depression or dysthymia. By another report, suicidal behavior was present in 78% of adults and 89% of adolescents with adjustment disorders. However, even with this latter report hospitalization was brief. A 5-year follow-up of patients diagnosed with adjustment disorder demonstrated that 2% had committed suicide (Casey, 2001). In short, although nurses need to address and respond to the presence of suicidal ideation, the risk is less when compared with another Axis I disorder.

The prognosis for individuals with adjustment disorders is positive. In comparison with mood disorders, one study reported that individuals with adjustment disorders tended to require less treatment, were able to return to work sooner, and were less likely to experience a recurrence. Whereas the hospital admission rate for adjustment disorders is higher than for dysthymia or anxiety disorders, the readmission rate has been significantly lower than for major depression, dysthymia, or anxiety disorders (Jones et al., 2002). At the end of the treatment, it is important that the patient express the absence of thoughts to harm self or others. A plan of action for addressing the current stressor, as well as strategies for coping with new stressors, will inoculate the patient against a recurrence of the adjustment disorder.

EVALUATION

Nurses evaluate clients' progress by measuring their achievement of identified outcomes. Nurses collect data that support or refute achievement of outcomes from personal observations, clients, clients' family and friends, and other health care providers. Evaluation occurs throughout hospitalization, and often community mental health providers continue evaluation after clients have been discharged. Nurses working in community settings, such as psychiatric home care, sometimes evaluate outcomes for clients who have never been admitted to an inpatient setting.

With decreasing lengths of stay in hospitals, nurses in inpatient psychiatric units do not always see dramatic changes in clients' symptoms. However, they do see some clear progress related to priority short-term outcomes such as absence of imminent suicidal intent, a plan for addressing the potential return of suicidal ideation after discharge, and the ability to conduct self-care activities. Nurses also observe some alleviation of the neurovegetative symptoms of depression (sleep, loss of appetite, fatigue, psychomotor retardation), alleviation of the severe hyperactive behavior of mania, improvement in cognitive functioning and communication, and initial understanding of the disorder and its treatment, including necessary self-care management. In this setting, nurses make referrals to therapists, psychiatrists, home care and community

Text continued on p. 245

NURSING CARE PLAN

Kayla is a 49-year-old married female, mother of two teenagers, who had seven previous episodes of major depression, with the most recent 2 years ago. She comes to the mental health clinic with the following signs and symptoms: crying for no apparent reason, sad mood, irritability, inability to concentrate that interferes with her secretarial job, extreme fatigue, self-blame for being a "bad mother," inability to attend to her children, loss of appetite, inability to make meals, lying on the couch for hours at a time, and loss of 12 pounds in the past 6 weeks. She has not showered in 10 days and her hair appears unbrushed and greasy. Kayla sleeps only 3 hours each night. Her continuing thoughts of driving her car off a bridge frighten her. She had two previous suicide attempts. One was during her most recent depression in which she overdosed on aspirin. She was originally prescribed Prozac, and she reports it "helped slightly." During her previous episode, venlafaxine (Effexor) 200 mg daily was prescribed with good results. Six months after starting the Effexor, she stopped the medication. Kayla reports that she has had marital difficulties over the past year, and recently her 15-year-old son was arrested for possession of marijuana. She reports a history of migraine headaches that are controlled with Midrin as needed. Kayla appears fatigued and is dressed casually in rumpled jeans and a blouse. She is admitted to the psychiatric inpatient unit.

DSM-IV-TR Diagnoses

Axis I	Major depressive disorder: recurrent, severe
Axis II	Deferred
Axis III	History of migraine headaches
Axis IV	Marital difficulties; son's legal and drug problems
Axis V	GAF = 30 (current); GAF = 70 (past year)

Nursing Diagnosis *Risk for suicide. Risk factors: past suicide attempts; suicidal thoughts; self-deprecating thoughts; severely depressed mood; inability to contract for safety; reduced coping ability and coping skills, loss of energy and will to live; migraine headaches, as evidenced by verbalizing not wanting to live; blaming self for being a "bad mother"; refusing food; sleep deprivation; messy appearance; and neglecting home, job, and family*

NOC Risk Detection, Risk Control, Impulse Self-Control, Suicide Self-Restraint, Depression Level, Mood Equilibrium, Social Support, Will to Live

NIC Suicide Prevention, Mood Management, Impulse Control Training, Environmental Management: Safety, Patient Contracting, Therapy Group, Coping Enhancement

CLIENT OUTCOMES	NURSING INTERVENTIONS	EVALUATION
Kayla will remain free from self-harm while on the unit and after discharge.	Conduct suicide risk assessments with Kayla while hospitalized and initially at home. *Early comprehensive assessment of self-harm or assault risk will prevent harm or injury.* Maintain safe hospital environment by frequent observation of client and removing dangerous objects. Intervene with hospital approved suicide prevention procedure, such as medication, seclusion or restraint, if other less restrictive interventions fail to maintain the client's safety. *Safety is the highest priority in client care.*	Kayla expressed feeling safer and exhibited no self-harm.
Kayla will contract for safety and will verbalize any suicidal thoughts or feelings to health care providers or adult family members.	Encourage Kayla to verbalize all suicidal thoughts to health care provider or to adult family member. Assist Kayla to sign a contract to refrain from hurting self. *Verbal and written expression of intent to remain safe, reinforce client commitment to safety.*	Kayla discussed her thoughts and feelings with nurses and family. She expressed relief that family still cared about her and wanted to help.
Kayla will discuss feelings and thoughts, reasons for living, and express hopefulness about the future.	Encourage Kayla to express all feelings and thoughts. *Expression provides relief from pent-up feelings or guilt and assists client to problem solve.* Assist Kayla to verbalize reasons for living *to help client focus on healthy aspects of her life.*	Kayla described her thoughts and feelings to staff and voiced relief and hopefulness about the future.
Kayla will use cognitive restructuring techniques to increase positive thinking patterns and reduce cognitive (thought) distortions.	Assist Kayla to identify distorted thinking patterns. Role-play thought stopping and thought substitution techniques. *Cognitive restructuring techniques help client to change negative thought patterns by replacing negative thoughts with realistic ones.*	Kayla was able to identify distorted thinking and negative thoughts and begin to replace those with realistic thoughts.
Kayla will participate in her treatment, including taking medications as prescribed.	Describe benefits of treatment and actions and side effects of medications to Kayla and family and the importance of staying on the medications as prescribed. *Client adherence increases when they understand benefits of the treatment program and taking medications.* Encourage family to assist Kayla to take medication when at home and monitor for drug admixtures. *Family involvement increases success of medication regimen.*	Kayla attended scheduled activities and followed treatment plan including medications, voicing the importance and rationale for both.

Nursing Diagnosis *Ineffective coping related to suicidal thoughts, depressed mood, fatigue, sleep deprivation, and inability to concentrate, as evidenced by inability to work or care for home and family, lying on couch for hours at a time, not eating or sleeping, and neglecting to bathe or groom*

NOC Suicide Self-Restraint, Depression Self-Control, Coping, Decision-Making, Sleep, Knowledge: Health Resources, Role Performance, Self-Esteem, Quality of Life

NIC Behavior Management: Self-Harm, Mood Management, Coping Enhancement, Decision-Making Support, Sleep Enhancement, Support System Enhancement, Therapy Group

Continued

NURSING CARE PLAN—cont'd

CLIENT OUTCOMES	NURSING INTERVENTIONS	EVALUATION
Kayla will verbalize her need for ongoing professional help.	Encourage Kayla to verbalize thoughts and feelings related to her illness, condition, and family and work situation. *Expression provides relief and beginning of problem solving.*	Kayla expressed concern over inability to function and take care of family and welcomed the assistance.
Kayla will actively participate in the prescribed treatment program including medications.	Administer medications and monitor client's adherence.	Kayla took medications as prescribed.
	Reinforce Kayla's attendance and participation in therapeutic activities. *Assistance by the nurse reinforces the importance of treatment adherence.*	Kayla attended group and other unit activities.
Kayla will demonstrate problem-solving strategies to help manage her problems.	Help Kayla to establish realistic goals, break down complex goals into small manageable steps, identify and develop strengths, discuss strategies to manage parenting responsibilities, ask for help when needed. *Techniques and strategies are tools that guide progress toward wellness.*	Kayla established goals for her recovery and identified strategies to achieve those goals. She identified her strengths to help in her recovery. With her husband's help, she developed strategies to use when interacting with her teenagers and their problems.

Nursing Diagnosis *Self-care deficit (bathing/hygiene, dressing/grooming) related to depressed mood and fatigue secondary to major depression, as evidenced by disheveled appearance and lack of attention to bathing and grooming*

NOC Self-Care: Bathing, Self-Care: Hygiene, Self-Care: Dressing, Self-Care: Activities of Daily Living, Psychomotor Energy, Motivation, Client Satisfaction: Physical Care

NIC Bathing, Dressing, Caregiver Support, Energy Management, Self-Responsibility Facilitation, Self-Esteem Enhancement

CLIENT OUTCOMES	NURSING INTERVENTIONS	EVALUATION
Kayla will bathe daily and dress herself in clean clothes.	Offer client assistance as needed, and encouragement to bathe and dress in fresh clothes. Provide articles for grooming (e.g., using soap, shampoo, deodorant). *Severely depressed clients frequently require help with grooming, but the activity often improves mood and initiates an increase of function.*	Kayla successfully initiated and maintained bathing and grooming.

NURSING CARE PLAN

Ryan is a 45-year-old insurance salesman. He is married, but separated, and has two children. He was diagnosed with bipolar disorder when he was 23 years old. He has a college degree in business and functions well between episodes of his illness. Over the past month, Ryan became increasingly hyperactive, starting new projects every day but not completing any, such as painting the garage, setting up a mail-order business for his insurance company, and writing stories he plans to publish. He has been calling his clients trying to sell them additional insurance, and he becomes angry with them when they decline. He plans to risk investing his life savings to open multiple offices for his business and hiring 10 to 15 new employees. He currently earns no income and has spent much of his savings account. He sleeps only 3 hours a night and is unable to sit still for a full meal or even stand still to drink a beverage. Ryan exhibits flight of ideas; his thoughts come quickly with minimal connection between them. His speech is rapid, and verbalization is difficult to follow. His wife left him, citing his irritability, angry outbursts, and lack of financial responsibility. Ryan has been visiting bars, picking up women, and having unprotected sex that resulted in genital herpes. He stopped taking his lithium 2 months ago. Ryan's friend and his parents brought him to the psychiatric emergency room.

DSM-IV-TR Diagnoses

Axis I	Bipolar I disorder: manic episode
Axis II	Deferred
Axis III	Sexually transmitted disease (genital herpes)
Axis IV	Marital stress; financial difficulty
Axis V	GAF = 25 (current); GAF = 75 (past year)

Nursing Diagnosis *Disturbed thought processes related to ineffective processing and synthesis of stimuli (secondary to brain chemistry changes in bipolar mania) and exaggerated responses to psychosocial stressors (secondary to bipolar mania), as evidenced by flight of ideas, grandiosity, initiating multiple simultaneous projects, poor judgment and insight, and intrusion in others' lives*

NOC Personal Safety Behavior, Distorted Thought Self-Control, Cognition, Information Processing, Communication, Medication Response, Safe Home Environment

NIC Environmental Management: Safety, Behavior Management: Overactivity/Inattention, Reality Orientation, Delusion Management, Mood Management, Medication Management

CLIENT OUTCOMES	NURSING INTERVENTIONS	EVALUATION
Ryan will communicate using logical and appropriate language and controlled speech (rate, tone, amount).	Actively listen and calmly respond to Ryan. *Shows respect for client and encourages him to express concerns in interactive process.* Demonstrate appropriate role modeling. *Helps to promote change by examples.*	Day 1: Ryan's speech was rapid, pressured, and demanding. Day 3: Ryan quietly and appropriately communicated with clients and staff.
Ryan will refrain from being intrusive, impulsive, and grandiose; he will use appropriate language; and he will engage in appropriate physical activities.	Instruct Ryan to think before interrupting. *Assists client to curb impulsivity.*	Ryan responded to staff approach by controlling outbursts and speaking appropriately by the end of the second day.
	Redirect behaviors in calm, firm, nondefensive manner by suggesting a walk, or other activity. *Provides healthy channels for excess energy and impulses and prevents escalation of behavior.*	Ryan used suggestions for engaging in activities and demonstrated behavioral control by the second day.
	Praise client for all attempts to use socially appropriate language and behaviors. *Provides positive feedback, promotes expected behaviors, and increases self-esteem.*	Ryan apologized for being out of control and thanked staff for helping him maintain his behavior.
Ryan will demonstrate accurate interpretation of self and the environment.	Teach Ryan to correct misinterpretations using problem solving and recalling actual events. *Promotes client's reality orientation.* Accept client's need to hold onto false beliefs while not agreeing with delusions. *Builds trust and maintains client's dignity.*	Day 1: Ryan continued to express grandiose delusions.
	Tell Ryan to notify staff when troubling thoughts occur. *Helps client to break illogical thought patterns. Assistance from staff reinforces client's efforts.*	Day 3: Ryan engages staff in discussions about his thinking and is increasingly logical.
	Encourage Ryan to stay involved in the milieu and real events. *Reinforces reality.*	Day 5: Absence of delusional thinking. Ryan engages in milieu activities.
Ryan will actively participate in his treatment plan, including medication, and will involve family in his care, as appropriate.	Administer mood stabilizing medications and monitor Ryan's symptoms. *Maintenance of effective medication regimen helps to reduce manic symptoms.*	Day 1: Ryan reluctantly took medications, stating, "I don't need anything but myself to get better." Day 3: Ryan displays calmer speech and behavior.
	Encourage Ryan to attend scheduled activities and groups. Engage family in client's care. *Family awareness of client's problems results in more effective responses and interactions.*	Day 5: Ryan attended all groups, stating logical thoughts and goals. He agrees to include family in treatment plan.

mental health agencies, and partial hospitalization programs for continued care in the community.

Nurses working with clients in the community see improvement in longer term outcomes such as improved socialization, return to usual activities, reduction in negative thinking, increased self-esteem, and the use of new coping strategies. Nurses also see improvement in areas such as resumption of family/work roles, continued improvement in cognitive processes (e.g., attention and concentration), decreased or absence of fatigue, and adherence to treatment plans. For some clients, these outcomes become evident within weeks of starting psychotherapy or somatic treatment regimens. For others, improvement requires months before clients achieve longer term outcomes. Data suggest that return to previous levels of functioning after an episode of depression takes longer than previously thought, particularly if clients have had multiple episodes (Greden, 2001; Klerman and Weissman, 1992).

Clients with mania present a unique evaluative situation, because episodes of mania are often followed by episodes of depression. Therefore, although clients have returned to a hypomanic or euthymic state at the time of hospital discharge, nurses must be alert to any indications of depression. Careful follow-up monitoring after discharge into the community is imperative for clients with bipolar disorders.

CHAPTER SUMMARY

- Mood disorders are a major public health problem, and depression is the fourth leading cause of "burden," including morbidity and mortality, in the world.
- Major depression is currently occurring at younger ages, and those most at risk are women with a family history of mood disorders.
- Mood disorders are usually recurrent and require lifelong management. Manifestations and treatment concerns vary across the life span.
- Two broad types of mood disorders include unipolar depressive and bipolar disorders.
- Multiple theories, including biologic, ethologic, cognitive, psychodynamic, and personality theories, attempt to explain mood disorders. Theories for etiology of

mood disorders are multiple, including a genetic, biologic predisposition for risk.

- Mania and depression are manifested by symptoms involving the affective, cognitive, physical, social, and spiritual aspects of the individual.
- Mania and depression occur in any setting and not only in psychiatric units.
- Comorbidity between medical and mood disorders is high.
- The nursing care of persons experiencing depression or mania consists of thorough assessment and subsequent planning and interventions for a range of nursing diagnoses related to physical, psychosocial, and spiritual needs.
- Nurses collaborate with other mental health care providers for care related to somatic, family, and group interventions.
- Adjustment disorders are passing episodes of clinically significant emotional or behavioral nonpsychotic symptoms in response to identifiable psychosocial stress or stressors. Symptoms develop within 3 months after the stressful event.
- The diagnosis of adjustment disorder means the client's behaviors or symptoms are different from usual patterns of response and the symptoms have persisted for less than 6 months (acute), unless symptoms are in response to an ongoing stressor or stressors (chronic).
- The severity of the reaction to the stressor is not predictable from the stressor and is unique to the individual.
- Clients with adjustment disorder are often treated as outpatients because the severity of their symptoms or subjective distress does not require inpatient hospitalization.
- Supportive psychotherapy is the most frequently used treatment method with clients with adjustment disorders.
- Attempting to understand the client's experience from his or her point of view fosters the therapeutic process.

REVIEW QUESTIONS

1 A client says to the nurse, "I had my first depression after my father died about 10 years ago, but I didn't get any treatment. Now it seems even little life events cause me to get depressed again." Which theory of neurotransmission may explain this client's complaint?

1. Stress increases the activity of monoamine oxidase.
2. Dysfunctional grieving inhibits metabolism of serotonin.
3. Prolonged grief depletes neuronal supplies of G-proteins.
4. Kindling may alter neuronal cell structure and function.

2 Which individual has the highest risk for major depression?

1. 8-year-old girl
2. 16-year-old boy
3. 35-year-old woman
4. 60-year-old man

3 A nurse assesses an elderly person for depression. Select the best question for the nurse to ask.

1. "How do you compare your activities and health now to 6 months ago?"
2. "Would you say you are currently having a major depressive episode?"
3. "What is your family history related to depressive illnesses?"
4. "Are you having crying spells every day?"

4 A nurse prepares the plan of care for a person having a manic episode. Which nursing diagnosis is most likely to apply? You may select more than one answer.

1. Imbalanced nutrition: more than body requirements
2. Sleep deprivation
3. Risk for deficient fluid volume
4. Social isolation
5. Disturbed thought processes

5 A client says to the nurse, "Life doesn't have any joy in it anymore. Things I once did for pleasure aren't fun." How would the nurse document this complaint?

1. Dysthymia
2. Anhedonia
3. Euphoria
4. Psychomotor retardation

6 A client with an adjustment disorder participates in a series of outpatient therapy sessions. The goals of the therapy are stress inoculation and assisting the client with self-management. Place these statements by the nurse in the correct sequence for this treatment modality.

1. "Let's talk while you make a list of the biggest problems in your life and discuss some possible solutions for each problem."
2. "Choose one problem-solving technique to decide how to handle arguments with your spouse."
3. "The purpose of our group today is to understand stressful events and how they affect one's abilities to manage life."

Additional self-study exercises and learning resources are available to you on the ***Companion CD*** *at the back of the book and on the* ***Evolve website*** *at* ***http://evolve.elsevier.com/Fortinash/.***

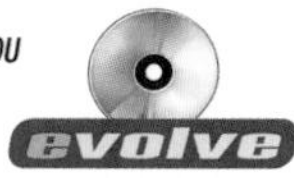

ONLINE RESOURCES

American Association of Suicidology: **www.suicidology.org**

American Foundation for Suicide Prevention: **www.afsp.org**

Child and Adolescent Bipolar Foundation: **www.bpkids.org**

Depression and Bipolar Support Alliance: **www.dbsalliance.org**

National Alliance on Mental Illness: **www.nami.org**

National Institute of Mental Health: **www.nimh.nih.gov**

Mental Health America: **www.nmha.org**

National Suicide Prevention Lifeline: **www.suicidepreventionlifeline.org**

Suicide Prevention Resource Center: **www.sprc.org**

REFERENCES

Abramson LY, Seligman MEP, Teasdale JD: Learned helplessness in humans: critique and reformulation, *Abnorm Psychol* 87:49, 1978.

Alexopoulos GS et al: Assessment of late life depression, *Biol Psychiatry* 52:164, 2002a.

Alexopoulos GS et al: Clinical presentation of the "depression-executive dysfunction syndrome" of late life, *Am J Geriatric Psychiatry* 10:98, 2002b.

American Psychiatric Association: *Diagnostic and statistical manual of mental disorders*, ed 4, text revision. Washington, DC, 2000, American Psychiatric Association.

Angelino AF, Treisman GJ: Management of psychiatric disorders in patients infected with human immunodeficiency virus, *Clin Infect Dis* 33:847, 2001.

Barnow S et al: The importance of psychosocial factors, gender, and severity of depression in distinguishing between adjustment and depressive disorders, *J Affect Disorders* 72:71, 2002.

Barondes S: *Mood genes: hunting for the origins of mania and depression*, New York, 1998, WH Freeman.

Beck AT: *Depression: clinical, experiential, and theoretical aspects*, New York, 1967, Hober.

Bohachick P et al: Social support, personal control, and psychosocial recovery following heart transplantation, *Clin Nurs Res* 11:34, 2002.

Bowlby J: *Attachment and loss*. vol. 1: *attachment*, New York, 1969, Basic Books.

Brown GW, Harris T: *Social origins of depression*, New York, 1978, The Free Press.

Casey P: Adult adjustment disorder: a review of its current diagnostic status, *J Psychiatr Pract* 7:32, 2001.

Casey P, Dowrick C, Wilkinson G: Adjustment disorders: fault line in the psychiatric glossary, *Br J Psychiatry* 179:479-481, 2001.

Chemerinski E, Robinson RG, Kosier JT: Improved recovery in activities of daily living associated with remission of poststroke depression, *Stroke* 32:113, 2001.

Clark NM, Gong M, Kaciroti N: A model of self-regulation for control of chronic disease, *Health Educ Behav* 24:28, 2001.

Consensus Development Panel: Mood disorders: pharmacological prevention of recurrences, *Am J Psychiatry* 142:469, 1985.

Eisch AJ et al: Brain-derived neurotrophic factor in the ventral midbrain-nucleus accumbens pathway: a role in depression, *Biol Psych* 54:994, 2003.

Fergusson DM, Woodward LJ: Mental health, educational, and social role outcomes of adolescents with depression, *Arch Gen Psychiatry* 59:225, 2002.

Fitzgerald PB et al: A randomized, controlled trial of sequential bilateral repetitive transcranial magnetic stimulation for treatment-resistant depression, *Am J Psychiatry* 163:88, 2006.

Frank E et al: Efficacy of interpersonal psychotherapy as a maintenance treatment of recurrent depression, *Arch Gen Psychiatry* 48:1053, 1991.

Freud S: Mourning and melancholia. In *The complete psychological works of Sigmund Freud*, London, 1957, Hogarth Press.

Gagnon LM, Patten SB: Major depression and its association with long-term medical conditions, *Can J Psychiatry* 47:149, 2002.

George MS, Lisanby SH, Sackeim HA: Transcranial magnetic stimulation: applications in neuropsychiatry, *Arch Gen Psychiatry* 56:300, 1999.

George MS et al: Vagus nerve stimulation and deep brain stimulation. In *Textbook of mood disorders*, Arlington, Va, 2006, American Psychiatric Association.

Gillespie CF, Nemeroff CB: Early life stress and depression, *Curr Psychiatry*, 4:15, 2005.

Greden JF: *Recurrent depression*, Washington, DC, 2001, American Psychiatric Publishing.

Gupta A, Bhatia S: Depression in Parkinson's disease, *Clin Gerontol* 22:59, 2000.

Hagerty BM, Williams RA, Liken S: Prodromal symptoms of recurrent major depressive episodes: a qualitative analysis, *Am J Orthopsychiatry* 67:308, 1997.

Hameed U et al: Antidepressant treatment in the primary care office: outcomes for adjustment disorder versus major depression, *Ann Clin Psychiatry* 17:77, 2005.

Hamet P, Tremblay J: Genetics and genomics of depression: a review, *Metab Clin Exp* 54:10, 2005.

Hammerly M: *Depression. How to combine the best of traditional and alternative therapies*, Avon, Mass, 2001, Adams Media.

Hankin BL, Abramson LY: Development of gender differences in depression: an elaborated cognitive vulnerability-transactional stress theory, *Psych Bulletin* 127:773, 2001.

Hirschfeld RMA et al: The National Depressive and Manic-Depressive Association consensus statement on the undertreatment of depression, *JAMA* 277:333, 1997.

Hirshfeld-Becker DR et al: Temperamental correlates of disruptive behavior disorders in young children: preliminary findings, *Biol Psychiatry* 51:563, 2002.

Holmes T, Rahe R, The social readjustment rating scale, *Jr Psychosomatic Res* 12:213, 1967.

Hollon SD, Haman KL, Brown LL: Cognitive-behavioral treatment of depression. In Gotlib IH, Hammen CL, editors: *Handbook of depression*, New York, 2002, Guilford Press.

Horwath E et al: Depressive symptoms as relative and attributable risk factors for first onset major depression, *Arch Gen Psychiatry* 49:817, 1992.

Johnson JG et al: Hopelessness as a mediator of the association between social support and depressive symptoms: findings of a study of men with HIV, *J Consult Clin Psychol* 69:1056, 2001.

Jones R, Yates WR, Zhou MH: Readmission rates for adjustment disorders: comparison with other mood disorders, *J Affect Disorders* 71:199, 2002.

Katon W et al: A randomized trial of relapse prevention of depression in primary care, *Arch Gen Psychiatry* 58:241, 2001.

Kendler KS: Twin studies of psychiatric illness: an update, *Arch Gen Psychiatry* 58:1005, 2001.

Kendler KS et al: The identification and validation of distinct depressive syndromes in a population-based sample of female twins, *Arch Gen Psychiatry* 53:391, 1996.

Kendler KS et al: A Swedish national twin study of lifetime major depression, *Am J Psychiatry* 163:109, 2006.

Kendler KS, Karkowski LM, Prescott CA: Causal relationship between stressful life events and the onset of major depression, *Am J Psychiatry* 156:837, 1999.

Kendler KS, Thornton LM, Gardner CO: Stressful life events and previous episodes in the etiology of major depression in women: an evaluation of the "kindling" hypothesis, *Am J Psychiatry* 157:1243, 2000.

Kendler KS, Thornton LM, Prescott CA: Gender differences in the rates of exposure to stressful life events and sensitivity to their depressogenic effects, *Am J Psychiatry* 158:587, 2001.

Kessler RC et al: The epidemiology of major depressive disorder, *JAMA* 289:3095, 2003.

Klerman GL, Weissman MM: The course, morbidity, and costs of depression, *Arch Gen Psychiatry* 49:831, 1992.

Kraepelin E: *Manic-depressive insanity and paranoia*, Edinburgh, UK, 1921, E&S Livingstone.

Kuehner C: Gender differences in unipolar depression: an update of epidemiological findings and possible explanations, *Acta Psychiatr Scand* 108:163, 2003.

Leonhard K: Aufteilung der endogenen Psychosen. Cited in Buher J: *Depression: theory and research*, New York, 1974, Winston Wiley.

Lewinsohn PM et al: Age cohort changes in the lifetime occurrence of depression and other mental disorders, *J Abnorm Psychiatry* 102:110, 1993.

Malkoff-Schwartz S et al: Social rhythm disruption and stressful life events in the onset of bipolar and unipolar episodes, *Psychol Med* 30:1005, 2000.

Mufson L et al: A randomized effectiveness trial of interpersonal psychotherapy for depressed adolescents, *Arch Gen Psychiatry* 61:577, 2004.

Murr C, Ledochowski M, Fuchs D: Chronic immune stimulation may link ischemic heart disease with depression, *Circulation* 105:83, 2002.

Murray CJL, Lopez AD: Alternative projections of mortality and disability by cause 1990-2020: global burden of disease study, *Lancet* 349:1498, 1997.

Murray M: *The pill book guide to natural medicines*, New York, 2002, Bantam.

Nesse RM: Evolutionary biology: a basic science for psychiatry, *World Psychiatry* 1:7, 2002.

Papadopoulos FC et al: Prevalence and correlates of depression in late life: a population-based study from a rural Greek town, *Intl J Geriatr Psychiatry* 20:350, 2005.

Pelkonen M et al: Suicidality in adjustment disorder: clinical characteristics of adolescent outpatients, *Eur Child Adolesc Psychiatry* 14:174, 2005.

Perlis RH et al: Clinical features of bipolar depression versus major depressive disorder in large multicellular trials, *Am J Psychiatry* 163:225, 2006.

Pollack LE: Inpatient self-management of bipolar disorder, *Appl Nurs Res* 9:71, 1996.

Post RM: Transduction of psychosocial stress in the neurobiology of recurrent affective disorders, *Am J Psychiatry* 149:999, 1992.

Ravindran AV et al: Stress, coping, uplifts, and quality of life in subtypes of depression: a conceptual frame and emerging data, *J Affect Disord* 71:121, 2002.

Regenold WT et al: Increased prevalence of type 2 diabetes mellitus among psychiatric inpatients with bipolar I affective and schizoaffective disorders independent of psychotropic drug use, *J Affect Disord* 70:19, 2002.

Righette-Veltema M et al: Postpartum depression and mother-infant relationship at 3 months old, *J Affect Disord* 70:291, 2002.

Rush AJ et al: Comorbid psychiatric disorders in depressed outpatients: demographic and clinical features, *J Affect Disord* 87:34, 2005.

Sapolsky RM: Glucocorticoids and hippocampal atrophy in neuropsychiatric disorders, *Arch Gen Psychiatry* 57:925, 2000.

Schmaling K, Becker J: Empirical studies of the interpersonal relations of adult depressives. In Becker J, Kleinman D, editors: *Psychosocial aspects of depression*, Hillsdale, NJ, 1991, Erlbaum.

Scott J: Cognitive therapy of affective disorders: a review, *J Affect Disord* 37:1, 1996.

Seligman MEP: *Helplessness: on depression development and death*, New York, 1975, WH Freeman.

Sharma P et al: Depression among hospitalized medically ill patients: a two-stage screening study, *J Affect Disord* 70:205, 2002.

Solberg LI, Trangle MA, Wineman AP: Follow-up and follow-through of depressed patients in primary care: the critical missing components of quality care, *J Am Board of Fam Practice* 18:520, 2005.

Steffens DC et al: Sociodemographic and clinical predictors of mortality in geriatric depression, *Am J Geriatr Psychiatry* 10:531, 2002.

Strik JJM et al: Clinical correlates of depression following myocardial infarction, *Int J Psychiatry Med* 31:255, 2001.

Struder HK, Weicker H: Physiology and pathophysiology of the serotonergic system and its implications on mental and physical performance: part I, *Intl J Sports Med* 22:467, 2001.

Tateno A, Kimura M, Robinson RG: Phenomenological characteristics of poststroke depression, *Am J Geriatr Psychiatry* 10:575, 2002.

Van den Berg MD et al: Depression in later life: three etiologically different subgroups, *J Affect Disord* 65:19, 2001.

van den Bree MB, Owen MJ: The future of psychiatric genetics: a review, *Ann Med* 35:122, 2003.

Van der Klink JJL et al: Reducing long term sickness absence by an activating intervention in adjustment disorders: a cluster randomized controlled design, *Occup Environ Med* 60:429, 2003.

Van der Klink JJL, van Dijk FJH: Dutch practice guidelines for managing adjustment disorders in occupational and primary health care, *Scand J Environ Health* 29:478, 2003.

Watson PJ, Andrews PW: Toward a revised evolutionary adaptationist analysis of depression: the social navigation hypothesis, *J Affect Disord* 72:1, 2002.

Yamanda M, Yamanda M, Higuchi T: Antidepressant-elicited changes in gene expression: remodeling of neuronal circuits as a new hypothesis for drug efficacy: a review, *Progress in Neuro-Psychopharmacol Biol Psychiatry* 29:999, 2005.

Young EA et al: HPA axis activation in major depression and response to fluoxetine: a pilot study, *Psychoneuroendocrinology* 29:1198, 2004.

Zahourek R: Alternative, complementary, or integrative approaches to treating depression, *J Am Psychiatric Nurs Assoc* 6:77, 2000.

Chapter 12

Schizophrenia and Other Psychotic Disorders

DIANE L. PAVALONIS

If a man does not keep pace with his companions, perhaps it is because he hears a different drummer.

HENRY DAVID THOREAU

OBJECTIVES

1. Identify the various theories and models explaining schizophrenia that have evolved over time.
2. Relate the significance of the biologic theory and its current role in the development of schizophrenia.
3. Discuss advancements in research that link genetic factors to schizophrenia.
4. Compare and contrast the course of illness, symptoms, and nursing interventions for the subtypes of schizophrenia and for associated disorders such as schizoaffective disorder.
5. Apply the nursing process to clients experiencing the positive, negative, cognitive, and depressive symptoms of schizophrenia.
6. Assess the situation of persons with schizophrenia and their families in the community.
7. Develop nursing care plans for prevention, aftercare, and psychoeducation for clients and families.
8. Evaluate the effectiveness of the various treatment modalities for schizophrenia in the clinical setting.

KEY TERMS

affect, p. 251
ambivalence, p. 251
anhedonia, p. 250
apathy, p. 250
autistic thinking, p. 251
avoliton, p. 250
cognitive symptoms, p. 250
delusion, p. 251
depressive symptoms, p. 250
dereism, p. 251
echolalia, p. 259
echopraxia, p. 259
hallucination, p. 251
loosening of associations, p. 251
negative symptoms, p. 250
paranoia, p. 250
perseveration, p. 266
positive symptoms, p. 250
poverty of thought, p. 250
premorbid phase, p. 257
prodromal phase, p. 257
psychotic phase, p. 257
residual symptoms, p. 260
thought blocking, p. 251

Schizophrenia is one of the most complex and debilitating mental disorders. It is not a single disorder, but a syndrome (group of diseases), with a wide range of severity and symptoms among individuals. It is a brain disease because symptoms occur from a number of factors that affect the brain's neurotransmitter system resulting in impaired thoughts, perceptions, cognitive functions, mood, and motivation (Sadock et al., 2004). Schizophrenia is a universal disorder that exists in all cultures and in all socioeconomic groups (National Institute of Mental Health [NIMH], 2005). It is often called a psychotic disorder meaning that people with schizophrenia have periods when they lose touch with reality and exhibit various kinds of psychotic symptoms. All symptoms of schizophrenia are debilitating, but not all symptoms are psychotic. The symptoms seem to come from different mechanisms, perhaps because different brain regions or circuits are affected. Therefore, symptoms respond to a variety of psychosocial and psychopharmalogic treatments discussed in this chapter and in Chapters 23 and 24 (Lieberman, 2006b).

Symptoms of schizophrenia are divided into four main groups:

1. **Positive symptoms** are psychotic symptoms, often called *florid symptoms* because of their dramatic nature. They include the presence of unusual sensations and perceptions such as hallucinations (false perceptions), delusions (false beliefs), **paranoia** (irrational suspicion), bizarre (odd or eccentric) behavior, and confused or obsessive thoughts that seem to return periodically, usually provoked by a variety of stressors. Because of the acute (sudden) onset of positive symptoms and their obvious detachment from reality, they grab our attention the most. Long-term studies and treatments, however, indicate that these florid, dramatic symptoms may not be as debilitating as the negative symptoms described next. Positive symptoms generally respond favorably to hospitalization, medication, reduced stimuli, and interactive therapy (Lewis and Lieberman, 2000).
2. **Negative symptoms** are more complex and difficult to treat and are present in all phases of the illness. They include **apathy** (indifference), withdrawal, **avolition** (lack of motivation), blunted or flat affect (reduced emotional expression), loss of warmth or vibrancy, **poverty of thought** (absent or reduced thoughts), and **anhedonia** (loss of pleasure in things previously enjoyed). They are not as obvious as positive symptoms and their onset is insidious (slow), but they may be more debilitating in the long run because of their paralyzing effect on the person's thoughts, emotions, and motivation (Beng-Choon et al., 2004). The persistence of negative symptoms can immobilize these individuals, making it difficult for them to relate to others in normal social situations. They tend to miss common social cues that most of us take for granted (Lieberman, 2006b). Negative symptoms have a poor response to the older, typical antipsychotics and may worsen when these drugs are used to treat the positive symptoms, making medication compliance an issue for client and family (Thornton et al., 2001a). Newer, atypical antipsychotic drugs, however, have promised better results for negative symptoms (see Chapter 24).
3. **Cognitive symptoms** are believed to be central to disturbed behaviors and functional disabilities and affect 40% to 60% of persons with schizophrenia. They include impaired memory (mainly working memory), inability to maintain attention over time, and disturbances in executive functioning (planning, organizing, reasoning, abstract thinking, and problem solving). The cognitive symptoms of impaired memory, inattention, and disturbances in executive functioning seem to be associated with the negative symptoms of apathy, poverty of thought, and avolition. Both sets of symptoms make it difficult for individuals to care for self, live independently, hold a job, or maintain a social life. Individuals with good verbal memories are better able to learn and retain the cognitive and social skills necessary to live a more productive life within the limitations of their illness (Beng-Choon et al., 2004) (see Chapter 15).
4. **Depressive symptoms** include anxiety, dysphoria (anguish), and irritability, and co-occur often in schizophrenia (see Chapter 11). These symptoms contribute to the 10% lifetime incidence of suicide in persons with schizophrenia (Lewis and Lieberman, 2000); 20% to 40% of individuals with schizophrenia attempt suicide at least once during their illness. Many suicides occur during periods of remission (when symptoms are reduced), after 5 to 10 years of living with this devastating illness (American Psychiatric Association [APA], 2004). Also, schizophrenia often coexists with drug dependence (alcohol, nicotine, cannabis, and cocaine, and medical conditions such as obesity and type 2 diabetes mellitus). Mortality caused by natural and unnatural causes is considerable, and the projected life span for people with schizophrenia is about 15 years less than the general population (Sullivan, 2005).

Symptoms of schizophrenia negatively affect all areas of the person's ability to function as a productive member of society, and the burden on the family and the community is enormous.

Schizophrenia has "ebbs and flows," meaning there are periods of relapse when symptoms are most obvious and periods of remission when symptoms are reduced. Persons who are treated, therefore, may not show obvious, positive signs of the disorder such as hallucinations or delusions. If negative symptoms are present, we may view apathy as shyness, lack of motivation as laziness, withdrawal as rudeness, poverty of thought as ignorance, and poor grooming as sloppiness, all of which add to the stigma of schizophrenia. The following examples describe behaviors that indicate the presence of schizophrenia in people in the community (Maguire, 2002):

- The unkempt middle-aged woman talking to herself while pushing a shopping cart filled with objects that look like junk to us but have special meaning for her
- The young man with a disheveled look cursing to himself and frantically searching for cigarettes in the gutter

These individuals may have other problems as well, including drug or alcohol abuse, mood disorders, and malnutrition. Many of them, however, are also struggling with untreated schizophrenia, and they represent that group of unfortunate individuals who cannot get the help they need to treat their mental illness. They are generally left alone to wander aimlessly until they commit a crime or social injustice that brings them to the attention of the psychiatric or legal system. They may then be hospitalized or jailed for a time, receiving treatment randomly, until they are once again released to the streets. Their families and friends have long since abandoned them, and with no support system and no insurance, prospects for recovery present special challenges (see Chapter 29).

For other more fortunate individuals who receive treatment early in the course of schizophrenia and have a strong support network, there is hope, if not yet a cure. For example, there is a young first-year college student with a strong familial history of schizophrenia experiencing his first psychotic break. He tried to kill both parents with a knife, believing they were plotting against him. With newer medications and early interventions, this young adult will probably be able to manage his symptoms of *paranoid schizophrenia* and possibly finish college. This is a very different outcome from what might have happened in the past, when people with schizophrenia were institutionalized for many years. Today, most people with schizophrenia are living in community settings.

Despite their prevalence, chronicity, and pervasive symptoms, the schizophrenias did not have the benefit of a scientific, biologic approach until the mid-nineteenth century. The research supporting the relationship of these complex disorders with the structure and function of the brain has produced more effective treatments and outcomes that one hopes will continue to improve in the years ahead. Also, advancements in genetic research are helping scientists to understand how specific genes relate to the cause, pathophysiology, and treatment of schizophrenia, offering even more promise in the next decade (National Institute of Mental Health, 2005; Sullivan, 2005).

HISTORIC AND THEORETIC PERSPECTIVES

From a historical perspective, schizophrenia was described as a complex, multifaceted disorder that goes beyond the hallucinations, delusions, or decreased motivation and drive that are most commonly associated with it (Sadock et al., 2004; Maguire, 2002). Until recently, science knew little about the cognitive function of the brain. The term *schizophrenia* has described this type of mental disorder only since the 1800s (Sadock et al., 2004).

In the late 1800s, prominent psychiatrist Emil Kraepelin (1856-1926) identified the cognitive impairment of schizophrenia (memory impairment); at the same time, he labeled the disorder *dementia praecox*. This term referred to the psychosis that ended in severe intellectual deterioration (dementia) and that had a premature (praecox) onset (Emery, 2004). Dementia praecox has two hallmark symptoms:

Hallucination, a subjective sensory-perceptual disorder involving all of the five senses, most commonly the auditory type. For example, a person hears voices criticizing him or commanding him to act when no actual presence exists.

Delusion, a fixed belief held by the individual that does not change with reason or logic (APA, 2004). For example, a person believes he is being followed by the CIA or that he is a famous historical figure or a fictional character.

A condition known as **dereism** often precedes these symptoms. Dereism is a loss of connection with reality and logic, where thoughts become private and idiosyncratic (odd or peculiar). The person also often experiences **thought blocking**, which is an abrupt blocking of the flow of thoughts or ideas.

BOX 12-1

Bleuler's Four As: Fundamental Symptoms of the Thought Disorder

- **Affect**: Observable, outward, bodily expression of emotions such as joy, sorrow, and anger. *Blunted affect*: Restricted expression of emotions. *Flat affect:* Lack of expression of emotions. *Inappropriate affect*: Affect that does not match the emotion being felt (e.g., laughing when sad). *Labile affect*: Rapid changes in emotional expression.
- **Autistic thinking**: Disturbances in thought resulting from the intrusion of a private fantasy world that is internally stimulated, resulting in abnormal responses to people and events in the real world.
- **Ambivalence**: Simultaneously holding two different attitudes, emotions, thoughts, or feelings about a person, object, or situation.
- **Loosening of associations** (LOA): Thought disturbance in which the speaker rapidly changes from one subject to another in an unrelated, fragmented manner.

From Sadock BJ, Kaplan HI, Sadock VA: *Kaplan and Sadock's comprehensive textbook of psychiatry*, ed 8, 2005, Lippincott Williams & Wilkins.

At about the same time, renowned Swiss psychiatrist Eugene Bleuler (1857-1939) identified the four As of schizophrenia as *autism*, *ambivalence*, and disturbances in affect and *associations* (loosening of associations [LOA]) (Maguire, 2002; Sadock et al., 2004) (Box 12-1). Bleuler also was the first to coin the term *schizophrenia*, which means "split mindedness." According to historical sources, the word comes from the Greek *skhizo* (split) and *phren* (mind). It is this meaning that is possibly responsible for confusing the disorder of schizophrenia with *dissociative identity disorder*, or multiple personality disorder, in which the personality "splits" off into different parts (see Chapter 13). In schizophrenia Bleuler saw the split as an inconsistency between emotion, thought, and behavior, with the personality remaining intact. Bleuler was also the first to redefine schizophrenia as a thought disorder, which is a more refined and accurate description (Maguire, 2002).

As mentioned earlier, hallucinations and delusions are symptoms of psychotic behavior. Therefore, individuals experiencing these symptoms have limited or absent capacity to recognize reality. During psychotic episodes, some clients are particularly troubling to society because of their bizarre behavior and their inability to meet the challenges of life's demands. Throughout the ages, however, persons with severe mental illness have influenced society and the world in remarkable ways. For example, the famous Dutch painter Vincent van Gogh (1853-1890) went on to create one of his most noted paintings, *The Starry Night*, while institutionalized with a mental illness. More recently, John Nash, genius mathematician and Nobel Prize winner in 1994, was diagnosed as having paranoid schizophrenia. The disease incapacitated Nash for many years. His life story was depicted in the film *A Beautiful Mind.*

Harry Stack Sullivan (1882-1949), a psychiatrist and social learning theorist, emphasized the importance of interpersonal relationships and believed that social isolation was the key in schizophrenia (Sullivan, 1953). Kurt Schneider described various delusional and hallucinatory experiences as first-rank symptoms, currently known as *positive symptoms*, and labeled the less decisive symptoms, such as perceptual disturbances, confusion, mood changes, and emotional impoverishment, as second-rank symptoms. Most of the second-rank symptoms are now called *negative symptoms*. His explanation goes beyond the DSM-IV-TR definition (Sadock et al., 2004; Maguire, 2002).

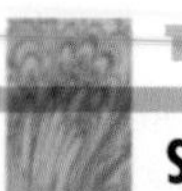

TABLE 12-1

Schizophrenia and Genetic Risks

RELATIONSHIPS TO PERSON WITH SCHIZOPHRENIA	GENETIC RISK OF DEVELOPING SCHIZOPHRENIA (%)
Identical twin	46
Child (both parents have schizophrenia)	50
Child (one parent has schizophrenia)	12
Brother, sister, or parent	12
Nephew, niece, or grandchild	5
First cousin	2

From Amenson CS: The family's role in recovery: *Pacific Clinics Institute: The Journal,* 1999, and guest speaker on schizophrenia: *Grand Rounds Conference, Sharp HealthCare,* San Diego, Calif, 2001.

ETIOLOGY

Research into the etiology of schizophrenia has never been more exciting or challenging, particularly regarding the roles heredity and genes play in the etiology of this complex disorder of the mind and brain (Sullivan, 2005).

Heredity/Genetic Factors

Although the precise cause of schizophrenia is still unknown, research suggests that vulnerability to schizophrenia is clearly related to genetic factors. Studies also show that a number of factors interact to produce the illness. These factors include heredity, events during fetal development that affect the developing brain (such as viral infections in the mother during pregnancy), environmental stressors (such as exposure to pollutants, toxins, and other substances), and stress (NIMH, 2005). Although the brain continues to be the focus of both diagnosis and treatment, current research into the mapping of the human genome has become equally critical in the understanding of schizophrenia. Family and twin studies show the tendency to develop schizophrenia is at least 60% inherited. A person has a 10% chance of developing schizophrenia if a parent or sibling has schizophrenia. For the general population, the chance is only 1%. If an identical (monozygotic) twin has schizophrenia, the probability rises to between 40% and 65%. In nonidentical (dizygotic) twins, the incidence is 17% (NIMH, 2005). Studies of families, adopted children, and twins have been widely used to try to understand how genetics and the environment affect the risk of schizophrenia, but the results provide no conclusive information about the location of the genes or the identity of the environmental factors that predispose or protect against schizophrenia. Studies show evidence that supports 12 potential candidate genes for schizophrenia (Sullivan, 2005). Recent research suggests a possible link to an infectious agent in the human genome that may play a role in schizophrenia (Lencz et al., 2007).

Some genes associated with schizophrenia code for enzymes and proteins that help cells in the brain communicate. These enzymes and proteins are involved in neurotransmitter systems such as dopamine, glutamate (GLU), and γ-aminobutyric acid (GABA). Other genes code for proteins involved in brain development (NIMH, 2005). Although the evidence for several genes is encouraging, none show a clear-cut cause of schizophrenia, although the findings provide a solid foundation for the next generation of studies in this compelling area (Sullivan, 2005). Whatever results new research brings, nurses are continuously challenged to treat the person with schizophrenia as a whole human being, combining the biologic sciences with the caring, interpersonal concepts of the psychosocial models. Table 12-1 lists the genetic risks though these vary slightly depending on the study. Figure 12-1 reveals structural changes in twins with schizophrenia.

Dopamine Hypothesis

Researchers believe dopamine, a catecholamine type neurotransmitter, acts within certain brain cells and nerve tracts to help regulate movement as well as emotions. Dopamine, therefore, affects mood, affect, thoughts, and motor behavior. The *dopamine hypothesis*, a major hypothesis in the etiology of schizophrenia, suggests that persons with schizophrenia have an increased level of dopamine in certain areas of the brain such as the nigrostriatal tract, which runs from the substantia nigra to the basal ganglia (Figure 12-2). This is a main dopamine tract responsible for normal execution of motor and cognitive functions. A certain amount of dopamine is thus necessary for smooth motor movements and clear thought processes. Excess dopamine, however, causes symptoms of psychosis, such as hallucinations and delusions, as it disrupts cognition and thought. Postmortem data support this theory, showing a 66% increase in the number of dopamine receptors in persons with schizophrenia. Thus, researchers think that schizophrenia results from too much dopamine-dependent neuronal activity in the brain. This means that there is an abundance of nerve cells that crave dopamine and overreact in a way that produces psychotic symptoms. Researchers believe that there is also an excess in the production or release of dopamine at nerve endings, increased receptor sensitivity, or decreased activity of dopamine antagonists (drug or substance that blocks or counteracts dopamine) (Figure 12-3). Some studies suggest that abnormalities in dopamine storage, vesicular transport, and release or uptake by the presynapic neuron may be the

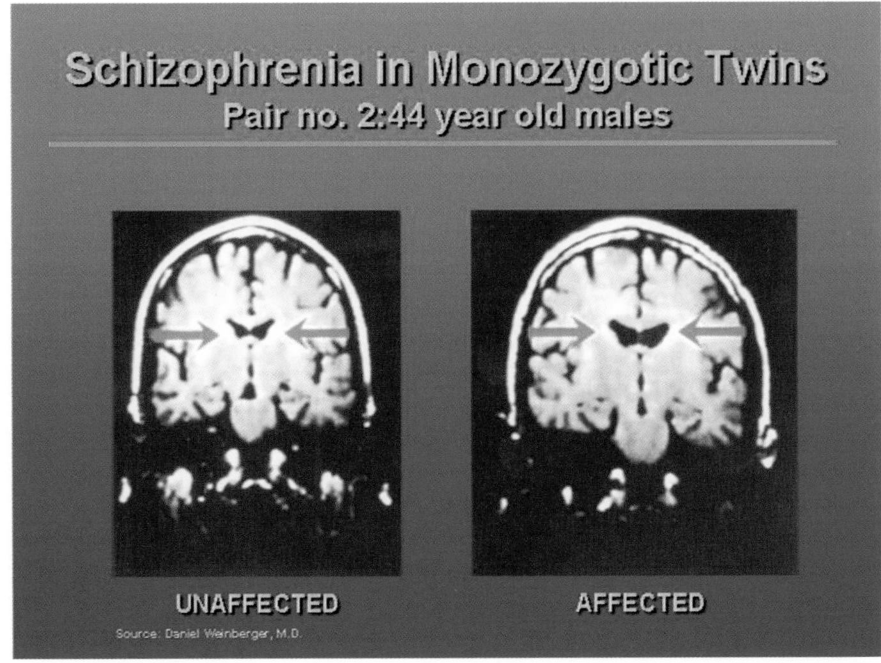

FIGURE 12-1 Loss of brain volume associated with schizophrenia is clearly shown by magnetic resonance imaging (MRI) scans comparing the size of ventricles (butterfly-shaped, fluid-filled spaces in the midbrain) of identical twins, one of whom has schizophrenia *(right)*. The ventricles of the person with schizophrenia are larger, suggesting structural brain changes associated with the illness. Note that such MRI scans cannot be used to diagnose schizophrenia in the general population because of normal genetic variation in ventricle size; many unaffected people have large ventricles. (Courtesy Daniel Weinberger, MD, Clinical Brain Disorders Branch, Division of Intramural Research Program, NIMH, 1990, updated, Dec 11, 2000.)

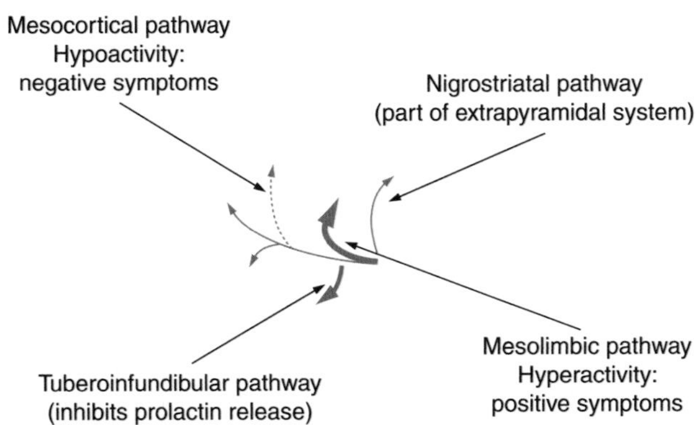

FIGURE 12-2 The four main dopaminergic tracts. (Courtesy David G. Daniel, MD, Bioniche Development, Inc., 2001.)

proximal cause of psychotic symptoms and may contribute to the risk of schizophrenia (Lewis and Lieberman, 2000).

Dopamine Hypothesis and Illicit Drugs

Cocaine and amphetamines are *dopaminergic compounds* (meaning their chemical structure is dopamine-like; therefore, they are dopamine agonists). They also increase psychosis, which supports the dopamine hypothesis that too much dopamine produces psychosis. Individuals with Parkinson's disease have reduced levels of dopamine. Sometimes these individuals take levodopa, a type of dopamine, and experience psychosis as a side effect.

Another hypothesis states that lysergic acid diethylamide (LSD) causes or increases hallucinations by its effects on serotonin. This indicates that the newer generation antipsychotics achieve a synergistic, therapeutic effect by blocking both dopamine and serotonin (Maguire, 2002). Persons with schizophrenia who take street drugs are at risk because of the unpredictable effects caused by these illicit substances. Consciousness-altering drugs, such as marijuana, tend to counteract the effects of antipsychotic medications by inducing the effects of the illness again (Thornton et al., 2001b).

Other Neurotransmitters Associated With Schizophrenia

Six other neurotransmitters that are also relevant by themselves or in conjunction with dopamine are serotonin, acetylcholine, norepinephrine, cholecystokinin, glutamate (GLU), and γ-aminobutyric acid (GABA) (Table 12-2).

Neurodevelopmental Hypothesis

Most people who develop schizophrenia do not show symptoms until later in their adolescence. Studies in teens who develop schizophrenia provide clues about this process. Normally, teens lose some unused neural connections as their brains mature. However, MRI scans reveal that teens with schizophrenia lose the connections at an accelerated rate (NIMH, 2005).

Faulty wiring is possibly responsible for genes creating too many or too few of the proteins needed to help neurons develop and migrate in the developing brain. Viruses or parasites the pregnant mother catches also possibly affect these processes. Toxin exposure through breathing, eating, drinking, and smoking are also perhaps responsible (NIMH, 2005).

Environmental Factors

Environmental factors associated with schizophrenia include toxins, pollution, infections, and viral exposure; malnutrition; being born in winter; being born in a city; and childhood brain injury. Interactions between the en-

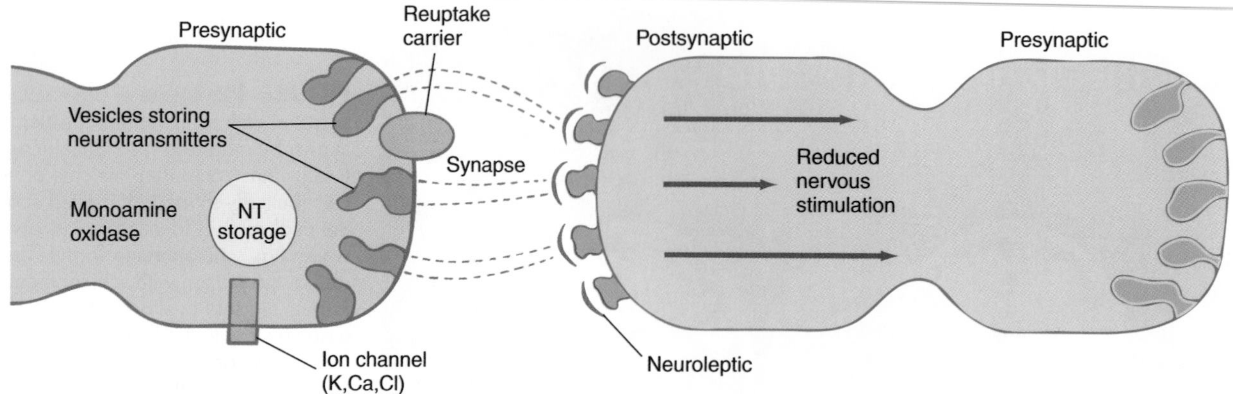

FIGURE 12-3 Neuroleptic (antipsychotic) action. Neurotransmitter action at the synapse is modified by neuroleptics, which block postsynaptic receptor sites to reduce nervous stimulation (reducing symptoms of schizophrenia).

TABLE 12-2

Neurotransmitters in Schizophrenia

NEUROTRANSMITTER	TYPE	FUNCTION
Dopamine	Catecholamine	Regulates motor behavior in extrapyramidal nerve tracts and also transmits in the cortex. Increases vigilance and may increase aggression. Too much produces psychosis; too little causes movement disorders (extrapyramidal symptoms [EPS]).
Serotonin	Indolamine	Brainstem transmitter; modulates mood; lowers aggressive tendencies. A deficiency is likely responsible for some forms of schizophrenia.
Acetylcholine	Cholinergic	Transmits at nerve-muscle connections (central nervous system and autonomic nervous system). A deficiency increases confusion and acting out behavior. Controls extrapyramidal symptoms (EPS).
Norepinephrine	Catecholamine	Transmits in the sympathetic nervous system. Induces the flight-or-fight syndrome (hypervigilance). Is sometimes insufficient in clients with schizophrenia who display anhedonia (loss of pleasure).
Cholecystokinin	Peptide	Excites the limbic neurons. A deficiency is related to avolition (lack of motivation) and a flat affect.
Glutamate	Amino acid	Excitatory neurotransmitter. Impairment in the *N*-methyl-D-aspartate, or NMDA, affects glutamate, which leads to problems in cognition, delusions, and possibly some negative symptoms of schizophrenia (Maguire, 2002).
γ-Aminobutyric acid (GABA)	Amino acid	Inhibitory neurotransmitter; predominantly a brain transmitter. Promotes a balance between dopamine and glutamate and thus inhibits impulsive behaviors.

vironmental factors and brain conditions affect the developing mind (NIMH, 2005).

Other Biologic Research

Extensive research on the neuroendocrine mechanisms underlying the stress response influenced psychiatrists to view these mechanisms as a possible explanation for several forms of psychotic states. This foundation remains a part of the theoretic framework explaining psychopathology even today.

Immunologic Factors

Viral exposure, particularly exposure to influenza during pregnancy, is a risk factor for developing schizophrenia. Scientists theorize that the influenza virus creates maternal antibodies. In the fetus, these become autoantibodies, which are an external source of developmental change. The mother's exposure to a virus during pregnancy possibly explains why some siblings develop schizophrenia and others do not (Maguire, 2002). There are few immunologic studies of schizophrenia, and they depend on epidemiologic data for their hypotheses.

Structural and Functional Factors

This theory states that the structure of the nervous system includes both gross and microanatomic defects. Studies used to examine structural and functional impairment of the brain are discussed in the next paragraphs.

Magnetic Resonance Imaging. Magnetic resonance imaging (MRI), a brain imaging technique available today, is used at the time of diagnosis to rule out structural causes of psychosis in clients with schizophrenia (Maguire, 2002). MRIs are internal snapshots of the brain taken slice-by-slice by using magnets instead of radiation. These snapshots or images are transmitted over a time sequence onto a monitor screen where they can be examined in depth. A review of 193 MRI studies from 1988 to 2000 showed some consistent structural abnormalities including ventricular enlargement, abnormalities of the medial and superior temporal lobes, and frontal, parietal, and cerebellar abnormalities (Lieberman, 2006b) (see Figure 12-1).

Positron Emission Tomography. Unlike MRI scans, PET scans use radioactively labeled probes to track blood flow changes or metabolic or other chemical changes in the brain. Researchers study these brain functional changes to find information about cognitive functioning in schizophrenia.

PET studies are also useful to track the action of various medications used to treat schizophrenia. By binding a radioactive tracer with a medication, researchers are able to study the specific sites the medications affect (Lieberman, 2006b).

Stress and Stress Models

For clients with chronic schizophrenia, environmental stress-producing events and situations are always present. The life events and subsequent stress increase dopaminergic transmission and cause a high level of arousal, leading to specific episodic recurrences of the illness. The high level of arousal results in intense hallucinatory experiences (Sadock et al., 2004).

In Hans Selye's stress model (1978), the individual interacts with the environment while various stimuli, or life events, occur. This creates stress, which differs in size and meaning for each individual. For some, the stress of life is capable of producing disease.

In Callista Roy's nursing adaptation model (1976), the person continually adapts to internal and external stimuli (some of which is stress producing), using both physiologic (biologic) and psychosocial modes of adaptation. Several nursing theorists (i.e., King, Levine, and Neuman) have examined the relationship between stress and illness, both physical and mental, using this theory.

Disease and Trauma

Some studies support the idea that schizophrenia is developmentally related to disease and trauma occurring during the prenatal period or in early childhood (Maguire, 2002). Complications that possibly increase risk for schizophrenia include viral infections during pregnancy, rhesus incompatibility, maternal preeclampsia, anemia, and diabetes mellitus (APA, 2004).

Substance Abuse

Substance abuse is a common co-occurring condition in persons with schizophrenia. More than 75% of this population is addicted to nicotine, 30% to 50% are addicted to alcohol, 15% to 25% are addicted to cannabis, and 5% to 10% are addicted to cocaine and amphetamines (Maguire, 2002). Research suggests that substance use disorders in schizophrenia are especially common among men with a history of childhood conduct disorder problems (Swartz et al., 2006). Thirthalli and Benegal (2006) cited studies with an association between adolescent use of cannabis and later development of schizophrenia or schizophreniform disorder. Depending on the person's genes, there is an increased vulnerability to psychosis after cannabis use. Cocaine initiates neurochemical changes in the brain by substituting for the natural endorphins, creating an intense craving for the drug. Eventually the long-term user experiences apathy, depression, and anhedonia, as often seen in clients with chronic schizophrenia.

Maguire (2002) noted that persons with schizophrenia often indulge in substances such as nicotine, caffeine, and cocaine to self-medicate and perhaps help improve their attention span, as they attempt to deal with competing stimuli that is a constant disruption in their lives. In addition, there is accumulating evidence that certain drugs used in pregnancy are linked with later schizotypal illnesses in childhood and adolescence.

Psychologic Theories

Many biologic factors predispose an individual to schizophrenia; however, psychosocial considerations are significant as well. Most models indicate that a person's vulnerability interacts with stressful environmental influences to produce the symptoms of schizophrenia (Sadock et al., 2004). Psychosocial stressors include stressful life events such as interpersonal losses, sociocultural stresses such as poverty or homelessness, or a stressful emotional situation where one lives (APA, 2004). Before the explosion in biologic theories, many thought schizophrenia was partially the result of individual or family faults. Some of these flaws included mother or father personality characteristics, marital discord, hostile dependency traits of mother or caregivers, poor infant-mother bonding, and interpersonal communication problems. With advances in biology, these theories have lost some credibility.

Some studies conclude that persons with schizophrenia have better outcomes when they come from families where there is little criticism and anger, where emotional bonds are relatively distant (not enmeshed), and where family members interact less. Outcomes related to family climate studies, however, have been defined only in terms of rehospitalization frequency and symptom intensity (Thornton et al., 2001c).

Cultural and Environmental Theories

Although schizophrenia exists in all socioeconomic groups, persons with schizophrenia more commonly inhabit the lower socioeconomic group. There are various explanations for this condition, one having to do with a *downward drift hypothesis* (Sadock et al., 2004). According to this hypothesis, the client with schizophrenia who possesses low social skills either moves into a lower socioeconomic group or fails to rise to a higher group (Maguire, 2002). People with schizophrenia also tend to be more numerous in urban and selected immigrant populations (Lewis and Lieberman, 2000).

Currently, about 800,000 Americans are homeless on any given night. Schizophrenia is a risk factor for homelessness, and estimates are that 11% of homeless people suffer from schizophrenia. Homeless people with schizophrenia live on the streets for many reasons. Some lack affordable housing or have difficulties with public funding. There is also some difficulty coordinating the necessary services for this population, including accessing the medication necessary to relieve their troubling symptoms and behaviors. Homeless persons with schizophrenia often have additional stressors such as substance abuse, infectious diseases, and the social isolation problems described earlier (APA, 2004) (see Chapter 29).

EPIDEMIOLOGY

In the United States, schizophrenia has a lifetime prevalence of 0.7 years and affects 1% of the general population (Csernansky et al., 2002) (Box 12-2). The prevalence of schizophrenia is equal in both men and women, and the peak age of onset is usually 15 to 25 years for men and 25 to 35 years for women (Maguire, 2002). Although equal numbers of males and females are affected, some data suggest that males may have more severe manifestations of schizophrenia, including an earlier age of onset (by 2 to 4 years), more marked neuropathologic abnormalities, poorer response to treatment, and less favorable outcome (Lewis and Lieberman, 2000). The incidence of schizophrenia, or the frequency of newly diagnosed cases in a specified population during a certain time period, is between 0.3% and 0.6% per 1000 persons per year in the United States. The prevalence and prognosis of the disease vary according to socioeconomic, geographic, and cultural factors. Although symptoms of the disorder have common universal characteristics, schizophrenia presents itself in different ways, depending on the clients' situations and demographic backgrounds (Sadock et al., 2004).

BOX 12-2

Epidemiology of Schizophrenia

- New diagnoses of schizophrenia occur between 0.3% and 0.6% per 1000 persons per year in the United States.
- 1.5% of the U.S. population has schizophrenia.
- The age of onset is later in females than in males.
- Paranoid-type schizophrenia occurs earlier in males than in females.
- Disorganized-type schizophrenia occurs earlier in females than in males.
- Prevalence is equal for males and females.
- Childhood-onset affects 1 in 40,000 children.
- The oldest age-of-onset group is after age 60.
- A female fetus exposed to influenza has a higher risk for schizophrenia than a male fetus.
- Males show significantly more structural brain abnormalities from perinatal or early childhood trauma than females.

Schizophrenia accounts for 20% of all hospital bed-days and 50% of all psychiatric beds in the United States. Schizophrenia is the most costly mental illness and roughly accounts for 2.5% of annual health care cost in the United States. In 1995, researchers estimated that the economic burden of schizophrenia in the United States was 65 billion (APA, 2004). Much of this cost was due to the relapse of psychosis and rehospitalization, as most clients experience a chronic course even though it varies from client to client (Csernansky et al., 2002). Loss of work and productivity is also a reason for the high cost.

Childhood-Onset Schizophrenia

Schizophrenia affects approximately 1 in 40,000 children compared to 1 in 100 adults. Like adults, children experience psychotic symptoms, social withdrawal, loss of social and personal care skills, flattened emotions, and an increased risk of suicide (NIH, 2003). The diagnostic criteria are the same as for adults but the symptoms appear before age 12 (Rapoport, 2000). These children see or hear things that do not exist. They sometimes have paranoid or bizarre thoughts and often have difficulty with paying attention. Impairments in memory and reasoning, speech, social skills, and emotional expression along with depressed mood are present. Children with prepuberty psychosis show abnormal brain development. MRI scans reveal fluid filled cavities in the middle of the brain enlarging abnormally between ages 14 and 18. This increase in fluid-filled cavities coincides with brain tissue volume shrinkage. These children lose gray matter beginning in rear structures involved in attention and perception. This loss of gray matter spreads to frontal areas responsible for executive functions. Causes for this illness include genetic predisposition, prenatal factors, and stressful life events (NIH, 2003).

Late-Onset Schizophrenia

Persons who first experience schizophrenia later in life have better outcomes in all areas. This is possibly because the person was able to be productive and acquire coping skills before the onset of schizophrenia. Better outcomes depend, in part, on their premorbid functioning (how they functioned before the illness). For example, if a client developed good social skills, had a satisfying sex life, and succeeded in academic or vocational achievements before the onset of schizophrenia, the chances for a successful outcome after the illness improve significantly (Thornton et al., 2001a).

With the overall increase in longevity, there will be more older clients with schizophrenia in our midst. Approximately 80% of people with schizophrenia had early-onset, whereas 20% have late-onset (after age 40) and very late onset (after age 60) according to the DSM-IV (APA, 2004).

Course of Illness

The course of illness generally includes recurrent, acute exacerbations of psychotic symptoms (hallucinations and delusions). Preventing relapse is critical, because each time relapse occurs there is an increased risk in deterioration of the individual's functions. Schizophrenia develops through premorbid, prodromal, and psychotic phases and follows a stereotyped pattern (APA, 2004).

The **premorbid phase** describes features that contribute to later development of the illness and includes mild deficits in social, motor, and cognitive functions occurring during childhood and adolescence, such as subtle motor abnormalities during infancy, and deficits in social functioning, organizational ability, and intellectual functioning around ages 16 to 17. Also, some minor physical anomalies such as variations in limb length and angle, and fingerprint patterns may be present in a subgroup of individuals but have a low predictive validity (Lewis and Lieberman, 2000).

The **prodromal phase** includes symptoms and behaviors that signal the approaching onset of the illness. This phase may last 2 to 5 years with psychotic symptoms emerging late in this phase marking the beginning of the psychotic phase. Symptoms include the following:

- Mood symptoms (e.g., anxiety, irritability, and dysphoria or anguish)
- Cognitive symptoms (e.g., distractibility, concentration difficulties, disorganized thinking)
- Obsessive behaviors
- Social withdrawal and role functioning deterioration
- Sleep disturbances
- Attenuated (weaker) positive symptoms (e.g., illusions [misinterpreting actual stimuli], ideas of reference [belief that all events refer to the client, for example, "the man on TV is speaking to me"], magical thinking [belief that one's thoughts produce outcomes, for example, "my bad thoughts were responsible for her illness"], superstitiousness)

The **psychotic phase** progresses through an acute phase, a recovery or maintenance phase, and a stable phase (APA, 2004):

- *Acute phase.* Individuals experience florid positive symptoms such as delusions, hallucinations, and negative symptoms such as apathy, withdrawal, and avolition. They are unable to perform self-care activities and may need brief hospitalization to provide safety and treatment.
- *Recovery or maintenance phase.* Occurs 6 to 18 months after acute treatment. Symptoms are present but less severe than in the acute phase. By 5 to 10 years after onset, most clients have a leveling off of their illness and functioning (APA, 2004). They are generally able to care for themselves with some supervision.
- *Stable phase.* The time in which symptoms are in remission, although some symptoms may persist or remain present in milder forms (residual symptoms). Some people are able to live independently in the community during this time (see Chapter 29).

In most Western countries, 1 to 2 years elapse between the onset of psychotic symptoms and the first treatment (APA, 2004). The long-term outcome varies widely from incapacitation to recovery. Approximately 10% to 15% of clients remain free of future episodes. Another 10% to 15% remain both chronically and severely psychotic. Better outcomes are associated with the following characteristics (APA, 2004):

- Female gender
- Lack of family history of schizophrenia
- Good preillness social and academic functioning
- Higher IQ
- Married status
- Later age of onset
- Fewer co-occurring factors
- Predominately positive symptoms

CLINICAL ALERT

Suicide is the leading cause of premature death among people diagnosed with schizophrenia. Up to 30% attempt suicide, whereas 4% to 10% die by suicide. Suicide is most common within the first 6 years after initial hospitalization and then again during periods of remission after 5 years of illness (APA, 2004).

Specific risk factors for suicide among individuals with schizophrenia include young age and a high socioeconomic status background. Additionally, the person experiencing schizophrenia sometimes considers suicide if he or she has a high IQ and a high level of achievement and has set goals high before symptoms occurred and is aware of perceived future losses. Earlier onset and multiple relapses add to suicide risk. People with severe depressions who feel hopeless are at risk. People who have expressed suicidal thoughts are also at risk. Despite identification of these risk factors, it is often difficult to predict whether an individual will attempt suicide. Professionals need to evaluate patients for suicide risk at all stages in the person's illness (APA, 2004).

Socioeconomic Class

The portion of schizophrenia that is attributed to the social problems of the underprivileged class remains controversial (Fortinash and Holoday Worret, 2007; Sadock et al., 2004). The overcrowded poor neighborhoods and the homeless mentally ill persons receiving inadequate follow-up care are burdens on this vulnerable population and on society.

Culture and Geographical Influences

The manifestations of schizophrenia and its prognosis vary in different cultures. In less-developed nations, the prognosis for schizophrenia is better than in the technologically advanced cultures, although severe cognitive impairment is rare in Western nations. Clients in developing countries tend to have a more acute onset, fewer episodic occurrences, and less frequent problems with affect. Also, cultures in developing countries are more accepting of the illness, because persons with schizophrenia are more readily welcomed back into the family and community following an acute episode (Sadock et al., 2004).

CLINICAL DESCRIPTION

According to the DSM-IV-TR classification, a diagnosis of schizophrenia must meet the following criteria: (1) it lasts at least 6 months, at least 1 month of which includes *active-*

DSM-IV-TR CRITERIA

Schizophrenia

A *Characteristic symptoms.* Two (or more) of the following, each present for a significant portion of time during a 1-month period (or less if successfully treated):
1 Delusions
2 Hallucinations
3 Disorganized speech (e.g., frequent derailment or incoherence)
4 Grossly disorganized or catatonic behavior
5 Negative symptoms (i.e., affective flattening, alogia, or avolition)
NOTE: Only one criterion A symptom is required if delusions are bizarre or hallucinations consist of a voice keeping up a running commentary on the person's behavior or thoughts, or two or more voices conversing with each other.

B *Social/occupational dysfunction.* For a significant portion of the time since the onset of the disturbance, one or more major areas of functioning, such as work, interpersonal relations, or self-care, are markedly below the level achieved before the onset (or when the onset is in childhood or adolescence, failure to achieve expected level of interpersonal, academic, or occupational achievement).

C *Duration.* Continuous signs of the disturbance persist for at least 6 months. This 6-month period must include at least 1 month of symptoms (or less if successfully treated) that meet criterion A (i.e., active-phase symptoms) and may include periods of prodromal or residual symptoms. During these prodromal or residual periods, the signs of the disturbance may be manifested by only negative symptoms or two or more symptoms listed in criterion A present in an attenuated form (e.g., odd beliefs, unusual perceptual experiences).

D *Schizoaffective and mood disorder exclusion.* Schizoaffective disorder and mood disorder with psychotic features have been ruled out because either (1) no major depressive, manic, or mixed episodes have occurred concurrently with the active-phase symptoms; or (2) if mood episodes have occurred during active-phase symptoms, their total duration has been brief relative to the duration of the active and residual periods.

E *Substance/general medical condition exclusion.* The disturbance is not due to the direct physiologic effects of a substance (e.g., a drug of abuse, a medication) or a general medical condition.

F *Relationship to a pervasive developmental disorder.* If there is a history of autistic disorder or another pervasive developmental disorder, the additional diagnosis of schizophrenia is made only if prominent delusions or hallucinations are also present for at least a month (or less if successfully treated).

Classification of longitudinal course (can be applied only after at least 1 year has elapsed since the initial onset of active-phase symptoms):
Episodic with interepisode residual symptoms (episodes are defined by the reemergence of prominent psychotic symptoms); also specify if it presents with prominent negative symptoms
Episodic with no interepisode residual symptoms
Continuous (prominent psychotic symptoms are present throughout the period of observation); also specify if it presents with prominent negative symptoms
Single episode in partial remission; also specify if it presents with prominent negative symptoms
Single episode in full remission
Other or unspecified pattern

From American Psychiatric Association: *Diagnostic and statistical manual of mental disorders*, ed 4, text revision, Washington, DC, 2000, American Psychiatric Association.

phase symptoms, and (2) the active-phase symptoms include at least two of the following manifestations: hallucinations, delusions, disorganized or catatonic behavior, or disorganized speech (see the DSM-IV-TR Criteria box).

Subtypes and Related Disorders

There are five major subtypes of schizophrenia and eight closely related disorders. The five subtypes of schizophrenia are as follows:

1. Paranoid
2. Disorganized (formerly called *hebephrenic*)
3. Catatonic
4. Undifferentiated
5. Residual

The closely related disorders include the following:

- Schizophreniform disorder
- Schizoaffective disorder
- Delusional disorder
- Brief psychotic disorder
- Shared psychotic disorder *(folie a deux)*
- Psychotic disorder due to a general medical condition
- Substance-induced psychotic disorder
- Psychotic disorder not otherwise specified (NOS)

Subtypes

Paranoid Schizophrenia

Paranoid schizophrenia results in less neurologic and cognitive impairment and a better prognosis for the individual. However, in the active phase of the disorder, the afflicted individual is extremely ill, and the symptoms often make the person a danger to self or others.

Delusions tend to be persecutory or grandiose and have a consistent theme. The persecutory delusions generate anxiety, suspiciousness, anger, hostility, and violent behavior. Auditory hallucinations are common and are related to the delusionary theme. Interactions with others are rigid, intense, and controlled (Fortinash and Holoday Worret, 2007; Sadock et al., 2004; APA, 2000).

According to the DSM-IV-TR criteria for schizophrenia, a diagnosis of paranoid schizophrenia must meet two of the symptoms in criterion A: the presence of delusions and hallucinations. The other diagnostic criteria for paranoid schizophrenia—disorganized speech, behavior, and other negative symptoms—are not prominent. The delusions and hallucinations must be present for a significant portion of time over a period of 1 month. This period is shorter if the condition is successfully treated. Also, if delusions are unusually bizarre or if the hallucinations involve commanding or commenting voices, only one of the criteria needs to be met. Paranoid schizophrenia often has a sudden onset, sometimes triggered by severe stressors (Fortinash and Holoday Worret, 2007; APA, 2004).

Prognosis. The course of paranoid schizophrenia is varied but tends to be more hopeful than the courses of other subtypes. Of all the schizophrenias, paranoid schizophrenia often has a better prognosis, particularly in the areas of occupational function and independent living (APA, 2000).

Disorganized Schizophrenia

The *disorganized* type of schizophrenia was formerly known as hebephrenic schizophrenia because of its early, dangerous onset and silly, childish affect. Severe disintegration of the personality characterizes this form of schizophrenia. Speech is disorganized and includes word salad (communication that includes both real and imaginary words in no logical order), incoherent speech, and clanging (rhyming). Behavior is odd, encompassing grimacing, grunting, sniffing, posturing, rocking, stereotyped behaviors, and uninhibited sexual behaviors such as masturbating in public. Socially the client with disorganized schizophrenia is withdrawn and incompetent. There are many cognitive and psychomotor defects, such as concrete thinking, the literal interpretation and use of language or inability to abstract, and poor coordination. *Primary process thinking*, or prelogical thought that aims for wish fulfillment associated with the pleasure principle characteristic of the id portion of the personality, is also a common defect (Fortinash and Holoday Worret, 2007; APA, 2000).

The client with disorganized schizophrenia has poor personal grooming and is often unable to complete activities of daily living (ADLs) without constant structural reminders, because the behavior is aimless and without goals (Sadock et al., 2004). Many negative (type II) symptoms are present.

Prognosis. Prognosis for the client with disorganized schizophrenia is poor, stemming from an early premorbid history of impaired adjustment that continues after the active phase of the disorder.

Of all the subtypes, paranoid schizophrenia and disorganized schizophrenia have the most clearly defined clinical criteria and have been studied the most. Studies have indicated a wide interest in the cognitive symptoms of schizophrenia, which include memory impairment and lack of problem-solving skills. Negative symptoms, such as emotional blunting, apathy, withdrawal, and avolition (lack of motivation), also remain a focus of concern. After all, it is the residual negative symptoms and the cognitive impairment that prevent individuals with this type of schizophrenia from holding jobs and forming lasting, satisfying relationships. Continued research, new medications, and innovations in therapy all offer hope for a brighter prognosis. Box 12-3 lists positive and negative symptoms.

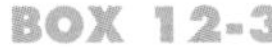

BOX 12-3

Positive (Type I) and Negative (Type II) Symptoms of Schizophrenia

POSITIVE

Delusions, persecutory or grandiose
Delusions of being controlled
Mind reading or thought insertion ideas
Hallucinations, auditory or other sensory modes
Bizarre dress and behavior
Thought disorganization and tangential (superficial) speech
Aggressive, agitated behavior
Pressured speech
Suicidal ideation present
Ideas of reference

NEGATIVE

Flat or inappropriate affect
Poor eye contact
Anhedonic attitude (loss of pleasure) and asocial behavior; withdrawal
Poverty of speech; blocking and lack of inflection
Poor grooming and hygiene
Decreased spontaneity in behavior
Lack of expressive gestures
Avolition (lack of motivation); apathy
Severely disturbed relationships with family, friends, peers
Inattentiveness

Catatonic Schizophrenia

Catatonic schizophrenia has, as its predominant feature, intense psychomotor disturbance. This disturbance often takes the form of stupor (psychomotor retardation) or excitement (psychomotor excitation). Manifestations of psychomotor disturbance include posturing, immobility, catalepsy (waxy flexibility), mutism, and negativism. There is sometimes automatic obedience, then excessive and purposeless movement. Other symptoms include **echopraxia** (imitating the movements of others), **echolalia** (repeating what was said by another), grimacing, and stereotypic movements. Often there is rapid alteration between these extremes (Fortinash and Holoday Worret, 2007; Sadock et al., 2004; APA, 2000).

The onset of catatonic schizophrenia often occurs with dramatic suddenness. An earlier withdrawal sometimes precedes catatonic stupor. It reflects the individual's reduced neurologic ability to filter out stimuli. There is no significant difference in age, sex, or education in the incidence of catatonic schizophrenia. To meet the DSM-IV-TR criteria for catatonic schizophrenia, the client must exhibit two of the following behaviors: motor immobility or excessive motor activity; extreme negativism (resistance to all instructions and attempts to be moved); peculiar voluntary movements such as grimacing, stereotyped movements, or posturing; and echolalia or echopraxia (APA, 2004).

The person with catatonic schizophrenia presents a nursing challenge. While in a state of psychomotor excitement, the client develops hyperpyrexia or collapse from extreme exhaustion. Close watch is necessary to prevent harm to self or others. Conversely, while in a stuporous state, the disease is life threatening because the person approaches a vegetative condition, will not eat, and is in danger of malnutrition or even starvation. Other complications include pressure ulcers from lack of mobility or strange posturing, constipation, or even stasis pneumonia in the older client.

Delusions often persist throughout the withdrawn state. For example, a client believes that he has to hold his hand out flat in front of him because the forces of good and evil are warring on the palm of his hand and he will upset the balance of good and evil if he moves his hand. Oddly enough, although this individual does not seem to attend to the environment around him, when he later returns to a normal state of consciousness, he will remember in detail what has occurred. Nurses need to be aware of this factor and not say or do anything within the stuporous client's hearing that they would not say or do when the client is in a normal state of consciousness.

Prognosis. The prognosis for catatonic schizophrenia varies depending on the age of onset, which is often in the early 20s to 30s. It tends to begin with an acute episode having an identifiable precipitating factor. If the client has developed a good support system before the illness, he or she will probably recover from the acute phase and have a partial or complete remission. More research is needed for this particular type of illness, especially as it seems to have decreased in Western nations. However, it is more prevalent in developing nations, where remission is usually complete.

Undifferentiated Schizophrenia

Undifferentiated schizophrenia meets criterion A for schizophrenia but cannot be classified as paranoid, disorganized, or catatonic. It does not clearly meet the criteria necessary for a diagnosis in any of these conditions, but it has some aspects of each type. The psychotic manifestations are extreme, including fragmented delusions, vague hallucinations, bizarre and disorganized behavior, disorientation, and incoherence (Fortinash and Holoday Worret, 2007; Sadock et al., 2004). Affect is usually inappropriate rather than flat, and catatonic symptoms are not present. Figure 12-4 shows a clinical pathway for a client presenting with psychosis.

The onset is usually acute, with excited behaviors such as aggressive hitting or biting. Some clients have chronic schizophrenia, with behavior that no longer fits a specific type but is a mixture of positive and negative symptoms. Usually the prodromal symptoms have developed over a period of years. Often growth and development milestones have been delayed. Thought processes are fragmented and have high fantasy content (primary process thinking). The individual has few or no friends, and family relationships are strained because of odd and restless behaviors. Dress and grooming are careless, and the individual seems bored with life. Nightmares and early morning awakening disturb sleep patterns.

Prognosis. The prognosis for the client with undifferentiated schizophrenia is generally poor, and the course is usually chronic. There are periods of exacerbation and remission where many negative symptoms prevent the patient from doing productive work, pursuing normal relationships, or enjoying life (Sadock et al., 2004).

Residual Schizophrenia

If an individual has had at least one acute episode of schizophrenia and is now free of prominent positive symptoms but has some negative symptoms, he or she is diagnosed with *residual schizophrenia*, or **residual symptoms**. In some clients, this pattern continues for years, with or without exacerbations. In others it seems to decrease to a complete remission. The usual signs of the illness that persist for the chronic or subchronic individual are mild loosening of associations, illogical thinking, emotional blunting, social withdrawal, and eccentric behavior. Diagnostic criteria for the client with residual schizophrenia are (1) absence of prominent delusions, hallucinations, disorganized speech, and disorganized or catatonic behavior and (2) continuing evidence of the presence of negative symptoms or reduced positive symptoms.

Prognosis. Prognosis is varied and unpredictable. It depends largely on premorbid history and the adequacy of support systems (Sadock et al., 2004; APA, 2000).

Related Disorders

Schizophreniform Disorder

The defining characteristics of *schizophreniform disorder* are the same as for schizophrenia, with two exceptions. The first is the duration, and the second is impairment of function. The duration is at least 1 month but less than 6 months. If symptoms persist for 6 months or longer, the diagnosis changes to schizophrenia. Social or occupational functioning sometimes does not occur in this disorder, unlike the diagnosis of schizophrenia, where functional disturbance (relationships, school or work, self-care) will be present.

Prognosis. It is estimated that one third of these individuals recover completely, whereas two thirds are likely to develop schizophrenia.

Schizoaffective Disorder

Schizoaffective disorder is a closely related disorder of schizophrenia, but the onset of illness generally occurs later in life. It presents with severe mood swings of either mania or depression and also with some of the psychotic symptoms. Most of the time, mania or depression coexists with the psychotic symptoms, but there must be at least one 2-week period in which there are only psychotic episodes. Researchers still do not know the cause of schizoaffective disorder, but most believe that the etiology is related to a combination of biologic, genetic, and environmental factors.

Text continued on p. 264

Psychosis

	Interval	Day of Admit	Day 2	Day 3	Day 4	Day 5	Day 6	Day 7	Day 8
	Location								
OUTCOMES	Physiologic	*Takes adequate fluid/nutrition with assistance *Tolerates meds *Is pain free	*Takes adequate fluid/nutrition with assistance *Increased sleep/rest time *Adequate elimination *Is pain free	*Adequate nutrition with reminders *Adequate elimination *Is pain free	*Sleeps 3-6 hours *Adequate elimination *Is pain free	*Takes adequate nutrition/fluids *Drug levels therapeutic range *Is pain free	*Sleeps 5-8 hours *Absence drug toxicity side effects *Is pain free	*Sleeps 5-8 hours *Is pain free	*Sleeps 5-8 hours *Able to manage food/activity requirements independently *Is pain free
	Psychologic	*Tolerates orientation to unit within capacity	*Oriented ×2	*Oriented ×3 *Demonstrates reduction in hallucinations and delusions	*Oriented ×4 *Reality testing with staff *Increased trust demonstrated	*Demonstrates more reality-based thoughts	*Able to focus on one topic 5-10 minutes	*Able to complete unit assignments and activities	*Able to complete unit assignment and activities independently *Able to plan/structure day
	Functional Status/Role	*Refrains from harming self or others with assistance *Takes direction from staff	*Refrains from harming self *Attends to basic ADLs *Seeks staff when anxious	*Refrains from harming self *Increased trust demonstrated *Increased ADLs *Complies with meds with reminders	*Increased ADLs *Controls impulses with assistance *Utilizing basic stress management techniques with assistance	*Demonstrates less psychosis and intrusive behavior	*Interacts with peers *Able to make decisions	*Able to maintain safety *Demonstrates safe behaviors	*Able to maintain safety *Independently complies with medical regimen
	Family/Community Reintegration	*Family/significant other aware of treatment program goals *Family/significant other provide history including meds	*Identifies family/significant other to staff	*Attends community meetings/milieu activities with staff supervision *Identifies family/significant other *Communicates with SW for increased understanding of Treatment goals/DC plans	*Family/significant other included in treatment/DC plans	*Identifies DC needs	*Identifies DC needs	*Identifies DC needs *Able to identify supports and how to use them	*Able to utilize supports and list ways to access them *States specific plans to manage symptoms, complies with meds and aftercare

NOTE: This Clinical Pathway is a tool to assist health care providers in achieving quality client outcomes by providing appropriate and timely client care. It is not intended to establish a community standard of care, replace a clinician's medical judgment, establish a protocol for all clients, or exclude alternative therapies. (See Variances at end of figure.)

CBC, Complete blood chemistry; *DC,* discharge; *ELOS,* estimated length of stay; *eval,* evaluation; *H/O,* history of; *I&O,* intake and output; milieu, therapeutic client environment; *OT,* occupational therapist; *Reiseurit,* hearing to determine if client is cognitively able to make a decision to refuse psychotropic medication; *S&R,* seclusion and restraint; *SW,* social worker; *UR,* utilization review.

FIGURE 12-4 Clinical pathway for psychosis. *Continued*

	Interval	Day of Admit	Day 2	Day 3	Day 4	Day 5	Day 6	Day 7	Day 8
	Location								
PROCESSES	Discharge Planning	*(SW) initiate assessment *Identify DC placement ELOS contact family/significant other (nursing) initiates assessment *Identify H/O med compliance, knowledge deficit, and chronicity	*Team involved in DC planning *Discussed with MD *UR notify managed care	*SW evaluation completed *Specific DC plan identified *Treatment team meeting #1	*Involve family/significant other in DC plan *Review with client	*Client, family/significant other communicate understanding DC plan and follow-up *UR contact manage care	*Reinforce client, family/significant other understanding DC plan and follow-up	*Transition to day treatment if indicated *Continue to identify/reinforce support system	*DC to least restrictive environment
	Education	*Orient to unit *Client's rights *Assess client/significant other *Assess knowledge of meds and chronicity	*Assist client with symptom recognition and importance of compliance *Include family/significant other as necessary	*Continue with symptom recognition *Continue to assess level of knowledge re: disorder and meds	*Assist in linking symptoms with precipitating event	*Assist in linking symptoms with precipitating events (noncompliance, drug abuse)	*Reinforce med education *Importance of compliance	*Develop aftercare plan to manage symptoms *Contact supports	*Develop aftercare plan to manage symptoms and contact supports
	Psychosocial/Spiritual/Legal	*Assess: Safety issues Mental status Spirituality Voluntary status	*Continue to assess: Safety issues Mental status Spirituality Voluntary status	*Continue to assess: Safety issues Mental status Spirituality Voluntary status	*Complete assessments and confirm: Safety Mental status Spirituality Legal status	*Continue to assess: Safety issues Mental status Spiritual Voluntary status	*Continue to assess: Safety issues Mental status Spiritual Voluntary status	*Continue to assess: Safety issues Mental status Spirituality Voluntary status	*Legal, psychosocial, spiritual evaluation completed
	Consults	*Physical exam within 24 hours ( )	*Other consults as needed	*Other consults as needed	*Other consults as needed	*Other consults as needed	*Other consults as needed	*Arrange aftercare consults as ordered	*Complete all consults
	Tests/Procedures	*Med levels ( ) *Drug screen ( ) *CBC ( ) *Thyroid function ( ) *SMAC ( )	*Other test/procedures as ordered	*Other test/procedures as ordered	*Other test/procedures as ordered	*Other test/procedures as ordered	*Other test/procedures as ordered *Check drug levels in therapeutic range	*Other test/procedures as ordered	*Test procedures as ordered outpatient
	Treatment	*Monitor I&O *Monitor sleep/rest patterns *Level of observation 1:1 ( ); every 15 min ( ); every 30 min ( ) *Reduce milieu stimulation *Treatment as ordered *S&R ( ) yes ( ) no ( )	*Monitor I&O *Monitor sleep/rest patterns *Level of observation 1:1 ( ); every 15 min ( ); every 30 min ( ) *Treatment as ordered	*Monitor I&O *Monitor sleep/rest patterns *Level of observation 1:1 ( ); every 15 min ( ); every 30 min ( ) *Treatment as ordered	*Monitor I&O *Monitor sleep/rest patterns *Level of observation 1:1 ( ); every 15 min ( ); every 30 min ( ) *Continue treatment plan as ordered	*Level of observation: 1:1 ( ); every 15 min ( ); every 30 min ( ) *Treatment plan as ordered *Monitor sleep/rest pattern	*Level of observation: 1:1 ( ); every 15 min ( ); every 30 min ( ) *Treatment plan as ordered *Monitor sleep/rest pattern	*Level of observation: 1:1 ( ); every 15 min ( ); every 30 min ( ) *Treatment plan as ordered *Monitor sleep/rest pattern	*Discharge with specified treatment confirmed for aftercare

	Interval	Day of Admit	Day 2	Day 3	Day 4	Day 5	Day 6	Day 7	Day 8
	Location								
PROCESSES	Medications (IV & Others)	*Meds as ordered *Protocols for anti-psychotic med management *Monitor side effects *Toxicity *Pain	*Meds as ordered *Protocols for anti-psychotic med management *Monitor side effects *Toxicity *Pain	*Meds as ordered *Protocols for anti-psychotic med management *Monitor side effects *Toxicity *Pain	*Meds as ordered *Protocols for anti-psychotic med management *Monitor side effects *Toxicity *Pain	*Meds as ordered *Contact managed care with med changes *Protocols for anti-psychotic med management *Monitor side effects *Toxicity *Pain	*Meds as ordered *Protocols for anti-psychotic med management *Monitor side effects *Toxicity *Review meds with family/significant other *Pain	*Meds as ordered *Protocols for anti-psychotic med management *Monitor side effects *Toxicity *Pain	*Discharge with meds and instructions as ordered *Discharge pain free
	Activity	*OT assessment *1:1 reality orient/brief contact *Assist with ADLs *Interventions to control self/other harm/impulses	*Continue OT eval *Engage in groups as tolerated *Assist with ADLs *Interventions to control self/other harm/impulses	*OT eval *Engage in groups as tolerated *ADLs with reminders *Interventions to control self/other harm/impulses	*Engage in 2 groups as tolerated *Interventions to control self/other harm/impulses	*Independent ADLs *Engage in 2 groups per day *Provide opportunity for simple decision making	*Independent ADLs *Engage in all unit activities *Provide opportunity for simple decision making	*Independent ADLs *Engage in all unit activities *Encourage independent decision making	*Independent ADLs *Engage in all unit activities *Confirm decision making *Confirm safety
	Diet/Nutrition/ Weight	*Nutritional screening *Elicit food preference *Offer adequate nutrition/fluids *Baseline weight (weekly unless otherwise ordered)	*Offer adequate nutrition/fluids *Provide simple meals: Finger foods Room-temperature drinks	*Offer adequate nutrition/fluids *Encourage meals in milieu as tolerated with staff supervision	*Offer adequate nutrition/fluids *Encourage meals in milieu as tolerated with staff supervision	*Offer adequate nutrition/fluids *Teach family/significant other importance of adequate nutrition/fluids	*Offer adequate nutrition/fluids *Teach family/significant other importance of adequate nutrition/fluids	*Reinforce adequate nutrition/fluids *Weekly weight	*Confirm patient family/significant other knowledge adequate nutrition/fluids *Confirm adequate nutrition/fluids

Pathway Variances: P1. CP completed early P2. Client off CP P3. Pathway Completed & Client Not Discharged P4. Initial Interval Not Appropriate

Element Variances:

1. Client/Family:
   1. Client physiologic status
   2. Client psychologic status
   3. Client/family refusal
   4. Client/family unavailable
   5. Client/family other
   6. Client/family communication barrier
   7. Element met early
2. Clinician:
   1. Order differs from CP
   2. Action differs from CP
   3. Response time
   4. Clinician other
   5. Court/guardianship
3. Operating Unit
   1. Bed/appointment not available
   2. Lack of data
   3. Supplies/equipment not available
   4. Department overbooked/closed
   5. Court/guardianship
   6. Operating unit other
4. Community
   1. Placement not available
   2. Home care not available
   3. Ambulance delay
   4. Transportation not available
   5. Community other
5. Payer
   1. Delayed giving authorization number
   2. Payer limitations
   3. Payer other

FIGURE 12-4, cont'd Clinical pathway for psychosis.

Symptoms that may occur during the depressed phase are similar to those occurring in major depression and include the following:

- Poor appetite
- Weight loss
- Inability to sleep
- Agitation
- General slowing down
- Loss of interest in usual activities (anhedonia)
- Lack of energy or fatigue
- Feelings of worthlessness
- Self-reproach (criticism)
- Excessive guilt
- Inability to think or concentrate, or thoughts of death or suicide

Symptoms that may occur during the manic phase are similar to those occurring in bipolar mania and include the following:

- Increase in social, work, or sexual activity
- Increased talkativeness
- Rapid or racing thoughts
- Grandiosity
- Decreased need for sleep
- Increased goal-directed activity
- Agitation
- Inflated self-esteem
- Distractibility
- Involvement in self-destructive activities

Symptoms that may occur during psychotic episodes are similar to those occurring in other psychotic disorders and include the following:

- Delusions (fixed beliefs—altered thought processes)
- Hallucinations (sensory/perceptual alterations)
- Incoherence
- Severely disorganized speech or thinking
- Grossly disorganized behavior
- Total immobility
- Lack of facial emotional expression (flattened or blunted affect)
- Lack of speech or motivation

Treatment. The following methods are useful for the treatment of schizoaffective disorder and other related disorders:

- *Psychotherapy*. The nurse and client work together to establish goals.
- *Medications*. Antipsychotics, antidepressants, lithium, or other mood stabilizers. Often several medications are used in combination.
- *Skills training*. Focuses on interpersonal skills, grooming and hygiene, budgeting, grocery shopping, job seeking, cooking, and other similar activities.

Self-Management. Give the following instructions to the client to help maximize the prognosis:

- Recognize that this is a prolonged illness.
- Identify strengths and limitations.
- Set clear, realistic goals.
- Develop a set of wellness strategies to help with daily living.
- Identify several people that will offer support as needed.
- Plan a regular, consistent, predictable, daily routine.
- Identify external stressors that possibly trigger illness.
- Identify internal symptoms that possibly trigger illness.
- Develop an action plan to deal with external and internal stressors.
- Make only one change in life at a time.
- Work toward an active, trusting relationship with nurses and treatment staff.
- Take medication regularly, as prescribed.
- Identify early signs of relapse and develop an early warning list.
- After a relapse, slowly and gradually return to responsibilities.
- Avoid street drugs.
- Discuss intake of alcoholic beverages with your physician.
- Eat a well-balanced diet.
- Get sufficient rest.
- Exercise regularly.
- Check reality with a trusted individual if you are unsure of the nature of your thoughts or feelings.
- Contrast your behavior with others if you are unsure of the nature of your actions.
- Accept that there will be occasional setbacks.

Managing Relapse. Give the following instructions to the client for managing a relapse:

- Develop a plan of action with your nurse or therapist if relapse signs appear. (Do this during well periods.)
- Involve a friend, family member, or other trusted individual to help in times of relapse.
- Your plan should include specific warning signs of relapse, an agreement to notify the nurse or therapist as soon as relapse warning signs appear, an agreement to contact those individuals who will help reduce stress and stimulation, and a list of specific ways to decrease stress and stimulation and increase structure.

Prognosis. This disorder often has a better prognosis than schizophrenia but a less positive prognosis than depression. It is a lifelong illness for most individuals, although the precise course of illness differs for each person. Symptoms tend to worsen during times of stress and limit functioning, resulting in hospitalization.

Symptoms of the Schizophrenias

Neuropsychiatrists have tried to find common threads that link the schizophrenias or areas of differentiation that separate them. There is a common underlying theme in schizophrenic disorders that is connected to certain symptom profiles of a perceptual, thought, emotional, cognitive, behavioral, or social nature (see the Clinical Symptoms box).

CLINICAL SYMPTOMS

Schizophrenia

PERCEPTUAL

Hallucinations:
- Auditory: May be commanding; content matches delusions
- Visual: May see images not actually present
- Tactile: For example, may feel like being surrounded by spider webs
- Olfactory and gustatory: Client may refuse to eat because food seems to smell or taste bad

Illusions: False perceptions caused by misinterpretations of real objects

Altered internal sensations:
- Formication: Sensation of worms crawling around inside one
- Chill: Feeling of chills in the marrow of one's bones

Agnosia: Perceptual failure to recognize familiar environmental stimuli, such as sounds or objects seen or felt; sometimes called "negative hallucinations"

Distortion of body image: With respect to size, facial expression, activity, amount and nature of detail, exaggeration or diminution of body parts

Negative self-perception: With respect to ability and competence

THOUGHT

Delusions: Unusual ideas, not reality based:
- Omnipotence: Perception of unrealistic power
- Persecution: Perception that someone is out to harm or kill the individual
- Controlling or being controlled: With respect to an outside force or entity

Derealizaiton: Loss of ego boundaries; cannot tell where own body ends and environment begins; feeling that the world around one is not real or is distorted

Ideas of reference: Perception that other people or the media are talking to or about the individual

Incorrect use of language:
- Neologisms: Invented words
- Incoherence: Nonsensical thoughts
- Echolalia: Imitating others' words
- Word salad: Mixed up words
- Concrete, restricted vocabulary: Unable to use abstract reasoning or to conceptualize
- Perseveration: Persistent repetition of the same ideas

Obsessive thoughts: Recurring thoughts

Poverty of thought: Reduction of thoughts

Thought blocking: Abrupt disruption of flow of thoughts or ideas

Loosening of associations: Fragmented thoughts noted in incoherent speech

Flight of ideas: Abrupt change of topic in a rapid flow of speech

EMOTIONAL

Labile affect, range of emotions:
- Apathy: Indifferent or dulled response
- Flattened affect: Restricted facial expression
- Reduced responsiveness
- Exaggerated euphoria
- Rage

Inappropriate affect: Laughing at sad events, crying over joyous ones

Disruption in limbic functioning: Inability to screen out disruptive stimuli and loss of voluntary control of response

COGNITIVE

Errors in memory recall and retention, especially working memory

Difficulty in comprehending, processing, and categorizing information

Difficulty sustaining attention: Unable to complete tasks, errors of omission

Lack of judgment: Unable to assess or evaluate situations or make rational choices

Lack of insight: Unable to perceive and understand cause and nature of own and others' situations (e.g., own illness)

Difficulty in executive functioning (e.g., planning, decision-making, problem-solving)

BEHAVIORAL

Little impulse control:
- Sudden scream as a protest of frustration
- Self-mutilation, to substitute physical for emotional pain
- Injury to a body part believed to be offensive
- Response to command hallucinations

Inability to cope with depression:
- Depressed client has a 50% risk for suicide
- Frequent exacerbations and remissions in one who has insight
- Lack of social support to help

Inability to manage anger: Anger and lack of impulse control lead to violence—verbal aggression, destruction of property, injury to others, homicide

Substance abuse as coping: Dulls painful psychologic symptoms

Noncompliance with medication: May feel it is not needed or has too many side effects

SOCIAL

Poor peer relationships:
- Few friends as a child or adolescent
- Preference for solitude

Low interest in hobbies and activities:
- Daydreamer
- Not functioning well in social or occupational areas
- Preoccupied and detached
- Behavioral autism: Marked impairment in social and behavioral functioning

Loss of interest in appearance:
- Careless grooming
- Introversion

Not competitive in sports or academics:
- Poor adjustment to school
- Withdrawal from activities

May suffer from the following:
- Attention deficit disorder
- Somatic symptoms (multiple physical problems)
- Schizoid or schizotypal traits: Solitary, detached, self-absorbed, social anxiety

Perceptual

Hallucinations occur in any of the five receptive senses (auditory, visual, tactile, olfactory, or gustatory), but the auditory area is most common, with over 50% of patients with schizophrenia reporting auditory hallucinations (hearing voices that are troubling for the client) (Lieberman, 2006b). Researchers believe that a left hemisphere brain abnormality causes hallucinations because the left hemisphere contains Broca's area, the language-processing center. From assessment procedures, researchers determined that the left hemisphere responded to hallucinations as if it were hearing real voices, which may be an indication that the hallucinations are a reflection of the actual delusional thinking of the person with schizophrenia (Green et al., 1994).

Clients and families must recognize that hallucinations are symptoms of the illness and are real to the client. Because of this, family attempts to force the truth on the client are not therapeutic and are sometimes even demeaning. Hallucinations respond to a reduction of stress and an increase in antipsychotic medication. They often become less troubling when clients are distracted. For example, some time-proven methods, such as keeping the client busy, using competing stimuli to drown out the voices (whistling, clapping, shouting the word *stop*), and teaching the client not to wait for the voices to occur, help occupy the mind with some other activity (Thornton et al., 2001c).

Thought

Even adults have a tendency to personalize and misinterpret events, most notably in times of stress or fatigue. It is self-fulfilling to occasionally escape from reality and imagine ourselves as more powerful or successful than we really are. For those of us without schizophrenia, however, these periods of fantasy are generally short lived and well within our control. What is different in the client with schizophrenia who is experiencing a delusion during an acute period is that the conviction is fixed, and a person with schizophrenia will reject any attempt by well-meaning individuals to explain reality during this time. Arguing with a client experiencing a delusion leads to further mistrust or anger. Families and friends need to realize that delusions are a result of the illness and not stubbornness or stupidity on the part of the client. Avoid emotional reactions, sarcasm, and threats. An empathetic response is always possible no matter what the delusion or conviction is.

For example, the client believes he is at the center of a government plot and cannot sleep at night. There are possibly underlying feelings of worthlessness or fear, and the delusion fills the need to be important and protected. An empathetic response is "It must be difficult not to be able to get some sleep at night and to feel afraid. You are safe here in the hospital, and the care you get will help you feel better." This type of response builds trust, rapport, and, possibly adherences to the treatment plan that will help the client improve (Thornton et al., 2001c). Implications for the psychoeducation of persons with schizophrenia include the following:

- Teaching at times when symptoms are relatively stable
- Simplifying instructions and reducing distractions (or providing distractions to offset symptoms as necessary)
- Providing both visual and verbal information
- Using direct, clear terms versus abstractions or concepts
- Teaching in small segments with frequent reinforcement
- Not offering choices that often confuse the individual, yet offering more choices as client improves

As a result of thought disturbance, speech is affected. Subtle forms of speech disorders are *circumstantiality*, in which the person digresses to unnecessary details, and *tangentiality*, or responding in a manner irrelevant to the topic at hand. If the person is less impaired, listening for themes helps to identify client concerns (Sadock et al., 2004).

Thought processes in schizophrenia change with the individual's clinical status. As clinical status worsens, sometimes thoughts evolve into a world of fantasy or are expressed as autistic thinking (internally stimulated thoughts not based in reality), **perseveration** (persistent repetition of the same idea in response to different questions), poverty of thought (lack of ability to produce thoughts), and loosening of associations (LOA) (fragmented, incoherent thoughts) (Sadock et al., 2004).

It is difficult to communicate with the client during these acute phases, which is frustrating to family and friends. Sometimes nonverbal communication, such as writing, is an effective way to communicate, as thoughts are usually more organized in writing. Do not force yourself to listen, as it will only frustrate both the client and the listener. Also, do not speak to others about the client as if the client were not there. Determine where the client's interests and strengths are, and use music, art, exercise, or movement to communicate during this period (see Chapter 23). Even if the language side of the brain is not functioning, the client is still able to focus on other activities. In the client with chronic disease, there is a general decline in intellectual functioning over the years, which presents a real challenge to nurses, families, and caregivers (Thornton et al., 2001c). Clients with chronic schizophrenia have little insight into their illness and, as such, experience impaired judgment. Patience, empathy, and understanding are critical factors in caring for clients with chronic schizophrenia.

Emotional

Emotional blunting and lack of displaying emotions are examples of negative symptoms in schizophrenia. Some people show few emotions while others show a total lack of facial expression. Some clients also avoid eye contact and have reduced verbal and nonverbal contact with others. The person's speech also lacks inflection so the person speaks in a monotone. Some have a lack of gestures (Lieberman, 2006b). This decrease in expressed emotions coupled with a monotone and lack of gestures when speaking makes it difficult to fully appreciate the interaction with the person.

Cognitive

Cognitive disturbances in people with schizophrenia affect everyday functioning. One area that is affected is vigilance. Vigilance is the ability to maintain attention over time. People who are unable maintain this attention have difficulty following instructions critical to their care. Not being able to maintain attention along with having difficulty with verbal fluency also has a negative impact on social and work related interactions. Other cognitive deficit areas include learning, reasoning, and problem solving. Difficulties in these areas hinder the person's ability to adapt to a rapidly changing everyday world (Lieberman, 2006b).

Behavioral

The behavioral disturbance of greatest concern in schizophrenia is the possibility of violence. The risk of violence increases if the client also has coexisting alcohol abuse, substance abuse, antisocial personality, or neurologic impairments (APA, 2004). However, these factors do not identify persons who will actually become violent. The challenges for nursing is to note changes in client behavior, read the situation accurately, interact according to the client's level of crisis, and intervene at a level that meets the client's need (Johnson, 2004). It is important to ask about thoughts of violence and determine who the intended victim is. Setting limits and using the behavioral approach are two strategies used to manage persistently violent clients. Clients in the community who are more likely to be violent with relapses need mandatory outpatient treatment programs. Mandatory outpatient treatment (MOT) is court-ordered treatment for those clients with mental illness who may not use services without a court order. Use MOT as a last resort (American Psychiatric Nurses Association, 2003). (See Chapter 22.)

Social

Poor social competence is one of the hallmarks of schizophrenia as seen in many of the negative symptoms described earlier in this chapter. Typically, people with schizophrenia have a history of a schizoid or schizotypical personality, which includes solitary behaviors, detachment, constricted or inappropriate affect, passive or indifferent responses, and lack of strong emotions. It is difficult for them to respond to normal social cues, initiate conversations, develop relationships with others, or become productive members of society. (See Chapter 13.)

In spite of research into the biologic causes of schizophrenia, the issue of nature versus nurture still poses questions. There is speculation that children raised by parents with schizophrenia may emulate the parent's poor social behaviors. Also, parents with children with schizophrenia may be turned off by their child's inability to relate or display normal emotions. Although many of the older theories of mother and child detachment and poor bonding have lost credibility, these factors linger as a result of mental health's strong affinity for the psychosocial therapies as a viable method of treatment (see Chapter 23). Studies show that persons with good verbal memories are better able to learn and retain social skills and therefore have more hope for a productive life within the limitation of their illness. Sadock et al. (2004) state that of all the diagnostic profiles used to describe schizophrenia, the early works of Bleuler and Schneider are the most common (Box 12-4).

Biologic Profiles

Neurologic examinations, neuropsychologic tests, and various brain-scanning techniques (neuroimaging) support symptom profiles and are relevant for clients with schizophrenia. Table 12-3 presents some of these examinations. In general, the tests verify findings that schizo-

BOX 12-4

Diagnostic Profiles of Bleuler and Schneider

BLEULER

Characteristics of Schizophrenia

Incongruence between feelings and thoughts
Incongruence in the behavioral expression of feelings and thoughts

Four Primary Symptoms of Schizophrenia (see Box 12-1)

Affect is disturbed
Autism is present
Ambivalence is common
Associations are loosened

Accessory Symptoms

Hallucinations
Delusions

SCHNEIDER

First-Rank Symptoms of Schizophrenia

Hallucinations
Thought withdrawal (belief that one's thoughts have been removed from one's head)
Thought broadcasting (belief that one's thoughts are broadcast from one's head)
Delusions
Somatic experiences

Second-Rank Symptoms of Schizophrenia

Perceptual disorders
Perplexity
Mood changes
Feelings of emotional impoverishment

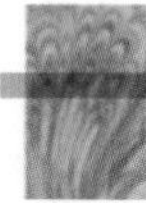

TABLE 12-3

Biologic Profiles in Schizophrenia

TEST	FUNCTION
NEUROLOGIC EXAMINATIONS	
Apgar rating of the newborn	To rate functioning of the newborn nervous system
Physiologic and anatomic testing of the nervous system (general)	To discover infections, lesions, or metabolic problems that affect the nervous system
NEUROPSYCHOLOGIC TESTS	
Halstead-Reitan battery	To test higher cortical functioning To detect early signs of memory and cognitive dysfunction To design and evaluate remediation programs (Osmon, 1991)
Luria-Nebraska test battery	To predict behavior by examining neurologic functioning (Meador and Nichols, 1991) To assess client progress in various areas
Eye-tracking and auditory tests	To discover information-processing deficits (Perry and Braff, 1994)
NEUROIMAGING STUDIES	
Magnetic resonance imaging (MRI)	To determine structural and functional changes in the brain, which confirm specific anomalies in the brains of individuals diagnosed with schizophrenia
Positron emission tomography (PET)	To determine effects of antipsychotic medications on certain neurotransmitter receptor sites and their various rates of occupancy by studying sections of the brain
Bioelectron activity measure (BEAM)	To measure activity of the brain in clients with schizophrenia by using colorized topography

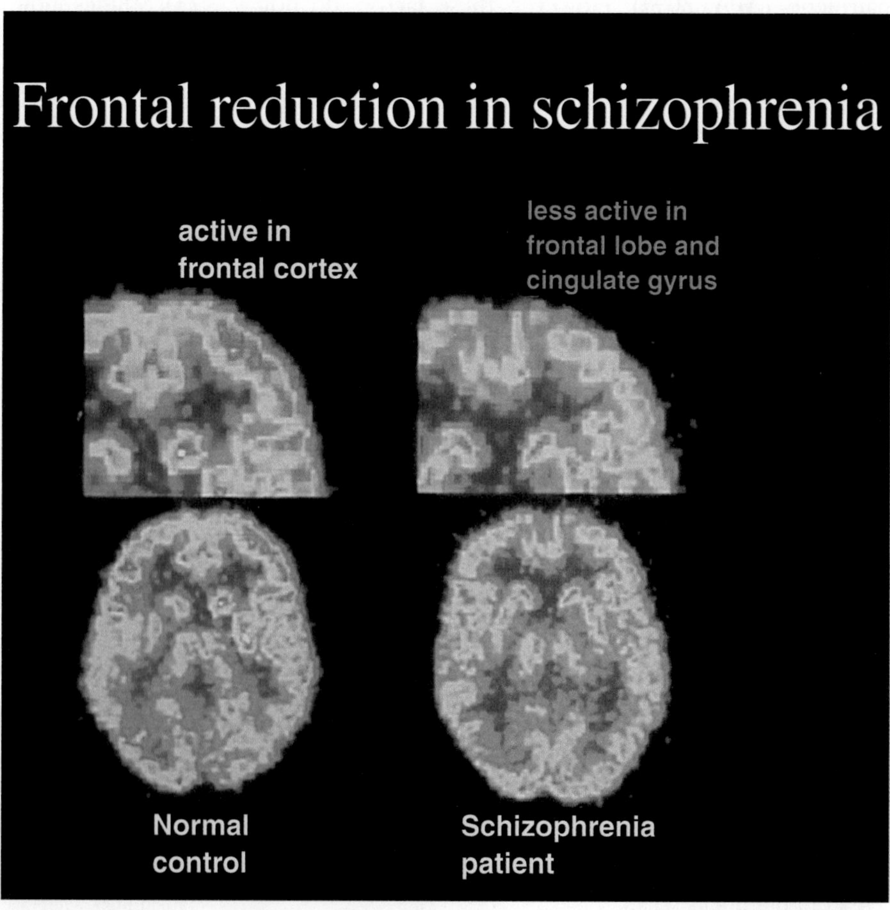

FIGURE 12-5 Positron emission tomography (PET) scan with 18F-deoxyglucose shows metabolic activity in a horizontal section of the brain in a control subject *(left)* and in an unmedicated client with schizophrenia *(right)*. Red and yellow indicate lower activity in the white matter areas of the brain. The frontal lobe is magnified to show reduced frontal activity in the prefrontal cortex of the client with schizophrenia. (Courtesy Monte S. Buchsbaum, MD, Mt. Sinai School of Medicine, New York.)

phrenia has diffuse, nonlocalizable areas of dysfunction. Evidence of generalized impairment is in persons with a first episode, as well as chronic schizophrenia, although the degree of impairment usually differs with subtypes. Individuals with schizophrenia seem to have impairments in the stimulus inhibition (gating) circuitry of the brain, sometimes leading to stimulus overload. Thus, they are handicapped in sorting out and paying attention to the information necessary to solve a problem.

Modern brain-scanning technology has enabled scientists to assemble not only a structural image of the brain but also a functional image that indicates activity in various areas (Figure 12-5). Forthcoming functional MRI studies, mentioned earlier (see Figure 12-1), will improve this contemporary area of research, as modern technology will enable the rapid transmission of information via the Internet.

DISCHARGE CRITERIA

For the client with schizophrenia to be discharged to the community, the following criteria need to be met. Client will:

- Demonstrate absence of suicidality.
- Verbalize control of hallucinations.
- Identify events or episodes of increased anxiety that worsen symptoms.
- Have family or a significant other willing to serve as a support network.
- Accept referral of self or a significant other to a physician, therapist, or agency for help and monitoring.
- Accept responsibility for own actions and self-care.
- Verbalize ways of coping with anxiety, stress, and problems encountered in the community.
- Have access to a safe living environment in the community: own home, board-and-care facility, or halfway house.
- Use known community resources, such as support groups, day care centers, and vocational or rehabilitation programs.
- Explain the following about medication: importance, expected effects, adverse effects, prescribed dose and time of taking the medication, and effects of the interaction of the medication with other substances such as food or alcohol.

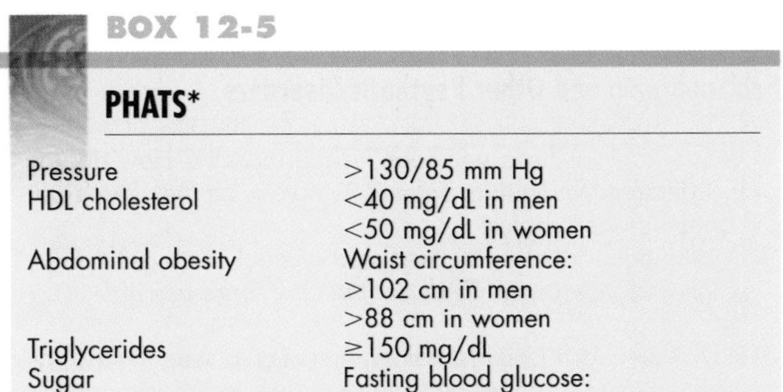

BOX 12-5

PHATS*

Pressure	>130/85 mm Hg
HDL cholesterol	<40 mg/dL in men <50 mg/dL in women
Abdominal obesity	Waist circumference: >102 cm in men >88 cm in women
Triglycerides	≥150 mg/dL
Sugar	Fasting blood glucose: ≥110 mg/dL

From Grove GA: Beware of PHATS in metabolic syndrome, *Curr Psychiatr* 5: 2006.
*Three of five positive criteria indicate metabolic syndrome.

The Nursing Process

ASSESSMENT

Assessment of the individual with schizophrenia is complicated because of the different symptom profiles for the various subtypes of the condition. Nurses obtain subjective data through symptom reporting and by the behavioral descriptions of significant others. Nurses perform objective assessment observation by using rating scales and by checking biologic indicators, as described in earlier sections. For psychiatric mental health nurses, it is important not to lose sight of the biologic focus so prevalent in the other specialties. For nurses, one of the critical components of assessment is what the client says in the interview. However, for people with psychotic disorders, there is impaired processing of perceptual information. As a result, physical symptoms such as pain are misperceived or misread. Likewise, for the nurse it is difficult to tell the difference between a genuine complaint and a delusion (Reeves and Torres, 2003). For example, the client who tells you she is pregnant and about to deliver a baby may have menstrual cramps, endometriosis, a sexually transmitted disease, constipation, or any number of ailments she interprets as a pregnancy. Likewise, a client who tells you his heart is broken could have angina, acid reflux, or other real complaints. Listening attentively to the client as well as completing a physical assessment is necessary for an adequate assessment. Furthermore, attention to vital signs as well as nutrition, exercise, and sleep patterns is necessary.

Clients with schizophrenia are at increased risk for the metabolic syndrome, and nurses need to assess for this syndrome. The metabolic syndrome is a cluster of findings including increased visceral adiposity, which the nurse measures by waist circumference, hyperglycemia, hypertension, and dyslipidemia (Meyer, 2005). PHATS is a mnemonic that helps monitor metabolic syndrome risk factors quickly (Box 12-5). The symptoms come from the National Cholesterol Education Program criteria.

Along with the biologic components, the nursing assessment includes psychologic ratings such as the mental status examination rating scale to organize data (see Chapter 3). The mental status examination considers the categories of appearance, behavior, orientation, memory, thought processes, perceptual processes, intellectual functioning, feelings (mood) and affect, insight, and judgment. Four of these categories are particularly important in schizophrenia: disturbances in perception, thought, feelings, and behavior (see the Nursing Assessment Questions box).

For children and adolescents, take into consideration the developmental status of the individual when assessing the positive and negative symptoms. Remember that in children normal patterns of thinking are concrete, not abstract. Likewise, consider the client's age when assessing impulse control because it is not normally developed until adolescence (Fields et al., 1994).

NURSING ASSESSMENT QUESTIONS

Schizophrenia and Other Psychotic Disorders

1 What problems have you been having recently? How do you feel differently now than before? *To determine the client's perception of the problem*
2 Do you now or have you ever used alcohol or drugs? If so, when and how often? *To determine the client's use of substances*
3 Have you heard (sounds, voices, messages), seen (lights, figures), smelled (strange, bad, good odors), tasted (strange, bad, good tastes), or felt (touching, warm, cold sensation) anything that others who were present did not? *To determine if the client is having hallucinations*
4 What are the voices like that you hear? What do they say? Are they troubling for you? *To determine if they instruct the client to harm self or other*

QUESTIONS TO DETERMINE IF THE CLIENT IS EXPERIENCING DELUSIONS

1 Do you believe that someone or something outside of you is controlling you in some way? Are you able to control other people?
2 Do you believe you are being watched? Followed?
3 Are people talking about you? If yes, explain how you know this.
4 Are you experiencing guilt? Do you believe you have anything to be guilty about? Do you think you are a bad person? If yes, what makes you believe this?

NURSING DIAGNOSIS

Nursing diagnoses are formulated from the information obtained during the assessment phase of the nursing process. The accuracy of each diagnosis depends on a careful in-depth assessment. Nursing diagnoses are prioritized according to client needs, from urgent to least urgent. Some of the more common diagnoses applicable to schizophrenia include the following:

- Risk for suicide
- Risk for self-directed violence
- Risk for other-directed violence
- Disturbed sensory perception
- Disturbed thought processes
- Impaired verbal communication
- Ineffective coping
- Interrupted family processes
- Self-care deficit (bathing/hygiene, dressing/grooming, feeding, toileting)
- Social isolation
- Risk-prone health behavior

OUTCOME IDENTIFICATION

Outcome identification is an estimate of the behavioral changes anticipated after interventions. The severity of the symptoms, the cultural setting, and the prognosis for the particular diagnosis all influence outcomes. The outcomes of schizophrenia therefore result from complex interactions. Outcomes are prioritized according to client needs, from most urgent to least urgent. Client will:

- Demonstrate an absence of suicidal behaviors or violent behaviors toward others.
- Demonstrate an absence of self-mutilating behaviors.
- Demonstrate significant reduction in hallucinations and delusions.
- Demonstrate reality-based thinking and behavior.
- Engage in own hygiene, grooming, and ADL skills.
- Socialize with peers and staff and participate in all groups.
- Adhere to medication regimen and verbalize an understanding of the role of medications in reducing psychotic symptoms.
- Demonstrate more functional coping and problem-solving methods.
- Participate in discharge planning with family/significant others.

PLANNING

Planning nursing interventions and treatment geared to the whole person and his or her social environment, including the family, is challenging. Because behavioral problems come from many sources and range from less serious to extremely serious, nurses needs to consider interventions at a variety of levels and prioritize according to client needs from the most urgent to the least urgent. Medical interventions generally focus on underlying biologic factors and involve diagnostic procedures such as neuroimaging, somatic strategies, and treatment with medication. The nurse's role at this level is to prepare the client and family by explaining the rationale for the interventions and assisting with treatment adherence. The nurse also uses nursing measures at this level based on his or her knowledge of basic biologic functions and needs.

Interpersonally and socially, clients with schizophrenia are disadvantaged by being unable to view things from the perspective of others. Because of the inability to abstract and correctly interpret, the individual with schizophrenia sees others as unpredictable and often misinterpret others' words and actions. Role-playing scenarios, which help clients to see things from another person's perspective, are helpful. Socialization is often a focus of the treatment plan because it includes the client in activities that are supportive and nonthreatening and that provide helpful feedback on how the client presents to others. Social skills groups are useful in helping the individual build interpersonal skills. Nurses need to avoid power struggles (see the Case Study).

Family interactions are particularly difficult for the client with schizophrenia. If the treatment team does not

CASE STUDY Lance, a 35-year-old man with chronic schizophrenia, was living in a single room in a downtown hotel that houses people with mental illness. Lance was never able to budget his minimal income to last the whole month. He had a fixed delusion that he owned the hotel where he lived, but that the manager and the government were defrauding him of his rent money. When Lance was short of cash at the end of the month, he became abusive and aggressive. When Lance was assaultive, the manager called the police, and Lance was readmitted to the psychiatric hospital involuntarily for dangerousness to others. In about 10 days he was discharged to the same hotel where he would live quietly for a while, helping the manager with tasks until the next delusional episode. This was a repetitive pattern for Lance, who had no support from relatives or friends.

CRITICAL THINKING

1. What is the significance of Lance's delusion?
2. Lance received good care at the psychiatric hospital. Standard outcome criteria for discharge were always met. If this pattern continued, what would the chances be that Lance would hold onto his delusion?
3. Why might a nurse's attempt to challenge the delusion be risky? What are some teaching strategies that nurses could use with Lance? In what form would they best be implemented? When Lance is stable, can he identify any early warning signs that things are starting to break down for him? Is Lance willing to accept/identify someone as a supporter who can help him?
4. If you were a community mental health nurse, how would you do follow-up care for Lance? Consider his money management issues and how these may affect Lance in obtaining his medications, food, and other necessities at the end of each month.
5. What signs of escalating anxiety would you look for in Lance's behavior? How would you manage his anxiety?

involve the family or significant supporters in the treatment planning for services after discharge, the family will be unable to help the clients maintain community support, thus leading to a relapse and rehospitalizations.

IMPLEMENTATION

It is important to involve the client and family in the treatment process, explaining all interventions and reasons for care. Well-planned interventions will still be challenging for the nurse if there are misunderstandings about what to expect or if there is resistance from client, family, or others. Financial or environmental limitations will also be problematic to interventions. As much as possible, clients need to set their own goals and pace for treatment and progress.

In the beginning, some clients are so ill that they cannot understand or accept an appropriate effort to help. In that case, the nurse needs to work on establishing a therapeutic relationship first before the client will accept the well-meaning interventions.

An existing therapeutic relationship between the client and nurse will be expanded later to include the client's family or significant others for lasting effectiveness of the interventions. In some cases, the nurse will need to make interventions at yet another level, the level of the school or the workplace. All involved need to be aware of the what, why, and how of the therapeutic plan so that they are able to work as a team.

When clients are in the most acute phase of their illness, choices are more limited and the structured interventions are most helpful. However, as the client's condition improves, the client can take advantage of more options and nurses are able to develop a recovery model of hope and care.

The family's economic situation also deserves attention. Health care personnel are not usually thinking of the cost of implementing a care plan that involves therapy, medication, diet, transportation access to outpatient care, or other factors creating unplanned expenses. It is important to assess for such expenses, problem-solve the issues, and include the solutions with the plan. Interventions are prioritized as much as possible according to client needs, from most urgent to least urgent.

Thornton et al. (2001c) identified four important Ss of schizophrenia—stimulation, structure, socialization, and support—to help families and caregivers help clients overcome negative symptoms (apathy, lack of motivation, lack of interest, lack of energy) (Box 12-6).

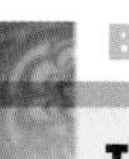

BOX 12-6

The Four Ss of Schizophrenia

Stimulation: Introducing, slowly and gradually, new routines, people, events, and situations to the client
Structure: Providing daily routine and expectations for every part of the day: waking, dressing, eating, activity
Socialization: Getting people in their lives to help with finances, health, food, socializing
Support: Offering encouragement to try new tasks; accompanying client to new places until the client makes friends

From Thornton JF et al: Schizophrenia: symptoms and management at home, *Internet Mental Health*, Jan 2, 2001.

Nursing Interventions

1. Observe and monitor risk factors, specifically for suicide or violence toward others. *This promotes safety of the client and others and reduces the risk for violence.*
2. Reduce/minimize environmental stimulation. *This promotes a quiet, soothing milieu (setting) that will lessen the client's impulsivity and agitation and prevent accident or injury.*
3. Provide frequent timeouts or brief, low-key interactions. *This calms the client by providing opportunities for rest, relaxation, and ventilation of impulsive feelings, which reduces the risk of acting-out behaviors.*
4. Support and monitor prescribed medical and psychosocial interventions. *This encourages the client and family to participate in the treatment plan and prevents the client's behavior from escalating to violence.*
5. Use clear, concrete statements versus abstract, general statements. *The client is not always able to understand complex messages, and, as such, the client sometimes*

has misperceptions or hallucinations. Individuals with schizophrenia generally respond better to concrete messages during the acute phase.

6. Attempt to determine factors that worsen the client's hallucinatory experiences (e.g., stressors that trigger sensory-perceptual disturbances). *Although hallucinations have a biochemical etiology, outside stressors sometimes intensify hallucinations in a vulnerable client, and identifying such stressors will help to prevent the severity of the hallucinatory experience.*
7. Praise the client for reality-based perceptions, reduction/cessation in aggressive/acting-out behaviors, and appropriate social interaction and group participation. *Warranted praise reinforces repetition of functional behaviors when given at appropriate times during the treatment plan, such as when medication has begun to take effect.*
8. Educate the client and family/significant others about the client's symptoms, the importance of medication compliance, and continued use of therapeutic support services after discharge. *This facilitates learning and increases the client and family/significant other knowledge base, ensures the client's continued therapeutic support, and possibly prevents relapse after discharge from the hospital.*
9. Distract the client from delusions that tend to exacerbate aggressive or potentially violent episodes. *Engaging the client in more functional, less anxiety-provoking activities increases the reality base and decreases the risk for violent episodes that troubling delusions cause.*
10. Focus on the meaning of the client's delusional system rather than focusing on the delusional content itself. *This helps to meet the client's needs, reinforces reality, and discourages the false belief without challenging or threatening the client.*
11. Accompany the client to group activities, beginning with the more structured, less threatening ones first and gradually incorporating more informal, spontaneous activities. *This promotes the client's socialization skills and expands the reality base in a nonthreatening way.*
12. Assist with personal hygiene, appropriate dress, and grooming until the client is able to function independently. *This helps to prevent physical complications and preserve self-esteem.*
13. Establish routine times and goals for self-care and add more complex tasks as the client's condition improves. *Routine and structure tend to organize and promote reality in the client's world.*
14. Spend intervals of time with the client each day, engaging in nonchallenging interactions. *This helps to ease the client into the community by first developing trust, rapport, and respect.*
15. Assess the client's self-concept. *A low self-concept results from social isolation.*
16. Act as a role model for social behaviors in interactions by maintaining good eye contact, appropriate social distance, and a calm demeanor. *This helps the client to identify appropriate social behavior.*
17. Keep all appointments for interactions with the client. *This promotes client trust and self-esteem.*
18. Listen actively to the client's family/significant others, allowing them to express fears and anxieties about mental illness, giving them support and empathy, and emphasizing client's strengths. *This helps the client to express emotions and assists in calming the client's irrational fears while acknowledging realistic concerns; it also promotes hope and bonding between the family/significant others and the client.*
19. Hold onto hope for clients until they are able to have hope for themselves. Increase the client's level of participation in his or her care as the client's condition improves to the extent the client is able. Allow the client choices within limits of the setting. Identify the client's strengths/assets and incorporate these into plans. Focus on activities/tasks that the client can do versus focusing on the client's limitations. *These interventions promote the client's hope and strengths and empower the client as he or she strives to achieve mental and emotional health.*

Additional Treatment Modalities

It is important that the mental health interdisciplinary treatment team work together to manage each client's mental and emotional disorder and symptoms. Consequently, team meetings are common in the psychiatric setting. Psychiatric mental health nurses, psychiatrists, psychologists, social workers, occupational therapists, recreational therapists, pharmacologists, nutritionists, primary care providers, special education teachers (for children and adolescents), and other support staff come together to communicate their expertise regarding the client's diagnosis, problems, and treatment plans. Briefly described next are the various goals and activities of these collaborative professionals in their respective disciplines (see the Additional Treatment Modalities box).

Psychopharmacology

Psychopharmacology is the somatic treatment of choice for schizophrenia. The pharmacist gives medications for clients with psychiatric disorders according to the physician's prescription and stays informed on new developments in psychotropic drugs. The pharmacist also, in collaboration with the physician and advanced practice nurses, educates the staff regarding the actions and side effects of the newer neuroleptic drugs. The pharmacist also consults with the psychiatrist regarding chemical properties of the medications and their interactions with food and other drugs. In many institutions, the pharmacist also takes some responsibility for client and family education.

Antipsychotic drugs are indicated for schizophrenia. Typical or first-generation antipsychotic drugs are high affinity antagonists of dopamine D2 receptors and are most effective in reducing the positive (psychotic) symptoms such as hallucinations and delusions. These same medications, however, have high rates of neurologic side effects such as extrapyramidal symptoms and tardive dyskinesia, because they block dopamine, which is a neurotransmitter responsible for smooth muscle movement in the extrapyra-

ADDITIONAL TREATMENT MODALITIES

Schizophrenia

- Therapeutic methods to prevent and manage violence
- Psychopharmacology
- Somatic therapy
- Milieu therapy
- Behavior modification
- Specific psychosocial rehabilitation interventions:
  Assertive community treatment
  Family interventions
  Supported employment
  Cognitive behavior therapy
  Social skills training
  Early intervention programs
- Personal therapy
- Group therapy
- Patient education
- Case management
- Guided imagery
- Assertiveness training
- Exercise, movement therapy, and dance therapy
- Occupational and recreational therapy
- Community client-family programs

midal nerve tracts. These are serious movement disorders that must be assessed and treated as soon as possible. The second-generation or atypical antipsychotics drugs promised increased efficacy and safety. The atypical drugs generally have a lower affinity for dopamine D2 receptors so may not produce the severe movement disorders that occur with the typical antipsychotics. The atypicals also have greater affinities for other neuroreceptors such as serotonin and norepinephrine and target negative symptoms more effectively (Leiberman et al., 2005).

Psychotropic drugs often have serious side effects (see the Research for Evidence-Based Practice box, on p. 275). Three of the most serious are akathisia (extreme restlessness), tardive dyskinesia (late-occurring EPS, which may be irreversible), and neuroleptic malignant syndrome (NMS), which can be potentially fatal. Acute dystonic reaction (neck or nuchal rigidity) is another troubling side effect commonly seen in the clinical setting (see Chapter 24).

Future Directions in Pharmacology. NIMH established the Measurement and Treatment Research to Improve Cognition in Schizophrenia (MATRICS) program. The MATRICS program researchers look at the brains of both healthy people as well as people with schizophrenia to see how they function. The information obtained during problem-solving tasks identifies potential molecular targets for new cognition-enhancing medications. Additionally, MATRICS supports the development of a new test to measure cognition in people with schizophrenia. The results from using the new tests will help determine whether the cognitive enhancing medications are working (NIMH, 2005).

The Role of the Nurse in Pharmacotherapy. The role of the nurse, in collaboration with the physician and pharmacist, is to support or participate in drug research that leads to effective treatment outcomes for clients with schizophrenia but with minimal or no debilitating side effects. Although the newer, atypical antipsychotics show promise in improving positive symptoms and an even greater advantage in improving negative symptoms, there are still many challenges in treating clients with schizophrenia and helping their families to understand and cope with the illness. These challenges include ongoing adherence to drug therapy, promoting medication education, and providing lifelong skills for reintegration into the community (Boyd, 2002; Guthrie, 2002).

Quality-of-life issues are also important in the long-term drug treatment of clients with schizophrenia. Nurses, the health care team, and families need to consider and manage potential adverse effects such as weight gain, diabetes mellitus, sexual dysfunction, cardiac effects, cognitive impairment, and first and foremost risk for suicide (Boyd, 2002). As drug research continues to evolve, most nurses, clinicians, and researchers agree that best treatment practice consists of medication in combination with other treatment modalities and ongoing community involvement.

When a client is discharged to the family and community, one important criterion is that he or she accepts responsibility for self-care, particularly with respect to medication. This has important implications for health teaching by nurses (see the Client and Family Teaching Guidelines box on p. 275 and the Research for Evidence-Based Practice box on p. 276).

Interventions for Agitation Symptoms. Research indicates that rapid control of acute agitation in schizophrenia is achieved through use of certain atypical antipsychotics, with a low incidence of extrapyramidal symptoms. However, researchers also indicate that more clinical experience is necessary to ensure safety and efficacy, especially with the older population and clients with renal or hepatic impairment (Murphy, 2002).

Pharmacotherapy is used in conjunction with physical or behavioral restraints for assaultive or combative clients when verbal interventions fail and client refuses to take oral medications. Health care providers apply restraints according to guidelines set forth by The Joint Commission (TJC) in conjunction with other accrediting bodies such as the Department of Health Services (DHS) and the Centers for Medicare and Medicaid Services (CMMS) (Murphy, 2002) (see Chapter 8).

Somatic Therapy

Electroconvulsive therapy (ECT), combined with atypical antipsychotic medications, is beneficial. This combination is useful for clients with schizophrenia or schizoaffective disorder who also have severe symptoms that have not responded to antipsychotic medications alone. Furthermore, clients with catatonic features also respond to this treatment (APA, 2004). Nursing implications for the client receiving ECT are clear explanation of the procedure, client and family education, renegotiation of the client's

MEDICATION KEY FACTS Schizophrenia

ANTIPSYCHOTICS (NEUROLEPTICS)
- Weight, body mass index (BMI), fasting blood glucose and lipids obtained at baseline and periodically during course of treatment recommended.

CONVENTIONAL ANTIPSYCHOTICS

Chlorpromazine (Thorazine), fluphenazine (Prolixin), perphenazine (Trilafon), thioridazine (Mellaril)
- Conventional agents have dropped dramatically with the advent of atypical (second and third generation) antipsychotic agents, although recent studies concluded that use of low-to-moderate doses of mid-potency first-generation antipsychotics should be considered more frequently.
- High incidence of tardive dyskinesia (TD)* and agranulocytosis (marked decrease in number of granulocytes).
- May cause seizures, neuroleptic malignant syndrome (NMS), cardiac arrest, tachycardia, and respiratory depression.
- Alcohol and other central nervous system (CNS) depressants may increase hypotensive effect, and CNS and respiratory depression.
- Lithium and epinephrine may increase neurologic toxicity.
- Monoamine oxidase inhibitors (MAOIs), tricyclic antidepressants (TCAs), anticholinergics may increase anticholinergic effects.
- Smoking decreases plasma levels.
- Children are more susceptible to dystonias.
- Elderly female patients have a greater risk of developing extrapyramidal side effects (EPSEs).†
- *Herbal considerations:* Betel palm and kava kava may increase risk for EPSE.†
- *Dietary considerations:* Caffeine may increase akathisia/agitation.

SECOND-GENERATION (ATYPICAL) ANTIPSYCHOTICS

Clozapine (Clozaril), olanzapine (Zyprexa), quetiapine (Seroquel), risperidone (Risperdal), ziprasidone (Geodon)
- Agranulocytosis may occur with clozapine.
- Alcohol and other CNS depressants may increase CNS depression.
- Extrapyramidal symptom-producing medications may increase extrapyramidal symptoms especially in olanzapine and risperidone.
- EPSE2 may occur; TD* and NMS‡ are rare. NMS‡ is greater in quetiapine, EPSE† is greater with higher doses of Risperidal.
- *Herbal considerations:* Betel palm and kava kava may increase risk for EPSE.†
- *Dietary considerations:* Caffeine may decrease clozapine level.

THIRD-GENERATION (ATYPICAL) ANTIPSYCHOTICS

Aripiprazole (Abilify)
- EPSE† and NMS‡ occur rarely.
- Lithium and other antipsychotics increase EPSE.†
- *Herbal considerations:* Cola tree, hops, nettle, and nutmeg increases neuroleptic effect. Betel palm and kava kava increase EPSE.†

MEDICATION FOR EPSE AND NMS

Dopamine Agonist

Amantadine (Symmetrel)
- Indicated for EPSE† and NMS.‡
- Anticholinergics, antihistamines, phenothiazine, tricyclic antidepressants may increase anticholinergic effects of amantadine.
- Hydrochlorothiazide may increase amantadine blood concentration and risk for toxicity.
- *Herbal considerations:* Belladonna and henbane increase anticholinergic effect.

Antihistamine

Diphenhydramine (Benadryl)
- Anticholinergics: May increase anticholinergic effects.
- MAOIs may increase the anticholinergic and CNS depressant effects of diphenhydramine.
- Not recommended for children, neonates, or premature infants because of the increased risk for paradoxical reactions. Overdosage in children may result in hallucinations, seizures, and death.
- *Herbal considerations:* Corkwood and henbane leaf increase anticholinergic effect.

Beta Blocker

Propranolol (Inderal)
- Abrupt withdrawal may result in sweating, palpitations, headache, and tremors.
- Diuretics and other antihypertensives may increase hypotensive effect.
- Nonsteroidal anti-inflammatory drugs (NSAIDs) may decrease antihypertensive effect.
- Selective serotonin reuptake inhibitors (SSRIs) decrease metabolism and increase propranolol effect.
- *Herbal considerations:* Aconite may increase toxicity and lead to death.

Benzodiazepines

Diazepam, lorazepam, clonazepam
- Have a beneficial effect on akathisia and acute dyskinesia.

Anticholinergic Agents

Benztropine (Cogentin)
- May produce severe paradoxical reactions, marked by hallucinations, tremor, seizures, and toxic psychosis.
- Amantadine, anticholinergics, MAOIs: May increase the effects of benztropine.
- Antacids, antidiarrheals: May decrease the absorption and effects of benztropine.
- Elderly are sensitive and are more likely to develop anticholinergic delirium.
- *Herbal considerations:* Kava kava, jaborandi, and pill-bearing spurge decrease benztropine effect.

* *Tardive dyskinesia (TD)* is a neurologic syndrome consists of abnormal, involuntary, irregular choreoathetoid movements of the muscles, head, limbs, and trunk caused by the long-term use of neuroleptic drugs, manifested as tongue protrusion, puffing of the cheeks, and chewing or puckering of the mouth; occurs rarely but may be irreversible.

† *Extrapyramidal side effects (EPSE)* are serious reactions that appear to be related to high dosages of neuroleptics. They are divided into three categories: (1) akathisia, the subjective feeling of muscular discomfort that causes patients to become agitated, pace, alternately sits and stands, feels lack of control; (2) Parkinsonian symptoms, which present as muscle stiffness, cogwheel rigidity, shuffling gait, perioral tremor, hypersalivation, and masklike facial expression; and (3) acute dystonias, which are spasmodic movements caused by slow, sustained, and involuntary muscle contractions such as torticollis, opisthotonos, and oculogyric crisis and can involve the neck, jaw, tongue, or entire body.

‡ *Neuroleptic malignant syndrome (NMS)* is a life-threatening neurologic disorder caused by an adverse reaction to antipsychotic drugs; it includes high fever, sweating, unstable blood pressure, stupor, muscle rigidity, and autonomic dysfunction.

RESEARCH for EVIDENCE-BASED PRACTICE

National Institutes of Mental Health (NIMH) Clinical Anti-Psychotic Trials of Intervention Effectiveness (1999-2006)

In 1999, NIMH began a 5-year funding project of the Clinical Antipsychotic Trials of Intervention Effectiveness (CATIE). In this study, researchers followed more than 1400 patients with schizophrenia at 57 sites across the country for up to 18 months. The purpose of the study was to learn whether there were differences among the newer antipsychotic drugs and whether these newer drugs (olanzapine, quetiapine, risperidone, and ziprasidone) held significant advantages over the older meds (perphenazine in this study). Summarizing the initial results, patients with chronic schizophrenia in this study discontinued their antipsychotic study medication at a high rate, indicating that there were substantial limitations in the effectiveness of the drugs. There were no significant differences in discontinuation because of the intolerable side effects. Olanzapine, however, was associated with greater weight gain and increases in glycosylated hemoglobin, cholesterol, and triglycerides (Lieberman, 2005).

Some patients who discontinued treatment with a newer atypical antipsychotic in the above mentioned phase 1 of the CATIE trial were invited to phase 2 of the trial where they were randomly assigned to clozapine (another atypical antipsychotic) or another atypical antipsychotic that they had not received in phase 1. The patients receiving clozapine were less likely to discontinue treatment because of inadequate therapeutic responses than were patients who received any of the newer atypical antipsychotic medications (McEvoy, 2006).

Analysis of the CATIE trials continues. Researchers observed differences in efficacy and side effects, so nurses need to consider these when individualizing patient care and treatment (Lieberman, 2006a). Nurses need to be aware of the different side effect profiles to provide adequate medication education.

CLIENT and FAMILY TEACHING GUIDELINES

Medications for Treatment of Schizophrenia

TEACH THE CLIENT AND FAMILY	STRATEGIES	RATIONALE
Right to informed consent and disclosure regarding benefits, side effects, anticipated prognosis with and without medication, alternatives	Initially and any time the medication or dosage is changed, written permission is obtained from the client. Items in the left column are discussed with the client. The nurse consults with the physician regarding disclosure beneficial to the client versus disclosure that is harmful.	The client has the right to choose how much society intervenes. The client experiences independence, self-esteem, and self-control. The client develops trust because of others' regard for his or her concerns.
Correct storage and administration of medications	Explain, demonstrate, and request return demonstration on handling and administration of medications. Work with the client to prepare a check chart on medication, dosage, and times Take control of the environment: reduce distractions, simplify instructions, teach in small segments, reinforce often.	Safety of client and others is ensured. The client who is involved develops ownership of process and adherence to treatment plan. The client will be able to better focus, minimize frustration, and feel successful.
Symptoms that are reduced or eliminated by the use of medication, action of medication	Encourage the client's own desire to prevent relapse; explain in a matter-of-fact way that many people have various illnesses and take medication for them.	Offers the client hope and reinforcement. Shares the rationale for treatment.
Side effects that may be experienced	Show the client how to use a journal to record feelings, thoughts, and behaviors over time.	Helps the client to assume responsibility for self-care; documents treatment effect.
Food and drug interactions to be avoided	Inform the client about symptoms and events to report, and who to tell.	Keeps side effects from getting out of control and causing complications.
How to use the support of family and friends	Include significant others in teaching sessions. Offer thorough education, answer questions, and engage in discussion.	Elicits the support of significant others, decreases family anxiety, and allows the nurse to be a client advocate.

consent, nurturance, monitoring, orientation, support, and analgesics for headache after treatment. Chapter 23 discusses ECT in more detail.

Milieu Therapy

Milieu therapy is a 24-hour environmental therapy that shelters, protects, supports, and enhances the client with mental illness within the psychiatric setting. This is the model currently in use on psychiatric units today. The model uses individualized treatment programs, self-governance, humanistic attitudes, an enhancing environment, and links to the family and community. The purpose of milieu therapy is to assist the client in learning to manage and cope with stress, as well as to correct maladaptive behaviors (see Chapter 23).

Behavior Modification

Behavior modification is a precise approach to bringing about behavioral change. Health care providers use several types of behavior modification for schizophrenia. For example, *operant conditioning* is widely used in child and adolescent units and is useful for anyone needing behav-

RESEARCH for EVIDENCE-BASED PRACTICE

Myers RE, Shepard-White F: Evaluation of reading level and readability of psychotropic medication handouts, *Journal of the American Psychiatric Nurses Association* 10, 2004.

Nurses routinely teach clients about their medications and the importance of taking an active role regarding medications. Nurses often use written materials as tools for this education, but the benefits depend on the learner's reading and comprehension levels. One study evaluated the adequacy of reading level and readability of client education handouts for 15 of the most frequently prescribed psychotropic medications. All the handouts were written well above the recommended eighth grade level for the general public and the recommended third to fifth grade level for low-literacy readers. As needed, nurses must modify current education materials to ensure that these materials are written at the correct reading level for their clients.

ioral controls. It operates on the principle of reinforcing desirable behaviors so that they will recur and ignoring negative behaviors. Techniques include relaxation and self-control procedures. Results from using this form of therapy indicate that intolerable behaviors such as withdrawal, screaming, incontinence, and incoherence lessen (Lieberman et al., 2006b).

Specific Psychosocial Rehabilitation Interventions

Rehabilitative efforts have become increasingly important in the management of long-term schizophrenia. Individuals who are well controlled on their medications but have difficulty with daily activities are excellent candidates for rehabilitative interventions. When these interventions are properly timed in the course of the illness, they often mean the difference between a good and a poor outcome (Thornton et al., 2001a). Research has shown that psychosocial treatments are effective for individuals with schizophrenia. This includes programs for assertive community treatment, family interventions, supported employment, cognitive behavior therapy, social skills training, and programs of early intervention to prevent relapse (APA, 2004).

Assertive Community Treatment. In assertive community treatment, each program is designed specifically for the individual's strengths and deficits. Treatment teams work 24 hours a day, 7 days a week to deliver care on an outpatient basis. The staff helps the person with activities of daily living such as shopping, grooming, budgeting, and taking medications. Teams also help with job-seeking skills and placement and with offering support. This treatment is most beneficial to people with schizophrenia who have a low level of functioning or who have difficulty with treatment compliance (APA, 2004).

Family Interventions. In family intervention, the main goal is to reduce the risk of client relapse through education, support, and training to all people the client broadly considers "family." Effective family interventions include educating concerned members about mental illness and the expected course of the illness, teaching members effective coping, stress reduction, and problem solving skills and helping all members improve their communication so all effectively participate in the treatment planning process (APA, 2004).

Supported Employment. Supported employment focuses on helping the person improve vocational functioning with the goal of working toward competitive employment. The person helps choose his job while the team offers ongoing, individualized support for mental health issues. Studies have shown that people with schizophrenia have difficulty keeping the jobs they obtain because of cognitive impairments (APA, 2004).

Cognitive Behavior Therapy. Cognitive-behavioral therapy explores the connection between distorted thinking and negative behavior. For example, the client who engages in all-or-nothing thinking does not participate in a craft session because "I can never do anything right." For high-functioning clients, homework is assigned to separate negative thoughts from negative feelings. Cognitive behavior therapy involves helping the person use his or her coping skills and supporting the patient as he or she rationally works on the symptoms (APA, 2004) (see Chapter 23).

Social Skills Training. Social skills training focuses on teaching clients specific behaviors that are necessary for success in social interactions. The therapist teaches these skills by demonstrating social skills or through role-playing. Research has shown that clients with schizophrenia are able to learn social skills and independent living skills and use these skills even if their psychiatric symptoms are unchanged (APA, 2004).

Early Intervention Programs. Intervening early when symptoms indicating relapse occurrence has helped prevent rehospitalizations. Health care providers teach clients and families to recognize the early signs of relapse before the crisis occurs (APA, 2004).

Limited Evidence-Based Strategies

In addition to evidence-based treatments, there are also some limited evidence-based stategies that have time-proven effectiveness. These treatment strategies include personal therapy, group therapies, programs to treat schizophrenia before the onset of illness, client education, case management, and cognitive remediation and therapy.

Personalized Therapy. Personalized therapy usually occurs weekly within a larger treatment program that includes medications, family involvement, and psychologic support. The primary purpose is to help the person achieve and maintain clinical stability. The person with schizophrenia meets with the therapist and the focus is the client's current level of functioning. As such, the therapist individualizes the therapy to meet the person's current needs (APA, 2004).

Group Therapy. Typical goals in group therapy include helping the client with problem-solving skills, setting goals, social interactions, and medication education and management. However, there is very weak evidence to support this therapy, and most of it is from the 1970s. Generally the groups consist of six to eight clients and are for clients with enough reality testing to participate in a meaningful manner (APA, 2004).

The type of group therapy suitable for clients with schizophrenia varies according to their level of functioning. Nurses generally use the Rogerian model, also known as client-centered therapy, developed by Carl Rogers (1902-1987), an American psychologist, in the 1940s. This is a humanistic therapy that helps clients to express and clarify feelings and promotes acceptance by the therapist. This therapy uses the technique of reflection and is not confrontational. It also allows the client to try out behaviors in a safe setting (Rogers, 1951) (see Chapter 23).

Client Education. Researches have not studied client education enough to determine how to best provide this service to most effectively meet clients' needs. Also, studies have not yet consistently shown that providing education improves clients' knowledge or changes their behavior. There are indications that this approach improves clients' social functioning (APA, 2004).

Case Management. A common problem with outpatient management is that client care is disorganized. Clients have multiple needs resulting from mental illness and physical illness needs to financial, employment, social, and housing needs. Case management coordinates these various needs. However, this approach has been difficult to study in a controlled manner and thus does not have a strong evidence base of support (APA, 2004) (see Chapter 28).

Self-Help Groups. Persons with schizophrenia are becoming increasingly active in their own care with the intent of decreasing dependence on professionals, decreasing stigma association with mental illness, and increasing an adequate support network (APA, 2004). Consumer models focus on recovery. Recovery models support more consumer involvement in care and focus on the person's strengths rather than only on symptoms. Individuals attempt to integrate their different life roles rather than seeing themselves as the illness. This movement fosters hope that change is possible. The person is able to make choices, thus feeling respected and self-directed. Empowerment and peer support are critical elements for success. Figure 12-6 illustrates treatment goals for people with schizophrenia.

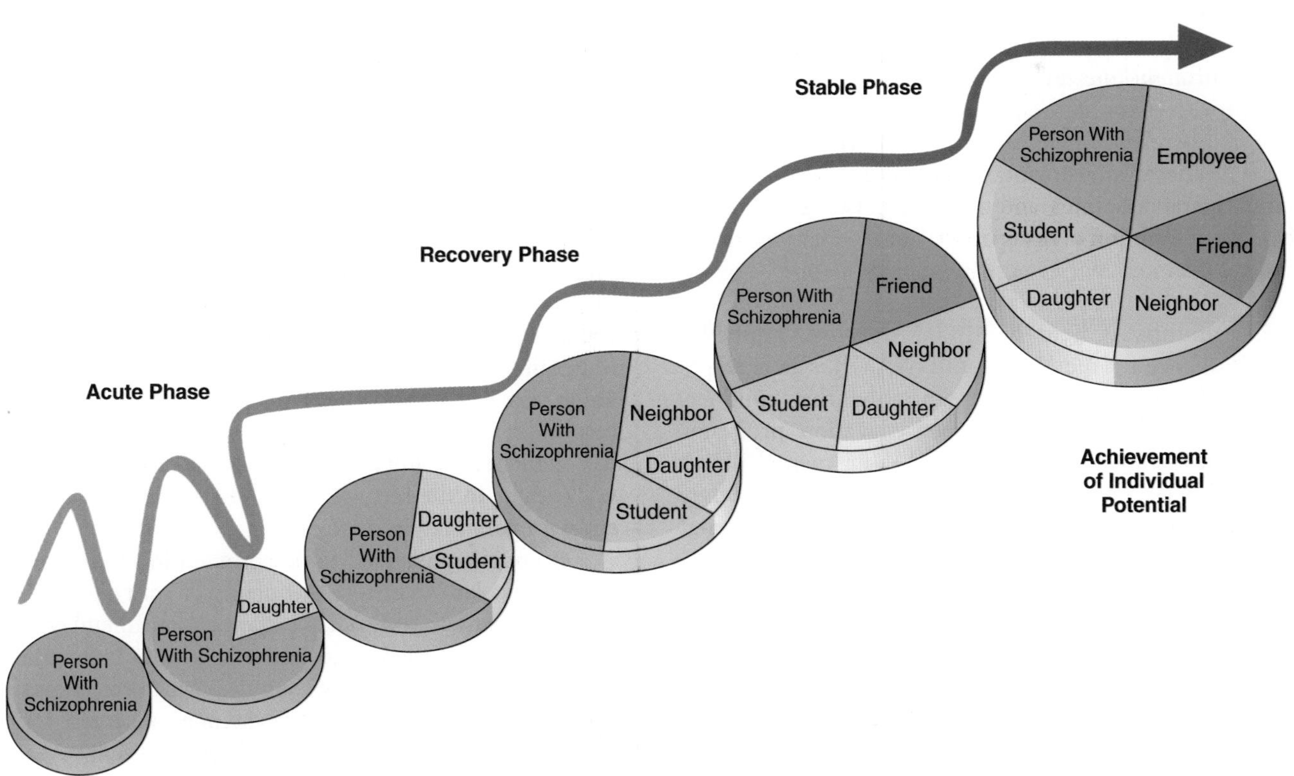

FIGURE 12-6 Treatment effectiveness: a growing personal journey. This figure demonstrates that as a person moves through the stages of schizophrenia recovery from the acute phase to the stable phase, she is able to focus on increasing her life roles. (Adapted from MHA Village: www.village-isa.org/Overview/psr_circle.htm; Lehman AF et al: Practice guideline for the treatment of patients with schizophrenia, second edition, *Am J Psychiatr* 161[2 suppl]:1-56, 2004.)

Guided Imagery. Guided imagery is a therapy in which the client pictures past pleasant memories. Therapists often combine it with relaxation therapy and use it with role-playing. However, it is not for clients who are experiencing psychosis because it confuses the client who is out of touch with reality and adds to the client's perceptual or thought disorder.

Assertiveness Training. Assertiveness training reduces the anxiety arising from interpersonal relationships, which are usually a problem for the client with schizophrenia. This training promotes expressive, spontaneous, goal-directed, self-enhancing behavior, such as learning to say no when necessary, rejecting unwanted behavior, and initiating conversations.

Occupational and Recreational Therapy. Occupational therapy is a diagnostic tool that assesses the functional level and progress of the client with schizophrenia. The occupational therapist uses crafts as a tool to check hand-eye coordination, perception, and fine muscle tone. Some occupational therapists visit the client's home to provide special equipment or needed therapy. In fact, today's psychosocial rehabilitation programs depend on active-directive learning principles designed to help the client regain or improve skills or to develop alternate compensatory skills useful for community living.

The recreational therapist's emphasis is on body kinesics, movement therapy, and resocialization through recreation and includes exercise, movement therapy, and dance therapy. These physical therapies promote body image through kinesthetic stimulation and provide ways to cope with stress. The emphasis is on cooperation rather than competition, especially for clients with schizophrenia. The therapist also works on client motivation, planning trips and outings and arts and crafts. For a more detailed description of occupational and recreational therapy, see Chapter 23.

Community Client-Family Programs. The National Alliance for the Mentally Ill (NAMI) is an example of an effective community organization that conducts family-to-family and peer-to-peer education programs that train members to teach others about mental illness and its effects on day-to-day living. NAMI also offers strategies for moving forward while coping with mental illness (NAMI Advocate, 2001).

Therapeutic Methods to Prevent and Manage Violence. The possibility of violent behaviors exists in seriously ill clients with schizophrenia, although there is no way to accurately predict who will become violent. Nurses and other clinicians need to be aware of the ways that anger, aggression, and violence are reinforced and take steps to prevent assault. Violence in interpersonal relationships happens as a result of differing expectations regarding therapeutic rules and their enforcement. Because of the nature of the illness, a client will misinterpret another person's intent, which will sometimes cause a violent response. A person in the acute stages of schizophrenia sometimes exaggerates another's irritation and misreads it as anger, or he or she misinterprets laughter as ridicule and strikes out in defense. Substance abuse also triggers violence.

De-escalation skills are effective techniques in interpersonal relationships in any context, but they are especially important for the psychiatric mental health nurse. De-escalation consists of less intrusive interventions, such as using nonthreatening verbal and nonverbal messages, or it requires a more hands-on method to safely disengage and control the aggressor physically. The choice to use the techniques set forth in Table 12-4 depends on the stage of the threat, the speed of escalation of the impending violence, and the feedback received from the client, which illustrates the effectiveness of the technique.

However, sometimes strategies fail and medication is the most effective treatment of choice to manage the emergency situation. A panel of experts has identified the oral types as the preferred alternate medications for acutely aggressive or agitated clients because of the traumatic effects of involuntary medication, especially when coupled with restraint. However, practitioners and regulatory standards concur that, if it is not possible to administer oral medications and the danger of the emergency situation exceeds the client's ability to demonstrate safe behaviors, intramuscular (IM) medications used in a limited manner (only for the emergency) are the safest choice (see Chapter 8). The expert panel identified the risk of side effects as the most important factor in the use of IM medications. Mental trauma experienced by the client and the risk of compromising the client-physician relationship were also important (Allen et al., 2001).

To prevent violence, it is important to avoid blame, ridicule, confrontation, teasing, or insult. Give the individual privacy and respect emotional boundaries. Be aware of your feelings and emotions and try to keep them neutral, as clients are generally sensitive to others' emotions. Maintain a calm, moderate demeanor, with a nonthreatening physical stance with arms unfolded, and remain a reasonable distance from the client. Keep your voice tone low to moderate, and refrain from whispering or laughing with others in the setting, especially within view of a client with paranoid tendencies.

Do not allow yourself to be cornered in the room of a client with a known history of violence or with one who has threatened others; always have another staff member with you, making sure there is an easy exit. Try not to be intimidated by violent outbursts, but take whatever measures necessary to secure the safety of everyone concerned. In the hospital this sometimes involves calling the assault response team, hospital security, or the local police department. In the community, try to secure help from friends or neighbors, and call the police if needed. The best way to prevent dangerous situations is to anticipate them and be prepared

Text continued on p. 281

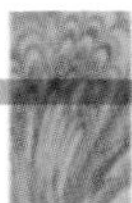

TABLE 12-4

Deescalation of Aggressive Behavior

CONCEPT	BEHAVIOR	RATIONALE
Managing the environment	Persuade the agitated/angry client to move to another area. Get help from colleagues to remove other clients, but have one colleague near you.	Prevents anxiety transference and protects others.
Showing confidence and leadership	*Hold regular drills with staff to practice strategies.* Give clear instructions. Be brief. Be assertive. Negotiate options. If the client has a weapon, instruct him or her to put it on the floor.	Prevents panic when crises occur. Avoids misunderstandings and not knowing what to do. Allows the client to feel that he or she has some room in exercising options.
Maintaining safety	Give signal to staff to call/phone assault team or police per policy (if verbal negotiations fail).	Protects client and others from harm or injury as a result of possible lethal attack.
Encouraging verbalization	Ask questions that are open ended and nonthreatening. Use "How?" "What?" "When?" to get details, but not "Why?" Keep voice calm and controlled.	Refocuses on the client's problem and not on his or her intent to act out the anger. Stops anger from escalating. ("Why" questions challenge client.)
Using nonverbal expression	Allow the client body space; do not stand closer than about 8 feet. Keep your body at a 45-degree angle. Have an open posture; hands at sides, palms outward.	Sends nonthreatening message, willingness to listen and accommodate the client.
Personalizing yourself and showing concern	Remind the client who you are; say words such as, "The world seems terrible now, but you haven't done any harm to him or her." Use words such as we or us. Use general leads such as "go on."	Shows empathy. Encourages and reflects cooperation. Shows that you are listening.
Using disengagement breakaways	Manage hair pulls, choke holds, grabs, and hugs according to safety instructions, videos, and return demonstrations.	Prevents injury to self, the client, and others.
Using removal, seclusion, and restraints	Rehearse these procedures regularly.	Allows the client to regain self-control.
Accurately documenting the event; holding a debriefing session with staff	Keep a detailed record: time, place, circumstances. Review and discuss the event.	Keeps an accurate account (e.g., for legal aspects). Helps staff to debrief, talk about feelings and learn what went right and how to improve.

Modified from *Assault response training and education manual,* San Diego, Calif, Sharp HealthCare, 2006.

NURSING CARE PLAN

Mark, a 30-year-old man, was estranged from his parents since age 18 years, when he was diagnosed with chronic undifferentiated schizophrenia. This resulted in his unpredictable and disruptive behavior at home, which finally became intolerable. Mark was sent to live in a board-and-care facility where he was maintained as long as he took his medications and complied with the program at the day treatment center he attended. The day treatment program provided Mark with the predictable structure, support, and guidance from staff, which he needed, as well as some affiliation and socialization with other clients. Because of his disorder, other clients easily influenced Mark. One day a group of clients he considered his friends persuaded him to take the government assistance check he had just received to "go party." Mark stopped taking his medications, took various street drugs, and did not return to the board-and-care facility or the day treatment center for a week. He showed up at the center one morning disheveled, dirty, incoherent, and frightened, stating, "I am really scared. Everybody left me. I'm hearing voices saying that I'm stupid and hopeless, and no one would help me because I'm not worth saving." Mark was admitted to the acute care unit in a psychiatric hospital for evaluation and treatment.

DSM-IV-TR DIAGNOSES

Axis I	Chronic, undifferentiated schizophrenia
Axis II	None
Axis III	None
Axis IV	Moderate to severe = 6 or 7; negative influence of friends, rejection by peers, ingestion of illicit drugs, lack of adequate support system (family, friends), economic issues (misuse of government assistance check)
Axis V	GAF = 10 (current); GAF = 30 (past year)

NANDA Diagnosis *Disturbed sensory perception (auditory hallucinations) related to client stopped taking medications, substance use, inability to process information (biologic factors) secondary to diagnosis of schizophrenia, rejection by peers, isolation and loneliness, low self-esteem, negative self-image/self-concept, and lack of adequate supports as evidenced by verbalization that he hears derogatory voices, fear that no one will help, anxiety, frustration, self-deprecation, and self-care deficit*

NOC Sensory Function: Hearing, Cognitive Orientation, Communication: Receptive, Distorted Thought Self-Control

NIC Hallucination Management, Cognitive Restructuring, Reality Orientation, Delusion Management, Environmental Management, Emotional Support

Continued

NURSING CARE PLAN—cont'd

CLIENT OUTCOMES	NURSING INTERVENTIONS	EVALUATION
Mark will not harm others and will demonstrate an absence of aggressive or violent behaviors while on the mental health unit.	Explore the client's hallucinations for command type content, intervening immediately if Mark demonstrates aggressive or violent behaviors that pose a risk for harm or injury toward himself or others. *Frustration, anger, dysfunctional coping, and command type hallucinations result in violence or injury to self or others, and the nurse needs to intervene at the first sign of aggression to protect client and others from harm.*	Mark remains calm on the unit with an absence of aggressive or violent behaviors. He states that "the voices are still troubling, but I know the staff will not let me harm myself or others."
Mark will demonstrate a reduction in symptoms with a decrease in the intensity of hallucinations and continued absence of aggressive or violent behavior while on the unit.	Focus on modifying and managing the symptoms of hallucinations through talk therapy, pharmacotherapy, and coping strategies such as clapping, whistling, or telling the voices to "go away!" *Interventions do not eliminate hallucinations initially. In the meantime, the client needs learned strategies to help cope with the intensity of the voices in order to reduce the risk of violence.*	Mark is using learned coping strategies to distract him from the hallucinations and to reduce the intensity of the voices. Mark continues to show no signs of violence toward himself or others.
Mark will verbalize reduced feelings of fear, isolation, loneliness, and rejection, and he will express a greater sense of control over his environment.	Identify, whenever possible, the need filled by Mark's hallucinations (dependency, loneliness, fear, rejection, loss of control). *Hallucinations fill the void created by the lack of human contact. Once the nurse identifies the need, the client generally experiences relief and anxiety reduction, and the nurse then uses the therapeutic alliance to assist the client with strategies for growth and change.*	Hallucinations increase when Mark's peers reject him, but brief, frequent discussions with nursing staff seem to reduce his anxiety and fear and enhance his sense of control over his environment.
Mark will verbalize that the voices are more under control ("The voices don't bother me as much," or "I don't hear the voices as often as I did.").	Monitor Mark's hallucinatory activity and observe for verbal and nonverbal behaviors associated with hallucinations (talking to himself, bolting and running out of the room, or striking out at others). *Assessment gives the nurse the opportunity to observe for behaviors that are associated with hallucinations, and to intervene early in the disturbance, which often prevent aggression and violence.*	Mark continues to respond to the voices in a nonthreatening way such as talking to himself on occasion. Mark does not demonstrate behaviors that pose a risk for harm or injury to himself or others, such as running through the unit or striking out in fear.
Mark will focus on real events and people in the environment.	Familiarize Mark with actual activities and events in the therapeutic setting when he is rested and stress-free. *Presenting reality in a nonthreatening way distracts Mark from his hallucinatory experience by focusing on actual events.*	Mark is better able to focus on events when gently oriented by the nursing staff after periods of rest and relaxation.
	Address Mark, other clients, and staff by name. *Using the real names of people in Mark's environment helps to orient Mark and reinforces reality.*	Mark responds to his own name when addressed.
Mark will participate in relevant conversations with staff and other clients.	Use simple, concrete, specific language (versus abstract, global language). *The client's misperceptions and altered perceptions influence the message and interfere with his understanding.*	Mark responds coherently when conversation is simple and not demanding or abstract.
	Use direct verbal responses versus unclear gestures (nodding head yes or no). *Gestures confuse the client and provide distorted perception or misinterpretation of reality.*	Mark misinterprets any subtle conversations or gestures by staff or peers.
Mark will slow down his speech and speak more coherently.	Help Mark to speak slowly and clearly if his speech is incoherent. *This will help Mark to organize his thought processes and increase his ability to be understood.*	Mark is able to slow down and make himself understood when encouraged by the nursing staff.
Mark will participate in planned treatment to decrease or eliminate hallucinations.	Assist Mark in stopping or managing hallucinations *to give him some control and increase his self-esteem.*	Mark begins to practice strategies to interrupt hallucinations, with prompting by staff as necessary.
	Teach strategies and activities that will help Mark to control hallucinations, such as contact staff when voices are bothersome, engage in a unit activity, exercise, or craft project when voices begin. *Providing strategies and alternatives to hallucinations gives the client some control and reduces fear and anxiety.*	
	Describe the hallucinatory behavior when the client appears to be hallucinating. "Mark, you seem distracted. Are you hearing voices?" *By reflecting on the client's behavior in an accepting way, the nurse facilitates disclosure and promotes trust.*	Mark accepts the nurse's observations and continues to use strategies to interrupt hallucinations.

CLIENT OUTCOMES	NURSING INTERVENTIONS	EVALUATION
Mark will progressively engage in more reality-based dialog with staff.	Refrain from arguing or discussing details of content. *When the nurse disagrees, the client will defend the content, which reinforces the importance of the hallucinations.*	Mark is beginning to discuss real events more often each day as staff members focus on reality and show acceptance of Mark.
	Voice the nurse's reality about Mark's hallucinations (without denying his experience; e.g., "I don't hear the voices you describe, Mark. The only voices I hear are those of the people in this room. I know how upsetting the voices are to you"). *Focusing on the client's feelings involved with the experience is appropriate. A realistic, yet nonthreatening, accepting response helps the client to distinguish actual voices from internal stimulation and increases trust.*	Mark states that he hears the voices less when he is engaged with staff.
	Do not use a judgmental attitude when interacting with Mark. *A nonjudgmental attitude will avoid diminishing the client's self-esteem and enhances rapport.*	Mark says he appreciates "not being ridiculed" during this troubling time.
Mark will adhere to medication regimen and verbalize understanding of its use to treat his symptoms.	Support the medical plan, including prescribed medications. *Medication assists in managing the biologic factors related to the hallucinations, and often makes it easier to engage the client in psychosocial and interactive therapies.*	Mark takes all prescribed medications; symptoms are decreasing.
	Discuss with Mark that sometimes the voices do not completely go away, but that he can learn to manage them. *This type of information will help the client to tolerate persistent, lasting hallucinations and continue learned techniques that relieve them (whistling, singing, clapping).*	Mark expresses hope that he can continue using learned strategies when discharged, such as whistling, singing, clapping, and so on.
Mark will name two precipitating events that occur just before the onset of hallucinations (e.g., frustration, fear).	Activate the client to name precipitants (stressors that trigger hallucinations). *Example:* "What happened just before you heard the voices?" *Anxiety-provoking situations may precede hallucinations. When the nurse identifies the situations, the client understands the connection and begins to manage, avoid, reduce, or eliminate them.*	Mark is able to reduce the frequency and intensity of hallucinations by using learned techniques (whistling, singing, clapping) and by identifying stressors that often occur before the onset of a hallucination.
	Continue to explore the content of the hallucinations for violence (command hallucinations to harm self or others). *Immediate intervention is necessary if this problem arises to protect the client or the environment from harm.* When the nurse determines that the client is not harmful to self or others, the nurse proceeds to use other therapeutic interventions relevant to the client's needs.	Mark shows no signs of violence toward self or others.
Mark will continue to express feelings of fear, anxiety, isolation, and rejection wherever they occur.	Continue the nurse-client therapeutic alliance to encourage sharing of areas that are problematic for the client. *Focusing on the client's immediate needs relieves client tension, fosters feelings of being understood and accepted, and encourages the client to remain engaged with the staff, right up until the client is discharged.*	Mark states that he feels understood and helped by staff, which will prepare him for discharge.
Mark will engage in the milieu schedule and activities, more frequently and willingly as he gets closer to discharge.	Provide environmental opportunities (groups and activities) to increase social contact and skills learning. *Involving the client in milieu and group activities promotes feeling of belonging, reduces feelings of fear and isolation and increases self-esteem and mastery of social skills.*	Mark engages in the same types of groups. He avoids discussion groups but likes occupational therapy. He states that the voices decrease when he is involved in activities or conversations with others. He says he will continue to try to get more socially involved.
	Activate Mark to attend to self-care activities (showers, mouth care, grooming). *Attention to self-care promotes acceptance by peers, enhances physical well-being, and increases self-esteem.*	Mark's self-care is improving every day and seems to be related to his reduction of hallucinations and other symptoms. Mark appears to be prepared for discharge.

with an effective plan of action per hospital or community procedure (Flowers, 2002) (see Chapter 22).

EVALUATION

Evaluation follows specific intervention statements and behavioral objectives, incorporating the concepts of quality, quantity, and time. For example, if a goal is to resocialize a client who has been isolating herself while on the unit, an intervention consists of having the client join the community meeting along with other clients on the unit. To evaluate the effectiveness of this intervention, nurses state specific behavioral client outcomes in measurable terms. For example, a beginning behavioral objective is "On her second day on the unit, Kayla will accompany the nurse to the community meeting, and she will remain with the group for 15 minutes."

Note that the outcome is criteria specific as to time (on the second day), quality of experience (going to the community meeting with the nurse), and quantity (for 15 minutes). These criteria are measurable. If all criteria are met, the minimal acceptable level of performance will progress, so that by the third day, the client outcome will read, "Kayla will go to the community meeting on her own, remain for 30 minutes, and make at least one comment."

The nursing process is dynamic and always changing. It is an ongoing design for interaction with the environment and is evaluated as such. For instance, if the nurse evaluates criteria and finds that it is not met on the second day, then the nurse will reconsider the client outcomes and nursing interventions and perhaps rewrite them at a level closer to the client's ability to perform. If a nurse revises the outcomes and they are still not met, the nurse needs to examine the rest of the nursing process in total. Thus, eventual success with the nursing process demands patience and persistence, and improvements occur in small steps, especially in clients with chronic schizophrenia (see Chapter 3).

CHAPTER SUMMARY

- Schizophrenia is one of the most complex and debilitating mental disorders.
- Schizophrenia is a not a single disorder but a syndrome (group of diseases) known as the schizophrenias.
- The schizophrenias are the largest group of mental disorders.
- Biologic factors are the primary focus in the research on etiology and treatment of schizophrenia.
- Five biologic models currently considered are heredity/genetic, neuroanatomic/neurochemical, neurotransmitter function (specifically the dopamine hypothesis), immunologic, and stress/disease/trauma/drug abuse.
- Advancements in genetic research hold promise for more effective treatment in the next decade.
- The five major subtypes of schizophrenia are paranoid, disorganized, catatonic, undifferentiated, and residual.
- Diagnostic criteria for schizophrenia include two or more symptoms of hallucinations, delusions, disorganized or catatonic behavior, or disorganized speech that are evident for at least 1 month.
- Involving the client with schizophrenia and the client's family or significant others in the client's treatment plan, as appropriate, is important and contributes to more effective treatment.
- Many practitioners use psychopharmacology as an intervention for many symptoms of schizophrenia. New medications with fewer side effects offer hope and more effective treatment outcomes for the complex symptoms of schizophrenia.
- Milieu therapy, psychosocial rehabilitation, client and family education, and behavior modification are some treatments used with clients with schizophrenia.
- Community resources are critical in rehabilitating clients and reintegrating them back into the community.

REVIEW QUESTIONS

1 **A nurse plans a series of psychoeducational groups for persons with schizophrenia. Which topic would take priority?**

1. How to complete an application for employment.
2. The importance of taking your medication correctly.
3. Ways to dress and behave when attending community events.
4. How to give and receive compliments.

2 **A young adult is hospitalized with undifferentiated schizophrenia. The parents are distraught and filled with guilt. An appropriate nursing response would be:**

1. "There are many theories about the cause of schizophrenia, but this illness is not your fault."
2. "Does anyone in your family have mental illness? Schizophrenia is a genetically transmitted disease."
3. "Look on the bright side. With the right medications and treatment, this disease can be cured."
4. "I'll recommend some excellent websites to learn about schizophrenia and other mental illnesses."

3 **A person with disorganized schizophrenia participates in a rehabilitative outpatient program. Select the most appropriate initial outcome for this individual. The individual will:**

1. Identify environmental triggers that produce feelings of fear.
2. Have increased organization of thought patterns.
3. Report the absence of auditory and visual hallucinations.
4. Set lunch tables correctly and fill cups with ice daily.

4 **Which statement by a person with paranoid schizophrenia most clearly indicates the antipsychotic medication is effective?**

1. "I used to hear scary voices but now I don't hear them anymore."
2. "My medicine is working fine. I'm not having any problems."
3. "Sometimes it's hard for me to fall asleep, but I usually sleep all night."
4. "I think some of the staff members don't like me. They're mean to me."

5 **Select the nursing diagnosis most likely to apply to a person with an acute exacerbation of schizophrenia, paranoid type.**

1. Social isolation related to impaired ability to trust others
2. Deficient diversional activity related to unstable control of hostile impulses
3. Impaired social interaction related to inadequately developed superego
4. Fear related to lack of confidence in significant others

6 **A client with catatonic schizophrenia has sat mute and rigid for 2 hours. Which nursing intervention would be most appropriate?**

1. Encourage the client to participate in a group sporting activity.
2. Put the client's extremities through passive range of motion exercises.
3. Seclude the client until voluntary movement is observed.
4. Offer short but frequent verbal phrases to communicate caring.

Additional self-study exercises and learning resources are available to you on the ***Companion CD*** *at the back of the book and on the* ***Evolve website*** *at* ***http://evolve.elsevier.com/Fortinash/.***

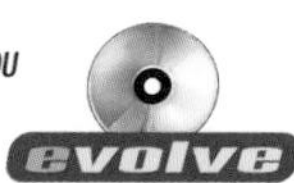

ONLINE RESOURCES

NARSAD, the Mental Health Research Association: **www.narsad.org**

National Schizophrenia Foundation: **www.nsfoundation.org**

National Alliance on Mental Illness: **www.nami.org**

National Institute of Mental Health: **www.nimh.nih.gov**

Mental Health America: **www.nmha.org**

REFERENCES

American Psychiatric Association (APA): *Diagnostic and statistical manual of mental disorders*, ed 4, text revision, Washington, DC, 2000, American Psychiatric Association.

American Psychiatric Association (APA): *Practice guidelines for the treatment of patients with schizophrenia*, ed 2, Washington, DC, 2004, American Psychiatric Association.

American Psychiatric Nurses Association: Position statement: mandatory outpatient treatment (MOT), *J Am Psychiatr Nurse Assoc* 10:247-253, 2004.

Allen MH et al: *The expert consensus guideline series: treatment of behavioral emergencies, a postgraduate medicine special report*, New York, 2001, McGraw Hill.

Beng-Choon H, Black DW, Andreasen NC: Schizophrenia and other psychotic disorders. In Hales RE, Yudofsky SC, editors: *Essentials of clinical psychiatry*, ed 2, p 200, Washington, DC, 2004, American Psychiatric Publishing.

Boyd M: Considerations for antipsychotic therapy: implications for the safe and appropriate management of patients, *J Am Psychiatric Nurses Assoc*, Aug, 2002; www.apna.org.

Csernansky R, Mahmoud R, Brenner R: A comparison of risperidone and haloperidol for the prevention of relapse in patients with schizophrenia, *N Engl J Med* 346:16-22, 2002.

Emery RE, Oltmanns TF: *Abnormal psychology*, ed 4, Upper Saddle River, NJ, 2004, Pearson Education.

Fields J et al: Assessing positive and negative symptoms in children and adolescents, *Am J Psychiatry* 151:249, 1994.

Flowers CJ: Antipsychotic polypharmacy in schizophrenia: *Eighth annual psychopharmacology update*, sponsored by Sharp HealthCare, San Diego, Calif, Sep 21, 2002.

Fortinash KM, Holoday Worret PA: *Psychiatric nursing care plans*, ed 4, St Louis, 2007, Mosby.

Green M et al: Dichotic listening during auditory hallucinations in patients with schizophrenia, *Am J Psychiatry* 151:357, 1994.

Guthrie SK: Managing psychiatric drug therapy across the continuum of care: focus on the schizophrenic patient: introduction, *Am J Health Syst Pharm* 59: 2002.

Johnson, ME: Violence on inpatient psychiatric units: state of the science, *J Am Psychiatr Nurses Assoc* 10:119, 2004.

Lencz T et al: Converging evidence for a pseudoautosomal cytokine receptor gene locus in schizophrenia, *Mol Psychiatry*, advance online publication, March 20, 2007.

Lewis DA, Lieberman JA: Catching up on schizophrenia: natural history and neurobiology, *Neuron* 28:325-334, 2000.

Lieberman JA et al: Effectiveness of antipsychotic drugs in patients with chronic schizophrenia, *New Engl J Med* 353:1209-1223, 2005.

Lieberman JA: The significance of CATIE: an expert interview with Jeffrey A. Lieberman, MD, *Medscape Psychiatr Ment Health* 11: 2006a.

Lieberman, JA et al: *The American Psychiatric Publishing textbook of schizophrenia*, Arlington, Va, 2006b, American Psychiatric Publishing.

Maguire GA: Comprehensive understanding of schizophrenia and its treatment, *Am J Health Syst Pharm* 59(suppl 5):S4-S11, 2002.

McEvoy, J et al: Effectiveness of clozapine versus olanzapine, quetiapine, and risperidone in patients with schizophrenia who did not respond to prior atypical antipsychotic treatment, *Am J Psychiatry* 163:600-610, 2006.

Meador K, Nichols F: The neurological examination as it relates to neuropsychological issues. In Hartlage L et al, editors: *Essentials of neuropsychological assessment*, New York, 1991, Springer.

Meyer JM: Schizophrenia and the metabolic syndrome, *Medscape Psychiatry Ment Health* 10, 2005; retrieved Apr 26, 2006, from www.medscape.com/viewarticle/506136.

Murphy MC: The agitated, psychotic patient: guidelines to ensure staff and patient safety, *J Am Psychiatr Nurses Assoc* 8(suppl 4): S2-S8, 2002.

Myers RE, Shepard-White F: Evaluation of adequacy of reading level and readability of psychotropic medication handouts, *J Am Psychiatr Nurses Assoc* 10:55-59, 2004.

NAMI's New Department of Education and Training: Advancing peer education and training, *NAMI Advocate*, Spring 2001.

National Institute of Mental Health (NIMH): Childhood-onset schizophrenia: an update, Publication No. 04-5124, Washington, DC, 2003, National Institute of Mental Health.

National Institute of Mental Health (NIMH): Schizophrenia research at the National Institute of Mental Health, 2005; retrieved Apr 5, 2006, from www.himh.nih.gov/publicat/schizresfact.cfm.

Osmon D: The neuropsychological examination. In Hartlage L et al, editors: *Essentials of neuropsychological assessment*, New York, 1991, Springer.

Perry W, Braff D: Information-processing deficits and thought disorders in schizophrenia, *Am J Psychiatry* 151(3):363, 1994.

Rapoport JL: *Childhood onset of "adult" pathology: clinical and research advances*. Washington, DC, 2000, American Psychiatric Press.

Reeves RR, Torres RA: Medical disorders among psychiatric patients, *Psychiatr Serv* 54:748, 2003.

Rogers CP: *Client-centered therapy*, Boston, 1951, Houghton Mifflin (classic).

Roy C: *Introduction to nursing: an adaptation model*, Upper Saddle River, NJ, 1976, Prentice-Hall (classic).

Sadock BJ, Sadock VA: *Kaplan and Sadock's comprehensive textbook of psychiatry*, ed 8, Philadelphia, 2005, Lippincott Williams & Wilkins.

Selye H: *Stress of life*, ed 2, New York, 1978, McGraw Hill (classic).

Sullivan H: *The interpersonal theory of psychiatry*, New York, 1953, WW Norton (classic).

Sullivan PF: The genetics of schizophrenia, *PLOS Med* 2:e212, 2005.

Swartz, MS et al: Substance use in persons with schizophrenia: baseline prevalence and correlates from the NIMH CATIE study, *J Nerv Ment Dis* 194:3, 2006.

Thirthalli J, Benegal V: Psychosis among substance users, *Curr Opin Psychiatry* 19:239-249, 2006.

Thornton JF et al: Schizophrenia: course and outcome, *Internet Mental Health*, Jan 2, 2001a; www.mentalhealth.com.

Thornton JF et al: Schizophrenia: the medications, *Internet Mental Health*, Jan 2, 2001b.

Thornton JF et al: Schizophrenia: symptoms and management at home, *Internet Mental Health*, Jan 2, 2001c.

Chapter 13

Personality Disorders

PAMELA E. MARCUS

Character develops itself in the stream of life.
GOETHE

OBJECTIVES

1. **Identify three elements of personality development as described by Freud in the psychosexual stages of development.**
2. **Discuss two contributions Margaret Mahler and Otto Kernberg made to object relations theory.**
3. **Name two biologic indices that are often abnormal in clients with a personality disorder.**
4. **Briefly explain behaviors that differentiate Clusters A, B, and C of Axis II in the DSM-IV-TR.**
5. **Recognize two nursing diagnoses for each cluster of the personality disorders.**
6. **Define splitting behaviors, and list two nursing interventions that effectively challenge the client's black-or-white view of the world.**
7. **Apply the nursing process in managing clients with personality disorders.**
8. **Develop a nursing care plan for different personality disorders.**

KEY TERMS

devaluation, p. 287
idealization, p. 287
milieu therapy, p. 298
object constancy, p. 287
object relations, p. 286
personality traits, p. 285
projective identification, p. 287
splitting, p. 287
state disorders, p. 285
trait disorders, p. 285
transitional objects, p. 287

Personality disorders, as classified by the DSM-IV-TR, are long-standing, pervasive, maladaptive patterns of behavior relating to others that are not caused by Axis I disorders. According to the DSM-IV-TR, a personality disorder is an "enduring pattern of inner experience and behavior that deviates markedly from the expectations of the individual's culture, is pervasive and inflexible, has an onset in adolescence or early adulthood, is stable over time, and leads to distress or impairment" (APA, 2000). All human beings have a personality made up of one's definition of self, skills used to relate to others, and a defense structure. When studying personality disorders, the nurse has to determine to what degree an individual compromises these qualities. Nurses determine these behaviors by observing how individuals relate to others, their perception of surroundings, and their ability to problem-solve. According to Manfield (1992):

> The term *personality disorder*, also called a "disorder of the self," refers to a lack of a genuine sense of "self" and a consequent impairment of self-regulating abilities. Instead of looking within themselves to locate feelings or to make decisions, persons with personality disorders look outside themselves for evaluations, directions, rules, or opinions to guide them.

When reviewing the diagnostic criteria for the various personality disorders (Axis II), it is important to differentiate personality traits from personality disorders. DSM-IV-TR has defined six general diagnostic criteria for a personality disorder and these are in the DSM-IV-TR Criteria box.

DSM-IV-TR CRITERIA

Personality Disorder

A An enduring pattern of inner experience and behavior that deviates markedly from the expectations of the individual's culture. This pattern is manifested in two (or more) of the following areas:

1 Cognition (i.e., ways of perceiving and interpreting self, other people, and events)

2 Affectivity (i.e., the range, intensity, lability, and appropriateness of emotional response)

3 Interpersonal functioning

4 Impulse control

B The enduring pattern is inflexible and pervasive across a broad range of personal and social situations.

C The enduring pattern leads to clinically significant distress or impairment in social, occupational, or other important areas of functioning.

D The pattern is stable and of long duration, and its onset can be traced back at least to adolescence or early adulthood.

E The enduring pattern is not better accounted for as a manifestation or consequence of another mental disorder.

F The enduring pattern is not due to the direct physiologic effects of a substance (e.g., a drug of abuse, a medication) or a general medical condition (e.g., head trauma).

From American Psychiatric Association: *Diagnostic and statistical manual of mental disorders,* ed 4, text revision, Washington, DC, 2000, American Psychiatric Association.

Personality traits are those behaviors, patterns of perceiving, relating to others, and thinking about the environment and oneself that are exhibited in a wide range of social and personal contexts (APA, 2000). These traits are either adaptive or maladaptive **trait disorders**, depending on whether the trait is inflexible or causes significant functional impairment or subjective distress. When this occurs, a person has a personality disorder. The symptoms of a personality disorder are not time limited nor do they occur only in a time of crisis (APA, 2000). Behaviors are long-standing, enduring, and not responsive to short-term psychotherapy or pharmacologic measures. Skodol, et al. (2000) studied functional impairment in individuals with several different types of personality disorders. They found that clients with schizotypal personality disorder and borderline personality disorder consistently had either moderate or poor functioning across several levels of psychosocial functioning, such as marital status, completion of school, and the ability to maintain employment. People who have avoidant personality disorder demonstrated an intermediate functional impairment.

Diagnoses made on Axis I are **state disorders**. These diagnoses constitute behavior patterns that are not as long in duration. Often health care providers are able to alleviate the symptoms of these disorders through the use of medication, psychotherapy, and milieu therapy for severe symptoms. Personality disorder diagnoses are on Axis II of the DSM-IV-TR in a cluster format as follows:

- *Cluster A:* Paranoid, schizoid, and schizotypal make up the odd or eccentric cluster. These diagnoses are more likely to be co-occurring (i.e., both diagnoses are present in the same individual with psychotic disorders).
- *Cluster B:* Antisocial, borderline, histrionic, and narcissistic constitute the dramatic and emotional cluster. The Cluster B group is often co-occurring with affective disorders.
- *Cluster C:* Avoidant, dependent, and obsessive-compulsive compose the anxious and fearful cluster. These diagnoses are often associated with anxiety disorders (APA, 2000).

Individuals with personality disorder diagnoses in each cluster are at risk for developing a co-occurrence with specific Axis I diagnoses. However, this is not a definite rule, and no consistent research findings demonstrate this (APA, 2000; Oldham and Skodol, 1992; Widiger and Rogers, 1989).

HISTORIC AND THEORETIC PERSPECTIVES

Freudian Theories

Sigmund Freud (1856-1939), noted psychoanalyst, was one of the early published students of human development and inner psychologic conflict. The two areas that this chapter covers are (1) Freud's structural theory, often referred to as the tripartite model of the hypothetical psychic structures of the id, ego, and superego, and (2) Freud's psychosexual stages of development.

Freud (1905) describes the psychosexual stages of development in his "Three Essays on the Theory of Sexuality." The first stage he describes is the oral stage. The traits associated with successful completion of this stage include the ability to relate to others without excessive dependency or jealously. Trust begins to develop, and with trust comes a sense of self-reliance and trust of self. Individuals who have difficulty with this stage often lack trust and are self-centered, dependent, and jealous (Tyson and Tyson, 1990).

The anal stage is the second stage described by Freud. This stage takes place during the time when the child begins to develop enough sphincter control to be able to control excretion of feces. This takes place approximately from ages 1 to 3 years. Adults demonstrate successful completion of this stage in their ability to manage ambivalence (uncertainty) by making decisions without shame or self-doubt. They show a sense of self-autonomy and independence. A person who finds it difficult to successfully complete this stage of development is unable to make decisions, withholds friendships or cannot share with others, is full of rage, is stubborn, and may have sadomasochistic tendencies (desire to hurt others or to be hurt by others) (Tyson and Tyson, 1990).

The phallic stage is the next stage identified by Freud. It is the period of development when the child becomes interested in his or her genitals. Freud understood this stage in terms of male development. According to his theory, the phallus (penis) is the principal organ of concern for both boys and girls. This stage occurs during the ages of 3 through 6 or 7 years. The child who successfully completes this stage masters his or her internal processes and impulses and gains a beginning sense of relating to other people in the environment. Individuals who are unable to resolve the conflict inherent in the phallic stage can experience multiple psychiatric disorders, particularly those that involve the superego function of guilt (i.e., the individual with an antisocial personality disorder does not have a well-developed superego).

According to Freud, the antisocial, borderline, histrionic, and narcissistic personality disorders involve individuals who experienced problems identifying with their sexual identity during the critical phallic stage. For example, an individual with a histrionic personality disorder who acts sexually provocative but denies that this behavior is sexually driven has experienced an internal conflict with his or her sexual identity.

The next stage of psychosexual development is the latency stage. During this stage, the child represses the libidinal (sexual) drives and turns her or his attention toward learning and industry. At this time there is further development of the ego in an effort to gain control over instinctual impulses. This stage takes place from the sixth or seventh year of life until puberty.

With this stage comes the exploration of the environment and play, when the child learns how to do things, to enjoy life and have fun, and continues to develop inner control over instinctive drives and emotions. This stage is important for later adult functioning, because the child with a sense of industry is able to delay gratification, which helps in areas of learning, work, and relating to others. Individuals who have problems successfully completing this stage have either too much or too little ability to develop inner control. Those who lack inner control have difficulty relating to others, because their emotions rule their interactions and problem-solving abilities. Individuals who have an excess of inner control have isolated their emotions and are more regulated, using repetition of thoughts or behavior to relate or problem-solve.

The genital stage is the last stage described by Freud in an individual's psychosexual development. This stage takes place during puberty. The importance of this stage is that there is an opportunity to rework earlier issues that the individual has not resolved, in the service of achieving a healthy, mature sense of sexual and adult identity. With the ability to work and learn, individuals establish goals and values within the context of their own unique personal identities.

If individuals have difficulty during the genital stage, this will compromise their sense of self and ability to relate to others. They will therefore be unable to attain their identified goals or form values. They will also experience difficulty in identifying their strengths and weaknesses, likes and dislikes, and types of skills they want to acquire. Some individuals who have difficulty resolving the genital stage manifest symptoms and behaviors that are within the whole range of personality disorders.

Object Relations

Object relations is the stability and depth of an individual's relations with significant others as manifested by warmth, dedication, concern, and tactfulness.

As theorists studied human behavior further, particularly observing development of personality structure and relatedness, the theory of **object relations** began to develop. Many have contributed to this theory, and it is being reevaluated and expanded as the study of human relations and personality development. Tyson and Tyson (1990) have clarified the difference between interpersonal relations and object relations in the following manner:

> The first (interpersonal relations) has to do with the actual interactions between people. Object relations (or "internalized" object relations) refers to the intrapsychic dimensions of experiences with others—that is, to the mental representations of the self and of the other and of the role of each in their interactions.

Separation-Individuation Phase

When studying object relations from a developmental standpoint, Margaret Mahler identified and studied the separation-individuation phase of development occurring between ages 3 and 25 months. Mahler's theory of separation and individuation evolved from a longitudinal study where she observed normal mothers and their babies during the child's first 3 years of life. The term *separation* in this context refers to the child's gradually developing self that is distinct and separate from the representation of the mother. The term *individuation* in this context means to recognize the infant's attempts to form a distinctive identity and to develop characteristics that are unique to that individual (Mahler, 1963).

Mahler (1963, 1972) described four stages of the process of separation-individuation: differentiation, practicing, rapprochement, and object constancy. These stages are presented in Box 13-1.

Kernberg's Theories

Otto Kernberg studied individuals with severe personality disorders, primarily borderline and narcissistic personality disorders. He formulated some ideas about these disorders and their development. According to Kernberg (1984), a person who is emotionally healthy has an integrated working structure of the id, superego, and ego. This means that the ego is intact, with sufficient ability to determine reality from fantasy and to separate self from another object. The superego is functional, not too rigid or punishing, but a filter for the ego. The id is integrated and not in conflict with the other two structures.

Kernberg identified two essential tasks that the early ego has to accomplish for the internalization of object relations. The first task involves the ability of the child to distinguish between self and other people to formulate healthy feelings about self and to identify with the other person. This is similar to Mahler's differentiation stage. The second task that Kernberg discussed in relation to

BOX 13-1

Mahler's Stages of Separation-Individuation

1. **Differentiation:** Occurs when the child is between 3 and 8 months old. During this stage, the child begins to differentiate his or her own image from that of the mother or significant nurturer.
2. **Practicing:** Occurs when the child is between 8 and 15 months old. The task of this stage is for the child to actively explore his or her world in a manner in which the child seems oblivious to the mother. This occurs when the child begins to walk and is able to explore the environment around him or her, as locomotion becomes more stabilized.
3. **Rapprochement:** Occurs when the child is between 15 and 22 months old. The child begins to return to the mother for emotional needs after completing the exploration of the surroundings (which occurs during the practicing phase). During this time the toddler becomes moody, is in distress, and exhibits temper tantrums, even when the mother is with the child. The child wishes to have things his or her way, which is not always what the mother had planned. The task is for the child to deal with the conflict between his or her wish for independence and individuation and with wanting love and comfort from the mother.
4. **The beginning of object constancy:** Occurs around 25 months. Object constancy involves the ability to maintain a relationship regardless of frustration and changes in the relationship. The toddler at 25 months is able to think about the mother even when the mother is not close to the child and therefore comforts himself or herself by the mother's representation. This comfort sometimes includes a blanket or stuffed toy that reminds the child of the mother.

Modified from Mahler MS: Thoughts about development and individuation, *Psychoanal Study Child* 18:307, 1963; Mahler MS: On the first three subphases of the separation-individuation process, *Int J Psychoanal* 53:333, 1972.

the internalization of object relations is that there is an integration of "good" and "bad" self-images, as well as an integration of "good" and "bad" object (the other person's) images. This consolidation of images leads to total self and object representations that are differentiated from one another and realistic. Both structures have good and bad, satisfaction and frustration, in their systems.

In the borderline personality disorder, or what Kernberg has called the *borderline personality organization*, this is a particularly important aspect. Kernberg identified splitting as a primary defense of the individual with borderline personality disorder. **Splitting** is the inability to synthesize the positive and negative aspects of self and others. The person with borderline personality disorder exhibits splitting by his or her difficulty in perceiving that he or she and other people have both good and bad aspects. There is a tendency to idealize persons or groups when those persons meet the needs of the individual with borderline personality disorder. This process is called **idealization**. At the other extreme, a person with borderline personality disorder devalues persons or groups when he or she perceives that needs are not being met. This process is called **devaluation**. The person with borderline personality disorder views self and others as either all good or all bad and is unable to reach a state of **object constancy**, which means that one is unable to hold the memory of significant others in mind. This individual is unable to use **transitional objects** that represent the significant other person and that help the individual remember the other person. For example, an individual with object constancy thinks of his or her loved one when experiencing something that reminds him or her of the other person, such as a favorite song or a tangible object. An individual who is unable to obtain object constancy cannot picture his or her loved one when that individual is away from him or her. Therefore the person views the absence of the significant other as abandonment.

Masterson (1976) identified four defenses that block the client's developmental growth from the stages of individuation-separation to autonomy: projection, clinging, denial, and avoidance. According to Masterson, the client with borderline personality disorder becomes stuck in the subphases of the individuation-separation stage. This leads to the client's failure to achieve object constancy.

A client with borderline personality disorder does not relate to people as wholes but as parts. He or she is unable to maintain a relationship through the frustration of everyday living and tends to experience anger and rage when feeling rejected or ignored. This individual is unable to evoke the image of the significant others when they are not present. If a significant person in the client's life dies, the client with borderline personality disorder cannot mourn but often exhibits one or more of the six constituent states: depression, anger and rage, fear, guilt, passivity and helplessness, and emptiness and void.

Another defense against the client's anxiety that is important for understanding the individual with a Cluster B personality disorder is **projective identification**. This defense is a primitive type of projection. Kernberg (1984) described this defense as having the following characteristics:

- The tendency to continue to experience the impulse that is simultaneously being projected onto the other person
- Fear of the other person under influence of that projected impulse
- The need to control the other person under the influence of this mechanism

For example, Allison is angry with her mother because her mother disapproves of her taste in clothes. She views her mother as having old-fashioned views. Allison begins to yell at her mother, telling her that she dresses like a little old lady *(projection)*. Allison's mother feels hurt and angry at her daughter and raises her voice, telling Allison that her dress is provocative and will bring unwanted attention *(mother reacts to the projection)*. Allison tells her mother that she refuses to talk to her anymore about how she feels unless the mother shows she cares about Allison *(controlling mother's response)*.

ETIOLOGY

As researchers in the biologic aspects of behaviors began to study some of the physiologic markers consistent with the Axis I diagnoses, they used some of the same studies with individuals with personality disorders, with consistent results. There have been family studies, including twin studies, that demonstrate a strong genetic influence, thus suggesting some ties between biologic factors and personality organization (Coryell and Zimmerman, 1989; Kavoussi and Siever, 1991; Marin et al., 1989; Siever, 1992; Siever and Davis, 1991).

One interesting aspect of this research occurred in the studies on individuals with schizotypal personality disorder who demonstrate impaired eye-tracking behavior. Impaired eye-tracking behavior is a person's inability to track a smoothly moving target (Siever, 1992). This is important for cognitive interpretation of information in the environment. Individuals with schizophrenia demonstrate difficulty with smooth-pursuit eye movements, and many believe this reflects disrupted neurointegrative functioning of the frontal lobes (Siever, 1992). The impaired eye-tracking studies are associated with the "deficit" traits of schizophrenia, namely the social isolation, detachment, and inability to relate to others.

Another biologic test indicative of cognitive-perceptual difficulties that occurs often in clients who have schizotypal personality disorder is *backward masking*. This test of neurointegrative functioning involves a "process in which a visual stimulus rapidly follows another visual stimulus and the subject has to identify the original stimulus" (Kavoussi and Siever, 1991). Siever (1985) found individuals with this personality disorder to have results similar to those noted in individuals with schizophrenia, but not as severe.

The ability to pay attention to stimuli is a biologic/cognitive marker that providers use to predict schizophrenia. The Continuous Performance Test, Identical Pairs Version, tests the ability to attend to stimuli. In their study of the schizotypal personality disorder, Roitman et al. (1997) reported that individuals demonstrated a verbal and spatial deficit when tested with the Continuous Performance Test, Identical Pairs Version, as compared with normal subjects and individuals who had other types of personality disorders. The test results were similar to the pattern usually seen in individuals with schizophrenia.

There are some neurochemical measures that are important indicators of biologic manifestations of the schizotypal personality disorder. Siever (1992) reported that cerebrospinal fluid homovanillic acid was increased in preliminary studies of schizotypal clients and correlated with positive psychotic-like criteria for schizotypal personality but without the negative or deficit symptoms. He also reported that plasma homovanillic acid was increased in clients with schizotypal personality disorder, as compared with client controls (Kavoussi and Siever, 1991). In 1988, researchers found that clients with borderline personality disorder who also had schizotypal personality disorder demonstrated evidence of a worsening of psychotic-like symptoms in response to an infusion of amphetamines.

In clients who have difficulty with affective regulation (mood), some biologic indices or tests are important to consider. The dexamethasone suppression test (DST), the thyrotropin-releasing hormone test (TRH), and electroencephalographic (EEG) sleep studies are biologic markers of affective disorders. Clients with borderline personality disorder had abnormal DST and TRH results, prompting researchers to question whether these clients have a variant of mood disorders. However, in studies that separated clients with borderline personality disorder into groups with and without depression, researchers reported that the nondepressed subjects had a higher percentage of normal DST and TRH results. Marin et al. (1989) have suggested that these results are related to depression rather than to the personality disorder.

Several studies demonstrate disturbances in central serotonergic neurotransmission, indicating that aggressive and suicidal behaviors in individuals with a personality disorder correlate with reduced levels of the cerebrospinal fluid 5-hydroxyindoleacetic acid (5-HIAA), a major metabolite of serotonin, which indicates a reduction in serotonin activity (Brown et al., 1982). Mann et al. (1986) found increased postsynaptic serotonergic receptors in suicide victims. Stanley and Stanley (1990) demonstrated information on both presynaptic and postsynaptic serotonergic markers, which suggests that a reduction in serotonin neurotransmission is an underlying biochemical risk factor for suicide. Marin et al. (1989) and Kavoussi and Siever (1991) surveyed several studies involving serotonin and its metabolites and found that there were serotonergic reduction in behaviors such as impulsiveness, motor aggression, and suicidal tendencies. Brown and Linnoila (1990) studied the cerebrospinal fluid metabolites of serotonin (5-HIAA), which indicated a relationship between reduced serotonergic activity and aggressive and impulsive behavior. Leyton et al. (2001) studied the relationship of 5-HT (serotonin) and brain regional alpha [11 C] methyl-L-tryptophan trapping in impulsive individuals. They found that individuals who have borderline personality disorder made more punishment reward commission errors on a psychologic test called the "go/no go task." This correlates with the behavior patterns of difficulty inhibiting or delaying responses and relates to the impulsive behavior common in this population. Low 5-HT synthesis capacity was in the corticostriatal pathways, which is possibly a factor to the development of impulsive behaviors in individuals with borderline personality disorder.

There is also a possible dysfunction of the brain system's ability to modulate and inhibit aggressive responses to environmental stimuli (Siever and Davis, 1991). Some data indicate that EEG slow-wave activity and a low threshold for sedation discriminate individuals with antisocial personality disorder from individuals with long-term depression (Siever and Davis, 1991).

The fact that individuals with personality disorders manifest some biologic markers is exciting for researchers and clinicians, as this information provides some suggestions that will be useful when treating this population. There is a need for future research in this area as the functions of the brain and the neurotransmitters become better known and understood.

EPIDEMIOLOGY AND CLINICAL DESCRIPTION

Cluster A Personality Disorders

Cluster A, often described as the odd or eccentric cluster, consists of the following personality disorders: paranoid, schizoid, and schizotypal. Clients in this cluster all have difficulty relating to others, isolate themselves, and are unable to socialize comfortably. Box 13-2 and the Clinical Symptoms box provide epidemiology and summaries of the clinical symptoms of each disorder.

Cluster B Personality Disorders

Cluster B personality disorders have components of dramatic behavior, a description widely used when describing individuals with a Cluster B personality disorder. The four diagnostic categories that make up this cluster are antisocial, borderline, histrionic, and narcissistic. Each personality disorder has unique features; each shares a dramatic quality in the way the individual lives his or her life. Box 13-3 and the Clinical Symptoms box on p. 290 provide epidemiology and summarize the key clinical symptoms of these disorders.

Cluster C Personality Disorders

Cluster C personality disorders are in the anxious or fearful cluster. They include avoidant personality disorder, dependent personality disorder, and obsessive-compulsive personality disorder. Box 13-4 and the Clinical Symptoms box on p. 291 provide epidemiology and summarize the key clinical symptoms of these disorders.

Unspecified Personality Disorders

The category of unspecified personality disorders describes individuals whose personality pattern meets the general criteria for a personality disorder but not the criteria for any specific personality disorder. It is also for an individual whose personality pattern meets the general criteria for a personality disorder, but the person has a personality disorder that is not in the current classification, such as passive-aggressive personality disorder.

PROGNOSIS

When providing nursing care to clients with personality disorders, it is important to consider the prognosis for improvement. This is especially important during the planning and evaluating portions of the nursing care plan. By definition, individuals with personality disorders have demonstrated pervasive and inflexible behaviors and thoughts that differ from their cultural expectations (APA,

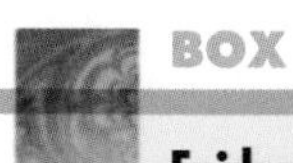

BOX 13-2

Epidemiology of Cluster A Personality Disorders

PARANOID PERSONALITY DISORDER

Diagnosed in 0.5% to 2.5% of the general population.
10% to 30% of the paranoid population is in inpatient psychiatric settings.
2% to 10% are in outpatient mental health clinics.
Families who have one or more members already diagnosed with paranoid personality disorder are at increased risk.
Males are diagnosed more often than females.
Substance abuse is common.

SCHIZOID PERSONALITY DISORDER

Males are diagnosed slightly more often than females.
Families with members who have schizophrenia or schizotypal personality disorder have increased prevalence.

SCHIZOTYPAL PERSONALITY DISORDER

Diagnosed in 3% of the general population.
30% to 50% also have major depression.
Individuals with schizotypal personality disorder seek treatment for anxiety or depression, not for the personality disorder features.
First-degree relatives of individuals with schizophrenia are at increased risk.
Males are diagnosed slightly more often than females.

CLINICAL SYMPTOMS

Cluster A Personality Disorders

PARANOID PERSONALITY DISORDER

Distrust, suspicion
Difficulty adjusting to change
Sensitivity, argumentation
Feelings of irreversible injury by others—often without evidence
Anxiety, difficulty relaxing
Short temper
Difficulty with problem solving
Lack of tender feelings toward others
Unwillingness to forgive even minor events
Jealousy of spouse or significant other—often without evidence

SCHIZOID PERSONALITY DISORDER

Brief psychotic episodes in response to stressful events
Lack of desire to socialize, enjoys solitude
Lack of strong emotions
Detached, self-absorbed affect
Lack of trust in others
Difficulty expressing anger
Passive reactions to crises

SCHIZOTYPAL PERSONALITY DISORDER

Incorrect interpretation of external events/belief that all events refer to self
Superstition, preoccupation with paranormal phenomena
Belief in possession of magical control over others
Constricted or inappropriate affect
Anxiety in social situations

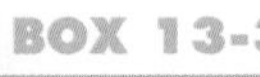

BOX 13-3

Epidemiology of Cluster B Personality Disorders

ANTISOCIAL PERSONALITY DISORDER

Usually diagnosed by age 18 years old.
Individuals have a history of conduct disorders before age 15 years old.
Males are diagnosed more often than females.
Characteristics are evident by early childhood in males and by puberty in females.
A high percentage of diagnosed individuals are in substance abuse treatment settings and prisons.
Incidence is more common in the lower socioeconomic classes.
Substance abuse is common.
Impulsive behavior is common.

BORDERLINE PERSONALITY DISORDER

Diagnosed in 2% of the general population.
10% of those in this population are in outpatient mental health clinics.
20% are in inpatient psychiatric settings.
75% of diagnosed individuals are female.
60% of those in the diagnosed disorder population have borderline personality disorder.
Diagnosed individuals have a history of physical and sexual abuse, neglect, hostile conflict, and early parental losses or separation.

HISTRIONIC PERSONALITY DISORDER

Females are diagnosed more often than males.
Diagnosed in 2% to 3% of the general population.
10% to 15% of the individuals who seek treatment have this disorder.

NARCISSISTIC PERSONALITY DISORDER

Diagnosed in less than 1% of the general population.
Diagnosed in 2% to 16% of the clinical population.
50% to 75% of those diagnosed are male.

CLINICAL SYMPTOMS

Cluster B Personality Disorders

ANTISOCIAL PERSONALITY DISORDER

Irresponsibility
Failure to honor financial obligations, plan ahead, provide children with basic needs
Involvement in illegal activities
Lack of guilt
Difficulty learning from mistakes
Initial charm dissolves to coldness, manipulation, blaming others
Lack of empathy
Irritability
Abuse of substances

BORDERLINE PERSONALITY DISORDER

Suicidal ideations
Self-mutilation
Impulsivity
Tendency to engage in impulsive acts (e.g., bingeing, spending money, reckless driving, unsafe sex)
Negative or angry affect
Feelings of emptiness and boredom
Difficulty being alone, feeling of abandonment
Difficulty identifying self
Perception of people as all good or all bad
Intense, stormy relationships

HISTRIONIC PERSONALITY DISORDER

Use of suicidal gestures and threats to get attention
Fluctuation in emotions
Attention-seeking, self-centered attitude
Sexual seduction and flamboyance
Attentiveness to own physical appearance
Dramatic, impressionistic speech style
Vague logic—lack of conviction in arguments, often switching sides
Shallow emotional expression
Craving for immediate satisfaction
Complaints of physical illness, somatization

NARCISSISTIC PERSONALITY DISORDER

Grandiose view of self
Lack of empathy toward others
Need for admiration
Preoccupation with fantasies of success, brilliance, beauty, ideal love

2000). These patterns first begin in adolescence or early adulthood and are stable over time. These symptoms lead to distress and functional and relationship impairment in the individual. With this definition in mind, the prognosis for individuals with personality disorders is guarded given the ingrained and pervasive nature of these disorders.

An example of how a personality disorder manifests in adolescence is made by examining the symptoms of conduct disorder in adolescence and the development of antisocial disorder in adulthood. Pajer (1998) studied the literature to determine if girls who displayed symptoms of conduct disorder continued the symptoms to demonstrate antisocial personality disorder as adults. Pajer concluded that the adults had higher mortality rates, an increase in criminal behavior, and many psychiatric co-occurring symptoms. They also had disturbed and sometimes violent relationships with a high rate of divorce and extramarital sexual activity, poor educational achievement, less stable work histories, and a high rate of using welfare systems and child protective agencies. Myers, Stewart, and Brown (1998) studied the progression of symptoms from those demonstrated in conduct disorder to antisocial personality disorder in adolescents who were seeking treatment for substance abuse. These studies concluded that early, structured therapy sometimes decreases the severity of the personality disorder in adult life (see Research for Evidence-Based Practice box).

In another study, Becker et al. (2000) investigated the co-occurrence of borderline personality disorder with other personality disorders with a group of adolescents who were hospitalized. The researchers compared this finding with adults who were admitted to the same hospital during the same period. They determined that in the adolescent group, schizotypal and passive-aggressive personality disorders occurred concurrently in a significant number of cases.

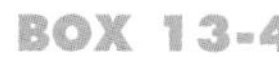

BOX 13-4

Epidemiology of Cluster C Personality Disorders

AVOIDANT PERSONALITY DISORDER

Diagnosis is equal for males and females.
Diagnosed in 0.5% to 1% of the general population.
10% are diagnosed in outpatient settings.

DEPENDENT PERSONALITY DISORDER

Most frequently diagnosed personality disorder.
More females are diagnosed than males.
Symptoms are demonstrated early in life.
Children or adolescents with chronic physical illness or separation anxiety disorder may be predisposed.

OBSESSIVE-COMPULSIVE PERSONALITY DISORDER

Diagnosed in 1% of the general population.
Diagnosed in 3% to 10% of the population who seek treatment.
Males are diagnosed twice as often as females.

CLINICAL SYMPTOMS

Cluster C Personality Disorders

AVOIDANT PERSONALITY DISORDER

Fearful of criticism, disapproval, or rejection
Avoidance of social interactions
Tendency to withhold thoughts or feelings
Negative sense of self, low self-esteem

DEPENDENT PERSONALITY DISORDER

Submissiveness, tendency to cling
Inability to make decisions independently
Inability to express negative emotions
Difficulty following through on tasks

OBSESSIVE-COMPULSIVE PERSONALITY DISORDER

Preoccupation with perfection, organization, structure, control
Procrastination
Abandonment of projects because of dissatisfaction
Excessive devotion to work
Difficulty relaxing
Rule-conscious behavior
Self-criticism and inability to forgive own errors
Reluctance to delegate
Inability to discard anything
Insistence on others' conforming to own methods
Rejection of praise
Reluctance to spend money
Background of stiff and formal relationships
Preoccupation with logic and intellect

Realistic expectations for improvement include a commitment by the client to explore and evaluate his or her thoughts and behaviors, especially when under stress. The nurse plays a powerful role by providing support, tools for this exploration, and client teaching. If the client is able to use the knowledge of his or her dysfunctional patterns to predict how he or she will respond when faced with a stressor, the nurse is able to plan innovative options for problem solving. In this way, the individual learns new responses and improves functioning. This process often needs to be repeated over time before behavioral and thought patterns change. Therefore, long-term treatment aimed at problem solving and cognitive reframing is indicated for these clients.

Linehan (1993) identified the repeating behavioral patterns of individuals with borderline personality disorder. She then began to study what interventions decrease the most destructive behavioral patterns, such as parasuicidal behavior, splitting, and intense emotional reactivity. This research yielded a treatment strategy called dialectical behavioral therapy (DBT). The principal assumption is to use the dialogue to assist the client in reworking destructive ways of dealing with crises. DBT teaches the client that there are choices in working through the crisis that decrease the suicidal thoughts or emotionally reactive patterns. The therapy focuses on the client's learning new patterns of thoughts and behaviors. Current research suggests that individuals who are treated with DBT have a decrease in hospitalizations because of a decrease in suicidal drive and a higher level of interpersonal functioning (Osboren and McCormish, 2006). (See Chapter 23.)

RESEARCH for EVIDENCE-BASED PRACTICE

Zanarini MC, Frankenburg FR, Hennen J, et al: Prediction of the 10 year course of borderline personality disorder, *American Journal of Psychiatry* 163(5): 827-834, 2006.

Zanarini et al. studied 293 individuals in a 10-year longitudinal research study to determine if symptoms of borderline personality disorder (BPD) are able to show remission. All of the original research participants were hospitalized in an inpatient unit at a New England psychiatric hospital for symptoms related to borderline personality disorder. Researchers gave the individuals several tools to verify the diagnosis of borderline personality disorder. Subjects were excluded from the research if they had a history of schizophrenia, schizoaffective disorder, bipolar I disorder, or an organic condition. Two interviewers determined the diagnosis. The individuals in the research were followed for 10 years, with interviews occurring every 2 years. Researchers defined remission as no longer meeting the criteria for borderline personality disorder in the Diagnostic Statistical Manual and the Revised Diagnostic Interview for Borderlines (DIB-R).

Of the 275 participants who initially were enrolled in the research; 242 reached remission from the symptoms of borderline personality disorder. The individuals who were able to achieve remission were younger when they were first diagnosed with BPD and had no psychiatric hospitalizations before the hospitalization that occurred when the initial research took place. These individuals had no history of childhood sexual abuse and had less severe childhood abuse or neglect. Their family history was negative for mood and substance abuse. There was an absence of PTSD and symptoms of the anxious Cluster C personality disorders. The individuals who achieved remission had low neuroticism (a predisposition toward negative affective states, such as depression, anxiety, and anger), high extroversion, high agreeableness, high conscientiousness, and a good vocational record.

This research is useful to therapists who provide care for individuals with BPD. It is helpful to be able to anticipate that a client can achieve remission if there is a combination of the characteristics mentioned here and psychotherapy.

DISCHARGE CRITERIA

Clients with personality disorders present in both inpatient and outpatient settings, such as day treatment facilities, partial hospital units, clinics, and private office practices. To determine when to discharge a client from an inpatient hospital setting, it is important to consider the risk factor of safety for the client and others. Some clients with personality disorders have suicidal ideas that are part of their day-to-day thought process. When evaluating clients with this ongoing theme, it is important to determine whether the client has a suicidal plan and if he or she intends to implement that plan (see Chapter 21).

Individuals with a personality disorder who are hospitalized often have more than one psychiatric diagnosis. Their lives are complex and chaotic. Psychiatric follow-up care, whether in a partial hospitalization program, a day treatment center, or with an outpatient psychotherapist, is important to help the client work through some of the issues that contributed to the crisis that culminated in the hospital stay. Before discharge from the hospital, it is important for the client to have a plan for outpatient follow-up care and the first posthospital appointment established.

Client teaching is a powerful tool to help the client understand the psychiatric problems that he or she is experiencing, as well as to help prevent a relapse of symptoms. Before discharge from the hospital, each client needs to receive education in the following areas:

- The need for follow-up care in an outpatient setting
- The psychiatric symptoms that indicate a need for emergent treatment
- An understanding of any medications that the client is receiving

This client teaching takes place in a group setting or on an individual basis. If one of the location activities is a relapse prevention group or a medication group, it is helpful for the primary nurse to review the material specific to each client before his or her discharge.

If the client in an outpatient setting, the nurse needs to consider the following issues before discharge from treatment:

- The client no longer has active thoughts of wanting to harm self or others.
- The client controls self-destructive impulses such as substance abuse when feeling upset or shoplifting when feeling empty.
- The client has an understanding of the symptoms that caused the need for psychotherapy.
- The client understands the types of symptoms that indicate a need for further treatment in the future.
- The client is able to use community 12-step groups if this is relevant to his or her problems, such as Alcoholics Anonymous, Narcotics Anonymous, Co-Dependents Anonymous, Incest Survivors Anonymous, and Overeaters Anonymous.

The Nursing Process

ASSESSMENT

When the nurse assesses a client for a personality disorder, the interview needs to take place in a comfortable, quiet, private, safe environment. Make sure there are no interruptions during the assessment. Individuals with these disorders are often withdrawn, defensive, guarded, and impulsive, or they are charming and friendly.

Do not be judgmental or confrontational during the interview. If the client demonstrates an escalation of anger or makes hostile, threatening comments to the assessment questions, a break will help the client regain composure. Do not threaten the client with seclusion or restraint, because this will provoke him or her to impulsively lose control.

The Nursing Assessment Questions box represents a comprehensive evaluation for clients who have a personality disorder. The five domains of human behavior examined are the physical, emotional, cognitive, social, and spiritual domains (see the Case Study, p. 294).

NURSING ASSESSMENT QUESTIONS

Personality Disorders

PHYSICAL DOMAIN

1 Is there evidence of appropriate activities of daily living?
2 Is the client neatly groomed?
3 Is the client dressed appropriately?
4 Does the client appear adequately nourished?
5 Is there evidence of a regular exercise program in his or her life?
6 Is there evidence of any physical illnesses?
7 Does the client concentrate on somatic concerns?
8 Is the client able to maintain eye contact?
9 Is the client experiencing tension?
10 Does the client demonstrate sympathetic stimulation, cardiovascular excitation, superficial vasoconstriction, or pupil dilation?
11 Does the client report trouble sleeping?
12 Is the client glancing about?
13 Is the client demonstrating extraneous movements, such as foot shuffling or hand and arm movements?
14 Does the client show facial tension?
15 Is his or her voice quivering?
16 Does the client report increased wariness?
17 Is the client having an increase in perspiration?
18 Does the client have a history of any of the following physical conditions?
Temporal lobe epilepsy
Progressive central nervous system disorder
Head trauma
Hormonal imbalance
Mental retardation
Abuse of alcohol or drugs

NURSING ASSESSMENT QUESTIONS

Personality Disorders, cont'd

PHYSICAL DOMAIN, cont'd

19 Is the client dressed inappropriately or in a seductive manner?
20 Does the client have a high incidence of accidents?
21 Is the client overly concerned with physical attractiveness?

EMOTIONAL DOMAIN

1 Does the client indicate having thoughts of harming self or others?
2 Does the client demonstrate demanding, hostile behavior?
3 Does the client have a history of aggressive actions?
4 Is the client emotionally volatile?
5 Does the client have poor impulse control?
6 Is the client suspicious of others?
7 Is the client fearful or highly anxious?
8 Does the client express feelings of helplessness?
9 Does the client appear apprehensive?
10 Does the client's thought pattern include feelings of uncertainty?
11 Does the client discuss concerns about unspecified consequences?
12 Does the client have persistent worries?
13 Does the client demonstrate critical behavior toward self and others?
14 Does the client have low self-esteem?
15 Is the client concerned about how others will evaluate him or her?
16 Does the client inflate his or her importance?
17 Does the client describe feelings of guilt or regret?
18 Does the client lack remorse and use excuses to justify hurting another?
19 Does the client lack empathy?
20 Is the client vindictive?
21 Does the client demonstrate a low frustration tolerance?
22 Does the client show a lack of motivation?
23 Is the client dependent on others to meet his or her needs?
24 Is the client's behavior passive?
25 Does the client discuss feelings of inadequacy?
26 Does the client deny strong emotions, such as anger and joy?
27 Does the client describe feelings of hopelessness?
28 Does the client demonstrate inappropriate sexually seductive behavior?
29 Does the client manifest a constricted affect?
30 Does the client exhibit an inappropriate affect, such as silly or vacant facial expressions?
31 Does the client display lability of his or her mood?

COGNITIVE DOMAIN

1 Does the client demonstrate inaccurate interpretation of stimuli, both internal and external?
2 Does the client have difficulty understanding abstract ideas?
3 Is the client able to identify problem areas?
4 Is the client able to identify options to solve the problems?
5 Does the client's identification of the problem area involve blaming others or self?
6 Is the client vindictive in his or her problem solving?
7 Does the client lie?
8 Is the client able to identify both good and bad traits in others?
9 Is the client able to distinguish positive and negative options to problem solving?
10 Does the client reflect too much on issues of concern?
11 Is the client's thought pattern redundant?
12 Is the client able to tolerate a delay in gratification?
13 Is the client able to identify his or her value system?
14 Does the client have difficulty learning from his or her mistakes?
15 Is the client impulsive?
16 Does the client manifest any deficits in long-term or short-term memory?
17 Is the client preoccupied?
18 Does the client have a lack of consensual validation?
19 Does the client describe any delusions?
20 Does the client experience any hallucinations? If so, what type: auditory, visual, tactile, gustatory, olfactory? What is the content of the hallucinations?
21 Does the client reveal any perceptual experiences?
22 Does the client confirm having any ideas of reference?
23 Does the client discuss any odd beliefs or magical thinking that influence his or her behavior?
24 Is the client's speech impoverished, digressive, vague, or inappropriately abstract?

SOCIAL DOMAIN

1 Does the client prefer to be alone?
2 Does the client express a desire to socialize but have concerns that others will not accept him or her?
3 Is the client dependent on others for meeting his or her needs?
4 Does the client participate in family activities?
5 Does the client have any friends?
6 Does the client have unstable relationships that consist of conflict and concerns about abandonment?
7 Is the client able to identify the dynamics of relationship problems?
8 Is the client using manipulative behavior as a means of getting needs met?
9 Does the client show evidence of splitting? Does the client place great value on relating with one person while becoming critical and angry with the other? Does the client devalue and complain about one individual to another person with whom the client has a positive relationship?
10 Does the client identify his or her sense of self by indicating membership in a relationship?
11 Is the client attention seeking, wanting to be the center of attention?
12 Is the client preoccupied with how others view him or her?
13 Is this client extremely sensitive to praise and criticism of others?
14 Is the client reluctant to give time, gifts, and support to his or her friends unless the client will profit?
15 Does the client choose solitary activities?
16 Does the client engage in any social activities?
17 Does the client feel increasingly anxious when in a social situation?
18 Does the client express no desire to have a sexual experience with another person?
19 Does the client have multiple sexual partners?
20 Is this client indifferent to praise and criticism of others?
21 Does the client expect others to exploit him or her?
22 Does the client exploit others to get his or her needs met?
23 Does the client question the loyalty or trustworthiness of friends or associates? Does the client question the loyalty of his or her spouse or sexual partner?
24 Does the client read hidden meanings into the harmless remarks of others?

Continued

NURSING ASSESSMENT QUESTIONS

Personality Disorders, cont'd

SOCIAL DOMAIN, cont'd

25 Does the client have grudges against others?
26 Is the client reluctant to confide in others?
27 Is the client preoccupied with self to the exclusion of others?
28 Does the client fail to honor financial obligations?
29 Does the client fail to plan ahead, such as traveling without a clear plan or quitting work without plans to begin another job?
30 Does the client provide his or her children with the basic needs for health?
31 Does the client engage in illegal activities?
32 Does the client abuse drugs or alcohol?
33 Does the client demonstrate a belief that he or she is owed a sense of entitlement?

SPIRITUAL DOMAIN

1 Does the client have a belief in a higher power?
2 Is the client able to state a meaning and purpose to his or her life?

CASE STUDY Ben, a 32-year-old single man, was evaluated by a nurse in an outpatient clinic at the recommendation of his father because of an increase in his isolative behavior. Ben did not want to come in for the interview, as he did not consider "being alone" a problem. He was oriented times three but was not spontaneous with answers to the nurse's assessment questions. His affect was flat, he averted his eyes, and his leg was shaking. He was unkempt, with a disheveled appearance and mismatched clothing. He had a vague, wandering, nonspecific way of discussing his problem and his lifestyle.

His mother had been recently hospitalized with pneumonia; however, Ben did not see that as part of his problem. He perceived his boss as disliking him, because the boss thought he was "weird." Ben said that he had no friends, found socializing difficult, and tended to withdraw further when forced to interact with others. He was suspicious of the interviewer and of his father's motives for asking him to seek psychiatric intervention.

The problem he identified was that he felt he had to "do more around the house" in his mother's absence. That seemed "unfair and like a burden" to Ben. "She just got sick so she wouldn't have to cook supper or do the laundry," Ben stated. "The doctors put her in the hospital so they will make more money off of her. Dad is in on it; he sent me here so you could make money."

Ben had not visited his mother in the hospital because he was afraid he would get germs there. Although he saw no reason for this interview, he consented to return to the clinic to "help" his father.

CRITICAL THINKING

1 What questions should the nurse ask Ben to determine symptoms in the physical domain?
2 How could the nurse assess the emotional domain?
3 How could the nurse assess Ben's problems in the cognitive domain?
4 What information about Ben helps to determine his functioning in the social domain?
5 What questions could the nurse ask Ben to assess how he functions in the spiritual domain?

NURSING DIAGNOSIS

Nurses develop a diagnosis based on the in-depth assessment of the client's health status. The nursing diagnosis is a statement that defines the problem and its characteristics and contributing factors and guides the development of the nursing care plan (see the Nursing Assessment Questions box). Nursing diagnoses are prioritized according to client needs and safety issues. The following nursing diagnoses (NANDA-I, 2007) are the most common when caring for clients with a personality disorder.

Paranoid, Schizoid, and Schizotypal Personality Disorders (Cluster A)

- Anxiety
- Ineffective coping
- Social isolation
- Disturbed thought processes

Antisocial, Borderline, Histrionic, and Narcissistic Personality Disorders (Cluster B)

- Risk for suicide
- Risk for other-directed violence
- Risk for self-mutilation
- Risk for self-directed violence
- Ineffective coping
- Disturbed personal identity
- Chronic low self-esteem
- Impaired social interaction
- Complicated grieving

Avoidant, Dependent, and Obsessive-Compulsive Personality Disorders (Cluster C)

- Anxiety
- Ineffective coping
- Chronic low self-esteem
- Impaired social interaction

OUTCOME IDENTIFICATION

An individual with a personality disorder has disturbances in self-image and relationships throughout life. Identifying outcomes includes the client's ability to demonstrate an understanding of problem areas and to display healthy and effective adaptive behaviors. The focus is on helping the individual to find patterns of maladaptive behavior, thoughts, and emotions that produce distress. The nurse and client work together to explore

NURSING ASSESSMENT QUESTIONS

Personality Disorders

These questions involve the nurse's observation of the client's appearance, general nutritional status, and level of observable anxiety manifestations:

1 Does the client appear appropriately dressed? Does the client maintain eye contact? Does he or she appear properly nourished? Does the client exhibit signs of anxiety, such as pacing, foot tapping, sighing, or facial tension? Does the client appear hypervigilant (overly watchful)? Does the client appear withdrawn?

The following questions will help the nurse to determine if there are disturbances in the client's relationships, thought processes, and behavior:

2 How would you describe yourself? What do you like about yourself? What would you like to change about yourself?

3 Describe your relationship with your spouse or significant other, your children, your parents, and other family members. Describe your relationship with your friends. What do you talk about? What types of activities do you do together?

4 How do you feel about your job? Do you get along with your boss and coworkers?

5 If you have a personal problem, whom do you trust to help you with it?

6 What are your main worries? How often do you think about them? Do you talk to anyone about these worries? Does that help?

7 Do you ever feel like hurting yourself or anyone else? Have you ever been suicidal? Have you ever hurt yourself by cutting your skin or burning yourself? How often does this occur?

8 Have you ever felt hopeless, helpless, worthless, and a burden? Do you feel this now? Are you getting any support from friends or family?

9 Do you ever use alcohol or illegal drugs? Have you ever gone to the doctor to get tranquilizers to reduce your nervousness? What did the doctor give you? What are you taking now?

10 What are your religious beliefs and practices?

options to change these maladaptive patterns to more effective coping strategies.

The outcome criteria come from the nursing diagnoses and are the expected client responses or behaviors that occur as a result of the plan of care. Nurses state outcomes in clear, measurable terms.

Client will:

- Demonstrate absence of active suicidal ideation.
- Stop having thoughts about harming others.
- Refrain from self-mutilation.
- Reach and maintain the highest functioning possible, as demonstrated by the ability to function at home, work, and in the community.
- Identify two impulsive behavior patterns that take place during times of stress.
- Recognize when he or she is experiencing cognitive distortions during a stressful period of time.
- Identify a cognitive distortion used most often during times of stress.
- Identify one new method of problem solving.
- Reward self, both with an item (such as some flowers) and a positive thought when able to successfully identify and change a cognitive distortion.
- Identify some patterns of isolative behavior.
- Tolerate short interactive periods with the nurse, family members, and peers (see the Case Study).
- Identify with positive role models.
- Contribute one statement in a group setting directed toward facilitating increased socialization.

CASE STUDY Lynn has been working with a nurse for the past 3 years in outpatient psychotherapy. She was recently arrested for stealing some candy and lipstick at a local department store after an argument with her boyfriend. During the session after the arrest, the nurse suggested to Lynn that she explore the dynamics of the incident and how this related to the argument with her boyfriend. Lynn became angry, then scared, expressing concern that she might lose the respect and the therapeutic relationship with the nurse. She ran out of the room, yelling that the nurse did not understand her pain, and slammed the door. Several minutes later, Lynn returned, apologized, and asked the nurse to forgive her.

CRITICAL THINKING

1 Which of Lynn's responses indicate that she had some insight into the dynamics of her impulsive stealing behaviors?

2 What changes in behavior are anticipated as a result of Lynn's gaining understanding about her impulsive behavior?

3 What two outcomes would be realistic for Lynn?

4 How should the nurse respond to Lynn's anger and subsequent apology?

PLANNING

When planning interventions with a client who has a personality disorder, it is important for the nurse to recognize that changes in behavior or thoughts often occur slowly. These changes are a result of the client's perception of the need for that change. Individuals with a personality disorder have disturbed interpersonal relationships and values that do not reflect the views held by the general population. Because of these disturbances, the nurse needs to collaborate with the client on the goals identified during treatment.

IMPLEMENTATION

Implementation of the plan of care for clients with personality disorders includes interventions focused toward modifying lifelong disruptive and dysfunctional behaviors and thoughts while promoting safety.

Nursing Interventions

1. Assess the client for suicidal ideation and determine the level of lethality *to prevent suicide, harm, or injury.*
2. If warranted, place the client on suicidal precaution, depending on his or her level of lethality (e.g., a client

CLINICAL ALERT

Clients with **personality disorders** have difficulty relating to others. As a consequence, these individuals have difficulty defining boundaries between self and others. Part of nursing care is to define boundaries within the therapeutic relationship in order to develop safe, client-centered therapeutic relationships. This is particularly important for the nurse to think about when he or she is feeling vulnerable, perhaps because of other personal or professional stressors. Smith et al. (1997) have highlighted ways to recognize and prevent sexually inappropriate behavior with a client. It is important that nurses assess their feelings toward the clients who are in their care, as well as nurses' own current stressors. Nurses need to ask the following questions: "Are the stressors interfering with my functioning on the job?" "In what ways can I deal with these issues without becoming vulnerable to the clients under my care?" If nurses recognize that they are experiencing special feelings for a particular client, they need to discuss these feelings with a colleague or obtain clinical supervision/assistance from the employee assistance program.

who has verbalized plans to hang himself or herself while on the unit needs close individual observation, even with no means or provisions to carry out the intent) *to prevent suicide.*

3. Establish a contract for safety with the client by asking the client to write a statement indicating that he or she will not harm himself or herself. If the suicidal impulse becomes too strong, encourage the client to seek out a staff member to discuss the increase in intensity of suicidal ideation *to protect the client from acting on suicidal impulses.*
4. Encourage the client to attend all unit group sessions *to receive support from peers and to provide opportunities for problem solving.*
5. Assess the client for an escalation of anger to rage and possible impulsive actions against others (obtain a history of violence if possible) *to prevent harm or injury to others.*
6. Contract with the client that he or she will no longer threaten staff or peers during hospitalization *to ensure the safety of others.*
7. Teach the client other options to manage angry, impulsive feelings and behavior such as leaving the room where the conflict is occurring or using a quiet area (e.g., an unlocked seclusion room) until the impulse to do harm passes. *Removing the client from a stimulating, provocative environment will decrease angry impulses.*
8. Discuss angry feelings in a group setting focused on exploring alternative problem-solving options. *Alternative actions will distract the client from angry feelings and help to focus energy on constructive activities.*
9. Assess the client for evidence of self-mutilation. *Clients who are self-destructive are likely to repeat such acts and may require further intervention.*
10. Obtain a contract from the client that he or she will approach a staff member when the urge to self-mutilate is present *to ensure the safety of the client.*
11. Place the client on an individual, close watch until the urge to harm self passes or until the client is able to identify another way to obtain emotional relief (e.g., wrapping in a sheet [Dresser, 1999] or participating in a movement therapy group) *to protect the client from harmful impulses and redirect the impulses toward alternative, constructive methods.*
12. If self-mutilation occurs, attend to the wounds in a matter-of-fact manner *to provide the client with safe care in a nonjudgmental manner.*
13. Encourage the client to keep a journal of thoughts and feelings the client had before experiencing the urge to self-mutilate *to help the client acknowledge feelings and thoughts and help decrease impulsivity.*
14. Medicate the client with an anxiolytic or antipsychotic medication, prn as ordered *to help the client control his or her intense anxiety or rage rather than self-mutilate.*
15. Use a time-out period, seclusion room, and physical restraints if all attempts of least restrictive measures have been unsuccessful *to protect the client.*
16. Assist the client in recognizing thought patterns that contribute to impulsive behavior. Nurses are able to do this by helping the client understand the role that intense feelings (e.g., abandonment, anger, rage, or anxiety) play in precipitating impulsive behavior or distorted thinking. Using a journal to document such feelings and thoughts and receiving feedback during group sessions are helpful, instructive methods. *Nurses teach clients to manage impulsive behavior and distorted beliefs through a variety of methods within the setting.*
17. Suggest alternative behaviors to deal with the intense feelings, such as the following:
    a. Recognizing the intense emotional state and writing in a journal or thinking about an action that helps to relieve the intensity of the feeling without resorting to impulsive or self-destructive acts
    b. Talking about the intense feeling while looking into a mirror, telling the mirror what the client would like to express to the object of anger
    c. Identifying healthy options to deal with the anger, such as discussing the issue with the person who is involved in the interaction
    d. Role-playing, with the nursing staff, different ways to approach the problem that precipitated the intense feelings
    e. Introducing the issue in the problem-solving setting or group meeting to receive feedback from peers
    f. Rewarding self with something that is pleasant and healthful, such as buying flowers or reading a novel
    g. Learning alternative ways to cope with intense feelings to thereby reduce anger/anxiety and provide constructive ways of managing life stressors
18. Help the client explore behavior that relates to the community, such as safe driving and responsibilities for

the environment, *to help the client focus on changes the client can make to live in a more healthy and responsible way.*

19. Evaluate the client's family system by observing the family dynamics and determining the client's role within the family. *How the client interacts within the family system and the role the client takes (e.g., victim, placater) offer the nurse insight into the client's self-perception* (see the Client and Family Teaching Guidelines box).
20. Engage the client in frequent short interactions several times during the shift *to illustrate the value of interacting with others.*

CLIENT and FAMILY TEACHING GUIDELINES

Set Method

Clients with personality disorders often have difficulties recognizing problem areas and identifying possible solutions. The nurse needs to incorporate teaching clients and family members to problem-solve more effectively as part of the care plan. One area of difficulty is communication. Kreisman and Straus (1989) have suggested using the SET method of communication. This was originally developed for clients with borderline personality disorder who were in crisis and were unable to communicate effectively. Kreisman and Straus's SET is a three-part system of communication. This is a particularly useful tool when the client is impulsive, is having outbursts of rage, is harmful to self or others, or is making unreasonable demands on others for care giving. In the SET method (Kreisman and Straus, 1989):

- The *S* stands for *support:* the nurse states a personal statement of concern for the client.
- The *E* is for *empathy:* the nurse acknowledges the individual's chaotic feelings in a neutral way, with the emphasis on the client's painful experience, not the staff member's feelings.
- The *T* is a *truth:* this statement is used to highlight the client's responsibility for his or her behavior and life.

For example, Charles had become angry when his wife, Nancy, did not go shopping and cook some meals for him before she went away for a business trip. His anger mounted, and he drank to deal with his intense feelings. He came to his partial hospitalization program, reporting a hangover.

His primary nurse led the following discussion about Charles' response to Nancy's travel on business:

Nurse: I know it is hard for you when Nancy has to go away. *[E]*

Charles: You got that right. It makes me so angry that she can't complete all her work here.

Nurse: Okay, I hear you *[S]*, but in her job, travel is a big part of business. *[T]*

Charles: Yeah, I know, and I think she's good at what she does. I just get so lonely, so empty, I then get angry and scared.

Nurse: Can you look at what type of things you can do when she is away that may help your feelings of emptiness? *[T]*

Charles: Like what?

Nurse: Like going to the movies on the night Nancy is out of town and seeing something she isn't interested in. Treat yourself to carryout Chinese or fast food, so that you have dinner without a lot of fuss. Does that sound like something that will help? *[T]*

Charles: I'll try.

From Kreisman JJ, Straus H: *I hate you—don't leave me: understanding the borderline personality,* Los Angeles, 1989, Body Press.

21. Use problem-solving groups and other groups that concentrate on self-care and community responsibilities *to help the client understand the value of interacting with others* (see Chapter 23).
22. Teach the client assertiveness techniques *to improve the client's ability to relate to others* (see Chapters 4 and 23).
23. Provide the client with direct feedback about his or her interaction with others in a nonjudgmental fashion *to facilitate learning new social skills.*

Additional Treatment Modalities

A team approach involving many disciplines provides the most comprehensive interventions for a client with a personality disorder in an inpatient, partial hospitalization, or day treatment setting (see the Additional Treatment Modalities box and Chapter 23).

Nurses are in a position to encourage and participate in research (see Online Resources). The more information the client and the client's family have, the more the choice about the use of treatment services and medication adherence makes sense. Research will assist the nurse in providing more comprehensive care and will aid in answering questions that will drive clinical practice.

Occupational Therapy

The occupational therapist assesses a client's abilities and disabilities and helps the client increase functioning and independent living skills in areas such as self-care, work, or leisure activity. The occupational therapist teaches adaptive skills for home, school, or job functioning. The occupational therapist often plans and leads groups that focus on areas such as stress management, enhancing parenting skills, conflict resolution, time management, money management, budgeting, feeling, and self-awareness.

Art Therapy

The art therapist uses art as a means of helping the client express thoughts and feelings he or she is not able to verbalize. This intervention helps the client to understand problem areas from a symbolic standpoint. The art therapist also teaches the client an alternative means of expression and self-soothing. For example, a client who is feeling intense rage and wants to self-mutilate will use art to express these feelings rather than act on them.

ADDITIONAL TREATMENT MODALITIES

Personality Disorders

- Occupational therapy
- Art therapy
- Music therapy
- Movement therapy
- Recreational therapy
- Medication therapy
- Individual therapy
- Cognitive behavioral therapy
- Dialectical behavioral therapy
- Group therapy
- Family therapy
- Milieu therapy

Music Therapy

The music therapist uses music to help the client express feelings and thoughts that are not easy to verbalize. Music helps the client relax and learn alternative self-soothing strategies.

Movement Therapy

Movement therapy teaches clients how they move their bodies when stressed and helps them learn methods of relaxation. Movement therapy is helpful for clients who become numb when experiencing intense feelings, such as abandonment or anger, to use methods of self-touching to reestablish a feeling state rather than self-mutilate.

Recreational Therapy

Recreational therapy helps clients with personality disorders explore ways to enjoy themselves without the use of self-destructive behaviors, such as abusing alcohol or drugs. This modality is helpful for clients who have difficulty socializing, because recreation strengthens social skills.

Medication Therapy

Medications often play a major role in helping the client with a personality disorder. Clients who are demonstrating violence against others sometimes require medications to gain emotional and behavioral control over their impulses. The practice guidelines for the treatment of individuals with borderline personality disorder (APA, 2004) suggest that clients who have affect dysregulation show a reduction in symptoms using a selective serotonin reuptake inhibitor (SSRI). If there is an anxiety component along with the affective dysregulation, this usually indicates a need for a benzodiazepine, such as clonazepam (Klonopin) along with the SSRI. Mood stabilizers such as lithium carbonate, carbamazepine (Tegretol), and valproate (Depakote) have been successful adjunctive treatments for affective dysregulation. For individuals who are demonstrating anger and impulsivity, an SSRI is the treatment of choice. The clinical practice guideline recommends using fluoxetine (Prozac) as the first line of treatment for this symptom. Clients who are very agitated or have psychosis sometimes respond to the use of a low-dose neuroleptic or antipsychotic class medication. Clients with extreme violence who are unable to control this impulse sometimes receive intravenous or intramuscular sedative-hypnotics, such as barbiturates, benzodiazepines such as diazepam (Valium), or antipsychotics such as haloperidol (Haldol) (Keltner and Folks, 2005). Monitoring side effects is an important nursing function (see Chapter 24).

Individual Therapy

Individual therapy helps the client explore problem areas, define new options, and discuss how the new behavior will help solve the original problem. With the emphasis in the health care system on short-term therapy, individual therapy is now problem-solving oriented as opposed to explorative based on early trauma. The use of Linehan's dialectical behavioral therapy (DBT) described earlier has an excellent rate of symptom reduction with the borderline individual (APA, Clinical Practice Guidelines, 2004; Osborne and McCornigh, 2006; Swarles et al., 2000).

MEDICATION KEY FACTS
Personality Disorders

- Pharmacologic interventions are symptom-oriented regardless of the type of personality disorder.
- Medications include short-term use of benzodiazepines and antipsychotics for aggressiveness and impulsivity.
- Mood stabilizers are used for dyscontrol, rage, violence, and impulsivity.
- Other medications include antidepressants and antianxiety agents.

Group Therapy

Group therapy is also problem-solving oriented. The work in group therapy is based on the repeated dynamics of the individuals in the group. This is especially beneficial for clients with a Cluster B personality disorder who are dramatic and require a lot of attention. The group members help the client to understand the effect his or her behavior has on each of them so that the client is able to use this information when relating to significant people in his or her everyday life.

Family Therapy

Family therapy is helpful for clients with a personality disorder because the dynamics of the family system are often repeated in other relationships in the client's life, such as with his or her boss or spouse. The family sessions consist of an assessment of the family system and an exploration of how the current problems that caused the client to seek care affect family dynamics. Because of the current philosophy of short-term therapy, exploration of earlier dynamics or trauma focuses on the current issue.

Milieu Therapy

When a client is hospitalized in an inpatient psychiatric setting or participates in a partial hospitalization program or a day treatment facility, the client becomes part of that milieu (environment). The purpose of **milieu therapy** is to re-create a community setting on these units so that the client is able to interact with other client peers to identify and problem-solve issues that occur while relating to others. Such relationship issues are discussed in community meetings or other problem-solving groups, such as a coping skills group.

The community meetings are for delegating tasks of the unit, such as cleaning off the tables at the end of the meal. This meeting is often used to ask each member to think through a daily goal for therapy and discuss how he or she plans to meet that goal. If something happens on the unit (e.g., if someone becomes aggressive or brings drugs or alcohol on the unit), the group discusses these concerns in the community meeting.

Problem-solving groups, such as coping skills groups, often pick a common area of concern, and the group works together to explore the issues and options necessary to solve the dilemma.

As in any other community, socializing is an important part of the interaction. In an inpatient, partial hospitalization program or day treatment milieu, socialization groups discuss problems with socializing. For example, the socialization group uses the discussion of a movie the group has just seen or current events read from a magazine or a newspaper to enrich the discussion.

NURSING CARE PLAN

Aaron was admitted to the psychiatric unit directly from the emergency department because he was involved in a fight with another man at a bar. He was under the influence of PCP, as well as alcohol, while at the bar. The emergency department staff assessed him as medically stable but suggested admission because of his potential for violence.

When Aaron arrived on the unit, he was angry, loudly stating that he had been treated unfairly in the emergency department and that he did not need to be admitted to the psychiatric unit "with all those nuts!" He demanded a TV in his room and a cigarette. When the staff denied his requests, he became louder and threatening. He told the charge nurse that he would get his way, that he had friends on the hospital board, and that there would be an investigation into the hospital treatment of his case if he was not allowed to smoke or to watch TV in private. He reminded the nurse that he was admitted for fighting in a bar, and stated, "I know how to get my way."

DSM-IV-TR DIAGNOSES

Axis I	Substance abuse: alcohol and PCP
Axis II	Antisocial personality disorder
Axis III	Medically stable, related to intoxication and withdrawal symptoms
Axis IV	Problems related to the social environment
Axis V	GAF = 40 (current); GAF = 60 (past year)

Nursing Diagnosis ***Risk for other-directed violence. Risk factors: a perception that others are denying him his rights and control over his environment; a history of violence against others; recent ingestion of PCP and alcohol; impulsivity; and an increase in verbal demands, a loud voice, and verbally threatening behavior***

NOC Aggression Self-Control, Abusive Behavior Self-Restraint, Impulse Self-Control, Stress Level, Risk Detection, Risk Control: Alcohol Use, Risk Control: Drug Use

NIC Anger Control Assistance, Environmental Management: Violence Prevention, Anxiety Reduction, Behavior Management, Surveillance: Safety, Security Enhancement, Medication Management

CLIENT OUTCOMES	NURSING INTERVENTIONS	EVALUATION
Aaron will be able to maintain control of his anger so that he will not threaten or harm others.	Monitor Aaron closely for escalation of the anger to rage or impulsive action. *Close monitoring will help predict any increase in impulsivity and prevent injury to self or others.* Contract with Aaron, if appropriate, that he will no longer threaten staff or client peers during the hospitalization. *Contracts used appropriately will assist Aaron with impulse control.*	Aaron was able to discuss his feelings about entering the hospital without exhibiting threatening or aggressive behavior.
Aaron will use the interactions with the nurse, members of the interdisciplinary team, and groups in the setting to discuss alternative options to deal with situations that provoke angry, potentially violent responses.	Teach Aaron other options to manage the angry feelings, such as leaving the area where the conflict is occurring or using a quiet area such as an unoccupied room until the impulse to do harm passes. *This will provide Aaron with other appropriate ways to handle angry feelings, rather than violence.* Discuss angry feelings in the group setting, how the anger escalates out of control, and what to do to control violent impulses. *Group input will provide alternative solutions to deal with angry feelings rather than resorting to violence.* (See Chapter 22.)	Aaron was able to control angry outbursts and ask for his needs in a calm manner during his hospital stay, and he shared his feelings with the group.
Aaron will comply with prescribed emergency medication as a last-resort therapeutic intervention if other interventions such as talking and stress-reducing strategies fail to contain aggressive behavior.	Administer medication as needed if all other therapeutic interventions fail to manage the client's anger and aggressive behavior. *Emergency medication is used only if the client's anger escalates out of control and presents an imminent danger to self or others in the psychiatric setting.* (See Chapters 8 and 24.)	Aaron was able to contain his aggressive behavior through a variety of interventions such as talking to the nursing staff individually and sharing feelings with others during group therapy. He adhered to the routine medication regimen but did not require the administration of emergency medication.

Continued

NURSING CARE PLAN—cont'd

Nursing Diagnosis *Ineffective coping related to intoxication and withdrawal from alcohol and PCP, as evidenced by the client's loud and threatening behavior, impulsivity and loss of control*

NOC Anxiety Self-Control, Aggression Self-Control, Impulse Self-Control, Coping, Social Support, Knowledge: Health Resources, Decision-Making

NIC Anxiety Reduction, Anger Control Assistance, Coping Enhancement, Substance Use Prevention, Teaching: Individual, Support System Enhancement, Decision-Making Support

CLIENT OUTCOMES	NURSING INTERVENTIONS	EVALUATION
Aaron will be able to determine his basic needs, make requests in a calm, thoughtful manner, and make some choices about his treatment and care.	The nurse will observe Aaron for symptoms of intoxication and withdrawal from alcohol and PCP, which require medication, and will administer medications as needed. *Symptoms of intoxication and withdrawal of both substances include irritability and loss of impulse control.*	Aaron was able to decrease his loud and threatening behavior after receiving medication to decrease withdrawal symptoms, and he was able to make some decisions regarding his care.
Aaron will become better adjusted to the psychiatric setting and more in control of his internal and external environment.	The nurse will assist Aaron in becoming adjusted to the unit by providing a tour, giving statements of support, telling Aaron how the hospitalization will help him, and providing Aaron with choices regarding his care when appropriate. *Aaron will feel more in control with a greater understanding of the environment and expectations, and he will be able to make some decisions about his care.*	Aaron is adjusting well to the therapeutic environment and continues to make decisions about his care. He states, "I feel that following the program in order to get well is my own choice" and "I realize it is my decision to quit alcohol and drugs."

Nursing Diagnosis *Chronic low self-esteem related to long-term negative feedback and the client's belief that he is unable to deal with problems, as evidenced by self-destructive behavior (drinking and physical fighting in the bar), inability to accept constructive limit setting from the nursing staff, and the tendency to demean others to increase his own feelings of self-worth*

NOC Self-Esteem, Motivation, Role Performance, Social Interaction Skills, Hope, Quality of Life

NIC Self-Esteem Enhancement, Support System Enhancement, Socialization Enhancement, Emotional Support, Counseling

CLIENT OUTCOMES	NURSING INTERVENTIONS	EVALUATION
Aaron will be able to discuss, during a one-to-one session with his primary nurse or in a problem-solving group, that his threatening behavior and demeaning behaviors toward others reveal his own feelings of low self-esteem.	Activate Aaron to attend all verbal groups for problem solving, particularly those that discuss behavior and feelings. *Aaron will obtain feedback from other group members about his threatening and demeaning behavior toward others, allowing him to hear the same feedback from several sources.*	Aaron identified a need during a process group without threatening anyone in the group. He verbalized other options to meet his identified need if the others chose not to assist him or were unable to help meet his need.
Aaron will be able to verbalize that his threatening and demeaning behaviors cause other people to distance themselves from him and will state how these negative responses from others reinforce his bad feelings about himself.	Discuss with Aaron how his threatening behavior and negative remarks toward others distance people. *This discussion will help Aaron become more aware of how his behavior contributes to others' unwillingness to attend to his needs, which reinforces his low self-esteem.*	Aaron is striving to cease his negative and demeaning behaviors toward others and states that he wants and needs approval from them to a certain degree so he will feel more worthwhile and accepted.
Aaron will be able to identify at least one positive attribute of his personality.	Assist Aaron in listing his strengths and areas that need adjustment as he views himself. *Aaron only identifies negative parts of himself. Listing both strengths and weaknesses helps Aaron have a more balanced view of himself.*	Aaron was able to identify two strengths in his character that he values and agreed to recognize these strengths in the future.
Aaron will be able to accept positive feedback about himself and demonstrate his positive self-regard by behaving in a more functional way.	Provide Aaron with positive feedback when he accomplishes something within the unit setting or in discussion with others. *Positive feedback reinforces functional behavior.*	Aaron demonstrates functional behavior in the psychiatric setting and has stated on several occasions that he feels good about himself and his accomplishments.

NURSING CARE PLAN

Kim is a 29-year-old single woman who became suicidal after her boyfriend, Greg, told her their relationship was over. She started to drink and use diazepam (Valium) to calm down after Greg left her. The relationship had become stormy, with frequent threats from Greg that he would stop seeing her. Kim became vengeful, went to Greg's parents' house where he was staying, and threw a rock into their living room window, shouting that she loved Greg and could not live without him. She shouted, "I don't want to hurt anyone. I just want to die!" and ran into the street in front of an oncoming car. The driver slammed on the brakes and hit Kim hard enough to knock her down and cause a pelvic fracture. She was admitted to the local hospital, still vowing to harm herself if Greg did not return to her.

DSM-IV-TR DIAGNOSES

Axis I	Substance abuse: alcohol and diazepam (Valium)
Axis II	Borderline personality disorder
Axis III	Pelvic fracture
Axis IV	Problems with primary support groups (except breakup with boyfriend)
Axis V	GAF = 30 (current); GAF = 60 (past year)

Nursing Diagnosis *Risk for suicide. Risk factors: Intense feelings of abandonment, increased anxiety level, impulsivity, and a history of suicidal attempts*

NOC Suicide Self-Restraint, Depression Level, Impulse Self-Control, Risk Control, Personal Well-Being, Social Support

NIC Suicide Prevention, Mood Management, Surveillance: Safety, Impulse Control Training, Patient Contracting, Support Group

CLIENT OUTCOMES	NURSING INTERVENTIONS	EVALUATION
Kim will not act on her suicidal thoughts.	Place Kim on suicide observations and assess her level of depressed thoughts. *Suicide observations will help prevent any further suicide attempts through early intervention.*	Kim decreased her suicidal ideation within 2 days of hospitalization.
Kim will honor the terms of her contract for safety.*	Help Kim to write a contract for safety that states she will inform the staff if her suicidal ideation increases. *Contracts sometimes result in early preventive measures to prevent a suicidal gesture.*	Kim was able to use the contract for safety to assist her with impulse control.
Kim will seek out the staff whenever she experiences suicidal thoughts.	Teach Kim to inform the staff if there is an increase in her suicidal ideation. *This will enable Kim to become an active participant in her suicide prevention and be more aware of how her thoughts and feelings influence her behavior.*	Kim contacted staff when she had suicidal thoughts, feelings of abandonment, impulsive urges, and other troubling feelings.

Nursing Diagnosis *Ineffective coping related to boyfriend ending a significant relationship, as evidenced by the client's vengeful behavior toward boyfriend, her impulsive behavior to do self-harm, and her use of drugs and alcohol*

NOC Suicide Self-Restraint, Impulse Self-Control, Coping, Information Processing, Social Support, Psychosocial Adjustment: Life Change, Personal Well-Being

NIC Coping Enhancement, Impulse Control Training, Teaching: Individual, Support System Enhancement, Decision-Making Support, Therapy Group

CLIENT OUTCOMES	NURSING INTERVENTIONS	EVALUATION
Kim will identify her impulsive behavior patterns that occur during times of stress, record these feelings in a journal, and share them in appropriate groups.	Teach Kim to link her feelings and behavior to how she responds to the events in her relationship by writing her thoughts and feelings in a journal, having one-to-one discussions with her assigned nurse, and listening to the input of the groups in the inpatient setting. *A journal will help Kim acknowledge her feelings and thoughts, determine her impulsive behavioral patterns, and decrease her reaction to those thoughts and feelings.*	Kim was able to talk with her assigned nurse and in the unit process groups about her intense feelings of loss and emptiness. She was able to use her journal as a coping mechanism when her emotions became overwhelming.
Kim will be able to identify at least one new method of problem solving to manage negative thoughts and impulses.	Teach Kim healthy ways to manage intense feelings of anger and sadness, such as expressing her feelings to supportive friends and family members. Teach her to use a coping behavior to help calm her intense emotions, such as listening to music, taking a hot bath, going to an exercise class, buying flowers, or writing in the journal. *These activities will help Kim to learn new coping patterns to deal with intense, painful emotions.*	Kim was able to use her journal by writing poetry to problem solve and calm herself when feelings became intense during the hospitalization.

*Use of contracts for client safety depends on nursing and physician assessment and does not replace vigilant observation by staff (Clinical Practice Guidelines, APA, 2004).

Continued

NURSING CARE PLAN—cont'd

Nursing Diagnosis *Complicated grieving related to boyfriend ending a significant relationship, as evidenced by the client's use of drugs and alcohol, vengeful behavior, suicidal ideation, and impulsive behavior to do self-harm*

NOC Grief Resolution, Coping, Communication, Depression Self-Control, Self-Esteem, Psychosocial Adjustment: Life Change

NIC Suicide Prevention, Grief Work Facilitation, Hope Instillation, Coping Enhancement, Support Group, Support System Enhancement

CLIENT OUTCOMES	NURSING INTERVENTIONS	EVALUATION
Kim will identify feelings generated by the ending of her relationship with Greg, such as anger, fear of being alone, and sadness.	Discuss with Kim in an open manner her feelings about the end of her relationship with Greg. *An open discussion with a trusted nurse will encourage Kim to share her hurt feelings, fear of loneliness, and abandonment issues, which will facilitate healthy mourning of the loss of the relationship.*	*At the end of the hospitalization, Kim was able to talk about the end of her relationship with Greg without suicidal thoughts or cravings for alcohol or diazepam (Valium).*
Kim will share her loss with group members who also experienced losses.	Encourage Kim to attend group problem-solving sessions on the unit to discuss her loss with other peers. *Sharing feelings in a safe setting will give Kim a better perspective on how others have dealt with losses.*	Kim shared her loss with appropriate group members.
Kim will use healthy methods to deal with her loss and not use alcohol or diazepam to mask her feelings.	Encourage Kim to write her thoughts and feelings about the end of the relationship in her journal. *Writing will help Kim to recognize her thoughts and feelings about the loss of the relationship, which will help her come to terms with the unresolved issues associated with the loss.*	Kim developed journal writing as a healthy method of dealing with her loss and working through painful issues.

EVALUATION

The evaluation stage of the nursing process is ongoing and takes place to ensure accountable, respectful, nonjudgmental nursing practice. There are two steps to the evaluation stage:

1. The nurse compares the client's current functioning with the identified outcome criteria.
2. The nurse asks questions to determine possible reasons if the outcome criteria were not met (Fortinash and Holoday Worret, 2007).

CHAPTER SUMMARY

- A personality disorder is a long-standing, pervasive, maladaptive pattern of behavior and relating to others that is not caused by an Axis I disorder.
- In psychodynamic theory there is a belief that an individual who develops a personality disorder has deficits in his or her psychosexual development or a failure to achieve object constancy.
- Research has hypothesized biologic considerations as possible causal factors for individuals developing personality disorders.
- The DSM-IV-TR Axis II is set up in a three-cluster format.
- Clients with personality disorders have difficulty relating to others at home, at work, and in the community.
- When working with individuals with personality disorders, it is most important to assess each client for the risk of violence toward self or others.
- Clients with personality disorders often exhibit self-destructive behaviors such as self-mutilation, eating disorders, alcohol or substance abuse, and shoplifting.
- Realistic expectations for improvement include a commitment by the client to explore and evaluate his or her thoughts, relationships, and behaviors, especially when under stress.

REVIEW QUESTIONS

1 The nurse explains to a client with a borderline personality disorder that the clinic's former psychiatrist resigned and a new psychiatrist has been hired. Which reaction is most likely?

1. Silence
2. Withdrawal
3. Rage
4. Anxiety

2 A nurse manages care for an individual with a personality disorder. Select the most attainable outcome for this client. The client:

1. Within 2 weeks, establish a satisfying intimate relationship with another adult.
2. Within 5 days, identify factors that led to development of the personality disorder.
3. Within 1 week, make a permanent commitment never to self mutilate.
4. Within 4 weeks, describe personal characteristics of reactions to stress.

3 An individual with an obsessive-compulsive personality disorder is consistently late for outpatient appointments as a result of repetitively checking whether appliances are unplugged before leaving home. Which nursing diagnosis applies?
1. Anxiety
2. Social isolation
3. Disturbed personality identity
4. Situational low self-esteem

4 An adult client with a borderline personality disorder vomits immediately after drinking 1 ounce of dishwashing soap in a suicide gesture. What should the nurse do first?
1. Assess and record the client's vital signs.
2. Promptly place the client on suicide precautions.
3. Immediately notify the attending psychiatrist.
4. Sit quietly with the client until the vomiting subsides.

5 A nurse assesses an individual with schizotypal personality disorder. Which characteristics are most likely? You may select more than one answer.
1. Male gender
2. Complaints of depression
3. Charges pending for assault
4. Chronic physical illness
5. Sibling diagnosed with schizophrenia

Additional self-study exercises and learning resources are available to you on the ***Companion CD*** *at the back of the book and on the* ***Evolve website*** *at* ***http://evolve.elsevier.com/Fortinash/.***

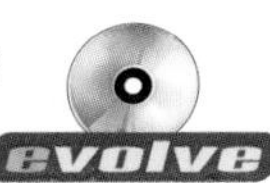

ONLINE RESOURCES

Borderline Personality Disorder Research Foundation: **www.borderlineresearch.org**

International Society for the Study of Personality Disorders: **www.isspd.com**

National Alliance on Mental Illness: **www.nami.org**

National Institute of Mental Health: **www.nimh.nih.gov**

Mental Health America: **www.nmha.org**

REFERENCES

American Psychiatric Association (APA): *Diagnostic and statistical manual of mental disorders*, ed 4, text revision, Washington, DC, 2000, American Psychiatric Association.

American Psychiatric Association (APA): Practice guideline for the treatment of patients with borderline personality disorder, www.psych.org/psych_pract/treatg/pg/borderline_revisebo, retrieved Mar 15, 2004.

Becker DF et al: Comorbidity of borderline personality disorder with other personality disorders in hospitalized adolescents and adults, *Am J Psychiatry* 157:2011-2018, 2000.

Brown GL et al: Aggression, suicide and serotonin relationships to CSF amine metabolites, *Am J Psychiatry* 139:741, 1982.

Brown GL, Linnoila MI: CSF serotonin metabolite (5-HIAA) studies in depression, impulsivity, and violence, *J Clin Psychiatry* 51(suppl):31, 1990.

Coryell WH, Zimmerman MBA: Personality disorder in the families of depressed, schizophrenia, and never-ill probands, *Am J Psychiatry* 146:496, 1989.

Dresser J: Wrapping: a technique for interrupting self-mutilation, *J Am Psychiatr Nurses Assoc* 1999 (April):67-70, 1999.

Fortinash KM, Holoday Worret PA: *Psychiatric nursing care plans*, ed 4, St Louis, 2007, Mosby.

Freud S: Three essays on the theory of sexuality, *Standard Edition* 7:125, 1905.

Kavoussi RJ, Siever LJ: Biologic validators of personality disorders. In Oldham JM, editor: *Personality disorders: new perspectives on diagnostic validity*, Washington, DC, 1991, American Psychiatric Press.

Keltner NL, Folks DG: *Psychotropic drugs*, St Louis, 2005, Mosby.

Kernberg OF: *Severe personality disorders: psychotherapeutic strategies*, New Haven, Conn, 1984, Yale University Press.

Kreisman JJ, Straus H: *I hate you—don't leave me: understanding the borderline personality*, Los Angeles, 1989, Body Press.

Leyton M et al: Brain regional alpha-{11C} methyl-L-tryptophan trapping in impulsive subjects with borderline personality disorder, *Am J Psych* 158:775-782, 2001.

Linehan MM: *Cognitive-behavioral treatment of borderline personality disorder*, New York, 1993, Guilford Press.

Mahler MS: Thoughts about development and individuation, *Psychoanal Study Child* 18:307, 1963.

Mahler MS: On the first three subphases of the separation-individuation process, *Int J Psychoanal* 53:333, 1972.

Manfield P: *Split self split object: understanding and treating borderline, narcissistic, and schizoid disorders*, Northvale, NJ, 1992, Jason Aronson.

Mann JJ et al: Increased serotonin-2 and beta-adrenergic receptor binding in the frontal cortices of suicide victims, *Arch Gen Psychiatry* 43:954, 1986.

Marin D et al: Biological models and treatments for personality disorders, *Psychiatr Ann* 19:143, 1989.

Masterson JF: *Psychotherapy of the borderline adult: a developmental approach*, New York, 1976, Brunner/Mazel.

Myers MG et al: Progression from conduct disorder to antisocial personality disorder following treatment for adolescent substance abuse, *Am J Psychiatry* 155:479, 1998.

NANDA International: *NANDA nursing diagnoses: definitions and classification*, 2007-2008. Philadelphia, 2007, NANDA-I.

Oldham JM, Skodol AE: Personality disorders and mood disorders. In Tasman A, Riba MB, editors: *American Psychiatric Press review of psychiatry*, vol 11, Washington, DC, 1992, American Psychiatric Press.

Osborne LL, McCornish, JF: Working with borderline personality disorder: nursing interventions using dialectical behavioral therapy, *J Psychosoc Nurs Ment Health Serv* 44:40-48, 2006.

Pajer KA: What happens to "bad" girls? A review of the adult outcomes of antisocial adolescent girls, *Am J Psychiatry* 155:862, 1998.

Roitman SE et al: Attentional functioning in schizotypal personality disorder, *Am J Psychiatry* 154:655, 1997.

Siever LJ: Biologic markers in schizotypal personality disorder, *Schizophr Bull* 11:564, 1985.

Siever LJ: Schizophrenia spectrum personality disorders. In Tasman A, Riba MB, editors: *American Psychiatric Press review of psychiatry*, vol 11, Washington, DC, 1992, American Psychiatric Press.

Siever LJ, Davis KL: A psychobiological perspective on the personality disorders, *Am J Psychiatry* 148:1647, 1991.

Skodol A et al: Functional impairment in patients with schizotypal, borderline, avoidant, and obsessive-compulsive personality disorder, *Am J Psychiatry* 159:276-283, 2000.

Smith LL et al: Nurse-patient boundaries crossing the line: how to recognize signs of professional sexual misconduct and intervene effectively, *Am J Nurs* 97:26, 1997.

Stanley M, Stanley B: Postmortem evidence for serotonin's role in suicide, *J Clin Psychiatry* 51(suppl):22, 1990.

Swarles M et al: Linehan's dialectical behavior therapy (DBT) for borderline personality disorder: overview and adaptation, *J Ment Health* 9:7-23, 2000.

Tyson P, Tyson R: *Psychoanalytic theories of development and integration*, New Haven, Conn, 1990, Yale University Press.

Widiger TA, Rogers JH: Prevalence and comorbidity of personality disorders, *Psychiatr Ann* 19:132, 1989.

Chapter 14

Substance-Related Disorders

MERRY A. ARMSTRONG

Evidence for addiction may be perfectly obvious to other people, but it is as if the addicted person is either completely blind or always looking in the other direction.

GERALD MAY

OBJECTIVES

1. Identify major theories related to substance use disorders and impulse control disorders.
2. Identify a multisystems approach to the etiology of addiction.
3. Describe the neurobiology of chemical addiction.
4. Define levels of substance use and abuse.
5. Apply the nursing process for clients with chemical use disorders.
6. Describe treatment options for clients with substance-related disorders.

KEY TERMS

addiction, p. 305
alcoholic blackouts, p. 317
alcoholism, p. 305
comorbid, p. 308
craving, p. 306
cross-tolerance, p. 328
detoxification, p. 328
dual diagnosis, p. 315
eating disorders, p. 305
fetal alcohol syndrome, p. 312
gateway drugs, p. 314
harm reduction, p. 333
misuse, p. 305
pathologic gambling, p. 305
prevention, p. 308
pseudoaddiction, p. 323
relapse prevention, p. 333
screening, p. 325
sexual addiction, p. 305
substance abuse, p. 316
substance dependence, p. 317
substance use disorder, p. 305
tolerance, p. 317
withdrawal, p. 317

The recognition of addiction as a process opened new doors to the identification of and treatment for the individual experiencing difficulties related to addiction. *Addiction* is a vague term often applied to chemical or substance use disorders, eating disorders, or impulse control disorders, like gambling. These disorders are in the *Diagnostic and Statistical Manual of Mental Disorders* (DSM-IV-TR) (American Psychiatric Association [APA], 2000) and are therefore within the domain of psychiatric mental health practice. Nurses need to be aware of the prevalence and stigma of these disorders in order to assess and intervene appropriately with many clients. For a variety of reasons, substance use is a significant contributor to health status and life satisfaction for all clients, from tiny neonates to the elderly. Substance use is a significant factor in dollars spent for illness care, loss of productivity, and disruption in family systems. According to the Robert Wood Johnson Foundation, addiction is the largest health care problem in the United States. Patients use or abuse of substances is a primary topic of concern. Addictions cross all specialties, age spans, and groups.

Health care professionals, including nurses, are instrumental in providing hope, encouragement, and effective treatment to patients. The goal for clients with substance use disorders is treatment, remission, and healing (Withers, 2001). The nurse's role is to be actively involved in the assessment, treatment, and prevention aspects of substance abuse. The nurse is often the first health care professional to become aware of a patient's problematic substance use, share this information with other members of the health care team, and coordinate subsequent nursing care or integrated care. The nurse is instrumental in making referrals to or working in intense rehabilitation and recovery programs and in assessing and treating symptoms of physical illness or addiction.

In 2004, the American Nurses Association (ANA), in conjunction with the International Nurses Society on Addictions (IntNSA), published the *Scope and Standards of Addictions Nursing Practice* (ANA, 2004). These standards set competencies for basic and advanced-level practitioners. Through research and scholarship, the International Nurses Society on Addictions advances the practice and the care of persons with addictive disorders. Nurses from all specialties become members of this organization, attend annual conventions, and read the organization's publication *The Journal of Addictions Nursing.* The organization has several publications, including a *Core Curriculum for Addictions Nursing* (Freeman, 2005b), and information regarding publications and organization activities are on the organization's website (www.intnsa.org). In addition, the organization offers certification to basic and advanced nurses in the area of addictions. Nursing roles and responsibilities in addictions are discussed more fully later in the chapter.

Debate still exists whether to refer to substance dependence (addiction) as a disease or a disorder, and the terms *addictive disorder* and *addictive disease* are often used interchangeably. Substance dependence, like alcoholism, cannot be transmitted from one person to another as in the classic transmission of disease, and some argue the term *disorder* is more accurate and common. However, disease sometimes occurs as the result of addiction, as cirrhosis of the liver for example. The core problem—addiction—is not exclusively a physical process. Addiction is, according to the National Institute of Drug Abuse (NIDA), a "complex, neurobehavioral disorder characterized by impaired control, compulsive use, dependency, and craving for the activity, substance, or food" (NIDA, 2002a). Further, "addiction is often (but not always) accompanied by physiological dependence, consisting of a withdrawal syndrome, and/or tolerance" (NIDA, 2002b). The spectrum of addictions covers substance use disorders, impulse control disorders such as **pathologic gambling** and **sexual addiction**, and **eating disorders** such as bulimia and anorexia. The purpose of this chapter is to discuss chemical or substance use disorders. Chapter 17 addresses eating disorders.

Addictions fall in the psychiatric domain instead of general medicine for the reasons outlined in the preceding paragraph. Within the spectrum, addictive disorders have physical consequences, but they are primarily psychologic occurrences. It is useful to remember, however, that schizophrenia and bipolar disorders were also once considered to be purely psychologic. Current knowledge about neurochemistry and genetics has placed addictive disorders at least partially in the neurobiologic or genetic category of disorders. One of the founders of Alcoholics Anonymous, Dr. Silkworth, thought that, because of the unique effect that alcohol had on some individuals, **alcoholism** was an allergy to alcohol. In 1939, Dr. Silkworth was correct in suspecting a physical cause for alcoholism and addiction. Although alcoholism is not an allergy, many now recognize it as a partially brain-based disorder and that some brains are more susceptible than others.

For the purposes of this chapter, the terms **addiction** and **substance use disorder** (SUD) or other dependency are interchangeable. **Misuse** is use of any illegal drug or legal drug for purposes other than which it was intended, or in excess such as using alcohol beyond the legal limit.

Addiction is a complex condition and situation. Individuals become addicted in various ways and over various periods of time. Therefore, recent thinking related to addiction does not place responsibility solely with the individual. Although all people share certain life experiences such as developmental milestones, physical health or illness, psychologic health or illness, the variations of individual responses are endless. Researchers believe that those with predisposition to SUDs have brains that are different before, during, and after exposure. Saying that, however, does not account for responses to those differences or to variations in coping abilities. Human brain chemistry is unique to each person as is life experience. It is not correct to say that because a person has alcoholic parents that he or she will or will not develop alcoholism later in life, because life is too complex for such broad statements. Scientists and researchers assess probability, which is different from certainty.

The statistical manipulation of data provides information that forecasts trends or probabilities relative to groups of individuals, but group probability does not apply to each person in the group. Scientists do not have adequate longitudinal data to predict with any confidence which individual person will develop an SUD. Many studies that describe characteristics of persons with SUDs are done after the person has exhibited symptoms of SUD, so their functioning and characteristics before the problem existed are unknown. Were the measured characteristics a product of addiction, or did they exist before addiction? To date, we have little longitudinal data (collected over many years of a person's life) to contribute to the identification of individual risk factors. We do, however, have grouped data that sorts out some of the factors that put people at risk for SUDs. These risk factors are addressed in a later section.

Adding to the complicated nature of the topic of addiction, some substances that are very addicting are legal, such as nicotine and alcohol. Using substances is not illegal, but possessing or selling illicit substances is illegal. Of course a person must possess a drug, if even briefly, before using it, so many gray legal areas exist in the interpretation of possession. State laws vary widely regarding drug possession and whether possession is a misdemeanor or a felony. State laws differ for different drugs, though federal standards apply everywhere. Mexico and Canada, which border the United States, also have different regulatory restrictions on the sale and distribution of substances.

HISTORIC PERSPECTIVES

Historically, worldwide substance use is well documented. People in most cultures either discovered or created intoxicating substances and used them for various reasons including ritual, ceremony, or for their healing properties. Some theorists believe that intoxication is a basic human need, required to relieve the suffering that is a part of all human existence. In the 1700s and 1800s, armies and groups who conducted other paramilitary efforts such as the Lewis and Clark expedition had to guarantee their recruits a specific amount of alcohol each day and a great deal of effort went into ensuring its availability under difficult circumstances.

The fly glyagaric mushroom *(Aminita muscaria)*, one of the earliest plants used for intoxication, was thought to have been documented, as *soma*, in a 3500-year-old Sanskrit text (Sadock and Sadock, 2000). In early Greek and Roman societies, as in many countries today, alcohol was routinely an important element of meals, celebrations, and other ceremonies. Before 1800 in the United States, alcohol and opium were readily available and used in combination for calming and sedating effects. In the 1800s and early 1900s, patent medicines contained cocaine, opium, morphine, or (after 1898) heroin, which led to addictions, accidental deaths, or poisonings of both adults and children. Hemp was grown in the American colonies, and smoking hemp became popular in the early 1900s. It is interesting to note that smoking a substance is the fastest way for the drug to enter the circulatory system.

The synthesis of drugs in the nineteenth century resulted in plentiful supplies of powerful habit-forming substances. Like many developments in health care, the need for such substances during war stimulated the development of these medications. In 1887, German scientists synthesized amphetamines, but there was not any research for practical use until the 1920s. Use of amphetamines was common during World War II by the military of various countries for increased vigilance and decreased need for sleep. The military still dispenses amphetamines for these purposes.

The hypodermic needle permitted direct injection into the body of powerful, purified substances such as heroin and later morphine. By 1900, the United States developed a substantial addicted population, with all the attendant social problems. This situation led to state and federal antinarcotics laws to regulate the sale and prescription use of narcotics, the most important of which was the Harrison Narcotic Act of 1914 (Sadock and Sadock, 2000). The Harrison Narcotic Act removed individual physician choice for treatment of patients and essentially put the federal government in control of one aspect of medical practice. Over the years, many thought prescribed substances (amphetamines, talwin, heroin, and others) were nonaddictive, but as more people used them, the data indicated otherwise.

To date, regulations, law enforcement, and many other efforts have not eliminated the use of illegal substances. People interested in using/abusing substances continue to actively search for new substances or new uses for known substances. As the use of a substance gains popularity and momentum, law enforcement initiates efforts to address that problem. Then users find a new substance, and the cycle continues, resulting in social dysfunction, addiction, and significant physical impairment. Many make money selling these compounds to a large marketplace, making it difficult to control use and abuse of substances.

Advertising reaches most of the U.S. population. Cigarettes and brands of distilled alcohol are widely advertised. Cigarette companies target adolescent and preteen populations, whereas marketing research heavily targets women (Carpenter et al., 2005). A quick review of a teen magazine and inspection of the ads demonstrates this effort in many subtle and some obvious ways, as the ads portray smoking and drinking alcohol as desirable behaviors.

The Drug Enforcement Administration (DEA) Schedule of Controlled Substances lists restricted substances. The entire schedule is presented on the DEA website at www.dea.gov, and a summary of the schedules appears in Box 14-1. Debate continues about placing various compounds on this list, because listing every substance or combination of chemicals that has addictive properties is not practically possible. Some drugs have no medical use and are therefore in an absolutely restricted category, meaning there is no legal access to that substance in the United States.

Neurobiologic Basis of Addiction

Addictive drugs (drugs of dependence) are categorized as depressants, stimulants, opiates, hallucinogens, inhalants, and nicotine. Nicotine and alcohol, though extremely high in addictive potential, are legal and therefore researchers have extensively studied them. They are not on the DEA list of controlled substances. Virtually all drugs of abuse evoke a rapid release of neurochemicals, followed by a reduced-from-baseline level of neurotransmitter when the effect of the drug wears off, creating a biologic need or **craving** for more of the drug. The drug serves as a reinforcer, increasing the probability of a repeat behavior and the use of that substance (Volkow et al., 2003).

Advances in knowledge of the effects of substances are a result of research technology such as positron emission tomography (PET), single photon emission tomography (SPEC), and functional magnetic imaging resonance (FMRI) scans, which allows researchers to actually visualize the neurobiologic effects of drugs. Other researchers developed "knockout mice" in which they remove a particular genetic component. These genetically altered mice, without particular glutamate (implicated in spatial learning and memory) receptors, do not become addicted to cocaine (Gatley and Volkow, 1998). These kinds of studies support acceptance of genetic influence on addic-

BOX 14-1

United States Drug Enforcement Administration Schedule of Controlled Substances

SCHEDULE I

Drug/substance has a high potential for abuse and has no currently accepted medical use in treatment in the United States.

Examples: Heroin, ibogaine, mescaline, marijuana

SCHEDULE II

Drug/substance has high potential for abuse but has currently accepted medical use with severe restrictions; abuse of the drug may lead to psychologic or physical dependence.

Examples: Cocaine, codeine, hydrocodone, methadone, morphine, meperidine

SCHEDULE III

Drug/substance potential for abuse less than for schedules I and; II and is currently accepted in medical practice, abuse of drug/substance leads to moderate or low physical dependence or high psychologic dependence.

Examples: Anabolic steroids, ketamine, thiopental

SCHEDULE IV

Drug/substance has low potential for abuse, is in current medical use, and abuse may lead to limited physical dependence or psychologic dependence, less than schedule III.

Examples: Benzodiazepines, stadol, darvon, ambien, sonata, meridia, chloral hydrate

SCHEDULE V

Only contains cough preparation with codeine up to 200 mg/100 ml, or 100 g.

From U.S. Drug Enforcement Administration; www.dea.gov.

tion. An individual with greater neuroplastic potential for glutamate and dopamine production and activation, for example, is more prone to addiction.

Dopamine is the primary neurotransmitter associated with reward. Dopamine levels normally increase during pleasurable sensory activities such as eating and sex. Drugs stimulate this same response, independent from the physical experience or cue. Glutamate, another important neurotransmitter, is important in memory formation, and is also associated with addiction. Over millennia, our brains have served to keep us alive and efficiently evolved to specifically "remember" what is pleasurable. Events that evoke dopamine release become powerful memories.

The creation of memory is largely unconscious, and we do not experience any physical sensation to tell us that our brains have created a memory. When a person learns a new behavior, like using a computer, and repeats the process a few times, the ability to do the same behavior is effortless. The memory pathway has been established, outside of conscious awareness. One cannot choose to not remember an event; the brain has created a memory, even if the individual cannot retrieve the memory. The same occurrence happens with using drugs: the brain remembers, and the behavior returns. The behavior is not completely outside of control, but the longer one uses a drug or repeats a behavior, the more strongly entrenched the behavior/memory becomes and the less volition the individual has with regard to that behavior. Some hypothesize that the same neural pathways are involved for impulse control disorders like gambling, sex addiction, and eating disorders that become habitual.

The process of memory formation involves sensation plus thought. The limbic system, which is the part of the brain containing a great deal of dopamine, is associated with emotion and memory. Dopamine and other neurotransmitter-releasing activities activate this part of the brain. Part of the limbic system dopamine pathway extends into the frontal region of the brain, the region responsible for prioritization, organization, and decision making. Because this portion of the brain is activated during addictive behavior, this greatly affects reasoning ability and the act of making responsible choices. The drug "hijacks" the brain. People who have been addicted over a long period of time have particular difficulty making decisions about their health or seeking treatment. Situational, individual, and environmental factors interact to sustain or restrain behavior. Researchers are still seeking a universal theory of addictions, and although key elements of the brain are involved, there will always be variances in individual neurologic functioning.

Advancements in knowledge of neurophysiology led to the development of the possibility of immunization for nicotine and amphetamines, although these are highly controversial measures. Issues of consent, effectiveness of immunization techniques, and many other topics are still unknown. Questions of informed consent and decisions about who would administer these inoculations are debated. Many arguments exist on all sides of these issues, including reimbursement for these vaccines (Harwood and Meyers, 2004). This type of immunization involves administration of a substance to which the molecules of a drug, such as nicotine, for example, would adhere. This molecular attraction renders the substance unavailable to brain receptors. It is possible, however, that an individual could override this effect by using great quantities of the substance. Current animal studies show promise for human application, and researchers have conducted some human trials of portions of the process. So far, immunization is promising for cocaine, nicotine, and other stimulants.

THEORETIC PERSPECTIVES

Early theorists focused on the individual who developed addictions. In the 1930s (long before the DSM criteria were developed), Jellinek was the premier researcher in the field of alcoholism and was a strong believer of alcoholism as a disease. He proposed that addictive processes have a biochemical basis and noted that people with alcoholism progress through four stages, with the two more severe stages resulting in dependence. The stages were the *prealcoholic symptomatic phase*, the *prodromal phase*, the *crucial phase*, and the *chronic phase*. His research led to the acceptance of Alcoholics Anonymous (AA) as a respected treatment modality. Almost every AA-based recovery center teaches the *Jellinek curve*, which describes the progression of alcoholism. Although this model is used less frequently as theory evolves, it is useful to understand that alcohol dependence is a complex process and not an isolated event.

At the turn of the century, many viewed alcoholism as a moral problem. However, considering alcoholism or drug addiction as a sign of moral corruption is not useful. Many prominent and respected people, including musicians, politicians, clergy, military, celebrities, students, professionals, and next-door neighbors, developed drug problems. Another view that is not useful is that drug addiction is due to a lack of intelligence. Historically, some very bright people have been dependent on drugs. Some of the problem stems from a belief by a person that they are too smart to get hooked. It's not so simple. Several individual factors contribute to addiction and are identified in this chapter.

Importantly, no single theory adequately explains substance abuse or addiction. Though scientists are unable to predict which person will develop alcoholism, genes and social and cultural factors interact in ways that place a person at high risk of developing the disease. As the relationship between these factors is further defined, researchers hope to take action to prevent the development of this disease (Sadock and Sadock, 2000).

ETIOLOGY

For years, researchers investigated the multiple and intersecting causes of SUDs and other addictions. Data yielded from research contributes to understanding vulnerability factors that predispose groups of persons to developing an SUD. **Prevention** efforts focus on factors known to have an impact on vulnerability. These efforts focus on one of three domains. *Individual*, *situational*, and *environmental* factors influence the development of addiction. No one factor is generally adequate to explain addiction phenomena, and overlapping areas exist between factors and categories.

Individual Factors

Demographic descriptors such as age, gender, and ethnicity are in this category. The individual's history of drug use, qualities of decision making, positive beliefs about the effects of drugs, availability of drugs and the money to purchase them, and an individual's physiologic response are all factors that contribute to the development of a substance use disorder. In addition, the person's appraisal and belief systems are considered, as is perceived risk of use and availability of friends who purchase drugs.

Research supports genetic predisposition for alcoholism. A threefold to fourfold risk exists for severe alcoholism in primary family members of a person who is alcohol dependent; it is 50% for men whose fathers were alcoholic. Twin studies done with women indicate 50% to 60% concordance (one twin being alcoholic predicts the other) (Kendler et al., 1992), indicating a significant genetic contribution to the susceptibility to alcoholism. The rate of problems with alcohol increases with the number of relatives with alcoholism, the severity of the disease, and the closeness of the genetic relationship to the person at risk. Genetic theories continue to evolve, and researchers are testing them primarily in animal models. Alleles (genes) ALDH2 and ALDH3 influence the predisposition to alcoholism (National Institute on Alcohol Abuse and Alcoholism, 2000). Dopamine and glutamate are neurotransmitters in various concentrations in different parts of the brain. Genetics influence the production and regulation of these and other neurotransmitters and plays an important role in addiction.

Studies of children of parents with alcoholism have led to predictions about who will develop alcoholism based on a lower level of response to alcohol. The lower level of response refers to tests that indicate that some individuals are more sensitive to the effects of alcohol than others (Schuckit, 2000). A reduced subjective response to alcohol is a risk factor for developing alcoholism. The person with a reduced subjective response has to drink more alcohol than others to feel the same effect. Researchers have reported the results of the first "genome scan" for drug abuse. The study provided evidence that specific regions of the human genome differ between abusers of illegal drugs and nonabusers. This study was an important step in identifying individuals who are at high risk for addiction. This knowledge makes it possible to direct appropriate preventive efforts and treatments to those individuals (NIDA, *NewsScan*, 2002).

Comorbid (co-occurring) mental illness is associated with greater rates of addiction and abuse. Posttraumatic stress disorder (PTSD) creates a risk for substance use or relapse. Some individuals begin to abuse substances after exposure to trauma. A total of 30% to 60% of persons with substance use disorders meet the criteria for comorbid PTSD. Persons with bipolar disorder also have increased risk for SUDs, as do patients with anxiety, depression, or schizophrenia disorders.

Along with the predisposition to addiction, researchers have also demonstrated a strong neurobiologic correlation between stress and drug use, especially in relation to relapse. Smokers experiencing stress, for example, sometimes relapse even after long periods of abstinence. Prolonged or chronic stress also fosters the continuation of addiction behaviors. Stress increases the hormone production of corticotropin-releasing factor (CRF), which in turn initiates the body's biologic response to stressors. After exposure to stress, CRF is in areas of the brain in increased amounts. Almost all drugs of abuse also increase CRF levels, which possibly indicate a neurobiologic connection between stress and substance abuse (NIDA, "Club Drugs," *Community Drug Alert Bulletin*, 2002).

Various psychologic theories explain substance use disorders. Some theories identify alcohol or other drugs as helping to decrease tension or feelings of psychologic pain. This hypothesis does not have data collected during real-life situations when heavy drinking or falling blood levels resulted in increased feelings of nervousness and tension to support it. Although researchers have studied addictive personality attributes carefully, no one unique personality profile is more prone to addiction than another (Sadock and Sadock, 2000). Theories of psychologic causation are insufficient to adequately explain the need for excessive substance use.

Situational Factors

Situational factors include peer influence, social norms, family influences, and social supports (Holder, 2000). Again, in real life these factors overlap with other situational, environmental, and individual influences.

Family systems theory is useful as a conceptual model to help promote understanding of emotional family functioning. Bowen's use of interrelated and interdependent concepts characterizes what happens in families when a member abuses substances (Bowen, 1978). Children from these families tend to become enmeshed in the family system. Their boundaries become blurred within the family and they live solely for each other. Family members use family secrets and myths as survival measures. These family members tend to cut off communication with those outside the family structure. The *multigenerational transmission process* traces the recurrence of the disease in the family in subsequent generations. The family conspires to maintain a system that supports addiction. The term *codependent* describes a person who helps another maintain his or her addiction by caring for them, handling their problems, and running interference. On the surface these efforts appear helpful, but they do not permit the affected individual the opportunity to experience the consequences of their behavior, an important agent for change. The term *codependent* is confusing and suggests the notion of blame for someone else's problems, creating a double victim situation. The terms *co-alcoholic* and *co-addict* have also been used. Because addiction carries stigma, the current thinking is to refrain from labeling individuals based on these behaviors.

Research about family influences on substance abuse led to interventions that strengthen the family unit. The social ecology model data suggest that parents have an early influence on development of drug use patterns of their children (Kumpfer and Turner, 1990/1991). Crespi and Sabatelli (1997) identified a connection between the developmental implications of parental alcoholism and achieving one's own independence. Some families tend to restrict the process of individuation and separation.

Healthy parental support is a strong predictor of decreased drug use in youth. Miller (1997) and others looked at family dynamics related to problem behaviors (e.g., academic failure, antisocial behavior, high-risk sex, and substance abuse). They designed treatment measures to improve family involvement, parenting skills, and parental monitoring with the goal of reducing adolescent drug use and associated behaviors.

Peer group pressures and the need to belong to the group are powerful positive reinforcers for youth (Newcomb, 1992; Oetting, 1992). Prevention efforts that target situational influences include changing perceptions in groups, promoting positive peer influence, bonding with non-using peers, and improved parenting skills. Modeling theory suggests that adolescents reared in homes where substances are readily available often repeat the behavior of adults and other role models who use substances to feel good. This is an example of overlapping areas, as modeling theory also applies to the environmental area of influence.

A related issue is the age at which persons begin drinking. The risk of developing an alcohol use disorder increases for those who start drinking before age 17 (24.5%) compared to those who start drinking at 21 or 22 (10%) or age 25 (less than 4%) (Grant and Dawson, 1997). Based on the results of one survey, the median age of the onset of alcohol abuse is 19 years (Kessler et al., 1997).

Environmental Factors

Environmental factors include access to and cost of desired substance, policies and policy enforcement, and severity of punishment for those who engage in illegal behavior to obtain substances or who sell to minors (Holder, 1999). Researchers based in community and public health disciplines determine the extent to which environmental factors influence addiction. A new method for obtaining substances has arrived via the Internet. Although law enforcement has been effective in limiting Internet prescribing, Internet purchase of controlled substances remains a problem (Cone, 2006). In 1 week in 2006, 185 Internet sites sold these drugs. The researcher found no evidence to block children from purchasing drugs online.

Community health researchers assess communities for risk factors, using several available models. One model is available through the National Institute of Drug Abuse (NIDA, 2000). Researchers use maps and mapping of neighborhoods to identify problem areas within communities and to then form action agendas for prevention and intervention.

Reimbursement is often poor for drug and alcohol treatment. The impression that addictions are self-created is partially true. So are some forms of diabetes, heart disease, respiratory disease, and others. There is no limit on treatment for chronic obstructive pulmonary disease (COPD), even though the patient has smoked for years. Reimbursement is available for the consequence of addiction, but prevention and treatment are expensive and not well funded.

Researchers conduct descriptive and analytical epidemiology studies in communities and across the nation to track alcohol and drug use trends. With the goal of prevention, they implement strategies to help individuals and communities. Intervention before dependence occurs is a secondary goal. The majority of adolescents who use drugs do not develop SUDS (Newcomb, 1995). The culture of early adulthood often includes alcohol use and drug experimentation, but most people stop this behavior when they enter the workforce and have families and financial obligations. Little data are available on impulse control disorders such as gambling, but studies are under way.

EPIDEMIOLOGY

Federal and individual state agencies concerned about drug use conduct many surveys to estimate drug use trends. Box 14-2 illustrates consumption standards for alcohol and classification for types of drinkers. The National Survey on Drug Abuse and Health (NSDAH) is a data set is a data set that helps researchers track the use of various substances in the United States. The 2004 report revealed that 19.1 million Americans, or 7.9% of the population ages 12 or older, used at least one illicit drug in the month before taking the survey (www.oas.samhsa.gov/nsduh/2k4overview/2k4overview.htm#toc).

Marijuana (classified as a hallucinogen) was the most common illicit drug in 2004, with a rate of 6.1% (14.6 million current users). There were 2.0 million current cocaine users, 467,000 of whom used crack. Approximately 929,000 persons used hallucinogens, and there were an estimated 166,000 heroin users. The number of current users of ecstasy had decreased between 2002 and 2003, but the number did not change between 2003 and 2004 (450,000). In 2004, 6.0 million persons were current users of psychotherapeutic drugs taken nonmedically (2.5%). These include 4.4 million who used pain relievers, 1.6 million who used tranquilizers, 1.2 million who used stimulants, and 0.3 million who used sedatives. These estimates are all similar to the corresponding estimates for 2003.

Researchers noted significant increases in the lifetime prevalence of use from 2003 to 2004 in several categories of pain relievers among those ages 18 to 25. Specific pain relievers with statistically significant increases in lifetime use were Vicodin, Lortab, or Lorcet; Percocet, Percodan, or Tylox; hydrocodone products; OxyContin; and oxycodone products.

Among youths ages 12 to 17, rates of current illicit drug use varied significantly by major racial/ethnic groups in 2004. The rate was highest among American Indian or Alaska Native youths (26.0%).

Approximately 121 million Americans, age 12 years and older, acknowledged current consumption of alcohol (50.3%). Fifty-five million participated in binge drinking, defined as five or more drinks on at least one occasion in the 30 days before taking the survey. About 17 million were heavy drinkers, defined as binge drinking on 5 or more days in the previous month. These numbers are similar to 2002 and 2003. The highest prevalence of binge and heavy drinking in 2004 was for young adults 18 to 25, with the peak at age 21. Young adults ages 18 to 22 in college full time were more likely than their peers not enrolled full time to use alcohol, binge drink, and drink heavily in 2004.

Approximately 24% currently used tobacco products, about 30% of the population ages 12 or older. Young adults ages 18 to 25 continued to have the highest rate of past month cigarette use (39.5%). The rate of cigarette use among youths ages 12 to 17 declined from 13% in 2002 to 11.9% in 2004.

BOX 14-2

Standard Drink and Consumption Levels

A STANDARD DRINK*
12 oz beer
5 oz wine
8 oz malt liquor
1.5 oz 80 proof spirits

CONSUMPTION DEFINITIONS

Abstinence
No drinking

Light Drinking
Less than 5 grams of alcohol per day

Moderate Drinking
Women: 1 drink of 15 grams of alcohol per day for women
Men: 2 drinks or 30 grams a day for men

Heavy or At-Risk Drinking
Women: More than 7 drinks per week or more than 3 drinks per occasion
Men: More than 14 drinks per week or 4 drinks or more per occasion
Any drinking by a minor
Any drinking by a pregnant woman
More than 15 grams a day if over age 65

Data from US Department of Health and Human Services, 2005; www.cdc.gov/alcohol/faqs.htm.
*All contain about 15 grams of alcohol.

Trends and initiation of use are another category in this data. From the same study, and based on a new approach to estimating incidence, the 2004 NSDAH shows that the illicit drug category with the largest number of new users was nonmedical use of pain relievers. In all, 2.4 million persons used these pain relievers for the first time within the previous 12 months. The average age at first use among these new initiates was 23.3 years. In 2004, 2.1 million persons had used marijuana for the first time within the previous 12 months. This estimate was not significantly different from the number in 2003 (2.0 million). The average age at first use among the 2.1 million recent marijuana initiates was 18.0 years. Most (63.8%) of the recent initiates were younger than age 18 when they first used. In 2004, 4.4 million persons had used alcohol for the first time within the previous 12 months. The number of alcohol initiates increased from 3.9 million in 2002 and 4.1 million in 2003. Most (86.9%) of the 4.4 million recent alcohol initiates in 2004 were younger than age 21 at the time of initiation. The number of persons who smoked cigarettes for the first time within the previous 12 months was 2.1 million in 2004, not significantly different from the estimates in 2002 (1.9 million) or 2003 (2.0 million). About two thirds of new smokers in 2004 were under the age of 18 when they first smoked cigarettes (67.8%).

The White House Office of National Drug Control Policy (ONDCP) and others have studied the total economic cost of alcohol, tobacco, and other drugs since 1985. According to estimates, the economic cost of substance abuse each year is about $400 billion, though others disagree with this figure. This estimate includes premature deaths, treatment and prevention costs, crime, social welfare programs, destruction of property, and costs associated with loss of jobs and earnings (Substance Abuse and Mental Health Service Administration [SAMHSA], 2002).

The United States government primarily funds the research on addictions. Resources developed by the Drug Abuse Warning Network, the Community Epidemiology Work Group, the Drug Enforcement Agency, and multiple other nongovernmental groups such as Erowid (www.erowid.org) provide nurses and other health care providers with databases and trends that influence the direction of education, prevention, and treatment. Regardless of the chosen practice area, nurses have a responsibility to update their information about drug use trends by using resources readily available on the Internet.

Substance Abuse in Special Populations

Although substance use disorders have a negative impact on all populations, researchers who study addiction recognize that for some people, substance abuse results in particularly negative consequences. These groups include women, pregnant women and the fetus, adolescents, older adults, and professionals.

Women

Research suggests that women are at higher risk than men for problems related to alcohol use, including organ damage and other problems (Stranges et al., 2004; Weschler and Austin, 1998). Women begin problem drinking later in life than men (late 20s or early 30s) and develop significant physical and psychosocial problems in a shorter period of time, often during childbearing years. This phenomenon is *telescoping*. Women more often than men cite an event such as divorce or separation that preceded drinking. Alcohol abuse also renders women more vulnerable than males to domestic violence (Norris, 1994) and completed suicide (Hill, 1995). Even lower rates of drinking predispose women for work-related problems, interpersonal relationship problems, and parenting problems (Chander and McCaul, 2003; Room, 1998). Treatment programs and 12-step programs originally developed to treat men because social norms did not acknowledge women's addiction. However, as times change, gender-specific programs developed and are being evaluated (see the Research for Evidence-Based Practice box).

Perinatal Conditions

Despite general knowledge about the danger of drinking alcohol while pregnant, binge drinking or frequent drinking continues to be a problem for this population. Pregnant women who reported any alcohol use, binge drinking, and frequent drinking were more likely to be less than 30 years old, employed, and unmarried (Center for Disease Control and Prevention [CDC], 2002). No drug is safe when used by a pregnant woman. Research through the years has shown that substances affect the mother and fetus in different ways when used during pregnancy. Many of the substances used by pregnant women are teratogens to the fetus, causing developmental malformations. Because many women abuse more than one drug, it is difficult to predict the damage to their babies. The effects of specific substances on fetuses is dependent on a number of factors including the type of drugs, amounts, patterns of maternal consumption, and the timing of exposure.

There is no strong evidence of teratogenicity for most of the currently used depressants, but pregnant women need to avoid these substances. Examples of depressants that cause changes in infants are thalidomide, phenobarbital, and benzodiazepines (in animals). The belief that caffeine is relatively safe in pregnancy is challenged by some because it readily crosses the placenta to the fetus (Schuckit, 2000).

RESEARCH for EVIDENCE-BASED PRACTICE

Grupp K: Women one year following gender-specific treatment for alcohol and/or other drug dependency, *Journal of Addictions Nursing* 17:5-11, 2006.

Fifty-three women who were 1 year post–substance dependence or abuse and who received gender-specific treatment in inpatient, outpatient, or a combination participated in a survey to measure their severity of addiction, satisfaction with treatment, and life satisfaction. Survey respondents were white (85%) and between 35 and 45 years old (45%); 36% were married, and 23% had never been married. Seventy-two percent lived in their own or family-owned homes, 36% reported chronic medical problems. Five of the women were in treatment because of legal difficulties. The treatment facility treated only women and offered a program that centered on the needs of women. A majority of women in the study experienced depression (89%) and anxiety (81%) during their lifetimes. Thirty-four percent had attempted suicide, and 40% reported past violent behavior.

At the time of the study, 76% of the women were not drinking or using drugs, and 12 (23%) of the women were drinking alcohol. Twenty-eight percent had maintained sobriety during the year after treatment. Eight of the 12 who were drinking had been drinking for at least 6 months, indicating relapse in the first 6 months after treatment. The women were satisfied with the treatment they received, and satisfaction with treatment correlated positively to satisfaction with life. Those with more significant psychiatric problems were less satisfied with their lives.

Nurses need to be aware that treatment and recovery are usually ongoing, lengthy processes and that relapse is common. Nurses offer hope to those in addiction that recovery is possible and that life can be satisfying without using substances, and they help to create treatment programs that address life issues as well as addiction, including efforts at reuniting families. Patients with comorbid conditions have a more difficult experience on the road to recovery. It is helpful for the nurse to share that information, and also that sobriety and satisfaction with life are within reach. Using the knowledge that comorbidity is common, nurses need to be alert for emerging symptoms of other psychiatric disorders and work with the health care team to effectively treat the client. Nurses are able to participate in research efforts to help those in addictions recover their lives.

Among women ages 15 to 44, combined data for 2003 and 2004 (National Survey 2004) indicated that 18.0% of those who were pregnant smoked cigarettes in the preceding month compared with 30.0% of those who were not pregnant. Rates of previous month cigarette smoking were lower for pregnant than nonpregnant women among those ages 26 to 44 (11.7 versus 29.1%) and among those ages 18 to 25 (28.0 versus 36.3%). However, among those ages 15 to 17, the rate of cigarette smoking for pregnant women was higher than for nonpregnant women (26.0 versus 19.6%), although the difference was not significant. Smoking in pregnancy accounts for an estimated 20% to 30% of low-birth-weight babies, up to 14% of preterm deliveries, and 10% of all infant deaths. Infants also have an increased risk of congenital abnormalities. Even healthy, full-term babies of mothers who smoke have been born with narrowed airways and curtailed lung function. Children of mothers who smoke during pregnancy sometimes exhibit hyperactivity and have an increased risk of cancer later in life (Schuckit, 2000). Studies show that babies born to marijuana users were shorter, weighed less, and had smaller head sizes than those born to mothers who did not use the drug. In addition, research reveals that children born to mothers who used marijuana also have difficulty concentrating when they are older (NIDA, *Frequently Asked Questions*, 2002).

Opioids present special problems in pregnant women and their offspring. Fetal damage is a result of genetic changes caused by the drug. Other medical problems include elevated rates of intrauterine death, low birth weight in infants, premature delivery, and a 2% to 5% risk of infant death (Schuckit, 2000). Newborns of opioid-dependent mothers exhibit withdrawal symptoms. At birth, children exposed to cocaine prenatally exhibited more abnormal reflexes, less motor maturity, and decreased ability to regulate their state of attentiveness than did unexposed children (Bauer et al, 2005).

Prenatal alcohol consumption continues to be a major concern. Drinking during pregnancy is the leading known cause of preventable birth defects and learning difficulties (Figure 14-1). These difficulties and defects are 100% preventable. Some general cognitive deficits were reported after an average of as little as three drinks per day during pregnancy (Schuckit, 2000). Drinking rates for pregnant women, though substantially lower than the rates for nonpregnant women of similar age, highlight a major concern because of the effects of alcohol on the fetus. The most severe effects of alcohol on the fetus are **fetal alcohol syndrome** (FAS) (Figure 14-2). The diag-

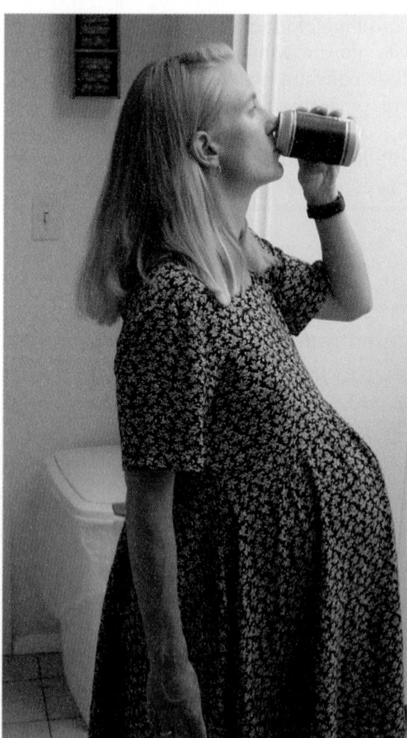

FIGURE 14-1 Alcohol and drug use during pregnancy interfere with normal fetal development.

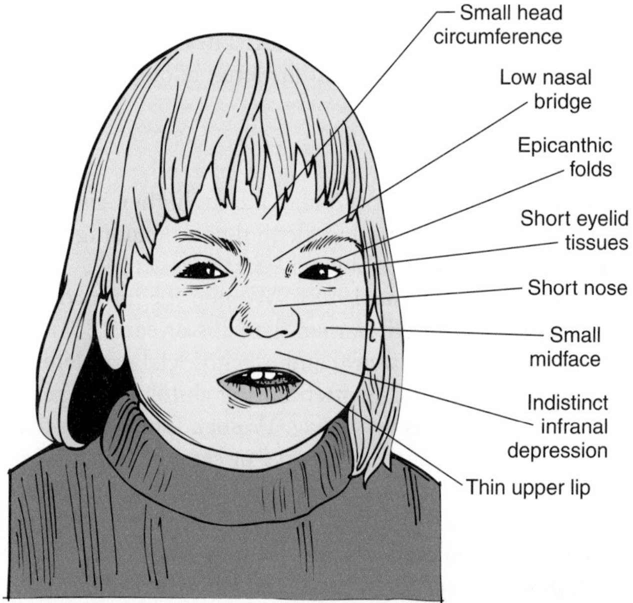

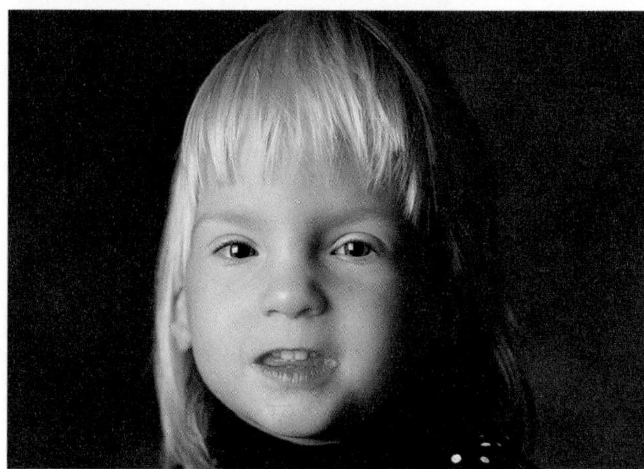

FIGURE 14-2 Fetal alcohol syndrome (FAS). Milder forms of alcohol-induced effects on the fetus and the infant are known as fetal alcohol effects.

nosis of FAS has three criteria: (1) growth retardation, (2) central nervous system involvement resulting in mental retardation and other learning difficulties, and (3) facial and other abnormalities (Bowden and Rust, 2000). FAS occurs in 1 to 3 per 1000 live births. Surviving infants exhibit any mixture of the syndrome, which includes a small head, small physical stature, mild to severe mental retardation, facial abnormalities including a flat bridge of the nose, an absent philtrum (medium groove between the upper lip and nose), an epicanthal eye fold (vertical skinfold over the angle of the inner canthus of the eye), an atrial or ventricular septal heart defect, syndactyly (malformations of the hands and feet with fusion of fingers or toes), and disorders of the temporomandibular joint.

Other signs of FAS include hearing loss or a developmental delay. As children reach school age, they have problems in reading, spelling, and arithmetic. As they grow older, they have an increased risk for developing alcohol abuse and dependence and some develop antisocial personality disorders and other psychiatric conditions (Schuckit, 2000).

Developments in the creation of maternal or neonatal biomarkers to detect alcohol use during pregnancy assist health care providers to detect exposure (Bearer, 2001; Savage, 2006). Many of these tests are not practical for routine use but help researchers study the effect of alcohol on developing fetuses and children. Nurses need to avoid victimizing women with substance use issues (Armstrong, 1992). Women sometimes do not know the facts about using drugs or alcohol while they are pregnant. Sources of factual information are scarce among some populations. Several states legislated mandatory incarceration for women who use substances while pregnant, but these programs have failed or have been ruled unconstitutional.

Adolescents

The term *problematic use* is often used with this age-group because adolescents often experiment or use drugs in conjunction with specific events such as parties, developmental or emotional crises, and peer group influences and pressures. The criteria presented in the DSM for symptoms of psychologic dependence or physical dependence may not apply to teenagers. Although peak use of alcohol and drugs is in late teens or early 20s, most people return to normal drinking patterns and do not progress to alcoholism or chronic abuse (Kessler et al., 1997; Newcomb 1995). Some adolescents go on to develop pervasive, recurrent patterns of use, which then result in serious consequences and diagnosable substance related disorders. Studies on vulnerability factors help researchers design prevention programs for at-risk youth. For example, one factor is age, because those who begin drinking before age 17 are more likely to develop an alcohol use disorder (24.5%) than those who drink at ages 21 or 22 (10%) or age 25 (less than 4%) (Grant and Dawson, 1997). Society considers experimenting with substances normative behavior for young adults. Many high school students drink or smoke cigarettes before age 13 (*Morbidity and Mortality Weekly Report*, 2005).

The popularity of substances rises and falls, with the use of hallucinogens declining in high schoolers (NIDA, 2006). The same data suggest that adolescent drug use is ubiquitous, found in rural, urban, and suburban populations. Of interest, and contrary to popular notions, researchers in this survey note that use of crack and heroin is not always in urban areas. A significant number of adolescents continue to use inhalants.

Males in this age-group have somewhat higher rates of illicit drug use than females, and much higher rates of smokeless tobacco and steroid use (NIDA, 2006). Students who are not college bound are more likely to use illicit drugs, drink heavily, and drink alcohol while in high school. In the lower grades, the college-bound showed a greater increase in cigarette smoking in the mid-1990s than did their non–college-bound peers.

The same study (Monitoring the Future) done in 2005 also revealed that the use of any illicit drug in the previous year was down by more than a third among eighth graders, down by under a quarter among tenth graders, and only 10% down among twelfth graders. Half of American secondary school students have tried an illicit drug by the time they reach graduation. Marijuana is the most prevalent of illicit drugs, and the 2005 survey indicated no significant decline in use of this substance. Annual use of ecstasy is declining since it peaked in 2001. Amphetamine use declined in upper grades but not in eighth grade. Tranquilizer use increased steadily from 1992 until 2000 and is now in decline. Prevalence rates for tranquilizer use is 2.8% in grade 8 and 6.8% in grade 12.

Among drugs that showed almost no change in 2005 were cocaine, crack, and heroin. The annual prevalence rate for powder cocaine is 1.7% in the eighth grade, 3% in tenth grade, and 4.5% in twelfth grade. Crystal methamphetamine prevalence is 2.3% in twelfth graders. Heroin use peaked in 2001 and is now slightly below 1% in all three grades. Narcotics other than heroin is reported only for the twelfth grade with the annual prevalence rate at 9%. Vicodin and OxyContin are the most common.

Alcohol and cigarettes are the most common substances youth use. Half of American youth have tried cigarettes by the twelfth grade, and 23% are current smokers. By the eighth grade, 26% have tried cigarettes, and 1 in 11 has become a current smoker. Cigarette use reached its peak in 1996. Declines in smoking among this age-group seem to have leveled; no significant declines occurred in 2005.

Seventy-five percent of high school seniors have tried alcohol (more than just a few sips), and 41% have done so by the eighth grade. More than half (58%) of seniors and 20% of eighth graders reported being drunk at least once, which causes concern given the fact that alcohol disorders develop faster when drinking begins early.

Three drugs that were used increasingly were sedatives, OxyContin, and inhalants. In each case, increases were modest and were confined to twelfth grade. Researchers speculate that some of these increases are due to respondents using drugs at one point (eighth grade) and continuing use through high school. Researchers do not know whether those reporting drug use had ever used the drug before. The same researchers believe that "generational forgetting" contributes to drug use—when drugs are reintroduced to young people. Researchers believe that when adverse effects of drugs become known, such as for LSD and methamphetamine, these particular drugs fall out of use. Both of these drugs had very bad reputations in the 1960s and 1970s. Over time, this information is forgotten, and young people begin to use the drug, only to rediscover unfortunate or fatal outcomes. Persons interested in preventing adolescent drug use focus on the "grace period" between when a drug becomes popular and then use falls off because of these negative consequences. Information campaigns to educate and publicize adverse effects are helpful during these times.

Of particular concern are prescription drugs, which have gained popularity. Use of these drugs is increasing, and the trend is rising among younger adolescents. Researchers believe this is partially due to the general practice of prescription drug advertising, which imparts the idea that drugs are safe. Prescription drugs have become gradually more popular over an extended period of time. Adolescents obtain them from friends, relatives, parents, or others who have usually obtained them legally. Nurses need to encourage everyone to dispose of medications when no longer in use.

Research conducted since the 1970s has produced a convincing body of evidence that the use of cigarettes, alcohol, and marijuana by children and adolescents is especially dangerous. These drugs impede social and intellectual development, cause disease or brain damage, and ruin or destroy lives. They often lead to dangerous activities such as driving under the influence, premature or unprotected sex, and violence. Eating disorders and impulse disorders occur more frequently with substance abuse disorders (Grilo et al., 2002).

There are three major surveys and systems that collect data on substance use by youth. Data from the National survey on Drug Use and Health indicate that more males than females ages 12 to 20 reported binge drinking (22.1% versus 17.0%) and heavy drinking (8.2% versus 4.3%). Among persons ages 12 to 20, past month alcohol use rates were 16.4% among Asians, 19.1% among blacks, 24.3% among American Indians or Alaska Natives, 26.4% among those reporting two or more races, 26.6% among Hispanics, and 32.6% among whites.

The Center on Addiction and Substance Abuse (CASA) at Columbia University analyzed the use of alcohol, cigarettes, and marijuana as entry or **gateway drugs** that lead to subsequent use of other illicit drugs, regardless of the age, ethnicity, or race of those involved. The highlights of their report emphasize the dangers that gateway drugs present to youth. They found that age at first use, frequency of use, and number of drugs used increase the probability of a youth becoming a regular drug user and addict. The implications of this comprehensive report are clear. If a child or adolescent makes it through the teenage years without smoking cigarettes and without repeatedly drinking beer or other types of alcohol, the odds are overwhelming that the child will never smoke marijuana. The Client and Family Teaching Guidelines box lists signs of substance abuse in children or adolescents and strategies to prevent substance abuse.

Developmentally, adolescents and children do not clearly understand what addiction means. When nurses interact with younger patients, they need to determine what the child knows in order to provide effective care and teaching. Children are afraid of addiction and worry about their families who smoke and worry that they also will become addicted (Miller and Armstrong, 2006).

CLIENT and FAMILY TEACHING GUIDELINES

SIGNS OF ADOLESCENT DRUG USE/ABUSE

- Bloodshot, red eyes, droopy eyelids
- Wearing sunglasses at inappropriate times
- Changes in sleep patterns (e.g., napping, insomnia)
- Unexplained periods of moodiness, depression, anxiety, or irritability
- Decreased interaction and communication with family
- Loss of interest in previous hobbies, sports, etc.
- Change in friends; will not introduce new friends
- Decline in academic performance, drop in grades
- Loss of motivation and interest in school activities
- Change in peer group
- Disappearance of money or items of value
- Use of eye drops/mouthwash
- Unfamiliar containers or locked boxes
- Money missing from the house

PREVENTION OF ADOLESCENT SUBSTANCE USE/ABUSE

- Ensure positive role modeling by parents and adults in the adolescent's world.
- Reinforce the dangers of substance use and teach positive behaviors.
- Provide support in coping with the social pressure exerted by peers.
- Establish limits, structure, and house rules for the adolescent's behavior.
- Help the adolescent to anticipate pressures, and reinforce positive coping behaviors.
- Engage the adolescent in life skills training programs where the emphasis is on positive skills training, resistance training, and group support.
- Monitor the adolescent's use of television, computer, movies, and video games, as media may portray legal and illegal substances as a part of daily life.

From The Clean Foundation, P.O. Box 28148, San Diego, Calif, 92198-0148.

Older Adults

Estimates about drug and alcohol abuse, and gambling problems, among older adults (over age 60) underrepresent the true numbers (Meninger, 2002); 16% of those 65 years and older experience alcohol use disorders (Meninger, 2002). In one study, approximately 70% of individuals older than 60 years admitted to hospitals had experienced health problems or accidents related to alcohol consumption (Colleran and Jay, 2002). Men in this age-group have increased rates of drinking, and females over age 60 have a 1% to 8% chance of having problem drinking patterns (Blow and Barry, 2003). The physiologic effects of aging intensify the effects of alcohol and other drugs (Menninger, 2002; Nguyen et al., 2001) because of decreased volume of body water, decreased body mass, central nervous system sensitivity, and decreased rate of metabolism of alcohol in the gastrointestinal tract. Relatively low levels of alcohol aggravate chronic health problems. Brennan et al. (2006) studied alcohol use by older adults and discovered that many adults age 55 to 65 use alcohol to manage chronic pain. Higher levels of pain were associated with increased use of alcohol for all drinkers, but problem drinkers used alcohol 31% of the time to manage mild pain and 56% of the time to manage moderate to severe pain. Nonproblem drinkers' rates were 18% for mild pain and 21% for moderate to severe pain. No major differences existed between sexes.

Caregivers need to carefully assess for these problems, and be alert for the possibility that an alcohol or other substance use disorder is creating some of the client's physical problems. For example, alcohol-induced cognitive changes mimic Alzheimer's disorder, and falls, assaults, and suicides are also correlated with alcohol use. According to estimates, the number of adults age 50 and older using illicit drugs will increase from 1.6 million in 1999 to 2001 to 3.5 million in 2020. Projected increases are due to a 52% increase in that age population and an increase in the number of persons from higher drug using groups who will reach the age of 50. Nurses entering the profession need to be cognizant of these trends.

Health Care Professionals

Health care professionals have the same prevalence of alcoholism and illicit drug use as the general population. Exact numbers are elusive because studies are limited, and underreporting is common. One estimate is that approximately 9% of physicians use drugs or alcohol. About 10% to 20% of nurses are identified as having substance abuse problems, and 6% to 8% of registered nurses have impaired practice as a result of their abuse of alcohol and drugs (Griffith, 1999). High-stress jobs (Trinkoff et al., 2000; Trinkoff and Storr, 1998), frequent contact with illness and death, and accessibility to prescription and controlled medications result in susceptibility to drug use, abuse, or dependence by those in the health care field. Physicians and nurses who practice in particular specialties such as anesthesiology have higher rates of substance abuse disorders than those who practice in other specialties. Some researchers hypothesize that repeated passive exposures to minute amounts of anesthetic agents sensitize workers in the operating rooms and sensitize brain pathways to opiates (Center for Substance Abuse Research [CESAR], 2005). The rate of addiction to opiates is high among anesthesiologists and surgeons.

Dual Diagnosis

Dual diagnosis, *comorbidity*, and *co-occurring disorders* are terms that describe concurrent mental illness and drug abuse or dependence. These disorders occur at the same time, or one follows the other, and eventually it is difficult to tell which came first. Even though the diseases of mental illness and drug abuse are comorbid, causality is not implied and either condition may precede the other. The symptoms of one condition often mask or conceal the symptoms of the other, and either condition assumes priority at any given time. Even though *dual* is common terminology, it is important to recognize that many individuals suffer from two *or more* disorders concurrently. For example, a person exhibits signs of severe psychosis, depression, and cocaine dependence. Approximately 30% of individuals diagnosed as mentally ill abuse drugs or alcohol; 37% of alcohol abusers and 53% of drug abusers also have at least one mental illness (National Mental Health Association [NMHA], 2002). The most prevalent psychiatric disorders among those with a history of substance abuse are antisocial personality disorder, bipolar disorder, and schizophrenia. Substances individuals most often abuse are alcohol, followed by marijuana and cocaine. Many patients with severe and persistent chronic mental illness are also addicted to nicotine.

As it is with the general population, substance abuse or dependence complicates almost every aspect of life. However, people with dual diagnoses are difficult to diagnose and to engage in treatment. Often they have lost their support systems and suffer from repeated relapses, hospitalizations, and involvement in the criminal justice system. National statistics indicate that a high percentage of incarcerated individuals have dual diagnoses.

Co-occurring Physical Conditions

The practice of sharing and reusing needles, syringes, and other types of drug injection equipment exposes individuals to risk of multiple infectious processes. Contact with injecting drug users often results in the transmission of human immunodeficiency virus (HIV), hepatitis B virus (HBV), and hepatitis C virus (HCV), among other diseases. There are no clear boundaries between major risk groups who engage in multiple types of drug abuse, unsafe sex practices, and contaminated equipment use. The increase of heterosexual HIV transmission among women, especially young women, has been linked to the mixing of drugs, alcohol, and unprotected sex. Injecting drug users have one of the highest HBV rates among all risk groups and account for at least half of all new HCV cases. Prevalence rates are as high as 50% for HBV and 65% for HCV among people who have injected drugs for less than a year. Co-infections of HBV, HCV, often cluster in injecting drug users (CDC, 1999).

CLINICAL DESCRIPTION

Most Americans try or use at least one substance that sometimes results in further use, abuse, or eventual addiction during their lifetime. Caffeine, tobacco products, and

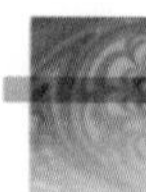

BOX 14-3

Classes of Substance Abuse

- Alcohol
- Amphetamines or similar acting drugs
- Caffeine
- Cannabis
- Cocaine
- Hallucinogens
- Inhalants
- Nicotine
- Opioids
- Phencyclidine (PCP) or similar-acting substances
- Sedatives, hypnotics, anxiolytics

From American Psychiatric Association: *Diagnostic and statistical manual of mental disorders*, ed 4, text revision, Washington, DC, 2000, American Psychiatric Association.

alcohol are the three most frequently used substances. Many people learn from negative experiences and do not continue to use the substance, or the lifestyle with many negative consequences of substance abuse deteriorates as one grows older. The substance-related disorders described in DSM-IV-TR include disorders related to the following:

- Use of drugs of abuse
- Medications
- Toxin exposures that may be accidental or intentional

There are 11 different classes of substances (Box 14-3). The DSM-IV-TR also addresses polysubstance dependence and other substance-related disorders.

The DSM-IV-TR divides substance-related disorders into two groups. One group contains the *substance use disorders*, and the other contains the *substance-induced disorders*. Each of these groups contains criteria for substance abuse, dependence, intoxication, and withdrawal that apply to the different classifications. The criteria for **substance abuse** and **substance dependence** are listed in the DSM-IV-TR Criteria box.

Specific Substances

Alcohol

Alcohol Use. Alcohol is the most widely used and most abused substance. About 9.6% of American males and 3.2% of American females are alcohol dependant (American Psychiatric Association, 2000). When those in good health use it sparingly, any changes in body function that occur are usually reversible. Likewise, some data reveal that alcohol under certain circumstances has beneficial effects. In limited amounts, alcohol increases socialization, stimulates the appetite, and decreases the risk for macular degeneration and gallstones. Research also indicates that it decreases the risk of cardiovascular disease by increasing high-density lipoproteins (HDLs) and decreasing platelet adhesion (Schuckit, 2000). When alcohol consumption exceeds two drinks daily, or when those in poor physical health drink, damage to body systems is more rapid and pervasive. Any amount of alcohol is considered harmful to developing fetuses, children, adolescents, and recovering alcoholics. It is also harmful to people taking medications that interact adversely with alcohol and for those with certain medical conditions or psychiatric disorders.

A telephone survey conducted between 2002 and 2003 revealed that 15% of U.S. workers (19.2 million people) reported using or being impaired by alcohol at work at least once in the preceding year. Impairment included being hung over (morning-after effects) at work (9.2%) and using alcohol during the workday (7.1%). Seventy percent of workers reported using or being impaired by alcohol less than monthly, 19% reported monthly impairment, and 11% weekly impairment (Frone, 2006).

Numerous studies document the relationship between violence and drugs. Persons in treatment for domestic violence and criminal offences have high rates of substance abuse problems. The severity of violence escalated when persons with higher drinking levels added another drug (Chermack and Blow, 2002).

Genetics partially determines the rate of metabolism of the substance, physiologic reactions, level of tolerance, and rates of elimination (Keltner and Folks, 2005). The liver metabolizes alcohol, where the enzyme alcohol dehydrogenase converts alcohol first to acetaldehyde. Then the enzyme aldehyde dehydrogenase converts acetaldehyde to acetate, and alcohol is ultimately metabolized to carbon and water.

Japanese, Chinese, and Korean men and women are more likely than whites to have an inactive form of alcohol dehydrogenase (ADH), which metabolizes alcohol in the liver. Another 40% of this population has active enzyme, but with decreased activity, resulting in an exaggerated response to alcohol (Li, 2000), which produces flushing, nausea, dizziness, and rapid heartbeat. The lack of this enzyme is protective against alcoholism. Native Americans, who are possibly genetically related to people of central Asian ancestry, do not lack this enzyme so do not have the benefit of protection.

The alcohol-deterrent drug Antabuse (disulfiram) also produces a flush reaction. Disulfiram inactivates aldehyde dehydrogenase in a person who carries the normal gene for that enzyme, in effect producing the same situation as in the Asians who have the inactive form of the gene. Acetaldehyde increases in the blood quickly, and the resulting discomfort serves as an effective deterrent to further drinking.

Alcohol Intoxication. Alcohol intoxication, as defined by DSM-IV-TR criteria, is based on evidence of clinically significant psychologic or maladaptive changes that occur during or shortly after the ingestion of alcohol. These changes include such behaviors as inappropriate sexual or aggressive actions, lability of mood, impaired judgment, and impaired social or work-related functioning. Associated signs related to these changes include slurred speech, incoordination, unsteady gait, nystagmus, the breath smell of alcohol, impaired attention and memory, and coma or stupor. Other medical or mental disorders must be ruled out.

DSM-IV-TR CRITERIA

Substance Abuse and Substance Dependence

SUBSTANCE ABUSE

A A maladaptive pattern of substance use leading to clinically significant impairment or distress, as manifested by one (or more) of the following and occurring within a 12-month period:
  1 Recurrent substance use resulting in a failure to fulfill major role obligations at work, school, or home (e.g., repeated absences or poor work performance related to substance use; substance-related absences, suspensions, or expulsions from school; neglect of children or household)
  2 Recurrent substance use in situations in which it is physically hazardous (e.g., driving an automobile or operating a machine when impaired by substance use)
  3 Recurrent substance-related legal problems (e.g., arrests for substance-related disorderly conduct)
  4 Continued substance use despite having persistent or recurrent social or interpersonal problems caused or exacerbated by the effects of the substance (e.g., arguments with spouse about consequences of intoxication; physical fights)

B The symptoms have never met the criteria for substance dependence for this class of substance.

SUBSTANCE DEPENDENCE

A maladaptive pattern of substance use, leading to clinically significant impairment or distress, as manifested by three (or more) of the following and occurring at any time in the same 12-month period:
  1 **Tolerance**, as defined by either of the following:
    a Need for markedly increased amounts of the substance to achieve intoxication or desired effect
    b Markedly diminished effect with continued use of the same amount of the substance
  2 **Withdrawal**, as manifested by either of the following:
    a The characteristic withdrawal syndrome for the substance
    b The same (or a closely related) substance is taken to relieve or avoid withdrawal symptoms
  3 The substance is often taken in larger amounts or over a longer period than was intended
  4 There is a persistent desire or unsuccessful efforts to cut down or control substance use
  5 A great deal of time is spent in activities necessary to obtain the substance (e.g., visiting multiple doctors or driving long distances), use the substance (e.g., chain-smoking), or recover from its effects
  6 Important social, occupational, or recreational activities are given up or reduced because of substance use
  7 The substance use is continued despite knowledge of having a persistent or recurrent physical or psychologic problem that is likely to have been caused or exacerbated by the substance (e.g., current cocaine use despite recognition of cocaine-induced depression or continued drinking despite recognition that an ulcer was made worse by alcohol consumption)

Specify if:

With physiologic dependence: evidence of tolerance or withdrawal or both (i.e., either item 1 or item 2 is present)

Without physiologic dependence: no evidence of tolerance or withdrawal (i.e., neither item 1 nor item 2 is present)

From American Psychiatric Association: *Diagnostic and statistical manual of mental disorders*, ed 4, text revision. Washington, DC, 2000, American Psychiatric Association.

Effects on the Neurologic System. Cellular damage and loss of brain tissue have been documented as a result of alcohol use. Some experience symptoms such as intense anxiety, psychoses, depressed mood, auditory hallucinations, or paranoia with intoxication after ingesting alcohol. Most individuals show a clearing of clouded consciousness within a few hours. Those with a previous history of severe alcohol abuse, brain damage or trauma, however, remain confused for days or weeks. This sometimes affects older individuals similarly.

Nurses should assess alcohol use in all cases of rapidly developing confusion. Assessment is imperative in the case of persons with known mental disorders so that providers do not confuse an alcoholic delirium with dementia or worsening mental disorder such as schizophrenia. Temporary or permanent signs of confusion are also associated with the direct effects of alcohol and with specific vitamin deficiencies. Wernicke-Korsakoff syndrome occurs as a consequence of a thiamine deficiency after many years of excessive alcohol consumption. Symptoms of Wernicke-Korsakoff syndrome related to this condition involve neurologic abnormalities including inflammatory hemorrhagic degeneration of the brain. Korsakoff's symptoms in the syndrome include a severe form of amnesia that is much more profound than usually occurs in early dementia. The person also exhibits an inability to learn new skills. Wernicke-Korsakoff syndrome has a mortality rate of more than 15% (Schuckit, 2000).

Marchiafava Bignami disease also occurs in some with alcohol abuse. Identification of this condition was rare before the routine use of neuroimaging. Atrophy of the corpus callosum and impaired cerebral blood flow characterize this disease. Studies suggest that there are possibly subtypes of this disease. Clinical presentation is acute, or chronic (Heinrich et al., 2004). The acute presentation includes dysarthria, impaired consciousness, tetraparesis, and symptoms of interhemispheric dysregulation; the acute presentation is associated with poor outcomes.

Alcoholic blackouts (also called *anterograde amnesia*) occur in individuals who have consumed sufficient alcohol such that the substance interferes with the acquisition and storage of new memories in the brain. The information is lost from memory within minutes of its occurrence. About one third of drinkers report at least one alcoholic blackout. Approximately 40% of teenage and young adult males have blackouts (Sadock and Sadock, 2000). The history of a blackout experience probably indicates at least one episode of a rapidly consumed excessive amount of alcohol. If there are no other symptoms of alcohol-related problems, a blackout is not indicative of alcohol dependence. Persons who have been alcohol dependent for many years have had blackouts after consuming only a small amount of alcohol. Blackouts are frightening and unpleasant, regardless of how long the person has been drinking.

Peripheral Neuropathy Peripheral nerve deterioration in both hands and feet result from chronic alcohol intake. Peripheral neuropathy occurs in about 10% of alcoholics after years of heavy drinking. Symptoms include numbness of hands and feet, often bilateral and often accompanied with tingling and paresthesias. Damage does not always improve with abstinence. Ulcerations develop from co-occurring circulatory problems related to alcohol use.

Effects on the Liver. The liver is particularly susceptible to damage by excessive use of alcohol because it processes alcohol. Increased alcohol use results in the accumulation of fats and proteins in liver cells, producing a (usually) reversible condition called fatty liver. Inflammation of liver cells along with an elevation of some liver function tests and other signs of alcoholic hepatitis such as fever, chills, nausea, abdominal pain, and jaundice result in excess deposits of hyaline and collagen near blood vessels, signaling early signs of cirrhosis of the liver. As damage progresses, normal blood flow through the liver decreases, dilated veins or varices develop, and fluid seeps from the liver and accumulates in the abdomen as ascites. As liver failure progresses, cognitive impairment also develops as a result of hepatic encephalopathy (Sadock and Sadock, 2000).

Effects on the Gastrointestinal Tract. Alcohol is associated with ulcers and gastritis or inflammation of the stomach. Alcohol stimulates gastric secretions and promotes colonization of a bacterium identified in the development of ulcers. Inflammation of the pancreas occurs as a result of blockage of pancreatic ducts along with simultaneous stimulation of the production of digestive enzymes. The result is either acute or chronic pancreatitis (Schuckit, 2000). Esophageal varices occur in cases of severe alcoholism and result from impaired liver circulation. These dilated and congested veins sometimes rupture and produce a fatal hemorrhage.

Nutrition. Alcohol has a profound effect on an individual's metabolism of carbohydrates because it impairs the function of the liver and pancreas to respond normally to insulin. This impairment results in very high or low levels of insulin in the blood and has a negative effect on the control of blood sugar in diabetics. Alcohol also interferes with the absorption, storage, and distribution of vitamins such as B_1, B_6, D, and E. Vitamins B_2, A, and K are often deficient in alcoholics (Schuckit, 2000).

Effects on the Cardiovascular System. Heavy consumption of alcohol increases blood pressure and elevates both low-density lipoprotein cholesterol and triglycerides. These changes in turn increase the risk for myocardial infarction and thrombosis. Alcohol at high doses also produces what is a reversible deterioration of the heart muscle. Wasting of the heart muscle results in cardiac arrhythmias and congestive heart failure or alcoholic cardiomyopathy (Sadock and Sadock, 2000). Higher levels of alcohol consumption are related to an increased risk for hemorrhagic stroke (Schuckit, 2000).

Effects on the Immune System. Researchers estimate that for some people, alcohol intake of between 4 and 8 drinks a day decreases the production of white blood cells and interferes with the ability of these cells to get to sites of infection. That amount of alcohol also interferes with red blood cell production, significantly increases the average size of red cells (the mean corpuscular volume [MCV]), and impairs the production and efficiency of clotting factors and platelets (Sadock and Sadock, 2000). A less effective immune system contributes to increased risks for contracting HIV, tuberculosis, and other infectious or noninfectious disease processes.

Sleep Disturbance. Alcohol intoxication often interferes with sleep. Persons under the influence fall asleep more quickly but have depressed levels of rapid eye movement (REM) and less stage 4 sleep. Interruptions between sleep stages, called sleep fragmentation, also occur (Sadock and Sadock, 2000). Although some people say they use alcohol to fall asleep, alcohol often interrupts their sleep architecture, meaning that they do not experience the normal pattern of light and deep sleep. An excitatory neurotransmitter, glutamate, increases as the initial depressant effect of alcohol wanes, causing irritability and inability to sleep. Glutamate rebound is also responsible for many hangover symptoms.

Hormonal Changes. Hormonal changes occur as a result of heavy alcohol consumption. Acute intoxication sometimes results in changes of prolactin, growth hormone, adrenocorticotropic hormone (ACTH), and cortisol. It also produces a reduction in parathyroid hormone associated with lowered levels of blood calcium and magnesium. Some of these changes result in symptoms of menstrual irregularity, decreased sperm production/motility, decreased ejaculate volume, decreased production of testosterone, and impotence.

Accidents. Accident rates resulting from alcohol consumption dramatically influence mortality and morbidity rates in the United States. In the year 2000, more than 1 in 10 Americans ages 12 years and older (22.3 million persons) stated that they drove under the influence of alcohol at least once in the previous 12 months (SAMHSA, 2001). Among young adults, ages 18 to 25 years, about 20% drove under the influence of alcohol in the year 2000. There is evidence that a blood alcohol level (BAL) as low as 15 mg/dl (0.01), or about one drink, significantly impairs a person's ability to drive an automobile. Alcohol also significantly contributes to bicycle and pilot errors, and to accidents in the home and workplace (Schuckit, 2000).

Prescription Drugs

Individuals use prescription medications that produce mind, mood, or behavior altering effects legally as prescribed or illicitly. Taken for nonmedical reasons, prescription opiates or other scheduled medications cause addiction, overdose, and death. Four categories of prescription drugs were researched in the 2005 NHSDA. These included pain relievers, tranquilizers, stimulants, and sedatives. In the latest survey, 3.8 million people reported using prescription drugs for nonmedical reasons, representing 1.7% of the population 12 years or older. Prescription drug use is designated as follows: pain relievers (2.8 million users), tranquilizers (1 million users), stimulants (0.8 million users), and sedatives (0.2 million users).

Some trends of concern are occurring among older adults, women, and adolescents. Misuse of prescription medications is the most common form of drug abuse in older adults. This population is especially vulnerable because of the multiple drugs that are often prescribed for medical conditions. Cognitive impairment and physical instability result in, or from, alterations of medication ingestion causing increased risk for automobile accidents and falls. Risks increase because older adults have a decreased capability of metabolizing many medications and often need a fraction of what a middle-aged person requires.

Because the frequency of adolescent prescription drug use is increasing, it is wise for parents and grandparents to be aware of prescription medications in their homes and to dispose of them properly when they are no longer needed. Take any medication no longer needed to a pharmacy for disposal.

Anxiolytic Drugs

Although classes of central nervous system (CNS) depressants work in different ways, they all produce drowsy, calming, sedating effects to help with sleep disorders or symptoms of anxiety. If an individual uses them over a long period, the body will develop tolerance because of the brain's adaptive mechanism called neuroplasticity. Many of these medications are lethal in overdose situations. Clients obtain them either by prescription or through other sources "on the street." As noted earlier, substances that are shorter acting with rapid onset such as lorazepam have higher addictive potential. When used as drugs of abuse, individuals often take them to reduce subjective unpleasant anxiety or used to manage withdrawal symptoms from other drugs such as alcohol, cannabis, heroin, methadone, cocaine, and amphetamines.

Medications in the *hypnotic* class include the carbamates, the barbiturates, the barbiturate-like hypnotics, all prescription sleeping medications, and almost all prescription antianxiety medications with the exception of a nonbenzodiazepine antianxiety agent like buspirone (BuSpar). Some medications in this class are anticonvulsants (see Chapter 24). Carbamates include medications such as meprobamate (Miltown, Equanil) and tybamate (Salacen, Tybatran), which are not common in the United States. They are lethal when taken in overdose amounts. The carbamates also seem to have a higher potential for dependence.

Barbiturates all end in *-al* in the United States. Examples include phenobarbital (Luminal) and secobarbital (Seconal). Barbiturate-like hypnotics include medications such as methaqualone (Quaalude), ethchlorvynol (Placidyl), and glutethimide (Doriden). Methaqualone is off the market because of its history of abuse. The class of hypnotics also includes chloral hydrate (Noctec). Benzodiazepines used as hypnotics include flurazepam (Dalmane), temazepam (Restoril), and triazolam (Halcion).

GHB is an illegal CNS depressant that relaxes or sedates the user. Individuals often use it in combination with alcohol and it is known as a *designer drug*. It has been involved in date rapes, poisonings, overdoses, and deaths. Individuals abuse GHB either for its intoxicating/sedative/euphoria producing properties or for its growth hormone-releasing effects, which build muscles. The effects last up to 4 hours, depending on the dose. In high doses, it depresses respirations and heart rates until death occurs. Overdose occurs quickly with nausea, vomiting, headache, loss of consciousness, and reflexes. The body metabolizes it rapidly, so it is difficult to detect in emergency rooms.

Antianxiety medications such as benzodiazepines include chlordiazepoxide (Librium), diazepam (Valium), lorazepam (Ativan), clonazepam (Klonopin or Clonopin), and alprazolam (Xanax). Benzodiazepines are relatively safe as far as overdose compared with most other types of sedatives and hypnotics. Used in high doses, benzodiazepines disturb sleep pattern and cause changes in affect (Schuckit, 2000). Withdrawal from benzodiazepines is lengthy, and rapid discontinuation of habitual use of large amounts often causes seizures.

Rohypnol is a benzodiazepine. It is not approved for prescription use in the United States, although it is used in Europe, Mexico, and more than 60 other countries for treatment of insomnia, sedation, and as a preoperative anesthetic. It is tasteless and odorless and dissolves easily in carbonated beverages. When used as a drug of abuse, alcohol accelerates its toxic and sedative effects. Rohypnol causes anterograde amnesia or blackouts. When used to victimize others, such as in cases of sexual assault or date rape, as little as 1 mg will impair a person for 8 to 12 hours. For this reason it is often called the forget-me pill.

Stimulants

This category of substances includes caffeine, ephedrine, propanolamine, amphetamines, and amphetamine-like substances. It also includes substances similar in action but with a different chemical structure such as diet pills. Stimulants are popular drugs of abuse because of their effects on the brain. People become addicted to the sense of high energy, alertness, and well-being that these drugs produce. These drugs act centrally, meaning that their effect is in the central nervous system mechanisms that control heart rate and respiration. Methamphetamine not only creates an immediate surge in dopamine, it blocks reuptake of dopamine, creating more available neurotransmitter in the synaptic spaces.

Individuals ingest stimulants orally, intranasally, by smoking, or by injection. "Ice" is a very pure form of methamphetamine. Individuals smoke it to produce an immediate and strong stimulant effect. Abusers of this stimulant have recovered from the damage to dopamine receptors substantially after 9 months of abstinence, but not from impairments in motor skills and memory (Mathias and Zickler, 2001). In 2004, 51% of methamphetamine treatment admissions came from the criminal justice system (SAMSHA, 2006).

Stimulants such as methylphenidine (Ritalin) and dextroamphetamine (Dexedrine) are for treatment of medical disorders such as narcolepsy, attention deficit disorder/hyperactivity disorder, and obesity. The effects of the stimulants are similar to cocaine, but they do not cause local anesthetic effects. In some instances, individuals take them on a regular schedule, similar to other medications, even when abused. Users sometimes binge and have brief drug-free times. These drugs raise blood pressure and body temperature to dangerous levels and elevate heart rate and respirations. Aggressive or violent behavior occurs with high-dose use, and anxiety, paranoia, and psychotic episodes occur with abuse and dependence of stimulants.

Caffeine-related disorders are in the DSM-IV-TR. Caffeine is the most widely consumed psychoactive stimulant in the world. It is a methylxanthine, as is theobromine (in chocolate) and theophylline (Theo-Dur). More than 80% of adults in the United States consume this substance regularly. Caffeine produces a wide variety of symptoms, depending on the individual and levels of consumption. Tolerance sometimes develops. Caffeine is in many beverages, including coffee, tea, chocolate, sodas, and as additive in some brands of bottled water. Caffeine is also in some medications. Some people who ingest large amounts of caffeine develop delirium. Cessation of caffeine causes withdrawal symptoms including headaches, but because a person's lifestyle is generally not centered around obtaining and using caffeine, it is not typically considered a drug of abuse.

Cocaine

Cocaine is an alkaloid stimulant that is similar in clinical pattern, intoxication, and treatment approaches to that of other stimulants such as the amphetamines. Cocaine is sold on the street as an impure powder mixed with glucose, mannitol, or lactose. Individuals usually inject the powder intravenously or snort it nasally. Individuals often sprinkle freebase cocaine (which has a lower melting point) over tobacco or smoke it in pipes designed for that purpose. The crystallized form of cocaine, also called "crack," has a relatively low melting point and is readily soluble in water. Freebase or crack cocaine is usually 40% or higher pure cocaine, whereas powdered cocaine is less pure. Intranasal use has an onset of about 3 to 5 minutes, with peak effects in 10 to 20 minutes. The high begins to fade in 45 minutes or less. Intravenous use gives a high that lasts 10 to 20 minutes or less. Peak blood levels usually develop quickly, within 5 to 30 minutes. The cocaine effects disappear relatively quickly over 2 hours, although some effect will remain for about 4 hours. Traces of cocaine are in the urine for at least 3 days and are sometimes in the urine for up to 14 days if high doses were used. As in all drugs with high abuse potential, tolerance develops quickly.

Changes such as euphoria or affective blunting, hypervigilance, agitation or anger, impaired judgment and social functioning, and anxiety characterize cocaine intoxication. Depressant effects such as sadness, decreased blood pressure, and psychomotor retardation occur with long-term, high-dose use. The course of intoxication is usually self-limiting to approximately 24 hours, after which withdrawal symptoms occur. These withdrawal symptoms are often referred to as the "crash" when the person is depressed, which stimulates a repeat cycle of use, withdrawal, and using again.

Opioids

Opioids include natural substances such as morphine, synthetics with morphine-like action, and semisynthetic drugs such as heroin. People have used opioids for at least 3500 years. Codeine and related medications such as oxycodone (OxyContin), hydrocodone (Vicodin), and hydromorphone (Dilaudid) are synthetics with morphine-like action. Fentanyl is a synthetic medication that individuals inject or use transdermally. Other opioids are either injected or taken orally. Other manufactured, synthetic opioids include meperidine (Demerol), methadone, and propoxyphene (Darvon). Opioids are anesthetic agents, antidiarrheal agents, cough suppressants, and pain relievers. Heroin is the most widely abused opiate alkaloid. It used to be prescribed in the United States to treat pain until its abuse potential was realized, but other countries still use it for pain control. Individuals either inject or smoke heroin and snort when a very pure form of the drug is available.

Like those addicted to any substance, people who use opioids center their lives on acquiring and using the drug. Morphine and heroin-dependent individuals consume huge amounts (as much as 5000 mg) of the drug. Fatal overdose is not unusual, caused by mistaking the strength of the drug or the quantity required for the desired effect. Signs of opioid intoxication include maladaptive behavioral or psychologic changes that develop during or shortly after use and pinpoint pupils. Euphoria is followed by apathy, dysphoria, psychomotor retardation or agitation, and impaired judgment or functioning. Cognitive changes such as drowsiness or coma, and slurred speech, are also evident.

Because opioids are pain-numbing analgesic drugs, persons using them routinely are not aware of their serious health problems. Intravenous drug users are at risk for subacute bacterial endocarditis (SBE) or other circulatory compromise created by foreign substances introduced in the process of intravenous use. A nurse working in any setting with a client with unexplained fever needs to ask the patient about IV drug use.

Steroids

Steroids, a topic of concern in substance use disorders, are manufactured substances related to male sex hormones. *Anabolic* refers to muscle building, and *androgenic* refers to increased masculine characteristics. Since the 1950s, athletes have used these steroids to boost their athletic performance. Individuals take anabolic steroids orally or by injection, usually in cycles of weeks or months rather than continuously. This type of schedule, called *cycling*, involves taking multiple doses of anabolic steroids over a specific period of time, stopping for a time, then starting again. Users also combine several types of steroids to maximize effectiveness while minimizing negative effects (called *stacking*). In *pyramiding*, a person starts with low doses of stacked drugs, then gradually increases the doses for 6 to 12 weeks. In the second half of the cycle, the individual gradually reduces the doses to zero.

Abuse of anabolic steroids is associated with higher risks for heart attacks and strokes, and increased risk of liver problems for those ingesting oral doses. Physical changes include breast development and genital shrinking in men plus increased risk of prostate cancer, infertility, and reduced sperm count. Women experience masculinization of their bodies with growth of facial hair and male-pattern baldness, changes in the menstrual cycle, enlargement of the clitoris, and a deepened voice. Effects on adolescents are to change growth hormones, resulting in arrested physical development. For all individuals, extreme mood swings occur, accompanied by violent behaviors. Depression, paranoid jealousy, delusions, and impaired judgment all occur as a result of anabolic steroid abuse (NIDA, "Anabolic Steroids," *Community Drug Alert Bulletin*, 2002).

Hallucinogens

Many different compounds are in this class of drugs. Hallucinogens alter perception, cognition, and mood. Lysergic acid diethylamide (LSD), one of the primary drugs in this class, was discovered in 1943. The widespread use of this semisynthetic drug, developed by the military for possible use as a chemical warfare agent, led to widespread use and abuse of hallucinogenic drugs. These drugs were made more cheaply and distributed more easily than the botanical versions such as psilocybin mushrooms and mescaline (peyote cacti). LSD is illegal and available in various forms.

Other drugs in this class include 3,4-methylenedioxymethamphetamine (MDMA, also called "ecstasy"); 3,4-methylenedioxyamphetamine (MDA); and 3,4-methylenedioxy-*N*-ethylamphetamine (MDEA, MDE). These are "club drugs" or "designer drugs" and are neurotoxic. Individuals usually take MDA and MDMA orally. Effects last between 3 and 6 hours, although confusion, depression, sleep problems, and paranoia often last weeks longer.

The use of MDA and MDMA sometimes results in deaths resulting from neurotoxicity, or serotonin syndrome. Symptoms include drug-induced anxiety or panic, hyponatremia, and hyperthermia (oral temperatures of more than 103° F). Autopsies show signs of rapid muscle destruction with massive hepatic necrosis, kidney failure, and heat stroke. Ecstasy causes neurons to release serotonin, leading to euphoria. Some individuals couple the use of ecstasy with antidepressants that block the reuptake of serotonin from the synaptic space, creating a substantial increase of serotonin in the brain, called serotonin syndrome. Individuals manufacture these drugs illegally in unregulated labs, so purchasers are never certain about the substances they are ingesting. Analysis of ecstasy has yielded amphetamines, ketamines, and other substances. For several years, this class of drug was imported to the United States primarily from Eastern Europe.

Clinical symptoms of hallucinogen use include panic attacks, flashbacks (unwanted recurrence of drug effects), psychosis, delirium, altered moods, and states of anxiety. Tolerance and dependence occur occasionally. Hallucinogens are different from other drugs of abuse because cessation of use after long-term use does not result in a distinct withdrawal syndrome. Hallucinogens also place a person at higher risk of suicide and trigger psychiatric disorders from as little as one dose of a hallucinogen (Sadock and Sadock, 2000).

Phencyclidine and Ketamine

Phencyclidine (PCP) is a hallucinogen, but it has its own set of CNS reactions. PCP interacts with a uniquely high-affinity binding potentials. It was initially an anesthetic, but providers discontinued its use because of severe reactions. It has a long duration of action and, because of potency, carries a high risk of toxicity. Individuals usually inhale or smoke it, although there are other routes of administration. Individuals often use PCP with other substances such as tetrahydrocannabinol (THC), cocaine, methamphetamine, or LSD. Clinical indications of significant neuronal hyperexcitability, hypertension, and hyperthermia are a potential medical emergency. As concentrations of PCP change, mixtures of symptoms of intoxication, delirium, psychosis, confusion, paranoia, hallucinations, and violent outbursts occur (Schuckit, 2000). Use of this drug has been popular in the southern states and Washington, D.C. (NIDA, "Frequently Asked Questions: What Is Drug Addiction?" 2002).

Ketamine, also known as "special K," or "vitamin K," is an anesthetic that was initially used illegally instead of PCP because it is less potent and has a shorter duration of action. About 90% of ketamine sold today is for veterinary use. Individuals often smoke it with marijuana or tobacco products for its effects of dreamlike states and hallucinations. In some cities, individuals inject it intramuscularly. At low doses, ketamine impairs attention, learning, and memory. In high doses, it causes delirium, amnesia, impaired motor function, elevated blood pressure, depression, and potentially fatal respiratory problems (NIDA, "Club Drugs," *Community Alert Bulletin*, 2002).

Nicotine

Nicotine dependence is the most deadly and costly dependence of all substance dependencies. Nicotine use is legal in the United States, and although use has declined, it remains a major contributor to disease and deaths. Approximately 50% of smokers die of smoking-related illnesses. An estimated 65.5 million Americans reported current use of a tobacco product in 2000. More than 6000 children die each year primarily as a result of sudden infant death syndrome (SIDS) and respiratory infections linked to parental smoking and to low birth weights associated with smoking during pregnancy. The types of tobacco products smoked include cigarettes (55.5 million people or 24.9%), cigars (10.7 million people or 4.8%), smokeless tobacco (7.6 million people or 3.4%), and pipes (2.1 million people or 1%). One trend is the increased recognition of the need for treatment of tobacco dependence. Individuals with other substance-abuse problems, especially alcohol abuse, are typically heavy smokers, as are people with psychiatric illnesses, including dual diagnoses.

Dependence on nicotine occurs in a relatively short time period. Reinforcement of smoking and the desire to continue using results from increases of norepinephrine, epinephrine, and serotonin caused by nicotine. The body rapidly absorbs nicotine into the circulation and it reaches the CNS is less than 15 seconds, and nicotine has both stimulant and depressive qualities. Smoking is also socially reinforcing for some individuals, particularly youth. The body metabolizes nicotine in variable times, which is why some people need cigarettes often and also go quite a while without nicotine. Because of this property, it is an intermittent reinforcer. According to behavioral theory, intermittent reward is the most compelling. Scientists do not yet know the mechanisms for variable times of metabolism.

Cannabis

This category includes marijuana and hashish, and both substances come from the Indian hemp plant. Marijuana typically refers to the upper leaves, flowering tops, and stems of the plant. Hashish comes from the dried resinous exudates from the tops and back side of the leaves of some plants. Cannabis, the bioactive substances extracted from the plant, remains the world's most commonly used illicit drug. It ranks fourth in the world after caffeine, nicotine, and alcohol. The active ingredient in these substances is tetrahydrocannabinol (THC), which produces most of the effects that lead to continued use. Hashish contains about 10% THC, while most marijuana purchased on the street contains from 1% to 5% THC. Some forms available today, however, contain up to 40% THC (Bennett and Bennett, 2002).

Individuals usually smoke cannabis in cigarettes or pipes, although some ingest it in food. Others combine it with other drugs such as opium, cocaine, or PCP. Symptoms of intoxication vary and include a "high" feeling of euphoria accompanied by inappropriate laughter and grandiosity, sedation, lethargy, impaired cognition, distorted sensory perceptions, impaired motor skills and performance, and a sensation of prolonged time sequences. The psychoactive effects are followed by other signs within 2 hours of use such as conjunctival injection (bloodshot eye appearance), increased appetite, tachycardia, and dry mouth. If the individual smokes cannabis, the effects develop within minutes and usually last 3 to 4 hours. Intensity of symptoms is related to several factors that include dose, method of ingestion, and the individual characteristics of the user. Cannabis is fat soluble, and high-dose effects sometimes persist for 12 to 24 hours longer as it is released from the tissues. Dependence and tolerance develop over time. One study showed that long-term users performed poorly on most memory, attention, time judgment, and information processing tests ("Long-Term Marijuana Use Affects Memory and Attention," SAMHSA, 2002).

Inhalants

This classification of substances includes products with breathable chemical vapors that produce psychoactive effects. More than a million people used inhalants to get high in the year 2000. For young people especially, these substances are cheap and easily accessible. Inhalants fall into three categories:

1. Solvents (paint thinners, degreasers, gasoline, and glues) include toluene, gasoline, ketones, chlorofluorocarbons, and others.
2. Gases (refrigerant gases; aerosol gases for whipping cream, spray paints, hair or deodorant sprays, and fabric protectors) include ether, chloroform, nitrous oxide (sold as poppers), butane, propane, gasoline, ketones, chlorofluorocarbons, ethyl chloride, and others. A common method of ingestion is the use "whippets," balloons filled with an inhalant and breathed for intoxicating effects.
3. Nitrites (aliphatic nitrites including cyclohexyl nitrite, amyl nitrite, and butyl nitrite [now illegal]).

Inhalants cause effects similar to anesthesia and slow body functions. Depending on dose, users experience slight stimulation, decreased inhibition, or loss of consciousness. Sniffing high concentrations induces heart failure, suffocation, and death. Other irreversible effects include hearing loss, peripheral neuropathies or limb spasms, CNS damage, or bone marrow damage. Reversible effects include liver and kidney impairment and blood oxygen depletion. Amyl and butyl nitrites have been associated with Kaposi's sarcoma. Long-term use leads to diffuse abnormalities in white brain matter (Rosenberg et al., 2002). Few formal human studies exist in this area as researchers cannot ethically conduct studies in which they ask a participant to do something injurious.

Club Drugs

As described earlier in the chapter, young adults at all-night parties called raves or trances are using club drugs (designer drugs). MDMA (ecstasy), GHB, Rohypnol, ketamine, methamphetamine, and LSD are some of the drugs ingested at these events. All club drugs have potential lethal effects or produce long-lasting or permanent damage to the human body. Uncertainties about drug sources, chemicals used, and possible contaminants make it difficult, if not impossible, to determine symptoms, toxicity, and consequences of use of these club drugs in any given community.

Pseudoaddiction

There is an important distinction between people who become addicted because of voluntary recreational use and those who become medically addicted because of the use of large amounts of opiates or other addicting drugs over a long period of time for legitimate medical reasons, resulting in **pseudoaddiction**. Even though these individuals become dependent on the drug, their lifestyle is not one of addiction. Those with chronic pain conditions fall into this category, which is not in the DSM. In addition, some people with an addiction have physical problems that necessitate pain relief. Some are anxious about obtaining the medication required for pain and are in psychologic and physical distress if the medication is not available. Undertreatment of pain sometimes leads to this phenomenon. Individuals with inadequate pain control sometimes horde (store) medications to use when they are in severe pain and have escalating anger and frustration when they are unable to obtain needed medication. Thus, they appear drug seeking. These individuals need a pain control management plan and access to medications to relieve their pain. Careful assessment is necessary to determine client needs (Freeman, 2005b).

Non–Dependence-Producing Drugs of Abuse

The *International Classification of Diseases*, tenth edition (ICD-10), has a category for these medications that physicians initially recommend but the client continues to use them even though they are medically unnecessary. Excessive dosage ranges occur. Medications in this category include antidepressants, analgesics, antacids, vitamins, steroids, hormones, laxatives, specific herbal or folk remedies, and diuretics. Usually the client has a strong motivation to take these drugs or to continue taking them, but no dependence or withdrawal symptoms develop. In 2002, the Food and Drug Administration announced plans to aggressively pursue the illegal marketing of non-herbal synthetic ephedrine alkaloid products. Herbal ephedrine alkaloids, known as ephedra, were sold in the United States as weight loss, energy, and sports supplements. Negative reactions to this drug include irregular or rapid heartbeat, chest pain, severe headache, shortness of breath, dizziness, loss of consciousness, sleeplessness, and nausea (Join Together Online, 2002). It is also an ingredient used to make methamphetamine.

Polysubstance Abuse and Dependence

Many people who use drugs try a variety of substances and settle on a "drug of choice," but use of multiple substances by those who use drugs is most common. Multiple drug use or abuse, commonly referred to as *polysubstance use or abuse*, is also likely to occur in individuals who progress through use or dependence on a variety of drugs over time. For example, some people start use/abuse with nicotine, caffeine, or alcohol. If they continue on to use other drugs, they often try cannabis, followed by stimulants, hallucinogens, or other CNS depressants. This differs from young people who consume any drug readily available at a party. The ingestion of multiple substances at the same time creates additional risks because of chemical drug interactions or potentiating effects.

Although individuals mix any combination of substances, some drug mixtures are more likely to occur. Those individuals with alcohol dependence are more likely to use or develop nicotine dependence. Those who are cocaine dependent are more likely to become dependent on alcohol. Some people who use opioids combine heroin and cocaine in a mixture called a *speedball*. The combination both enhances the effects and decreases the side effects of both drugs. Other combinations of multiple drug ingestion exist (Schuckit, 2000).

PROGNOSIS

Becoming dependent on drugs is usually a gradual process. Contributing elements related to individual, environmental, and situational factors influence this process. It is the same for the recovery process. One of the most prominent factors that leads an individual to recovery is the client's recognition that substance use has caused or influenced life's problems and interrupted functioning. Recognition of serious problems takes a long while, partially because of the frontal lobe involvement in addiction, mentioned earlier. Treatment professionals refer to the recognition of serious problems as "hitting bottom," meaning the individual is now without options for basics such as shelter and food, or is unwilling to tolerate their lifestyle because of negative consequences. The steps individuals take differ, but ultimately the goal is to change patterns of functioning to maintain sobriety. Sobriety is the goal for complete abstention from drugs, alcohol, and addictive behaviors. The client has to learn how to prevent or minimize relapses and get back on course toward achievement and maintenance of abstinence. Most people who seek recovery from substance use disorders succeed, especially those who are motivated and capable of functioning at a high level (Schuckit, 2000). It often involves several attempts, and many clients relapse nine or ten times before achieving and sustaining sobriety. A relapse or slip is not a failure but an expected part of the recovery process. Compare the recovery process to the commitment to a particular behavior exercise. It is difficult to maintain the activity without lapses. Addiction is not an intellectual process. Some are intellectually brilliant and still become addicted. Addiction is insidious and puzzling. It is a difficult challenge and people who have addictions are opposing a powerful force.

The course of substance use, intoxication, dependence, abuse, and withdrawal varies with the class of substance, route of administration, other factors as discussed under the specific substances, and each individual's internal and external factors. Nevertheless, there are some generalizations about prognosis and recovery. Intoxication usually develops rapidly after use and continues as long as the individual uses the substance. When use declines or stops, withdrawal develops and continues for varying lengths of time, depending on the half-life of the substance and related factors. Persons whose use of substances is recent typically receive a diagnosis of *substance abuse*. For many, abuse of particular substances progresses into *substance dependence* for the same substances.

The course of substance dependence varies. It is usually chronic, lasting 6 months or more, with periods of heavy intake that are sometimes stress related and periods of partial or full remission. During the first year after clients achieve sobriety, they are particularly vulnerable to relapse. Individuals with a history of earlier onset use, higher levels of substance intake and greater numbers of substance-related problems who also exhibit a past history of tolerance or withdrawal have a more difficult course of recovery. In a similar way, persons who exhibit comorbid serious mental disorders such as conduct disorders, antisocial personality disorder, untreated major depression, or bipolar disorder are more likely to experience ongoing impairments and, ultimately, a poorer outcome. A supportive community that includes family and friends, who are often lost during addiction, take a while to re-create. Recovery groups and their members frequently become the recovering addict's primary social support, at least in early recovery phases.

DISCHARGE CRITERIA

The following are examples of treatment outcome criteria that determine discharge readiness. Client will:

- Maintain abstinence or reduce harm (more applicable to some substances than others) from substance use.
- Admit to potential or actual lifelong dependence on psychoactive substances.
- Express knowledge of the continual process of recovery ("one day at a time").
- Verbalize realistic goals.
- Maintain attendance in a support group (Alcoholics Anonymous, Narcotics Anonymous, or others).
- Express increased self-esteem.
- Demonstrate new, constructive coping mechanisms and strategies to manage anxiety, stress, frustration, and anger.
- Engage in use of substitutes to replace drug-seeking, drug-taking behaviors such as hobbies, school, employment, spiritual support, volunteer work, social relationships.
- Express the feeling of being in control of one's life.
- Express hope for the future.
- Abandon people and situations that influence and contribute to drug-taking behaviors.
- State consequences of psychoactive substance use on biopsychosocial/cultural/spiritual well-being.
- State names and phone numbers of resources to contact when unable to cope, or when experiencing a need to relapse to substance-taking behaviors.
- Investigate substance abuse assistance programs in the workplace, such as the employee assistance program (EAP).
- Ask family or significant others to attend Al-Anon/Alateen support groups.

The Nursing Process

ASSESSMENT

The nurse maintains a professional, nonjudgmental attitude toward the client or significant others. The development of a beginning trusting nurse-client relationship is a priority with any clients but particularly clients with SUDs. Clients often hide, deny or minimize substance abuse though they are desperately in need of treatment. Because of the social stigma associated with SUDs, the professional needs to be successful in gathering information and building trust by firmly and gently questioning the client about potential substance use problems. Persons who abuse substances often have negative experiences with judgmental health care professionals. Though understandable, this type of judgmental or negative approach discourages the client's involvement in health care systems. Nurses have the choice to reinforce this stereotype of the rejecting health care professional or form a new relationship with the client based on insights and an understanding of the client's situation.

The identification of substance-related symptoms is usually based on self-report. The nurse's awareness of what the client does *not* say as well as what the client says is important. The nurse makes decisions about when to ask questions, what questions to ask, and when to seek more information from those who know the client (see the Case Study). In many instances, the nurse confirms the history with family members, significant others, and previous treatment facilities. The nurse also assesses the client's readiness for change because motivation plays a key role in the success or failure of treatment efforts. By remembering that assessment is an ongoing process, the

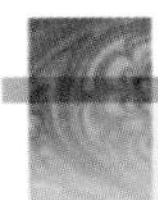

BOX 14-4

Drug Categories Considered in an Assessment

Nicotine: Cigarettes, chewing tobacco, pipe smoking, snuff, etc.
Alcohol: Beer, wine, whiskey, gin, etc.
Cannabis: Marijuana, pot, hashish
Cocaine: Crack, freebase
Central nervous system depressants: Sedatives, hypnotics, and anxiolytic-related drugs
Central nervous system stimulants: Caffeine, ephedra, amphetamines, diet pills, benzedrine inhalers
Opioids: Heroin, codeine, methadone, oxycodone (OxyContin), hydrocodone (Vicodin), morphine
Hallucinogens: Lysergic acid diethylamide (LSD), mescaline, phencyclidine (PCP), mushrooms, peyote
Inhalants: Solvents (glue, paint, gasolines), aromatic hydrocarbons (aerosols, gases, hair spray), nitrites
Anabolic-androgenic steroids
Synthetics: Meperidine hydrochloride (Demerol), propoxyphene hydrochloride (Darvon)
Over-the-counter (OTC) drugs: Antihistamines, cough syrups, sleeping pills, hormones, laxatives, herbal products
Designer/club drugs: Ecstasy, MDMA, MDEA, MDA, GHB, Rohypnol, ketamine

CASE STUDY Grace is a 32-year-old white woman admitted to the emergency department in a local hospital at 0200 hours following an assault near a tavern where she had spent the evening drinking. Though she never drank as a young adult, vowing she would never be an alcoholic like many in her family, Grace began drinking heavily at age 28 and was in a treatment program following a DUI 1 year ago. Her drinking began after a divorce. Grace is now a single parent of two children, ages 10 and 7.

She presented with facial lacerations and possible other blunt trauma head injuries, saying that a man she did not know assaulted her when she did not want to go home with him. She was incoherent and confused. The nurse noted that Grace's temperature was 99° F, blood pressure was 160/60 mm Hg, and respirations were 28. A packet of white powder found in Grace's pocket was sent to the laboratory for analysis.

CRITICAL THINKING

1 What is Grace's most immediate problem?
2 What would you assess first?
3 What physical findings (other than alcohol) might indicate drug use?
4 What drug screen tests would be appropriate, if any?
5 What nursing diagnoses would be relevant at this time?
6 What complications might exist if Grace needs medical/surgical procedures?

nurse will obtain critical assessment data, even when the client limits disclosure.

When gathering information about drug use, the nurse uses a systematic approach by integrating questions regarding legal and illicit substances into the general history. The nurse also assesses age, ethnicity, and demographic factors related to drug use at this time. In addition, the nurse obtains information about use in other drug categories listed in Box 14-4. A client's positive response regarding any drugs alerts the interviewer to obtain further information about the specific drug or drugs used. The nurse focuses on the age of first use, the period of heaviest lifetime use, patterns of use, the presence or absence of binges, and any occurrence of blackouts. The nurse assesses use during the immediate past to determine the possibility of withdrawal symptoms or toxicity. The other components of a complete health history include a psychosocial history, family history, risk for suicide or violence (toward self or others), and a mental status examination.

Collaboration among the nurse, client, family, and treatment team is essential in the assessment, planning, and implementation of the plan of care. For the client who abuses or is dependent on substances, the path to treatment and recovery requires hope, realistic outcome criteria, and a comprehensive plan of care.

Physical Examination

On examination, identification of specific physical health findings associated with alcohol or drug dependence suggests the possibility of a substance abuse problem. For alcohol abuse, signs and symptoms include the following:

- Jaundice
- Arcus senilis (an opaque ring, gray to white in color, that surrounds the periphery of the cornea)
- Acne rosacea (facial redness)
- Palmar erythema
- Enlarged liver
- Cigarette burns and stains on fingers
- Upper abdominal pain resulting from inflammation of the pancreas
- Decreased sensation in the feet or hands resulting from peripheral neuropathy
- Positive stool guaiac (gastrointestinal bleeding)
- Hypertension
- Tremor
- Tachycardia

For drug abuse, signs and symptoms may include the following:

- Cardiac arrhythmias
- Needle tracks
- Cellulites
- Conjunctivitis
- Poor dentition
- Rapid weight loss
- Changes in pupil size

In addition, signs of withdrawal or intoxication specific to each drug class are sometimes present. During the assessment process, the nurse observes for and questions the client regarding the incidence of accidents and injuries that are related to substance use.

Screening Instruments

A wide variety of instruments are available for screening of substance-related or induced disorders. The CAGE questionnaire is a well-validated, brief screening instrument that is easy to memorize and use (Box 14-5). A positive response to two of the four items of the CAGE

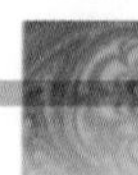

BOX 14-5

CAGE Screening Test for Alcoholism

1. Have you ever felt you ought to **C**ut down on your drinking?
2. Have people **A**nnoyed you by criticizing your drinking?
3. Have you ever felt **G**uilty about your drinking?
4. Have you ever had a drink first thing in the morning to steady your nerves or get rid of a hangover (**E**ye-opener)?

From Ewing JA: Detecting alcoholism: the CAGE questionnaire, *JAMA* 252:1905, 1984.

indicates a potential problem for alcoholism. The Drug Abuse Screening Test (DAST) contains 28 self-reported items and is easy to answer. The Alcohol Use Disorders Identification Test (AUDIT) is useful in identifying both drug and alcohol abuse disorders. If screening test scoring shows that problems possibly exist, the nurse follows up with questions about withdrawal symptoms, tolerance, legal and social complications, and work history. The diagnostic criteria for substance abuse and substance dependence are in the DSM-IV-TR Criteria box on p. 317).

Laboratory Tests

In addition to the history and physical examination and screening tools, part of the assessment process includes laboratory testing for drug use. Ethical issues continue to be a concern with drug testing, such as potential infringement of civil rights and the issue of obtaining the client's informed consent. The use of laboratory tests for diagnosing substance abuse continues to become more complex and sophisticated. A large number of variables affect the results, including the type of the drug, dosage ingested, frequency of use, type of body fluid tested (urine, blood, stool), differences in drug metabolism, half-life of the drug, sample collection time and relationship to the time of use, and the sensitivity of the test itself. A negative drug test may not mean that the metabolites of the drug are not present, but that the levels are not sufficient for reporting. For example, a person close to someone else smoking marijuana inhales some of the product. That person's lab test is positive for THC, but not at the level the government sets for reportability.

Laboratory tests do not always detect alcohol or the presence of substances. Relying solely on the results of laboratory tests are therefore misleading. However, abnormal laboratory test results often suggest substance abuse or dependence problems. They are also useful in tracking relapse or compliance successes of individuals in treatment or recovery. Blood tests are clinically useful in determining light or heavy alcohol or drug use. These are quantitative measures because they measure serum levels of intoxication. The disadvantages of blood testing include increased expense, the use of an invasive procedure, a narrow window of time for detection of drugs, and lack of usable veins in intravenous drug users. One of the most commonly used laboratory tests is the blood alcohol level (BAL). In most states, the BAL is determines legal

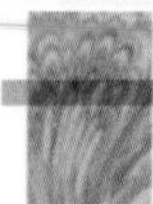

TABLE 14-1

Alcohol Intoxication

BLOOD ALCOHOL LEVEL (BAL)	CONSEQUENCES
20-50 mg/dl blood (0.02-0.05)	No legal consequences, some impaired coordination, potential changes in behavior
80-100 mg alcohol/dl blood (0.08-0.1)	Legal intoxication, impaired ability to drive, slurred speech, staggered gait, impaired sensory function
100-150 mg alcohol/dl blood (0.1-0.15)	Markedly uncoordinated balance, gross cognition and judgment distortions
Levels above 200 mg/dl blood (0.2-0.3)	Notable impairment in all sensory and motor functions
Levels above 300 mg/dl blood (0.3 and above)	Potential for cardiovascular and respiratory collapse; coma and death can occur if lifesaving measures are not initiated

Data from Schuckit MA: *Drug and alcohol abuse: a clinical guide to diagnosis and treatment*, ed 5, New York, 2000, Kluwer Academic/Plenum.

NOTE: States may differ in defining blood levels for legal intoxication and traffic violations. For example, Colorado has defined a blood alcohol level of 0.02 to 0.05 as a traffic violation if the driver is under 21 years of age (2000).

intoxication. Table 14-1 provides information on blood alcohol levels and extent of impairment.

Other laboratory test results used as markers include elevated liver enzymes and macrocytic anemia. Elevation of the liver enzyme gamma-glutamyl transpeptidase (GGT) is the most sensitive marker; an increase in the level indicates recent alcohol use. However, GGT is rarely elevated in persons younger than 30 years old. It is also a less sensitive marker in women than in men. More than half of alcoholic clients tracked have elevated GGT, red blood cell mean corpuscular volume (MCV), uric acid, triglycerides, aspartate aminotransferase (AST), and urea. Another indicator of recent heavy drinking (five or more drinks) is an elevated carbohydrate deficient transferring. The presence of hepatitis C antibody raises questions regarding substance use, though individuals can acquire hepatitis C many ways other than intravenous drug use.

Urine drug screens provide help in detecting the presence of drug/alcohol consumption within a specified time frame. Urine testing is qualitative and notes the presence or absence of the substance. Many report a significant number of false-positive and false-negative findings. Urine specimen tests vary, but most are low cost and have well accepted and monitored standards, and the samples can be retested or saved, if necessary. Typical urine drug screens that an emergency department performs include morphine, codeine, amphetamine, methamphetamine, cocaine metabolite (benzoylecgonine), THC metabolite, benzodiazepines, barbiturates, and alcohol. Many of these tests are also available for job testing or for home or private use. Shortcomings of urine samples include privacy issues surrounding the sample collection and possibilities of sample dilution, substitution, or alteration by deceptive clients. Many drugs are not included in either blood or

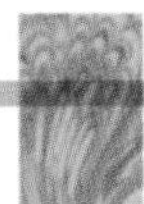

TABLE 14-2

Substance Detection in Urine

SUBSTANCE	DAYS AFTER LAST USE
Alcohol	0.5
Amphetamine	1-2
Barbiturates (short acting)	3-5
Barbiturates (long acting)	10-14
Benzodiazepines (Diazepam)	2-4
Cocaine	0.3
Opioids (codeine/morphine)	1-2
Opiates (heroin)	2-3
Phencyclidine (PCP)	2-8
Cannabis (THC)	2-8 (acute); 14-22 (chronic)

Data from Withers NW: Deceptions in addiction psychiatry, *Am J Forensic Psychiatry* 22:7-28, 2001.

urine laboratory detection measures. To determine heroin or cocaine abuse, many recommend collecting a urinalysis three times weekly. However, random, intermittent, interval screening also works and is less expensive. Table 14-2 gives a guideline for the length of time a substance remains detectable in urine. However, rates of excretion depend on multiple variables, so some figures vary from those in the table.

NURSING DIAGNOSIS

The nurse identifies nursing diagnoses from the information obtained during the assessment phase of the nursing process. The accuracy of diagnoses depends on a careful, in-depth assessment. Input from the client, family, significant others, and treatment team members is helpful in determining which nursing diagnoses are most relevant in treatment planning. It is the nurse's responsibility to prioritize nursing diagnoses for each client according to client needs. The most frequently used nursing diagnoses when caring for clients with substance-related disorders include the following:

- Acute confusion
- Anxiety
- Chronic confusion
- Disturbed sensory perception
- Disturbed thought processes
- Dysfunctional family processes: alcoholism
- Hopelessness
- Hyperthermia
- Imbalanced nutrition: less than body requirements
- Imbalanced nutrition: more than body requirements
- Impaired memory
- Impaired social interaction
- Ineffective coping
- Ineffective denial
- Ineffective health maintenance
- Insomnia
- Interrupted family processes
- Readiness for enhanced spiritual well-being
- Risk for injury
- Risk for poisoning
- Risk for posttrauma syndrome
- Risk for suicide
- Risk for trauma
- Risk for other-directed violence
- Risk for self-directed violence
- Sexual dysfunction

OUTCOME IDENTIFICATION

Outcome criteria for clients with substance-related disorders come from nursing diagnoses and are the expected responses the client will achieve. Nurses direct outcomes toward short- or long-term changes in behaviors and lifestyle. Nurses select outcomes depending on the particular characteristics of the substance(s) abused, the degree of dependence, the client's age, and other relevant demographic characteristics of the user. Outcomes provide the nurse and client with definitive, measurable steps to achieve before attaining desired discharge criteria. Examples of outcome criteria are listed here. Client will:

- Maintain sobriety.
- Maintain vital signs within normal range.
- Maintain normal fluid hydration.
- Remain free of seizure activity.
- Verbalize the ability to sleep without sedation.
- State that there is a reduction in symptoms of withdrawal (which may occurs weeks or months after last use).
- Verbalize a reduction in delusional thinking, absence of hallucinations or illusions, absence of suicidal or homicidal ideation.
- Verbalize a desire to stop drinking or using drugs, or in some instances to decrease/limit use.
- Verbalize, "I feel safe in my environment."
- Maintain a well-balanced diet of sufficient calories to meet prescribed nutritional needs.
- Participate in the therapeutic activities of the treatment plan (individual/group/family).
- Express a need to contact family members or significant others regarding support.
- Explore factors that interfere with the treatment plan (e.g., lack of social or family support, lack of financial resources, seeking old drinking buddies or drug-using peers).
- Verbalize that recovery is a lifelong process, which occurs one day at a time.
- Express the desire to establish relationships with nondrinking or nondrugging friends and avoid situations that previously invoked alcohol or drug use.
- Identify realistic goals for rehabilitation (e.g., continue with the 12-step program, random urine drug screens).
- Use community resources to establish and maintain recovery.
- Reestablish structure in lifestyle that limits opportunities for drug or alcohol use (e.g., work, school, or family activities).
- Substitute healthy coping mechanisms and activities for drug use behavior.

PLANNING

Nurses address many aspects of care when planning for the client with an SUD. Often, basic needs such as housing, employment, and nutrition enter the plan. If the client is hospitalized, discharge plans include sobriety support as well as resources to help the client obtain and sustain housing and income. Many have debated the topic of addiction being a disability, and because addiction is such a complex situation, there has been no lasting, good answer. Clients in early recovery clearly need a great deal of assistance, but as with any chronic disorder, stability is achievable.

As has been discussed, relapse is part of recovery, and the nurse and client need to develop a plan of care that meets the individual's ongoing needs. As in any nursing situation, the nurse bases care on the data gathered during the assessment process and also on a revision of that data as new information becomes available. Nurses consider the client's immediate needs, often of an emergent nature, as well as the long-range goals of treatment and aftercare. Collaboration with clients and others who care for them is essential in developing, revising, and evaluating the plan of care. For the client who abuses substances or has an impulse control disorder like gambling, the road to abstinence and recovery requires realistic outcome criteria and a consistent plan of care.

IMPLEMENTATION

The nurse working with a client who abuses alcohol and drugs develops a prioritized plan of care for each stage of the recovery process. *Client safety and health are always the first priority*, so the nurse focuses on treating and supporting the client through the drug withdrawal process called detoxification. Nutritional support, including protein-rich diets and supplementation with vitamin B, occurs in this first stage. If violence or threats toward self or others are a problem, the nurse and staff intervene to provide safety for clients and the environment.

In subsequent stages of recovery, the nurse and health team members focus on education concerning the drug abuse/dependence process; physical, psychologic, and psychosocial consequences of continuing to use drugs; relationship skills training; anger management; and self-esteem building. The nurse assists the client in identifying healthy supports and in developing a new support system that does not include drug-taking activities or friends. Abstaining from the substance is often the least complicated part of recovery. The final stage focuses on the client's life after drugs. To attain and maintain sobriety, people in recovery often must give up acquaintances and friends who regularly use drugs. They also frequently have to change living situations, get new clothing, learn to manage money, reconcile long-standing issues such as outstanding debts and warrants, and most especially deal with the emotional realities of life as a sober person. Without the buffering effects of substances, even small problems seem like major crises until the individual has been sober long enough to gain perspective and stability. Nurses help clients make long- and short-term goals and address vocational rehabilitation. It is essential to provide some sort of posttreatment contact with the client to monitor progress and provide ongoing support. Twelve-step programs such as Alcoholics Anonymous, Narcotics Anonymous, and Cocaine Anonymous can provide the individual with a framework and network of support for ongoing recovery, hope that sobriety is achievable, and contacts who understand the process of withdrawal and recovery. Other groups such as Rational Recovery are also available. For families, Al-Anon or Alateen are 12-step model programs available and provide support to those affected by addiction.

Acute Treatment: Withdrawal and Detoxification

Individuals vary greatly in response to substances, and their symptoms vary during withdrawal. The amount of drug that creates withdrawal symptoms in one person is sometimes different for another person. These variations are due to individual neurochemistry, tolerance, and many other factors. Predicting exactly what amount of drug will cause an overdose is also individual, though there are limits. Also, because street drugs vary in strength and purity, it is difficult to know the exact amounts a person has taken.

Sudden withdrawal or rapid decreases in amounts of certain substances in an individual who is physically dependent often require immediate medical intervention. Withdrawal states related to depressants like alcohol and stimulants are the most likely to lead to emergency treatment situations. Withdrawal from opiates is unpleasant but not usually life threatening. As in other types of emergencies, initiation of life-support measures is a first priority. These measures include maintenance of respirations and cardiac function and control of hemorrhage or seizures. A client who is debilitated before going through withdrawal is more at risk of complications from withdrawal processes.

If a client needs medications during withdrawal, providers often administer adequate doses to prevent the dangerous or problematic effects of withdrawal. Nurses who lack experience sometimes fail to give adequate doses of medication when a dosage range is prescribed. In the process of **detoxification**, the nurse gives enough of the drug (or one to which the person has **cross-tolerance**) to relieve the withdrawal symptoms. This substance, such as Librium or Ativan, is then decreased gradually over a period of days (Schuckit, 2000). Benzodiazepines like lorazepam (Ativan) have a cross-tolerance with alcohol, so they are used to manage withdrawal symptoms. Providers also use barbiturates. After stabilization has occurred, accurate history taking, physical evaluation, and laboratory testing will help to identify additional priorities for care. If an individual is withdrawing from multiple substances, he or she is at increased risk of serious outcomes. The Clinical Indicators for Withdrawal Scale–Revised (CIWA-R) is useful in many institutions to guide the amount of medication needed. The provider assesses the client on a variety of criteria and medicates the person based on a total score. This scale is typically used during alcohol withdrawal with a revised version for use with opiate withdrawal.

CNS Depressants

As with stimulants, symptoms of withdrawal are usually the opposite of the acute effects of that drug. The length of the withdrawal period is the half-life of the drug of abuse. Many individual variables influence this as well. Withdrawal symptoms from CNS depressants include insomnia, high levels of anxiety, elevated body temperature, pulse and respiratory rates, fine tremors, gastrointestinal upset, muscle aches, diaphoresis, and labile blood pressure. Confusion and other cognitive changes such as delirium, hallucinations, or delusions have occurred in some clinical cases of depressant drug withdrawal. With alcohol and barbiturates especially, grand mal seizures sometimes develop. Withdrawal from depressants lasts from 3 to 7 days for short-acting drugs and up to 3 to 6 months for longer acting drugs. Withdrawal from benzodiazepines results in characteristic symptoms similar to those that occur in or during alcohol withdrawal.

Alcohol

For 95% of those experiencing withdrawal from alcohol, symptoms are mild to moderate in severity and include those similar to depressant withdrawal. Withdrawal symptoms include two or more of the following: autonomic hyperactivity (pulse rate greater than 100 or sweating); increased hand tremor; insomnia; psychomotor agitation; anxiety; nausea or vomiting; and occasionally grand mal seizures or transient visual, auditory, tactile hallucinations, or illusions. Alcohol withdrawal begins within 12 hours of stopped or decreased alcohol consumption, peaks in 48 to 72 hours, and usually decreases by 4 to 5 days. Some symptoms last several weeks or months longer. They cause clinically significant impairment or distress in areas of the individual's life that are important to usual functioning. The mortality rate is typically low for those experiencing alcohol withdrawal (Schuckit, 2000). As with intoxication, other disorders need to be ruled out. Alcohol withdrawal delirium (delirium tremens [DTs]) occurs in less than 10% of those who experience the alcohol withdrawal syndrome. Alcoholic hallucinosis occurs more frequently and often includes frightening visual hallucinations such as worms or bugs. Though the person has perceptual disturbances, they are generally oriented to time, place, and person. Disorientation characterizes impending DTs. Adequate and rapid medical intervention in clients who are withdrawing from alcohol should eliminate these more severe symptoms. Clients experiencing severe withdrawal symptoms from alcohol usually require B vitamins, including thiamine (vitamin B_1), folic acid, and vitamin B_{12}, as a result of inadequate dietary intake and malabsorption. If alcohol withdrawal delirium is diagnosed, other general medical conditions such as liver failure, pneumonia, or recent head trauma sometimes also exist. If the person has been drinking heavily, withdrawal symptoms can start within 4 hours after stopping alcohol intake.

Pharmacologic intervention is not necessary for all cases of alcohol withdrawal. In some instances, general support measures will improve comfort. Although any depressant medication works, providers most often use the benzodiazepines because they are less likely to cause neurotoxicity and decreases in vital signs, and they are consistently effective. Short-acting benzodiazepines such as oxazepam (Serax) or lorazepam (Ativan) are given to clients with severe liver failure or those with severely impaired cognition. Longer acting drugs such as chlordiazepoxide (Librium) are for most others undergoing severe withdrawal from alcohol (Schuckit, 2000). If the client has had withdrawal seizures before, antiseizure medication such as clonidine is necessary. The history of withdrawal seizures is an important part of an intake assessment for an individual withdrawing from alcohol.

Acamprosate (Campral) is a medication used to treat craving in early sobriety. Clinical studies are in progress, and clients report mixed results. Other medications are in the development stage.

Opioids

Beginning withdrawal from the last dose ranges from 4 to 12 hours for heroin and up to 1 to 3 days for methadone. Peak intensity occurs within 48 to 72 hours. Acute withdrawal symptoms from heroin last about 5 days, and those for methadone last several weeks. Sometimes withdrawal symptoms last longer, and sometimes they do not completely end for several months. Symptoms of morphine and heroin withdrawal include craving and irritability, lacrimation (tearing of the eyes), rhinorrhea (runny nose), diaphoresis, and yawning. As withdrawal progresses the following occur: restless sleep, involuntary leg movements, restlessness, hypertension, tachycardia and temperature irregularities, dilated pupils, loss of appetite, gooseflesh, back and other muscle or bone pain, and tremors. Finally, insomnia, yawning, and a flulike syndrome also occur. Clonidine (Catapres) is the most commonly used nonopioid medication used to treat withdrawal symptoms from opioid use. Side effects from clonidine include sedation and hypotension, so nurses need to monitor blood pressure. Methadone has been the treatment of choice for morphine and heroin addicts, although new technologies are emerging (see the NIDA website). L-Alpha-acetyl methadol (LAAM) is another drug used in opioid withdrawal. It is longer acting and is useful in communities that are far from methadone clinics. Methadone and LAAM are synthetic opioids given to addicts to suppress withdrawal symptoms. Methadone or LAAM maintenance continues until the person is able to withdraw from these substitute drugs. Methadone and LAAM are addicting, but individuals withdraw from them by gradually decreasing the total daily dose until they are methadone or LAAM free. Careful monitoring of methadone or LAAM levels is necessary in addition to monitoring vital signs. Overdose of these substances leads to cardiovascular collapse and death.

Suboxone (buprenorphine) is a new long-acting medication used in maintenance therapy, people can obtain this at a qualified physician's office instead of a clinic. Suboxone (known on the street as "boop") has a high street value and abuse potential. Providers often give naltrexone (narcan is the IV form, Revia is the oral form) to people in recovery to block opioids from reaching receptors in the brain. A new implant has been developed that delivers a steady dose of the drug.

Stimulants

For cocaine, amphetamines, and other CNS stimulants, the physical signs of withdrawal are limited. Because of tolerance, withdrawal may develop while the person is still taking the drug and includes nonspecific aches and pains. The clinical syndrome includes intense craving and drug-seeking behaviors, agitation, temporary intense depression, and a loss of appetite that gives way over time to fatigue with associated insomnia, continued depression, and a decrease in craving. Sometimes cocaine-related stimuli, such as seeing a white powder substance, trigger cravings for cocaine. These conditioned responses probably contribute to relapse and are difficult to eliminate. Symptoms related to the final phase of withdrawal from stimulants include exhaustion, a rebound in appetite, and a need to sleep and occur during the first 9 hours to 14 days. Normalization of sleep patterns, decrease in craving, and a more normal mood follow. Withdrawal then progresses to recurrence of fatigue, anhedonia, and anxiety. Treatment focuses on treating the symptoms and providers generally avoid using medications. An inherent danger is that clients will seek other mood-altering substances, including alcohol and benzodiazepines, to fill the void they experience from giving up stimulants.

Emerging data suggests that it is best to treat persons with methamphetamine addiction for at least 3 months to a year in an intensive, comprehensive, and highly structured living environment. Clients also participate in a long-term and intensive outpatient program that provides information on structure and life skills, and instruction and education focused on managing triggers and cravings. Relapse prevention includes providing educational, vocational, and employment opportunities and involvement in 12-step programs with the recommendation of life-time enrollment in such programs. No one treatment or protocol works for everyone (SAMHSA) (retrieved July 2006 from www.nida.nih.gov/Infofacts/methamphetamine.html).

Caffeine

Withdrawal from caffeine-related disorders usually occurs with relatively low doses of caffeine in both adults and children. Caffeine withdrawal occurs around 12 to 24 hours after consumption ends and usually resolves in 2 to 7 days. Symptoms include headache, fatigue, yawning, nausea, or more disturbing symptoms such as muscle tension, irritability, anxiety, and cognitive changes. Because the symptoms of caffeine withdrawal often overlap with other medical conditions, psychiatric disorders, and drug withdrawal states, a careful assessment of recent caffeine use is an important consideration. If a client consumes caffeine and this relieves the symptoms, this will clarify the diagnosis (Sadock and Sadock, 2000).

Nicotine

Nicotine withdrawal has characteristic features of dysphoric or depressed mood, insomnia, irritability, frustration or anger, anxiety, difficulty concentrating, restlessness or impatience, decreased heart rate, and increased appetite or weight gain. Craving is a common occurrence after quitting. Most withdrawal symptoms peak in 1 to 3 days, but withdrawal symptoms often last 4 to 6 weeks or more. Craving and weight gain continue even longer. Symptoms are most acute among those who smoke cigarettes. Nicotine replacement therapies, including gum, patches, sprays, and inhalers, help lessen the impact of withdrawal symptoms and double the cessation rates of tobacco use. Non-nicotine medications such as bupropion (Zyban or Wellbutrin) and clonidine (Catapres) also treat withdrawal symptoms (Sadock and Sadock, 2000). Without medical assistance, 80% of smokers who quit will relapse within the first 2 years. Studies indicate that remaining in a smoking cessation program for at least a year significantly improves success rates. These programs involve phoning the patient or having he or she check in online, always offering the patient the option to return to a cessation class when necessary.

Hallucinogens and Inhalants

There is no clinically significant withdrawal syndrome for hallucinogens or inhalants. Treatment facilities for inhalant users are difficult to find. Research suggests that chronic users are the most difficult to treat and exhibit numerous social and psychologic problems. Users often suffer withdrawal symptoms such as hallucinations, nausea, excess sweating, hand tremors, muscle cramps, headaches, chills, and delirium tremens. Relapse is common.

Other categories of illicit or legal drugs are generally associated with mild to moderate withdrawal symptoms. Symptoms of cannabis withdrawal such as irritability, tremor, perspiration, nausea, appetite change, and sleep disturbances have been documented with high doses, but the clinical significance is uncertain. Withdrawal therefore is not a criterion in the DSM-IV-TR (Sadock and Sadock, 2000). Treatment is supportive.

Nursing Interventions

In acute situations:

1. Maintain a patent airway in the client, monitor vital signs, and intervene in situations involving client hemorrhage, seizures or cardiac arrest *to address the client's life-threatening problems.*

For all clients:

2. Maintain the safety of the client and others (chemical or mechanical restraint is sometimes necessary) *be-*

cause some clients exhibit unanticipated, out of control, violent, or assaultive behaviors.

3. Observe for additional signs and symptoms of substance overdose, withdrawal, and drug-to-drug interactions *to prevent complications.*
4. Assess the physiologic and psychologic symptoms of withdrawal and the effects of medications prescribed during the withdrawal process *to provide safe, effective treatment during withdrawal.*
5. Initiate therapeutic interventions to treat withdrawal symptoms, including anxiety and other complications, *to help the client safely withdraw from the addictive substance.*
6. Provide emotional support to the client, family, and significant others *to establish trust and include those important to the client in the treatment process.*
7. Support the client in meeting nutritional/metabolic needs either orally or intravenously, depending on the client's ability to take and retain fluids, *to provide adequate hydration and food as needed.*
8. Refer to a nutritionist as needed or engage the family in identifying and meeting the client's personal, cultural, or spiritual preferences *to offer holistic and interdisciplinary care.*
9. Increase carbohydrate intake and offer straws or other edible or nonedible but safe objects/foods to chew on (e.g., sugar-free hard candies, trail mix, toothpicks, straws, and gum) *to decrease some of the client's cravings for illicit substances and satisfy the client's oral needs.*
10. Initiate a vitamin and mineral replacement therapeutic regimen as prescribed *because low levels of vitamin B and other vitamins and minerals such A, C, D, E, and K, iron, magnesium, and zinc are common with chronic alcohol ingestion.*
11. Provide support to the client/family in acknowledging deception and denial. *A variety of psychotherapeutic techniques are useful for the client/family because interventions involving support and empathy, while not enabling the client, assist the individual/family to work through the denial process and develop awareness that many life problems are related to substance-abuse* (see Chapter 23).
12. Intervene with secondary medical complications or residual effects of substance use exhibited by the client *because the prolonged use/abuse of alcohol or other drugs sometimes cause a variety of complications and temporary or permanent damage to major body systems.*
13. Establish a trusting, caring, empathic yet firm therapeutic relationship with the individual *to help the client improve self-esteem and deal with thoughts of guilt and remorse.*
14. Encourage the client's efforts to establish, reestablish, or strengthen family/significant other supports through a variety of measures such as role-playing and providing a quiet and private environment for the client to meet with or telephone family *because clients who abuse substances frequently have lost meaningful contact with their family/significant others.*
15. Teach the client, family, and significant others about substance abuse, symptoms, management, treatment, and prevention, individually and as group members. Assess the style of learning that works best for the client to meet learning needs (i.e., verbal, visual, or written communication). Use materials in the language the client is most comfortable with, if possible. Provide factual information about prevention measures that work. *The nurse acts as an advocate and as a resource person regarding successful treatment and prevention efforts and the need for a healthy lifestyle for clients and their families/significant others.*
16. Support the client and family in maintaining active involvement with 12-step or alternative support groups, such as AA, Al-Anon, Al-a-Teen, Narcotics Anonymous (NA), and Rational Recovery. *Past experience in working with substance abuse clients indicates that lifelong membership in a 12-step or alternative recovery program is, for many individuals, the key to remaining sober. Families also benefit from groups that help them to change previous patterns of relating to the client and others.*
17. Encourage the family to be flexible and supportive regarding the client's participation in support groups *because establishing a new lifestyle, such as engaging in a support group network, takes time, effort, and motivation.*
18. Assist the client in establishing a new social support system by putting him or her in touch with community organizations where the client will find alternative housing, make new friends, and experience opportunities to build inner strength and develop drug-free coping measures. *The client often faces the enormous task of establishing a new social network that is drug free; knowledge and guidance regarding resources and recovery programs will provide invaluable assistance in making the client's efforts successful.*

Additional Treatment Modalities

Rehabilitation for substance disorders is a vital part of treatment. Now, more than ever before, researchers are evaluating treatment outcomes through funded studies. In 2002, SAMHSA launched a new program called "Changing the Conversation: The National Treatment Plan Initiative to Improve Substance Abuse Treatment." The goal of this program was to ensure that quality treatment services and programs were available to all that needed them. In this initiative, five key guidelines were identified:

1. There is "no wrong door" to treatment (i.e., anyone needing treatment is identified and receives it).
2. Invest for results (i.e., use treatment and services wisely to produce desired results).
3. Commit to quality (i.e., continually strive to improve treatment).
4. Change attitudes (i.e., challenge stigma and misinformation regarding addiction treatment and the nature of the recovery process).
5. Build partnerships (i.e., work together to make needed changes).

Treatment programs offer a wide variety of services and goals. Likewise, clients have different motivations and reasons for seeking treatment. It is important to recognize that there will be no perfect match of client and program. Instead, it is the genuineness, interest, and preparation of the staff and the approaches they use that will help the client to achieve recovery. Collaborative team interventions enhance successful treatment and rehabilitation outcomes. Providers need to use all available resources. Ultimately, it will be the client's decision and responsibility to achieve and maintain a life of sobriety and recovery. People often make the following assumptions about treatment (NIDA, 1999):

- Treatments are aimed at reducing the prevalence of a disorder.
- No single treatment is effective for all individuals.
- Effective treatment focuses on multiple needs.
- Remaining in treatment for an adequate time is critical for treatment effectiveness.
- An individual's treatment plan requires continual assessment and modification as necessary.
- Multiple types of treatment are necessary for most people and include medication; individual, group, family therapies; and other treatment modalities.
- The majority of individuals needing alcohol and drug treatment are likely to have a co-occurring psychiatric disorder (dual diagnosis).
- Recovery from addiction is a long-term process and frequently requires multiple episodes of treatment.

Psychotherapy

Psychotherapy for individuals with addictions is usually successful and addresses the client's addiction as well as any comorbid (co-occurring) disorders or life-interfering behaviors that are present. For example, therapy models and interventions for individuals with personality disorders will be different from therapies for persons with depression or anxiety. In general, clients with addictions are actively involved in a recovery program as well as participate in individual or group therapies.

Individual Therapy. One type of individual psychotherapy is for clients who have high levels of anxiety, inadequate coping mechanisms, and a low tolerance for frustration. The primary focus is on the here and now of the client's life as he or she learns to relate to others and adjust to a life without reliance on drugs. Some clients communicate more effectively in a one-on-one relationship versus a group setting. Cognitive behavioral therapy (CBT) is an evidence-based approach to therapy for substance using/abusing clients (Freeman, 2005a). Dialectical behavioral therapy (DBT) is also research based and has been adapted for use with substance use disorders. Research has also found motivational interviewing techniques to be effective with persons with addictions (Miller and Rollnick, 2002). Providing therapy to adult children of alcoholics based on developmental theories has also been described (Brown, 1988).

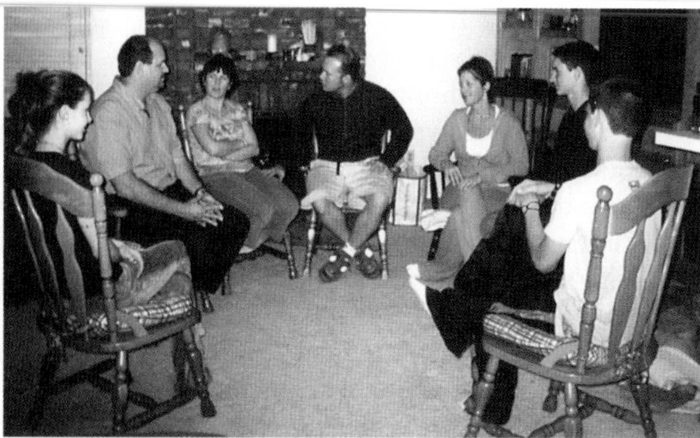

FIGURE 14-3 Family therapy is an important factor when one member is in recovery for substance abuse.

Therapists need to address the client's protective patterns of denial and deception during the course of therapy. Like many other clients, these individuals often test the therapeutic bond between client and therapist. They often address issues such as relapse, onset of depression, and resistance to continuation of therapy.

Group Therapy. Most therapies conducted on an individual basis are also adaptable to a group mode. Group therapy is typically more cost effective and reaches greater numbers of people. Group therapy has certain advantages for clients with substance-related disorders that are difficult to achieve in individual therapy. In a group setting, clients with similar experiences and problems confront or support each other in a relatively safe environment. The role of the nurse or therapist is to facilitate group members' participation and assist in clarifying interpersonal interactions within the group. In addition to discussions, the group also shares didactic or educational information regarding substance use and recovery. Clients in recovery who have maintained sobriety share experiences and serve as role models for newly admitted clients.

Family Therapy. Family therapy has gained credibility in treatment programs designed for both adults and adolescents. Family therapy is based on family systems theory. The genogram (Bowen, 1978) is a useful instrument for tracing the intergenerational use of substances. Researchers are scanning genomes to identify which members in a family are more likely to use illicit drugs. Recently, researchers working with teenagers isolated a particular gene that influences susceptibility to smoking. If the teen is also depressed, this increases the genetic effect. Other genetic and environmental research studies are under way to link family members with specific types of substance use. Some researchers believe that from 60% to 80% of addiction is related to genetic susceptibility.

Recognition and acceptance of alcoholism as an illness that affects all members of the family supports a need for family therapy (Figure 14-3). When the family member who abuses alcohol suddenly attains sobriety, the dynamics of the entire family change. Some clients experience relapse if the family does not know how to relate to the person when he or she is sober. Family members in alcoholic families often have a tendency to lack trust for one another, feel unloved and unwanted, and carry a heavy burden of guilt.

Behavioral Therapy. Some programs use behavioral approaches such as relaxation therapy or biofeedback to teach clients how to manage everyday stressors or insomnia. Usually behavioral modification approaches are used in addition to other forms of education and counseling. Approaches include assertiveness training or aversive conditioning.

Aversive conditioning is used with nicotine-dependent clients to develop learned negative associations with cigarettes. Aversive conditioning with disulfiram (Antabuse) is one technique of behavior therapy used for alcoholics. This treatment is not used extensively in the United States. Claims for lasting success are questionable because long-term studies are rare. The client is conditioned by pairing the sight, smell, and taste of alcohol with an emetic. Induced nausea and vomiting subsequently result in aversion to alcohol. After the conditioning experience, the client is given disulfiram, which inhibits the enzyme aldehyde dehydrogenase; even a small amount of alcohol causes a toxic reaction because of acetaldehyde accumulation in the blood.

Clients in treatment for aversive conditioning need to be in good health, highly motivated, and cooperative. Providers warn them about the consequences of using the drug disulfiram if and when even small amounts of alcohol are ingested. If ingestion occurs, clients experience flushing and feelings of heat in the face, chest, and upper limbs. Other symptoms include pallor, hypotension, nausea, general malaise, dizziness, blurred vision, palpitations, air hunger, and numbness of the upper extremities.

Rapid Detoxification Procedures

Rapid detox lasts about 3 days and involves heavy sedation to shorten opiate withdrawal and is usually accomplished in a hospital under the continual supervision of an anesthesiologist. Ultra brief detox lasts approximately 4 to 6 hours or less. Sometimes done in a doctor's office, providers have used the ultra rapid anesthesia detoxification method in the United States since 1995, and it has come under criticism for deaths during the procedure. Both procedures include administering the client naltrexone, sometimes in combination with midazolam. As mentioned, naltrexone blocks the narcotic molecule from the receptor sites in the brain and nervous system, thereby ending the effect of opiate drugs. However, because the life of addiction has not been addressed in this method, clients return home to their previous situations without other supports in place. Although the client is in fact detoxed from the substance, he or she is still in active addiction because the person's behaviors have not changed.

Oral naltrexone has few side effects and is the treatment of choice for highly motivated clients such as addicted professionals or individuals in the criminal justice system. Revia, the oral form of naltrexone, is like Antabuse, preventing persons from having any effect from opiates if they use them. Some clinical trials suggest that clients in early sobriety who are depressed have a better response to treatment and remain sober longer if they also take oral naltrexone. Providers need to warn clients that if they are taking this medication and they injure themselves, they will not respond to a narcotic analgesic agent until the naloxone is cleared. Some researchers believe that naltrexone reduces cravings; research is under way. Bodily implants are available in some areas.

Relapse Prevention

The principles of **relapse prevention** are used throughout the rehabilitation process to help clients avoid or take control of situations in which relapse is possible. The client practices steps to take if relapse occurs and develops a comprehensive plan to follow. The individual identifies situations in which he or she is most likely to relapse or use drugs and makes lifestyle changes including living areas, shopping, and selection of friends and family who will support a life of abstinence.

Harm Reduction

Harm reduction techniques help an individual to change patterns of use to decrease the risk of harm and to adapt a healthier lifestyle. For example, acknowledging that some persons are addicted and will use intravenous drugs, needle exchange programs were created to reduce the rates of AIDS and hepatitis C. In addition, providing opiate replacements (methadone, LAAM, or buprenorphine) eliminates the necessity of illegal activities like burglary to fund an addiction. Does this exchange one addiction for another? Yes, but harm-reduction techniques allow addicts to work, live relatively stable lives, and create support systems to improve the probability they will be able to live without illegal drugs. Other examples of risk reduction include designated driver programs, cigarettes with lower levels of tar and nicotine, and hepatitis B vaccination programs for drug users who inject drugs (Heather et al., 1993).

12-Step Support Groups

For decades, Alcoholics Anonymous (AA) and similar groups were the only widely available treatment programs. These groups still provide support and reinforcement in recovery for a large number of individuals. More recently, other programs of treatment based on other principles and research have become available. For those who benefit from groups, options are available to meet a wide variety of needs. Individuals who have been active in a 12-step program or in Al-Anon serve as sponsors (mentors) for those who are involved in earlier stages of recovery. Help is available 24 hours a day and every day of the week. Although the 12-step programs do not keep statistics because they do not see that as their role, anecdotal information suggests that the greater the level of participation in the groups and the greater the intensity of exposure, the more successful the outcomes. Participants in these programs see recovery as a lifetime process. They do not promote harm reduction; sobriety is the accepted goal. Contrary to popular opinion, AA has never supported aggressive confrontation. The goal has been to establish a safe and welcoming community with many resources where the individuals who abuse alcohol are able to turn.

AA is the original self-help group for recovering alcoholics. AA was founded in 1935 and was built on the foundation that support and encouragement from others with alcoholism aid persons on the road to recovery. AA encourages new members to work with a sponsor (a recovering alcoholic) who negotiates with the newcomer about working the 12 steps (sometimes a yearlong process) and other goals of the sponsor-sponsee relationship. Women sponsor women, and men sponsor men. Relationships in early recovery are not recommended, for a variety of reasons. The goal of sobriety is to create a life outside of addiction and to give back to the recovery community through service. The Twelve Steps of AA are listed in Box 14-6.

AA groups are available in each community. Meetings are open or closed. During open meetings, anyone with an interest, including spouses, friends, and significant others, are able to attend. Closed meetings are only for individuals in the recovery process. Groups are available for specific populations such as women, nonsmokers, businesspeople, and professionals. Some groups use American Sign Language, and many provide access for the handicapped. Many AA groups now accept the need for those with dual diagnoses to take prescribed psychotropic medications to keep their illnesses stabilized. AA is an international organization with a growing presence in many countries.

Narcotics Anonymous (NA) embraces a philosophy similar to that advocated by AA. It is a support group for individuals addicted to narcotics. Because many individuals are polysubstance abusers or dependent on multiple drugs, attendees often have problems with one or more substances. Cocaine Anonymous (CA) is another variant. Sometimes persons with multiple addictions attend AA, acknowledging that they are addicted to alcohol; persons who exclusively use alcohol are in the minority, though many people recognize that alcohol was their first problem substance.

Al-Anon and *Al-a-Teen* self-help groups operate independently from AA groups. Al-Anon is a support group for spouses and friends of individuals with alcoholism. There are opportunities to learn about alcohol as a disease and to share common problems and solutions with other spouses. These groups also discuss behaviors and issues common to the disease process, such as boundary setting, avoidance, enabling, self-inflicted guilt, and shame. Al-a-Teen is a nationwide support group for teens (children more than 10 years old) who have alcoholic parents. Similar to Al-Anon, the group helps children realize they are not the cause of their parent's drinking. Sharing experiences and feelings normalizes experiences that children think are theirs alone.

Adult Children of Alcoholics (ACoA) is a support group for adults who were raised in alcoholic homes. Adult children of alcoholics manifest behaviors of control, enabling, making excuses for others' behaviors (especially the behavior of alcoholic individuals), inability to trust one's self, and feelings of inadequacy and insecurity. Individuals learned these patterns in childhood, often from parents who themselves were products of alcoholic households. Individuals in these situations develop constant patterns of assuming responsibility for and taking care of others' needs. The support groups provide opportunities to discuss problems and feel acceptance from others with similar experiences. Sometimes people with these patterns are drawn to the helping professions.

Some people object to the faith orientation of traditional 12-step programs, which asks that members identify a "Higher Power." Though this power is defined in whatever terms the individual chooses, inclusion of Christian prayer in most meetings suggests support for traditional Christian orientation. Alternative groups to AA include Rational Recovery, which uses more behavioral approaches, Secular Organization for Sobriety (SOS), and Women for Sobriety (WFS).

BOX 14-6

The Twelve Steps of Alcoholics Anonymous

1. We admitted we were powerless over alcohol, that our lives had become unmanageable.
2. Came to believe that a Power greater than ourselves could restore us to sanity.
3. Made a decision to turn our will and our lives over to the care of God as we understood Him.
4. Made a searching and fearless moral inventory of ourselves.
5. Admitted to God, to ourselves, and to another human being the exact nature of our wrongs.
6. Were entirely ready to have God remove all these defects of character.
7. Humbly asked Him to remove our shortcomings.
8. Made a list of all persons we had harmed, and became willing to make amends to them all.
9. Made direct amends to such people wherever possible, except when to do so would injure them or others.
10. Continued to take personal inventory, and when we were wrong promptly admitted it.
11. Sought through prayer and meditation to improve our conscious contact with God as we understood Him, praying only for knowledge of His will for us and the power to carry that out.
12. Having had a spiritual awakening as the result of these steps, we tried to carry this message to alcoholics and to practice these principles in all our affairs.

MEDICATION KEY FACTS Substance-Related Disorders

ALCOHOL DEPENDENCE

Acamprosate calcium (Camprel) (for abstinence), disulfiram (Antabuse) (deterrent to alcohol use/abuse)

- Cyclic antidepressants may cause neurotoxicity.
- MAOIs may cause delirium and psychosis with combination use.
- Acamprosate is not recommended in children.
- *Herbal considerations:* St. John's wort may cause alcohol-like reactions.

ALCOHOL/OPIOID DEPENDENCE

- Naltrexone (ReVia, Trexan) works as adjunct in treatment of alcohol dependence and opiate addiction by decreasing cravings.
- Must be drug-free before beginning treatment.

OPIOID DEPENDENCE

Buprenorphrine/nalaxone (Narcan, Suboxone), levomethadyl acetate (LAAM, ORLAAM)

- Methadone is a substitute drug in narcotic analgesic dependence therapy and treatment of severe pain.
- Methadone has a high physical and psychologic dependence liability, and withdrawal symptoms will occur on abrupt discontinuation.
- Alcohol and other CNS depressants may increase CNS or respiratory depression, and hypotension may cause fatal reactions with high doses.
- MAOIs may produce a severe, sometimes fatal reaction; do not use together.
- Children are more prone to experience paradoxical excitement. Nalaxone and LAAM are not recommended for children younger than 16 years.
- These medications are not recommended for the elderly.
- *Herbal considerations:* Valerian, chamomile, kava kava, and poppy may increase CNS depression.

NICOTINE DEPENDENCE

- Bupropion (Zyban) is for smoking cessation.

OTHER DRUGS FOR TREATMENT OF ALCOHOLISM

Diazepam (Valium), clonazepam (Klonopin) for alcohol intoxication or withdrawal, and chlordiazepoxide (Librium) for alcohol withdrawal and anxiety

- The drugs are contraindicated in acute alcohol intoxication and acute angle-closure glaucoma.
- Abrupt or too-rapid withdrawal may result in pronounced restlessness, irritability, insomnia, and seizures.
- Alcohol and CNS depressants increase CNS depression.
- These medications are not indicated for children under 6 years old.
- *Herbal considerations:* Cowslip, kava kava, and valerian may increase CNS depression.

Inpatient Care

Inpatient hospitalization provides a structured treatment program for those who are severely impaired or debilitated, those who fail in outpatient treatment efforts, and those who have serious medical or psychiatric problems and/or are in an acute state of crisis. The hospital stay is typically short term, about 2 to 4 weeks, and it is best when followed by extended aftercare for 6 to 12 months.

Outpatient Care

Outpatient treatment centers teach the client to change and adjust to life without drugs while living in a real-life situation. It is less expensive than inpatient hospitalization and can be just as effective in many cases. Outpatient care generally continues until the client is ready for a less intensive level of care.

Halfway Houses

Halfway houses provide shelter as well as support, group therapy, and direct access to AA meetings. These living situations provide opportunities for gradual reentrance into the family and progressive reentry into the work environment and society. Halfway house placement is for clients who have been alienated from their families or are homeless.

Day or Night Hospitalization

Partial hospitalization is for clients who need additional professional support. Some clients resume employment and spend the night in the hospital, whereas others spend the day at the treatment center and go home at night. As with the halfway house, partial hospitalization provides additional therapeutic support during early or difficult phases of rehabilitation.

Previous research has shown that a minimum of 90 days of treatment for residential and 21 days for short-term inpatient programs is predictive of positive treatment outcomes for adults. Unfortunately, many long-term treatment programs have been cut or eliminated because of managed care. In the first large-scale study designed to focus on drug abuse treatment outcomes for 1167 adolescents, researchers found that longer stays in treatment programs effectively reduce substance abuse, symptoms of mental illness, and criminal activity (Hser et al., 2001).

Medications

Researchers search for the magic bullet drug that will cure craving and prevent a relapse. The best way to cure addiction is to avoid addictive substances altogether. However, as this chapter has demonstrated, avoidance frequently does not always work.

No one drug guarantees recovery. Therefore medications are typically an adjunct to other therapies. These include acamprosate (Campral), a promising medication used in Europe to calm the withdrawal effects of alcohol and produce an effect of lessening the preference for alcohol, and naltrexone (ReVia, Trexan), a medication whose clinical usefulness has been demonstrated in some studies.

Methadone and LAAM Treatment Programs. Methadone is a long-acting opioid similar to heroin in its properties. LAAM is an analog of methadone that has a 72- to 96-hour half-life. Providers give these drugs for similar reasons: to serve as substitutes for other opioids

CLINICAL ALERT

All clients taking **naloxone** (Revia) need to carry a card or wear a metal bracelet stating that they are taking naloxone and, if injured, will not respond with analgesia from narcotics. This information is critical in the event of a traumatic injury and important for emergency personnel to know.

such as heroin, to reduce criminal activity, and to decrease drug craving.

Methadone and LAAM maintenance for opioid dependence are only administered in facilities that are licensed, that offer counseling services including outreach, and that have security measures in place to minimize illegal use of opioids. The client must have been opioid dependent for a year or more and must not have benefited from drug-free treatment approaches. Some clients stay on these substitutes for 10 years or longer.

Opiate antagonists such as naloxone (Narcan) and naltrexone (Trexan, ReVia) block the effects of heroin and other opioids in rehabilitation and overdose. Most clients are then tested periodically for the resumption of opioid use. Treatment occurs along with other approaches and has varying degrees of success (Schuckit, 2000).

Community-Based Organizations and Faith and Spiritual Communities

These organizations often address the needs of families and have a positive impact on the problem of substance abuse. Social support from outside influences moderate or influence the effects of a family history of drug and alcohol problems. Many communities have developed after-school programs, mentoring activities, sports and educational programs, and other funded or nonfunded programs to provide opportunities for healthy relationships and activities.

Spirituality is an important part of recovery for many individuals. For 6 out of 10 Americans, religious faith is the most important influence in their lives, and for 8 out of 10, religious beliefs provide comfort and support (*Alcohol, tobacco and other drugs*, 1995). Teens who never attend religious services are at above-average risk for drug and alcohol problems, whereas those who attend at least weekly have a lower than average risk (*National survey of American attitudes*, 2001). Factors that foster teen abilities to resist drugs include positive peer affiliations, bonding in school activities, relationships with caring adults, opportunities for school success and responsible behavior, and the availability of drug-free activities.

NURSING CARE PLAN

Andre is a 45-year-old Bosnian immigrant, recently separated from his wife and two grown children. He was admitted to a psychiatric acute care unit with recurring symptoms of major depression (feeling sad and hopeless) and possible abuse of alcohol and hydrocodone (Vicodin). Andre sustained a back injury 5 years ago before leaving Bosnia when his family was forced to quickly abandon their home and he tried to carry his valued objects with him. He took pain medication (Vicodin) as prescribed, but sometimes it was not effective and he had trouble sleeping. He then began drinking alcohol to alleviate the pain and help with sleep. He is requesting more pain medication. Since admission, Andre reports insomnia, nervousness, and loss of appetite. He expresses despair about his constant back pain. This is his second hospital admission in the past year. The first admission was 3 months ago for suicidal depression. He was discharged on antidepressants but stopped taking them because he could not afford the prescription. He denies any suicidal plans or intentions now. Andre says he drinks "a pint or so" of vodka a day, or more when he can afford it. He is afraid of what happens to him when he tries to stop drinking and admits he needs help to withdraw from alcohol. He would also like to stop taking Vicodin but his work, which is stocking shelves, is hard on his back and he is often in pain at the end of the day. He was an electrician in Bosnia but does not have the credentials to work as a licensed electrician in the United States. His wife also works and does not want a divorce. There is some hint of domestic violence, but Andre will not talk about it. Both he and his wife are employed full time but have no insurance. They have been active in a local church, which Andre says is important to him and his family. *

DSM-IV-TR DIAGNOSES

Axis I	Recurrent major depression, alcohol dependence, opioid dependence (with physiologic dependence)
Axis II	None
Axis III	Back pain
Axis IV	Severity of psychosocial stressors (extreme = 4) inadequate finances, no health insurance, disruption in relationship, situational stressors secondary to immigration
Axis V	GAF = 15 (current); GAF = 45 (past year)

Nursing Diagnosis *Risk for injury. Risk factors: combined effects of alcohol and pain medication and risk for injury secondary to substance withdrawal (seizures, aspiration, falls)*

NOC Seizure Control, Aspiration Prevention, Fall Prevention Behavior, Knowledge: Personal Safety, Risk Control

NIC Seizure Management, Fall Prevention, Medication Management, Teaching: Disease Process, Risk Identification, Health Education

*Further assessment is necessary to detect if Andre has a pseudoaddiction, though the nurse suspects this when the client is admitted. Because of his limited financial resources and lack of health care insurance, Andre's back injury may not have been pursued as aggressively as possible, although alternative non-narcotic pain relief measures were included in his treatment regimen. Once pain is adequately controlled, it is likely that Andre's need for alcohol would be eliminated, as there is no history of a drinking problem before his back injury. It is important for the nurse to ensure that arrangements are made for Andre to receive outpatient care, which is challenging in a no-insurance situation. In this case, nurses need to collaborate with social workers who may be able to find low-cost insurance or arrange for temporary public assistance until Andre's problems are stabilized. This would prevent readmission and further difficulties with depression and pain control. Andre should always be assessed for recurring depression, risk for suicide, and the need for antidepressant therapy, given his history, even though he denied suicidality on this admission. (See Chapter 11 for more on depression and suicide.)

CLIENT OUTCOMES	NURSING INTERVENTIONS	EVALUATION
Andre will verbalize symptoms of withdrawal from alcohol (rapid heart rate, sweating, tremors, insomnia, agitation) and Vicodin (craving, irritability, restlessness), he will and comply with the prescribed medication protocol to manage these symptoms, especially withdrawal from alcohol, which can be life threatening.	Administer prescribed medication according to Andre's mental and physical status, *to relieve initial signs of withdrawal, and to prevent or limit the development of life-threatening withdrawal symptoms.*	Client verbalizes willingness to go through withdrawal in order to stop feeling "so sad and hopeless." He also acknowledges the need for help in managing his back pain other than using Vicodin, which he knows is an addictive substance.
Andre will be free from episodes of life-threatening symptoms related to substance withdrawal such as seizures, aspiration, or falls that can lead to head injury and death. He will trust the staff and the treatment protocol used to maintain his safety.	Reassure the client that he will be safe and free from harm or injury *to develop trust and decrease feelings of anxiety by explaining that he will be monitored continually and that his symptoms can be controlled with appropriate treatment interventions.*	Client states he is able to verbalize withdrawal symptoms and ask for support as soon as they occur. He expresses trust in the staff and the treatment protocol used to control his symptoms safely.
Andre and his wife will verbalize knowledge of the following: Alcohol and narcotic dependence and withdrawal symptoms The risk for injury or death The need for medical intervention, especially for alcohol withdrawal Available community support networks Importance of their church and faith	Educate client and spouse about alcohol and drug dependence, risk for injury or death, symptoms of withdrawal, importance of medication for safe withdrawal, and aftercare support *to help prevent relapse, injury, or death and to empower client and spouse through education.*	Andre and his wife are able to verbalize knowledge of alcohol and narcotic dependence and withdrawal symptoms, the risk for injury or death, and the need for medical interventions at first signs of alcohol withdrawal. They are able to list available community support networks and have made plans to attend one of them and to continue attending their church.

Nursing Diagnosis *Ineffective coping related to chronic pain, depressed state, and inadequate use of coping methods, as evidenced by dependence on alcohol and narcotic pain medication, necessitating medical withdrawal*

NOC Risk Control: Alcohol Use, Risk Control: Drug Use, Impulse Self-Control, Coping, Anxiety Self-Control, Depression Self-Control, Decision-Making, Quality of Life

NIC Substance Use Treatment: Alcohol Withdrawal, Substance Use Treatment: Drug Withdrawal, Medication Management, Coping Enhancement, Anxiety Reduction, Impulse Control Training, Mood Management, Emotional Support, Decision-Making Support

CLIENT OUTCOMES	NURSING INTERVENTIONS	EVALUATION
Andre will verbalize that he (1) has a problem with escalating narcotic drug use, (2) will comply with efforts to control pain with non-narcotic analgesia, and (3) will identify problems created by alcohol and narcotic pain medications.	Support client statement that he is dependent on drugs for pain control and offer hope that he can withdraw safely while symptoms are managed. *Additional support by the nurse can help client to achieve the first step toward abstinence.*	Client verbalizes that he is frightened and depressed and wants help from his family and the health care system.
Andre will practice effective coping skills that were previously used during difficult times and learn new skills to manage problems related to pain control.	Evaluate client's usual coping style by using interview/counseling techniques *to establish attainable goals and coping methods to achieve them.* Help client explore strengths and areas for growth *to assist in developing new coping skills and build on previously effective coping methods while discarding ineffective ones.* Collaborate with other health care professionals to explore continuation of non-narcotic pain treatment after discharge and pursue work evaluation for skills for nonphysical labor *to ensure that client continues to pursue effective coping skills and prevent relapse.*	Client is effectively integrating existing coping skills with newly acquired coping methods at the time of discharge. Andre identified the following effective coping methods: Perform exercises to reduce back spasms (with doctor's approval). Use only non-narcotic pain treatments. Find work that does not contribute to back pain or injury. Participate in alcohol and drug support groups (e.g., AA, NA). Meet with trusted clergy or therapist regularly. Client and staff are meeting to discuss pending discharge goals, and contact resources for reintegration with family and community. Client is actively seeking alternative work that will not result in pain or injury to back. Client will participate in community support groups for alcohol and drug abuse, and continue with church activities.

Continued

Irreversible Dementias

Alzheimer's Disease

Alzheimer's disease (AD) is an irreversible, progressive disease that ultimately leads to death. It is usually diagnosed after ruling out other etiologies (see the DSM-IV-TR Criteria box below). AD is not a normal part of aging. It affects approximately 4.5 million people in the United States (Lingler and Kaufer, 2002). According to estimates, there will be between 11 million to 16 million people with AD by the year 2050 (Hebert et al., 2003). Factors that contribute to the development of the late-onset form of AD include (1) socioeconomic, (2) lifestyle, (3) environmental, (4) illnesses, (5) medical conditions, and (6) medical treatments for these conditions (Katzman, 2004; Papassotiropoulos et al., 2006). A familial pattern is not evident with late-onset AD. On the other hand, the less common, early-onset form of AD that occurs before the age of 65 does show a familial pattern (Marin et al., 2002).

Several factors described next are associated with the development of AD. These include the accumulation of abnormal proteins, genetic mutations, neurotransmitter deficiency, and diminished blood-brain barrier competence.

DSM-IV-TR CRITERIA

Dementia of the Alzheimer's Type

A The development of multiple cognitive deficits manifested by both of the following:
- **1** Memory impairment (inability to learn new information and to recall previously learned information)
- **2** One (or more) of the following cognitive disturbances:
  - **a** Aphasia (language disturbance)
  - **b** Apraxia (inability to carry out motor activities despite intact motor function)
  - **c** Agnosia (failure to recognize or identify objects despite intact sensory function)
  - **d** Disturbance in executive functioning (e.g., planning, organizing, sequencing, abstracting)

B The cognitive deficits in criteria A1 and A2 each cause significant impairment in social or occupational functioning and represent a significant decline from a previous level of functioning.

C The course is characterized by gradual onset and continuing cognitive decline.

D The cognitive deficits in criteria A1 and A2 are not the result of any of the following:
- **1** Other central nervous system conditions that cause progressive deficits in memory and cognition (e.g., cerebrovascular disease, Parkinson's disease, Huntington's disease, subdural hematoma, normal pressure hydrocephalus, brain tumor)
- **2** Systemic conditions that are known to cause dementia (e.g., hypothyroidism, vitamin B12 or folic acid deficiency, niacin deficiency, hypercalcemia, neurosyphilis, HIV infection)
- **3** Substance-induced conditions

E The deficits do not occur exclusively during the course of delirium.

F The deficits are not better accounted for by another Axis I disorder (e.g., major depressive disorder, schizophrenia).

From American Psychiatric Association: *Diagnostic and statistical manual of mental disorders,* ed 4, text revision, Washington, DC, 2000, American Psychiatric Association.

Abnormal Proteins and Their Products

Amyloid Plaques. The classic characteristics of AD are the accumulation of amyloid plaques outside of and between neurons and the development of neurofibrillary tangles within the cells. **Amyloid plaques**, also called *senile plaques* or *neuritic plaques*, are formed of amyloid proteins and surround affected neuronal cells. The amount of plaques is related to the degree of mental deterioration. Amyloid plaques interfere with cell-to-cell communication, resulting in decreased availability of acetylcholine (ACh) (a neurotransmitter and chemical messenger of the central nervous system that plays a role in learning and memory). Decrease of ACh is associated with Alzheimer's and Parkinson's diseases. Amyloid plaques also result in the degradation of the gray matter of the brain (neuron cell bodies concentrated in the cerebral cortex and generally associated with cognition and intellect) (Taber's, 2005). These plaques develop when a substance known as an amyloid precursor protein (APP) is split by enzymes (proteins that change the rate of chemical reactions) to form short peptide chains called oligomers. (A peptide is a compound containing two or more linked amino acids.) Whereas these peptides are often 38 to 43 amino acids in length, it is the 42 amino acid peptide that contributes the most to the formation of plaques (Katzman, 2004).

Neurofibrillary Tangles. Neurofibrils or neurofibrilla are tiny fibrils that extend in every direction in the cytoplasm of the neuron cell body, maintaining the shape of the neuron and extending into the axon and dendrite (Taber's, 2005). Neurofibrils are critical to neuronal synapse and intercellular communication. **Neurofibrillary tangles**, commonly associated with AD, first form in the neurons of the hippocampus, an area of the brain responsible for short-term (recent) memory. They also contain paired helical filaments (PHF), which come from a tau protein. These proteins are associated with microtubules found in the glial cells of people affected by AD. Tau protein is structurally important for neurons, and when high enzyme activity causes tau protein to dissociate from the cell microstructure, PHF forms. PHF interferes with protein transport resulting in impaired cellular metabolism and ultimately, death of the neuron (Katzman, 2004).

The development of PHFs is actually the result of AD and not a cause of it. Moreover, neurofibrillary tangles are associated with tau protein formation in many other neurodegenerative disorders without the presence of beta-amyloid proteins (the main component of amyloid plaques, discussed above). In fact, 10% to 15% of clients with AD have Lewy bodies present within the cells, rather than neurofibrillary tangles (Katzman, 2004). Lewy bodies and Lewy body disease are described next.

Lewy Bodies and Lewy Body Disease. Frederic Lewy, a German neurologist (1885-1950), first described Lewy bodies in 1913 in association with Parkinson's disease. Lewy bodies are neuronal cells or lesions with colored bodies found in the substantia nigra (nuclei of the midbrain that help regulate unconscious muscle activity). Although Lewy bodies are present in the gray matter of clients with Parkinson's disease, the location of the lesions and the neurodegenerative process of Lewy body disease are different (see Parkinson's dementia, discussed later).

Diffuse Lewy body disease (LBD) is a late-life primary degenerative dementia. It affects mostly men. Pure dementia caused by LBD is quite rare. Most people who suffer from LBD have simultaneous LBD and AD. In this case, the onset is 60 years of age and autopsy generally indicates that Lewy bodies, senile plaques, and neurofibrillary tangles are all present.

Genetic Mutations. Researchers estimate that 10% to 40% of AD cases are genetic. Some scientists believe that eventually all cases of AD will show a genetic determination (Selkoe, 2004). The identification of abnormal proteins and neurofibrillary tangles associated with AD helped researchers to identify the respective genes associated with its development. Early-onset AD has been frequently associated with mutations in one of three genes: (1) amyloid-precursor protein on chromosome 21, (2) presenlin-1 on chromosome 14, and (3) presenlin-2 on chromosome 1 (Reiman, 2006). Chromosome 19, which codes for the apolipoprotein E (apo E) type 4 allele, is a common susceptibility gene associated with late-onset AD. This gene possibly accounts for 30% of the cases of late-onset dementia. New research has identified a genetic link between aging and the onset of AD. Scientists discovered two genes named HSF-1 and DAF-16, which they believe prevent the accumulation of beta-amyloid plaques, the main suspect in AD. These two "housekeeping" genes are like janitors that sweep away the buildup of the "gooey" beta-amyloid protein, but the genes become less active with age. Future research will pave the way for new drug treatment (Cohen, 2006). A recent international study has identified a gene named *SORL1* that apparently raises the risk of developing the most common form of AD (*LA Times*, 2006). It is doubtful that *SORL1* or any other gene will play as big a role in causing the disease as apo E does.

Neurotransmitter Deficiencies. Cholinergic neurons normally decrease in number as people age, making less ACh available (Gustavson and Cummings, 2003). Neurons that produce ACh are destroyed early in AD (Keltner and Folks, 2005). The nucleus basalis of Meynert contains many cholinergic pathways that are responsible for the production of approximately 90% of ACh production in the brain (Keltner and Folks, 2005). ACh conducts impulses between the neurons of the frontal cortex. The frontal cortex is responsible for complex thought, and the hippocampus is responsible for memory and cognition. Cholinergic cell loss and a decrease in available ACh are directly associated with memory and cognitive impairment.

Angiopathy and Blood-Brain Barrier Incompetence. The neurovascular model of AD development describes a compromised blood-brain barrier that results in dysregulation of brain interstitial fluid, and injury to neurons. In AD, capillary wall changes are often in the brains of persons with AD on autopsy. The changes, caused by atherosclerotic plaques, lead to nodular vessels with lumpy thickening of the basement membrane accompanied by thinning of the endothelium and loss of the fine network that normally cover the blood-contact surfaces. The result is the destruction of the barrier that prevents many blood serum components from entering the brain (the blood-brain barrier). Consequently, amyloid proteins are deposited in the walls and blood vessels of the cerebral cortex (Zlokovic, 2005).

Vascular Dementia (Multiinfarct Dementia)

Vascular dementia, formerly called multiinfarct dementia, is a change in cognition caused by the effects of one or more strokes on cognitive function. Nutrients are not able to nourish the brain because of the occlusion or obstruction of small arteries or arterioles in the cerebral cortex (see the DSM-IV-TR Criteria box below).

Parkinson's Dementia

Parkinson's disease (PD) is a neurologic disorder that causes tremors, rigidity (inflexibility), bradykinesia (slow motor movements), abnormalities of posture, a grave or mask-like facial expression, and a shuffling gait (way of walking). Dopamine producing nerve cells in the substantia nigra develop the pigmented Lewy body lesions that

DSM-IV-TR CRITERIA

Vascular Dementia

A The development of multiple cognitive deficits manifested by both of the following:
- **1** Memory impairment (impaired ability to learn new information or to recall previously learned information)
- **2** One (or more) of the following cognitive disturbances:
  - **a** Aphasia (language disturbance)
  - **b** Apraxia (impaired ability to carry out motor activities despite intact motor function)
  - **c** Agnosia (failure to recognize or identify objects despite intact sensory function)
  - **d** Disturbance in executive functioning (i.e., planning, organizing, sequencing, abstracting)

B The cognitive deficits in criteria A1 and A2 each cause significant impairment in social or occupational functioning and represent a significant decline from a previous level of functioning.

C Focal neurologic signs and symptoms (e.g., exaggeration of deep tendon reflexes, extensor plantar response, pseudobulbar palsy, gait abnormalities, weakness of an extremity) or laboratory evidence indicative of cerebrovascular disease (e.g., multiple infarctions involving cortex and underlying white matter) that is judged to be etiologically related to the disturbance.

D The deficits do not occur exclusively during the course of a delirium.

From American Psychiatric Association: *Diagnostic and statistical manual of mental disorders,* ed 4, text revision, Washington, DC, 2000, American Psychiatric Association, 2000.

NURSING CARE PLAN—cont'd

DSM-IV-TR Diagnoses

Axis I	Dementia of the Alzheimer's type with cognitive-perceptual disturbances Dementia of the Alzheimer's type with behavioral disturbances
Axis II	Rule out dependent personality disorder (traits)
Axis III	Diabetes type 2, controlled
Axis IV	Client is occasionally aware of her decline and expresses frustration. Client misses her husband whenever she can remember their life together.
Axis V	GAF = 35 (current); GAF = 45 (past year)

Nursing Diagnosis *Disturbed thought processes related to inability to process and synthesize information as evidenced by recent memory loss (becoming progressively worse), decreased ability to reason and form judgments, and interruption in logical stream of thought*

NOC Cognitive Orientation, Concentration, Memory, Information Processing, Communication: Expressive, Communication: Receptive, Medication Response, Safe Home Environment

NIC Cognitive Stimulation, Memory Training, Dementia Management, Reminiscence Therapy, Medication Management, Family Support, Environmental Management: Safety

CLIENT OUTCOMES	NURSING INTERVENTIONS	EVALUATION
Amelia will use her intellect and judgment to the best of her ability with the help of family/caregivers.	Develop a stimulating therapeutic activities program. *Cognitive stimulation in deficit areas and positive reinforcement promote self-esteem and encourage Amelia to attain the highest functional level possible.*	Otto and Elsa find that Amelia enjoys walks, and they establish routines. Amelia recognizes some previously familiar birds and indicates she wants birdseed to feed them. She also enjoys simple puzzles and assists Elsa in laundry tasks.
Amelia will retain some control in her life by exercising her right to choose.	Monitor Amelia's environment and activities and collaborate with all caregivers to do the following: Simplify choices in food, clothes, colors, and activities. Use multiple sensory cues, especially auditory, visual, and tactile senses, to indicate choices. *Choices, even simple ones, give control back to Amelia and improve her self-esteem, making her more willing to try to participate in daily activities.*	Amelia is responding to the use of multiple cues by increasingly exercising her right to choose. During the first week, Amelia makes an independent choice five times. During the second week, she makes seven choices.
Amelia will be oriented to place, time of day, scheduled activities, and family members.	Develop simple calendars with daily routines and easy-to-read clocks. Encourage family members to repeat their names and relationships often in conversations. *These actions assist in overcoming recent memory loss. Establishing routine decreases the stress of making decisions; verbal cues reinforce recognition and eliminate the need to chat.*	After 2 weeks, Amelia knows the time for her walks with Otto and indicates that she wants her supply of birdseed. She is less frequently confused regarding the identification of persons and never fails to recognize Otto and Elsa.
Amelia will use remote memory during periods of reminiscence.	Make time each day for periods of reminiscence using old photos, specially designed picture books, and rummage boxes. *The use of multiple sensory cues to stimulate remote memory is building on the retained strength of habitual skills to stimulate use of remote memory.*	Amelia looks at old photographs with Otto and Elsa and indicates her recognition with short phrases or smiles. She independently finds the box of various colored and textured yarns and handles them with satisfaction, indicating that she remembers knitting when she was well.
Amelia will have decreased catastrophic reactions (see Box 15-3).	Analyze with all caregivers what the previous causes of catastrophic reactions have been. Simplify the environment (evaluate furniture and objects, colors, noise level). *Analyzing and simplifying the environment maximizes the client's safety and reduces the stressors causing the catastrophic incidents. Collaborative planning ensures consistent successful approaches to tasks and reduces client and caregiver stress.*	Amelia has two catastrophic reactions during the past 2 weeks. Otto and Elsa analyze each incident and discover that the underlying causes were (1) increased noise from street repairs in front of the house and (2) being rushed to leave for a dental appointment.

Nursing Diagnosis *Self-care deficit (bathing/hygiene, dressing/grooming) related to perceptual and cognitive alterations secondary to neurologic damage in the brain as evidenced by inability to recognize the need for self-care (bathing, changing clothes), inability to dress in the right order, and inability to reason and judge (inappropriate choice of clothing)*

NOC Self-Care: Bathing, Self-Care: Hygiene, Self-Care: Oral Hygiene, Self-Care: Dressing, Coordinated Movement, Self-Direction of Care, Self-Care: Activities of Daily Living, Client Satisfaction: Physical Care

NIC Dementia Management: Bathing, Self-Care Assistance: Bathing/Hygiene, Oral Health Maintenance, Self-Care Assistance: Dressing/Grooming, Teaching: Individual, Self-Care Assistance: Instrumental Activities of Daily Living, Self-Responsibility Facilitation, Body Image Enhancement

CLIENT OUTCOMES	NURSING INTERVENTIONS	EVALUATION
Amelia will bathe three times a week with prompting from family/caregivers.	Determine habitual time and manner of bathing. *Establishing a pattern based on Amelia's previous habits will use her retained remote memory.* Ensure privacy *to preserve dignity and self-esteem.* Determine room and water temperature. *Comfort and safety will encourage positive client response.* Reduce sensory stimulation (e.g., noise from TV, radio, other people) to enable client to attend to the task at hand. Mirrors need to be covered if the client incorrectly interprets the reflection to be an observer. *Limiting the number of responses required by Amelia facilitates her cooperation and independence.* Provide a home health aide three times a week for 2 weeks. *Caregivers, Elsa and Otto, will increase their knowledge and skills and thus enhance their confidence and ease in assisting Amelia. The home health aide (HHA) will teach the caregivers ways to maintain skin integrity and general health. The supervising nurse will check on Amelia's general health status and type 2 diabetes.*	The home health aide successfully bathes Amelia twice in the first week with Elsa's help. During the second week, Elsa is successful on two occasions with the HHA assisting. Extend HHA assistance for 1 more week and reevaluate.
Amelia will be well groomed with assistance of family/caregivers and will comply with dental and hygiene care.	Determine areas of dysfunction in grooming. Set adequate routines of visual and verbal cues to assist in grooming routines. Assist directly only as necessary to complete task. Use positive reinforcement. Refer for dental prophylaxis and assist the family in preplanning with the dentist and hygienist for a successful visit. Assist Otto and Elsa in formulating follow-up plan for daily oral hygiene. *These interventions reduce stress for client and caregivers, avoid excess disability, provide a positive environment, avoid unnecessary physical disabilities, and promote physical well-being.*	Elsa and Otto are successful on 5 out of 7 successive days in cueing Amelia to complete her dental hygiene and in helping with combing her hair. An appointment is made with the dentist who previously cared for her, and Otto informs the dentist of the present situation. Evaluate success of visit later.
Amelia will dress herself appropriately with assistance from family/caregivers as needed.	Check Amelia's clothing supply. Simplify dressing choices for Amelia by the following: Remove clothes not currently being worn. Assemble coordinated outfits on one hanger and limit these to six to eight choices. Stack clothes in the order in which they are to be put on. Sort clothes and assist family in choosing those that are appropriate yet easy for Amelia to put on (e.g., eliminate buttons, buckles, pantyhose, etc., and replace with elastic waists, snaps, Velcro fasteners, knee- or thigh-high hose). *Amelia will retain control and independence by making some simple clothing decisions and will be socially appropriate in her attire, thus increasing her self-esteem and reducing stress for all.*	Family/nurse/HHA see the improvement in Amelia's appearance, and Amelia is responding with smiles at the compliments about her appearance. Otto is having some problems adjusting to the change in her dress style (not putting on hose and heels as she had) and in moving some of his favorite outfits of Amelia's out of the closet. Elsa comments favorably on the ease of dressing Amelia now and on Amelia's increased comfort, evidenced by her willingness to participate in activities and her calmer interactions.

Continued

NURSING CARE PLAN—cont'd

Nursing Diagnosis *Compromised family coping related to inadequate understanding of the process of Alzheimer's disease by the caregivers, inability of the spouse to adequately manage the emotional conflicts, role changes, temporary abandonment, weak support systems, and ineffective communication/relationship with the secondary caregiver as evidenced by Otto's being away from home more and Elsa's loss of weight and social withdrawal*

NOC Family Coping, Family Support During Treatment, Family Participation in Professional Care, Caregiver Stressors, Caregiver Emotional Health, Caregiver-Patient Relationship

NIC Family Support, Family Mobilization, Family Involvement Promotion, Respite Care, Decision-Making Support, Mutual Goal Setting

CLIENT OUTCOMES	NURSING INTERVENTIONS	EVALUATION
Otto and Elsa will verbalize realistic perception of their roles and responsibilities in caring for Amelia and will share their limitations and knowledge with other concerned family members and caregivers.	Facilitate meeting with all family members. *Sharing knowledge of status and prognosis of Amelia's illness establish the core of a support system based on mutual respect and understanding.* Address the family's knowledge deficits and obtain feedback from participants. *Education calms fears and promotes rational planning; each person retains knowledge in unique ways, and sharing a common understanding is vital to successful planning and implementation.* Collaborate in developing roles for each caregiver. *Understanding each one's role, including expectations and limitations, reduces behaviors that lead to abuse or abandonment of the client and elicits positive care outcomes for the client.*	Elsa meets with other family members who live in the area, and the family members express gratitude for being educated and included in Amelia's care; they offer assistance with outings and evening care. On two consecutive nursing visits, Otto and Elsa successfully review information on the pathologic and neurologic deficits of Alzheimer's disease and are coping well with Amelia's behavior manifestations. Interventions have been successful on four occasions. Otto and Elsa congratulate each other on their accomplishments.
Otto and Elsa will express their feelings in a mutually supportive manner.	Facilitate sessions directly for caregivers or provide referrals to appropriate health professionals. *Caregivers need permission to express themselves in a nonjudgmental, supportive environment.*	Otto and Elsa join each other for breakfast on most weekdays to plan for the day and critique the previous day's activities. Revisions of plans have been accepted in most cases.
Otto and Elsa will collaborate with all family/support persons in planning, problem solving, and decision making regarding Amelia's care and Otto and Elsa's personal needs as well.	Inform family of support services in the community. Encourage attendance at support groups or individual counseling sessions. *Support services and groups provide external assistance and concern for the caregiver's needs.* Facilitate positive methods (e.g., calendars, defining responsibilities and problem-solving tasks). *Sharing and preplanning will avoid conflict and pursue positive outcomes.*	Otto and Elsa attend an Alzheimer's disease support group together while an adult grandchild stayed with Amelia. Otto is late one evening but later apologizes to Elsa for the incident.
Otto and Elsa will exhibit effective coping strategies in managing Amelia's care.	Promote healthful methods of caregiver self-care (e.g., socialization, exercise, adequate diet, and time for personal renewal). *Developing effective coping strategies restores positive physical and mental health and promotes a functional family unit.*	Elsa has regained only 2 pounds but admits to eating better and feeling more energetic. She attends a sewing class, resuming a previous social activity. Otto is having dinner with an old friend before attending a pharmacy seminar while Elsa stays with Amelia for the evening.

EVALUATION

Evaluating the client's progress and how much nurses have achieved satisfactory client and caregiver outcomes are especially challenging with clients with AD and other cognitive disorders. Factors that influence success vary greatly with each person. Here are some questions that the nurse needs to clearly answer and understand before addressing specific topics:

- Is the cognitive impairment reversible or irreversible?
- For reversible dementias, has the underlying medical condition of substance use been identified and resolved?
- Is the client experiencing delirium, depression, dementia, an amnestic disorder, or a combination of these?
- What is the setting (i.e., acute care, long-term care, home)?
- Is the living situation adequate for the client's needs?
- Are the needs for activities of daily living, nutrition, safety, emotional and activity needs adequate for that person's condition or stage of progression?
- What is the caregiving situation?

- Are caregiver resources, knowledge, and understanding adequate? Are additional resources or training needed?
- What medical and psychiatric problems have been identified in the nursing assessment and history?
- What is the current medication profile?
- Is medication adherence a problem?
- Have medications for the treatment of AD been ordered? If so, are side effects a problem?
- Are there difficulties obtaining adequate medical supervision?
- What behavioral problems have been identified?
- What behavioral interventions have been effective?
- What is the client's functional status?
- What is the interdisciplinary plan of care?

When the nurse has answered the preceding questions satisfactorily, the interdisciplinary team will be better able to determine how the specifics of the client outcomes have been achieved.

CHAPTER SUMMARY

- The prevalence of dementia increases with age.
- Alzheimer's disease is the most common form of dementia.
- The cause of Alzheimer's disease is unclear. Current theories include genetics, abnormal proteins and their products, neurotransmitter and receptor deficiencies, and angiopathy and blood-brain incompetence.
- The key pathologic process is abnormal amyloid in the brain, which alters the brain's metabolism and results in neuronal death.
- The pathologic process of cognitive disorders results in neurologic deficits such as reduced ability to perceive the environment and organize appropriate responses, decreased attention span, language deficits, memory loss, changes in emotional responses, and a decline in the ability to reason and form judgments.
- Alzheimer's disease has three stages: mild, moderate, and severe.
- A variety of cognitive assessment tools determine medical and nursing diagnoses.
- The nurse plans and supervises therapeutic activity programs to achieve the highest possible functional status for the client and prevent excess disability.
- Caring for a person with a cognitive disorder is a significant physical and emotional burden for caregivers.
- All nursing care for clients with cognitive disorders occurs in collaboration with the client's caregivers.
- Nurses formulate care plans that are based on assessment of both the client's and caregiver's needs.
- Successful care plans are based on successful functional status and not on a curative basis.

REVIEW QUESTIONS

1 A nurse assists a client with moderate stage Alzheimer's disease at mealtime. Which statement should the nurse use?

1. "Would you like beans or potatoes?"
2. "Why aren't you eating your dinner, honey?"
3. "Your food is getting cold. Eat your dinner now."
4. "If you don't eat, you could get dehydrated."

2 A nurse counsels family members of a client with early Alzheimer's disease regarding the stages of the disease. Order these symptoms in the sequence they are most likely to occur.

1. Urinary incontinence
2. Neologisms
3. Apraxia

3 An elderly client is hospitalized with pneumonia and treated with multiple antibiotics. After 2 days, the client becomes irritable and restless, and says to the nurse, "My pet parakeet flew across the room." A family member says the client has been healthy and living independently but does not own a pet. Select the most likely analysis of this scenario.

1. The client is delusional and likely experiencing depression.
2. The client is experiencing illusions secondary to delirium.
3. Dementia has emerged as the result of the stress of the physical illness.
4. The antibiotic doses have been inadequate to treat the infection.

4 A nurse prepares the plan of care for a 79-year-old client with late-stage Alzheimer's disease. Which nursing diagnoses would be priorities to include? You may select more than one answer.

1. Risk for infection
2. Acute confusion
3. Risk for aspiration
4. Impaired verbal communication
5. Hopelessness

5 A nurse administers medications to four clients with Alzheimer's disease. Which medication would be expected to interfere with glutamate rather than cholinesterase?

1. Donepezil (Aricept)
2. Rivastigmine (Exelon)
3. Galantamine (Razadyne)
4. Memantine (Namenda)

*Additional self-study exercises and learning resources are available to you on the **Companion CD** at the back of the book and on the **Evolve website** at **http://evolve.elsevier.com/Fortinash/**.*

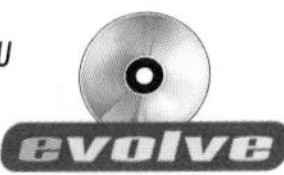

ONLINE RESOURCES

Alzheimer's Association: www.alz.org

Alzheimer's Association: Brain Tour: www.alz.org/brain/01.asp

Alzheimer's Disease Education and Referral Center: www.alzheimers.org

American Health Assistance Foundation: Amyloid Plaques and Neurofibrillary Tangles: www.ahaf.org/alzdis/about/AmyloidPlaques.htm

American Health Assistance Foundation: How the Brain and Nerve Cells Change during Alzheimer's Disease: www.ahaf.org/alzdis/about/Brain_Neurons_AD_Normal.htm

National Alliance on Mental Illness: www.nami.org

National Institute of Mental Health: www.nimh.nih.gov

Mental Health America: www.nmha.org

Rush Alzheimer's Disease Center: The Rush Manual for Caregivers: www.rush.edu/cms_docs/rushdoc_26.pdf

REFERENCES

Adeleman AM, Daly MP: Initial evaluation of the patient with suspected dementia, *Am Fam Physician* 71:1745-50, 2005.

Alzheimer's Association: *Alzheimer's disease facts and figures*, 2007. Available at http://www.alz.org/national/documents/Report_2007FactsAndFigures.pdf.

Alzheimer's Association: Facts about dementia: Korsakoff's; www.alzheimers.org.uk/ Facts_about_dementia/What_is_dementia/info_korsakoffs.htm, 2003.

American Psychiatric Association: *Diagnostic and statistical manual of mental disorders*, ed 4, text revision [DSM-IV-TR], Washington DC, 2000, American Psychiatric Association.

American Society of Health Systems Pharmacists: Reminyl to become Razadyne; www.ashp.org/news/ShowArticle.cfm?id=10515, 2005.

Aupperle PM: Navigating patients and caregivers through the course of Alzheimer's disease, *J Clin Psych* 67(suppl 3):8-14, 2006.

Boroson S et al: The mini-cog as a screen for dementia: validation in a population based sample, *J Am Geriatr Soc* 51:1451-1454, 2003.

Camp CJ et al: Use of nonpharmacologic interventions among nursing home residents with dementia, *Psychiatr Serv* 53: 1397-1401, 2002.

Center for Disease Control and Prevention: vCJD (Variant Creutzfeldt-Jakob disease); www.cdc.gov/ncidod/dvrd/vcjd/, 2005.

Clarfield AM: The decreasing prevalence of reversible dementias, *Arch Intern Med* 163:2219-2229, 2003.

Clark CM, Ewbank DC: Performance of the dementia severity rating scale: a caregiver questionnaire for rating severity in Alzheimer disease, *Alz Dis Assoc Dis* 10:173-178, 1996.

Clary GL, Krishnan KR: Delirium: Diagnosis, neuropathogenesis and treatment, *J Psych Pract* 7:310-323, 2001.

Cohen E et al: Opposing activities protect against age onset proteotoxicity, *Science*, 313:1604-1610, 2006.

Cole MG: Delirium in elderly patients, *Am J Geriatr Psychiatry* 12:7-12, 2004.

Cotter VT et al: Cognitive function assessment in individuals at risk for Alzheimer's disease, *J Am Acad Nurse Pract* 15:79-86, 2003.

Doody RS: Practice parameter management of dementia (an evidenced based review), report of the Quality Standards Subcommittee of the American Academy of Neurology, *Neurology* 56:1154-1166, 2001.

Dwolatzky T, Clarfield AM: Reversible dementias [letter], *J Neurosurg Psychiatry* 74:1008, 2006.

Edwards N: Differentiating the three D's: delirium, dementia, and depression, *Medsurg Nurs* 12:347-357, 2003.

Feldman HH, Jacova C: Mild cognitive impairment, *Am J Geriat Psychiat* 13:645-655, 2005.

Ferri CP et al: Global prevalence of dementia: a Delphi consensus study, *Lancet* 366:2112-2117, 2005.

Folstein MF et al: "Mini-mental state": a practical method for grading the cognitive state of patients for the clinician, *J Psychiatric Res* 12:189-198, 1975.

Forbes.com: Novartis says new Exelon patch as efficient as capsules in treating Alzhemier's; www.forbes.com/markets/feeds/afx/2006/07/19/afx2889835.html, 2006.

Foreman M et al: Assessing cognitive function, *Geriatr Nurs* 17:228-233, 1996.

Gustavson AR, Cummings JL: Cholinesterase in non-Alzheimer dementias, *J Am Med Dir Assoc* 4:S165-S169, 2003.

Hebert LE et al: Alzheimer disease in the U.S. population: prevalence estimates using the 2000 census, *Arch Neur* 60:1119-1122, 2003.

Herr K: Pain assessment in cognitively impaired older adult, *Am J Nurs* 102:65-68, 2002.

Holtzer R et al: Depressive symptoms in Alzheimer's disease: natural course and temporal relation to function and cognitive status, *J Am Geriatr Soc* 53:2083-2089, 2005.

Katzman R: A neurologist's view of Alzheimer's disease and dementia, *Inter Psychoger* 16:259-273, 2004.

Keltner NL, Folks DG: *Psychotropic drugs*, ed 4, St Louis, MO, 2005, Mosby.

Kertesz A et al: The evolution and pathology of frontotemporal dementia, *Brain* 128:1996-2005, 2005.

Knopman DS et al: Essentials of the proper diagnosis of mild cognitive impairment, dementia, and major subtypes of dementia, *Mayo Clin Proc* 78:1290-1308, 2003.

Kopelman MD: Disorders of memory, *Brain* 125:2152-2190, 2002.

Kovach J et al: The serial trial intervention: an innovative approach to meeting needs of individuals with dementia, *J Gerontol Nurs* 32:18-25, 2006.

Launer LJ: Nonsteroidal anti-inflammatory drug use and the risk for Alzheimer's disease: dissecting the epidemiological evidence, *Drugs* 63:731-739, 2003.

Lingler JH, Kaufer DI: Cognitive and motor symptoms in dementia: focus on dementia with Lewy bodies, *J Am Acad Nurs Prac* 14:398-404, 2002.

Luchsinger JA et al: Antioxidant vitamin intake and risk of Alzheimer disease, *Arch Neurol* 60:203-208, 2003.

Luis CA et al: Mild cognitive impairment: directions for future research, *Neurology* 61:438-444, 2003.

Marin DB et al: Alzheimer's disease: accurate and early diagnosis in the primary care setting, *Geriatrics* 57:36-40, 2002.

Martin A: Antioxidant vitamins E and C and risk of Alzheimer's disease, *Nutr Rev* 61:69-73, 2003.

Masterman D: Treatment of the neuropsychiatric symptoms in Alzheimer's disease, *J Am Med Dir Assoc* 4:S146-S154, 2003.

McCusker J: The delirium index, a measure of the severity of delirium: new findings on reliability, validity, responsiveness, *J Am Geriatr Soc* 52:1744-1749, 2004.

Medline Plus: Huntington's disease; www.nlm.nih.gov/medlineplus/ ency/article/000770.htm, 2005.

Mendez MF et al: Acquired sociopathy and frontotemporal dementia, *Dement Geratr Cogn Disord* 20:99-104, 2005.

Merino JG, Luchsinger JL: Parkinson's disease dementia; www.emedicine.com/med/topic3110.htm, 2004.

Moretti R et al: Cholinesterase inhibitors as a possible therapy for delirium in vascular dementia, *Am J Alzheimers Dis Other Demen*, 19:333-339, 2004.

Nath et al: Clinical features and natural history of progressive supranuclear palsy: a clinical cohort study, *Neurology* 60:910-916, 2003.

National Institute of Neurological Disorders and Stroke (NINDS): Cruetzfeldt-Jakob fact sheet; www.ninds.nih.gov/disorders/cjd/detail_cjd.htm, 2006a.

National Institute of Neurological Disorders and Stroke: Frontotemporal dementia information page; www.ninds.nih.gov/disorders/picks/picks.htm, 2006b.

National Institute of Neurological Disorders and Stroke: Huntington's disease: hope through research; www.ninds.nih.gov/disorders/huntington/detail_huntington.htm #53543137, 2006c.

National Institute of Neurological Disorders and Stroke: Multi-infarct dementia information page; www.ninds.nih.gov/disorders/multi_infarct_dementia/multi_ infarct_dementia.htm, 2006d.

National Institute of Neurological Disorders and Stroke: Progressive supranuclear palsy; www.ninds.nih.gov/disorders/psp/psp.htm, 2006e.

National Institute on Aging: Alzheimer's disease fact sheet; www.nia.nih.gov/Alzheimers/ Publications/adfact.htm, 2006.

Panza F et al: Current epidemiology of mild cognitive impairment and other predementia syndromes, *Am J Geri Psych* 13:633-644, 2005.

Papassotiropoulos A et al: Genetics, transcriptomics, and proteomics of Alzheimer's disease, *J Clin Psych* 67:650-651, 2006.

Paulsen JS et al: Neuropsychiatric aspects of Huntington's disease, *J Neurol Neurosur Psychiatry* 71:301-314, 2001.

Radiology Info: Functional MR imaging—brain; www.radiologyinfo.org/en/info.cfm?pg=fmribrain, 2006.

Reiman EM: In this issue: the genetic, transcriptomic, and proteomic study of Alzheimer's disease, *J Clin Psychiatry* 67:650-651, 2006.

Reisberg B et al: Practical geriatrics: an ordinal functional assessment tool for Alzheimer's type dementia, *Hosp Community Psych* 36:593-595, 1985.

Report: More than 5M have Alzheimer's, *The Californian*, 2007.

Richardson S: Delirium: assessment and treatment of the elderly patient, *Am J Nurse Pract* 7:9-15, 2003.

Schneider LS et al: Effectiveness of atypical antipsychotic drugs in patients with Alzheimer's disease, *N Engl J Med* 355:1525-1538, 2006.

Selkoe DJ: Alzheimer disease: Mechanistic understanding predicts novel therapies, *Ann Intern Med*, 140:627-38, 2004.

Smith M, Buckwalter K: Behaviors associated with dementia, *Clin J Oncol Nurs* 10:183-191, 2006.

Stahl S: *Essential psychopharmacology: the prescriber's guide*, New York, 2005, Cambridge University.

Tariot PN: Memantine treatment in patients with moderate to sever Alzheimer disease already receiving donepezil: a randomized controlled trial, *JAMA* 291:317-324, 2004.

Tost H et al: Huntington's disease: phenomenological diversity of a neuropsychiatric condition that challenges traditional concepts in neurology and psychiatry, *Am J Psychiatry* 161:28-34, 2004.

Twedell D: Clinical updates: delirium, *J Cont Educ Nurs* 36:102-103, 2005.

Wang L et al: Performance-based physical function and future dementia in older people, *Arch Int Med* 166:1115-1120, 2006.

Warren NM et al: Cholinergic systems in progressive supranuclear palsy, *Brain* 128:239-249, 2005.

Webster J, Grossberg GT: Strategies for treating dementing disorders, *Nurs Home Med* 6:161, 1996.

White S: The neuropathogenesis of delirium, *Rev Clin Gerontol* 12:62-67, 2002.

Yesavage et al: Development and validation of a geriatric depression screening scale: a preliminary report, *J Psychiatr Res* 17:37-49, 1983.

Zgola J: Doing things: *A guide to programming activities for persons with Alzheimer's disease and related disorders*, Baltimore, 1987, Johns Hopkins University Press.

Zlokovic BV: Neurovascular mechanisms of Alzheimer's neurodegeneration, *Trends Neurosci* 28:202-208, 2005.

Chapter 16 Disorders of Infancy, Childhood, and Adolescence

CHANTAL M. FLANAGAN

Behavior in the human being is sometimes a defense, a way of concealing motives and thoughts, as language can be a way of hiding thoughts and preventing communication.

ABRAHAM MASLOW

OBJECTIVES

1. Describe symptomatology for infants, children, and adolescents with each of the following: mental retardation, autism, separation anxiety disorder, attention deficit hyperactivity disorder, intermittent explosive disorder, oppositional defiant disorder, and conduct disorder.
2. Differentiate symptoms a child or adolescent exhibits compared to an adult for major depressive disorder, bipolar disorder, schizophrenia, and anxiety.
3. Discuss the components of a thorough nursing assessment and application of the nursing process for infants, children, or adolescents.
4. Identify nursing interventions relevant for children and adolescents with behavioral disorders.
5. Identify three effective ways to include the family in the treatment process.

KEY TERMS

assent, p. 382
behavior contract, p. 387
behavior modification, p. 386
catastrophic reaction, p. 370
coprolalia, p. 373
echolalia, p. 373
echopraxia, p. 373
palilalia, p. 373
stereotypic motor activities, p. 370
therapeutic play, p. 387
tic, p. 373

Infants, children, and adolescents are faced with challenges that are increasing in intensity and quantity. Since the 1980s, children and adolescents have been exposed to rapidly changing technology such as the Internet, chat rooms, video games and cell phones. The family system has dramatically altered from two-parent homes to homes where a single parent, same-sex parents, or grandparents serve as the caregivers. Youth violence is widespread, with gang activities and children bringing weapons to school. Parental and adult supervision is diminishing as the schools become overcrowded and both parents need to work. These factors make it difficult for the child to achieve the expected developmental, cognitive, and emotional milestones required to succeed later on in life. The inability for a child to achieve these milestones impairs the child's ability to function at home or in the school setting, and it hinders the child from developing healthy peer relationships, resulting in a mental disorder.

Mental disorders are more common in children and adolescents than ever before. The National Institute of Mental Health (2005) identified that 1 out of every 10 children in the United States suffer from a mental disorder impacting their ability to function in at least one environmental setting such as school. This impairment will sometimes recur, continue, or worsen as the child grows into adulthood, affecting the individual's ability to function in society. Nurses have the opportunity to assess and treat infants, children, and adolescents in diverse health care settings. Some infants will present with colicky behavior, feeding and sleeping problems, and failure to thrive. Some toddlers will need treatment for behavioral problems such as aggression and impulsivity. Children and adolescents frequently present with medical problems when in fact the underlying problem is a mental disorder. Symptoms are often misdiagnosed because children and adolescents often present symptoms differently than adults. The nurse's assessment needs to be comprehensive to identify children, adolescents, and their families in need of mental health referrals and early intervention. The earlier the diagnosis is identified, the sooner the client and the family are able to receive necessary treatment and obtain community resources. Because of the limited research studies conducted for this population, the efficacy and safety of treatment, specifically medications, have not been adequately established.

Nurses treat children and adolescents within the context of the family system. One cannot be separated from the other. It is important for the nurse to understand the mental health problems and needs that infants, children, and adolescents face and the effect these issues will have on their growth and development. This chapter discusses the major mental disorders affecting infants, children, and adolescents and provides direction for applying the nursing process in the assessment, diagnosis, and treatment of this population.

HISTORIC AND THEORETIC PERSPECTIVES

The first juvenile court was established in Chicago, Illinois, in 1899. In 1909, a group of socially concerned women created the Juvenile Psychopathic Institute. They hired a neurologist, William Healy, to be the first director. He then created a team that included a neuropsychiatrist, a psychologist, and a social worker. This became the model for future treatment programs. Psychoanalysts and behavioralists made up the staff at child guidance clinics.

President Harry Truman signed the National Mental Health Act on July 3, 1946. The National Institute of Mental Health (NIMH) was formed in 1949. During this time, many believed that mothers were responsible for their child's emotional and psychologic well-being. Psychiatrists and pediatricians started to train as child psychiatrists, and the American Academy of Child Psychiatry was formed in 1953 (Schowalter, 2005). NIMH funded programs for advanced education in infant, child, and adolescent psychiatric mental health nursing in the early 1950s.

MENTAL RETARDATION

Etiology and Epidemiology

Mental retardation is evident and diagnosed before age 18. The hallmark of mental retardation is below-average intellectual function, accompanied by impaired learning, communication, interpersonal interactions, and an inability to function independently. Levels of impaired function are related to the level of mental retardation, as described below.

Despite extensive evaluations, no definitive etiology can be found in 58% to 78% of individuals with mild mental retardation and 23% to 43% of individuals with severe or profound mental retardation. When found, the etiology is genetic, medical, environmental, or a combination. Researchers estimate the prevalence of mental retardation at 1% of the U.S. population (Szymanski, 1999).

Clinical Description

Subtypes. Approximately 85% of individuals with mental retardation have *mild retardation.* These children typically develop social and communication skills during the preschool years, have only minimal sensorimotor problems, and often are not identified until a later age. They generally acquire academic skills up to approximately the sixth-grade level. In adulthood, they generally achieve social and vocational skills adequate for minimum self-support. They usually require some level of supervision, guidance, and assistance. In most cases, however, they live successfully in the community—some independently and some in supervised settings (American Psychiatric Association [APA], 2000).

About 10% of the population with mental retardation has *moderate retardation.* Most individuals with moderate mental retardation acquire some communication skills during early childhood and benefit from vocational training, but they seldom advance academically beyond the second-grade level. With moderate supervision, they are usually able to provide for their own personal care and learn to travel in familiar areas. Peer relationships often decline in adolescence because of problems in recognizing and acquiring socially correct interactions. During adulthood they generally perform unskilled or semiskilled work and live and function in the community in supervised settings (APA, 2000).

About 3% to 4% of individuals with mental retardation have *severe retardation.* They typically acquire little if any communicative speech during early childhood, but they sometimes learn to use basic communication and develop elementary self-care skills in the school-age period. They may benefit from learning to sight-read some "survival" words. As adults, some are able to perform simple skills in closely supervised settings. They generally live in some protected environment within the community such as group homes or with their families unless some other handicaps require specialized nursing or other care (APA, 2000).

Only 1% to 2% of mentally retarded individuals suffer from *profound retardation.* Most also have an identified neurologic condition such as cerebral palsy, sensory deficits, epilepsy, and other neurologic disorders causing their retardation. They have considerable sensorimotor problems recognized in early childhood such as poor head control, feeding problems, and the inability to roll over. They require a highly structured setting with constant monitoring and assistance for the best possible development. Under this level of care, some develop enough motor skills, self-care skills, and communication to perform simple tasks in a closely supervised and sheltered setting (APA, 2000).

Prognosis

The prognosis reflects the interaction of biomedical, psychologic, and environmental factors. Studies show that those with severe to profound mental retardation have a shortened life expectancy as a result of medical conditions such as epilepsy and feeding problems and limitations of self-care and communication (Szymanski, 1999).

PERVASIVE DEVELOPMENTAL DISORDERS

Pervasive developmental disorders are a collection of neuropsychiatric disorders in which the child manifests deficits in a broad range of developmental areas such as communication, social interactions, cognitive skills, and behavior that often is stereotypical. Autism is the most prevalent of these disorders (Volkmar, 1999).

Autistic Disorder

Etiology

Scientists offer several theories on the causes of this disorder. Possible causes include genetic, neurologic, metabolic, immunologic, and environmental factors, as well as complications from birth. The most accepted theory is that an abnormality in the structure and functioning of the brain causes autism. Excessive sugar, food sensitivity, food additives, vaccines, or allergies do not cause autism (Valente, 2004).

Epidemiology

Studies suggest that the rate of autistic disorder is as high as 1 in 500 or fewer, whereas other sources such as the DSM-IV-TR report 5 cases per 10,000. Rates are three to four times higher in males than in females. Females, however, tend to have more severe mental retardation. Siblings of individuals with the disorder have an increased risk of developing autistic disorder (APA, 2000; Volkmar, 1999). Family members of the autistic child sometimes have other behavioral and developmental disorders such as attention deficit disorder or Asperger's disorder (Valente, 2004).

Clinical Description

A variety of behavioral symptoms are often present, including any of the following: hyperactivity, short attention span, impulsivity, aggressivity, self-injurious behaviors, and temper tantrums. Abnormal eating patterns (e.g., limiting intake to a few foods or eating non-nutritious objects) or sleeping patterns (e.g., recurrent awakenings with rocking) are present as well. Individuals often have restricted, repetitive, and stereotyped patterns of behavior, interest, and activity. They become preoccupied in ways that are extreme, either in intensity or focus, and they rigidly follow specific, nonfunctional routines or rituals. In some cases, they use stereotypic and repetitive mannerisms or become persistently preoccupied with parts of objects. For example, a client with autism insists on lining up objects over and over again to maintain sameness and orderliness. They are often unable to tolerate even minor changes in the environment and have an intense or **catastrophic reaction** to minor changes such as a new chair or new seating arrangement at dinner. Some demand maintaining nonfunctional and unreasonable adherence to rituals and routines. For example, if a child is used to brushing his teeth before he gets into his pajamas, he will become very upset if he is asked to change the order and put on his pajamas first and then brush his teeth.

Autistic children often demonstrate **stereotypic motor activities** (e.g., clapping or flapping of hands, spinning, rocking, swaying) and posture (e.g., walking on tiptoes, odd postures, or strange hand movements). Play cannot be disrupted, and they often show intense preoccupation with objects such as buttons or zippers. They frequently are fascinated with movement of such things as fans, revolving objects, or the opening and closing of doors or drawers or constantly turning the light switch on and off. Some become attached to unusual objects, such as a piece of string or rubber band, and ignore typical items children usually attach to, such as a blanket or teddy bear.

Individuals with autistic disorder typically lack emotional reciprocity or do not actively participate in simple social play or games. Instead they prefer solitary activities or only attempt to involve others as objects of their play (e.g., position another child as bench to sit on). Mood or affective abnormalities are often present, such as giggling or weeping for reasons that are not apparent to the observer or showing no emotional reaction when a situation normally calls for a reaction. They often have inappropriate responses to danger, such as showing no fear of real danger or excessive fear of harmless objects. Some also injure themselves by head banging or biting various body parts. These individuals respond oddly to sensory stimuli. For example, some have a high pain threshold, oversensitivity to sound or touch, or exaggerated response to light or color. Others have a fascination with a particular sensory stimulation, such as constantly rubbing a hard surface or a specific piece of furniture.

Approximately 80% of individuals with autistic disorder have some degree of mental retardation, approximately 50% have severe or profound retardation, and 30% have mild retardation (Volkmar, 1999). Autism also affects other cognitive areas, such as insight, reasoning and judgment. Communication problems usually present so severely in both verbal and nonverbal areas that spoken language is often absent. Individuals who do speak are not always able to begin or keep up a conversation with others, or they use such stereotyped and repetitive language that others find it difficult to continue a conversation with them. Speech often contains abnormal pitch, intonation, rate, and rhythm (e.g., monotonous or inappropriate sing-song pitch and rhythm or question-like raises of tone at the end of declarative sentences). Grammar is often immature, stereotyped, and repetitive (e.g., inappropriate repetition of jingles or commercials, regardless of meaning). Sometimes

DSM-IV-TR CRITERIA

Autistic Disorder

A A total of six (or more) items from criteria 1, 2, and 3, with at least two from criterion 1 and one each from criteria 2 and 3:
 1 Qualitative impairment in social interaction, as manifested by at least two of the following:
  a Marked impairment in the use of multiple nonverbal behaviors such as eye-to-eye gaze, facial expression, body postures, and gestures to regulate social interaction
  b Failure to develop peer relationships appropriate to developmental level
  c A lack of spontaneous seeking to share enjoyment, interests, or achievements with other people (e.g., by a lack of showing, bringing, or pointing out objects of interests)
  d Lack of social or emotional reciprocity
 2 Qualitative impairments in communication as manifested by at least one of the following:
  a Delay in, or total lack of, the development of spoken language (not accompanied by an attempt to compensate through alternative modes of communication such as gesture or mime)
  b In individuals with adequate speech, marked impairment in the ability to initiate or sustain a conversation with others
  c Stereotyped and repetitive use of language or idiosyncratic language
  d Lack of varied, spontaneous make-believe play or social imitative play appropriate to developmental level
 3 Restricted repetitive and stereotyped patterns of behavior, interests, and activities, as manifested by at least one of the following:
  a Encompassing preoccupation with one or more stereotyped and restricted patterns of interest that is abnormal either in intensity or focus
  b Apparently inflexible adherence to specific, nonfunctional routines or rituals
  c Stereotyped and repetitive motor mannerisms (e.g., hand or finger flapping or twisting, or complex whole-body movements)
  d Persistent preoccupation with parts of objects

B The client shows delays or abnormal functioning in at least one of the following areas, with onset before age 3 years: (1) social interaction, (2) language as used in social communication, or (3) symbolic or imaginative play

C The disturbance is not better accounted for by Rett's disorder or childhood disintegrative disorder.

From American Psychiatric Association: *Diagnostic and statistical manual of mental disorders,* ed 4, text revision, Washington, DC, 2000, American Psychiatric Association.

grammar is metaphorical so that only those familiar with the individual's use of language understand what the autistic child is communicating. Some individuals are not able to understand simple questions, directions, or jokes, whereas others develop excellent long-term memory of insignificant data such as train schedules, baseball statistics, songs, or dates (APA, 2000; Volkmar, 1999) (see the DSM-IV-TR Criteria box). Some individuals with autistic disorder develop exceptional but circumscribed skills that are commonly referred to as "islands of genius." For example, a person may not be able to count appropriate change in a store but is able to quote and solve complicated mathematical formulas. Or the individual with autism may not be able to read sheet music but can play complex symphonic pieces after hearing them only once.

Prognosis

There is no cure for autism. Language skills and overall intellectual level are the strongest factors related to the ultimate prognosis. Available studies that have followed the course of this disorder suggest that only a small percentage of individuals with the disorder go on to live and work independently as adults. In about one third of the cases, some degree of partial independence is possible. The highest-functioning adults with autistic disorder typically continue to exhibit problems in social interaction and communication together with restricted interests and activities. Evidence demonstrates that early, intense educational interventions using highly structured programs help the client achieve the highest level of functioning in social, communication, and cognitive skills (Volkmar, 1999).

Asperger's Disorder

Asperger's disorder contains many similar features of autistic disorder: self-injurious and aggressive behavior; impairment in social interaction; and restricted, repetitive patterns of behavior, interests, and activities. These produce significant impairment in social, occupational, or other important areas of functioning. However, in contrast to autistic disorder, no clinically significant delays in language, cognitive development, age-appropriate self-help skills, adaptive behavior, or curiosity about the environment occur (APA, 2000). This disorder follows a continuous course, and usually the duration is lifelong. There is a better long-term outcome for individuals with Asperger's than there is for those with autism. Prognosis is best if treatment begins by 24 to 36 months of age (Tanguay, 2000; Volkmar, 1999).

DISORDERS OF INFANCY OR CHILDHOOD

Reactive Attachment Disorder

Etiology and Epidemiology

Children who are exposed to extreme poverty, parental physical and emotional abuse or neglect, or institutionalized care are at risk for developing a reactive attachment disorder. Although there have been limited studies describing prevalence of this condition, reactive attachment disorder appears to be rare (less than 1%).

Clinical Description

This disorder usually begins within the first few years of life and typically results from abusive or neglectful caregiving. Reactive attachment disorder has two subtypes: inhibited and disinhibited. In the *inhibited type,* the child is unable to interact socially for the child's developmental level. Because of the lack of early healthy bonding and intimacy, the child fails to initiate or respond to social

DSM-IV-TR CRITERIA

Reactive Attachment Disorder

A Markedly disturbed and developmentally inappropriate social relatedness in most contexts, beginning before age 5 years as evidenced by either of the following:
  1 Persistent failure to initiate or respond in a developmentally appropriate fashion to most social interactions, as manifest by excessively inhibited, hypervigilant, or highly ambivalent and contradictory responses (e.g., the child may respond to caregivers with a mixture of approach, avoidance, and resistance to comforting, or he or she may exhibit frozen watchfulness)
  2 Diffuse attachments as manifest by indiscriminate sociability with a marked inability to exhibit appropriate selective attachments (e.g., excessive familiarity with relative strangers or lack of selectivity in choice of attachment figures)

B The disturbance in criterion A is not accounted for solely by developmental delay (as in mental retardation) and does not meet criteria for a pervasive developmental disorder.

C Pathogenic care is evidenced by at least one of the following:
  1 Persistent disregard of the child's basic emotional needs for comfort, stimulation, and affection
  2 Persistent disregard of the child's basic physical needs
  3 Repeated changes of primary caregiver that prevent formation of stable attachments (e.g., frequent changes in foster care)

D There is a presumption that the care in criterion C is responsible for the disturbed behavior in criterion A (e.g., the disturbances in criterion A began following the pathogenic care in criterion C).

Specify type:

Inhibited type: if criterion A1 predominates in the clinical presentation

Disinhibited type: if criterion A2 predominates in the clinical presentation

From American Psychiatric Association: *Diagnostic and statistical manual of mental disorders,* ed 4, text revision, Washington, DC, 2000, American Psychiatric Association.

cues (e.g., fails to seek being comforted or to engage in social interactions). Some are even fearful of accepting comfort from others. In the *disinhibited type*, the child lacks appropriate boundaries and is unable to differentiate between strangers and safe attachment relationships. These children often inappropriately seek comfort and attention from unknown adults or will become distressed when separated from strangers (Boris et al., 2005; APA, 2000) (see the DSM-IV-TR Criteria box).

Often the caregiver brings the child to the pediatrician with problems of severe colic or feeding difficulties, failure to gain weight, detached and unresponsive behavior, difficulty being comforted, or avoidance of social interactions (Maldonado-Duran et al., 2005).

Prognosis

Sometimes symptoms of this disorder will lessen if the child is placed in a supportive and loving environment where the adults provide and encourage healthy and nurturing relationships.

Separation Anxiety Disorder

Etiology and Epidemiology

Separation anxiety disorder is more common in first-degree relatives and is possibly more common in children whose mothers have panic disorder. It usually develops after a stressful event (e.g., death of a close and valued relative or pet, illness in the child or parent, or a major change in the environment, such as a move to a new neighborhood). This disorder occurs in approximately 4% of children and adolescents and is more common in females. It typically presents before late adolescence (APA, 2000).

Clinical Description

With an excessive need to know the whereabouts of their parents or others, individuals with separation anxiety often try to stay in touch with frequent telephone calls. Because they experience discomfort in being away from home, some become resistant to traveling alone and are hesitant to attend activities that other peers enjoy, such as camp, school, and sleepovers at friends' houses. Some will not stay in a room alone. Children with separation anxiety disorder demonstrate clinging behavior. They attempt to shadow their parents inside and outside the home and with increasing frequency and intensity. Bedtime is difficult, with the child or adolescent insisting that the parent remain with him or her until he or she falls asleep. During the night, these individuals often try to get into bed with the parents or another significant figure. Some will even sleep outside the parent's door if they are unable to enter the room.

Physical complaints often appear during actual or anticipated separation and frequently include stomachaches, headaches, nausea, and vomiting. Older children and adolescents experience a racing or pounding heart, dizziness, and faintness. The somatic complaints often lead to numerous trips to physicians and subsequent medical procedures.

Individuals with this disorder often experience recurrent, excessive distress when they are away from home or major attachment figures. Some become extremely upset and miserable away from home and are preoccupied with reunion fantasies. Some become extremely fearful that imagined harm will happen to the significant other(s). Fears about danger to themselves or their families sometimes present as fears of animals, monsters, the dark, muggers, burglars, kidnappers, accidents, or plane or train travel. Some fears also present as concerns about death and dying. They show various moods, such as excessive worry that no one loves them and they therefore want to die, or unusual anger when someone tries to separate them from their parent or significant other. At times, the depressed mood justifies a diagnosis of major depression. When they reach adulthood, some of these individuals develop panic disorder with agoraphobia.

Nightmares often contain elements of the individual's fears, such as family death through fire, murder, or other

DSM-IV-TR CRITERIA

Separation Anxiety

A Developmentally inappropriate and excessive anxiety concerning separation from home or from those to whom the individual is attached, as evidenced by three or more of the following:

1. Recurrent excessive distress when separation from home or major attachment figures occurs or is anticipated
2. Persistent and excessive worry about losing or possible harm befalling major attachment figures
3. Persistent and excessive worry that an untoward event will lead to separation from a major attachment figure (e.g., getting lost or being kidnapped)
4. Persistent reluctance or refusal to go to school or elsewhere because of fear of separation
5. Persistent and excessive fear or reluctance to be alone or without major attachment figures at home or without significant adults in other settings
6. Persistent reluctance or refusal to go to sleep without being near a major attachment figure or to sleep away from home
7. Repeated nightmares with the theme of separation
8. Repeated complaints of physical symptoms (such as headaches, stomachaches, nausea, or vomiting) when separation from major attachment figures occurs or is anticipated

B The duration of the disturbance is at least 4 weeks.

C The onset is before age 18.

D The disturbance causes clinically significant distress or impairment in social, academic (occupational), or other important areas of functioning.

E The disturbance does not occur exclusively during the course of a pervasive developmental disorder, schizophrenia, or other psychotic disorder and, in adolescents and adults, is not better accounted for by panic disorder with agoraphobia.

From American Psychiatric Association: *Diagnostic and statistical manual of mental disorders*, ed 4, text revision, Washington, DC, 2000, American Psychiatric Association.

catastrophe. Academic difficulties result from refusal to attend school and thus increase the problem with social avoidance. School refusal occurs in about 5% of all school-aged children. It usually occurs between ages 5 and 6 and 10 and 11 (King, 2001) (see the DSM-IV-TR Criteria box).

Prognosis

Typically there are periods of severity and reduction of symptoms. Both the anxiety about possible separation and the avoidance of situations involving separation may persist for many years.

TIC DISORDERS

Tourette's Disorder

Etiology and Epidemiology

Tourette's disorder is most often a genetic neurologic disorder, although other factors are responsible in 10% to 15% of children. This includes head trauma, carbon monoxide poisoning, and complications from pregnancy. Tourette's disorder occurs in approximately 5 to 30 children per 10,000 and 1 to 2 per 10,000 in adults. It is approximately two times more common in males than in females. Other disorders associated with Tourette's disorder include attention deficit/hyperactivity disorder (ADHD), obsessive-compulsive disorder, and learning disorders (APA, 2000).

Clinical Description

A **tic** is a sudden, rapid, involuntary, repetitive movement or vocalization (APA, 2000). Although experienced as irresistible, some clients are able to suppress it for a varying length of time. Stress typically exacerbates tics, and distracting activities such as reading or sewing may reduce them. Tics are often markedly decreased or absent during sleep.

Some simple motor tics include eye blinking, neck jerking, shoulder shrugging, facial grimacing, and coughing. Simple vocal tics include throat clearing, grunting, sniffing, snorting, and barking. Complex motor tics are facial gestures, grooming behaviors, jumping, touching, stamping, smelling an object, and **echopraxia**, or the imitation of another's movements. Complex vocal tics include coprolalia, palilalia, and echolalia. **Coprolalia** is repeating socially unacceptable words, typically obscene words. **Palilalia** is repeating one's own sounds or words. **Echolalia** is repeating the last-heard words, sounds, or phrases from another person.

In Tourette's disorder, the number, type, frequency, complexity, and severity of the tics vary over time. The most common tics in Tourette's disorder involve the head and parts of the body such as the torso and limbs. Common vocal tics include clicks, grunts, barks, sniffs, snorts, and coughs. Coprolalia occurs in less than 10% of the cases. Complex motor tics reported in Tourette's disorder include touching, squatting, deep knee bends, retracing steps, and twirling during walking. The most frequent initial tic is blinking. Other initial tics reported include tongue protrusion, squatting, sniffing, hopping, skipping, throat clearing, stuttering, uttering sounds or words, and coprolalia. Other relatively common symptoms include hyperactivity, distractibility, and impulsivity. Obsessions and compulsions are common in a client with Tourette's disorder. In some cases, these tics lead to physical injuries. For example, head banging sometimes results in retinal detachment, or knee and neck jerking lead to orthopedic problems. Some clients obsessively pick at their skin, leading to potential infections or mutilation.

Shame, self-consciousness, and depressed mood occur as a secondary result of problems from Tourette's disorder. Various learning disabilities such as dyslexia are common in individuals who have Tourette's disorder. Frequently reported associated symptoms include social discomfort and rejection by others that interfere with social, academic, and occupational functioning. In severe cases, tics interfere with activities of daily living, such as reading or eating, or cause medical complications (APA, 2000) (see the DSM-IV-TR Criteria box on p. 374).

DSM-IV-TR CRITERIA

Tourette's Disorder

A Both multiple motor and one or more vocal tics have been present at some time during the illness, although not necessarily concurrently. (A *tic* is a sudden, rapid, recurrent nonrhythmic, stereotyped motor movement or vocalization.)
B The tics occur many times a day (usually in bouts) nearly every day or intermittently throughout a period of more than 1 year, and during this period there was never a tic-free period of more than 3 consecutive months.
C The disturbance causes marked distress or significant impairment in social, occupational, or other important areas of functioning.
D The onset is before age 18.
E The disturbance is not due to the direct physiologic effects of a substance (e.g., stimulants) or a general medical condition (e.g., Huntington's disease or postviral encephalitis).

From American Psychiatric Association: *Diagnostic and statistical manual of mental disorders*, ed 4, text revision, Washington, DC, 2000, American Psychiatric Association.

Prognosis

Tourette's disorder begins as early as 2 years of age, but it typically presents during childhood or early adolescence. Although it is almost always a lifelong disorder, in most cases symptoms diminish during adolescence and adulthood (APA, 2000).

ATTENTION-DEFICIT AND DISRUPTIVE BEHAVIORAL DISORDERS

Attention-Deficit/Hyperactivity Disorder

Etiology

Researchers do not know the etiology of ADHD, but studies suggest an interaction between psychosocial and biologic factors. There is a strong correlation between genetic factors and ADHD. Concordance is 51% in monozygotic twins and 33% in dizygotic twins. Adoption studies also support genetics over environmental etiology (Cantwell, 1996). ADHD occurs more often in the first-degree relatives of children with ADHD (APA, 2000).

Epidemiology

Rates of attention-deficit/hyperactivity disorder (ADHD) in school-age children are estimated at 3% to 7% of the population. As many as two thirds of those diagnosed with ADHD also meet the criteria for another mental disorder, including up to 50% for oppositional defiant disorder or conduct disorder. Other disorders that frequently occur with ADHD include mood disorders, anxiety disorders, Tourette's and chronic tic disorders, substance abuse, speech and language delays, and learning disorders.

Clinical Description

Behavioral manifestations usually occur in various or multiple environments within the child's life, such as the school, home, church, or recreational activities. The level of problems typically varies from time to time in the same or different settings. Symptoms generally worsen in situations that require sustained attention or lack interest to the child or adolescent, such as listening to teachers, performing repetitive tasks, or reading lengthy materials. Symptoms actually disappear or become minimal when under strict control, such as during a diagnostic interview or when receiving frequent rewards for appropriate behavior. Symptoms tend to worsen in unstructured, group situations such as the typical classroom and playground.

Hyperactivity presents in many forms: fidgeting or squirming in a seat, getting up when one is expected to remain seated, excessive running or climbing when it is dangerous or inappropriate, loud and disruptive play during quiet activities, demonstrating a driven verbal or motor quality. Even though toddlers developmentally present with a lot of activity and inquisitiveness, toddlers with ADHD present qualitatively different. They are always moving, running, jumping, and climbing on furniture, or are unable to remain still for completion of simple tasks such as putting on a coat or listening to a simple story.

Some school-age children settle down somewhat but still display excessive overactivity. Some demonstrate difficulty remaining seated by hanging onto the edge of their seats, squirming constantly, playing with objects, or tapping their hands and feet. They stay focused for activities they enjoy, such as watching TV or playing video games, but cannot maintain attention or focus for activities they find boring or difficult. At home they frequently do not finish meals or even finish activities that they have begun. They make excessive noise, interrupting others during quiet times and talking constantly, such as giving a running commentary on a television show. Adolescents often express a subjective feeling of restlessness and often report a preference to engage in active rather than sedentary activities.

Impulsivity manifests itself in the following ways:

- Impatience
- Failing to delay responses
- Shouting out answers before the question has been finished
- Difficulty waiting for one's turn or problems waiting in line without pushing and shoving
- Frequently interrupting others to the point of social, academic, or occupational problems
- Making comments out of turn
- Failing to listen to directions
- Initiating inappropriate contact with others by interrupting conversations
- Grabbing others by their clothing, limbs, or belongings
- Touching things that are off limits to them
- Clowning around at times of expected quiet

Accidents often result from knocking over objects, running into people, grabbing dangerous objects such as a hot pan, or taking dangerous risks without consideration of the consequences, such as riding a bicycle at night without reflective lights. They often exhibit temper outbursts, bossiness, stubbornness, and excessive and frequent insistence for their requests to be met.

DSM-IV-TR CRITERIA

Attention-Deficit/Hyperactivity Disorder

A Either criterion 1 or 2 is present:

1 Six (or more) of the following symptoms of inattention have persisted for at least 6 months to a degree that is maladaptive and inconsistent with developmental level:

INATTENTION

- **a** Often fails to give close attention to details or makes careless mistakes in schoolwork, work, or other activities
- **b** Often has difficulty sustaining attention in tasks or play activities
- **c** Often does not seem to listen when spoken to directly
- **d** Often does not follow through on instructions and fails to finish schoolwork, chores, or duties in the workplace (not the result of oppositional behavior or a failure to understand instructions)
- **e** Often has difficulty organizing tasks and activities
- **f** Often avoids, dislikes, or is reluctant to engage in tasks that require sustained mental effort (such as schoolwork or homework)
- **g** Often loses things necessary for tasks or activities (e.g., toys, school assignments, pencils, books, or tools)
- **h** Is often easily distracted by extraneous stimulus
- **i** Often forgetful in daily activities

2 Six (or more) of the following symptoms of hyperactivity/impulsivity have persisted for at least 6 months to a degree that is maladaptive and inconsistent with developmental level:

HYPERACTIVITY

- **a** Often fidgets with hands or feet or squirms in seat
- **b** Often leaves seat in classroom or in other situations in which remaining seated is expected
- **c** Often runs about or climbs excessively in situations in which it is inappropriate (in adolescents or adults, may be limited to subjective feelings of restlessness)
- **d** Often has difficulty playing or engaging in leisure activities quietly
- **e** Is often "on the go" or often acts as if "driven by a motor"
- **f** Often talks excessively

IMPULSIVITY

- **g** Often blurts out answers before questions have been completed
- **h** Often has difficulty awaiting turn
- **i** Often interrupts or intrudes on others (e.g., butts into conversations or games)

B Some hyperactive-impulsive or inattentive symptoms that caused impairment were present before age 7 years.

C Some impairment from the symptoms is present in two or more settings (e.g., at school [or work] and at home).

D There must be clear evidence of clinically significant impairment in social, academic, or occupational functioning.

E The symptoms do not occur exclusively during the course of a pervasive developmental disorder, schizophrenia, or other psychotic disorder and are not better accounted for by another mental disorder (e.g., mood disorder, anxiety disorder, dissociative disorder, or personality disorder).

Code based on type:

Attention-deficit/hyperactivity disorder, combined type: If both criteria A1 and A2 are met for the preceding 6 months

Attention-deficit/hyperactivity disorder, predominantly inattentive type: If criterion A1 is met but criterion A2 is not met for the preceding 6 months

Attention-deficit/hyperactivity disorder, predominantly hyperactive-impulsive type: If criterion A2 is met but criterion A1 is not met for the preceding 6 months

From American Psychiatric Association: *Diagnostic and statistical manual of mental disorders*, ed 4, text revision, Washington, DC, 2000, American Psychiatric Association.

Individuals with ADHD may also develop a number of other problems and symptoms as a result of the underlying attention and hyperactive-impulsive problems. These include low frustration tolerance, demoralization, low self-esteem, mood lability, and depressed mood.

Inattention occurs in various settings. Schoolwork or other activities often contain careless errors showing lack of close attention to details. Work is messy, with evidence of not thinking through the project or schoolwork. Often it appears that the child is daydreaming and not listening to what is being said or asked. Trivial stimuli such as household noises often distract these individuals, who then leave their assigned task to attend to the interrupting stimuli. The child moves from one unfinished task to another, leaving increasing clutter in the child's path. Materials needed for specific tasks typically become scattered, lost, or carelessly handled and damaged. They often forget and miss appointments, fail to meet schoolwork deadlines, or forget lunch money. As a result, academic achievement is often low. Children with ADHD are often regarded as lazy, unmotivated, and believed to have below-average intelligence. Studies have demonstrated that 10% to 20% of children with ADHD also have a learning disorder and are, in fact, of normal intelligence (Nearns, 1997).

Social problems occur as a result of losing the train of conversation and changing topics inappropriately, not following expected rules of games or activities, and appearing uninterested in others. Family members frequently develop resentment, particularly when the variability of symptoms leads parents to believe that their children's troublesome behavior is willful. Families of these children likely have more stress, experience feelings of inadequacy and parental incompetence, have marital discord and disruption, and experience increased social isolation (Dulcan et al., 1997) (see the DSM-IV-TR Criteria box).

Prognosis

ADHD features continue into adolescence in the majority of children diagnosed as hyperactive and generally decrease during late adolescence and early adulthood. A family history of ADHD, psychosocial adversity, and comorbidity with conduct, mood, and anxiety disorders increase the risk of continued ADHD. Specific predictors of poor outcome include oppositional and aggressive behavior directed at adults, low IQ, poor peer relations, and continuing ADHD symptoms. Comorbid oppositional defiant disorder raises the risk of conduct disorder. Behavioral management is the best psychosocial intervention. Structure and consistency in home and school is of particular importance for a positive outcome (Pliszka, 2000). Many adults who were diagnosed with ADHD in childhood report a decrease of behavioral hyperactivity but a continuation of difficulty concentrating for long periods of time or attending to complex projects.

Oppositional Defiant Disorder

Etiology

Oppositional defiant disorder occurs more often in families where the child care is disrupted by a succession of different caregivers, or where harsh, inconsistent, or neglectful child-rearing practices occur. The disorder occurs more commonly when serious marital problems are present (APA, 2000).

Epidemiology

Rates vary considerably, from 2% to 16%, based on the nature of the population sample and method of assessment. Oppositional defiant disorder occurs more frequently in males before puberty and with approximately equal frequency after puberty. The disorder also occurs more commonly when at least one parent has a history of one of the following: mood disorder, oppositional defiant disorder, conduct disorder, ADHD, antisocial personality disorder, or a substance-related disorder. ADHD commonly occurs, and learning disorders and communication disorders tend to be associated with oppositional defiant disorder (APA, 2000).

Clinical Description

The essential features of negativism, defiance, disobedience, and hostility toward authority figures typically present with persistent stubbornness, resistance to directions, and unwillingness to compromise or negotiate with adults. Evidence of defiance also presents as deliberate and persistent testing of limits, typically by ignoring directions, arguing, and refusing to accept responsibility for misbehavior. Hostility is usually directed at adults or peers and includes deliberately annoying others verbally. Symptoms invariably present at home but are sometimes absent or minimal at school and are generally directed toward those the child knows best. Individuals with oppositional defiant disorder do not regard themselves as troublesome but blame others for making unreasonable demands or blame the circumstances.

During early childhood, some show evidence of difficult temperament (e.g., high reactivity, difficulty in being soothed) or high motor activity. During the school years, the following problems often occur: low self-esteem, mood lability, and low frustration tolerance. Swearing and use of alcohol, tobacco, or illicit drugs that impact peer relationships and disrupt adult relationships are also common. Cognitive and perceptual symptoms are not usually present in oppositional defiant disorder (APA, 2000) (see the DSM-IV-TR Criteria box).

DSM-IV-TR CRITERIA

Oppositional Defiant Disorder

A A pattern of negativistic, hostile, and defiant behavior lasting at least 6 months, during which four or more of the following are present:
  1 Often loses temper
  2 Often argues with adults
  3 Often actively defies or refuses to comply with adults' requests or rules
  4 Often deliberately annoys people
  5 Often blames others for his or her mistakes or misbehavior
  6 Is often touchy or easily annoyed by others
  7 Is often angry and resentful
  8 Is often spiteful or vindictive
  NOTE: Consider a criterion met only if the behavior occurs more frequently than is typically observed in individuals of comparable age and developmental level.
B The disturbance in behavior causes clinically significant impairment in social, academic, or occupational functioning.
C The behaviors do not occur exclusively during the course of a psychotic or mood disorder.
D Criteria are not met for conduct disorder, and, if the individual is age 18 years or older, criteria are not met for antisocial personality disorder.

From American Psychiatric Association: *Diagnostic and statistical manual of mental disorders*, ed 4, text revision, Washington, DC, 2000, American Psychiatric Association.

Prognosis

The onset is typically gradual, usually occurring over the course of months or years. In a significant number of cases, oppositional defiant disorder develops into conduct disorder. This disorder tends to persist over time in approximately half of the cases (Loeber, 2000).

Conduct Disorder

Etiology

The following factors put the child at risk for conduct disorder:

- Parental rejection and neglect
- Difficult infant temperament
- Inconsistent child-rearing practices with harsh discipline
- Physical or sexual abuse
- Lack of supervision
- Early institutional living
- Frequent changes of caregivers
- Large family size
- Association with a delinquent peer group
- Certain family psychopathology

Conduct disorder occurs more frequently when a biologic or adoptive parent has antisocial personality disorder; a biologic parent has alcohol dependence, a mood disorder, schizophrenia, or a history of ADHD or conduct disorder; or a sibling has conduct disorder. Although definitive etiology for conduct disorder is inconclusive, one current and widely accepted model proposes that the disorder is linked to genetic predisposition triggered by environmental risk and low stress tolerance coupled with inadequate coping skills (APA, 2000; Steiner et al., 1997).

Epidemiology

According to DSM-IV-TR, rates appear higher in urban than in rural settings and vary depending on the nature of the population sampled and methods of research used (APA, 2000). Bauermeister et al. (1994) found the pattern of conduct disorder was highest in 13- to 16-year-olds, with a sharp decline thereafter. In boys, the prevalence reached a high point from 10 to 13 years of age, with a gradual decline from ages 13 to 20. In girls, a gradual increase occurred in late childhood and early adolescence, peaking at age 16, and was followed by a sharp decline.

Clinical Description

Conduct disorder presents mainly with a repetitive and persistent pattern of behavior that violates both the basic rights of others and major age-appropriate societal norms or rules. The behaviors typically present in a variety of settings, including home, school, and the community. Because the child or adolescent tends to minimize the problems with adults who do not adequately supervise the child or adolescent, the behaviors are sometimes difficult to detect (Loeber, 2000).

Clients with conduct disorder manifest aggressive behavior and react aggressively toward others. They bully, threaten, and intimidate; initiate physical fights; use weapons in ways that could lead to injury; act cruelly to people or animals; steal; and force sexual activity. The severity of these behaviors sometimes involves rape, assault, or (rarely) homicide. Deliberate destruction of property results in fire damage, vandalism, and destruction of others' property for simple vengeance. In addition to theft or robbery, the child or adolescent is often deceitful, demonstrating frequent lying or breaking promises to obtain goods or favors or to avoid obligations or responsibility.

These clients also frequently attempt to avoid consequences by blaming others. Early onset of problematic behavior usually includes sexual activity, drinking, smoking, use of illegal substances, and other high risk–taking acts. Behaviors usually persist into adulthood. These behaviors frequently lead to school suspensions, unplanned pregnancy, physical injury, sexually transmitted diseases, legal problems, dismissals from work or other activities, and the inability to attend regular schools.

Children or adolescents with conduct disorder generally do not empathize with other people's feelings and are unconcerned with other's situations or needs. They exhibit uncaring behavior but will often express words of guilt or remorse because they have learned that it reduces or prevents punishment. This stated sense of remorse is usually fabricated and insincere.

Although they project an image of "toughness," they often experience low self-esteem with poor frustration tolerance, irritability, temper outbursts, and reckless behavior. There are two subtypes of conduct disorder: overt and covert. Overt behavior is confrontational and includes fighting and aggression. Covert disruptive behaviors manifest as concealing and theft. The behaviors associated with conduct disorder often impair peer relationships (Loeber, 2000) (see the DSM-IV-TR Criteria box on p. 378).

Prognosis

An onset of conduct disorder before age 10 (childhood-onset type) generally indicates a more severe and persistent type that often develops into adult antisocial personality disorder. These individuals typically are male, display more physical aggression, are more likely to have oppositional defiant disorder during childhood, and meet full criteria for conduct disorder before puberty. Individuals in the adolescent-onset group (no symptoms of conduct disorder before age 10) display less aggression, are likely to have better peer relationships, and display conduct problems in groups (APA, 2000; Loeber, 2000).

Intermittent Explosive Disorder

Etiology and Epidemiology

Research is limited, but there is some evidence that the neurotransmitter serotonin plays a role in the development of intermittent explosive disorder. This disorder is usually diagnosed in childhood through early adulthood and is rare. Intermittent explosive disorder is more common in males than females.

Clinical Description

The child is unable to resist aggressive impulses that result in severe acts of aggression. This includes destroying property, striking or hurting others, and threatening to harm a person. The degree of violence is disproportionate to the precipitating event. For example, the child destroys his room after being told to put his clothes in the hamper. The violence will last minutes or hours. The child describes the aggressive acts as "spells" or "attacks." The child will feel an immediate tension release followed by feelings of remorse or embarrassment (APA, 2000).

During the aggressive episode, the child experiences feelings of rage, racing thoughts, and increased energy. After the aggressive act, the child reports feelings of depression and fatigue. Some have reported tingling sensations, tremors, palpitations, chest tightness, pressure in the head, or hearing an echo preceding the aggressive attack (APA, 2000) (see the DSM-IV-TR Criteria box on p. 378).

Prognosis

Children with intermittent explosive disorder may experience school problems such as suspension or detention and may encounter impaired relationships with peers. They

DSM-IV-TR CRITERIA

Conduct Disorder

A A repetitive and persistent pattern of behavior in which the basic rights of others or major age-appropriate norms or rules are violated, as manifested by the presence of three (or more) of the following criteria in the preceding 12 months, with at least one criterion present in the preceding 6 months:

Aggression to people and animals:

1 Often bullies, threatens, or intimidates others
2 Often initiates physical fights
3 Has used a weapon that can cause serious physical harm to others (e.g., a bat, brick, broken bottle, knife, gun)
4 Has been physically cruel to people
5 Has been physically cruel to animals
6 Has stolen while confronting a victim (e.g., mugging, purse snatching, extortion, armed robbery)
7 Has forced someone into sexual activity

Destruction of property:

8 Has deliberately set fires with the intention of causing serious damage
9 Has deliberately destroyed others' property (other than by setting fires)

Deceitfulness or theft:

10 Has broken into someone else's house, building, or car
11 Often lies to obtain goods or favors or to avoid obligations (i.e., cons others)
12 Has stolen items of nontrivial value without confronting a victim (e.g., shoplifting, but without breaking and entering; forgery)

Serious violations of rules:

13 Often stays out at night despite parental prohibitions, beginning before age 13 years
14 Has run away from home overnight at least twice while living in parental or parental surrogate home (or once without returning for a lengthy period)
15 Is often truant from school, beginning before age 13 years

B The disturbance in behavior causes clinically significant impairment in social, academic, or occupational functioning.

C If the individual is age 18 years or older, criteria are not met for antisocial personality disorder.

Code based on age at onset:

Conduct disorder, childhood-onset type: Onset of at least one criterion characteristic of conduct disorder before age 10 years

Conduct disorder, adolescent-onset type: Absence of any criteria characteristic of conduct disorder before age 10 years

Conduct disorder, unspecified onset: Age at onset is not known

Specify severity:

Mild: Few if any conduct problems in excess of those required to make the diagnosis *and* conduct problems cause only minor harm to others

Moderate: Number of conduct problems and effect on others intermediate between mild and severe

Severe: Many conduct problems in excess of those required to make the diagnosis *or* conduct problems cause considerable harm to others

From American Psychiatric Association: *Diagnostic and statistical manual of mental disorders,* ed 4, text revision, Washington, DC, 2000, American Psychiatric Association.

DSM-IV-TR CRITERIA

Intermittent Explosive Disorder

A Several discrete episodes occur that suggest a failure to resist aggressive impulses that result in serious assaultive acts or destruction of property.

B The degree of aggressiveness expressed during the episodes is grossly out of proportion to any precipitating psychosocial stressors.

C The aggressive episodes are not better accounted for by another mental disorder (e.g., antisocial personality disorder, borderline personality disorder, a psychotic disorder, a manic episode, conduct disorder or attention-deficit/hyperactivity disorder) and are not due to the direct physiologic effects of a substance (e.g., a drug of abuse a medication) or a general medical condition (e.g., head trauma, Alzheimer's disease).

From American Psychiatric Association: *Diagnostic and statistical manual of mental disorders,* ed 4, text revision, Washington, DC, 2000, American Psychiatric Association.

also may become physically injured as a result of their aggressive outbursts. There is limited data on the prognosis of intermittent explosive disorder, but the course appears to be chronic or episodic, lasting from the childhood years into the early 20s.

DISCHARGE CRITERIA

Client will:

- Demonstrate safe conduct toward self and others.
- Engage in self-care within level of capability.
- Demonstrate emotional and behavioral control within capacity.
- Attend to tasks, schoolwork, and performance without unnecessary anger or frustration.
- Exhibit healthy self-concept and self-esteem in words and actions.
- Demonstrate functional eating habits and behaviors appropriate for age and stature.
- Use cognitive, communication, and language skills to make him or herself understood and to get needs met.
- Demonstrate interactive skills appropriate for level of development.
- Verbalize satisfaction with gender identity and sexual preference.
- Interact meaningfully with staff, peers, and family within capability.
- Seek attention and assistance appropriately from significant persons and refrain from unnecessary interactions with strangers.

- Adhere to treatment regimen, including medications as needed.
- Play appropriately with peers according to age and unit guidelines.
- Engage in educational and vocational programs as prescribed for each individual.
- Use adaptive coping techniques and stress-reducing strategies.
- Respond satisfactorily to others' attentions and requests.
- Use community resources to enhance quality of life.
- Engage in ongoing individual and family therapy.
- State specific reasons that demonstrate readiness for discharge.

ADOLESCENT SUICIDE

Adolescent suicide does not neatly fall under any diagnostic category. Adolescent suicides have quadrupled since 1950 from 2.5 to 11.2 per 100,000 and currently represent 12% of all deaths in this age-group. Approximately 2 million U.S. adolescents attempt suicide, 700,000 receive medical attention, and 2000 die each year. It ranks third as the leading cause of death in adolescents. For every completed suicide researchers estimate that there are 20 to 200 attempts. Between 80% and 90% of the attempters have a diagnosable psychiatric disorder. Reported factors include anxiety, disruptive disorder, bipolar disorder, substance abuse and personality disorders, a family history of mood disorders, a family history of suicidal behavior, exposure to family violence, impulsivity, abuse and molest, stress events (real or perceived), and the availability of methods (Shaffer, 2001). Substance abuse/dependence enhances the risk of suicidal thoughts and suicide attempts (Gould, 1998). Wagner et al. (2000) found that nearly half of the children and adolescents hospitalized for suicidal ideation had attempted suicide at least once in the past.

Hanging was the most common method in the 10- to 15-year-old age-group, whereas firearms were the most common method in later adolescence. Fewer warning signs and fewer precipitating events preceded the suicide in children and young adolescents. Intoxication and romantic failure were not a risk in those younger than 15, as so often occurs in older adolescents. Self-destructive behavior in the form of self-injury is of growing concern. Significant risk factors for suicide include the following: males with a prior attempt who are older than 16 with an associated mood or substance disorder, females with a mood disorder and prior attempt. Clients with a diagnosis of major depression and agitation are at high risk for suicide (Shaffer, 2001).

CLINICAL ALERT

Older children and adolescents engage in self-injurious behavior as a way to cope with their painful feelings or situation, to feel that they are in reality, or to communicate their feelings of hopelessness and helplessness. Self-injurious behavior affects approximately 1% of the population. The act of **self-injury** is defined as damaging bodily tissue to alter one's mood. Types of injury include cutting, burning, biting, head banging, bruising, picking at the skin, and hair pulling. Teenagers learn this behavior from their peers as an immediate release of emotional tension. There are also websites that describe techniques to "cut" and methods to hide the wounds. Self-injurious behavior is not suicidal behavior, but may be rehearsal behavior, and some teenagers accidentally commit suicide in the process. Repeated acts of self-injury also desensitize the individual who may subsequently find it easier to commit suicide. The nurse needs to assess for signs of self-injurious behavior, educate the family, and help the teenager to develop adaptive strategies and techniques for coping with anxiety and stress.

YOUTH VIOLENCE

Youth violence is becoming more common with younger children committing more aggressive acts than ever before. Early childhood aggression has a relatively high likelihood of persistence over time (Vance, 2002). Students bringing guns and knives to school have prompted the school systems to have stricter "no tolerance" rules and higher security such as metal detectors and on site police officers. The surgeon general published a report on youth violence ("Youth Violence," 2001) summarizing research studies that discussed possible risk factors, interventions, and preventions for youth violence.

There was an epidemic of violence in the United States during 1983 to 1993 because of an increase in gang violence, drug usage, and easier access to guns. From 10% to 15% of high school seniors admitted to committing at least one serious violent act the previous year. Approximately 30% to 40% of males and 15% to 30% of females have committed a serious violent act at some point in their lives. There were more arrests for violent crimes committed by African Americans and Hispanics but confidential surveys completed by adolescents demonstrated a more narrow racial disparity ("Youth Violence," 2001).

Risk Factors

During childhood, the greatest risk factor for committing violent acts are being male, having a low IQ, ADHD, delinquent behavior, substance use, poverty, abuse, or neglect, parents with antisocial personality, and single-parent homes. The strongest risk factors in adolescence are being male, peer rejection or isolation, substance use, gang involvement, and associating with peers who commit crimes. Other factors identified include parental divorce, separation, negative parent-child interaction, witnessing domestic violence, and physical and sexual abuse.

Studies have shown that exposure to violence on TV, the Internet, and video games increases aggressive behavior in children. Continued research is necessary to study the long-term effects of exposure to violence ("Youth Violence," 2001; Rae-Grant, 1999). Other research has studied particular violent interactive entertainment as increasing risk taking and self-defeating behaviors. These include the use of substances and alcohol, accelerated onset of sexual activity, lower grades in school, less exercise, read-

RESEARCH for EVIDENCE-BASED PRACTICE

Dunbar B: Anger management: a holistic approach, *Journal of the American Psychiatric Nurses Association* 10:16-23, 2004.

Many adolescents struggle with expressing their anger safely. Dunbar studied a holistic treatment approach to anger by incorporating 12 concepts of anger in a 16-week course. The concepts included the following:

- Open-mindedness
- Anger does not equal bad
- Responsibility for managing own anger
- Physical cues
- Relaxation
- Underlying emotion
- Negative thoughts
- Assertive responses
- Physical activity
- Self-esteem
- Should system
- Resentment

Participants completed the Anger Management Self-Assessment Scale created by Dunbar before the first group session, 4 weeks into the program and again within 2 weeks of completing the program. The groups met for 1 hour each week. After the course, the participants evaluated themselves as having an increased ability to recognize anger cues, to identify and act on primary emotions with increased feelings of assertiveness, and to recognize feelings of self-worth. They all agreed that they learned healthy anger management techniques.

ing fewer books, being desensitized to violence and the suffering of others, and more fearful of the world. Children with emotional problems appear especially vulnerable (Villani, 2001; American Academy of Child and Adolescent Psychiatry, 2000, 2001; American Psychological Association, "Family and Relationships," 2000).

Protective Factors

On the more positive side, researchers have identified some protective factors. These include positive and consistent parental discipline, daily structure, positive parent-child relationships, and family church involvement. Children whose parents have a high school or higher education, who have family support, and who have good problem-solving abilities are less at risk for developing violent behaviors. Living at home, having an internal locus of control, use of faith as a coping method, competence in daily life, and good interpersonal skills are also other protective factors (Vance, 2002) (see the Research for Evidence-Based Practice box).

ADULT DISORDERS IN CHILDREN AND ADOLESCENTS

Substance Abuse

Although a large number of adolescents try drugs or alcohol, the majority do not progress to abuse or dependence. In 1996, the annual Monitoring the Future Study found that nearly one third of high school seniors reported having been drunk in the before taking the survey month and one fifth reported marijuana use. Nearly 5% reported daily marijuana use (Weinberg et al., 1998). By the end of high school, approximately 90% of students have tried alcohol and 40% have tried an illicit drug, typically marijuana (Bukstein et al., 1997).

Many believe that drug use is more a function of social and peer factors, whereas abuse and dependence are more related to biologic and psychologic processes. Risk factors for dependence include the following:

- Executive cognitive dysfunction
- Disorders of behavioral self-regulation
- Difficulties with planning, attention, abstract reasoning, foresight, judgment, self-monitoring, and motor control
- Need for sensation seeking
- Difficulties with affect regulation
- Drug-abusing parents
- Maternal depression
- Anxiety

Factors that protect against substance use include adequate intelligence and problem-solving ability, positive self-esteem, supportive family relationships, positive role models, and intact affect regulation (Weinberg et al., 1998).

Depression

Population studies report a prevalence of major depression and dysthymia of approximately 0.4% to 2% in children and 4% to 8% in adolescents, with a lifetime prevalence of major depression in adolescents of 15% to 20%. Children with at least one depressed parent are three times more likely to develop major depression. Symptoms include changes in appetite, sleep, energy level, and concentration. Some children exhibit a depressed or irritable mood, behavioral problems such as temper tantrums, low frustration tolerance, and manifest anxiety symptoms accompanied with somatic symptoms. Adolescents typically exhibit more sleep and appetite disturbances, suicidal ideations and attempts, and difficulties functioning in relationships in school and at home (Birmaher et al., 1996) (see the Case Study on p. 381, left column).

Other problems often accompany depressive disorders. This includes substance abuse, suicidal tendencies, and behavioral problems. Children and adolescents with depression have a comorbid diagnosis in 40% to 70% of cases; those with dysthymic disorder or anxiety have a comorbid diagnosis in 30% to 80% of cases (Birmaher et al., 1996).

Bipolar Disorder

Health care providers often miss the diagnosis of pediatric bipolar disorder because of the overlapping of symptoms. Children frequently present with atypical symptoms that are often markedly labile and irregular and are irritable, aggressive, or mixed rather than euphoric. Reckless behavior often leads to school failure, fighting, dangerous play, and inappropriate sexual activity. Youths diagnosed with bipolar disorder are more likely to have rapid cycling or mixed episodes with a greater risk of suicide. These symptoms are different from common childhood phenomena of boasting, imaginary play, overactivity, and youthful indiscretions (Beiderman, 1998; McClellan et al., 1997).

CASE STUDY A mother brought her 15-year-old son for evaluation. She reported that he lost 10 pounds in the past month and failed two classes when normally he is a B student. She further stated she hears him on his computer for hours at a time late a night. She complained that he is moody, irritable, and argumentative. She separated from her husband 4 months earlier, and since that time her son has been isolative and withdrawn. He is gone for hours after school, and when his mother asks where he was he states that he was out walking or at the library. He has been concerned with his appearance for the past week.

CRITICAL THINKING

1 What further questions would you ask to identify the diagnostic criteria the client would meet?
2 What lab tests would be helpful in identifying the appropriate diagnosis?
3 Is the client at risk for suicide? State reasons to support answer.
4 What is the most appropriate treatment recommendation at this time?

CASE STUDY Jake, a 10-year-old, was admitted to the children's unit after becoming increasingly aggressive at home. He was suspended from school after threatening to blow up the school with a bomb. He had been admitted 6 months earlier with a diagnosis of ADHD. His mother reported that Jake was prescribed methylphenidate (Ritalin). She admitted that she did not give him the medication consistently because Jake continued to be impulsive and aggressive whether or not he was taking the medication. She also reported that his moods were labile and unpredictable. She reported that he would be laughing and loving one minute and then the next minute he would have a temper outburst that could last up to an hour. During one temper tantrum on the day before his admission, he screamed, "Just kill me with a knife." His sleep has also been affected with intermittent insomnia and early morning awakening. His mother expressed concern that Jake spends a few hours a day on the computer, which interferes with his homework and doing chores at home.

CRITICAL THINKING

1 What are important questions to ask Jake and his mother?
2 What level of nursing supervision is appropriate at this time?
3 Do Jake's symptoms meet criteria for any other disorder?
4 What would you teach the family?

A child with bipolar disorder often appears amusing and shows misleading infectious cheerfulness in the midst of significant problems such as school suspensions and family fights. The thinking of these children is frequently illogical and grandiose. These children or adolescents often tell teachers how to teach the class. They often fail intentionally because they believe they are being taught incorrectly. They hold a belief that they will achieve in a prominent profession despite failing grades. Some believe that stealing is legal for them. They often overreact to minor irritations in the environment, and they frequently have inappropriate sexual behaviors such as propositioning teachers, making overt comments to peers, or calling sex phone (1-900) lines. Some individuals become overly interested in money and purchase items from (1-800) lines with others' credit cards and take more dangerous dares, believing that they are above the possibility of danger (see the Case Study above, right column). A major problem exists when bipolar disorder is present at the time an adolescent begins to drive and has increased autonomy. Automobile accidents take a heavy toll on the lives of this age-group, and the rate of accidental deaths is compounded when insight, reasoning, and judgment are clouded by mental disorders or when drugs are involved.

Psychosis

Schizophrenia rarely presents before 13 years of age, although cases have been documented as young as 3 and 5 years of age. An onset before age 13 (very early onset schizophrenia) usually is insidious and includes withdrawal, poor hygiene, odd behaviors such as hoarding or storing food and other objects, and a decline in academic functioning. Other developmental delays occur as well, including delays in cognitive, motor, sensory, and social functioning. Communication and interaction with family members and peers is problematic.

The presence of psychosis in preschool-age children presents an extremely difficult problem. Brief hallucinations under stress, imaginary friends, and fantasy figures are common. By the school-age years, persistent hallucinations are associated with serious disorders. Delusional content and hallucinations usually reflect developmental concerns. Hallucinations often include monsters, pets, or toys, and delusions typically revolve around identity issues and are less complex. After age 7, loose and illogical thinking does not usually occur in normal children (McClellan et al., 1997).

Anxiety Disorders

A pediatric primary care sample revealed a 1-year prevalence of anxiety disorders of 15.4% in 7 to 11-year-olds. Epidemiologic studies in nonreferred 11-year-olds documented the following prevalences: separation anxiety, 3.5%; overanxious disorder, 2.9%; simple phobia, 2.4%; social phobia, 1%. Risk factors for developing anxiety disorders in children include behavioral inhibition, insecure attachment, cognitive factors, developmental events, traumatic events, and access to support systems (Bernstein et al., 1996).

Developmental differences exist in the symptoms of anxiety. Children ages 5 to 8 most commonly report unrealistic worry about harm to parents and attachment figures and school refusal. From ages 9 to 12, children report excessive distress at times of separation. Adolescents typically report somatic complaints and school refusal. School refusal is present in three quarters of those identified with separation anxiety disorder.

In a community sample, more than two fifths of youths met criteria for exposure to at least one major trauma by age 18. Six percent met the criteria for a lifetime diagnosis of posttraumatic stress disorder. Symptoms for children under the age of 5 years included excessive clinging, crying, and withdrawal. Children between the ages of 6 to 11 years exhibited disruptive behavior, difficulty paying attention, loud outbursts, difficulties in school, feelings of depression and anxiety, and somatic complaints. Teenagers exhibited flashbacks, emotional numbing, sleep problems, substance abuse, risk-taking behaviors, suicidal thoughts, and isolation. Following a natural disaster, separation from parents, ongoing maternal preoccupation with the event, and altered family functioning were greater predictors of symptom development than exposure alone (Cohen, 1998). Pilowsky et al. (1999) found that adolescents with panic attacks were three times more likely to verbalize suicidal thoughts and two times more likely to have attempted suicide in the past than adolescents without panic attacks.

Obsessive-compulsive disorder (OCD) has a 6-month prevalence of 1 in 200 children and adolescents. OCD has been reported in children as young as 5 years with the mean age of 10 years. Children typically demonstrate normal age-dependent obsessive-compulsive behaviors such as wanting things done "just so" and sometimes insist on elaborate bedtime rituals. These behaviors usually stop by middle childhood and are replaced by collections, hobbies, and focused interests. Frequently observed symptoms in children and adolescents include obsessions (contamination fears), worry about harm to self or others, aggressiveness, sexual ideas, scrupulosity/religiosity, forbidden thoughts, the need to tell, ask, or confess, and compulsions (washing, repeating, checking, touching, counting, ordering/arranging, hoarding, praying).

The Nursing Process

The nursing process is applicable to children and adolescents in the psychiatric setting. Knowledge of growth and development is essential, as is the ability to do a thorough clinical assessment, including both medical and psychosocial aspects. The nurse assesses the child or adolescent within the context of the entire family structure and dynamics, including the cultural and socioeconomic situation.

Parents often seek treatment for the child or adolescent after being referred by the school system or after their own multiple attempts to change the child or adolescent have been unsuccessful. It is often difficult for adults to comprehend that children, especially young children, have mental disorders. As a result, parents delay treatment for years in the hope that the child will "grow out of it." Although it is common for a family to present a child or adolescent as the "identified client" (family member with the problem), it is important to remember that children will often act out the underlying family dynamics or family psychopathology. In addition, families are often in denial that the child may have a disorder that has been identified in other family members, such as tic disorders, obsessive-compulsive disorders, mood disorders, or psychosis.

Some families are skeptical of proposed treatment recommendations and discredit the therapeutic interventions. They continue to use unhealthy multigenerational parenting techniques. Families see initial improvement in a child or adolescent who is in treatment and then prematurely discontinue newly adopted interventions. This inevitably results in the relapse of the child or adolescent's condition and family dysfunction. Treatment success and outcome depend on family commitment to learning new skills and consistently applying them. Early assessment and intervention from all caregivers and educators is the most ideal treatment goal.

> **CLINICAL ALERT**
>
> When working with children, the nurse needs to remember that the child or adolescent is a minor and that the primary caregiver/guardian has legal rights in addition to the child's rights. Children and adolescents are able to give assent, and caregivers/guardians give informed consent. This applies to all forms of treatment such as medications and research studied. In the inpatient setting, this applies to all client rights, including admission to the mental health units, and seclusion and restraint. The nurse obtains the child or adolescent's signature, according to policy, on all assent and consent forms in addition to the caregiver/guardian's signature.

ASSESSMENT

A thorough physical assessment involving all body systems and a thorough mental status exam helps the nurse to identify potential physical or emotional problems that contribute to the overall health and well-being of the child or adolescent (Box 16-1). It is essential to obtain a thorough alcohol and drug history including the amount used, length of use, and the date and time of use. A drug history consists of questions that cover all potential methods of drug use such as sniffing paint thinners and other similar intoxicating chemicals, glue, or the contents of aerosol cans; smoking; drinking; or injecting.

Developmental Stage

Because each child and adolescent has unique strengths and weaknesses, this challenges the nurse to assess the client in the context of the family culture and socioeconomic circumstances while considering the phases of normal growth and development. Infants, children, and adolescents experience developmental delays as a result of family traumas, social deprivation, abuse, neglect, or complications from a major mental disorder. Children and adolescents are sometimes advanced in some developmental phases of their life but are delayed in other areas. For example, a client is advanced for his age in his development of cognition, but he is behind in developing social skills.

Family Life

The child or adolescent's family life and home environment are crucial aspects of assessment that lead to comprehensive understanding of the presenting mental health problems. The nurse needs to have an understanding of the types of interactions within the family relationships and each member's perception of the family dynamics, successes, and problems. It is important for the nurse to

BOX 16-1

Mental Status Exam for an Infant/Toddler

Appearance: level of nourishment, hygiene, and dress
Reaction to situation: initial reaction to strangers and reaction to transition of nurse playing with infant during assessment
Self-regulation: Level of alertness including crying and the ability to be soothed and to soothe self; reactions to sensory stimulation (sounds, touch, etc.); unusual behaviors such as head banging, hair pulling, spinning objects, flapping hands, walking on toes; activity level such as sitting quietly, climbing on furniture, exploring the room; attention span (e.g., following object with eyes, exploration of an object with hands, playing with toy); frustration tolerance such as the ability to persist in a difficult task, crying, tantrums; aggressiveness including appropriate assertiveness or excessive aggressiveness
Motor: Muscle tone and strength, movement of face, tongue, swallowing, drooling, unusual tics, seizures; gross motor including picking head up, rolling over, standing up, walking, running, hopping; fine motor including grasping finger, pincer (thumb to index finger) grasp, stacking, scribbling, puzzles
Speech and language: Vocalization and speech production such as quality, rate, volume; receptive language including comprehension of language, responding to questions and commands appropriately; expressive language including child's effectiveness of communicating, babbling, imitation, vocalization of single words, complete sentences
Thought*: Fear, such as a feared object, fear of being separated from caregiver; dreams including nightmares; dissociative state including sudden withdrawal and inattention, glazed eyes, tuning out

Modified from Thomas J et al: Practice parameters for the psychiatric assessment of infants and toddlers (0-36 months), *J Am Acad Child Adolesc Psychiatry* 36:21-36, 1997.
*Taking into consideration the age and developmental level of the client, this category may not apply; however, symptoms may precede thought disorders later in life, such as looseness of associations and echolalia.

understand characteristics of the home environment, including cleanliness and the size of the home, where and with whom the child or adolescent sleeps, patterns for meals, pet care, chores, homework, times and frequencies of recreational activities, and bedtime rituals.

NURSING DIAGNOSIS

All currently used North American Nursing Diagnosis Association International (NANDA-I) nursing diagnoses are applicable to children and adolescents (NANDA-I, 2007). However, because of the tendency for children and adolescents to act out the many problems with which they struggle, some diagnoses are more important. Safety issues are most significant and a first priority with any client in the mental health setting.

Family problems and conflicts may be equally or more relevant for the nurse to consider than other client needs or problems. Ineffective role performance, impaired parenting, and interrupted family processes are all important diagnoses for the nurse to consider. Always consider the needs of the family in the process of assigning nursing diagnoses.

OUTCOME IDENTIFICATION

Outcome criteria come from the nursing diagnosis in the nursing process. The nurse prioritizes outcomes and states them in simple terms. The outcome criteria for children and adolescents will consider and focus on promotion of normal growth and development in an effort to improve areas of current developmental deficits in addition to improving any identified dysfunction. The outcome criteria include the treatment goals of the child or adolescent, the nurse, the interdisciplinary team, and the caregivers. Children and adolescents are more likely to participate in the treatment process when they are included in decisions about their care and progress. Examples of outcome criteria are listed here. Client will:

- Demonstrate a decrease or elimination of aggressive behaviors toward self and others.
- Seek assistance and support from adults before losing self-control.
- Identify triggers that provoke negative behavioral responses.
- Demonstrate age-appropriate relationships with adults.
- Demonstrate age-appropriate relationships with peers.
- Use age-appropriate play and recreational activities to express self.

PLANNING

In the beginning phases of the nursing process, the nurse sets realistic expectations based on the child or adolescent's developmental level of ability and function. The nurse is aware that negative behavioral patterns have been part of the family dynamics and often have occurred for long periods of time. Ideally, the nurse plans for small, incremental changes in behavior with obtainable goals. The nurse's effort for mutual goal setting will demonstrate respect and trust with the child or adolescent. The nurse explains the plan to the child or adolescent in simple terms, requesting the client's active participation and best effort, with the understanding that the nurse will work in a cooperative effort with the client and family to obtain stated treatment goals.

IMPLEMENTATION

As the nurse implements the individualized and prioritized care plan, the nurse's role is to support the child or adolescent and the family through the behavioral change process. The child or adolescent will try to continue using previously established behaviors, many of which are negative. The nurse will demonstrate clear, consistent, and realistic expectations using role-modeling and therapeutic communication skills. The nurse will set consistent boundaries and limits as the child or adolescent questions authority and struggles to learn adaptive age-appropriate functioning.

Nursing Interventions

1. Conduct a thorough assessment with the parents/guardians and the client *to observe interactions*, and then assess them separately if appropriate.

2. Assess for the presence of suicidal ideation and for past aggressive behaviors including triggers *to aggressive behavior to ensure the client's safety and to prevent harm to others.*
3. Maintain a safe environment by continually assessing for contraband (objects that are sharp, alcohol, or illicit drugs) and being aware of any behavioral changes or signals that may indicate increasing anger or aggression *to prevent violence and maintain a safe environment.*
4. Establish a therapeutic alliance and maintain appropriate boundaries *to ensure consistency and security.*
5. Help the client to identify strengths and positive qualities *to foster self-esteem, self-assurance, and confidence.*
6. Demonstrate, teach, and reinforce cooperative, respectful and positive behaviors *to assist the client in developing and redefining successful and positive relationships.*
7. Set clear and consistent limits in a calm and nonjudgmental manner *to promote a safe environment and to develop trust.*
8. Redirect disruptive behavior with recreational activities *to channel excess energy and to prevent escalation.*
9. Inform the client of the consequences for not adhering to the limits *to allow the client the opportunity to respond and to express feelings and cognitively process options.*
10. Use timeouts or quiet time when the client does not respond to limits *to give the client time to deescalate in a quiet environment and process the event.*
11. Role-play situations that trigger aggressivity or self-mutilation or encourage alcohol or illicit drug use *to explore and reinforce alternative methods of coping.*
12. Teach anger management techniques *to lessen the feelings of powerlessness and prevent future escalation.*
13. For the younger child, initiate therapeutic play *to encourage the client to express thoughts and feelings in alternative ways in the absence of adequate language and to reestablish healthy boundaries.*
14. Establish a behavior modification program for the preschool and the school-aged child that rewards the client for expressing self-safely *to reinforce positive behaviors and to enhance self-esteem and sense of self-accomplishment.*
15. Involve the adolescent in developing a behavioral contract by identifying expected behaviors and privileges *to reinforce positive behaviors and to enhance self-esteem and independence.*
16. Engage the client in group therapy and recreational activities *to assist the client in developing positive peer communication and to improve social skills and motor skills.*
17. Provide positive feedback and recognition when the client adheres to the behavioral program and treatment plan *to promote self-esteem and to reinforce positive behaviors.*
18. Teach the parents/guardians about the disorder, the importance of consistency and structure, and the significance of medication compliance if indicated *to minimize guilt, increase the knowledge base about the disorder and realistic expectations and reinforce the consequences of medication noncompliance.*
19. Assess the parents/guardians for available support systems and refer to support groups and individual and family therapy as needed *to increase the parents' ability to cope and minimize feelings of isolation and guilt.*

Additional Treatment Modalities

Nurses use a variety of collaborative interventions with children and adolescents in the mental health setting. Recreational, occupational, music, and art therapies, in addition to school, group, family, and individual therapies, are treatment modalities that to promote overall health and well-being for the child and adolescent. Cognitive behavioral therapy groups have demonstrated effectiveness in teaching the adolescent to manage symptoms, utilize problem-solving skills, and change negative thought patterns and emotional reactions.

Pharmacologic Interventions

Many medications for adults are also used for children and adolescents. The predominant classifications include stimulants, antidepressants, antianxiety agents, anticonvulsants, and antipsychotics. The nurse plays a crucial role in administering the medication, monitoring for clinical effectiveness and adverse reactions, and assessing compliance. The nurse communicates these findings to the multidisciplinary treatment team and to the primary care provider. The nurse remains current in the knowledge of medications and continually seeks education regarding newly developed medications and their clinical effects on this population.

Group Activities

Group play and recreational activities are important when assisting the child or adolescent to develop positive peer communication and improve interpersonal relationships. Group play offers an excellent opportunity for the nurse to role model and teach new age-appropriate skills, reinforce positive behaviors, and promote nurturing peer relationships. The nurse will set limits in group play to promote a safe environment and to demonstrate ways to show cooperation with and respect for peers. Children and adolescents often have learned to tease and provoke peers in group settings. The nurse will nonjudgmentally assist them in redefining successful relationships.

Interventions are often more difficult with adolescents than with children, depending on the clinical presentation. It is normal for adolescents to question authority and test limits and rules. The nurse needs to establish rapport and a therapeutic alliance with the adolescent early in the course of treatment. Adolescents need and look for role models, so it is imperative that the nurse maintain appropriate boundaries and not seek to behave as an adolescent or a friend to gain their acceptance.

Group activities provide an excellent opportunity for the nurse to interact with adolescents during treatment.

NURSING CARE PLAN

Michael, a 9-year-old boy, was admitted to the children's unit after he attempted to stab his teacher with a pencil. He has a history of poor peer and sibling relationships and frequently is placed on detention at school for fighting with peers during recess. He has been taking Ritalin for the past year after he was diagnosed with attention deficit hyperactivity disorder. His mother complains that Michael continues to have a low frustration tolerance, often displaying temper outbursts when he does not get his way or when he is asked to do his homework or chores. He physically assaulted his 6-year-old sister when she was playing with his toy and then proceeded to break her toys. There are marital problems between Michael's parents related to his father's excessive drinking. Michael's mother acknowledges that she has difficulty being consistent and firm with Michael. She thinks that her husband is too strict and tries to compensate by being more flexible. The mother related that she has suffered from depression the past 2 years and has been taking Paxil. The family has recently started family therapy.

DSM-IV-TR DIAGNOSES

Axis I	Attention deficit hyperactivity disorder; rule out intermittent explosive disorder
Axis II	None
Axis III	Asthma
Axis IV	Severity of stressors = 3 (moderate): school detentions, alcoholism of biologic father, mother's depression
Axis V	GAF = 35 (current); GAF = 45 (past year)

Nursing Diagnosis *Risk for other-directed violence. Risk factors: a positive history of aggression toward peers, sibling and teacher (e.g., attempted to stab his teacher with a pencil, detentions at school)*

NOC Abuse Protection, Abuse Cessation, Abuse Behavior Self-Restraint, Hyperactivity Level, Impulse Self-Control, Fear Level

NIC Abuse Protection Support, Anger Control Assistance, Anxiety Reduction, Impulse Control Training, Behavior Modification: Social Skills, Support Group

CLIENT OUTCOMES	NURSING INTERVENTIONS	EVALUATION
Michael will demonstrate safe behaviors.	Provide close observation as indicated *to ensure the client's safety and to maintain a safe environment.*	Michael continues aggression, pushing peers and throwing objects when he is angry, requiring time out in his room.
	Set firm limits and consequences for aggressive behaviors. *Structure and clear expectations clarify boundaries for improved self-control.*	
	Help Michael to identify situations that precipitate his aggressive outbursts *to help the client identify sources of frustration.*	Michael identifies precipitants for his behavior only after aggressive acts and is working on recognizing triggers before he acts on feelings.
Michael will demonstrate alternative behaviors to violent outbursts.	Help Michael to identify three alternative behaviors to use when he becomes frustrated or angry.	Michael seeks staff when he is feeling angry and on the verge of losing control 75% of the time.
	Give Michael stickers for the star program every time he uses alternative behaviors *to reinforce appropriate behaviors and build self-esteem.*	Michael is currently on the silver level of the program, earning the use of his Game Boy and privilege of eating in the cafeteria with peers.
	Encourage Michael to play nerf football when he is frustrated or angry *to promote socially acceptable and safe ventilation of negative feelings.*	Michael plays nerf football when he feels frustrated 80% of the time.
	Encourage Michael to draw his feelings on a daily basis *to express his hostile feelings in safe manner.*	Michael draws pictures to help identify his feelings daily. His insight is improving slowly.
Michael will identify three situations that precipitate violent outbursts.	Encourage the client to verbalize feelings in daily one-to-one conversations *to ventilate emotions and receive encouragement and reinforcement from staff.*	Michael verbalizes when he feels angry with peers and with staff 50% of the time.
	Discuss possible situations that precipitate Michael's violent outbursts *to connect negative feelings with aggressive actions.*	Michael identifies situations that cause him to get angry (when he doesn't win at a game, when peers make fun of him, and when he's told he's done something wrong).
Michael will follow the unit rules and maintain the silver or gold level on the star program.	Explain the unit's rules and the star program *to clarify information and expectations for client.*	Michael demonstrates an understanding of the unit rules and the star program.
	Provide consistent staffing *to build a trusting relationship.*	Michael is beginning to respond positively to his designated staff.
	Set firm limits and consequences for breaking the unit rules. *Structure and clear expectations clarify boundaries for improved self-control.*	Michael continues to provoke peers, and he requires frequent timeouts during the shift. He continues to be on bronze level with no privileges.

Continued

NURSING CARE PLAN—cont'd

Nursing Diagnosis *Impaired social interaction related to low self-esteem, lack of positive peer and sibling relationships as evidenced by physical altercations with peers and sibling*

NOC Psychomotor Energy, Stress Level, Fear Level: Child, Play Participation, Social Interaction Skills, Self-Esteem, Family Functioning

NIC Behavior Management: Overactivity/Inattention, Behavior Modification: Social Skills, Socialization Enhancement, Self-Esteem Enhancement, Therapy Group

CLIENT OUTCOMES	NURSING INTERVENTIONS	EVALUATION
Michael will interact with peers and sibling without exhibiting aggressive behaviors.	Give Michael a sticker every time he verbalizes his anger and frustration appropriately *to reinforce appropriate behaviors and build self-esteem.*	Michael has verbalized to peers when he was angry 90% of the time and is currently on the gold level of the star program. His bedtime has been extended and he has earned snack privileges.
Michael will demonstrate good sportsmanship by not crying, yelling, or becoming aggressive when he does not win a game or arguing over the rules of the game.	Engage Michael in activities with peers that encourage teamwork and good sportsmanship.	Michael was able to accept that his team lost in a game of kickball and received positive recognition from his peers and staff.
	Give Michael a sticker every time he demonstrates good sportsmanship *to reinforce acceptable social interactions.*	
	Provide multiple role modeling incidents during activities *to demonstrate alternative ways to manage frustration.*	Michael attempts to act maturely 25% of the time when frustrated.

MEDICATION KEY FACTS Attention-Deficit/Hyperactivity Disorder

Pharmacologic therapy for ADHD includes psychostimulants (dextroamphetamine [Dexedrine], methylphenidate [Ritalin, Concerta], dextroamphetamine/amphetamine salts [Adderall]), noradrenergic specific reuptake inhibitors (NSRIs) (atomoxetine [Strattera]), adrenergic agents (clonidine [Catapres]), and some antidepressants such as bupropion (Wellbutrin) and selective serotonin reuptake inhibitors (SSRIs) (citalopram [Celexa], fluoxetine [Prozac], fluvoxamine [Luvox], paroxetine [Paxil], sertraline [Zoloft], venlafaxine [Effexor]).

PSYCHOSTIMULANTS/NSRI

- Hypertensive crisis may occur if combined or used within 14 days of MAOIs.
- Abrupt withdrawal after prolonged use of high doses may produce lethargy lasting for weeks.
- There is an increased risk of seizures (methylphenidate).
- Prolonged administration to children with ADHD may inhibit growth.
- *Herbal considerations:* St. John's wort may produce serotonin syndrome (characterized by a number of mental, autonomic, and neuromuscular changes).

ADRENERGIC AGENTS

- Abrupt withdrawal may result in rebound hypertension.
- Life-threatening elevations of BP with tricyclic antidepressants and beta-blockers.
- *Herbal considerations:* Aconite increases toxicity and may lead to death.

NEW AGENT (MODAFANIL)

- Central nervous system stimulants may potentiate action.

CLINICAL ALERT

The nurse needs to carefully observe the child or adolescent who has **ADHD** and who is taking medications. Children or adolescents taking stimulant medications such as methylphenidate hydrochloride (Ritalin) demonstrate adverse changes in appetite, sleep, and levels of restlessness. In addition, children or adolescents sometimes develop new tics, or previously existent mild tics exacerbate. Atomoxetine (Strattera) also increases suicidal thoughts in some children and adolescents. If this occurs, it is important that the nurse hold the medication, ensure safety, document the findings, and notify the provider of the clinical observations. Often, changes in dosage or discontinuance of the medication are required.

Group activities enable the adolescent to develop interpersonal skills, give and accept feedback during communication with peers, practice more adult-like relationships, listen with empathy, achieve success, and learn appropriate ways to interact with the world.

Behavior Modification Programs

For the child approximately 3 to 11 years old, a behavior modification program is frequently used in treatment plans. **Behavior modification** involves a systematic and structured program that identifies developmental and age-appropriate goals that are observable and measurable within an established time frame. The goals often focus on activities of daily living (ADLs), impulse control, and peer and sibling relationships. The child is rewarded for accomplishment of each goal. A chart lists each goal, and the child is rewarded with stars, stickers, or colors to signify progress. Many school systems use colored charts. Sometimes a behavior program is implemented in the home to correlate with the school program and thereby promote consistency.

Preadolescents and adolescents often use a **behavioral contract.** These contracts emphasize one to three goals that are more complex in nature (e.g., will speak to others with respect; will actively participate in group activities).

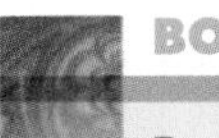

BOX 16-2

Example of a Behavioral Contract

Contracts are effective tools for compliance with desired behaviors if they are (1) *realistic,* (2) *age appropriate* (younger children require simple, single-level expectations), (3) *consistently maintained* (parent cannot change from contract by telling child he or she can play first then fulfill expected behaviors after play), and (4) *valued* by all parties involved.

BEHAVIORAL CONTRACT PRINCIPLES

- Criteria of the contract are determined through negotiation by all parties.
- The contract is most effective if written.
- *Short-range,* attainable goals are defined.
- Behaviors are rehearsed before final commitment to the contract.

PROCEDURE

1. Write a clear, brief but detailed description of the client's desired behavior.
2. Set the time and frequency of expected behaviors.
3. Specify positive reinforcements dependent on fulfilling items 1 and 2.
4. Specify adverse consequences dependent on nonfulfillment of items 1 and 2.
5. Add a bonus clause that includes additional positive reinforcements if the client exceeds initial minimal demands.
6. Specify how responses will be observed, measured, and recorded (e.g., a chart on the refrigerator) and specify the procedure for informing the client about achievement.
7. Deliver reinforcement soon after the response (do not wait to give an earned reward).

SCENARIO

Daniel, 10 years old, scatters his clothing and belongings in his room and every room in the house. He drops what he does not want to use at that moment on the floor or furniture. He then spends large amounts of time asking where his belongings are. His parents are exasperated, so they begin a contract with Daniel, which implies that Daniel and his parents are involved in the behavior change rather than Daniel alone.

Daniel and his parents sit down at a quiet time to calmly discuss the problematic behavior. Daniel usually plays an interactive television game every afternoon after school and almost any time he wants on weekends. Mom, Dad, and Daniel decide together, through negotiation, how much Daniel is able to do to keep the house and his room clean. If he complies, Daniel will have access to his TV game as a reward. Mom writes the contract, and all agree to 1 week of rehearsal before they sign it.

SAMPLE CONTRACT

1. and 2. (See the procedure noted above.) Daniel will do the following:
   a. Dress or undress *only* when in his room and no other room in the house.
   b. Use one game or toy at a time, putting all other games and toys that he is not using in specific, labeled, designated place in his room (at all times).
   c. Put all clean clothes on hangers or in drawers in his room (by bedtime at 8 PM).
   d. Put all dirty clothes in the bathroom hamper (before school by 7:30 AM and before bedtime at 8 PM).
   e. Place backpack next to desk and books on top of desk in his room (immediately after school by 3 PM).
   f. Look over entire house for any of his belongings, picking up any items he finds (before bedtime at 8 PM every evening).
3. If items 1 and 2 are fulfilled, Daniel will play with his TV game each day from 4 to 5 PM on school days and any 2 hours he chooses on weekends and holidays (log of hours will be posted on the refrigerator for Daniel to complete with one parent).
4. If items 1 and 2 are unmet, Daniel loses his TV game privilege (on that day if unmet in the morning *or* on the next day if unmet at bedtime).
5. *Bonus:* If Daniel meets the contract each day for total of 5 days, he can choose one place from a prepared list for the family outing on Saturday or Sunday.
6. Mom will mark with an X and sign initials on the refrigerator poster (every morning); Dad will mark and sign (every evening). If one parent is away, the other will sign off. The family will discuss and review the contract and performance at dinner each evening. There will be no delayed reinforcements (TV or no TV) at any time or on any day.

Signed (Daniel) ____________________ Date __________
(Mom) ____________________
(Dad) ____________________

From Fortinash KM, Holoday Worret PA: *Psychiatric nursing care plans,* ed 5, St Louis, 2007, Mosby.

The nurse will usually place a checkmark after each goal to signify that the adolescent has accomplished that goal. Rewards in the form of increased privileges such as a later bedtime or curfew or an activity with a parent or friend are an outcome of maintaining the contract. A sample behavioral contract appears in Box 16-2.

Therapeutic Play

For the younger child, nursing interventions frequently occur in activities of **therapeutic play**. Play is the work of children. Children are able to use recreational and creative play activities in relationships with peers and adults as they work to master new developmental tasks. Children express their thoughts, feelings, frustrations, fears, and hopes through therapeutic play. The perceptive nurse observes and guides the child in play and interacts to modify distortions and reestablish healthy boundaries and safe limits as the child redefines behaviors through play.

EVALUATION

The evaluation phase of the nursing process documents the treatment progress, as evidenced by actual outcomes. The observant nurse objectively reviews the evaluation phase to determine the effectiveness of the treatment plan. In addition to outcomes, the nurse examines other factors. For instance, were the treatment goals cognitively and developmentally appropriate for the child or adolescent? Are there other stressors within the family or social support system that are adding to the presenting problems, thus contributing to unrealistic expectations for the child or adolescent (e.g., health, financial, or placement problems)?

The interdisciplinary team coordinates any care plan modifications in an effort to maintain cohesiveness within the treatment implementation. It is also important to continually communicate the treatment evaluation with the caregivers. This helps to reinforce treatment gains, reinforce new methods of parental interventions, and assist the caregivers in monitoring and reestablishing new and realistic expectations.

For inpatient hospitalization it is important that the nurse begin, early in the course of treatment with the family, to prepare them for the potential and pending discharge. Work that initially begins in an inpatient setting is usually transitioned to home or other outpatient placements, such as day treatment, residential care, or a group home. In the evaluation phase, the nurse encourages the child or adolescent and the family to make healthy transitions to the ongoing therapeutic relationship with the next primary mental health provider (i.e., nurse specialist, social worker, psychologist, or psychiatrist).

CHAPTER SUMMARY

- Of mentally retarded individuals, 85% are mildly retarded, 10% are moderately retarded; 3% to 4% are severely retarded, and 1% to 2% are profoundly retarded.
- Children with autistic disorder present with repetitive movements, no emotional reciprocity, impaired communication (both verbal and nonverbal), and an indifference to affection. Seventy-five percent have some degree of mental retardation.
- The most commonly diagnosed mental disorders are attention-deficit/hyperactivity disorder (ADHD), mood disorder, and pervasive development disorder.
- Some children with ADHD have the following histories: child abuse or neglect, multiple foster placements, neurotoxin exposure, infections, drug exposure in utero, low birth weight, and mental retardation.
- ADHD causes problems in academics, social relationships, self-esteem, and occupation because of its demanding, impulsive, and seemingly lazy manifestations.
- Separation anxiety is a disruptive disorder that prevents children from engaging in normal activities because of constant fear that their loved ones will be harmed in their absence.
- Like autistic disorder, Tourette's disorder involves repetitive movements, sounds, and actions; however, unlike autistic disorder, these symptoms diminish during adolescence and adulthood, and the disorder is not pervasive.
- One of the main characteristics of conduct disorder is the client's violent or aggressive behavior with little concern of how it affects others.
- Behavior modification programs are systematic structured plans with specific goals and time frames. The client is rewarded for attaining goals.
- Early identification and treatment of the child and adolescent are crucial in assisting the client in the home, school, and social setting for both the short and long term.
- Nursing interventions with children and adolescents are intense and challenging. The nurse works closely with the family and the multidisciplinary team to provide care.

REVIEW QUESTIONS

1 A nurse assesses a 9-year-old female for the risk of violence. School officials report that although the client is very intelligent, she was suspended for bringing illicit drugs on campus. The child has lived with her mother since the parents were divorced 2 years ago. Her father is in prison. How many risk factors for committing a violent act are present for this child?
1. One
2. Two
3. Three
4. Four

2 A nurse prepares the plan of care for an adolescent with moderate mental retardation. Select the highest level achievable outcome(s) for this client. You may select more than one answer. Within 5 years, the client will:
1. Complete high school or GED.
2. Safely use local public transportation.
3. Live independently in an apartment.
4. Correctly use a telephone.
5. Attain employment in a sheltered workshop.

3 A nurse counsels the parents of a child with autistic disorder. The parents say, "We are going to completely redecorate our child's room. We think that will help." Select the nurse's best response.
1. "Children with autistic disorder usually prefer that things stay the same."
2. "Bright colors are often stimulating for children with autistic disorder."
3. "Remember to not use rugs so that your child will not slip and fall."
4. "New toys and games will help develop your child's intellectual abilities."

4 A nurse suggests activities for a 7-year-old child with autistic disorder. Which activity is most likely to engage this child?
1. Playing checkers with one other child
2. Building with blocks alone
3. Playing kickball with a small group of children
4. Having a birthday party with six to eight other children

5 The parent of a child with Tourette's disorder says to the nurse, "I think my child is faking the tics because they're absent during sleep." Select the nurse's accurate response.
1. "Perhaps your child was misdiagnosed."
2. "This finding indicates a worsening of the child's condition."
3. "Your observation indicates the medication is effective."
4. "Tics are often reduced or absent during sleep."

*Additional self-study exercises and learning resources are available to you on the **Companion CD** at the back of the book and on the **Evolve website** at **http://evolve.elsevier.com/Fortinash/**.*

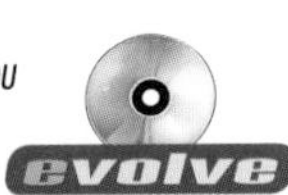

ONLINE RESOURCES

American Academy of Child and Adolescent Psychiatry: **www.aacap.org**

American Academy of Pediatrics: **www.aap.org**

Association of Child and Adolescent Psychiatric Nurses: **www.ispn-psych.org/html/acapn.html**

Attention Deficit Disorder Resources: **www.addresources.org**

Autism Society of America: **www.autism-society.org**

Child Abuse Prevention Association: **www.childabuseprevention.org**

Federation of Families for Children's Mental Health: **www.ffcmh.org**

National Alliance on Mental Illness: **www.nami.org**

National Institute of Mental Health: **www.nimh.nih.gov**

Mental Health America: **www.nmha.org**

National Youth Violence Prevention Resource Center: **www.safeyouth.org**

SAMHSA's National Mental Health Information Center: Caring for Every Child's Mental Health Campaign: **www.mentalhealth.samhsa.gov/child**

REFERENCES

American Academy of Child and Adolescent Psychiatry: AACAP joins health organizations' consensus on entertainment violence danger, *News Release*, 2000.

American Academy of Child and Adolescent Psychiatry: Children and watching TV, *Facts for families* #54, Washington, DC, 2001, AACAP.

American Psychiatric Association: *Diagnostic and statistical manual of mental disorders*, ed 4, text revision, Washington, DC, 2000, American Psychiatric Association.

American Psychological Association: *Family and relationships: children and television violence*, Washington, DC, 2000, APA.

Bauermeister J et al: Epidemiology of disruptive behavior disorders, *Child Adolesc Psychiatry Clin North Am* 3:177-194, 1994.

Biederman J: Resolved: Mania is mistaken for ADHD in prepubertal children: affirmative, *J Am Acad Child Adolesc Psychiatry* 37:1091-1096, 1998.

Bernstein GA et al: Anxiety disorder in children and adolescents: a review of the past 10 years, *J Am Acad Child Adolesc Psychiatry* 35:1110-1119, 1996.

Birmaher B et al: Childhood and adolescent depression: a review of the past 10 years, part I, *J Am Acad Child Adolesc Psychiatry* 35:1575-1583, 1996.

Boris N et al: Practice parameter for the assessment and treatment of children and adolescents with reactive attachment disorder for infancy and early childhood, *J Am Acad Child Adolesc Psychiatry* 44:1206-1219, 2005.

Bukstein O et al: Practice parameters for the assessment and treatment of children and adolescents with substance use disorders, *J Am Acad Child Adolesc Psychiatry* 44:609-621, 1997.

Cantwell DP: Attention deficit disorder: a review of the past 10 years, *J Am Acad Child Adolesc Psychiatry* 35:978-987, 1996.

Cohen J et al: Summary of the practice parameters for the assessment and treatment of children and adolescents with posttraumatic stress disorder, *J Am Acad Child Adolesc Psychiatry* 37: 997-1001, 1998.

Dulcan M et al: Practice parameters for the assessment and treatment of children, adolescents, and adults with ADHD, *J Am Acad Child Adolesc Psychiatry* 36(10 suppl):855-1215, 1997.

Dunbar B: Anger management: a holistic approach, *J Am Psychiatr Nurses Assoc* 10:16-23, 2004.

Gould MS: Psychopathology associated with suicide ideation and attempts among children and adolescents, *J Am Acad Child Adolesc Psychiatry* 37:915-923, 1998.

King NJ: School refusal in children and adolescents: a review of the past 10 years, *J Am Acad Child Adolesc Psychiatry* 40:197-205, 2001.

Loeber R: Oppositional defiant disorder and conduct disorder: a review of the past 10 years: part I, *J Am Acad Child Adolesc Psychiatry* 39:1468-1684, 2000.

Maldonado-Duran M et al: Child abuse & neglect: reactive attachment disorder, *eMedicine*, 2005; retrieved on Jan 9, 2006, from www.emedicine.com/ped/topic2646.htm.

McClellan J et al: Practice parameters for the assessment and treatment of children and adolescents with bipolar disorder, *J Am Acad Child Adolesc Psychiatry* 36(10 suppl):1775-1935, 1997.

National Institute of Mental Health: Child and adolescent mental health, 2005; retrieved Oct 17, 2005, from www.nimh.nih.gov/healthinformation/childmenu.cfm.

Nearns J: Attention deficit/hyperactivity disorder, *CME Resource*, 1-28, 1997.

North American Nursing Diagnosis Association International: *NANDA nursing diagnoses: definitions and classifications, 2007-2008*, Philadelphia, 2007, North American Nursing Diagnosis Association.

Pilowsky E: Panic attacks and suicide attempts in mid-adolescence, *Am J Psychiatry* 156:1545-1549, 1999.

Pliszka S: The Texas children's medication algorithm project: report of the Texas consensus conference panel on medication treatment of childhood attention deficit/hyperactivity disorder: part II tactics, *J Am Acad Child Adolesc Psychiatry* 39:920-927, 2000.

Rae-Grant N: Violent behavior in children and youth: preventive intervention from a psychiatric perspective, *J Am Acad Child Adolesc Psychiatry* 38:235-241, 1999.

Schowalter J: A history of child and adolescent psychiatry in the United States, *Psychiatric Times*, 2005; retrieved on January 9, 2006, from www.psychiatrictimes.com/p030943.html.

Shaffer D et al: Practice parameters for the assessment and treatment of children and adolescents with suicidal behavior, *J Am Acad Child Adolesc Psychiatry* 40:24-51, 2001.

Steiner H et al: Practice parameters for assessment and treatment of children and adolescents with conduct disorder, *J Am Acad Child Adolesc Psychiatry* 36:1482-1485, 1997.

Szymanski L et al: Practice parameters for the assessment and treatment of children, adolescents and adults with mental retardation and comorbid mental disorders, *J Am Acad Child Adolesc Psychiatry* 38:5-31, 1999.

Tanguay PE: Pervasive developmental disorders: a 10-year review, *J Am Acad Child Adolesc Psychiatry* 39:1079-1095, 2000.

US Surgeon General: *Youth violence: a report of the surgeon general.* Retrieved April 24, 2002 from www.surgeongeneral.gov/library/youthviolence.report.html.

Valente S: Autism, *J Am Psychiatr Nurses Assoc* 10:236-243, 2004.

Vance JE et al: Risk and protective factors as predictors of outcome in adolescents with psychiatric disorder and aggression, *J Am Acad Child Adolesc Psychiatry* 41: 36-43, 2002.

Villani S: Impact of media on children and adolescents: a 10-year review of the research, *J Am Acad Child Adolesc Psychiatry* 40:391-401, 2001.

Volkmar FR: Practice parameters for the assessment and treatment of children, adolescents, and adults with autism and other pervasive developmental disorders, *J Am Acad Child Adolesc Psychiatry* 38:32-54, 1999.

Wagner K et al: Cognitive factors related to suicidal ideation and resolution in psychiatrically hospitalized children and adolescents, *Am J Psychiatry* 157:2017-2021, 2000.

Weinberg NZ et al: Adolescent substance abuse: a review of the past 10 years, *J Am Acad Child Adolesc Psychiatry* 37:252-261, 1998.

Chapter 17

Eating Disorders

ANNE CLARKIN-WATTS

You gain strength, courage, and confidence by every experience in which you really stop to look fear in the face . . . you must do the thing you think you cannot do.

ELEANOR ROOSEVELT

OBJECTIVES

1 Identify the behavioral and psychologic symptoms of anorexia nervosa and bulimia nervosa.
2 Compare and contrast the medical complications of anorexic and bulimic behavior.
3 Analyze the biologic, sociocultural, familial, and psychologic factors that contribute to the etiology of eating disorders.
4 Explain the vicious cycle of eating disorder behavior.
5 Discuss the psychologic issues associated with eating disorder behaviors.
6 Describe the type of therapeutic relationship that is most effective with clients who have eating disorders, including the approach and attitude the nurse demonstrates to achieve this relationship.
7 Apply the nursing process for clients with eating disorders.

KEY TERMS

alexithymia, p. 393
anorexia nervosa, p. 390
binge eating disorder, p. 395
body image disturbance, p. 369
bulimia nervosa, p. 390
comorbidity, p. 395
dichotomous thinking, p. 393
emotional dysregulation, p. 393
enmeshed families, p. 393
interoceptive deficits, p. 397
purging, p. 397
secondary gains, p. 393

Eating disorders are serious psychiatric illnesses with devastating, potentially fatal medical complications. Eating disorders have the highest mortality rate of all mental illnesses and often become chronic, lifelong conditions. In **anorexia nervosa,** a pathologic drive for thinness and a disturbed body image lead to self-starvation. In **bulimia nervosa,** a similar drive for thinness exists, but dietary restraint leads to cycles of binge eating and purging, usually with self-induced vomiting.

The epidemic of eating disorders in the late twentieth century happened at the same time as cultural trends in three major industries: the fashion industry, the diet and fitness industry, and the women's movement. A shift toward thinness in fashion, the emergence of the diet and fitness industry, and changes in women's roles created a climate for an outbreak of eating disorders. Box 17-1 summarizes these cultural trends.

This epidemic of eating disorders got the public's attention. The media are still fascinated with eating disorders, which has helped raise awareness about eating disorders worldwide. An explosion of literature since the 1980s includes medical and psychiatric research, sociocultural essays, biographies, and popular press.

HISTORIC AND THEORETIC PERSPECTIVES

The drastic increase in eating disorders in the late twentieth century suggests that it is a fad, or trend, of modern, fashion-conscious young women and, more recently, body-conscious young men. However, self-starvation, bingeing, and purging have existed for centuries. Throughout history, food has always been a compelling cultural symbol, so denial of appetite

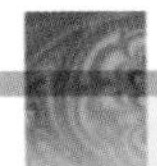

BOX 17-1

Cultural Trends and Eating Disorders

FASHION INDUSTRY

Cultural ideals of beauty have always been reflected in current fashion. The trend in fashion since the 1960s has been increasingly toward thinness. By the late twentieth century, fashion had become a huge industry, fueled by advertising dollars and exerting great influence on the public, especially women. The media are full of images of the thin, fit, "perfect" body, an ideal that is unattainable for most people. Epidemiologic studies show that 0.1% of people have a natural body type that matches the ideal. This leads most people to believe that their normal, healthy shape is too fat. The pervasiveness of this trend is reflected in the dieting behavior and body dissatisfaction among high school, elementary school, and middle school children.

DIET AND FITNESS INDUSTRY

The second trend is the creation of the diet and fitness industry. Weight management has moved out of the doctor's office and into multibillion-dollar businesses run by opportunistic, business-minded people who are not part of the health professions. The media flood the public with an array of products such as pills, powders, packaged food, diet books, videos, and a variety of health club and diet program memberships designed to help us attain the "perfect body." Men have become more obsessed with an ideal, lean, and muscular body, which is equally unattainable for the average guy, leading men to buy into the diet and fitness industry. Eating disorders have become much more common in males.

WOMEN'S MOVEMENT

A third trend is the ongoing women's movement. Although women's struggles for equality are not new, women's roles have changed dramatically since the early 1980s. Pressure to balance motherhood, marriage, and career has influenced women of all generations. The need for women to achieve success both academically and professionally while still fulfilling their traditional female roles creates conflicts, even as it affords women greater societal rights and freedom.

Professional women need to be aggressive to successfully compete in the business world, yet women are still socialized to be passive and accommodating. Some feminists view the drive for thinness as symbolizing a woman's attempt to destroy her femininity to compete in a man's world or as male society's reaction to the women's movement. Pressuring women to strive for an impossible ideal of thinness promotes feelings of inadequacy that drive women to constantly diet and exercise.

and rejection of food are always attention-getting behaviors. Earlier in history, cases of anorexia nervosa were rare and poorly understood.

Incidence in History

Brumberg, in *Fasting Girls* (1989), and Bell, in *Holy Anorexia* (1987), noted that medieval women commonly starved themselves in devotion to Christ. Both authors detail the case of Saint Catherine of Siena of Italy (1347-1380), who kept an extensive diary of her fasting and self-induced vomiting. Her piety also included self-flagellation and other self-punishing behavior, not very different from the self-destructive behavior common today among clients with anorexia and bulimia. This demonstrates the connectedness of anorexic and bulimic behaviors from the beginning of their known existence.

Few clinical accounts of normal-weight bulimia nervosa existed until case histories began to appear in psychoanalytic literature in the 1950s. In "The Case of Ellen West," American psychoanalyst Binswanger (1958) described a woman he treated in 1915 who starved herself, binged and purged with self-induced vomiting, exercised excessively, and used laxatives. Obsessed with food and clinically depressed, she committed suicide 13 years later. In *The Fifty Minute Hour*, psychiatrist Robert Lindner (1955) described the case of "Laura," a client with bulimia nervosa.

These psychoanalytic case studies focus on symptoms as manifestations of intrapsychic issues such as oral impregnation fears, oral eroticism, rejection of femininity, and unconscious hatred of the mother, ignoring cultural or biologic factors. Lesser-known case studies noted bulimic behavior among young girls in boarding schools and refugee children, suggesting a connection to separation fears, a theory held today regarding the onset, or beginning, of eating disorders during adolescence (Johnson and Connors, 1987).

The term *compulsive overeating* was first used in the 1950s to describe binge eating among the overweight and obese population (Stunkard, 1959; Hamburger, 1951). Compulsive eating was compared with alcoholism, with its similar cravings and secret binges followed by shame and guilt. *Binge eating disorder* is currently being considered as a new diagnosis for this disorder.

In the mid-1970s psychologist Marlene Boskind-Lodahl described a group of normal-weight women she saw at Cornell University's mental health clinic who shared the anorectic individual's fear of fat and drive for thinness. These women also regularly binged and purged. In her 1983 book, the author described her clinical experience and new research with this group, who represented the first wave of the current outbreak of eating disorders (Boskind-Lodahl and White, 1983). Russell (1979) coined the term *bulimia nervosa*, linking bulimia to anorexia nervosa.

ETIOLOGY

Researchers have studied a variety of etiologic theories regarding eating disorders from biologic, psychologic, psychoanalytic, behavioral, and addiction viewpoints. Currently there is no clear agreement on what causes eating disorders. However, many opposing theories have come together to form a framework that better explains eating disorders as multidetermined syndromes. Now, researchers believe that eating disorders are caused by an interaction of biologic susceptibility, including genetic markers for both neurobiologic vulnerability and personality traits, and environmental influences, including family, social, and cultural environments. A predisposed individual experiences stress, often related to the developmental tasks of adolescence, and decides to diet, which triggers the eating disorder (Box 17-2).

BOX 17-2

Etiologic Factors Related to Eating Disorders

BIOLOGIC FACTORS
Family history of eating disorders
Genetic predisposition for high-risk personality traits
Premorbid neurobiologic dysregulation, causing anxiety or depression

SOCIOCULTURAL FACTORS
Diet and fitness industry
Changes in women's and family roles
Fashion industry
Stress related to developmental tasks of adolescence

PSYCHOLOGIC FACTORS
Low self-esteem
Perfectionism
Emotional immaturity
Interoceptive deficits
Ineffectiveness
Compliance, conflict avoidance

FAMILIAL FACTORS
Enmeshment, poor conflict resolution skills
Focus on social acceptance, achievement, ideal body image, parental dieting
Separation/individuation issues
Some incidence of alcoholism or physical or sexual abuse

Biologic Factors

The many physiologic abnormalities found in anorexia nervosa and bulimia nervosa suggest a biologic etiology. The homogeneity, or sameness, of the symptoms is striking; anorexic clients express remarkably similar thoughts and beliefs and engage in identical odd behaviors, suggesting a genetic etiology. A confounding factor is that extreme behaviors of starving, bingeing, and purging themselves cause a range of neurobiologic, metabolic, and behavioral abnormalities. Some of these effects make the client continue the behavior. For example, starving decreases appetite and delays gastric emptying, resulting in less desire to eat (Polivy and Herman, 2002). Many of these changes reverse with refeeding and the end of purging, but not all.

Significant research into the genetics of eating disorders is currently taking place, including a study by the National Institutes of Mental Health (NIMH), and an international, multisite project sponsored by the Price Foundation. Twin and family studies suggest that up to 50% of the risk for eating disorders is possibly genetic. Relatives of anorexic clients are twelve times more likely to develop anorexia nervosa and four times more likely to develop bulimia nervosa. Researchers believe a gene on chromosome 1 increases risk for anorexia nervosa and a gene on chromosome 10 increases risk for bulimia nervosa (Grice et al., 2002; Klump et al., 2001; Fairburn et al., 1999). It is not likely that a single gene causes eating disorders. The concept of genetic markers for high-risk personality traits and neurobiologic dysfunction is a more significant theory.

The comorbidity (co-occurrence) of mood disorders and eating disorders also suggests a neurobiologic link in the pathogenesis of anorexia nervosa and bulimia nervosa. New research shows significantly high basal serotonin and oversensitivity in the serotonin system in anorexic clients. Researchers wonder if this creates constant anxiety, which is relieved by starving, which decreases serotonin. Bulimic clients show low basal serotonin, associated with depression. Serotonin levels and mood both improve with bingeing. Serotonin dysregulation is often present premorbidly and persists in many clients after recovery, suggesting a fundamental biologic dysregulation that the person tries to modulate with eating disorder behaviors (Bailer et al., 2004, 2005; Kaye et al., 2001a). Research with recovered anorexic clients also shows overactive dopamine receptors, related to excessive worry and a lack of positive response to common comforts and pleasures, such as food (Kaye et al., 1999; Kaye, 2005).

Sociocultural Factors

By adolescence, everyone has been exposed to countless advertisements by the diet and fashion industries that encourage them to strive for an idealized body and promise that dieting and exercise will achieve that goal. This "ideal" body shape is unrealistically thin for girls and equally unrealistically lean and muscular for boys. Most normal-sized adolescents feel dissatisfied with their bodies (Groesz et al., 2002). Teenagers from families who nurture and reward them with food; equate food with pleasure, comfort, and love; or use food as punishment by imposing dieting and food restrictions may view food as damaging or bad. The preanorexic or prebulimic person often observes her mother's struggles to balance all of society's expectations. Some have watched their mothers try to maintain a feminine image while striving to achieve in the business world. Some boys also observe their dieting parents and listen to their parents' self-criticism about weight and shape.

Another risk factor is participation in sports that encourage weight loss, such as cheerleading, wrestling, or running track. Participation in intensely competitive sports that encourage perfectionism and compulsive exercise are also high risk.

Psychologic Factors

Although the same sociocultural pressures challenge all adolescents, only a few, approximately 8%, develop eating disorders. Some teens have personalities and coping styles that seem to protect them from eating disorders, whereas other teens have personalities and coping styles that put them at risk. Some high-risk personality traits are common to all eating disorders, whereas some personality traits are more specific to anorexia nervosa or bulimia nervosa (Box 17-3).

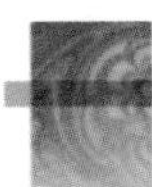

BOX 17-3

High-Risk Personality Traits for Development of Eating Disorders

ALL EATING DISORDERS
Low self-esteem
Compliance, conflict avoidance
Sense of ineffectiveness
Alexithymia (difficulty naming and expressing emotions)
Interoceptive deficits (inability to accurately identify and respond to bodily cues)

ANOREXIA NERVOSA
Perfectionism
Emotional immaturity
Risk/harm avoidance

BULIMIA NERVOSA
Impulsivity
Emotional dysregulation (oversensitivity to and difficulty modulating emotions and behavior)

Cognitive therapy literature describes certain distorted thinking patterns as characteristic of people who have eating disorders (Lock and le Grange, 2005a and 2005b). They include **dichotomous thinking** (individuals view situations as either all good or all bad), control fallacies (individuals feel solely responsible for the happiness and failure of others), and personalization (individuals compare themselves endlessly with others and perceive others' behavior as a direct reaction to them) (see Chapter 13).

Familial Factors

Personality traits are sometimes genetic, but researchers believe the environment greatly affects the personality as well. Families are a strong environmental influence. In 1978, Minuchin, Rosman, and Baker described a stereotypical "eating disorder family" as Caucasian, upper-middle class, intact, enmeshed, rigid, and hostile. Nowadays, eating disorders occur in all socioeconomic levels, races, and cultures, with a range of interactive family styles. **Enmeshed families** have poor boundaries, expect conformity, and discourage individuality and direct expression of feelings. Parents are often controlling, critical, and demanding. They sometimes demonstrate poor conflict-resolution skills, which is displayed as denial of disagreement, conflict avoidance, or constant, unproductive arguing. The result is tension and fear of conflict.

These families often put a lot of importance on body image, social acceptance, and achievement. Research demonstrates the powerful influence of parental encouragement of dieting and preoccupation with body image (Davis et al., 2004). Maternal comments about children being overweight sometimes cause body dissatisfaction and dieting (Smolak et al., 1999). Girls who do not identify with their mothers are at higher risk for low self-esteem and eating disorders (Hahn-Smith and Smith, 2001). A poor marital relationship increases the risk of eating disorders in children (Wade et al., 2001). If a child sees the drive for thinness, dieting, or other extreme behaviors in her role models, he or she is likely to try dieting as an attempt to improve self-esteem (Agras et al., 1999).

In extremely dysfunctional families, the damage is often severe. Alcoholism and physical and sexual abuse have devastating effects. Emotional abuse is subtly damaging. In some cases, parents do not encourage the child to be independent, to develop self-trust, or to have pride in his or her individuality. If the child learns to avoid conflict to please others and learns to fear adult responsibilities, adolescence is a crisis. The sense of self never fully develops, and the pressures to separate and be an individual in adolescence are terrifying, not only to the child but also to the parents.

Confronted with this crisis, it is not surprising that the adolescent feels overwhelmed and out of control. The myth of thinness as the key to confidence, success, and control is compelling. The adolescent begins dieting, loses weight, begins to feel better, continues dieting and losing weight, and experiences a sense of control and accomplishment. Unfortunately, **secondary gains** such as attention and envy from peers, and often from parents, reinforce this behavior. Later, when people tell her she is getting too thin, the adolescent feels a sense of power and control that she has never felt before. By losing weight, she not only has gotten attention, but she also has frustrated those who try to make her eat normally. These secondary gains are often very rewarding, especially to a compliant, conflict-avoidant individual with low self-esteem. The diet has distracted her from her actual conflicts and given her a sense of mastery. Although this mastery is false, the adolescent does not want to lose it.

Sometimes the individual is unable to stick to the diet. Binge eating often begins as a reaction to the deprivation of dieting. Bingeing not only relieves hunger but also numbs pain and distracts from actual conflicts. It sometimes represents an angry rebellion against the pressure to be thin. The relief of a binge is temporary, quickly followed by guilt about eating and panic about loss of control and weight gain. Purging reverses the binge—and the guilt. Figure 17-1 illustrates the interrelationship of all the etiologic factors in the cycle of eating disorders.

EPIDEMIOLOGY

Eight million women and 1 million men currently suffer from eating disorders. Studies using strict DSM-IV-TR criteria estimate that 3% to 10% of adolescent and college-age women and 2% of adolescent males are bulimic. The rate is 2% among the general population. Disturbed eating patterns, including dieting with occasional use of diet pills, laxatives, or vomiting, occurs in 13% of young women. Binge eating without purging at least once a week occurs in approximately 5% to 20% of all women and slightly fewer men. Studies show anorexia nervosa to be consistent at a rate of 0.5% to 1% in adolescent and college-age women. Anorexia nervosa is much less common in males.

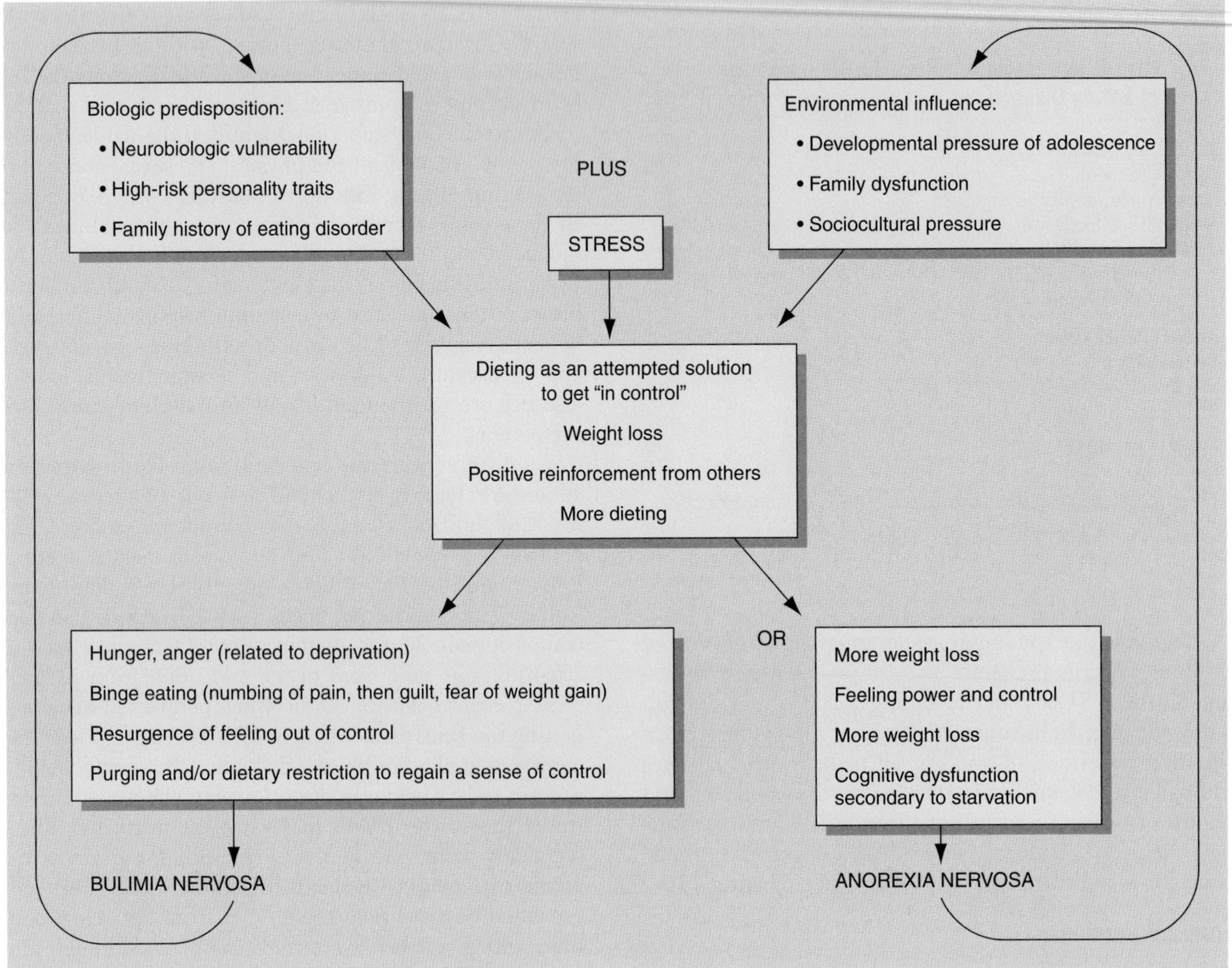

FIGURE 17-1 The cycle of eating disorders.

Box 17-4 summarizes the incidence and prevalence of eating disorders.

Sex Ratio

Eating disorders mostly affect females, although more cases in men are emerging. Since the early 1980s, the ratio of male to female cases of all three eating disorders have increased from 1:100 to 1:10. A few gender differences have emerged, specifically showing that eating disordered men are more likely to have premorbid obesity and are more likely to exercise excessively (Fernandez-Aranda et al., 2004; Lewinsohn et al., 2002b).

Age of Onset

Most eating disorders begin in adolescence. About 86% of those with eating disorders report an onset before age 20. The average age of onset of bulimia nervosa is 18 years, with 80% of cases reported with an onset between ages 15 and 30 years. In anorexia nervosa, the peak age range of onset has decreased from 14 to 18 years to ages 11 to 18 years. Many cases of anorexia nervosa have occurred in children as young as 8 years old. The range of onset ages for both disorders is 8 to 70 years.

Cross-Cultural Studies

The incidence and prevalence of eating disorders around the world are similar among European countries, the United States, Canada, Mexico, Japan, Australia, and other Westernized countries with plentiful food supplies. In the United States, there is no difference in incidence among racial, ethnic, or socioeconomic groups.

Mortality

The mortality rate in anorexia nervosa is higher than in any other psychiatric diagnosis, reported at 6% to 20% (Agras, 2001). Mortality rate increases with each year the illness persists, with a 20% death rate for those with anorexia for 20 years or more. Estimates of mortality rates from bulimia nervosa range from 2% to 19%. Suicide is frequently the cause of death in persons with eating disorders (Lowe et al., 2001; American Psychiatric Association [APA], 2000; Emborg, 1999).

BOX 17-4

Epidemiology for Eating Disorders

- 7 million women and 1 million men suffer from eating disorders in the United States.
- Average age of onset is 11 to 18 for anorexia nervosa, cases as young as 8 years old; average age of onset is 17 for bulimia nervosa.
- 5% to 8% of adolescent and college-age women and 2% of adolescent men have bulimia nervosa.
- 2% of women and less than 1% of men in the general population have bulimia nervosa.
- Less than 1% of the general population has anorexia nervosa.
- 10% of adolescent and college-age women have subclinical anorexia nervosa; 15% have subclinical bulimia nervosa.
- 5% to 20% of the general population (male and female) binge regularly (but do not purge).
- 90% of clients with eating disorders are female, a decrease from 95% to 99% in past studies.
- 50% of those with eating disorders recover; 77% report a duration of 1 to 5 years.
- Mortality rates for bulimia nervosa are 2% to 19%; for anorexia nervosa, mortality rates are 6% to 20%. The rate increases to 20% for those who have had anorexia nervosa for 20 years.
- Similar incidence and prevalence rates are found among Western countries where food is abundant and dieting is common.
- Comorbidity (co-occurrence): Axis I: mood disorders (dysthymic disorders, major depressive disorder), anxiety disorders (generalized anxiety disorder, social phobia, obsessive-compulsive disorder, posttraumatic stress disorder), dissociative identity disorder, substance-related disorders. Axis II: personality disorders (borderline personality disorder, avoidant personality disorder, obsessive-compulsive personality disorder).

Comorbidity (Co-occurrence)

Comorbidity is the concurrent existence of two or more disorders. Depression is diagnosed in 40% to 75% of individuals with eating disorders, more frequently with bulimia nervosa than with anorexia nervosa. Two thirds of eating disorder clients are diagnosed with comorbid (co-occurring or coexisting) anxiety disorders, specifically generalized anxiety disorders, obsessive-compulsive disorder, and social phobia (Kaye et al., 2004; Milos et al., 2002). In anorexia nervosa, obsessive-compulsive disorder is the most frequent co-occurring diagnosis, followed by mood disorders, posttraumatic stress disorder, social phobia, and dissociative disorder (Milos et al., 2002; Lewinsohn et al., 2000a). Substance use disorders coexist more with bulimia nervosa than with anorexia nervosa (von Ranson et al., 2002; Lewinsohn et al., 2000a). A careful diagnosis is necessary to separate the side effects of starvation and purging from symptoms of co-occurring mood disorders.

The occurrence of *comorbid (co-occurring) personality disorders* is well known to clinicians dealing with eating disorders. Three fourths of clients with eating disorders have an Axis II diagnosis. Borderline personality disorder is the Axis II diagnosis most commonly associated with eating disorders. Avoidant and obsessive-compulsive personality disorders are also prevalent (Rosenvinge et al., 2000). A quarter to a third of eating disorder clients report a history of childhood sexual abuse. These individuals had a higher incidence of co-occurring dissociative disorders and impulsive, self-injurious behavior (Paul et al., 2002; Wonderlich et al., 2001).

CLINICAL DESCRIPTION

Eating disorders are an easily recognizable group of psychiatric diagnoses. Refusal to eat, severe weight loss, and self-induced vomiting are unmistakable indicators of an eating disorder. However, making a precise DSM-IV-TR diagnosis and determining specific nursing diagnoses to reflect a particular client's case are challenging and complicated tasks.

Anorexia nervosa and bulimia nervosa are the two specific eating disorder diagnoses in the DSM-IV-TR classification. The category of eating disorder not otherwise specified (EDNOS) is provided to diagnose individuals with disordered eating who do not meet the criteria for anorexia nervosa or bulimia nervosa. The DSM-IV-TR Criteria boxes detail the criteria for these three diagnoses. The clinical symptoms of anorexia nervosa and bulimia nervosa are in the Clinical Symptoms boxes.

Obesity is not included as an eating disorder in the DSM-IV-TR classification because all cases of obesity do not involve psychiatric illness. Obesity itself is classified in the *International Statistical Classification of Diseases and Related Health Problems* (ICD-10) as a general medical condition (APA, 2000).

Inclusion or exclusion of **binge eating disorder** (BED) in the DSM-IV-TR classification has been a controversial issue. BED is cited as an example of an EDNOS and is included in the DSM-IV-TR as a proposed diagnosis for further study. BED is described specifically as recurrent episodes of binge eating, in which the individual eats more than most people eat during a similar period and feels out of control while eating. Other criteria include distress, guilt, and disgust regarding the behavior (APA, 2000).

Anorexia nervosa and bulimia nervosa are distinct diagnoses but have many of the same features. Many underweight clients with anorexia nervosa binge and purge, and many clients with bulimia nervosa use fasting or exercise, but not purging, to compensate for binges. The subtypes as well as the EDNOS category assist in making the most precise diagnosis. For example, if an individual meets the criteria for both bulimia nervosa and anorexia nervosa, the diagnosis of anorexia nervosa, binge eating/purging type is made, because it is the only category that includes *all* of the symptoms (neither subtype of bulimia nervosa deals with weight loss). Half of individuals with eating disorders "migrate" from one diagnosis to another over time. This finding indicates that eating disorder diagnoses need further refining (Milos et al., 2005).

DSM-IV-TR CRITERIA

Anorexia Nervosa

A Refusal to maintain body weight at or above a minimally normal weight for age and height (e.g., weight loss leading to maintenance of body weight less than 85% of that expected, or failure to make expected weight gain during period of growth leading to body weight less than 85% of that expected)

B Intense fear of gaining weight or becoming fat even though underweight

C Disturbance in the way in which one's body weight or shape is experienced, undue influence of body weight or shape on self-evaluation, or denial of the seriousness of the current low body weight

D In postmenarchal females amenorrhea (i.e., the absence of at least three consecutive menstrual cycles) (A woman is considered to have amenorrhea if her periods occur only after hormone [e.g., estrogen] administration.)

Specify type:

Restricting type: During the current episode of anorexia nervosa, the person has not regularly engaged in binge eating or purging behavior (i.e., self-induced vomiting or the misuse of laxatives, diuretics, or enemas).

Binge-eating/purging type: During the current episode of anorexia nervosa, the person has regularly engaged in binge-eating or purging behavior (i.e., self-induced vomiting or the misuse of laxatives, diuretics, or enemas).

From American Psychiatric Association: *Diagnostic and statistical manual of mental disorders,* ed 4, text revision, Washington, DC, 2000, American Psychiatric Association.

DSM-IV-TR CRITERIA

Bulimia Nervosa

A Recurrent episodes of binge eating. An episode of binge eating is characterized by both of the following:

1. Eating, in a discrete period of time (e.g., within any 2-hour period), an amount of food that is definitely larger than most people would eat during a similar period of time and under similar circumstances
2. A sense of lack of control over eating during the episode (e.g., a feeling that one cannot stop eating or control what or how much one is eating)

B Recurrent inappropriate compensatory behavior to prevent weight gain, such as self-induced vomiting; misuse of laxatives, diuretics, enemas, or other medications; fasting; or excessive exercise.

C The binge eating and inappropriate compensatory behaviors both occur, on average, at least twice a week for 3 months.

D Self-evaluation is unduly influenced by body shape and weight.

E The disturbance does not occur exclusively during episodes of anorexia nervosa.

Specify type:

Purging type: During the current episode of bulimia nervosa, the person has regularly engaged in self-induced vomiting or the misuse of laxatives, diuretics, or enemas.

Nonpurging type: During the current episode of bulimia nervosa, the person has used other inappropriate compensatory behaviors, such as fasting or excessive exercise, but has not regularly engaged in self-induced vomiting or the misuse of laxatives, diuretics, or enemas.

From American Psychiatric Association: *Diagnostic and statistical manual of mental disorders,* ed 4, text revision, Washington, DC, 2000, American Psychiatric Association.

DSM-IV-TR CRITERIA

Eating Disorder Not Otherwise Specified

The *eating disorder not otherwise specified* category is for disorders of eating that do not meet the criteria for a specific eating disorder. Examples include the following:

1. For females, all of the criteria for anorexia nervosa are met except that the individual has regular menses.
2. All of the criteria for anorexia nervosa are met except that, despite significant weight loss, the individual's current weight is in the normal range.
3. All of the criteria for bulimia nervosa are met except that the frequency of binge eating and inappropriate compensatory mechanisms occurs less than twice a week or for less than 3 months.
4. The regular use of inappropriate compensatory behavior by an individual of normal body weight after eating small amounts of food (e.g., self-induced vomiting after the consumption of two cookies).
5. The individual repeatedly chews and spits out, but does not swallow, large amounts of food.
6. Binge-eating disorder: recurrent episodes of binge eating in the absence of the regular use of inappropriate compensatory behaviors characteristic of bulimia nervosa.

From American Psychiatric Association: *Diagnostic and statistical manual of mental disorders,* ed 4, text revision, Washington, DC, 2000, American Psychiatric Association.

CLINICAL SYMPTOMS

Anorexia Nervosa

BEHAVIORAL SYMPTOMS

Self-starvation—reported intake restriction and refusal to eat

Rituals or compulsive behaviors regarding food, eating, or weight loss

Engages in self-induced vomiting, laxatives, diuretics, or excessive exercise to lose weight

Wears baggy or inappropriate layers of clothing

PHYSICAL SYMPTOMS

Weight loss 15% below ideal weight

Amenorrhea—absence of three or more menstrual cycles when expected to occur (primary or secondary)

Slow pulse, decreased body temperature

Cachexia (muscle wasting), sunken eyes, protruding bones, dry skin

Growth of lanugo (fine hair) on face and body

Constipation

Cold sensitivity

In adolescence, weight loss may delay puberty and retard growth

PSYCHOLOGIC SYMPTOMS

Denial of the seriousness of current low weight, denial of hunger

Body image disturbance (seeing self as unrealistically fat when the person is actually at or near ideal weight, or experiencing parts of the body as unrealistically fat or out of proportion) (Figure 17-2)

Intense and irrational fear of weight gain that does not diminish as weight is lost

Constant striving for the "perfect" body

Self-concept unduly influenced by shape and weight

Preoccupation with food, cooking, nutritional information, and feeding others

Shows delayed psychosexual development or lacks age-appropriate interest in sex and relationships

CLINICAL SYMPTOMS

Bulimia Nervosa

BEHAVIORAL SYMPTOMS

Recurrent episodes of binge eating (consumption of a large amount of food in a discrete period of time)

Engages in **purging** behaviors, such as self-induced vomiting, use of laxatives, diuretics, diet pills, ipecac, enemas, excessive exercise, or periods of fasting, to compensate for the binge

PHYSICAL SYMPTOMS

May experience fluid and electrolyte imbalances from purging:
- Hypokalemia (low potassium)
- Alkalosis (high alkaline in body fluids)
- Dehydration
- Idiopathic edema (tissue swelling)

Cardiovascular
- Hypotension (low blood pressure)
- Cardiac arrhythmia/dysrhythmia (irregular heartbeat)
- Cardiomyopathy (heart muscle problem)

Endocrine
- Hypoglycemia (low blood sugar)
- May experience menstrual dysfunction

Gastrointestinal
- Constipation, diarrhea
- Gastroparesis (delayed gastric emptying)
- Esophageal reflux (backflow of food from stomach)
- Esophagitis (inflammation of the esophagus)
- Mallory-Weiss syndrome (tears in esophagus)
- Dental enamel erosion
- Parotid gland enlargement (glands situated below/in front of each ear)

PSYCHOLOGIC SYMPTOMS

Body image disturbance

Persistent overconcern with body weight, shape, and proportions

Mood swings and irritability

Self-concept unduly influenced by body weight and shape

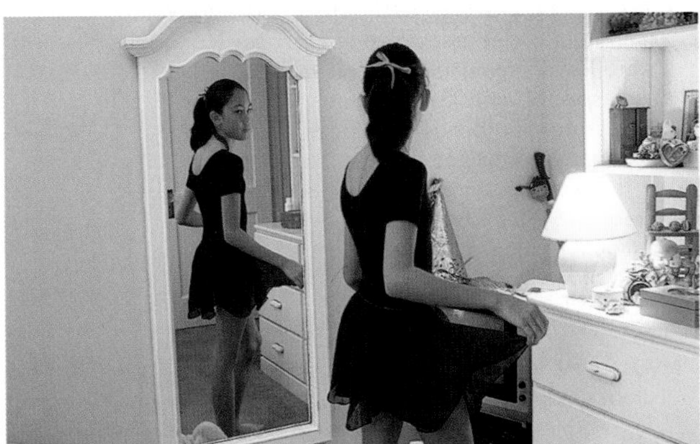

FIGURE 17-2 An individual's appearance influences self-concept. Clients with eating disorders often have a distorted view of their physical appearance, perceiving themselves as unrealistically large. (From Sorrentino SA: *Mosby's textbook for nursing assistants,* ed 6, St Louis, 2004, Mosby.)

PROGNOSIS

The course of the illness in eating disorders is variable. Some individuals recover fully from a single, time-limited episode of anorexia nervosa or bulimia nervosa. Many teens with anorexia nervosa who recover their normal weight later develop bulimia nervosa. Many individuals with eating disorders follow a chronic course or a pattern of relapses and remissions. Others show slow improvement after several years of treatment.

Long-term outcome studies show a more promising prognosis for those clients who continue treatment. More than 50% show improvement after 5 years (Lowe et al., 2001; Polivy and Herman, 2002). Weight restoration is necessary but not sufficient for recovery. Individuals need to resolve core problems related to eating behavior and underlying psychologic issues as well (Sysko, 2005). Outcome literature indicates that long-term cognitive-behavioral, family, or interpersonal therapy, often combined with antidepressant medication, results in the most sustained improvement (Keel et al., 2002; Dare et al., 2001; Lowe et al., 2001; Mitchell et al., 2001).

DISCHARGE CRITERIA

Client will:
- Be free from self-harm.
- Achieve minimum (within 10%) normal weight as determined by the treatment team.
- Consume adequate calories to maintain a minimum normal weight.
- Demonstrate ability to follow the treatment regimen recommended for postdischarge (i.e., compliance with medication, food plan, control over binge/purge behavior, plan for follow-up care).
- Verbalize awareness and understanding of the psychologic issues related to the eating disorder behavior and the maladaptive use of food and weight control to try to cope with these issues.
- Demonstrate the use of improved coping abilities to respond to stress and to manage emotional issues.
- Exhibit developmentally appropriate boundaries within the family system.
- Attend group therapy sessions that encourage healthy eating patterns and positive self-image and self-concept.
- Interact with peers who support the client in maintaining healthy behavior.
- Keep follow-up appointments with therapist, psychiatrist, and dietitian.

The Nursing Process

ASSESSMENT

The nursing assessment of clients with eating disorders involves sensitivity, thoroughness, and sharp observation skills. The first few minutes of the interview are essential, as first impressions set the tone for the entire treatment experience. Clients with eating disorders are sensitive to others and are quick to judge whether others are trust-

CASE STUDY Sarah is a 20-year-old college student who was brought to the emergency department by her boyfriend after she fainted in the shower. The boyfriend took the nurse aside and confided that Sarah was bulimic and that he was concerned that her eating disorder was related to the fainting episode. He said that Sarah was secretive and somewhat defensive about the bulimia. The initial physical examination showed no injuries from the fall, and Sarah's vital signs were normal. Her parotid glands appeared enlarged. Her weight appeared within a normal range. Her affect was tense and anxious. She avoided eye contact with the nurse and mumbled that she had recently been up late studying and had not been getting enough sleep.

CRITICAL THINKING

1 How should the nurse approach Sarah? How can the nurse bring up the subject of bulimia nervosa?
2 If Sarah responds defensively or with denial, how should the nurse respond?
3 What further physical assessments should be done?
4 What other information is needed to complete the nursing assessment?

worthy. If the nurse forms a therapeutic alliance immediately, this will prevent many of the power struggles that are common (see the Case Study at left and the Nursing Assessment Questions box). Because many clients with eating disorders have one or more coexisting disorders, it is critical for the nurse to assess for the co-occurring disorders (see Box 17-4).

NURSING DIAGNOSIS

Nursing diagnoses are made from the information obtained during the assessment phase of the nursing process. The accuracy of diagnosis depends on a careful, in-depth assessment. Nursing diagnoses are prioritized according to client needs from most urgent to least urgent.

Anorexia Nervosa

Safety or health risks:

- Risk for self-mutilation
- Risk for imbalanced body temperature
- Deficient fluid volume
- Risk for imbalanced fluid volume

NURSING ASSESSMENT QUESTIONS

Eating Disorders

1 How do you feel about being here today? *To determine if self-referred or forced into treatment and to assess willingness to participate in treatment*
2 Have you ever talked with anyone before about your eating disorder? *To assess level of self-disclosure and to reduce anxiety and feelings of shame*
3 Have you been in therapy before? *To assess treatment history and get details of previous treatment, including the name of clinician, dates of treatment, outcomes, and client's experience of the treatment*
4 Describe your weight throughout your life. Include the following factors when discussing weight:
   Current weight, including fluctuations during past 6 months
   Desired weight
   Lowest and highest weight (excluding pregnancy)
   Perception of childhood and adolescent size and shape
   Perception of current size and shape
   Family history of eating disorders or obesity
   Family history of dieting or preoccupation with thinness
   Childhood experiences related to weight and eating
   To determine premorbid weight and perceptions of body
5 How do you feel about the way your body looks? *To assess body dissatisfaction and body image distortion*
6 Assess dieting history:
   When did you first diet?
   What started your dieting?
   What happened when you dieted?
   Did you lose or gain weight?
   Has anyone encouraged you to lose weight?
   What dieting behaviors have you used?
   To determine use of fasting, structured diet, restriction, diet products/programs
7 Assess binge eating:
   Do you binge eat?
   When was the first time you binged?
   Get details about typical binge eating, including when, where, duration, frequency, type and amount of food, any rituals or patterns involved. Ask if secrecy, hiding, stealing, or lying is involved. Assess control (i.e., can client interrupt a binge once it has begun?). *To determine the nature of bingeing in order to plan effective treatment; habits that are long-lasting are usually more challenging*
8 Help client identify feeling states associated with the binge: before bingeing, in the planning stages, and during and after the binge. Ask client to focus on past binge episodes and answer this question: "Did you feel angry or anxious?" *To determine client's feelings regarding binge behaviors*
9 Assess food cravings (e.g., time of day, weekends, where in menstrual cycle, associated with places [car, work, home, store]). *To determine if client is able to associate cravings with specific times/situations*
10 Assess purging behavior. Include the following:
   Type (e.g., vomiting, diuretics, laxatives, diet pills, ipecac, thyroid pills, amphetamines, cocaine, exercise)
   Frequency (times/week)
   Amount of food purged
   Age of first purging episode
   Date of last purging episode
   To identify client's usual methods of purging
11 Assess menstrual history (onset of menses, regularity, premenstrual syndrome, menstrual dysfunction, any hormone therapy). *To determine effect of dysfunctional behaviors on menses*
12 Assess medical side effects of eating disorder. *To identify any concomitant medical problems*
13 Assess comorbidity (co-occurring) factors (e.g., mood disorders, anxiety, substance abuse). *To determine if there are other factors that will complicate the problem*

- Constipation
- Perceived constipation
- Imbalanced nutrition: less than body requirements
- Delayed growth and development

Perceptual/cognitive/emotional disturbances:
- Anxiety
- Disturbed body image
- Hopelessness
- Powerlessness
- Chronic low self-esteem

Problems in communicating and relating to others:
- Sexual dysfunction
- Impaired social interaction
- Social isolation

Disruptions in coping abilities:
- Ineffective coping
- Disabled family coping
- Ineffective denial

Client and family teaching needs:
- Deficient knowledge regarding nutrition and medical side effects of anorexic behavior
- Noncompliance with refeeding process

Bulimia Nervosa

Safety or health risks:
- Risk for self-mutilation
- Risk for imbalanced fluid volume
- Constipation
- Perceived constipation
- Imbalanced nutrition: less than body requirements

Perceptual/cognitive/emotional disturbances:
- Anxiety
- Disturbed body image
- Hopelessness
- Chronic low self-esteem

Problems in communicating and relating to others:
- Sexual dysfunction
- Impaired social interaction
- Social isolation

Disruptions in coping abilities:
- Compromised family coping
- Disabled family coping

Client and family teaching needs:
- Deficient knowledge regarding nutrition and side effects of bulimic behavior
- Noncompliance with treatment program

OUTCOME IDENTIFICATION

Outcome criteria come from nursing diagnoses and are the expected client responses to be achieved (see the Case Study above, right column). Outcomes are prioritized according to client needs from most urgent to least urgent.

Anorexia Nervosa

Client will:
- Participate in therapeutic contact with staff.
- Consume adequate calories for age, height, and metabolic need.
- Achieve minimum normal weight.
- Maintain normal fluid and electrolyte levels.
- Resume normal menstrual cycle.
- Demonstrate improvement in body image with a more realistic view of body shape and size.
- Demonstrate more effective coping skills to deal with conflicts.
- Manage family conflicts more effectively.
- Verbalize awareness of underlying psychologic issues.
- Achieve ideal body weight for age, height, and metabolic need.
- Perceive body weight and shape as normal and acceptable.
- Resume sexual interest and age-appropriate sexual behavior.
- Demonstrate absence of food rituals, preoccupation with food, or fears of food.

CASE STUDY Laura is a 27-year-old married mother of a 3-year-old child. Laura has been hospitalized after a suicide attempt, in which she overdosed on a combination of 100 laxatives and a full bottle of her antidepressant medication. She is currently seeing a psychiatrist for depression and bulimia nervosa. The nursing assessment reveals that Laura currently binges and purges up to three times per day. Purging consists of self-induced vomiting, as well as the use of laxatives (usually 5 or 6 pills every day). She is within normal weight range at 140 pounds and 5 feet 9 inches. Laura is participating in unit activities willingly, although her affect is depressed. She is eating very little at meals and has agreed not to purge while in the hospital.

CRITICAL THINKING

1. How will the nurse determine Laura's therapeutic involvement with staff and peers?
2. What are realistic expectations of Laura for eating regular meals? What data should be monitored to track her improvement in nutritional status?
3. How will the nurse recognize improvements in eating behavior and cessation of purging?
4. How will Laura demonstrate awareness of any psychologic issues underlying her bulimia?

Bulimia Nervosa

Client will:
- Participate in therapeutic contact with staff.
- Maintain normal fluid and electrolyte levels.
- Consume adequate calories for age, height, and metabolic need.
- Cease binge/purge episodes while in inpatient setting; cease dieting.
- Demonstrate more effective coping skills to deal with conflicts.
- Demonstrate age-appropriate boundaries with family.
- Verbalize awareness of underlying psychologic issues.
- Demonstrate improved awareness of body sensations and emotional states.
- Perceive body shape and weight as normal and acceptable.

PLANNING

The nurse's attitude toward the client with an eating disorder is as critical in the plan of care as any specific therapeutic intervention. Clients with eating disorders appear fragile, and although they are vulnerable, they are often quite rigid and frustrating. If the nurse does not form a good working alliance with a firm, yet compassionate approach, client care quickly turns into a series of power struggles, and the treatment will fail. The plan of care has to include consistent, collaborative efforts by the client, family, and interdisciplinary staff.

IMPLEMENTATION

For the client with an eating disorder, the nurse needs to implement a balanced plan of action that includes behavioral interventions to interrupt the cycle of eating disorder behavior, and psychologic interventions to improve emotional regulation, interpersonal skills, and awareness of other psychologic issues. A safe, structured environment is essential to prevent self-harm, promote weight gain or nutritional restoration, and help the client express in words what the client is acting out with the behavior. A safe environment is necessary to teach more effective coping skills, monitor the use of medications, and coordinate the multidisciplinary efforts of the treatment team.

Nursing Interventions

Nursing interventions are prioritized according to client needs, from most urgent to least urgent.

1. Provide a safe, nonthreatening environment. *This ensures safety and prevents violence.*
2. Assess any risk of suicide (suicidal ideation, gesture, plan). *This prevents self-harm* (see Chapter 21).
3. Engage the client in a therapeutic alliance. *This encourages expression of a wide range of thoughts and feelings, including any self-destructive urges.*
4. Restore minimum weight and nutritional balance through a behavioral program. For anorexia, this includes refeeding with food, food supplements, and tube feedings when necessary. For bulimia, this includes eating meals prescribed by a dietitian and avoiding purging by having the nurse remain with the client for at least 1 hour after each meal. *This promotes health and wellness.*
5. Create a structured, supportive environment with clear, consistent, firm limits. *This helps to establish a predictable routine and promotes internal control that the client currently lacks.*
6. Coordinate with the dietitian to construct a behavioral plan that includes weight-gain goals of approximately 3 pounds per week, specific eating goals of eating 90% to 100% of meals, and reinforcements of increased privileges for compliance and goal achievement. *Structure helps the client to gain self-control and reduces the anxiety generated by noncompliance and an unpredictable routine.*
7. Encourage the client to express thoughts, feelings, and concerns about body and body image. *Verbalization helps the client transform a sense of shame, guilt, and fear into specific areas of conflict, and it clarifies the original issues (self-esteem, intimacy, sex, adult responsibility, identity).*
8. Continue to help the client increase understanding of body image distortion. *The goal is for the client to recognize that preoccupation with perceived flaws is a distraction from more complex issues that will not resolve by changing body size or shape.*
9. Assist the client in recalling positive eating experiences, such as a time when the client was able to eat a normal portion of sweets and stop without bingeing. *This emphasizes the fact that the client is capable of engaging in successful episodes of eating and promotes hope.*
10. Assume a caring, yet matter-of-fact approach without being overly sympathetic or overly confrontational or authoritarian. *This assists the client in maintaining clear boundaries and avoids power struggles.*
11. Normalize the client's lack of appetite and feelings of fullness as typical of the early refeeding process. Normalize fears of obesity as part of the distorted thinking typical of eating disorders. *This helps the client to accept the treatment plan and not set up power struggles based on distorted thinking and distorted body cues.*
12. Intervene with the client's anxiety by helping the client associate the experience of anxiety as a signal of unrecognized feelings and needs. *The client's recognition that anxiety is a defense against deeper conflicts will bring relief and start the process of problem solving* (see Chapter 9).
13. Offer positive feedback when the client follows the treatment plan and works to maintain the goals of the individual contract. Examples: "You have eaten three new foods this week." "You listen attentively in group." *Praise increases self-esteem, promotes compliance, and encourages repetition of positive behaviors.*
14. Engage the client in therapeutic interactions and groups (e.g., individual therapy, group therapy, family therapy, occupational/recreational therapy). *This will encourage the client to express feelings and conflicts created by eating disorder behaviors in a supportive environment and reduce anxiety* (see Chapter 23).
15. Assist the client in identifying issues of low self-esteem, separation and individuation, family dysfunction, and fear of maturity. *This will help the client to reveal and process any psychologic conflicts related to the eating disorder.*
16. Discuss with the client how obsession with food and weight is a way to avoid more difficult life problems and challenges. *This will help the client increase awareness and gain insight about the dynamics of the eating disorder.*
17. Collaborate with the dietitian to teach the client about adequate nutrition for the client's height and body type. Educate the client about metabolic adaptations characteristic of starvation and refeeding, such as the need to increase kilocalories as energy expenditure increases. *This will counter the client's erroneous*

information about ideal weight and size and nutritional requirements to restore health.

18. Collaborate with the social worker, family therapist, physician, and other members of the interdisciplinary team. *This will promote consistency in implementing the treatment plan.*
19. Teach adaptive therapeutic strategies (cognitive, behavioral, assertive). *This will promote realistic thoughts, feelings, and coping behaviors and help the client realize that it is irrational to believe that losing weight will solve the client's problems* (see Chapter 23).
20. Educate the family about healthy boundaries and the importance of normal client separation and individuation versus overprotection and family enmeshment. *Education about these issues will promote mutually satisfying interpersonal relationships among family members* (see the Client and Family Teaching Guidelines box).

CLIENT and FAMILY TEACHING GUIDELINES

Eating Disorders

TEACH THE FAMILY

- Stress that the cycle of eating disorder behaviors is life threatening and must be interrupted.
- Emphasize that eating disorder behaviors are hard to change and the idea of gaining weight or stopping purging is terrifying to the client.
- Explain that the client experiences common underlying issues such as low self-esteem, separation/individuation conflicts, interoceptive deficits, fear of maturity, and conflict avoidance.
- Activate the client to share what has been learned in group and individual therapy about the particular psychologic issues related to the eating disorder.
- Encourage the client to directly verbalize thoughts and feelings about family interactions.
- Promote, calmly and firmly, normal eating and weight gain as prescribed in the treatment plan, and recognize eating disorder symptoms and signs of relapse.
- Recognize how client's anxiety promotes controlling behaviors that can set up a power struggle and client rebellion. This reinforces and worsens the eating disorder.
- Decrease enmeshment: stop preparing separate meals, set age-appropriate limits, and expect the client to follow family rules.
- Understand that family's well-intentioned attempts to be supportive will sometimes backfire by sending the message that the client is helpless and therefore not held to age-appropriate responsibilities.

TEACH THE CLIENT

- Expect to not feel hungry as a result of starvation or purging, but to follow the meal plan, in spite of feeling full.
- Expect to feel fat and uncomfortable because of the distorted thinking and interoceptive deficits that are characteristic of eating disorders.
- Increase tolerance for these distressing feelings.
- Express thoughts and feelings in therapeutic interactions.
- Transform various feelings about one's body into concrete concerns.
- Be specific about thoughts and feelings: "What exactly are you afraid will happen?" or "What does, 'I'm freaking out,' mean specifically?"

21. Collaborate with the occupational therapist to teach the client about appropriate exercises. *This will reduce compulsive behavior and encourage the client to exercise in moderation.*

Additional Treatment Modalities

Interdisciplinary Treatment Team

The interdisciplinary team consists of representatives from the fields of nursing, psychiatry, medicine, psychology, pharmacology, dietary education, social work, occupational therapy, and chaplain or spiritual guidance as needed. Interdisciplinary treatment team meetings are the opportunity for sharing assessment information and developing the multidisciplinary treatment plan. Nurses often coordinate this plan and make sure that it is implemented. As managed health care has taken over more of the mental health care industry, hospital stays have become shorter, and fewer specialty units such as eating disorder units exist. Clients with eating disorders are often admitted to general psychiatric units or medical units, putting nurses in a leadership role in the coordination of the treatment team. A successful treatment outcome depends on how well team members work together.

Biologic Modalities

Clients with anorexia nervosa who are more than 15% below ideal body weight need close medical monitoring. After the initial assessment and treatment for the effects of starvation, such as amenorrhea, osteopenia and osteoporosis, and vitamin and mineral deficiencies, nurses need to monitor the client closely while refeeding takes place. Refeeding with meals, supplements, or nasogastric tube normally begins with approximately 1000 to 1600 kcal/day and slowly increases to 2000 to 4000 kcal/day, depending on the client's ideal weight. A goal of 2 to 3 lb/week is considered safe. Self-starvation results in energy-conserving metabolic changes, which shift quickly as refeeding progresses. Rapid increases in energy expenditure necessitate the continued increase of kilocalories to achieve weight gain. The risk of refeeding syndrome, a possibly life-threatening complication, is high in the early phase of treating a severely malnourished client. Nurses are able to prevent edema, congestive heart failure, hypophosphatemia (low phosphate), and other serious electrolyte imbalances with slow refeeding and careful monitoring (APA Work Group on Eating Disorders, 2000).

Clients with bulimia nervosa need initial assessments for acute fluid and electrolyte imbalance, particularly serum potassium, and for any of the dangerous side effects related to their individual purging behaviors. Bone mineral density screening for osteopenia and osteoporosis and assessment for amenorrhea are necessary as well. If purging is not completely stopped, electrolytes need continual monitoring.

There are many other modalities, or methods, of treatment for eating disorders. The Additional Treatment Modalities box on p. 402 lists these methods, and the next section discusses them in greater detail.

CLINICAL ALERT

If the client is compliant with the contract but does not make the expected weight gain, the nurse will suspect that the client is **purging** and report this to the treatment team, who will probably recommend that the nurse confront the client with the purging behavior. Increased supervision after meals and during administration of supplements to prevent purging will follow. The nurse will remain in the room with the client for an hour after eating or will have the client sit at the nursing station for that period. The contract may be amended to include these changes. If weight gain does not occur in a few days, the nurse will initiate tube feeding.

ADDITIONAL TREATMENT MODALITIES

Eating Disorders

- Biologic
- Pharmacologic
- Psychotherapeutic
  - Individual psychotherapy
  - Behavioral therapy
  - Cognitive therapy
  - Family therapy
  - Group therapy
  - Expressive therapies
- Adjunctive therapy
  - Occupational therapy
  - Nutrition education and counseling
  - Social work

MEDICATION KEY FACTS

Eating Disorders

There is empirical evidence for selective serotonin reuptake inhibitors (SSRIs) (fluoxetine [Prozac], sertraline [Zoloft], fluvoxamine [Luvox], citalopram [Celexa]), and selective norepinephrine reuptake inhibitor (SNRIs) (venlafaxine [Effexor]) to be effective in **binge-eating disorder** and **bulimia nervosa.** The first-line strategy for **anorexia nervosa** is SSRI. Fluoxetine is helpful in preventing relapse.

See Chapter 11 for Medication Key Facts related to SSRIs and SNRIs.

Pharmacologic Modalities

Data show that selective serotonin reuptake inhibitor (SSRI) medications, particularly fluoxetine (Prozac), are effective in treating bulimia nervosa, although the dose needed for the "antibulimic" effect is usually 60 mg or more. No medication directly treats anorexia nervosa, but fluoxetine (Prozac) is effective in preventing relapse in weight-restored clients (Zhu and Walsh, 2002; Kaye et al., 2001b; Mitchell et al., 2001). Atypical antipsychotic agents have shown some success in helping low-weight anorexic clients tolerate the extreme agitation related to weight gain and also in treating obsessive-compulsive behaviors (Mitchell et al., 2001).

SSRI medications treat co-occurring mood disorders in clients with eating disorders. This helps treat the eating disorder by relieving depression and anxiety enough for the client to do the work of psychotherapy. Bupropion (Wellbutrin) is contraindicated because of its tendency to lower the seizure threshold in clients with eating disorders. Antianxiety medication is used sparingly and is not generally useful.

Medical side effects of eating disorders require the use of medication. Nurses treat hypokalemia (low potassium) with oral or intravenous potassium supplements. Nutritional anemia is treated with iron supplements. Gastroparesis, or delayed gastric emptying, is treated with metoclopramide (Reglan). Infected parotid glands are usually treated with antibiotics. Laxative dependence is often treated with a combination of stool softeners, bran, fiber, fluids, and decreasing doses of laxatives (if taking very high doses, such as 50 to 100 laxatives at a time, abrupt withdrawal is dangerous and gradual withdrawal is done under close supervision) (see Chapter 24).

Psychotherapeutic Modalities

Individual Psychotherapy. Individual psychotherapy is the preferred treatment for eating disorders. Psychodynamically oriented therapists recommend long-term, insight-oriented therapy to repair early developmental failures or traumas and teach adaptive coping skills. Most therapists recommend active therapies such as behavioral techniques for symptom management and cognitive restructuring to change distorted thinking patterns. Cognitive therapists are likely to recommend structured, short-term therapy with more focus on changing thought patterns and less on insight. Most therapists, whatever their orientation, use hospitalization as a means to manage acute exacerbations (worsening) of either the eating disorder symptoms or the associated mood disorder symptoms.

Behavioral Therapy. Behavioral therapy looks at the behavior that needs to be changed. Self-monitoring of eating behaviors and eating disorder symptoms is an effective behavioral intervention. Behavioral contracts for weight gain, for regulating eating and exercise, and for extinguishing binge/purge behaviors are also useful. Exposure to the problem (bingeing) with response prevention (stopping the purge) is an effective behavioral intervention for bulimia nervosa. For example, a client eats "scary" or binge foods, and the nurse prevents the purge behavior by remaining with the client for one hour after the binge.

Cognitive Therapy. Cognitive therapy helps clients reframe negative or distorted thoughts with more realistic thinking. Most clients with eating disorders have distorted thoughts and beliefs related to food, weight, self-concept, and interpersonal relationships. Cognitive therapy techniques such as keeping a thought record, reframing thoughts, and cognitive restructuring help change these cognitive distortions. Cognitive therapy modified for the young adolescent population is showing positive results (Wilson, 2006). Sometimes therapists pair cognitive therapy with behavioral therapy. This is called cognitive-behavioral therapy (see Chapter 23).

Family Therapy. The primary goal of family therapy is to actively involve the entire family in changing the person's eating disorder behaviors. Improving family interactions is a longer term goal. This is a new approach to family therapy that research has shown to be very effective. Adolescents with eating disorders are expected to participate in family therapy. Educating the family about eating disorders is essential, as the eating disorder behavior often becomes the focus of the family, leading to power struggles that reinforce the behavior (see the Research for Evidence-Based Practice box).

Group Therapy. Group therapy is a way for clients to discuss problems with other members who share the same experiences. Clients with anorexia nervosa and bulimia nervosa often set themselves apart from others. They avoid eating with others, secretly binge and purge, and lie about their behaviors. This often results in feelings of isolation and shame and, with anorexia nervosa, reinforces negative secondary gains related to feeling "special." Being in an eating disorders group offers clients a safe place to self-disclose and be understood, while preventing secondary gains related to being "different."

Expressive Therapies. Expressive therapies are the nonverbal activities of art, music, dance, journal writing, and poetry. Clients with eating disorders have alexithymia (difficulty naming feelings) and interoceptive deficits (inability to accurately identify and respond to bodily cues) and often have difficulty finding the words needed for "talk" therapy. The use of expressive therapies, therefore, allow for greater self-disclosure and exploration of fundamental issues.

RESEARCH for EVIDENCE-BASED PRACTICE

Lock J, le Grange D: Family-based treatment of eating disorders, *International Journal of Eating Disorders* 37(suppl):S64-S67, S87-S89, 2005; Lock J, le Grange D: *Help your teenager beat an eating disorder,* New York, 2005, Guilford Press.

Family therapy has always been a vital component of eating disorder treatment. Because most eating disorders begin during adolescence, including parents in treatment is the standard of care. A well-researched, family-based approach is the Maudsley method, developed at the Maudsley Hospital in London in the 1980s and used at Stanford University and the University of Chicago. The Maudsley method represents a very different approach from traditional family therapy for anorexia nervosa, which believed dysfunctional family systems caused eating disorders and focused on separating the client from the family. The theory was that by giving the client more control over eating, normal autonomous behavior would emerge, and as the client completed the developmental task of separation/individuation, she would give up the eating disorder behaviors. The Maudsley group does not hold these assumptions about the etiology or psychodynamics of eating disorders. The group believes that the causes of eating disorders are unknown. The Maudsley group tells families that they are not to blame and focuses on anorexia nervosa as a life-threatening mental illness that must be interrupted. The group points to evidence that early, aggressive intervention leads to better outcomes and prevents the more severe, chronic form of the illness. The Maudsley method sees parents as the main agent of change in the treatment process. Parents implement the behavioral contract designed by the treatment team, especially the meal plan. The team members instruct parents on how to get their child to eat. They also teach siblings how to support the client to eat. To prevent counter-productive power struggles, the treatment team closely observes the family's efforts and coaches them. The team offers constant support to keep the family from giving up on the treatment goals. Outcome studies of this approach with anorexia show a 90% improvement rate compared to 18% improvement in those receiving individual therapy. Five-year follow-up studies show that 70% of clients remained in recovery. This method also shows promising results in treating bulimia. The National Institutes of Mental Health is currently conducting a 5-year outcome study of this approach.

Adjunctive Therapy

Occupational Therapy. Occupational therapy helps clients with eating disorders learn how to plan meals, shop, and cook for themselves, especially if they have not eaten properly for many years. Although the dietitian will do the actual meal planning, occupational therapy will help the client carry out the plan. Education concerning healthy moderate exercise is also necessary to alter compulsive exercise patterns (see Chapter 23).

Nutrition Education and Counseling. Nutritional education and counseling includes (1) calculating the client's ideal weight range using the basal metabolic index and other methods, (2) planning a refeeding program, and (3) meal planning. Although clients with eating disorders are obsessed with food, most have distorted information about nutrition. A registered dietitian conducts nutritional education and counseling with the nurse's input.

Social Work. Hospital social workers are helpful in finding community resources such as day treatment services, board and care homes, group homes, residential treatment facilities, or vocational rehabilitation. They also provide individual and family therapy with the nurse's input. Clients with chronic eating disorders often do not function well in society, and social workers help them make the transition from the hospital to the community.

NURSING CARE PLAN

Samantha is a 19-year-old college sophomore who is hospitalized for severe cachexia (95 pounds, 5 feet 7 inches) with hypokalemia (low potassium), nutritional anemia, and cardiac dysrhythmia. She arrived home complaining that she was too tired to concentrate on her studies. Her parents, who had not seen her in several months, were stunned at her weight loss and immediately took her to the family physician, who hospitalized her. Samantha's physician reports that she has been dieting and excessively exercising for the past 2 years, but that she had always stayed within 10% of ideal body weight. Samantha had been in individual psychotherapy during her first year of college but now states that she did not continue with therapy as she had promised. As her self-image deteriorated, her bingeing and purging episodes became more frequent. Samantha minimizes her weight loss, complains of feeling fat, is sullen and angry, and wants to be discharged.

DSM-IV-TR Diagnoses

Axis I	Anorexia nervosa, binge eating/purging type
Axis II	Rule out borderline personality disorder
Axis III	Deferred
Axis IV	Moderate (3) (unable to meet college demands; lives away from family)
Axis V	GAF = 50 (current); GAF = 65 (past year)

Nursing Diagnosis *Imbalanced nutrition: less than body requirements related to self-starvation and possible purging behavior, as evidenced by severe weight loss, hypokalemia, and cardiac dysrhythmia*

NOC Nutritional Status: Food and Fluid Intake, Nutritional Status: Biochemical Measures, Weight Control, Symptom Control, Body Image, Knowledge: Diet

NIC Eating Disorders Management, Weight Gain Assistance, Nutrition Management, Weight Management, Teaching: Prescribed Diet

CLIENT OUTCOMES	NURSING INTERVENTIONS	EVALUATION
Samantha will consume adequate calories for age, height, and metabolic need (e.g., 75% of each meal will be consumed by the end of the hospital stay).	Initiate refeeding in collaboration with treatment team (Box 17-5). *Starving behavior is out of control, and Samantha cannot begin eating again on her own.*	Samantha eats only 25% of meals on day 1, but on day 2, she eats 50% and drinks all three dietary supplements. After 7 days, she is eating 75% of all meals and the supplements are discontinued.
	Encourage Samantha to choose her own menu. *Samantha will possibly be more cooperative if she feels she has some control over the refeeding process.*	Samantha selects her own meals on day 3.
Samantha will achieve minimum normal weight (less than 15% below ideal weight for 5 feet, 7 inches, approximately 115 pounds).	Weigh daily with the client's back facing the scale. *Knowledge of daily weight changes will reinforce Samantha's obsession with weight. Not knowing will help her tolerate weight gain and help her to let go of overcontrol of her body.*	Samantha achieves her goal weight by discharge.
Samantha will gain an average of 4 pounds per week.	Continue to implement the refeeding plan and contract as needed *to maintain the client's expected weight.*	Samantha maintains her expected weight.

Nursing Diagnosis *Disturbed body image related to psychologic conflicts (fear of growing up, fear of sexuality), as evidenced by complaints of body dissatisfaction, fear of weight gain, and minimizing weight loss when more than 15% below minimal normal weight (e.g., 95 pounds, 5 feet 7 inches)*

NOC Body Image, Identity, Sexual Identity, Self-Esteem

NIC Body Image Enhancement, Self-Esteem Enhancement, Anxiety Reduction, Truth Telling

CLIENT OUTCOMES	NURSING INTERVENTIONS	EVALUATION
Samantha will demonstrate realistic perceptions of body shape and size.	Encourage expression of thoughts and feelings regarding body. *Verbalizing specific concerns will help Samantha uncover psychologic issues related to her body image.*	Samantha verbalizes awareness that she is underweight and that her dissatisfaction with her body has to do more with psychologic issues than with her weight.
Samantha will demonstrate increased insight into body image distortion.	Collaborate with dietitian to give fact-based information to counter Samantha's irrational beliefs about body size and shape (e.g., "You are 20 pounds below minimum healthy weight for your age and height"). *Factual information given by more than one team member reinforces the difference between Samantha's perception of her weight and her actual weight.*	Samantha verbalizes that she perceives herself as being heavier than her actual weight.
Samantha will demonstrate an enhanced self-concept based on positive characteristics, rather than based totally on her body shape.	Give Samantha truthful feedback about the positive qualities she demonstrates on the unit. *Samantha's self-concept is influenced by her body rather than who she is as a person and she needs to view herself in terms of her true qualities.*	Samantha verbalizes positive, truthful qualities about herself that were unrelated to her body, such as "I know I'm a worthwhile person because people like me" or "Many people say that I have a talent for art."

Nursing Diagnosis *Noncompliance with the treatment plan related to psychologic conflicts (control issues and/or separation issues), as evidenced by anger, refusal to self-disclose to the staff, and requests to be discharged*

NOC Acceptance: Health Status, Health Beliefs: Perceived Control, Caregiver-Patient Relationship, Knowledge: Disease Process, Will to Live

NIC Health System Guidance, Self-modification Assistance, Support System Enhancement, Patient Contracting, Mutual Goal Setting, Teaching: Procedure/Treatment

CLIENT OUTCOMES	NURSING INTERVENTIONS	EVALUATION
Samantha will participate in therapeutic interactions with staff and will engage in less power struggles.	Develop a therapeutic alliance with Samantha by using her input in her treatment plan. *Including Samantha as a part of the treatment team increases her sense of control and decreases power struggles, strengthening the therapeutic alliance.*	Samantha participates as part of the treatment team and has not had any major power struggle with the staff.
Samantha will comply with the interdisciplinary treatment plan.	Use contracts written by the team with clear expectations and consequences *to increase Samantha's compliance and further reduce power struggles.*	Samantha complies with the expectations of her behavioral contract.
Samantha will acknowledge her condition and the need for treatment.	Use reality orientation to challenge Samantha's minimization of the seriousness of her condition. Give information about laboratory results, medical status, and so on. *Samantha's denial will decrease when she is given concrete information.*	Samantha verbalizes awareness of her need for hospitalization and treatment. She admits that in order to succeed in life and in college, she will need to follow the prescribed therapeutic plan.

BOX 17-5

Refeeding Procedure

If Samantha does not eat 90% of her meals on day 1, she will receive three dietary supplements on day 2. Supplements will continue daily until she eats 90% of her meals.

If she does not finish her supplements on day 2, she will be tube fed on day 3. Tube feeding will continue until she eats 90% of all meals for 1 day.

If she refuses tube feeding, she will be discharged.

CASE STUDY

Eileen is a 16-year-old young woman admitted to the hospital for increasingly out-of-control bulimic symptoms, including bingeing and purging up to 10 times a day and abuse of laxatives. During her first week of hospitalization, the primary focus was to correct Eileen's fluid and electrolyte balance and monitor her to prevent purging. Eileen slept for long periods of time during the first week. She participated superficially in group sessions, complaining mainly of physical discomfort related to the cessation of her purging behavior and use of laxatives. During the second week of treatment, the team set goals to help Eileen become more involved in the psychologic issues related to her bulimia. The interventions included encouraging Eileen to work on underlying issues of self-esteem and family dysfunction.

CRITICAL THINKING

1. How will the nurse evaluate Eileen's progress in working on underlying issues? What three specific client outcomes would indicate such progress?
2. What specific observations should the nurse make during group sessions to evaluate Eileen's progress?
3. What verbalizations expressed by Eileen would indicate progress in her work on underlying issues?

EVALUATION

The nurse evaluates the progress of the client with an eating disorder in an organized, timely manner, according to the outcomes identified in the care plan. For the client with an eating disorder, the evaluation includes physiologic, behavioral, psychologic, social, and cultural assessments. Laboratory values, vital signs, weight, and food/fluid intake provide the data used to evaluate physiologic responses to treatment. Observing and recording the client's affect, level of program participation, specific eating behaviors, peer interactions, and responses to staff provide evaluative data that help the team track the client's behavioral responses to treatment. The use of active listening while interacting with the client in group therapy, during activities, and during individual interactions provides additional data from which to evaluate the client's psychologic and behavioral responses to treatment. Evaluation of outcomes also reveals the effectiveness of the interventions used by nursing and the treatment team (see the Case Study).

CHAPTER SUMMARY

- Eating disorders are syndromes with physiologic, behavioral, and psychologic features.
- Self-starvation, binge eating, and purging behaviors have existed for many centuries, but until recent times, eating disorders were rare.
- The reasons for the recent outbreak of eating disorders are unclear, but many believe they are related to current cultural trends in the fashion industry, the diet industry, and the women's movement.
- Eating disorders have a multidetermined etiology, including biologic, genetic, sociocultural, psychologic, and familial factors.

- There is a high incidence of depression among clients with eating disorders and their families.
- Personality traits that are common among individuals with eating disorders include low self-esteem, perfectionism, interoceptive deficits, harm avoidance, ineffectiveness, alexithymia, and compliance.
- Common dynamics in families of origin in persons with eating disorders include a focus on achievement, body image and social acceptance, enmeshment, poor conflict resolution skills, and difficulty with age-appropriate separation/individuation.
- Most individuals with eating disorders are female, although the incidence among males is increasing. Bulimia nervosa is more common than anorexia nervosa. Eating disorders are most common among high school and college students, although the incidence is growing among younger children.
- Clients with eating disorders often have other psychiatric diagnoses. Common Axis I diagnoses are mood and anxiety disorders. Common Axis II diagnoses are borderline, avoidant, and obsessive-compulsive personality disorders.
- Anorexia nervosa and bulimia nervosa are distinct diagnoses in the DSM-IV-TR classification, but they have many of the same features.
- The course of the illness is either chronic or episodic, requiring long-term or repeated episodes of treatment.
- Interdisciplinary treatment is indicated to deal with the multifaceted nature of eating disorders.
- Medical complications from eating disorders are life threatening. Self-induced vomiting and abuse of laxatives and diuretics cause serious electrolyte imbalances that lead to cardiac dysrhythmias and cardiac arrest.
- Nurses need to take a firm, professional, yet compassionate approach to avoid the power struggles that commonly undermine treatment of individuals with eating disorders.
- The plan of care needs to balance behavioral interventions that interrupt the cycle of behavior with psychologic interventions that deal with fundamental issues and promote positive coping skills.
- A safe, structured environment is necessary to prevent self-harm, promote nutritional restoration, and help the client understand the meaning of his or her behavior and learn more effective coping skills.
- Nurses need to refeed in a structured manner, with clear expectations and consequences. Positive reinforcement is more effective than punishment. Consistency is essential.
- The client needs to understand how he or she is using the eating disorder to avoid psychologic issues. The nurse assists the client in balancing attention between restoring nutritional health and dealing with fundamental conflicts.
- SSRI antidepressants are used to treat the coexisting depression in clients with eating disorders and often help decrease binge urges in clients with bulimia.
- Therapists usually recommend long-term individual psychotherapy of various modalities or methods for all clients with eating disorders. Family therapy is essential for adolescents. Group psychotherapy is also a widely used treatment method.

REVIEW QUESTIONS

1 A nurse assesses an adolescent female with anorexia nervosa. Which physical findings support the diagnosis? You may select more than one answer.
1. Temperature of 96.9°
2. Pulse rate of 48
3. Sensitivity to heat
4. Oily skin
5. Facial lanugo

2 If a client's ideal body weight is 124 lbs., which current weight meets diagnostic criteria for anorexia nervosa?
1. 105 lbs.
2. 109 lbs.
3. 112 lbs.
4. 119 lbs.

3 A client with an eating disorder has a history of taking 20 to 30 laxative products per day. Which intervention(s) should be added to the plan of care? You may select more than one answer.
1. Immediate discontinuation of all laxative products
2. Daily oral stool softener medications
3. Intake of fiber and bran products
4. Liberal oral intake of fluids
5. Gradual downward titration of laxative medications

4 Prioritize these nursing diagnoses for a client with bulimia nervosa.
1. Imbalanced nutrition: less than body requirements
2. Powerlessness
3. Social isolation
4. Risk for imbalanced fluid volume

5 A nurse assesses personality traits of a client with an eating disorder. Which comment by the client indicates bulimia nervosa rather than anorexia nervosa?
1. "I try to do what my parents want, but I usually don't get things right."
2. "I feel good. I feel just fine. I don't have any problems."
3. "I don't look as good as most of my friends. That's why I don't have many dates."
4. "If I want to do something, I just do it. I don't like to analyze things too much."

Additional self-study exercises and learning resources are available to you on the ***Companion CD*** *at the back of the book and on the* ***Evolve website*** *at* ***http://evolve.elsevier.com/Fortinash/.***

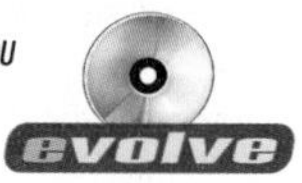

ONLINE RESOURCES

Academy for Eating Disorders: **www.aedweb.org**

Anorexia Nervosa and Related Eating Disorders: **www.anred.com**

National Alliance on Mental Illness: **www.nami.org**

National Association of Anorexia Nervosa and Associated Disorders: **www.anad.org**

National Eating Disorders Association: **www.nationaleatingdisorders.org**

National Institute of Mental Health: **www.nimh.nih.gov**

Mental Health America: **www.nmha.org**

REFERENCES

Agras W: The consequences and costs of the eating disorders, *Psychiatr Clin North Am* 24:371, 2001.

Agras S, Hammer L, McNicholas F: A prospective study of the influence of eating-disordered mothers on their children, *Int J Eat Disord* 25:253, 1999.

American Psychiatric Association: *Diagnostic and statistical manual of mental disorders*, ed 4, text revision. Washington, DC, 2000, American Psychiatric Association.

American Psychiatric Association Work Group on Eating Disorders: Practice guideline for the treatment of eating disorders (revision), *Am J Psychiatry* 157(suppl 1):1-39, 2000.

Bailer U et al: Altered 5-HT2a receptor binding after recovery from bulimia-type anorexia nervosa: relationships to harm avoidance and drive for thinness, *Neuropsychopharmacology* 29:1143-1155, 2004.

Bailer U et al: Altered brain serotonin 5-HT 1a receptor binding after recovery from anorexia nervosa measured by positron emission tomography and (carbonyl11c)way-100635, *Arch Gen Psychiatry* 62:1032-1041, 2005.

Bell R: *Holy anorexia*, Chicago, 1987, University of Chicago Press.

Binswanger L: The case of Ellen West. In May R, Angel E, Ellenburger H, editors: *Existence*, New York, 1958, Basic Books.

Boskind-Lodahl M, White W: *Bulimarexia: the binge/purge cycle*, New York, 1983, WW Norton.

Brumberg J: *Fasting girls*, New York, 1989, New American Library.

Dare C et al: Psychological therapies for adults with anorexia nervosa: randomized controlled trial of outpatient treatment, *Br J Psychiatry* 178:216, 2001.

Davis C et al: Looking good-family focus on appearance and the risk for eating disorders, *Intl J Eat Disord* 35:136-144, 2004.

Emborg C: Mortality and causes of death in eating disorders in Denmark 1970-1993: a case register study, *Int J Eat Disord* 25:243, 1999.

Fairburn C et al: Twin studies and the etiology of eating disorder, *Int J Eat Disord* 26:349, 1999.

Fernandez-Aranda F et al: Personality and psychopathological traits of males with eating disorders, *Eurpoean ED Review* 12:367-374, 2004.

Grice D et al: Evidence for a susceptibility gene for anorexia nervosa on chromosome 1, *Am J Hum Genet* 70:787, 2002.

Groesz L, Levine M, Murnen S: The effect of experimental presentation of thin media images on body satisfaction: a meta analytic review, *Int J Eat Disord* 31:1, 2002.

Hahn-Smith A, Smith J: The positive influence of maternal identification on body image, eating attitudes and self esteem of Hispanic and Anglo girls, *Int J Eat Disord* 29:428, 2001.

Hamburger W: Emotional aspects of obesity, *Med Clin North Am* 35:483, 1951.

Johnson C, Connors M: *The etiology and treatment of bulimia nervosa*, New York, 1987, Basic Books.

Kaye W et al: Altered dopamine activity after recovery from restricting-type anorexia nervosa, *Neuropsychopharmacology* 21:503-506, 1999.

Kaye W et al: Altered serotonin 2A receptor activity in women who have recovered from bulimia nervosa, *Am J Psychiatry* 158:1152, 2001a.

Kaye W et al: Double-blind, placebo controlled administration of fluoxetine in restricting and restricting-purging- type anorexia nervosa, *Biol Psychiatry* 49:644, 2001b.

Kaye W et al: Comorbidity of anxiety disorders with anorexia nervosa and bulimia nervosa, *Am J Psychiatry* 161:2215-2221, 2004.

Keel P et al: Long-term impact of treatment in women diagnosed with bulimia nervosa, *Int J Eat Disord* 31:151, 2002.

Klump K, Kaye W, Strober M: The evolving genetic foundations of eating disorders, *Psychaitr Clin North Am* 24:215, 2001.

Lewinsohn P, Striegel-Moore R, Seeley J: Epidemiology and natural course of eating disorders in young women from adolescence to young adulthood, *J Am Acad Child Adolesc Psychiatry* 31:284, 2002a.

Lewinsohn P et al: Gender differences is eating disorder symptoms in young adults, *Int J Eat Disord* 32:426-440, 2002b.

Lindner R: The case of Laura. In *The fifty minute hour*, New York, 1955, Holt, Rinehart & Winston.

Lock J, le Grange D: Family-based treatment for eating disorders, *Intl J of Eat Disord* 37(suppl): S64-S67, S87-S89, 2005a.

Lock J, le Grange D: *Help your teenager beat an eating disorder*, New York, 2005b, The Guilford Press.

Lowe B et al: Long-term outcome of anorexia nervosa in a prospective 21-year follow-up study, *Psychol Med* 31:881-890, 2001.

Minuchin S, Rosman B, Baker L: *Psychosomatic families: anorexia nervosa in context*, Cambridge, Mass, 1978, Harvard University Press.

Milos G et al: Comorbidity of obsessive-compulsive disorders and duration of eating disorders, *Int J Eat Disord* 31:284, 2002.

Milos G et al: Instability of eating disorder diagnoses: prospective study, *British J Psychiatry* 187:573-578, 2005.

Mitchell J et al: Combining pharmacotherapy and psychotherapy in the treatment of patients with eating disorders, *Psychiatr Clin North Am* 24:315, 2001.

Paul T et al: Self-injurious behavior in women with eating disorders, *Am J Psychiatry* 159:408, 2002.

Polivy J, Herman P: Causes of eating disorders, *Annu Rev Psychol* 53:187, 2002.

Rosenvinge J, Martinussen M, Ostensen E: The comorbidity of eating disorders and personality disorders: meta-analytic review of studies published between 1983 and 1998, *Eat Weight Disord* 5:52, 2000.

Russell G: Bulimia nervosa: an ominous variant of anorexia nervosa, *Psychol Med* 9:429, 1979.

Smolak L, Levine M, Schermer F: Parental input and weight concerns among elementary school children, *Int J Eat Disord* 25:263, 1999.

Stunkard A: Eating patterns and obesity, *Psychiatry Q* 33:284, 1959.

Sysko R et al: Eating behavior among women with anorexia nervosa, *Am J Clin Nutr* 82:296-301, 2005.

von Ranson K, Iacono W, McGue M: Disordered eating and substance use in an epidemiological sample. I. Associations within individuals, *Int J Eat Disord* 31:389, 2002.

Wade T, Bulik C, Kendler K: Investigation of quality of the parental relationship as a risk factor for subclinical bulimia nervosa, *Int J Eat Disord* 30:388, 2001.

Wilson G et al: Cognitive-behavioural therapy for adolescents with bulimia nervosa, *European Eat Dis Review* 14:8-16, 2006.

Wonderlich S et al: Eating disturbance and sexual trauma in childhood and adulthood, *Int J Eat Disord* 30:401, 2001.

Zhu A, Walsh B: Pharmacologic treatment of eating disorders, *Can J Psychiatry* 47:227, 2002.

Chapter 18

Sleep Disorders

NANCY STARK NAPOLITANO

Sleep is that golden chain that ties health and our bodies together.
THOMAS DEKKER

OBJECTIVES

1. Describe the major categories of sleep disorders.
2. Discuss the factors and presenting signs and symptoms of each sleep pattern disturbance.
3. Develop an understanding of the assessment tools that identify sleep disorders in clients across the life span.
4. Discuss how nursing and medical experts make differential diagnoses as they relate to problems of sleep pattern disturbance among their clients.
5. Apply the nursing process to clients who are experiencing major alterations in their sleep-wake cycles.
6. Formulate relevant nursing diagnoses for clients who demonstrate significant abnormalities in their sleep-wake pattern.
7. Design comprehensive nursing care plans that reflect guiding practices for restorative sleep for clients in acute care, long-term care, and community-based settings.
8. Evaluate the effectiveness of interdisciplinary interventions to promote restorative sleep in clients who are experiencing sleep pattern disturbances.

KEY TERMS

Sleep is a basic human need, fundamental for human survival. Although an individual's sleep pattern typically changes as he or she progresses through the life span, adequate amounts of restorative sleep are necessary in each phase of human development to maintain the best level of physical and psychologic functioning. People are not always aware of the essential role that restorative sleep plays in their everyday life until sleep becomes disrupted because of an acute or chronic sleep pattern disturbance. Psychiatric nursing practice frequently involves the management of clients with sleep pattern disruptions, as these disruptions often coexist with some types of mental disorders. Sometimes clients experience a disruption in mental health functioning as a result of a sleep pattern disturbance.

Approximately 47 million to 70 million Americans suffer from some type of chronic sleep disorder (National Institutes of Health [NIH] 2006; Walsh, 2004). These sleep disturbances account for a large percentage of the complaints of daytime sleepiness experienced by persons as they age (National Sleep Foundation, 2005). The average nightly sleep duration for the average adult has fallen from approximately 9 hours per night to 7 hours per night. This common problem results from many sleep pattern disturbances that are either self-imposed or occur as a result of a primary or secondary sleep pattern disorder. Some causes of sleep deprivation include insomnia, narcolepsy, breathing-related sleep disorders, circadian rhythm sleep disturbances, recurrent nightmares, sleep terrors, and sleepwalking disturbances. The resulting sleep deprivation often presents significant health and safety concerns for the affected individual.

Excessive sleep loss is catastrophic and has far-reaching consequences. Current data from the National Transportation Safety Board indicate that fatigue from sleep deprivation accounts for more than 100,000 highway accidents and 1500 deaths every year (American College of Physicians, 2005; NIH, 2006). Sleep deprivation also leads to increased risks for having both work-related accidents and substandard work performance on the job. This is especially true when a client has a job with nighttime work assignments or rotating shift work.

Ongoing sleep deprivation also significantly impacts the overall quality of physical and psychologic health. Persistent sleep deficits are an increased risk factor for coronary heart disease (Ayas et al., 2003), impaired cognitive functioning (Von Dongen et al., 2003), obesity (Spiegal et al., 2004), diabetes (Ayas et al., 2003), and altered immune function (Bryant et al., 2004). Additionally, sleep pattern disturbances coexist with such mood disorders as major depression, bipolar disorder, and generalized anxiety disorder (American Psychiatric Association [APA], 2000).

THEORETIC PERSPECTIVES

Physiologic and Homeostatic Sleep Regulation

Sleep is a temporary state of unconsciousness that many think restores and repairs the body (Guyton and Hall, 2006; Kaplan and Sadock, 2002). Although research has not identified a specific sleep neurotransmitter, several interconnected, complex biochemical and neurologic processes work together to directly or indirectly influence the sleep-wake cycle (First and Tasman, 2004). Most researchers agree that neurotransmitters act on certain areas of the brain to control sleep and wakefulness. Researchers also think that neurotransmitters such as adenosine, acetylcholine, and melatonin have a sleep-promoting function, whereas serotonin and norepinephrine most likely maintain arousal (First and Tasman, 2004; Sadock and Sadock, 2004).

The regular recurrence of the sleep-wake cycle is one example of a physiologic **circadian rhythm** that is highly influenced by the body's internal biologic clock. Located in the hypothalamus of the brain, this biologic clock or regulator known as the suprachiasmatic nucleus is able to adjust sleep-wake intervals in a cyclical 24-hour pattern because of its sensitivity to the external cues of light and darkness. Researchers postulate that the presence of sunlight and other types of artificial light creates the necessary neurosensory stimulation of the photoreceptors in the retina that will eventually suppress the release of melatonin (a chemical mediator that promotes sleep) from the pineal gland. When this takes place, a state of wakefulness occurs during daylight hours. In contrast, a state of darkness promotes sleep as a result of melatonin release. Thus, in a 24-hour period, the biologic clock suppresses and then stimulates the release of melatonin to synchronize sleep and wakefulness using the external cues of light and darkness (Guyton and Hall, 2006; Kaplan and Sadock, 2002).

An individual who has a relatively normal day-night sleep pattern typically goes through a recurrent cycle of sleep and wakefulness within a defined 24-hour period because of the influence of the body's biologic clock. However, if the cues for light and darkness are disrupted in some way (i.e., as a result of night shift work, travel across several time zones), the individual will most likely experience some type of sleep disturbance because of the interruption of sleep regulating cues of light and darkness from the external environment.

When an individual progresses from a state of wakefulness to a stage of sleep, there are changes in the brain wave activity. This is evident when using an electroencephalogram (EEG) recording. These changes occur according to states of sleep and wakefulness. There are four distinct types of brain waves that include alpha, beta, theta, and delta waves. Each of these categories contains brain wave activity that has a distinct range of brain wave amplitude and frequencies, depending on the activity of the cerebral cortex during the various stages of the sleep cycle (Guyton and Hall, 2006; Saladin, 2004) (Figure 18-1).

Alpha waves occur at a frequency of 8 to 13 Hz and occur most often in adults who are awake but are resting and not attending to any particular mental task (Guyton and Hall, 2006). Beta waves occur at a frequency of 14 to 30 Hz and occur when an individual is mentally active and receptive to sensory stimulation (Saladin, 2004). Theta and delta waves are low-frequency waves and both occur in adults experiencing sleep states. Theta recordings are usually at frequencies of 4 to 7 Hz and also occur in children during awake states. Delta waves are slower wave frequencies, when compared to theta recordings, and usually occur at frequencies below 3.5 Hz (Saladin, 2004). Delta waves occur in adults who are in deep sleep stages and in infants during states of wakefulness (Saladin, 2004).

Normally, a restorative sleep pattern has two distinct stages of sleep: **non–rapid eye movement (NREM) sleep** and its associated four sleep stages (stages 1, 2 , 3, and 4) and **rapid eye movement (REM) sleep** (Kaplan and Sadock, 2002) (Figure 18-2). During the NREM sleep cycle, an individual initially enters the first of four stages of sleep, repeating them in a cyclical fashion throughout the sleep episode. The individual first enters into stage 1 NREM sleep upon closing his or her eyes and drifting into a light sleep state (Kaplan and Sadock, 2002; Saladin, 2004). The EEG of an individual who is in stage 1 NREM shows many alpha waves. The person is able to be aroused easily during this state of the sleep cycle (Saladin, 2004). If not awakened during stage 1 NREM sleep, the individual will enter stage 2 NREM sleep where he or she will become less easily aroused. The predominant EEG recording during this stage reflects high K-complexes and spindle-like tracings at frequencies of 12 to 14 Hz (Kaplan and Sadock, 2002). Soon thereafter, the individual will enter stage 3 NREM sleep where theta and delta wave activity will appear on the EEG recordings (Saladin, 2004). During this stage of NREM sleep, the vital sign recordings (body tempera-

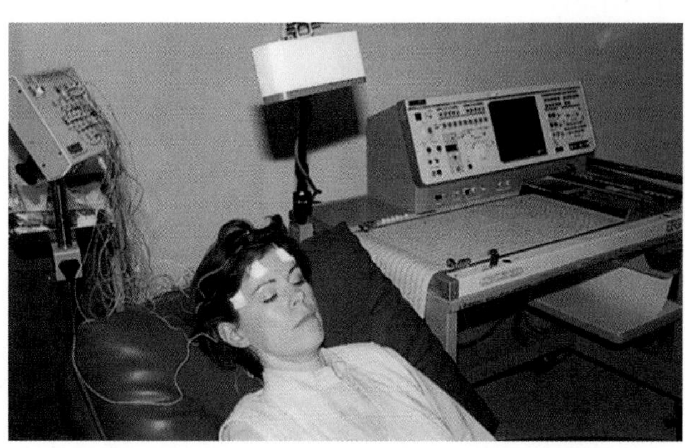

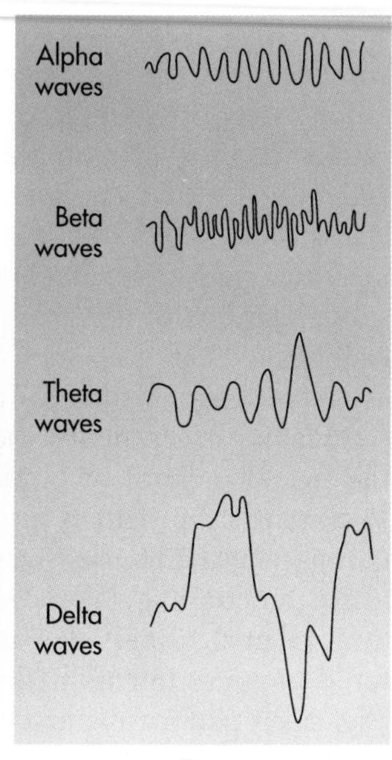

A B

FIGURE 18-1 The electroencephalogram (EEG). **A,** Photograph showing a person undergoing an EEG test. Notice the scalp electrodes that detect voltage fluctuations within the cranium. **B,** Examples of alpha, beta, theta, and delta waves seen on an EEG. (From Lewis SM: *Medical-surgical nursing: assessment and management of clinical problems,* ed 7, St Louis, 2007, Elsevier.)

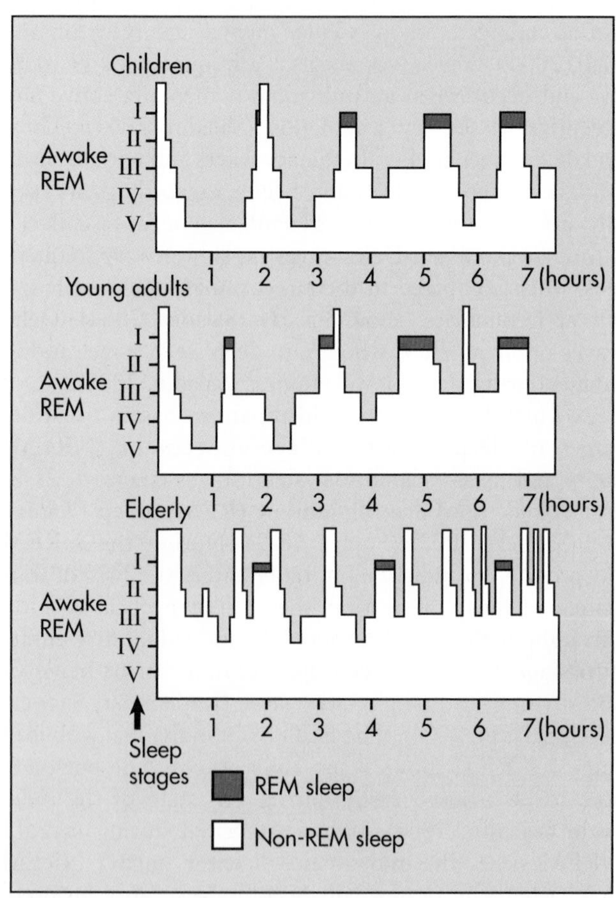

FIGURE 18-2 Normal sleep cycles. Rapid eye movement (REM) sleep occurs cyclically throughout the night at intervals of approximately 90 minutes in all age-groups. REM sleep shows little variation in the different age-groups, whereas stage 4 sleep decreases with age. In addition, elderly persons awaken frequently and show a marked increase in total time awake. (From McCance KL, Huether SE: *Pathophysiology: the biologic basis for disease in adults and children,* ed 5, St Louis, 2006, Elsevier.)

ture, pulse, respiration, and blood pressure) usually reflect a decline from baseline values, and the individual is in a deeper sleep state when compared to the two previous NREM stages. Progressively, the individual will enter stage 4 NREM sleep, where arousal is difficult. Vital sign recordings are usually at their lowest level from baseline recording, the muscles are very relaxed, and the EEG brain wave activity reflects a predominance of delta wave, or slow wave, activity (Kaplan and Sadock, 2002; Saladin, 2004).

After moving from wakefulness through stages 1 through 4 NREM sleep, the person then goes back from stage 4 NREM to stage 2 NREM sleep. Then the individual enters the active sleep stage known as REM sleep (Saladin, 2004). The first REM period of the sleep episode takes place approximately 90 minutes after the individual first falls asleep, with subsequent REM periods occurring four to five times, at 90-minute intervals, throughout the sleep episode (Kaplan and Sadock, 2002; Saladin, 2002). The duration of each REM period usually lasts from 5 to 30 minutes, depending on the individual. For example, if the individual is extremely tired, REM sleep is shorter or does not occur at all during the sleep episode. However, once the individual becomes less fatigued, the REM periods typically increases in frequency and duration throughout the sleep cycle (Guyton and Hall, 2006).

REM sleep is an active cerebral state. During this stage of sleep, there is an increase in cerebral metabolism with brain waves paralleling those of an awake state (Guyton and Hall, 2006). This stage of sleep is also called paradoxical sleep because of the seemingly contradictory findings of active brain wave activity in a difficult-to-arouse person (Saladin, 2004). The individual has decreased muscle tone and has irregular muscle movements during this stage of sleep. Active dreaming also takes place that is usually associated with the presence of rapid eye movements.

Normal sleep patterns/requirements vary across the life span. On average, the newborn sleeps approximately 16 hours a day, with 50% of total sleep time spent in REM sleep (Kaplan and Saddock, 2002). Over the course of the first 6 months of life, the infant's sleep patterns continually change so that by the end of the first 6 months, it will closely resemble an adult's sleep pattern. The infant also typically develops more consolidated sleep patterns within the first few years of life and usually have uninterrupted blocks of sleep without the need for a daytime nap by the age 4. As the child ages, his or her nighttime sleep requirements usually decrease so that by the adolescent period, the sleep requirements are the same as an adult's (Thiedke, 2001). Although adolescents require approximately 9 to 10 hours of sleep per night, they still experience daytime sleepiness because of a phase delay in their sleep-wakefulness pattern (First and Tasman, 2004). The adolescent typically does not experience sleepiness until the early morning hours and does not wake up naturally until the late morning or early afternoon (First and Tasman, 2004). Adolescents therefore experience sleep disturbances for activities that require them to wake early, such as school or social obligations. Sleep patterns of young adults show that they spend 25% of total sleep time in REM, whereas middle and older adults spend even less time in REM sleep than young adults. Thus, in middle and older adulthood, a person experiences more fragmented sleep with the development of a daytime napping pattern, especially in the older adult who has difficulty with uninterrupted nocturnal sleep (First and Tasman, 2003).

HISTORIC PERSPECTIVES

Historically, the ancient Greeks theorized that a benevolent force known as "hypnos," or the god of sleep, controlled sleep. The dreams that took place during the sleep state were symbolic messages sent from the Greek gods. During the second century AD, the professional diviner Artemidorus Daldianus was responsible for interpreting the meaning of these messages and eventually wrote a five-volume Greek work titled *Oneirocritic*, or *The Interpretation of Dreams*. It was Daldianus' belief that if a person's dreams were linked to his or her previous life experiences, then the dream was insignificant and not symbolic of a message from the Greek gods. Throughout this time period, dreaming was generally thought to be an outward manifestation of the internal mental acts that took place throughout the previous day (Klosch and Ulrich, 2005).

Some 1700 years later, the Viennese physician Sigmund Freud (1856-1939) challenged Daldianus' conclusions in his 1899 publication of *The Interpretation of Dreams*. Freud postulated that dreams were, in fact, very significant and were symbolic of unconscious desires. It was Freud's belief that dreams were an outward expression of the unconscious mind and they could be accurately analyzed through the use of free association. In essence, one could uncover the individual's unconscious desire for wish fulfillment through dream analysis (Freud's dream theory, 2006).

Around the same time, renowned Austrian psychiatrist Alfred Adler (1870-1937) developed a general theory of dream analysis that would later lay a foundation for other neo-Freudian theorists who would follow. One of the basic views of Adler's theory was that dream content could be linked to individual mastery and the dream's mood or feeling state could prepare an individual for current and future problem-solving needs. The dream content was an expression of the individual's character and his or her ongoing challenge to overcome inferiority (Adler's dream theory, 2006).

Carl Gustav Jung's (1875-1961) dream theory eventually became one of the most influential theories in analytic psychology. Jung viewed dreams as being representative of the individual's mental world, expressed in a symbolic language that characterized both the objective and subjective nature of the dream experience (Jung's dream theory, 2006).

There was no support for sleep research until the 1950s, when Nathaniel Kleitman and Eugene Aserinsky began recording the eye movements of sleep subjects. Kleitman and Aserinsky uncovered the physiologic processes associated with rapid eye movement (REM) sleep. During their laboratory analysis, these researchers observed that the young sleep subjects had cyclical periods of rapid eye movement during certain stages of their sleep cycle. They eventually determined that these REM periods of the sleep cycle were associated with a relatively high percentage of self-reported dream states, high brainwave activity, and little or no skeletal muscle movement during these REM episodes. This discovery was a significant breakthrough in sleep research and was the basis for future theories related to sleep (Klosch and Ulrich, 2005).

Almost 10 years after this REM sleep discovery, French neurophysiologist Michael Jouver discovered an association between pontine stimulation (brain stem stimulation) in the brains of cats and the associated onset of REM phases of sleep. His research, however, did not find any link between REM sleep and higher order brain activity; the brain stem, specifically the pons varolii (part of the brain stem), appears responsible for stimulating REM activity, at least in cats (Klosch and Ulrich, 2005).

In the 1970s, the research of Allan Hobson and Robert W. McCarley of Harvard Medical School provided further support for a biochemical basis for sleep and dreaming. Hobson and McCarley presented two complementary theories (reciprocal-interaction and activation-synthesis) that attempted to explain how REM phases were activated and inhibited during the sleep cycle. In reciprocal interaction, the researchers asserted that the REM phases of the sleep cycle and the dreaming that takes place during this time are turned on and off throughout the night by neurons in the brain stem (pons). The activation-synthesis theory explains how the higher brain centers operate in the dream experience.

These researchers claimed that the chemical messenger acetylcholine was responsible for sending impulses to various brain regions (pons, cortex, and limbic areas), resulting in the initiation of REM activity and the associated dream state. Cessation of the REM sleep state, and thus dreaming, took place through the release of "REM off" chemical messengers, norepinephrine and serotonin. Unlike Jouver's findings, Hobson and McCarley found higher brain centers participating in dreaming (Klosch and Ulrich, 2005).

Although previous theoretic and empirical data have contributed greatly to our current understanding of the nature of sleep, much is still unknown. The prevalence of sleep pattern disturbances has generated an increased public awareness of this problem. Consequently, current research continues in this area as the search for a deeper understanding of sleep becomes known.

ETIOLOGY

There are many complex, multifaceted causes of sleep disturbances. In some instances, it is difficult to find strong evidence to support some causes, as many areas of sleep research are still in the beginning stage. Additionally, a sleep disorder such as insomnia sometimes begins as a result of precipitating factors such as genetics or stress and continues to become a chronic condition because of perpetuating circumstances (contextual conditioning).

According to the DSM IV-TR (APA, 2000), sleep disorders are either primary or secondary, depending on their presumed etiology (Box 18-1). Primary sleep disorders include the dyssomnias and parasomnias. The **dyssomnias** include sleep disorders that occur because of abnormalities of the physiologic mechanisms that regulate sleep and wakefulness. **Parasomnias**, on the other hand, are primary sleep disorders that occur as a result of the activation of physiologic systems at incorrect times during the sleep-wake cycle, resulting in abnormal behavior or physiologic events during the sleep state. Parasomnias are often paroxysmal sleep disturbances that are more common in children (Thiedke, 2001). Secondary sleep disorders are most often related to psychiatric illnesses (i.e. mood disorders), the effect of substances, or they are secondary to a general medical condition (Neil, 2005).

BOX 18-1

Primary Sleep Disorders

Primary sleep disorders are presumed to arise from endogenous abnormalities in sleep-wake generating or timing mechanisms, often complicated by conditioning factors.

DYSSOMNIAS

Characterized by abnormalities in amount, quality, or timing of sleep:

- Primary insomnia
- Primary hypersomnia
- Narcolepsy
- Breathing-related sleep disorder
- Circadian rhythm sleep disorder (formerly *sleep-wake schedule disorder*)
  - Jet lag type
  - Shift work type
  - Delayed sleep phase type
- Dyssomnia not otherwise specified

PARASOMNIAS

Characterized by abnormal behavior or physiologic events occurring in association with sleep, specific sleep stages, or sleep-wake transitions:

- Nightmare disorder (formerly *dream anxiety disorder)*
- Sleep terror disorder
- Sleepwalking disorder
- Parasomnia not otherwise specified

Data from American Psychiatric Association: *Diagnostic and statistical manual of mental disorders*, ed 4, text revision, Washington, DC, 2000, American Psychiatric Association.

Biologic Factors

Biochemical alterations in neurotransmitters such as serotonin, melatonin, norepinephrine, and dopamine may play a major role in the deregulation of sleep and wakefulness (Sadock and Sadock, 2004). An inherent physiologic imbalance of these chemical mediators or the use of substances that influence sleep increases an individual's chance of a developing a sleep pattern disturbance. For example, such substances as tricyclic antidepressant drugs interfere with REM sleep (Wilson and Argyropoulos, 2005). Additionally, the development of a substance-induced sleep disorder syndrome sometimes occurs in individuals who use certain prescribed drugs and over-the-counter medications at the same time. Clients who stop taking these medications are also at risk for a substance-induced sleep disorder because these people are often incapable of restoring healthy sleep patterns (APA, 2000). Examples of substances that influence sleep include alcohol, stimulants such as caffeine, amphetamines, and cocaine, and the sedative effects of opiates, hypnotics, and antianxiety medications.

Researchers believe narcolepsy results from a deficiency of hypocretin-1 and hypocretin-2, neurotransmitters produced by the hypothalamus. The deficiency results from an autoimmune response caused by genetic or environmental factors (Quillen, 2005).

Genetic/Hereditary/Familial Factors

There has been a connection between a genetic predisposition or familial association and some types of sleep disturbances. For example, there is a fairly consistent association between a familial predisposition and primary insomnia (APA, 2000). Although some research suggests a genetic link to insomnia, data from twin studies have shown inconsistent findings (APA, 2000, Bastien and Morin, 2000). A genetic association to narcolepsy is in the adolescent population. Additionally, the type of circadian rhythm sleep disturbance called delayed sleep phase is associated with a genetic predisposition to this disorder (Ancoli-Israel et al., 2001). Obstructive sleep apnea also has a familial association (APA, 2000).

Psychiatric/Cognitive/Behavioral Factors

Some sleep pattern disturbances also occur with some mood and anxiety disorders (APA, 2000). In some instances, it is difficult to determine whether the sleep pattern disturbance is a precursor to the onset of the psychiatric illness or whether the illness, in some significant way, influenced the development of a sleep pattern disturbance. In particular, clients with insomnia usually report the onset of sleep problems after experiencing a fairly sudden onset of psychologic stressors (APA, 2000). Clients with a chronic problem with insomnia have ruminative thoughts that play a role in maintaining nighttime hyperarousal (Buysse, 2004). Additionally, insomnia is also a diagnostic criterion for several psychiatric disorders, including depression, dysthymia, mania, and generalized anxiety disorder (McCall, 2004; APA, 2000). Lastly, substance use/abuse and discontinuance also impact an individual's ability to obtain restorative sleep.

General Medical Condition

Sleep disturbances, such as insomnia, daytime sleepiness, and sleep fragmentation, may also be due the direct physiologic effects of a general medical condition on the sleep-wake system (APA, 2000). For example, sleep fragmentation often occurs in clients experiencing chronic pain (Iber, 2004). Sleep abnormalities resulting from a medical illness do not always reflect the severity or intensity of the disease process (Iber, 2004). For example, the severity of the sleep disturbance in clients with chronic lung disease or a cardiac condition varies according to the nature of the specific disorder and severity of the impairment (Iber, 2004). Sleep pattern disturbances are also present when a client has a biochemical alteration resulting from a medical illness such as an endocrine disorder.

Sociocultural and Environmental Factors

Self-induced sleep deprivation is the cause of sleep problems in both adolescents and adults. The delayed onset of nocturnal sleep in adolescents, demanding work and school schedules, and social demands are a few of the many factors that pose a challenge in attaining and maintaining the necessary amount of restorative sleep.

EPIDEMIOLOGY

Because of the temporary nature of many sleep disturbances, and the lack of formal diagnoses, some sleep disorders go unreported. The true prevalence of sleep disorders, therefore, is difficult to determine, but epidemiologic surveys suggest that they are becoming more common than ever before. Approximately 47 million to 70 million people in the country do not get adequate sleep because of some type of sleep disturbance (NIH, 2006; Walsh, 2004). Half of these individuals report chronic sleep pattern disturbances (NIH, 2006). In a survey conducted by the National Sleep Foundation, 75% of respondents reported that they had experienced some type of sleep disturbance for a few nights a week, or more, over the preceding year (National Sleep Foundation, 2005). The data reflect a growing trend in sleep disturbances among adults in the United States.

Dyssomnias

Insomnia is one of the most common sleep disorders in the United States. Although some individuals experience brief periods of insomnia throughout their lifetime, it is estimated that 30 million adults have a persistent problem with insomnia, which can disrupt daily functioning (NIH, 2006). The prevalence of this disorder increases with age and is more common in women across all age-groups (Buysse, 2004). There is also a link between insomnia and psychiatric illness, most commonly depression, in 40% to 50% of the population (Roth, 2004).

Narcolepsy and *hypersomnias* are two types of primary sleep disturbances characterized by excessive daytime sleepiness (Mignot, 2005). Narcolepsy is the most studied of all hypersomnias and is more prevalent than once thought. Between 135,000 and 250,000 people have narcolepsy, although the average time between symptom onset and formal diagnosis is approximately 10 to 15 years (NIH, 2006; Quillen, 2005). Delay in a formal diagnosis is most likely due to this disorder being mistaken for other common causes of excessive daytime sleepiness, such as insomnia (Quillen, 2005). Narcolepsy is not common in children and is generally initially recognized during the adolescent years (Thiedke, 2001).

Breathing-related sleep disorders are a group of disorders characterized by excessive daytime sleepiness caused by a sleep-related breathing condition such as obstructive or central **sleep apnea** syndrome (the temporary cessation or absence of breathing) (APA, 2000). Epidemiologic data indicate that 18 million Americans have obstructive sleep apnea (OSA) (National Institutes of Health, 2006; Holman, 2005; Willard and Dreher, 2005). Men, ages 30 to 60, are twice as likely as premenopausal women to have this disorder. The estimated prevalence of this disorder is 4% of the adult male population and 2% of the adult female population (Willard and Dreher, 2005; Quan, 2004). Obstructive sleep apnea also occurs in children and affects 1% to 3% of children. When found in this population, OSA is usually due to adenotonsillar hypertrophy, craniofacial abnormalities, and allergic conditions, all of which result in airway obstruction during sleep (Thiedke, 2001).

Individuals with *circadian rhythm sleep disturbance* rarely seek medical treatment. Therefore, the true prevalence of this sleep disturbance is difficult to estimate. The delayed sleep phase subtype of the disorder impacts up to 4% of adults and up to 7% of adolescents (APA, 2000). The shift work and jet lag subtypes of the disorder often result in more severe symptoms for late-middle-aged and elderly people. Up to 60% of night shift workers have the shift work subtype of circadian rhythm sleep disorder (APA, 2000).

Parasomnias

Sleep terror disorder occurs in 1% to 6% of the childhood population and is more common in boys than in girls (Kaplan and Sadock, 2004). These sleep pattern disturbances typically occur in children ages 3 to 8, with the episodes usually taking place during NREM sleep cycles.

Nightmares happen at any age to any gender. The child with nightmares usually is able to recall the event (not typical in a child with sleep terrors) and is usually arousable during the nightmare event (Thiedke, 2001).

Sleepwalking disorder (somnambulism) typically occurs around the ages of 4 to 8 with the peak prevalence being at 12 years of age. This disorder, like sleep terror disorder, is more common in boys than in girls (Kaplan and Sadock, 2004). Both sleep terror disorder and sleepwalking disorder tend to run in families (Kaplan and Sadock, 2004).

CLINICAL DESCRIPTION

According to the DSM-IV-TR, sleep disorders are best classified according to their presumed cause or etiology (APA, 2000). The primary sleep disorders are caused by alterations in internal processes that influence sleep and wakefulness. Secondary sleep disturbances generally develop as a result of medical or mental conditions, or they occur from the use of substances (Neil, 2005).

Dyssomnias

Insomnia

The dyssomnia known as **insomnia** is characterized by a predominant complaint of difficulty initiating or maintaining sleep, or experiencing nonrestorative sleep, for at least 1 month. This sleep disturbance typically leads to excessive daytime sleepiness and causes significant impairment in daily functioning (APA, 2000). Transient periods of insomnia can occur throughout an individual's lifetime and may be attributed to anxiety-producing situations that are self-limiting for the affected individual. The anxiety can occur either in response to an anxiety-producing situation or in anticipation of an anxiety-provoking experience (Kaplan and Sadock, 2004). In this situation, once the anxiety decreases, the sleep pattern disturbance typically lessens or abates and no treatment would be indicated. On the other hand, persistent insomnia is characterized by the inability to initiate or maintain restorative sleep for at least 1 month. The sleep pattern disturbance often interferes with the individual's social or occupational functioning (see the Case Study).

Narcolepsy

Narcolepsy is the sudden onset of brief sleep attacks, lasting 10 to 20 minutes, that typically take place two to six times per day (Kaplan and Sadock, 2004). Thus, a person with narcolepsy will suddenly fall asleep while engaging in meaningful activities such as driving a car, eating, or interacting with people (Quillen, 2005). Symptom onset for narcolepsy typically manifests during puberty or adolescence (Kaplan and Sadock, 2004).

CASE STUDY Hazel is a 42-year-old woman who has insomnia. She gives a history of having frequent awakenings during the night, usually starting about 1½ hours after she goes to sleep. Hazel states she initially started having sleep problems when she was under an immense amount of stress from her job. She is no longer stressed by her job, but she continues to have problems maintaining a continuous pattern of sleep on a regular basis.

CRITICAL THINKING

1. What factors support a diagnosis of insomnia?
2. Formulate two nursing diagnoses that may be relevant to Hazel's plan of care.
3. What can the psychiatric nurse teach Hazel about her illness? What lifestyle changes can Hazel make that may improve her sleep quality and limit the progression of her problem?
4. What treatments are typically employed to treat this type of sleep disturbance?
5. How will the health care team members know if Hazel's condition is improving?

CLINICAL ALERT

Clients with **narcolepsy** experience excessive daytime sleepiness that results in multiple sleep attacks, typically taking place at inappropriate times during the client's normal period of wakefulness. Clients with this disorder also experience cataplexy (the sudden but temporary loss of bilateral muscle tone) and the presence of dreamlike hallucinations. The psychiatric nurse needs to teach the client to manage narcolepsy by discussing the triggers that provoke it (strong emotional stimuli, sleep deprivation) and the available treatment strategies that may help prevent it (forced daytime napping, adherence to medical treatment).

Approximately 70% of people with narcolepsy also experience **cataplexy**, a common sign of this disorder (APA, 2000). Cataplexy is the sudden loss of muscle tone and voluntary muscle movement. Strong emotional experiences such as laughing or crying cause this reaction (Quillen, 2005). Persons with narcolepsy also report **sleep paralysis**, where they are not able to speak or move just before the onset or upon awakening from the brief sleep attack. Additionally, some report hallucinations and experiencing vivid sensory perceptual experiences either upon awakening (hypnopompic hallucinations) or when entering the brief sleep episode (hypnagogic hallucinations) (APA, 2000; Kaplan and Sadock, 2004).

Breathing-Related Sleep Disorders

Breathing-related sleep disorders are a group of disorders resulting from a sleep-related breathing condition such as obstructive or central sleep apnea syndrome or central alveolar hypoventilation (APA, 2000).

Persons with obstructive sleep apnea typically have some degree of narrowing or complete obstruction of the upper airway (Quan, 2005), which results in loud snoring episodes and regular apneic periods during sleep that last

CASE STUDY John is a 35-year-old obese man who presents to an outpatient treatment facility with complaints of excessive daytime sleepiness. He states he sleeps an average of 9 hours per night but he never feels rested. His wife states that John has periods of loud snoring during his sleep and even periodically stops breathing for short periods throughout the night. After a thorough medical evaluation, he was diagnosed with sleep apnea. John also gives a history of regular alcohol use and has been in treatment for alcohol dependence in the past.

CRITICAL THINKING

1. What factors may have led the physician to believe John has obstructive sleep apnea?
2. Describe the diagnostic tests that are typically done to diagnose a person with obstructive sleep apnea.
3. Formulate two nursing diagnoses that may be relevant to John's plan of care.
4. What can the psychiatric nurse teach John about his illness? What lifestyle changes can John make that may improve his sleep quality and limit the progression of his illness?
5. What treatments are typically employed to treat obstructive sleep apnea?
6. How will the health care team members know if John's condition is improving?

CLINICAL ALERT

Obstructive sleep apnea is a type of breathing-related sleep disorder (BRSD) where the airflow through the oral or nasal passages stops during sleep. This type of BRSD results from obstruction of the airways and is common in overweight individuals and in people who use alcohol or other sedative/hypnotic drugs. The apneic periods usually last 10 seconds or more and account for many unexplained deaths and disabilities throughout the life span (Sadock and Sadock, 2004). The psychiatric nurse needs to immediately manage the apneic periods by assessing the frequency and duration of these episodes and administering oxygen or continuous positive airway pressure (CPAP) therapy according to the clinical condition of the client. The nurse also needs to teach the client about the precipitating factors that play a role in the onset of apneic episodes (being overweight, use of sedative drugs) and also teach the client about the treatment strategies that are available for long-term management.

10 to 30 seconds (American Academy of Sleep Medicine, 2004). Many affected individuals have a large neck circumference and are obese with a body mass index measurement of 30 or greater (Willard and Dreher, 2005). These individuals often wake up briefly during the night and experience excessive daytime sleepiness because of the periods of breathing cessation experienced during the night (see the Case Study).

Circadian Rhythm Sleep Disorder

Circadian rhythm sleep disorders are a group of sleep pattern disturbances with a persistent or recurrent pattern of sleep disruption that result from a difference in an imposed sleep-wake cycle and the individual's own circadian sleep-wake pattern requirements (Kaplan and Sadock, 2004). Circadian rhythm sleep disorders result from a delayed sleep phase, jet lag, shift work, or an unspecified source (APA, 2000; Kaplan and Sadock, 2004). Daytime sleepiness is common because of the delayed sleep onset and the mandatory early awakening related to employment or social obligations. Insomnia also occurs.

Jet lag type of the circadian rhythm sleep disorder has periods of sleepiness and alertness that occur at an inappropriate time of day relative to local time (APA, 2000). These patterns of sleep and wakefulness occur after repeated travel across more than one time zone.

Shift work type of the circadian sleep disorder is usually the result of night shift work or frequently rotating shift work (APA, 2000). It also takes place in individuals with irregular sleep schedules (Kaplan and Sadock, 2004). The individual with this type of sleep pattern disturbance typically experiences insomnia during the major sleep period or excessive sleepiness during the major awake period (APA, 2000). These symptoms are usually most pronounced right after the individual changes schedules, but, in some cases, the symptoms do not improve with the passage of time.

The *delayed sleep phase* of the circadian rhythm sleep pattern disturbance occurs when the individual has a persistent pattern of late sleep onset and late awakening times and is unable to fall asleep and wake up at the desired earlier times (APA, 2000). Once sleep can be maintained, however, it may be uninterrupted until the normal awakening period.

Parasomnias

In general, parasomnias are the presence of abnormal behavior or physiologic events that occur in association with sleep, specific sleep stages, or sleep-wake transitions (APA, 2000).

Nightmare Disorder

Nightmare disorder is one type of parasomnia that usually takes place during the REM period late in the sleep cycle. Individuals with this disorder frequently experience fragmented sleep as a result of waking up during the night with frightening dreams that threaten their survival, security, or self-esteem. Clients are usually able to recall the nightmares in vivid detail (APA, 2000).

Sleep Terror Disorder

An individual with sleep terror disorder experiences arousal during non-REM sleep. This individual will typically awaken during the early part of the night. The awakening is usually caused by manifestations of extreme anxiety or panic (Kaplan and Sadock, 2004). It is not unusual for the person to scream or cry and appear disoriented during a sleep terror episode. As with sleepwalking, the individual with sleep terror disorder is usually not able to recall the event.

CLINICAL ALERT

Episodes of complex motor activity that take place during slow wave sleep characterize **sleepwalking.** Some examples of sleepwalking activities include waking from sleep during the first third of the night and walking around inside the home or unlocking doors and going outside. This presents a safety risk because the individual also engages in dangerous activities such as operating machinery during the sleepwalking phase. The psychiatric nurse needs to teach the client and family members about the factors that increase the likelihood of a sleepwalking episode (e.g., distended bladder, environmental noise, psychosocial stressors, alcohol and sedative/hypnotic use) and develop a plan to minimize its occurrence. Patient safety is the number one priority in planning care for this client.

Sleepwalking Disorder

Sleepwalking disorder (somnambulism) is also considered a parasomnia (APA, 2000). Individuals with a sleepwalking disorder typically will repeatedly engage in such complex behaviors as walking, dressing, toileting and driving, all while they are in a deep non-REM stage of sleep (Kaplan and Sadock, 2004). While sleepwalking, the individual appears to be in a trance, and arousal is difficult. At times, the individual awakens while performing complex tasks, but most frequently he or she returns to sleep and later awakens without any recall of the events that took place during the sleepwalking episode (APA, 2000).

Parasomnia Not Otherwise Specified

Sleep disorder related to another mental disorder involves a prominent complaint of a sleep disturbance, such as insomnia or hypersomnia that results from a diagnosable mental disorder, such as a mood disorder or anxiety disorder (APA, 2000).

Sleep disorder that results from a general medical condition involves a prominent complaint of sleep disturbance that results from the direct physiologic effects of a general medical condition on the sleep-wake system (APA, 2000).

Substance-induced sleep disorder involves prominent complaints of sleep disturbance that result from the use, or recent discontinuation of use, of a substance (including medications). Specific substances include alcohol, amphetamines and related stimulants, caffeine, cocaine, opioids, sedatives, hypnotics, and anxiolytics, or other substances (APA, 2000).

PROGNOSIS

In general, the prognosis for the majority of sleep disorders is good provided the problem is diagnosed and accurately identified in a timely manner. The clinical courses for sleep pattern disturbances are variable, with some presenting as self-limiting occurrences and others resulting in recurring, persistent health challenges. For example, such disorders as insomnia and circadian rhythm sleep disorders have a high rate of recurrence and relapse, whereas narcolepsy and some types of breathing-related sleep disturbances are manageable with treatment. Of all types of sleep disturbances, researchers have studied insomnia and obstructive sleep apnea the most.

DISCHARGE CRITERIA

Most people with sleep pattern disturbances are not hospitalized for the sleep disorder unless the particular disorder is life threatening (i.e., breathing-related sleep disorder with extensive periods of apnea). In these instances, the criteria for discharge relate to the particular situation under consideration. For example, a client with a serious breathing-related sleep disorder develops a variety of problems (i.e., hypoxia, arterial hypertension, cardiac dysrhythmias) because of prolonged periods of apnea. Therefore, the client needs to have these problems resolved in order to be safely discharged to the community or home setting. Clients with a sleep disorders and a coexisting psychiatric or medical condition that are hospitalized need to meet the discharge criteria, which is standard for the co-occurring psychiatric or medical condition.

A large percentage of primary sleep disorders also go undiagnosed, generally because the affected individuals attribute their symptoms to factors other than the sleep pattern disturbance itself and do not seek treatment for the disorder until late into the disease process. In instances where a health care provider identifies a sleep problem during the course of the illness, the affected individual is usually treated in an out patient setting.

Client will:

- Demonstrate satisfactory understanding of his or her illness and the common strategies for appropriate management.
- Identify physical and psychosocial stressors that exacerbate the sleep disturbance.
- Identify signs and symptoms of the sleep pattern disturbance, focusing on the initial clinical manifestations that indicate the need for early intervention.
- Identify a social support network that will be instrumental in helping the client to achieve his or her previous or highest level of functioning.
- Verbalize adequate knowledge of the predisposing, precipitating, and perpetuating factors commonly associated with sleep pattern disturbances.
- Demonstrate sufficient understanding of the treatment plan, including prescribed medications (intended use, action, dose, side effects, contraindications, interactions with other substances).

The Nursing Process

ASSESSMENT

Assessment of the individual with a sleep pattern disturbance is a complex process because of the various symptom profiles that present. For example, an individual with primary insomnia minimizes his or her symptoms of daytime fatigue, excessive sleepiness, or mental sluggishness. It is important that the nurse obtain both subjective reporting data from the affected individual and his or her

BOX 18-2

Assessment of Sleep Patterns and Routines

- Number of hours of sleep per night
- Time of day/night that client goes to bed or falls asleep
- Any recent changes to established sleep patterns and routines (if changes are stated, determine what factors seem to affect sleep; assess for both inhibiting and enhancing factors)
- Regularity of sleep routine (regular or irregular)
- Night time awakenings (describe)
- Presence of daytime napping (describe)
- Use of sleep aids or substances that disrupt sleep (e.g., sleep medications, stimulants, antidepressants, alcohol)
- Present stressors and those from recent or remote past
- Objective reporting: from bed partner (e.g., snoring, apneic periods); from parents (e.g., sleepwalking, nightmares, sleep terrors)

bed partner as well as a comprehensive database from objective and quantifiable data sources. The data obtained from the sleep history will determine if the client has a significant problem with his or her sleep pattern and if referral to a sleep specialist is necessary.

The nurse obtains subjective data by using a sleep history questionnaire or by having the client keep a sleep diary (Box 18-2). The observations of the bed partner or parents are also beneficial in the data-gathering process. The nurse will use rating scales such as the Epworth Sleepiness Scale to gain objective data on the clients sleep habits (Neil, 2005). The nurse also obtains data by checking for physiologic indicators of sleep pattern disturbances while the individual sleeps. Nurses today are able to assess the quality of sleep cycles in a sleep laboratory by monitoring multiple physiologic processes while the client sleeps. This includes observing electroencephalographic (EEG) (brain wave) activity, electrooculographic (extra ocular eye movements) activity, electromyographic (EMG) activity (muscle movement), heart rate and rhythm, respiratory rate, and blood pressure, through the use of polysomnography testing (multiple sleep testing). Health care providers are able to do additional testing if they suspect the individual has a problem with a particular disorder. For example, if they suspect a client has a breathing-related sleep disorder, then they will measure such factors as oxyhemoglobin saturation (presence of oxygen in the blood), exhaled carbon dioxide ($CO2$) levels (changes in carbon dioxide levels that can adversely affect breathing), breathing effort (labored breathing indicates a problem), airflow measurements, and muscular efforts during breathing (Neylan et al., 1999).

NURSING DIAGNOSIS

Nurses formulate diagnoses based on the information from the client assessment. Once formulated, the diagnoses will direct the development of a comprehensive treatment plan that will be most effective in achieving the preestablished treatment goals for the client with sleep disorders. Nursing diagnoses are prioritized according to client needs, from most urgent to least urgent. The following nursing diagnoses are the most applicable for clients with sleep pattern disturbances (North American Nursing Diagnoses Association International [NANDA-I], 2007; Carpenito, 2002):

- Sleep deprivation
- Insomnia
- Ineffective breathing pattern
- Anxiety
- Fatigue
- Ineffective coping
- Ineffective role performance

OUTCOME IDENTIFICATION

Nurses develop realistic, client-centered treatment plan goals based on the appropriate outcomes. These outcomes are the anticipated behavioral responses to expect from a client with sleep pattern disturbances once he or she actively participates in the plan of care. Outcomes are prioritized according to client needs, from most urgent to least urgent. Following are several examples of client outcomes that address some of the expected behaviors of a client who demonstrates healthy and adaptive behavioral responses to sleep pattern disturbances. Client will:

- Identify the primary causes of the sleep pattern alterations.
- Communicate appropriate interventions for a particular sleep pattern disorder and implement them.
- Demonstrate a significant reduction of sleep pattern disturbances through self-reports and objective evaluation measures.
- Participate actively in discharge planning with members of the acute care and community-based practice health care team.

PLANNING

Collaborative planning requires active participation of the client with the multidisciplinary health care team members. Treatment considerations reflect evidenced-based health care practices and include the client. The treatment plan needs to be comprehensive and include relevant biologic, psychosocial, and cognitive treatment modalities. This approach will be most effective in helping restore sleep patterns in the affected client.

IMPLEMENTATION

Nurses develop an individualized plan of care for each client in order to achieve his or her anticipated behavioral outcomes. The plan needs to be comprehensive and appropriate to the level of care the client needs in the clinical setting. Most clients with sleep pattern disturbances present in the community practice setting unless the sleep disturbance is a co-occurring problem associated with a psychiatric condition or a medical disorder. In this latter instance, the client often presents in the acute care setting. In either case, nurses work directly with the client, the members of the multidisciplinary health care team, and the client's family and significant others in designing the plan of care.

Nursing Interventions

Nursing interventions are prioritized according to client needs, from most urgent to least urgent.

1. Monitor the client's sleep patterns and identify risks (breathing-related sleep disorder, sleepwalking, narcolepsy, daytime fatigue) *to prevent harm and injury to the client.*
2. Activate the client to keep a sleep diary *so that he or she will identify patterns that promote sleep pattern disturbance.*
3. Develop a sleep hygiene plan and educate the client about sleep hygiene practices *to promote rest and sleep in the sleep-deprived client.*
4. Teach the client about useful strategies for symptom management *to promote a sense of control over the problem.*
5. Help the client to structure and maintain a quiet, comfortable environment that is conducive to sleep *to promote sleep and rest during designated periods throughout the day/night.*
6. Help the client to identify specific stressors that affect his or her ability to obtain restorative sleep *to help the client avoid or reduce stressors and obtain restorative sleep.*
7. Promote the development of adaptive coping skills, such as relaxation techniques, through client and family education *to assist the client in managing the psychosocial stressors that negatively affect his or her ability to obtain restorative sleep.*
8. Identify the client's social support system *to foster use of this resource in the client's adaptation to perceived psychosocial stressors.*
9. Promote compliance with prescribed medication plans in the treatment of a co-occurring psychiatric illness or in the short-term treatment of a primary sleep disorder. The use of *medications is an effective intervention in the treatment of primary or secondary sleep pattern disturbances.*
10. Teach the client the importance of limiting the intake of substances that cause a substance-induced sleep disorder (such as alcohol, amphetamines and other stimulants, nicotine, caffeine). *Use of prescription medications such as opioids, sedatives, hypnotics, and anxiolytics also affect sleep quality, and the client should only use them when directed by the client's health care provider. Some substances negatively affect a client's ability to attain restorative sleep.*
11. Educate the client regarding the effect that (short term and long term) circadian rhythm disturbances have on restorative sleep patterns, and explore ways to establish regular sleep patterns when sleep routines are disrupted. *Knowledge will inform and empower the client to accept help and initiate learned strategies to restore regular sleep patterns.*
12. Refer the client to a sleep disorder specialist as needed *to determine if advanced practice interventions are necessary. Further testing, such as polysomnography, is sometimes necessary to arrive at a differential diagnosis for the client.*

Additional Treatment Modalities

Pharmacologic Modalities

Medications that treat primary sleep pattern disturbances are either sedative/hypnotic drugs or stimulants. The particular type of pharmacologic agent(s) prescribed to treat sleep problems is dependent on whether the goal of therapy is to induce sleep or to stimulate wakefulness. Additionally, the treatment plan sometimes includes other prescribed psychopharmacologic agents such as antidepressants and anxiolytics, especially if the sleep pattern disturbance occurs with another psychiatric illness. Clients also use over-the-counter medications in an attempt to manage symptoms of this illness. Many times, clients attempt to manage symptoms with over-the-counter medications before seeking treatment from the health care provider.

Dyssomnias

Insomnia. The benzodiazepine and nonbenzodiazepine hypnotics, along with other nonpharmacologic treatments, are used for a client with insomnia. In general, this treatment lasts no longer than 2 weeks, as tolerance and withdrawal syndromes result from long-term use (Kaplan and Sadock, 2004). This is especially true for the benzodiazepine drugs because of their high addictive potential. Benzodiazepine hypnotics, such as triazolam (Halcion), temazepam (Restoril) and flurazepam (Dalmane), have the greatest potential for psychologic and physiologic dependency and are not commonly the first-line treatment for this disorder. They also interfere with REM sleep.

Nonbenzodiazepine hypnotics, such as zolpidem (Ambien) and zaleplon (Sonata), have less abuse potential and have less of a problem with rebound insomnia and REM sleep when compared with the benzodiazepine drugs (Mauk, 2005). Eszopiclone (Lunesta) is a new nonbenzodiazepine hypnotic for insomnia (Laustsen, 2005). Lunesta has been effective in reducing sleep latency in patients with problems with insomnia and is also effective in helping the client to maintain sleep (Box 18-3).

Antidepressants are sometimes prescribed, especially for clients with coexisting problems with depression and insomnia. Most drugs in this category decrease REM sleep and are effective in treating depressed clients with marked insomnia (Wilson and Argyropoulos, 2005).

Many clients use over-the-counter medications that contain antihistamines, for symptom management. Such drugs as Sominex and Unisom contain diphenhydramine, an antihistamine that has both sedative and anticholinergic effects (dry mouth, blurred vision, constipation, nasal congestion, urinary retention).

Narcoplesy. Modafinil (Provigil) is the preferred treatment for excessive daytime sleepiness associated with narcolepsy (Quillen, 2005). Central nervous system (CNS) stimulants such as dextroamphetamine (Dexedrine, Dex-

MEDICATION KEY FACTS Sleep Disorders

Benzodiazepines (triazolam [Halcion], *temazepam* [Restoril], flurazepam [Dalmane]) and *nonbenzodiazepines* (zalepon [Sonata], *zolpidem* [Ambien], *eszopiclone* [Lunesta])

- Hypnotics for treatment of insomnia.
- Abrupt or too-rapid withdrawal of benzodiazepines may result in pronounced restlessness, irritability, insomnia, and seizures.
- Long-term administration in children associated with rickets because of altered vitamin D metabolism with benzodiazepines.
- Paradoxical central nervous system (CNS) excitation can occur with antihistamines with benzodiazepines.
- *Herbal considerations:* Kava kava, chamomile, and valerian may increase CNS depression.
- *Dietary considerations:* Caffeine may counteract sedation and increase insomnia with benzodiazepines. Grapefruit may alter absorption with benzodiazepines. High-fat, heavy meals may delay onset of sleep by approximately 2 hours with nonbenzodiazepines.

OTHER THERAPIES FOR INSOMNIA

Antidepressants (trazodone [Desyrel], *mirtazapine* [Remeron], *amitriptyline* [Elavil]), *antihistamines* (diphenhydramine [Benadryl]), *melatonin receptor agonists* (Ramelteon)

- In general, low rate of side effects and adverse events
- Amitriptyline not recommended for older adults because of anticholinergic effects.

OVER-THE-COUNTER (OTC) PRODUCTS

- OTC products, alternative treatments, and complementary therapies have not been systematically evaluated; efficacy data are lacking; and there are concerns about side effects.
- Herbal products (melatonin, valerian) are not regulated by the U.S. Food and Drug Administration (FDA), and preparations may vary. Avoid taking melatonin with antidepressants as melatonin is structurally related to serotonin. Valerian is possibly associated with hepatotoxicity.

STIMULANTS FOR HYPERSOMNIA

- Cerebral stimulants (psychostimulants) such as methylphenidate (Ritalin, Concerta) and dextroamphetamine (Adderall) are used for narcolepsy.
- Modafinil (Provigil) is indicated for narcolepsy and other sleep disorders. CNS stimulants may potentiate action of modafinil.

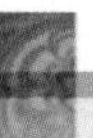

BOX 18-3

Eszopiclone (Lunesta)

- Categorized as a nonbenzodiazepine hypnotic drug (schedule IV controlled substance) indicated for the treatment of insomnia.
- Unknown how it works exactly, but researchers believe the effect on sleep induction and sleep maintenance is related to the drug's effect on GABA receptor complexes.
- Results of clinical trials of eszopiclone have indicated that it is effective in decreasing sleep latency (the amount of time an individual takes to fall asleep) and improving sleep maintenance (the amount of time an individual remains asleep once he or she enters the sleep cycle).
- Eszopiclone has central nervous system (CNS) depressant effects and therefore has synergistic effects when given with other CNS depressant drugs (psychotropics, anticonvulsants, antihistamines, and any other drugs/substances [e.g., alcohol] that may produce CNS depression).
- Caution clients who are taking eszopiclone about performing psychomotor tasks (driving a car, operating machinery) while on this medication.
- There are no known contraindications to the use of this drug at the present time. Side effects of this medication are similar to those associated with other hypnotics and are usually mild. These include drowsiness, dizziness, and lightheadedness. Adverse effects include unpleasant taste, dry mouth, dizziness, viral infections, infections, and a variety of abnormal thinking and behavioral changes.
- Recommended dose (for nonelderly clients) is 2 mg by mouth taken just before bedtime; 1 mg oral administration is recommended for elderly clients. If the client is having a problem maintaining sleep, the dose can be increased (3 mg for nonelderly clients and 2 mg for elderly clients) if necessary.
- Eszopiclone is categorized as a pregnancy category C drug. Data from long-term clinical trials in pregnant woman are not available.

Data from Sepracor Inc: Lunesta (eszopiclone) tablets (drug insert) 2005; retrieved Apr 24, 2006, from www.lunesta.com.PostedApprovedLabelingText.pdf.

trostat) and methylphenidate (Concerta, Ritalin) also manage the symptoms associated with narcolepsy. However, because of the potential for negative reactions of CNS stimulants, they are usually not the first choice for treatment (Quillen, 2005). Additionally, antidepressants such as the selective serotonin reuptake inhibitors (Prozac) and tricyclic drugs (Tofranil) are also effective in managing the cataplexy (Quillen, 2005; Kaplan and Sadock, 2004). Additionally, a sleep-wake schedule that includes regularly scheduled naps helps some clients with narcolepsy (Kaplan and Sadock, 2003).

Hypersomnia. The pharmacologic treatment of primary hypersomnia sometimes includes the use of central nervous system stimulant drugs such as amphetamines and modafinil (Provigil) (Kalpan and Sadock, 2004). Nonsedating antidepressants like bupropion (Wellbutrin) are also effective in symptom management in some clients with this disorder (Kaplan and Sadock, 2004).

Breathing-Related Sleep Disorders. Obstructive sleep apnea (OSA) syndrome is the most common type of breathing-related sleep disorder that often results in ineffective breathing patterns. Medications, such as selective serotonin reuptake inhibitors (SSRI) and tricyclic antidepressants, treat apnea, as they decrease the time the client spends in REM sleep, when apnea is most likely to take place. Health care providers usually discourage clients with this disorder from using sedating substances such as alcohol, as these types of sedatives often exacerbate the problem (Kaplan and Sadock, 2004). Sedating substances relax the airway, thus increasing the risk of longer apneic episodes through the night. See additional treatment modalities for OSA in the following sections.

Circadian Rhythm Sleep Disorders. The use of short-acting hypnotics that will induce sleep is also useful for the short-term treatment.

Parasomnias

Nightmare Disorder. Pharmacologic agents that suppress REM sleep, such as the tricyclic antidepressants and benzodiazepine hypnotic drugs, treat the symptoms associated with nightmare disorder (Kaplan and Sadock, 2004). This disorder is frequently self-limiting in children and is manageable with short-term psychotherapy and desensitization (First and Tasman, 2004).

Sleep Terror Disorder. In the rare instance that medication management is necessary, small doses of diazepam (Valium) administered at bedtime are effective in improving this condition (Kaplan and Sadock, 2004).

Sleepwalking Disorder. Drugs that suppress stages 3 and 4 sleep, such as benzodiazepine hypnotics, have been used in the management of this disorder (First and Tasman, 2004; Kaplan and Sadock, 2004). The primary concern is to provide for the client's safety while he or she is experiencing the sleepwalking episode. If possible, the affected individual needs to occupy the bedroom on the ground floor of the house to prevent falls. Locking windows and exterior doors and removing dangerous objects from the environment are also beneficial. (See Chapter 24 for more information on medication.)

Psychotherapeutic Modalities

In addition to pharmacologic treatment modalities, the psychiatric nurse also participates in the planning of interventions that focuses on the psychotherapeutic aspect of sleep disorder treatment. These modalities include client education on behavioral modification and cognitive reframing. For example, client education begins with an emphasis of sound sleep hygiene practices (Box 18-4) to promote the best possible conditions for restorative sleep. In instances where a sleep problem such as insomnia is of a chronic nature, the client is often conditioned to expect that he or she will have sleep problems, no matter what. In this situation, the use of techniques to decondition or unlearn previous behaviors with cognitive behavioral therapy will be effective (Jacobs et al, 2004; Kaplan and Sadock, 2004) (see the Research for Evidence-Based Practice box; see Chapter 23). Additionally, clients with chronic insomnia are sometimes discouraged because prior treatments are ineffective in symptom management. Hence, the nurse needs to provide the client with psychosocial support as the client participates in ongoing behavioral changes. It helps clients with transient problems with insomnia that results from stressful life events to know that

BOX 18-4

Sleep Hygiene Practices

- Go to sleep and awaken at the same time each day in order to promote a consistent sleep-wakefulness pattern. Try to avoid daytime napping.
- Reduce or eliminate the use of stimulants (caffeine, nicotine) and other substances (alcohol) that interfere with sleep.
- Avoid physical exercise or mental stimulation just before bedtime.
- Practice effective coping strategies to manage stress (e.g., progressive relaxation, deep breathing, listening to relaxing music).
- Create an environment that is conducive to restorative sleep (i.e., comfortable temperature, quiet environment, comfortable clothing, low-level lighting).
- Develop a bedtime routine that will be conducive to promoting sleep (e.g., taking a warm bath, reading a book, practicing meditation).

RESEARCH for EVIDENCE-BASED PRACTICE

Jacobs G et al: Cognitive behavior therapy and pharmacotherapy for insomnia: a randomized controlled trial and direct comparison, *Archives of Internal Medicine* 164:1888-1896, 2004.

The objective of this randomized, controlled clinical trial was to evaluate the effectiveness of cognitive behavioral therapy (CBT) and pharmacologic therapies in the management of chronic insomnia in young and middle-aged adults. Researchers assigned 63 study participants randomly to one of four treatment options; CBT (n = 15), pharmacotherapy (n =15), combination therapy (n =18) and placebo (n =15). Researchers used treatment outcome measures such as sleep diary entries, Nightcap sleep monitor recordings of sleep onset latency, sleep efficiency and total sleep time, and scores on the Beck Depression Inventory and Profile of Mood States scale to analyze the effectiveness of these various treatments in managing chronic insomnia. This study found cognitive behavioral therapy (CBT) was a more effective treatment for chronic insomnia than pharmacologic treatment with zolpidem (Ambien), when used alone or in combination with CBT, on most sleep outcome measures. Although the application of the research findings of this study is somewhat limited because of the small sample size, this study does provide important information for clinical consideration. Additional research examining the effectiveness of cognitive behavioral therapy in the treatment of insomnia is necessary. However, preliminary research findings do suggest that CBT is an effective treatment for some populations who suffer from chronic insomnia.

the sleep pattern disturbance will usually improve once the underlying cause is minimized or eliminated.

Additional treatment modalities for obstructive sleep apnea often include the use of continuous positive airway pressure (CPAP). This treatment requires the client to wear a mask during sleep. Positive pressure is applied to the airways, minimizing airway obstruction and improving ventilation. In some cases, clients use oral appliances to assist in clearing the airway passage. Overweight clients are also encouraged to lose weight. Lastly, some clients have a surgical intervention known as uvulopalatopharyngoplasty to minimize airway obstruction by removing the tonsils and excess tissue of the soft palate (Willard and Dreher, 2005).

The primary aim in managing a circadian rhythm sleep disorder is to establish some degree of regularity in the sleep-wake cycle by synchronizing sleep-wake patterns with typical daily schedules. The client benefits by identifying external environmental cues that he or she can link to a certain phase of the sleep-wake pattern. Trying to manipulate the sleep schedule by encouraging the client to sleep earlier than his or her previously established "late night" patterns usually helps with some circadian rhythm sleep disorders (delayed sleep phase type, jet lag type). By progressively delaying the bedtime and awakening times over a few weeks' duration, the client eventually attains a regular sleep-wake schedule that is more compatible with his or her lifestyle. Then the nurse assists the client in gradually adjusting the timing of the sleep-wake cycle by administering light therapy or encouraging the client to spend a certain amount of time out in the sunlight. Exposure to light is effective for advancing the delayed sleep phase and thus progressively shifting the sleep-wake cycle (First and Tasman, 2004). Synchrony of sleep-wake patterns to light and dark schedules is often beneficial for these types of sleep disorders. Sleep pattern disturbances that are caused by rotating shift work or night shift work are more challenging to manage. Anything the client is able to do, however, to establish some regularity in the sleep-wake pattern will be beneficial to the overall quality of sleep. Additionally, a client's adherence to sound sleep hygiene practices are very important. Treatment planning that requires the participation of a sleep care specialist is sometimes necessary, especially in instances when the client presents with many complex problems.

NURSING CARE PLAN

Ted, a 57-year-old moderately obese man with mild to moderate anxiety, had been experiencing excessive episodes of loud snoring, gasping, labored mouth breathing, and abnormal chest and abdominal movements during sleep, accompanied by periods of breathing cessation (sleep apnea). His symptoms continued for approximately 3 months' duration, interrupting Ted's and his wife's normal sleep patterns and leaving them both exhausted during the day. Ted insisted that his symptoms would all disappear when he lost some weight and exercised more, but his hectic work schedule and busy life prevented him from focusing on diet and exercise. When Ted refused to seek help, his wife, Karen, moved to another room to sleep, which created marital problems. Ted also suffered from daytime drowsiness and sleepiness as a result of his constant interrupted sleep patterns. His normal REM cycle was also interrupted, which compromised his biologic need for a sound, deep dream sleep. Additionally, Ted's condition seemed to exacerbate his usual mild anxiety, and he became more irritable, often without reason. When Ted became sleepy while driving his car, he and Karen realized that Ted's condition had placed them both in danger. One evening, after a close call while driving home from work, Karen finally convinced Ted to consult a physician, who referred Ted to a sleep apnea clinic for evaluation. Tests indicated that Ted was experiencing a breathing-related sleep disorder (obstructive sleep apnea), and continuous positive airway pressure (CPAP) was prescribed. After other physical causes were ruled out, Ted was instructed to engage in weight reduction and exercise/activity programs commensurate with his age and condition.

DSM-IV-TR DIAGNOSES

Axis I	Breathing-related sleep disorder (obstructive sleep apnea) Anxiety traits noted
Axis II	Deferred
Axis III	Moderate obesity
Axis IV	Moderate: 4 to 5 (anxiety/irritability, resistive to treatment, slight marital discord)
Axis V	GAF-71 (current); GAF-81 (past year)

Nursing Diagnosis *Ineffective breathing pattern related to inadequate ventilation, obesity, obstructive sleep apnea (OSA), and mild to moderate anxiety, as evidenced by loud, persistent snoring/gasping and labored mouth breathing during sleep resulting in periods of wakefulness for both Ted and Karen; unusual chest and abdominal movements; breathing cessation episodes that continue throughout the night; interrupted REM cycle (deep, dream sleep); daytime sleepiness, fatigue, and exhaustion; increased anxiety symptoms (restless, agitated) and irritability (angers easily)*

NOC Respiratory Status: Ventilation, Anxiety Level

NIC Airway Management, Ventilation Assistance, Anxiety Reduction, Nutrition Management, Exercise Promotion, Emotional Support

Continued

NURSING CARE PLAN—cont'd

CLIENT OUTCOMES	NURSING INTERVENTIONS	EVALUATION
Ted will demonstrate a regular, nonlabored breathing pattern during regular sleep hours, with normal chest movements on inspiration and expiration, and an absence of snoring, gasping, mouth breathing, or sleep apnea.	Support Ted in using the prescribed breathing treatment of CPAP every night during normal sleep hours. *CPAP is a time-tested breathing method specifically designed to regulate efficient ventilation and respiratory function and eliminate mouth breathing, snoring, gasping, and sleep apnea, resulting in a regular, nonlabored breathing pattern and REM sleep during normal sleep hours.*	Ted's breathing is regular with normal chest movements on inspiration and expiration. Snoring, gasping, and mouth breathing are reduced or absent. No sleep apnea has been noted.
Ted and Karen will both learn about the CPAP breathing equipment (how to apply the mask, plug in the unit, turn on the machine, and clean and care for the unit components).	Instruct Ted and Karen about the application of the CPAP unit, such as applying the mask properly and snuggly over the nose, plugging in the apparatus to a regular electrical wall outlet, and cleaning and caring for the unit. *Use of new equipment, especially one that involves breathing and respiratory function and use of a mask, is often scary and confusing for the first time. The nurse's teaching skills and professional approach will often calm client/family fears, anxieties, and confusion and result in greater compliance to treatment.*	Ted and Karen demonstrate effective application and care of the CPAP breathing equipment.
Ted will begin a weight reduction program with the help of nursing and nutritional services and will resume a weight recommended for his age and physical condition.	Activate Ted to engage in a safe, time-tested weight management program commensurate with his age, height, and physical condition. *Excess weight contributes to some forms of breathing-related sleep disorders and exacerbates snoring, gasping, mouth breathing, sleep apnea, and ineffective ventilation. Appropriate weight will help to eliminate or reduce symptoms and promote a healthier lifestyle.*	Ted has enrolled in a weight reduction program with professional recommendations.
Ted will begin an exercise/activity program with the recommendation of an exercise physiologist commensurate with his age, physical condition, lifestyle, and capabilities.	Engage Ted, with Karen's support, in the prescribed exercise/activity program that compliments his lifestyle. *Exercise and activity often expedite weight loss when accompanied by a nutritional/weight management program, which will reduce Ted's breathing-related sleep disorder symptoms in a timelier manner.*	Ted regularly participates in an exercise/activity and weight management program with Karen's support.
Ted and Karen will continue to comply with the treatment and enjoy uninterrupted sleep throughout each night with cessation of Ted's previous breathing-related sleep disorder symptoms and an absence of fatigue, exhaustion, or sleepiness during the day.	Praise and support Ted and Karen in Ted's continued use of the CPAP unit at night and adherence to his new nutritional/weight management program and activity/exercise regimen. *Praise and support of the client's treatment plan help the client and family connect the success of the client's treatment with the need for continued compliance and offers hope and confidence in the treatment as well.*	Ted continues to use the CPAP unit each night and to comply with the activity/exercise and weight management programs with Karen's support. Ted reports less fatigue, exhaustion, and daytime sleepiness.
Ted and Karen will contact appropriate professional and technical support persons for any questions or concerns about CPAP procedure or apparatus.	Construct a list of support contact persons for Ted and Karen. *Access to professional support persons to address questions/concerns or to help restore/replace faulty CPAP equipment will increase the client's confidence and allay fears and anxieties about the treatment.*	Ted and Karen contact CPAP professionals as appropriate and are aware that their insurance will pay for a new CPAP mask every 6 months.

Nursing Diagnosis *Anxiety related to breathing-related sleep disorder symptoms (inadequate ventilation, loud snores, gasps, labored mouth breathing, periods of breathing cessation [sleep apnea]) during normal sleep hours; fatigue, exhaustion, and sleepiness during daytime hours; wife forced to sleep in another room, as evidenced by agitation (angers easily); restlessness (unable to relax during the day or during periods of nighttime wakefulness); rapid heart rate during anxious periods; upset about wife's decision to sleep in another room*

NOC Anxiety Self-Control, Symptom Control, Vital Signs, Stress Level, Acceptance: Health Status, Coping

NIC Anxiety Reduction, Vital Signs Monitoring, Anger Control Assistance, Exercise Promotion: Stretching, Teaching: Procedure/Treatment

CLIENT OUTCOMES	NURSING INTERVENTIONS	EVALUATION
Client will demonstrate a reduction in anxiety to a tolerable level (decreased episodes of anger/agitation/restlessness) and normal heart rate after using CPAP for a period of 1 week to manage symptoms associated with his breathing-related sleep disorder.	Activate Ted, with Karen's help, to use prescribed CPAP treatment every night for as long as necessary. *Client's use of continuous positive airway pressure will reduce many of the physical symptoms known to exacerbate anxiety, such as ventilation problems, rapid heart rate, interrupted night time sleep, gasping for air, being aroused by a spouse, and sleep apnea. Additionally, improving client symptoms will encourage his wife to return to their shared bed and resume normal marital patterns.*	Ted demonstrates reduced anxiety, anger, agitation, and restlessness since using the CPAP unit. Heart rate is within normal limits.
Client will demonstrate a reduction in both physical and psychosocial symptoms of anxiety with decreased anger, agitation, and restlessness.	Teach the client some strategies to reduce symptoms of anxiety: simple breathing and relaxation techniques (deep breathing and tensing and relaxing the muscles), activities and exercises (simple stretching), cognitive-behavioral techniques (reframing converts words like *anxious* to less threatening terms such as *eager* or *curious*) (see Chapter 23). *Time-tested anxiety-reducing strategies decrease anxiety provoked by a variety of biologic and psychosocial stressors, most of which are usually unknown by the client. In this situation, the client's physical symptoms seemed to exacerbate his anxious nature and required both biologic and psychosocial interventions.*	Ted is using learned anxiety-reducing strategies on a regular basis and relates a significant reduction in physical and psychosocial symptoms of anxiety and a decrease in anger, agitation, and restlessness.
Client and spouse will seek counseling as necessary to ensure adherence to prescribed treatment for breathing-related sleep disorder symptoms and continued use of anxiety-reducing strategies.	Educate client and spouse about the importance of adhering to CPAP treatment and the continued use of anxiety-reducing strategies, as well as the benefits of counseling to assist in those areas when needed. *Counseling is often useful in the complex nature of a breathing-related sleep disorder and will help both client and spouse to manage the physical and psychologic components of the condition over time.*	Ted and Karen demonstrate adequate knowledge and understanding about Ted's need for continued CPAP treatments and anxiety-reducing strategies. Ted states, "CPAP treatments have really helped my breathing and snoring problems; Karen and I sleep so much better every night. The counseling sessions have helped us both to calm down by reducing my anxiety."

EVALUATION

Ongoing evaluation is crucial in determining whether the client is progressing toward the desired outcomes or if the nurse needs to revise the treatment plan. The psychiatric nurse and members of the health care team, including the client when appropriate, need to participate in both a formal and informal evaluation process to determine the client's progression along the health care continuum, such as whether desired outcomes are occurring in a timely manner and when modification of the plan is necessary at any point along the nursing process.

CHAPTER SUMMARY

- Sleep pattern disturbances continue to present health challenges to clients across the life span.
- The causes associated with sleep pattern disturbances are many, including familial, biochemical, psychiatric, sociocultural, and environmental considerations.
- The DSM-IV-TR categorizes sleep pattern disturbances according to their presumed etiology (dyssomnias and parasomnias).
- Detection and accurate diagnoses of sleep problems are crucial to the effective management of the disorders. Diagnostic tools include a sleep questionnaire/journal/diary, sleep rating scales, and polysomnography testing.
- Common treatment plans for sleep disturbances include psychopharmacology, cognitive behavioral therapy, contextual deconditioning, relaxation training, stimulus control, sleep restriction, surgery, and medical management of underlying medical causes.
- Client and family education is critical to the successful management of sleep disturbances. Education often includes topics on sleep hygiene, symptom identification and management, and treatment effectiveness.

REVIEW QUESTIONS

1 At a community health fair, an adult says to the nurse, "I think I need medication to help me sleep. I've seen a lot of commercials on television about sleep drugs." Select the nurse's initial response.

1. "Drugs help some people with sleep problems. Tell me more about how you get ready for bed and your sleep pattern."

2. "You should make an appointment with a psychiatrist. Sleep disturbances are often a sign of mental illness."
3. "The medications for insomnia are addictive. Are you sure you want to begin using them?"
4. "There are many over-the-counter medications that can help you sleep better. Talk to your pharmacist."

2 A client has a new prescription for eszopiclone (Lunesta). Which instruction(s) would the nurse give about taking this medication? You may select more than one answer.
1. "Take your medication after your evening meal."
2. "Take your medication just before you get ready for bed."
3. "There are some dangerous side effects with this drug."
4. "This drug will help you fall asleep faster and stay asleep."
5. "This drug works better if you take it with a glass of wine."

3 An adult with major depression complains of severe sleep disturbances, daytime drowsiness, and fatigability. How would the nurse classify this sleep problem?
1. Primary sleep disorder
2. Secondary sleep disorder
3. Dyssomnia
4. Parasomnia

4 Which individual(s) would be most likely to have obstructive sleep apnea? You may select more than one answer.
1. A 9-year-old child with chronic tonsillitis
2. An 18-year-old female with an eating disorder
3. A 26-year-old female with inflammatory bowel disease
4. A 35-year-old female with a fractured femur
5. A 45-year-old obese male

5 A nurse sees amitriptyline (Elavil) 25 mg at bedtime on the medication administration record of a client with multiple sclerosis. The nurse's drug handbook indicates 25 mg is a low dose for this antidepressant drug. What is the nurse's correct analysis of this situation?
1. An error on the medication administration record is likely. Recheck the physician's order.
2. A low dose of amitriptyline (Elavil) has been prescribed to improve the client's sleep.
3. A lower dose is needed because of the neurologic changes associated with multiple sclerosis.
4. Antidepressant medications are more effective when given in the evening.

*Additional self-study exercises and learning resources are available to you on the **Companion CD** at the back of the book and on the **Evolve website** at **http://evolve.elsevier.com/Fortinash/**.*

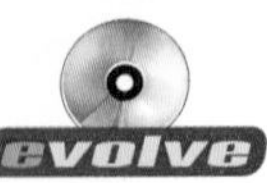

ONLINE RESOURCE

National Sleep Foundation: **www.sleepfoundation.org**

REFERENCES

Adler's dream theory; retrieved Mar 15, 2006, from http://dreamresearch.ca/enc/adler.pdf.

American Academy of Sleep Medicine: Sleep apnea believed to have contributed to the death of NFL legend Reggie White, Dec 29, 2004.

American College of Physicians: Current clinical issues: is sleep the new vital sign? *Ann Internal Med* 142:877-880, 2005.

American Psychiatric Association: *Diagnostic and statistical manual of mental disorders*, ed 4, text revision, Washington, DC, 2000, American Psychiatric Association.

Ancoli-Israel S et al: A pedigree of one family with delayed sleep phase syndrome, *Chronobiol Int* 18:831-840, 2001.

Ayas N et al: A prospective study of sleep deprivation and coronary heart disease in women, *Arch Intern Med* 163:205-209, 2003.

Bastien CH, Morin C: Familial incidence of insomnia, *J Sleep Res* 9, 49-54, 2000.

Bryant PA, Trinder J, Curtis S: Sick and tired: Does sleep have a vital role in the immune system? *Nat Rev Immunol* 4:457-467, 2004.

Buysse D: Insomnia: What is it; what needs translation. *Frontiers of knowledge in sleep disorders: opportunities for improving health and quality of life.* National Institutes of Health, 8/3/2004.

Carpenito LJ: *Nursing diagnosis: application to clinical practice*, Philadelphia, 2002, Lippincott.

First M, Tasman A: *DSM-IV-TR mental disorders: diagnosis, etiology, and treatment*, New Jersey, 2004, John Wiley & Sons.

Freud's dream theory; retrieved Mar 15, 2006, from http://dreamresearch.ca/enc/freud.pdf.

Guyton A, Hall J: *Textbook of medical physiology*, ed 11, Philadelphia, 2006, Saunders.

Holman M: Obstructive sleep apnea syndrome: implications for primary care, *Nurse Pract* 30:38-43, 2005.

Iber C: Normal and abnormal sleep: populations at risk: chronic medical disorders. *Frontiers of knowledge in sleep disorders: opportunities for improving health and quality of life.* National Institutes of Health, 8/3/2004.

Jacobs G, et al: Cognitive behavior therapy and pharmacotherapy for insomnia: a randomized controlled trial and direct comparison, *Arch Intern Med* 164:1888-1896, 2004.

Jung's dream theory; retrieved Mar 15, 2006, from http://dreamresearch.ca/enc/jung.pdf.

Kaplan HI, Sadock BJ: *Synopsis of psychiatry: behavioral sciences, clinical psychiatry*, ed 9, Baltimore, 2002, Lippincott, Williams & Wilkins.

Klosch G, Ulrich K: Sweet dreams are made of this, *Sci Am Mind* 18:39-45, 2005.

Laustsen G: Eszopiclone (Lunesta) for treatment of insomnia, *Nurse Pract* 30:67-68, 2005.

Mauk K: Healthier aging: Promoting sound sleep habits in older adults, *Nursing 2005* 35:22-25, 2005.

McCall W: Normal and abnormal sleep: populations at risk: psychiatric disorders. *Frontiers of knowledge in sleep disorders: opportunities for improving health and quality of life.* National Institutes of Health, 8/3/2004.

Mignot E: Narcolepsy/hypersomnia. Frontiers of knowledge in sleep disorders: opportunities for improving health and quality of life. National Institutes of Health, 8/3/2004.

National Institutes of Health (Department of Health and Human Services): Research on sleep and sleep disorders (reissue of PA-95_014), Bethesda, Md: Mar 2, 2006.

National Sleep Foundation: *2005 sleep in America poll*, Washington, DC, Mar 29, 2005.

Neil S: GP clinical viewpoint: primary sleep disorders, *General Practitioner*, pp 88-90, Oct 7, 2005.

Neylan TC, Reynolds CF, Kupfer DF: In RE Hales, SC Yudofsky, JT Talbott, editors: *American psychiatric press textbook*, ed 3, pp 955-982, Washington, DC, 1999, American Psychiatric Press.

North American Nursing Diagnoses Association International: *NANDA nursing diagnoses: definitions and classification 2007-2008*, Philadelphia, 2007, NANDA-I.

Quan S: Sleep disordered breathing. *Frontiers of knowledge in sleep disorders: opportunities for improving health and quality of life.* National Institutes of Health, 8/3/2004.

Quillen T: Sounding the alarm for narcolepsy, *Nursing 2005* 35: 74-75, 2005.

Roth T: Prevalence of sleepiness and sleep disorders. *Frontiers of knowledge in sleep disorders: opportunities for improving health and quality of life.* National Institutes of Health, 8/3/2004.

Sadock BJ, Sadock VA: *Concise textbook of clinical psychiatry*, ed 2, Philadelphia, 2004, Lippincott Williams & Wilkins.

Saladin K: Anatomy and physiology, ed 3, New York, 2004, McGraw-Hill.

Spiegel K et al: Brief communication: sleep curtailment in healthy young men is associated with decreased leptin levels, elevated ghrelin levels, and increased hunger and appetite, *Ann Intern Med* 141:846-850, 2004.

Thiedke C: Sleep disorders and sleep problems in childhood, *Am Fam Physician* 63:277-284 2001.

Von Dongen HP et al: The cumulative cost of additional wakefulness: dose-response effects on neurobehavioral functions and sleep physiology from chronic sleep restriction and total sleep deprivation, *Sleep* 26:117-126, 2003.

Walsh JK: *Testimony by James K. Walsh, Ph.D. Chairman, on behalf of the National Sleep Foundation: fiscal year finding for the Department of Health and Human Services, House Labor, Health and Human Services, Education and Related Agencies Appropriations Subcommittee*, Mar 30, 2004; retrieved Dec 17, 2005, from www.sleepfoundation.org/whatsnew/walsh_testimony.cfm.

Willard R, Dreher HM: Wake up call for sleep apnea, *Nursing 2005* 35:46-49, 2005.

Wilson S, Argyropoulos S: Antidepressants and sleep: a qualitative review of the literature, *Drugs* 65:927-947, 2005.

Chapter 19

Sexual Disorders

KATHRYN THOMAS AND SHELLY F. LURIE-AKMAN

The species that have evolved long-term bonds are also, by and large, the ones that rely on elaborate courtship rituals . . . Love and sex do indeed go together.

EDWARD O. WILSON

OBJECTIVES

1 Explore theories on the causation and incidence of sexual dysfunctions.
2 Identify categories of sexual dysfunction according to the DSM-IV-TR and NANDA.
3 Discuss effective interviewing and assessment techniques for clients with sexual disorders.
4 Demonstrate awareness of the primary treatment approaches used for sexual dysfunction, from medical, psychologic, and relational perspectives.
5 Apply the nursing process in caring for clients with sexual dysfunctions.
6 Describe the different diagnoses of the sex offender (paraphilic) population.
7 Discuss the focus of treatment for paraphilic disorders.
8 Explain at least two types of treatment and effects on illness symptomatology.
9 Analyze the relationship between treatment and recidivism.
10 Apply the nursing process in caring for clients with sexual (paraphilic) disorders.

KEY TERMS

ego dystonic pedophile, p. 439
ego syntonic pedophile, p. 439
EROS-CTD system, p. 433
exogenous testosterone, p. 432
intracorporeal injections, p. 433
Kegel exercises, p. 434
nocturnal penile tumescence, p. 432
paraphilias, p. 437
penile-brachial index, p. 433
pheromones, p. 433
plethysmography, p. 432
PT-141, p. 433
sensate focus, p. 434
sexual recidivisim, p. 438
sexual response cycle, p. 427
triggers, p. 440
vaginal dilator, p. 434
victimizer, p. 438
viropause, p. 432

This chapter explores two categories of sexual disorders: sexual dysfunctions and paraphilias.

SEXUAL DYSFUNCTIONS

The term *sexual dysfunction* has long described a range of troubling and dissatisfying complaints individuals have about their sexuality. Sexual dysfunctions include such issues as the lack of desire or interest in sex, the inability to get aroused or to be orgasmic, experiencing orgasm so quickly that it leaves the partner dissatisfied, having pain rather than pleasure with sex, and extreme vaginal constriction that does not allow for penetration. The reported incidence of sexual dysfunction is extensive. In a major national survey of men and women between the ages of 18 and 59, 31% and 43%, respectively, reported they had some problem with their sexual functioning (Laumann et al., 1999). The good news is that since the 1990s there has been enormous research interest in this area. New treatments are now available and even more proposed. There is much more help available for individuals and couples than there ever was before.

HISTORIC AND THEORETIC PERSPECTIVES

Historically, in the United States we have encouraged the belief that healthy and normal sex is heterosexual, married, monogamous, procreative, and noncommercial. Social norms regarding sexual behaviors were closely linked to medical and religious views. At the turn of the last century, many viewed sex as something to be restrained and controlled, especially for females. Women who enjoyed sex were pathologic, yet their problems with "hysteria" were treated with orgasmic release facilitated by medical doctors using a variety of devices. The Reverend Sylvester Graham (of Graham Cracker fame) and Dr. John Harvey Kellogg (of Kellogg's Corn Flakes) preached that male ejaculation reduced precious, health-preserving vital fluids and encouraged men to abstain from masturbation and any unnecessary sexual behavior (Abbott, 2000). They claimed that their food products facilitated this restraint. Despite these influences, Alfred Kinsey, American biologist (1894-1956), and colleagues found that Americans were being sexual, enjoying sex, and curious about it in record numbers (1948, 1953).

Much of our current perspective on sexual dysfunctions comes from Austrian psychologist, Sigmund Freud (1856-1939). According to Freud, childhood experiences had a subconscious influence on sexual behavior in adulthood. Infantile feelings such as the fear of castration and penis envy along with actual experiences combined to create sexual dysfunctions. He believed that sexuality was the cause of many of the difficulties people faced (Freud, 1977). As a result of Freud's theories, many used psychoanalysis, or the uncovering of old fears and traumas, in the treatment of sexual dysfunctions for more than 50 years.

In 1966, William Masters, a physician, and Virginia Johnson published their classic book, *Human Sexual Response*. Before its publication, they observed more than 10,000 male and female volunteers engaged in masturbatory and partnered sexual activity (Masters and Johnson, 1966). As a result of this research, they were able to describe exactly what happens to the body during erotic stimulation, from excitement to plateau to orgasm and, finally, to resolution. In 1970, they published a second text, *Human Sexual Inadequacy*, in which they discussed their work in helping others overcome sexual dysfunction. In this book, Masters and Johnson outlined the probable causes for dysfunction and gave detailed prescriptions for treatment. They shifted the emphasis of treatment to the behavioral area by recommending a series of specifically directed exercises, done in a 13-day intensive format and guided by a dual therapy team. In the course of this work, they developed many specific techniques, including sensate focus and the squeeze technique (Masters and Johnson, 1970).

Since the late 1960s, researchers have learned much about sexual dysfunctions and about sexuality in general. Structured treatment programs such as Masters and Johnson's did not always solve every problem. Sexuality is too complex to be reduced to a sex manual solution. Helen Singer Kaplan (1974) identified the need for behavioral techniques along with psychoanalysis in treatment. Kaplan is also responsible for the development of a model for the **sexual response cycle**, or the stages of desire, arousal, and orgasm. This model is the basis for the DSM-IV-TR designations for sexual dysfunction. These pioneer theorists and researchers are only some of many who have contributed to our knowledge of human sexuality.

In the mid-1990s, there was a great deal of research interest in male sexual function that led to the development of PDE5s (Viagra). By 1999, more were becoming interested in the field of female sexuality. Rosemary Basson proposed a new theory of the sexual response cycle most applicable to females (Basson, 2001). She suggested an intimacy-based sexual model whereby spontaneous sexual desire is not the only antecedent to sexual interaction, allowing that couples often have sex for nonsexual reasons. The model suggests that intimacy needs lead to sexual stimuli, which in turn lead to sexual arousal, desire, and finally enhanced intimacy. Sexual desire is not only spontaneous, but it can be produced by intimacy. Sex therapy today involves combinations of pharmacologic, physical, behavioral, educational, communication-enhancing, and psychodynamic techniques.

ETIOLOGY

Etiologies for sexual dysfunction cover a wide range of possibilities. Categories include physical/biologic, psychologic/emotional, cultural, and relationally oriented. Several factors often contribute to one person or one couple's inability to have satisfying sex (Box 19-1).

Physical/Biologic Factors

Interest in brain, neurochemical, and hormonal research and its relationship to sexual functioning is growing. For example, researchers know that testosterone stimulates sexual desire in males and females (Rogers, 2001). An understanding of the role of the two divisions of the central nervous system has helped our awareness of why stress reduces sexual arousal and interest. Vascular, neurologic, and endocrine disorders, as well as a range of problems such as cancer, connective tissue and pain disorders, depression, incontinence, and sexually transmitted diseases, all contribute to the development of sexual dysfunctions (Hillman, 2000). Substance abuse is epidemic in our society and seriously affects the ability to function sexually. Medications, especially antidepressants, antihypertensives, and hormonal treatments, also affect sexual satisfaction.

Psychologic/Emotional Factors

For a long time, many thought early childhood experiences influenced sexual development and sexual functioning. Indeed, many still believe that psychologic issues are more important in the etiology of sexual dysfunctions than any other factor (see the Research for Evidence-Based Practice

BOX 19-1

Etiologic Factors for Sexual Dysfunctions

PHYSICAL/BIOLOGIC FACTORS

Vascular
Cardiac disease
Diseases of the blood vessels

Neurologic
Stroke
Head injuries
Spinal cord disorders
Epilepsy
Parkinson's disease
Peripheral nerve disorders

Endocrine
Diabetes
Altered hormonal levels, especially testosterone

Pharmacologic
Antidepressants
Antihypertensives
Hormonal therapy
Mind and mood altering substances
Alcohol

Other Causes
Cancer
Connective tissue disorders
Pain disorders
Depression
Incontinence
Sexually transmitted diseases

PSYCHOLOGIC/EMOTIONAL FACTORS
Childhood experiences
Body image
Anxiety and stress
Learned pattern of response

CULTURAL FACTORS
Misinformation about sex
Lack of sex education
Different social standards of men and women
Sexual myths and attitudes

RELATIONAL FACTORS
Differences in sexual desire or interests
Lack of attraction
Lack of communication
Lack of trust

box). There is currently much literature and discussion about the effect of childhood sexual trauma on later sexual functioning (Berman et al., 2001). Anxiety, stress, and depression also contribute to changes in sexuality. Masters and Johnson (1970) created the term *spectatoring.* This psychologic phenomenon is the tendency to observe, monitor, and critique one's own sexual activity, thus detracting from the actual experience. Positive and negative perceptions of one's body image impact sexual interest and function. Reactions to body image impact sexuality more than hormonal changes for women at menopause (Koch et al., 2005).

Cultural Factors

A variety of cultural factors influence sexual functioning. Negative childhood learning, lack of sex education, and the different social standards of men and women all account for some degree of dissatisfaction. There is a connection between sexually dysfunctional beliefs and actual sexual dysfunction (Nobre and Pinto-Gouveia, 2006). Sexual myths influence attitudes toward sex—for example, the myth that men are always ready for sex—may give women the wrong idea about men, which in turn can lead them to behave sexually in ways that are not natural or gratifying for either partner.

Relational Factors

Unresolved relationship problems, including financial and family stress, often pull a couple apart and disrupt their sexual relationship. Couples often have poor or ineffective communication about their sexual likes and dislikes. Oftentimes, couples do not discuss what they do or do not enjoy sexually nor share their feelings about the experience. Differences in sexual drives and interests further complicate the relationship. Money (1986) used the term *lovemap* to describe one's idealized picture of who and what types of behaviors make up one's sexual arousal pattern. Lovemaps vary from individual to individual; therefore, a couple is sometimes not well matched in their attraction to one another or in the sexual activities that interest them. Gottman and Silver (2000) extensively studied relationship satisfaction and suggested that the best predictor of duration and happiness is the ratio of positive-to-negative interactions.

RESEARCH for EVIDENCE-BASED PRACTICE

Randolph ME, Reddy DM: Sexual functioning in women with chronic pelvic pain: the impact of depression, support and abuse, *Journal of Sex Research,* 43:38, 2006.

This 2006 study involved 48 females who were recruited through the Endometriosis Society and who reported chronic pelvic pain (dyspareunia). They ranged in age from 19 to 50, and the majority were married and predominantly of European American decent. The participants received a packet of self-report measures including the Derogatis Interview for Sexual Function, a pain inventory, a depression inventory, a sexual/physical abuse questionnaire, and a measure that assessed the quality of the individual's relationship with her partner. The authors hypothesized that the severity level of the pain experience and its interference in one's life (i.e., whether there was a history of sexual abuse and how much partnership mutual support there was) would indirectly predict sexual function through its relationship with depression. The reported aim of the study was "to construct an integrative model predicting sexual functioning for women with chronic pelvic pain." The authors suggested that theirs was the first study to address the interrelationships among all of the variables.

Results showed that women in the study reported a slightly statistically significant rate of sexual dysfunction. A total of 54% of the participants were possibly or probably suffering from depression. 64.5% of the women reported sexual abuse, with 8% reporting it in childhood, 36.5% in adulthood, and 19% in both adulthood and childhood. Randolph and Reddy had previously believed that the pain experience did not directly predict sexual dysfunction, and the results supported this hypothesis.

As the result of the findings, the researchers arrived at a model that did support their assumptions. Thus, they suggested that child sexual abuse, the pain experience, and relationship mutual support predicted depression, and it was the depression that led to sexual dysfunction. The findings reflect the factors that influence sexual function in individuals who have chronic pelvic pain. If the woman is depressed or without support in her relationship, she is more likely to have sexual functioning issues. Thus, in designing treatment, it is not only necessary to treat the sexual functioning issues but also to include depression assessment and treatment strategies related to sexual trauma healing and relational therapy. Otherwise, the chances of success are less. The authors concluded that this study offers hope because it found that those who are coping well in life cope with their pain better and report good sexual functioning despite the odds.

EPIDEMIOLOGY

The most widely cited study of sexual behavior and sexual dysfunction is the National Health and Social Life Survey (Laumann et al., 1999). In that study, 43% of women and 31% of men reported having sexual problems. However, the survey covered only women and men from ages 18 to 59. Because sexual problems often affect the elderly, the actual amount of people who experience sexual dysfunctions is probably greater. The survey asked questions about seven kinds of dysfunction. The most frequently reported dysfunction for women was the lack of sexual desire, whereas men frequently reported early ejaculation. Many have argued that these statistics reflect a growing "medicalization" of sex. Bancroft et al. (2003) suggested that the survey did not try to determine whether the causes of sexual dysfunction were relational or physiologic.

CLINICAL DESCRIPTION

The DSM-IV-TR divides sexual dysfunctions into sexual desire disorders, sexual arousal disorders, orgasmic disorders, sexual pain disorders, sexual dysfunction due to a general medical condition, substance-induced sexual dysfunction, and sexual dysfunction not otherwise specified (see the DSM-IV-TR Criteria box). The first three categories are based on Kaplan's (1974) stages of the sexual response cycle.

PROGNOSIS

Having an understanding of what types of treatment are available and how successful they are allows nurses to properly guide and instruct their clients. In some cases, treatment outcomes are excellent, whereas in others they are poor. For example, hypoactive sexual desire disorders tend to have a more negative prognosis than other disorders. This is partially due to the lack of physiologic factors and partly because some people who complain of low desire are actually responding to other factors, such as issues in the relationship. Current interest in this area will eventually lead to better understanding and more successful treatments. Testosterone therapy for women and men forms the basis for pharmacologic research, as decreased androgen levels contribute to the lack of desire (Guay, 2002).

Masters and Johnson (1970) estimated that on 5-year follow-up post treatment, only 5.1% of clients had relapsed. However, none have ever replicated their studies, and many have questioned their evaluation techniques. In general, many believe that sexual dysfunctions are difficult to treat. The literature is lacking in long-term follow-up studies, and thus estimating prognosis is difficult. The drug companies provide statistics on the efficacy of their products such as Viagra or Cialis. These products have been useful for men but much less so for women. The reasons for this are unclear, as male and female arousal happens similarly. Most therapy for sexual dysfunction involves the use of cognitive-behavioral techniques. The success of these techniques directly reflects the client's willingness and persistence in implementing them.

DSM-IV-TR CRITERIA

Sexual Dysfunctions

DESIRE PHASE DISORDERS

Hypoactive sexual desire disorder: A deficiency or absence of sexual fantasy or drive for sexual activity

Sexual aversion disorder: Aversion to or avoidance of genital sexual contact with a partner

AROUSAL PHASE DISORDERS

Female sexual arousal disorder: Inability to attain or maintain an adequate lubrication/swelling response of sexual excitement

Male erectile disorder: Inability to attain or maintain an adequate erection

ORGASM PHASE DISORDERS

Female orgasmic disorder: Delay in or absence of orgasm after sexual excitement phase (must be persistent or recurrent)

Male orgasmic disorder: Delay in or absence of orgasm following sexual excitement phase (must be persistent or recurrent)

Premature ejaculation: Onset of orgasm and ejaculation with minimal sexual stimulation (must be persistent or recurrent)

SEXUAL PAIN DISORDERS

Dyspareunia: Genital pain associated with sexual intercourse (not resulting from a general medical condition)

Vaginismus: Involuntary contractions of the perineal muscles with penetration (not resulting from a general medical condition)

SEXUAL DYSFUNCTION DUE TO A GENERAL MEDICAL CONDITION

Use same subtypes as above but indicate the underlying medical condition

SUBSTANCE-INDUCED SEXUAL DYSFUNCTION

Use same subtypes as above and indicate specific substance

SEXUAL DYSFUNCTION NOT OTHERWISE SPECIFIED

Does not meet criteria for the category of sexual dysfunction

Data from American Psychiatric Association: *Diagnostic and statistical manual of mental disorders,* ed 4, text revision, Washington, DC, 2000, American Psychiatric Association.

DISCHARGE CRITERIA

Following intervention, client will:

- Express increased satisfaction with sexual functioning.
- Develop better understanding of the etiology and the symptoms of the disorder.
- Demonstrate use of appropriate intervention techniques designed to alleviate the specific disorder.
- Develop communication strategies with his or her partner to express desires, likes, and dislikes.
- Develop appropriate coping strategies to deal with frustrations and setbacks.

Because sexuality is so essential to the well-being of individuals and of couples, nurses need to be aware that assisting their clients to achieve positive sexual expression is an important goal (see the Case Study). Facilitating this goal is a rewarding but difficult task. It demands that nurses reflect on their own attitudes, values, comfort, and knowledge of sexuality.

For any given client or couple, it is difficult to predict how long interventions and treatment will last. As previ-

CASE STUDY Teresa and Rory are a couple in their mid-30s. They have been together for 5 years, cohabiting for 3 years, and are considering marriage. However, Rory says that before they can marry, he wants to deal with their sexual issues. He says that Teresa is rarely interested in sex. He always has to initiate, and she often turns him down. Teresa admits that she never has had a strong sexual drive, possibly because she comes from a family that was religious and never discussed sex. She agrees that she often turns Rory down but says she has two reasons: The first is that Rory often wants to engage in what she refers to as "kinky sex," meaning that he likes to role-play and even tie her up at times. The second reason is that he often ejaculates quickly, leaving her unsatisfied. Rory says that it is important for him to be creative in the bedroom. He believes this is important for maintaining long-term sexual interest. He admits that at times he ejaculates shortly after entry and that this has been a long-standing issue. He never wanted to discuss it before because he was embarrassed. Both Teresa and Rory say there are so many good things in their relationship that they will do whatever it takes to work on these sexual issues.

CRITICAL THINKING

1. What symptoms of sexual dysfunction/dissatisfaction does this couple exhibit?
2. What are the precursors/antecedents to the couple's sexual problems?
3. Which nursing diagnoses are appropriate for this couple?
4. How would you help Teresa and Rory achieve greater sexual satisfaction?

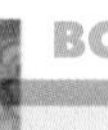

BOX 19-2

Principles of Sexual Assessment

- Before beginning a sexual assessment, examine your own feelings, attitudes, and level of comfort.
- Ensure a private, quiet space for assessment, ample time, and an unhurried attitude.
- Do not ask questions on sexuality first. Begin with background information and fit the sexual assessment into the overall assessment.
- Begin questioning about sexuality with the least sensitive areas and move to areas of greater sensitivity. For example, begin by asking, "Where did you first learn about sex?"
- Maintain appropriate eye contact and a relaxed, interested manner.
- Be professional and matter-of-fact about information asked or obtained. Avoid extreme reactions. Maintenance of an open, nonjudgmental attitude is essential.
- Use language that is professional but understood by the client(s) being interviewed. This is a good opportunity to teach about the words of sex.
- Remember, the nurse's tone of voice and manner reflect trust. If clients feel they can trust the nurse, they will be more open.
- Sex is not something most people are used to talking about, and this makes interviewing difficult. If the nurse has the right attitude, however, clients will generally be open, willing, and even eager to talk.

ously noted, some disorders are difficult to treat, whereas others are relatively simple. Individual factors sometimes speed up or complicate the recovery period. The astute nurse is consistently aware of these variables and needs to recognize the importance of flexibility. The overall goal of intervention is the achievement of sexual satisfaction, and the nurse recognizes that sexual satisfaction varies from individual to individual.

THE NURSING PROCESS

ASSESSMENT

Sexuality is clearly a difficult and sensitive topic for most people to address. When discussing sexuality with clients, nurses need to recognize that they are not immune to the feelings, beliefs, values, and attitudes that affect others. Therefore, when the nurse is dealing with client-related sexual issues, both the nurse and the client sometimes experience discomfort. A holistic nursing assessment includes sexuality as it relates to the importance of the client's well-being. A firm knowledge base, expert use of the nursing process, and a nonjudgmental attitude are necessary to work with this group of clients.

Assessment is always the beginning point and an essential phase in working with clients with sexual dysfunction. Nurses need a clear understanding of the complexity of the symptoms and areas of dysfunction. Sexual dysfunctions happen throughout various phases of the sexual response cycle. Some sexually based issues reflect individual functioning or are couple related. Sexual assessment includes all assessment factors, such as background, physical health, religious and cultural beliefs, education, occupation, significant relationships, and social relationships. In addition to the assessment of the specific complaint, the nurse also considers the individual or couple's perspective of the problem and their desire to change.

The sexual history is an important aspect of the assessment (Box 19-2). Alfred Kinsey (1894-1956) and his colleagues (1948) suggested beginning with the least awkward topic such as sex education and work toward more difficult and personal topics. The sex history includes early childhood experiences, history of masturbation, teenage experiences, use of erotica and fantasies, contraception history, relationship history, sexual orientation, satisfaction with sexuality, and an opportunity for questions and concerns. Nurses are not usually trained in taking a sexual history; however, it is a skill that nurses can learn using their already well-developed techniques of interviewing and communication.

NURSING DIAGNOSIS

Once the nurse has gathered assessment data, the nurse is in a position to analyze the findings and arrive at diagnoses. It is best to use DSM-IV-TR diagnoses of sexual dysfunctions with the North American Nursing Diagnosis Association International (NANDA-I)-approved nursing diagnoses to reflect specific problems. A combination of medical and nursing diagnoses helps to ensure that the nurse develops adequate plans for intervention. The nurse determines diagnoses on an individual basis and carefully selects them from the NANDA list (NANDA-I, 2007). Nursing diagnoses are prioritized according to client needs, from most urgent to least urgent. Nursing diagnoses common for sexual dysfunctions include the following:

- Sexual dysfunction
- Ineffective sexuality pattern
- Chronic pain
- Ineffective role performance
- Disturbed body image
- Anxiety
- Fear
- Risk-prone health behavior
- Impaired verbal communication
- Ineffective coping
- Defensive coping
- Hopelessness
- Deficient knowledge
- Situational low self-esteem
- Social isolation

OUTCOME IDENTIFICATION

This phase involves the nurse's determination of expected client outcomes from the nursing diagnoses. Outcomes are prioritized according to client needs, from most urgent to least urgent. Outcomes common for sexual dysfunction include the following:

Client will:

- Describe the specific sexual problem to the nurse by the second visit.
- Make an appointment for a physical examination (if appropriate) by the time of the third visit with the nurse.
- Discuss feelings associated with the identified sexual problem by the time of the third visit with the nurse.
- Participate in sex therapy sessions (if appropriate) by the time of the fourth visit with the nurse.
- Practice recommended strategies learned in sex therapy by the sixth week in therapy.
- Describe two strategies learned to enhance sexual functioning after the sixth week in therapy.
- Incorporate strategies learned in sex therapy into routine sexual activity by the end of therapy and on an as-needed basis after therapy.

PLANNING

Once the nurse has performed a thorough assessment, established the diagnoses, and identified outcome criteria, it is time to start the planning phase of the nursing process. Planning involves formulating an individualized plan of care designed to address all issues presented. Then, the nurse and the client work together to define realistic treatment goals. Individuals and couples dealing with sexual dysfunction need to carefully consider what they are willing to do to work toward these goals. The plan of care is often different for individuals with the same problem because of each person's values, beliefs, attitude, and perception of the problem. For example, a client with a primary orgasmic dysfunction has difficulty with masturbatory exercises as a particular treatment strategy because he believes that touching one's own genitals is unacceptable. When a client's individual beliefs prevent the implementation of a plan of care, treatment success depends on further exploration of the problem or an alternative plan of care.

CLIENT and FAMILY TEACHING GUIDELINES

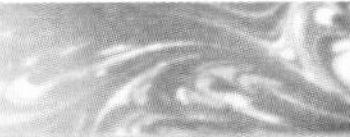

Sexual Dysfunctions

TEACH INDIVIDUAL CLIENTS

- Engage in breathing and relaxation techniques to reduce anxiety.
- Incorporate ways to increase comfort with and knowledge of one's body, using gradual and progressive touch. These exercises can be done in the shower or the bath or with the use of a mirror.
- Begin specific body image exercises involving positive affirmations and mirror work.
- Practice the use of fantasy, erotica, self-stimulation, and toys to enhance sexuality.
- Provide information about human sexual response principles and current knowledge of the hormonal and biochemical control of sexual functioning.

TEACH COUPLES

- Help couples develop communication skills that enhance the ability to openly discuss sexuality, including ways to express likes and dislikes.
- Suggest that couples take turns planning a favorite sexual/sensual scenario, then both act it out.
- Create a positive sexual atmosphere through the use of sexual humor, flirtation, touch, and enjoyment of one another. Help couples to have fun together.
- Inform couples of theories about the individuality and variance of sexual interest and levels of desire.
- Encourage couples to try something new, for example, a full body or genital massage, sexual play at spontaneous moments, or variations in time or location for sexual activity.

IMPLEMENTATION

To begin the implementation phase, the nurse needs to be aware of the specific nature of the problem and the possible etiologies. Implementation includes education, counseling, and assistance in identifying specific strategies, referral, and support (see the Client and Family Teaching Guidelines box). The nurse also needs to be aware of various treatment modalities and the prognosis for recovery with each intervention. The nurse's role is to help the client(s) express concerns about sexual functioning; express feelings about the impact of these concerns; and build a knowledge base, self-esteem, and communication skills. The nurse is also capable of recommending a physical examination or treatment and sex therapy. Nurses also monitor client compliance and progress in treatment and help develop appropriate discharge planning. Nurses need to stress to the client or couple that treatment success largely depends on following through with the plan of care.

To help clients with the exercises, knowledge, and interventions necessary to create more satisfying sexual relations, it is essential to first have a trusting, open, and comfortable relationship. It is difficult enough to discuss sexual difficulties with others, so without a comfortable relationship, many sexual problems will go unrecognized and untreated. Sexual issues and problems associated with the maturing process are increasingly common because the population that embraced the birth control pill must now cope with the complexities of acquired immunodeficiency syndrome (AIDS), menopause, and viropause, the male version of hormonal changes. Women may experience depression and a lack of sexual desire resulting from diminished hormone levels and related painful intercourse (dyspareunia). Men may feel trapped in their jobs/careers or relationships. Sexually active adults who are not in monogamous relationships may have concerns about sexually transmitted diseases (STDs), even though there are protective methods to reduce risk. It is important for the nurse to examine all of the individual's sexual issues and problems within the context of a relationship. Implementation of a plan of care most often involves a couple and not just one person. Placing the blame on either partner will prevent the couple's ability to heal. Working with each member of the couple as equals while doing sexual therapy is most effective.

Nursing Interventions

Nursing interventions are prioritized according to client needs from most urgent to least urgent.

1. Help client(s) to better understand human sexual response. Recommend appropriate reading materials such as Masters and Johnson's *Human Sexual Response* and Helen Singer Kaplan's *The New Sex Therapy*. Other reading materials to introduce include Rosemary Basson's intimacy-based model (Basson, 2001). *Knowledge of human sexual response forms a foundation for understanding other aspects of sexual functioning and their relationship to sexual disorders.*
2. Educate client(s) about sexual dysfunctions, including possible etiologies, symptoms, and treatment options. Include various methods of assessment such as physical, urologic, gynecologic, and laboratory examinations, as well as a psychosocial sexual assessment. *Through education, clients are able to understand why changes in sexual functioning are happening to them, and they are better able to identify symptoms that signal a sexual problem.*
3. Teach the client(s) positive communication and relationship skills. Support and reinforce client(s) in facilitating these skills. Provide communication and relationship-based homework assignments. Suggest bibliotherapy such as John Gottman's *The Seven Principles of Making Marriage Work*. *Problems in the relationship as well as the inability to communicate are often the cause of sexual dysfunctions. Positive communication and relationship skills enhance intimacy and sexuality.*
4. Assist client(s) in exploring their fears/anxieties related to sexuality. Do this in a private, trusting, and open atmosphere. Encourage them to talk about what they learned about sexuality and what their experiences were. Teach breathing and relaxation techniques to facilitate ease in dealing with these issues. *An open forum for discussing sexuality, accompanied by time proven strategies, helps clients overcome some of the repressed feelings they have and helps them be more open to satisfying sexual experiences.*
5. Help client(s) enhance self-esteem related to sexuality. Encourage positive self-talk such as affirmations, cognitive therapy exercise, and body image exercises (see Chapter 23). Discuss variations of sexual expression and treatment. *Lack of self-esteem is often a contributing factor in sexual dysfunction, and time-tested treatment and strategies will help to improve the client's self-esteem and self-image.*
6. Refer client(s) to physical treatment modalities or sex therapy as applicable. *These therapeutic interventions will help to maximize client success in dealing with sexual dysfunction.*

Additional Treatment Modalities

Once the nurse completes a careful assessment and determines a specific diagnosis of sexual dysfunction, several treatment modalities are available (see the Additional Treatment Modalities box). The history of sex therapy involved the use of cognitive-behavioral techniques, because originally theorists believed the reasons for sexual problems were psychologic in nature. The current emphasis, however, is on physiologic causation (although often causes are unknown) and on treatments that combine biologic, psychologic, and couples-related approaches.

Medically Based Interventions

There is a current interest in how testosterone levels affect sexual functioning in both males and females. Although decreasing levels of testosterone are more common in the elderly, this condition affects people in younger age groups as well. Studies show varied declines in testosterone levels in males as they age, and it remains controversial how these decreased levels or hypogonadism affect men. Endocrine testing is sometimes necessary. In general, researchers believe that **exogenous testosterone** used in males with hypogonadism improves sexual desire and possibly sexual function in general (Harman et al., 2001). This phenomenon is called **viropause** or andropause, and it increases abdominal weight gain and decreases bone and lean muscle mass.

Various other physiologic methods are used in both diagnosis and treatment of male sexual dysfunction. **Nocturnal penile tumescence** involves the use of a plethysmograph and determines erectile response during the sleep cycle when males are known to erect frequently. **Plethysmography** involves the use of a strain gauge that

ADDITIONAL TREATMENT MODALITIES

Sexual Dysfunctions

PSYCHOPHYSIOLOGIC MODALITIES

- Anxiolytics
- Atypical antidepressants such as bupropion
- Cialis
- EROS-CTD
- Estrogen replacement for women
- Intracavernosal injections
- Levitra
- Lidocaine-based topical cream
- MUSE
- Penile prosthesis
- Selective serotonin reuptake inhibitors (SSRIs)
- Exogenous testosterone therapy for men
- Viagra
- Vibrators

Possibilities on the Horizon

- DHEA
- Dopamine receptor agonists
- Oxytocin
- Pheromones
- PT-141
- Viagra cream
- Exogenous testosterone replacement for women

PSYCHOSOCIAL MODALITIES

- Body therapies (e.g., massage, chakra balancing, tantric yoga)
- Communication techniques
- Education
- Erotic stimuli training
- Gradual dilation of the vagina
- Masturbation training
- Semans's stop-start technique (Semans, 1956)
- Sensate focus

fits around the penis to detect erection. In some cases, daytime evaluation using visual erotic stimuli and the plethysmograph will determine erectile potential. A useful measure for monitoring the difference between penile and brachial blood pressures is the **penile-brachial index**. There are other invasive and noninvasive tests for evaluation of arterial and venous blood flow to the penis, including pulse-wave assessments, intracorporeal pharmacologic testing, ultrasound (the use of sound waves to evaluate structures and functions within the male genitalia), and cavernosography. Neurologic assessments that carefully evaluate various components of neural control of erection are also available.

In women, health care providers are also evaluating testosterone levels, because there is growing evidence that lowered levels of testosterone lead to hypoactive sexual desire and that replacement improves sexual functioning. However, researchers do not fully understand the relationship between testosterone levels and sexual desire in females (Bancroft, 2002). Lowered estrogen levels cause decreased lubrication, vaginal wall thinning, and vaginal pain. Thus, detecting levels of estradiol in the blood and estrogen replacement is sometimes necessary. Plethysmography determines blood flow to the vagina, which is an indicator of arousal; however, this procedure is inconsistent and invasive.

CLINICAL ALERT

Men taking Viagra, Levitra, or Cialis need to contact their physician immediately if they experience erections lasting longer than 4 hours, painful erection, chest pain, sudden loss of vision, fainting, rash, or urinary problems. Drugs are generally considered safe for erectile dysfunction as long as the client gives a complete medical and drug history.

Sildenafil (Viagra), a testosterone therapy, was approved for use in the spring of 1998 and led to immediate worldwide interest. Others have introduced similar PDE5 inhibitors, including vardenafil (Levitra) and tadalafil (Cialis). These work by blocking the enzyme that breaks down cyclic guanosine monophosphate to boost the chemical's relaxing effect on penile muscles. Combined with stimulation, these drugs have been helpful in achieving erection in a vast number of men (Jackson et al., 2005). Studies in women using PDE5 inhibitors have not proven as successful (Everaerd and Laan, 2000). There are a variety of selective serotonin reuptake inhibitors (SSRIs) that are useful in the treatment of premature ejaculation. Anxiolytics have been successful in the treatment of vaginismus.

Intracorporeal injections of vasodilators such as prostaglandins, papaverine, or combinations of these and other drugs are injected directly into the corpus cavernosum and produce erection. Intraurethral pharmacotherapy involving the introduction of vasoactive drugs through a system called MUSE is still available. In males, there is a surgery that will alter penile arterial blood flow or surgery can be used to implant prosthetic devices. Prosthetic devices come in two different general forms and have been developed over time with more satisfactory results. There is a semirigid rod made of silicone or metal, and there are inflatable pumps of varying degrees of sophistication.

In 2001, the Food and Drug Administration cleared the **EROS-CTD system** for use in treating the symptoms of female sexual dysfunction. This is a device that creates a gentle suction over the clitoris with the goal of bringing increased blood flow to the genitals. The blood flow then puts pressure on the nerves and causes a reaction in the clitoris. An autonomic reflex also results in increased lubrication and an increased ability to achieve orgasm (Women's Sexual Health, 2001).

Others are developing a variety of pro-sexual drugs to treat sexual problems. These include **pheromones**, or chemical odors that influence sexual attraction, and dopamine receptor agonists (drugs that enhance dopamine, a neurotransmitter), which show some promise as centrally acting agents. For women, there is current research using transdermal and gel-based testosterone. A new compound, **PT-141**, a melanocortin/oxytocin agonist that has central nervous system (CNS) effects, is showing promise for female arousal disorders (Palatin, 2006).

Psychologically Based Interventions

Sex therapy practitioners and clinical sexologists have utilized a wide range of psychologically based techniques. In general, homework assignments and supportive counseling form the basis of sex therapy. Sex therapy often involves weekly, bimonthly, or even monthly visits to the therapist, during which time the clients have the opportunity to discuss symptoms, progress, feelings, and observations.

The cognitive-behavioral techniques for sexual therapy Masters and Johnson developed have evolved over the years into more effective and comprehensive strategies. Masters and Johnson (1970) developed the **sensate focus** technique, which involves focusing on body sensations while shutting out other stimuli. Sensate focus is a way of developing relaxation, learning to tune in to the body rather than the thoughts, and creating an atmosphere where there is no demand for sexual pleasure or sexual release. The idea was that individuals often were so distracted with intellectual thought ("I have so much to do today"), self-deprecating thought ("My thighs are so huge, how can anyone think I'm sexy?"), and performance anxiety ("I wonder if I'm as good as her previous lover") that they lose touch with the actual experience.

Ideas for sensate focus include giving each other weekly massages, bathing one another, or gently caressing each other's bodies with a feather duster. The partner being massaged must only receive the sensations without feeling the need to reciprocate. There is no expectation of arousal or orgasmic response, just a need to enjoy the sensual pleasuring.

Masturbatory training exercises for women assist with developing better arousal response and better orgasmic capacity. Often, women perform **Kegel exercises,** which involve tightening the pubococcygeal (PC) muscle and bring blood and sensation into the genital region. They then begin a set of structured exercises to become familiar with the feelings associated with clitoral and labial touch. Males with erectile dysfunction perform masturbatory exercises using erotic focus and erotic stimuli to facilitate arousal and to decrease anxiety. Stop-start and squeeze techniques are helpful in training males with early ejaculation to be more sensitive to their genital sensations and thus delay ejaculation.

For vaginismus, the treatment involves the use of **vaginal dilators**. The gradual introduction of larger and larger dilators, coupled with relaxation techniques, will help women to overcome the fear and pain and help decrease involuntary spasm. Sets of dilators are available online for this purpose, but women have used fingers or other insertion-type objects as well. A cotton-tipped applicator usually serves as the first dilator because it is small, soft, and nonthreatening.

Specific sexually focused education and cognitive restructuring are two techniques highly used by therapists. Educational needs vary from specific ways to masturbate to theories about sexual response. Cognitive restructuring involves replacing negative or unpleasant thoughts about sexuality with more positive or realistic thoughts. An example is reframing one's sexual experiences in a more positive and pleasant light. Other helpful suggestions include using erotic materials to help train sexual focus and incorporate sexual thinking and feelings into the daily schedule. Males and females are also able to have masturbation training to help enhance their sensitivity to sexual stimulation. Masturbation training and practice facilitates and improves orgasm or orgasmic potential in both men and women. Masturbation training and the goal of becoming orgasmic also involves the use of cognitive restructuring as a method to replace old beliefs about sexuality and techniques with healthy, realistic beliefs, which reduce the fear of losing control (see Chapter 23 for more information on cognitive therapy).

The varieties of specific methods in sex therapy have proven helpful for individuals who develop sexual dysfunctions. However, without the sensitivity and attention to other factors in the client's life, these methods alone do not provide satisfactory results. Some of these factors include cultural and religious values, other psychologic disorders, poor sexual learning, and body image issues.

Relationally Based Interventions

One of the most difficult but important issues in working with clients is determining whether there is true sexual dysfunction or whether the problem really lies in the relationship. If there is a relationship problem, no amount of medically based or psychologically based therapy will be enough to facilitate success. Couple issues include role changes, the introduction of children, difficulty setting aside time for intimacy, loss of passion for the partner, anger toward the partner, a sexual desire discrepancy, or lack of trust. Communication is often at the heart of the problem. To improve couple's communication, there needs to be active listening as well as learning how to ask for what one wants and enjoys. (See Chapter 4 for more information on active listening and other therapeutic skills.) Gottman (1999) suggested that there are constructive and destructive communication techniques in relationships. Constructive tactics include leveling and editing, validating, and volatile dialogue. Volatile dialogue assumes that healthy couples argue, and in doing so, they discuss their problems openly rather than hold them inside, which will bring feelings of anger and resentment. Destructive tactics are criticism, contempt, defensiveness, belligerence, and stonewalling. Stonewalling is where a partner puts up a wall and refuses to communicate by remaining silent. The most significant predictor of the couple's prognosis to heal their sexual intimacy issues is in the respect, regard, and liking they have for one another.

EVALUATION

Evaluation of outcomes is a necessary step in determining the effectiveness of interventions. It is an ongoing process and not just facilitated at the end of the involvement with the individual or couple. If the nurse thoroughly and carefully defines outcome criteria, evaluation is a relatively simple process of deciding whether these outcomes were

NURSING CARE PLAN

Karla, a 42-year-old woman, mentions to the nurse during a routine history and examination that she has some sexual issues to discuss. She tells the nurse that her partner of 5 years recently broke off the relationship because of these sexual problems. Karla says that she is in generally good health. She was diagnosed with depression 3 years ago and has been taking paroxetine (Paxil), 20 mg daily. She is on no other medications except for a daily vitamin pill. She tells the nurse that when she and her partner were first dating, sex seemed good in the relationship. They were affectionate to each other and had sex approximately two to three times a week. Shortly after they began living together 4 years ago, sex dropped off to monthly and then became nonexistent. She says her partner tried to initiate sex but gave up after she continually refused him. Eventually the intimacy and closeness wore away and they fought more often. Without much discussion her partner announced that their relationship was over and promptly moved out. Karla said she was devastated at first but now believes it is a wakeup call to do something about her sexual problems.

Karla explained that she was born in Russia to a conservative Jewish family and that sexuality was never discussed. She had no formal sex education but recalls being interested in sex and reading books for information. She does not recall any early childhood sexual experiences and says that she has never masturbated. She did not date in high school, partly because of the strictness of her family. During college, she had a brief relationship with a man that she considered marrying. However, there was little attraction, and she decided to leave Russia to live in the United States. Since arriving in this country, she has had several other relationships, none of which was longer than 3 years.

According to the client, she experiences little sexual interest. She reports that she has never put much focus on sex but that in the past 4 years it has gotten less important. She says that she is concerned about this and would like to be "more normal" when it comes to sex. She says she is slow to get aroused, and sometimes she and her partner would give up after getting frustrated by the response. She rarely has orgasms. She believes that she has always had these problems to some degree but that they have gotten worse. Now that she is out of the relationship, she is not sure what to do about her sexuality but believes that in future relationships it will again be a factor. She reports being very stressed about this and says that she has been avoiding social commitments for fear she will meet someone.

Toward the end of the interview, Karla shyly and reluctantly reveals that she finds sex somewhat "dirty" and that she is a lesbian and has had sexual relationships only with women since she was in college. She says that her family still lives in Russia and is unaware of her sexual orientation.

DSM-IV-TR Diagnoses

Axis I	Hypoactive sexual desire disorder Major depression
Axis II	None noted
Axis III	None known
Axis IV	Moderate = 3 (primary relationships, socialization, anxiety)
Axis V	GAF = 55 (current); GAF = 65 (past year)

Nursing Diagnosis ***Sexual dysfunction related to deficient knowledge, beliefs about sexuality, side effects of medication, as evidenced by client's reported lack of sexual interest and arousal, and questions about source of sexual problems***

NOC Sexual Functioning, Sexual Identity, Role Performance

NIC Teaching: Sexuality, Sexual Counseling, Self-Awareness Enhancement, Role Enhancement

CLIENT OUTCOMES	NURSING INTERVENTIONS	EVALUATION
Karla will complete one factual book on sexuality by the next session with the nurse.	Suggest that Karla read *Women's Sexuality* by Ellison by next session. *This will help educate the client about human sexuality to overcome some of her deficits.* Schedule a follow-up appointment *to ensure continuity.*	Karla reports that she had read the book and was able to discuss what she read.
Karla will read women's erotica on a daily basis.	Suggest that Karla read female erotica by authors Barbach or Friday for a short time every day. *This will help to enhance her awareness of sexuality and help her overcome some of the previously learned messages.*	Karla did not buy a book on female erotica until 2 days earlier. She has read sexual stories since then.
By the next session with the nurse, Karla will make an appointment with her psychiatrist to discuss her medication.	Instruct Karla to discuss the potentially negative sexual side effects of paroxetine (Paxil). *The nurse is aware that SSRIs diminish sexual interest and affect arousal.*	Karla reports that after discussing the medication side effects, she and her physician decided to do a trial of bupropion (Wellbutrin) for depression.
Karla will agree to enter sex therapy with a qualified therapist by next session.	Activate Karla to receive treatment for sexual issues. *Sex therapy is helpful in overcoming sexual difficulty and anxiety.* Educate Karla about techniques of sexual therapy. *She will be better informed to make appropriate choices for herself.* Refer Karla to qualified sex therapist *for continued professional help.*	Karla reports that she has an appointment with the sex therapist in 2 weeks.

Continued

NURSING CARE PLAN—cont'd

Nursing Diagnosis *Anxiety related to stress from recent loss of relationship, fears about sexual functioning, perceived feeling of how others will respond to her sexual orientation, as evidenced by client's statements that she is anxious and unable to relate socially or sexually*

NOC Anxiety Level, Anxiety Self-Control, Symptom Control, Stress Level

NIC Anxiety Reduction, Simple Relaxation Therapy, Coping Enhancement, Teaching: Individual

CLIENT OUTCOMES	NURSING INTERVENTIONS	EVALUATION
Karla will be able to discuss her feelings of anxiety with the nurse by follow-up session.	Assist Karla to be aware of her anxiety and how it affects her sexually and in other areas of her life. *Knowing more about the nature of the anxiety will help the client find better ways to work with it.* Help Karla to describe situations that make her anxious. *This will help Karla better prepare for periods of anxiety and create strategies to overcome them.*	Karla is able to discuss her fears about entering another relationship and feelings about her sexual orientation with the nurse. Karla is able to relate that going to all-female events in the lesbian community made her anxious and she feared exposure. She decides in the future to go with a friend.
Karla will practice breathing and relaxation exercises during her periods of erotic reading and when confronted with social obligations.	Educate Karla on breathing and relaxation exercises (see Chapter 23). *This will help Karla focus on relaxation when she is confronted with sexuality and social contact instead of anxiety.*	Karla reports that she is able to focus on relaxation during the time she is reading erotic material.

Nursing Diagnosis *Hopelessness related to belief that she will be unable to overcome her sexual problems and may never have a healthy relationship, as evidenced by her statements that "things seem hopeless" and "my sex life may never get better"*

NOC Hope, Depression Self-Control, Motivation, Quality of Life

NIC Suicide Prevention, Hope Instillation, Mood Management, Socialization Enhancement, Emotional Support

CLIENT OUTCOMES	NURSING INTERVENTIONS	EVALUATION
Karla will verbalize that she is not feeling suicidal. Karla will be able to verbalize feelings of self-doubt and hopelessness with the nurse during follow-up session.	Evaluate Karla for any evidence of suicidal thoughts or behaviors *to ensure client safety.* Help Karla to express her feelings *to provide some relief and to allow her to feel validated.*	Karla does not show any signs of suicidal thoughts or behaviors. Karla is able to willingly discuss her feelings during the session.
Karla will report a feeling of hope after she sees her physician and the sex therapist and sees some progress in her sexual interest.	Activate Karla to follow up with her physician and the sex therapist. Ask her to report back on her progress, treatment, and strategies, and *to recognize that there are resources to help with the problems she faces. Also provide ongoing support for the work she is doing.*	Karla reports that she believes the change in medication and the sex therapy exercises she is using have helped to increase her interest in sex and her hope for continued progress.

met. The nursing process is cyclical so that if the nurse determines that outcome criteria were not met, the nurse will reexamine the assessment phase or any other phase of the nursing process to determine if some key underlying factors were overlooked.

To better understand the cyclic nature of the nursing process in the area of sexual dysfunction, the nurse needs to consider each phase. For example, suppose that during assessment the nurse learned that the client had decreased sexual desire. An important nursing diagnosis identified was sexual dysfunction resulting from a lack of knowledge, limited experience, and negative beliefs about sexuality. One of the outcome criteria that the nurse developed with the client was that she would acquire and read female erotica on a daily basis. The rationale was that consciously putting sex into one's life will enhance sexuality and that the practice of reading positive, erotic messages will counterbalance some of the previously learned beliefs. However, if the client does not buy the books or has left them on the table unread, the nurse needs to go back to the assessment phase and determine if something was missed. Was the client embarrassed and guilt ridden about the use of erotica? Perhaps the client's reluctance is due to some unresolved anger at her partner for leaving her, and she is trying to disrupt her treatment as a way to get back at her partner. If the nurse finds these or additional issues in assessment, the nurse will then revise the care plan to include them. Nursing diagnoses, outcome criteria, and interventions will then change as well. If the nurse did not miss anything in assessment, perhaps the outcome criteria were unrealistic. The issue of the client's anxiety is often complex and deep, and it is sometimes unrealistic to assume that she will be able to relax and read erotic stories. Evaluation needs to be ongoing as well.

PARAPHILIAS

HISTORIC AND THEORETIC PERSPECTIVES

Paraphilias is a common clinical term meaning sexual deviations/disorders. Paraphilias present inappropriate sexual fantasies involving deviant sexual acts, inappropriate sexual urges, and acting out of these fantasies and urges.

Once a psychiatric syndrome is described clinically, several steps are necessary to establish diagnostic validity, such as laboratory studies, delimitation from other disorders, follow-up studies, and family studies. No psychiatric syndrome has yet been fully validated by the complete series of these steps. However, many syndromes have had much data published in most phases of the validation but lack data in the other areas of validity. For instance, although there are some laboratory tests and follow-up studies of sexual deviance, there are few family studies of paraphilias.

The following questions remain prominent when managing this complex and challenging group of clients: Are all clients engaging in sexually inappropriate behaviors considered to have a paraphilic disorder or are they just "bad people" who act out in an inappropriate sexual manner? This chapter presents detailed concepts that will enable the reader to formulate a differential diagnosis after performing a comprehensive psychiatric assessment and psychosexual history.

LEGAL IMPLICATIONS

Forensic Psychiatry and Paraphilias

Forensic psychiatry is the application of psychiatry for legal purposes. This highly specialized area of psychiatry addresses issues related to criminal responsibility and competency to stand trial for various crimes. Formulating a forensic opinion regarding the paraphilias is difficult at best. A person who has committed a sexual crime in response to psychotic processes, such as hallucinations or delusions, is sometimes not criminally responsible (insanity plea); however, this individual is not always diagnosed with a paraphilic disorder. A person who commits a sexual crime in response to "recurrent, intense, sexually arousing fantasies, sexual urges or behaviors involving (1) nonhuman objects, (2) the suffering or humiliation of oneself or one's partner, or (3) children or other nonconsenting persons" (American Psychiatric Association [APA], 2000) meets the criteria of a paraphilic disorder and does not always include forensic issues as previously stated. An important aspect to explore during a forensic evaluation is the client's ability to recognize the criminality of the behavior (sexual crime) and the ability to conform the behavior to the requirements of the law, which is not intended to address the client's ability to control himself or herself. This is a part of the forensic opinion, and depending on the results of this assessment, the outcome is possibly a prison sentence or confinement to a maximum-security forensic psychiatric facility until assessment finds that the client is no longer a danger to society.

RESEARCH for EVIDENCE-BASED PRACTICE

Beauregard E, Lussier P, Proulx J: An exploration of developmental factors related to deviant sexual preferences among adult rapists, *Sexual Abuse: A Journal of Research and Treatment* 16:151-161, 2004.

The purpose of this study was to explore possible etiologic factors that contribute to the development of deviant sexual desires/behaviors. Researcher obtained information regarding developmental factors of 118 sexually aggressive clients via the Computerized Questionnaire for Sexual Aggressors (Proulx et al., 1994). Researchers determined sexual preferences via penile plethysmography. Exploration of the relationship between developmental factors and deviant sexual arousal was through multiple regression analyses.

The authors identified three developmental factors that related to deviant sexual preferences. They are a sexually inappropriate family environment, use of pornography during childhood and adolescence, and deviant sexual fantasies during childhood and adolescence. These results suggest that developmental factors play a part in the etiology of deviant sexual preferences. However, nurses need to be aware that these results are not all-inclusive. Other biologic factors play a role as well.

The authors have identified that a limitation to their study was the utilization of a small sample size, and they suggest that further studies are necessary in this area. Future studies need to also address other etiologic factors that contribute to the development of sexual deviance.

The Sexually Violent Predator Act

In 1990, the state of Washington's legislature enacted the Community Protection Act, which provided for the civil commitment of sexually violent predators. After a prison sentence, a sexually violent predator was able to be civilly committed against his will to a state psychiatric facility until he was found safe to return to the community. This was model legislation for the development of a similar law referred to as the Sexually Violent Predator Act, which 17 states across the United States have passed into legislation. This law established a civil commitment procedure for "any person who has been convicted or charges with a sexually violent offense and who suffers from a mental abnormality or personality disorder which makes the person likely to engage in the predatory acts of sexual violence" (Wash. Rev. Code Ann. §71.09.030, 1991). Washington state law defines a predatory act as "an act directed toward a stranger or an individual with whom a relationship has been established or promoted for the primary purpose of victimization" (Wash. Rev. Code Ann. §71.09.030, 1991). It is conceivable, therefore, that most sexually violent predators are either pedophiles or rapists.

ETIOLOGY

It is unclear as to what makes an individual develop a paraphilic disorder. Several studies have attempted to suggest etiologic factors and the prevalence of sexual deviancies (see the Research for Evidence-Based Practice box). Research has not concluded cause-and-effect etiology of paraphilias. It is important to acknowledge that people do not voluntarily decide what types of sexual arousal pat-

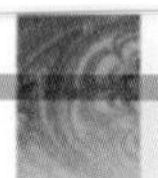

BOX 19-3

Etiologic Factors for Paraphilias

BIOLOGIC FACTORS
Chromosomal functioning
Hormonal levels

HEREDITARY/ENVIRONMENTAL FACTORS
Hereditary predisposition (familial transmission)
History of sexual abuse
Use of pornography during childhood and adolescence

terns they will have. Researchers suggest possible etiologies (Box 19-3).

Biologic Factors

In the biologic field, two areas are relevant: chromosomal functioning and hormonal levels. In 1942, Klinefelter and his colleagues described Klinefelter's syndrome as a condition characterized by (1) the development of gynecomastia (enlarged breasts) at the time of puberty, (2) aspermatogenesis (low sperm production), and (3) an increased secretion of follicle-stimulating hormone by the pituitary gland in the brain. In this particular syndrome, the client presents with 47 chromosomes instead of the normal 46; an extra X chromosome is present. The client is either a male (XY) with an extra X chromosome or as a female (XX) with an extra Y chromosome. Clients with this syndrome look like a male at birth. Hence, parents naturally raise them as males and assign them a male sex role. Money et al. (1957) described an otherwise normal 8-year-old boy with Klinefelter's syndrome who insisted he felt more comfortable dressed in girl's clothing. Klinefelter's clients have very small testes and produce little testosterone and virtually no sperm. They also experience problems with sexual orientation and the nature of their erotic desires.

Federhoff et al. (1994) reported the identification of clients with genetically based neuropsychiatric disorders who present with sexually deviant behaviors. Thirty-nine clients with Huntington's disease presented with a paraphilia and hypoactive sexual disorders. Similarly, clients with Tourette's disorder often have higher rates of paraphilic-like behaviors.

Hereditary/Environmental Factors

Gaffney et al. (1984) found evidence that suggests paraphilic disorders are hereditary. Groth (1979) found that children who were sexually active with adults during childhood were environmentally influenced and therefore potentially at risk for developing a pedophilic disorder. This is an example of victim turned **victimizer**, or sex offender.

EPIDEMIOLOGY

According to the DSM-IV-TR, although paraphilias are not generally diagnosed in clinical facilities, the sizable commercial market in paraphiliac pornography and paraphernalia suggests that its prevalence in the community is "likely to be higher" (APA, 2000). The paraphilias that most commonly present problems are pedophilia, voyeurism, and exhibitionism. About half of the clients with paraphilias who present are married (APA, 2000).

Some clinicians have addressed the presence of comorbidity (co-occurrence) in a certain percentage of the paraphilic population (Kafka and Hennen, 2002). Some of these clients also suffer from an unrecognized mental illness. Examples of comorbid (co-occurring) illnesses include mood disorders, anxiety disorders, substance use disorders, and personality disorders. The presence of a comorbid (co-occurring) illness that goes unnoticed sometimes has an effect on the client's course of treatment and prognosis (Seligman and Hardenburg, 2000).

The nurse needs to be aware of neuropsychiatric disorders or mental states associated with hypersexual behaviors. This includes frontal lobe damage, sexual deviancy, psychotic disorders, affective disorders, and cognitive disorders.

CLINICAL DESCRIPTION

The essential diagnostic features of a paraphilia are "recurrent, intense sexually arousing fantasies, sexual urges, or behaviors generally involving (1) nonhuman objects, (2) the suffering or humiliation of oneself or one's partner, or (3) children or other nonconsenting persons that occur over a period of at least 6 months" (APA, 2000). Another criterion is that "the behavior, sexual urges, or fantasies cause clinically significant distress in social, occupational, or other important areas of functioning" (APA, 2000). The DSM-IV-TR Criteria box summarizes the criteria and description of the paraphilias.

In 1994, Kafka introduced the term *paraphilia-related disorders* (PRD). These consist of a group of sexual syndromes characterized by hypersexual but culturally accepted behaviors. Some examples of PRDs as listed by Kafka (1994) are compulsive masturbation, telephone/cyber sex, pornography dependence, and the paraphilia-related disorders not otherwise specified (NOS).

PROGNOSIS

Nurses need to be cautious in attempting to predict **sexual recidivism**, or the chronic, repetitive inappropriate acting out of sexual behaviors considered unacceptable that have or have not resulted in criminal conviction. Clients currently undergoing treatment for a sexual disorder often have a lower level of sexual recidivism (Berlin et al., 1991). The Berlin et al. (1991) study revealed a higher reoffense rate for those clients who do not receive (or who have never received) treatment than for those engaged in treatment. Treatment compliance is a therapeutic issue that nurses have to address while treating this population (see the Case Study).

With continued treatment compliance and strict client monitoring, clients *may* present less of a risk to society. It is important for nurses to also acknowledge that treatment efficacy cannot be proven at this time. Further studies are needed in this area.

DSM-IV-TR CRITERIA

Paraphilias

EXHIBITIONISM
The exposure of one's genitals to an unsuspecting person(s) followed by sexual arousal

FETISHISM
Use of objects (e.g., panties, rubber sheeting) for the purpose of becoming sexually aroused

FROTTEURISM
Rubbing up against a nonconsenting person to heighten sexual arousal

PEDOPHILIA
Fondling or other types of sexual activities with a prepubescent child (usually under age 13 years who has not yet developed secondary sex characteristics). Heterosexual pedophiles are sexually attracted to female children under age 13 years. Homosexual pedophiles are sexually attracted to male children under age 13 years. **Ego syntonic pedophiles** do not view this type of behavior as troublesome and will not voluntarily seek treatment for it. **Ego dystonic pedophiles** are concerned and troubled with this type of behavior and sometimes voluntarily seek treatment to deal with it. There are several types of pedophiles:

- Homosexual
- Heterosexual
- Bisexual (sexual attraction to both males and females)
- Limited to incest (sexual attraction to a child in one's immediate family)
- Exclusive type (sexually attracted to children only)
- Nonexclusive type (may also be sexually attracted to adults of either sex)

SEXUAL MASOCHISM
Being the receiver of pain (either physical or emotional), humiliation, or suffering for the purpose of becoming sexually aroused

SEXUAL SADISM
The infliction of pain (either physical or emotional) or humiliation onto another person followed by sexual arousal

TRANSVESTIC FETISHISM
The act of cross-dressing (heterosexual males wearing female clothing) for the purpose of becoming sexually aroused

VOYEURISM
Observing unsuspecting persons who are naked, in the act of disrobing, or engaging in sexual activity ("peeping Tom") followed by sexual arousal

PARAPHILIA NOT OTHERWISE SPECIFIED
Disorders that do not meet the criteria for the aforementioned categories:

Telephone scatologia: Obscene phone calling; "900" sex lines
Necrophilia: Sexual activity with corpses
Partialism: Exclusive focus on a particular body part for sexual arousal
Zoophilia: Sexual activity involving participation with animals (bestiality)
Coprophilia: Sexual arousal by contact with feces
Klismaphilia: Sexual arousal generated by use of enemas
Urophilia: Sexual arousal by contact with urine
Ephebophilia:* Fondling or other types of sexual activities with postpubescent children (usually between the ages of 13 to 18 years) who are developing secondary sex characteristics (e.g., pubic hair, breasts)
Paraphilic coercive disorder:* Rape; aggressive sexual assault involving an act of sexual intercourse against one's will and without consent

Data from American Psychiatric Association: *Diagnostic and statistical manual of mental disorders,* ed 4, text revision, Washington, DC, 2000, American Psychiatric Association.
*Not included in DSM-IV-TR.

CASE STUDY

Tyler is a 24-year-old college student who attends the local university and lives at home with his parents and two older sisters. He was referred for treatment after conviction for raping a 22-year-old female. Tyler has been an active participant in an eight-member outpatient sex offender group for the past 5 years. The Department of Parole and Probation is about to release him back into the community without any further legal requirements. The nurse group leader is uncomfortable with Tyler's desire to be discharged outright from group. Her discomfort is related to the seriousness of the disorder, not to the amount of progress he has made. Tyler has been compliant with treatment during the past 5 years. His treatment consisted of weekly group attendance with participation, compliance with medications when prescribed, development and implementation of appropriate relapse-prevention strategies, and sound understanding of the nature of his disorder.

CRITICAL THINKING

1. What criteria does the nurse use to effectively evaluate Tyler's readiness for discharge from therapy?
2. What concerns might the nurse have regarding Tyler's prognosis after discharge?
3. With whom might the nurse consult in rendering her decision regarding Tyler's discharge from the therapy group?
4. Would family therapy be indicated on discharge from the group therapy session? What is the rationale for this intervention?
5. How could the nurse be responsible if Tyler relapses after discharge from the group?

DISCHARGE CRITERIA

Client will:

- State the nature of the specific paraphilic disorder and its impact on self and others (breakdown/ absence of cognitive distortions).
- Identify **triggers**—stimuli that heighten unacceptable sexual desires and provoke inappropriate sexual behaviors.
- Develop appropriate relapse-prevention strategies.
- Communicate and problem-solve effectively.
- Practice effective coping strategies.
- Identify support systems.

THE NURSING PROCESS

ASSESSMENT

The client with a sexual disorder exhibits a variety of behavioral symptoms, depending on the nature of the disorder. Some symptoms are more difficult to assess than others. The client with a pedophilic disorder sometimes exhibits perceptual disturbances. It is not uncommon to hear such a client state, for example, "The child looked older than he was." Sometimes this thinking is a cognitive distortion (errors in thinking).

Cognitive distortions are often present in the client with a sexual disorder. Two cognitive distortions most often present in this client population are denial and rationalization. *Denial* is a defense mechanism used to avoid dealing with problems and responsibilities related to one's behaviors. *Rationalization* is a defense mechanism used to justify upsetting behaviors by creating reasons (rationale) that allow the individual to believe that the behaviors were necessary or appropriate. These are the most critical issues that the nurse has to address early in the therapeutic process. A client making a statement such as "Well, the child didn't fight me and agreed to have sex with me" is a good indication that such cognitive distortions are present.

Another symptom that requires assessment is a disturbance in feeling. Clients with paraphilic disorders commonly lack remorse for their victims. If they do experience remorse, they are unable to acknowledge it as a result of cognitive distortions. Occasionally, clients with a pedophilic disorder claim to experience feelings of "being loved" by the child with whom they have had inappropriate sexual activity.

Nurses need to assess clients with a paraphilic disorder for the presence of behavioral and relating disturbances. These are assessed in the client's inability to develop age-appropriate relationships, altered relationships with others, and social withdrawal that occurs because of embarrassment or media attention (see the Nursing Assessment Questions box).

NURSING DIAGNOSIS

After collecting client assessment data, the nurse is ready to begin formulating diagnoses. In doing so, the nurse sometimes finds that the client has symptoms indicative of more than one diagnosis, such as a paraphilic disorder, a psychoactive substance disorder, or a personality disorder (see Chapters 13 and 14). This chapter does not discuss multiple diagnoses. However, it is important for the nurse to be aware of this possibility.

When addressing nursing diagnoses for the client with a paraphilic disorder, the nurse selects those that are specific and appropriate to each individual based on an analysis of comprehensive data collected during assessment. Nursing diagnoses are prioritized according to client needs, from most urgent to least urgent. Nursing diagnoses common for paraphilias include the following:

- Risk for other-directed violence
- Ineffective sexuality pattern
- Ineffective coping
- Ineffective denial
- Interrupted family processes
- Deficient knowledge (of illness and aspects of treatment)
- Noncompliance (with therapeutic regimen)
- Impaired social interaction

OUTCOME IDENTIFICATION

Client-centered outcomes relate to the client's nursing diagnoses and are the opposite of the defining characteristics. The nurse states outcomes in clear, measurable, behavioral terms and, when possible, includes a time frame in which the client is expected to achieve them. Outcomes are expected or anticipated and are specific goals the client will achieve through the implementation of the plan of care. Outcomes are prioritized according to client needs, from most urgent to least urgent. Behavioral terms the nurse needs to use in developing client-centered outcomes include words such as "Client will . . . state, list, perform, and participate."

Client will:

- Verbalize any feelings of harm toward others on day of admission.
- State two sexually inappropriate behaviors within 3 days of admission.

NURSING ASSESSMENT QUESTIONS

Paraphilias

1 What brings you here for treatment? *To assess client's level of insight*

2 Do you think you have a sexual disorder? *To determine if cognitive distortions are present*

3 Do you think you've caused any physical or emotional harm to your victims? *To determine if there are disturbances of feelings present*

4 How has this problem affected your lifestyle and relationships? *To determine the presence of disturbances in relationships*

- Write a list of triggers that provoke inappropriate sexual acting out within 1 week of admission.
- Describe two appropriate coping strategies within 1 week of admission.
- Participate actively in weekly group psychotherapy sessions for clients with sexual disorders within the first week of admission.
- Demonstrate knowledge of the effects of inappropriate sexual behavior on others within 2 weeks of admission.
- Verbalize two appropriate methods to meet sexual needs by the time of discharge.
- List several relapse-prevention strategies that are appropriate to client needs within the second week of admission and repeat at time of discharge.
- Explain the importance of medication compliance and follow-up care with outpatient group psychotherapy by the time of discharge.

PLANNING

After establishing diagnoses and identifying the client's problem, the nurse is ready to begin developing a plan of care specific to the individual client. Client care is based on mutually agreed on, realistic, client-centered outcomes. The nurse involves the client in the development of an individualized plan of care, with the expectation that the client will participate in the planning process.

In the population of clients with paraphilic disorders, it is not uncommon to find cognitive distortions. Nurses need to be aware of this possibility so as to include the client in the development of the plan of care. For example, a client who is in denial of a paraphilic disorder is not able to fully cooperate with the planning of care or view client-centered outcomes as realistic.

IMPLEMENTATION

The nurse works with the client to develop an individualized plan of care that will help the client identify the presence of cognitive distortions (if appropriate), prevent reoffending by identifying triggers that provoke inappropriate sexual activity, and develop effective relapse-prevention strategies (see the Client and Family Teaching Guidelines box). The nurse also explains the significance of treatment on recidivism and stresses the importance of medication compliance and follow-up care with outpatient group psychotherapy.

It is often difficult to provide nursing care to clients with inappropriate sexual behaviors because of the sensitive nature of the disorder. Nurses need to recognize this possibility and be aware of their own comfort level when discussing sexual issues with these clients. Identifying the presence of a paraphilic disorder often has devastating effects on clients and their significant others. It is important for nurses to include significant others in the interventions.

Nursing Interventions

Nursing interventions are prioritized according to client needs, from most urgent to least urgent.

1. Help the client to confront cognitive distortions through direct questioning methods that reveal the client's offending behaviors. Explain how these distortions affect treatment outcomes. Activate journaling to help the client track inappropriate sexual fantasies. *Clients need to be aware of the presence of a problem and be willing to acknowledge it for successful treatment outcomes. Journaling assists the client to break down sexual fantasies and see them more clearly.*
2. Educate the client and significant others about paraphilic disorders and aspects of treatment, such as identifying triggers that provoke inappropriate sexual activity and methods that help avoid relapse. Encourage active participation in the educational process by compiling lists in a journal for review by the client and the nurse. Place copies of these lists in the client's medical record to inform other team members about the client's progress. *This knowledge helps to provide a foundation for treatment.*
3. Enhance the client's compliance with treatment by openly discussing with him or her the effects of inappropriate sexual behaviors on others. Provide research studies regarding the effects of treatment on recidivism rates and handouts about the scope of treatment and how compliance assists in regaining control of sexual behaviors. *Compliance with treatment reduces the risk of relapse.*
4. Teach the client appropriate coping strategies, assertiveness skills, and problem-solving techniques. *Learned strategies help to prevent relapse.*
5. Promote the client's development of appropriate social skills and provide support and encouragement to the client for efforts to control the disorder. Peer-to-peer mentorship is sometimes appropriate to enhance appropriate social skills and feelings of acceptance. Some clients feel guilty over their behavior and become socially isolated. *Support and encouragement will signify to the client that there are healthy, functional, acceptable aspects of his or her personality.*

Additional Treatment Modalities

After careful assessment to determine the specific diagnoses of paraphilic disorder, the nurse is then able to begin a range of treatment modalities (see the Additional Treatment Modalities box).

CLIENT and FAMILY TEACHING GUIDELINES

Relapse-Prevention Strategies for Paraphilias

TEACH THE CLIENT AND SIGNIFICANT OTHER

- How to identify triggers that provoke inappropriate sexual thoughts and desires by listing the precursors to inappropriate sexual acting out (e.g., the client with a pedophilic disorder who claims he must drive by the schoolyard at 3 PM to get home [school yard = 5 trigger]).
- Relapse-prevention strategies are based on identification of triggers. Identifying triggers helps the client to avoid reoffending behaviors.

ADDITIONAL TREATMENT MODALITIES

Paraphilias

- Antiandrogenic medications
  - Depo-Provera
  - Lupron Depot
- Selective serotonin reuptake inhibitors (SSRIs)
- Individual and group psychotherapy/psychoeducation
  - Insight oriented
  - Goal directed
- Occupational/recreational therapy
- Family therapy/couples counseling

MEDICATION KEY FACTS

Sex-Drive Depressants

Sex-drive depressants are indicated for reduction of sexual arousal and libido and for inappropriate or disruptive sexual behavior in patients with dementia.

PROGESTOGENS

Medroxyprogesterone (Depo-Provera)

- Decreases sperm count, produces hot flashes, sweating, impotence, and insomnia.
- Smoking may increase risk for deep vein thrombosis.

LUTEINIZING HORMONE-RELEASING HORMONE (LHRH) AGONIST

Leuprolide (Lupron Depot), goserelin (Zoladex Implant)

- Leuprolide decreases sperm count, produces hot flashes, anxiety, and insomnia.
- Serious side effect is decrease in bone density with long-term use.
- Severe allergic reactions include rash, pruritus, urticaria, itching, flushing, and purpuric skin lesions.

ANTIANDROGEN/PROGESTOGEN

Cyproterone (Androcur)

- Causes atrophy of seminiferous tubules and gynecomastia with chronic use.
- *Dietary considerations:* May impair carbohydrate metabolism and fasting blood glucose. Hypercalcemia and changes in plasma lipids can occur.

Pharmacologic

The need for medications is based on the collaborative efforts of the multidisciplinary team to assess the intensity and impulsivity of the client's disorder and symptoms.

Antiandrogenic Medications

Medroxyprogesterone Acetate. Medroxyprogesterone acetate (Depo-Provera) 500 mg taken intramuscularly once a week has had some success for clients with paraphilic disorder (Berlin and Meineke, 1981). This form of external control helps clients to develop their own internal controls to avoid relapse. Clients have reported that this medication reduces the frequency and intensity of inappropriate sexual thoughts and fantasies.

The nurse needs to be aware of several side effects related to Depo-Provera. Because this type of medication decreases testosterone levels and sperm production, the client who is receiving Depo-Provera is less able to father a child. Common side effects include weight gain, increased blood pressure, and fatigue. The nurse needs to suggest a dietary consultation to help the client maintain weight and decrease the possibility of weight gain. The nurse also needs to take the client's blood pressure before each dose. In general, if the diastolic pressure is 100 mm Hg or greater, the nurse should withhold the medication. The nurse needs to discuss the client's blood pressure readings, and whether to administer the medication, with the client's physician.

The medication is thick, and a client should have doses no larger than 500 mg per muscle. The gluteal muscle is also used in administering Depo-Provera. It is not necessary to administer this medication via Z track (pulling the skin to one side tautly, in the shape of the letter Z, before injection to increase absorption of the medication), as there is no conclusive evidence that this method of injection increases absorption. Some clients complain of pain in the injection sites and need reassuring that the pain will go away within a day. If given in the deltoid muscle, the nurse will want to instruct the client to engage in range-of-motion exercises (moving the shoulder and arm in a circular motion) following injection.

Depo-Provera is not administered without informed consent and the client's signature on a consent form that explains about the medication and its therapeutic and nontherapeutic effects. The nurse reviews this form with the client as part of the client's individualized plan of care.

Leuprolide. Leuprolide (Lupron Depot) is a relatively new form of treatment used more frequently with the paraphilic population. This medication is a more powerful antiandrogenic drug. It acts similarly to Depo-Provera by lowering testosterone levels in the client with a paraphilic disorder. This medication is usually prescribed as 7.5 mg intramuscularly once a month. It is also available in a nondepo form; the usual prescribed dose is 1 mg/day subcutaneously.

Side effects include a decrease in libido (the desired result), bone pain, osteoporotic changes, gynecomastia, hair growth, weight gain, high blood pressure, dizziness, headaches, mood swings, and phlebitis. The nurse needs to assess for the presence of nontherapeutic effects.

In the beginning of treatment with Lupron Depot, clients are prescribed flutamide (Eulexin), 250 mg PO (by oral route) three times a day, to enhance the testosterone-suppressing aspects of Lupron Depot by blocking testosterone receptors. This is prescribed secondary to the increase in testosterone production within the first 2 to 4 weeks after having started treatment with Lupron Depot.

Again, it is important for the nurse to monitor the client's blood pressure before administering Lupron Depot. The same criteria apply to Depo-Provera.

Selective Serotonin Reuptake Inhibitors. Current literature contains several case reports regarding the

CLINICAL ALERT

Clients receiving Depo-Provera or Lupron Depot need monitoring for bone mass density, as these powerful antiandrogenic medications cause **osteoporotic changes.** Some clients are prescribed biphosphonate medications such as Fosamax to address this potentially dangerous side effect.

CLINICAL ALERT

The nurse needs to be alert for signs of **noncompliance with treatment** or signs indicative of **potential relapse,** as evidenced by such clues as the client's refusal to take medications or attend therapy sessions. Client statements such as "I don't know why I need this; I'm just here because the courts sent me," social withdrawal, presence of cognitive distortions, and lack of honesty are all risk factors for noncompliance.

treatment of paraphilic disorders with SSRIs such as fluoxetine (Prozac) or sertraline (Zoloft). These medications have fewer side effects than the antiandrogenic medications. Single case reports address the efficacy of paraphilic treatment with SSRIs by increasing serotonin activity, thereby decreasing sexual appetite. It is important to note that further research is necessary because of the absence of double-blind chart studies in this area (Kafka, 1997).

Individual and Group Therapies

Advanced practice nurses may be qualified to lead or co-lead psychotherapy/psychoeducation groups with the physician or another member of the treatment team. The purposes of group psychotherapy/psychoeducation are to (1) address cognitive distortions and (2) educate this client population regarding the identification of triggers, relapse-prevention strategies, the importance of treatment compliance, self-esteem issues, appropriate coping strategies, and problem-solving skills.

Recreational and occupational therapy are also provided to assist the client in time structuring, which is a relapse-prevention strategy (see Chapter 23 for further information about therapies). Family/couples therapy is sometimes recommended, depending on the individual client care needs. Usually the social worker or psychologist provides this type of therapy, but occasionally an advanced practice nurse or psychiatrist provides it.

EVALUATION

Nurses need to continually evaluate the effectiveness of their interventions on client behaviors in order to effectively treat this population. If the selected nursing interventions are not helping the client to achieve his or her outcomes, the nurse needs to revise the nursing care plan. Discuss the plan with the client and obtain his or her assistance in revising it. The areas in which client outcomes have been successfully achieved should be identified as "resolved." If newly identified problems occur, address these as well in the client's plan of care.

NURSING CARE PLAN

Martin is a 50-year-old vice president of a major corporation who has been diagnosed as having voyeurism. He occasionally acted out by engaging in voyeuristic activities at his country club in the ladies' locker room. He would secretly masturbate while "peeping." Martin's wife is currently unaware of his behavior but suspects something is wrong. When she confronted Martin regarding her suspicions, he denied the existence of any problems.

Martin voluntarily agreed to treatment primarily out of concern that his wife will discover his disorder. He also began to recognize that he spends a great deal of time on the job fantasizing or engaging in voyeuristic and masturbatory activities. Martin has been lying to his wife about his whereabouts for approximately 10 years.

The treatment team focused on assisting Martin in developing appropriate coping strategies. Treatment also included psychoeducation regarding trigger identification and appropriate relapse-prevention strategies. The need for couples counseling to disclose the secret of Martin's behavior was also addressed. Martin was given medroxyprogesterone (Depo-Provera), 500 mg IM q wk, to help him control his inappropriate sexual behaviors.

DSM-IV-TR Diagnoses

Axis I	Voyeurism
Axis II	Deferred—compulsive traits noted
Axis III	None
Axis IV	Moderate = 3 (marital conflict, job stress, anxiety)
Axis V	GAF = 61 (current); GAF = 61 (past year)

Nursing Diagnosis *Ineffective sexuality pattern related to use of cognitive distortions, presence of defense mechanisms (denial), as evidenced by engaging in socially unacceptable sexual behaviors (public masturbation) and voyeurism without regard for others*

NOC Sexual Identity, Role Performance, Self-Esteem

NIC Sexual Counseling, Behavior Management: Sexual, Coping Enhancement

Continued

NURSING CARE PLAN—cont'd

CLIENT OUTCOMES	NURSING INTERVENTIONS	EVALUATION
Martin will identify two sexual behaviors that are socially unacceptable within the first week of admission without the presence of cognitive distortions.	Monitor for the presence of cognitive distortions via a thorough sexual history. *The presence of cognitive distortions indicates if Martin is able to identify socially unacceptable behaviors and needs further treatment.*	Martin readily identifies his voyeuristic and public masturbatory behaviors as inappropriate within the first week of admission.
Martin will verbalize the effects that his behavior has on others within 2 weeks of admission. (*Examples:* "I know my behaviors cause other people pain." "I realize that my wife has also been a victim of my sexual behaviors.")	Educate Martin regarding the impact of his socially unacceptable behaviors on others, through individual and group therapy sessions. *The client's knowledge of the effects of his socially unacceptable behaviors on others is often the beginning of treatment compliance.*	Martin verbalizes an understanding of the effects of his behavior on others within 2 weeks of admission.
Martin will participate in group therapy sessions for clients with sexual disorders and will openly discuss his inappropriate sexual behaviors within 1 week of admission.	Encourage Martin's participation in a group for clients with sexual disorders. *These clients frequently believe that they are the only ones who engage in inappropriate sexual behaviors, which leads to feelings of hopelessness, embarrassment, and isolation. Group therapy provides confrontation, support, and hope.*	Martin actively participates in group therapy sessions within the first week of admission. He states that the group encouraged him to talk openly about his diagnosis within the second week.

Nursing Diagnosis *Ineffective coping related to inability to trust wife with his secret and inadequate problem-solving skills, as evidenced by use of maladaptive coping methods such as lying, denial, ineffective communication with wife (unable to discuss thoughts and feelings regarding disorder), anxiety, and fear that wife will discover his secret*

NOC Coping, Social Interaction Skills, Impulse Self-Control, Anxiety Self-Control

NIC Coping Enhancement, Behavior Management: Sexual, Impulse Control Training

CLIENT OUTCOMES	NURSING INTERVENTIONS	EVALUATION
Martin will effectively communicate his thoughts and feelings about his disorder and behaviors with his wife and selected staff within 1 week of admission.	Activate Martin to verbalize his thoughts and feelings concerning his current coping methods (lying, nondisclosure) by providing a nonjudgmental, supportive environment for disclosure to occur. *This will help Martin begin to understand the impact of his present coping strategies on himself and his wife.*	Martin verbalizes many thoughts and feelings about the impact his disorder has on his marriage within 1 week of admission.
Martin will identify concerns he has about disclosing his disorder and behaviors to his wife by the time of discharge.	Educate Martin and his wife about his disorder, its implications, and treatment. *Educating Martin and his wife about his disorder and aspects of treatment will calm their fears and anxieties and assist them in developing trust and establishing an effective, supportive relationship.*	At the time of discharge, Martin is able to share his secret with his wife, who is very supportive and eager to learn more about how she could help her husband cope with his disorder.
Martin will formulate two achievable relapse-prevention strategies by the time of discharge.	Help Martin to formulate appropriate strategies to use at significant times during his vulnerability *to assist in avoiding relapse and to prevent Martin from reoffending.*	Martin discusses two relapse-prevention strategies with the staff. He will call his wife before leaving work, and he will discuss inappropriate sexual thoughts or impulses with his wife or therapist when they occur.

Nursing Diagnosis *Deficient knowledge of illness and aspects of treatment related to cognitive distortions, anxiety, and uncertainty, as evidenced by failure to seek prior treatment for his disorder and inappropriate sexual behaviors*

NOC Knowledge: Sexual Functioning, Knowledge: Treatment Procedures

NIC Teaching: Sexuality, Teaching: Disease Process, Learning Facilitation

CLIENT OUTCOMES	NURSING INTERVENTIONS	EVALUATION
Martin will verbalize a basic understanding of his illness within 1 week of admission.	Evaluate Martin's current level of knowledge regarding his illness and readiness to learn by asking direct questions. *A client needs to demonstrate readiness to learn in order for learning to occur.* Create a climate conducive to learning such as a quiet, private, safe environment. *Learning has a better chance of actualizing when there are no distractions and the nurse has the client's complete attention.*	Martin is beginning to learn about his illness and the triggers that provoke his sexual thoughts and feelings. He says he is ready to learn how to deal with his inappropriate sexual impulses.
Martin will identify triggers that tend to provoke inappropriate thoughts and feelings within 2 weeks of admission. (*Example:* Having too much free or unstructured time.)	Educate Martin about the importance of trigger identification and use of relapse-prevention strategies as critical steps in treatment. *Use of effective treatment strategies will help Martin to gain more control of his inappropriate sexual behaviors.* Suggest that Martin write a list of triggers that provoke sexually inappropriate activity, and review this list with him. *This will help the nurse to evaluate Martin's insight into his disorder and symptoms, and the exercise of writing will help to reinforce learning.*	Martin continues to recognize the elements and situations that trigger his inappropriate sexual thoughts and feelings. He states he will take steps to obstruct them, such as filling in free time with appropriate activities. Martin is able to write a list of triggers that provoke his inappropriate sexual behaviors.
Martin will formulate two relapse-prevention strategies: construct a schedule of appropriate, planned activities to fill in free or unstructured time; and open the lines of communication with his wife. These strategies will be in place by the time of discharge.	Help Martin to develop at least two appropriate relapse-prevention strategies for his identified triggers. *A concrete, realistic plan will provide Martin with workable, achievable strategies to prevent relapse.*	Martin has successfully developed two relapse-prevention techniques that will help block triggers and prevent sexually offensive behaviors.
After discharge, Martin will join a community support group for clients with sexual disorders.	Help Martin join a community support group for clients with sexual disorders. *An outpatient peer support group will provide Martin with the continuity of care and realistic feedback he needs to prevent relapse.*	Martin agrees to join a community support group for clients with sexual disorders, and his wife supports the plan.

In treating the client with a paraphilic disorder, it is not unrealistic to expect the client to acknowledge the presence of the paraphilic disorder, identify triggers, develop relapse-prevention strategies, and state the importance of treatment compliance after discharge. If the client does not meet these outcomes by the time of discharge, the client is at a greater risk for reoffending. The need to protect both the client and society from possible relapse or recidivism is critical.

The minimal expected period for outpatient treatment is 2 years, although the actual time for treatment is considerably longer because treatment often depends on the client's probationary sentence. These clients need careful monitoring for any changes in their condition that will lead to relapse. Monitoring occurs through weekly outpatient group therapy or by periodic visits with the client's therapist. A client is formally discharged from outpatient treatment based on the level of progress and current status regarding the paraphilic behaviors.

CHAPTER SUMMARY

- Sexual dysfunctions include a wide range of problems that impact individuals and couples and lead to distress and dissatisfaction.
- Sexual dysfunctions are the most common of all sexual problems that come to the attention of health care practitioners. The prevalence of sexual dysfunctions is 43% of women and 31% of men.
- A history of sexual repression and incorrect information about sex contribute to the high incidence of sexual problems reported.
- Pioneers such as Freud, Kinsey, Masters and Johnson, Kaplan, and Basson have added to the understanding and acceptance of sexuality. Some have developed methods to help overcome the range of problems.
- Sexual dysfunctions are complex in nature and develop from many biologic, psychologic, cultural, and relational causes.
- The prognosis for treatment in individuals who experience sexual dysfunction is complicated by the lack of effective outcome studies. Each disorder has its own prognosis, and each situation is unique. Motivation, acceptance, commitment, and interest by the individual or the couple are necessary for treatment.
- According to Kaplan, sexual dysfunctions are categorized by the phase of the sexual response cycle. Thus, specific dysfunctions include desire, arousal, and orgasm phase disorders. Sexual pain disorders are also within the rubric.
- The nurse needs to have a sufficient understanding of human sexuality, an awareness of his or her feelings and values regarding sexuality, and a commitment to

include sexuality and sexual concerns into client care in a nonjudgmental manner.
- Establishment of a plan of care includes the significant other. When both members of the couple are involved, blame is less likely to occur.
- Assessment is holistic and includes the client's or couple's sexual history and interviewing, as well as the necessary laboratory and medical diagnostic techniques.
- Nursing diagnoses correlate with the DSM-IV-TR diagnoses for sexual dysfunctions. The blending of both medical and nursing diagnoses will help nurses to establish accurate and individualized client profiles that include specific sexual issues and also diagnoses such as anxiety, body image disturbances, and spiritual distress.
- Nursing interventions need to include client education about human sexual functioning, sexual response, and sexual dysfunctions; helping clients improve their communication; support for the clients' fears and anxieties; support for enhancement of the client's self-esteem; and referral for professional help.
- Many complex diagnostic and treatment modalities have been developed for sexual dysfunctions. These include medical, psychologic, and relational methods and involve neurologic, surgical, endocrine, and vascular treatments, as well as specific sex therapy techniques and couples-related therapy. There are more therapeutic modalities currently for males than for females.
- Paraphilias are sexual deviations/disorders presenting with inappropriate sexual fantasies involving deviant sexual acts, inappropriate sexual urges, and acting out of these fantasies and urges.
- Persons with a family history that is positive for the presence of a paraphilic disorder or history of victimization are at risk for developing a similar or different paraphilic disorder.
- Interventions should be based on the client's individual needs. The plan of care includes confrontation of cognitive distortions, exploration of the effects of inappropriate sexual behaviors on others, psycho-educational group therapy to teach the client how to identify triggers that provoke inappropriate sexual thoughts, development of relapse-prevention strategies and the effects of treatment on illness symptomatology, the importance of treatment compliance during and after the hospital stay, and development of appropriate coping strategies and problem-solving skills.
- The client with a paraphilic disorder who is compliant with treatment has a decreased risk of sexual recidivism.

REVIEW QUESTIONS

1 A nurse assesses four newly hospitalized clients. For which client would it be most important for the nurse to ask about sexual functioning?
1. An 8-year-old boy on chemotherapy for myelogenous leukemia
2. A 24-year-old woman having a laparoscopic appendectomy
3. A 35-year-old woman having a laparoscopic cholecystectomy
4. A 58-year-old man with a diabetic foot ulcer

2 A 56-year-old woman complains to the nurse, "My husband just isn't interested in sex anymore. I guess we're too old." Select the nurse's best response.
1. "As people get older, sex is less important. Develop other aspects of your relationship."
2. "Men experience hormonal changes, just like women. For men, it's called viropause."
3. "Have you talked to him about his sexual fantasies? Maybe that would pique his interest."
4. "There are other, more important things in life. Let's discuss your grandchildren."

3 A nurse counsels an adult with a 4-month-old ileostomy. The nurse asks about sexual activity since the surgery. The client says, "We haven't had sex. My spouse is afraid of hurting the stoma." Which comment by the nurse would be most therapeutic?
1. "You may engage in sexual activities now. Make sure the bag is sealed so it doesn't leak during sex."
2. "Try some new positions for sexual activities so you don't put any pressure on the stoma."
3. "The stoma is healed, but sexual intimacy can be psychologically difficult after an ileostomy."
4. "There are other ways than sex to have intimacy with your spouse. What other activities interest both of you?"

4 After discovering his wife masturbating, a husband tells the nurse, "I guess I just don't satisfy her anymore." Select the nurse's best response.
1. "Masturbation is a normal part of human behavior."
2. "How many times have you seen her masturbate?"
3. "Did she use any foreign objects to masturbate?"
4. "Let's refer you and your wife to a sex therapist."

5 Which statement(s) by a client with a paraphilia indicates treatment was effective? You may select more than one answer.
1. "I will come to the clinic for my leuprolide injections once a month."
2. "I will limit my sexual activities to watching pornographic videos."
3. "I volunteer at an elementary school, so I have supervision when I'm near children."
4. "I have new software that prohibits me from visiting sexually oriented chat rooms."
5. "When I get urges to have sex with children, it's best for me to stay at home."

*Additional self-study exercises and learning resources are available to you on the **Companion CD** at the back of the book and on the **Evolve website** at **http://evolve.elsevier.com/Fortinash/**.*

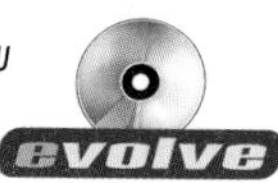

ONLINE RESOURCES

National Alliance on Mental Illness: **www.nami.org**

National Institute of Mental Health: **www.nimh.nih.gov**

Mental Health America: **www.nmha.org**

REFERENCES

Abbott E: *A history of celibacy*, Cambridge, Mass, 2000, Da Capo Press.

American Psychiatric Association: *Diagnostic and statistic manual of mental disorders*, ed 4. text revision, Washington, DC, 2000, American Psychiatric Association.

Bancroft J: Biological factors in human sexuality, *J Sex Res* 39: 15-21, 2002.

Bancroft J, Loftus J, Long J: Distress about sex: a national survey of women in heterosexual relationships, *Arch Sex Behav* 32:193, 2003.

Basson R et al: Report of the international consensus development conference on female sexual dysfunction: definitions and classifications, *J Sex Marital Ther* 27:83-94, 2001.

Berlin FS, Meineke CF: Treatment of sex offenders with antiandrogen medication: conceptualization, review of treatment modalities and preliminary findings, *Am J Psychiatry* 138:601, 1981.

Berlin FS et al: A five-year plus follow-up survey of criminal recidivism within a treated cohort of 406 pedophiles, 111 exhibitionists and 109 sexual aggressives: issues and outcomes, *Am J Forensic Psychiatry* 12:5, 1991.

Berman L et al: Pharmacotherapy or psychotherapy? Effective treatment for FSD related to unresolved childhood sexual abuse, *J Sex Marital Ther* 27:421-426, 2001.

Everaerd W, Laan E: Drug treatments for women's sexual disorders, *J Sex Res* 37:195-204, 2000.

Federhoff JP et al: Sexual disorders in Huntington's disease, *J of Neuropsychiatry Clin Neurosci* 6:147-153, 1994.

Freud S: *On sexuality*, New York, 1977, Penguin Press. (classic)

Gaffney GS et al: Is there familial transmission of pedophilia? *J Nerv Ment Dis* 172:546, 1984.

Gottman J, Levenson R: What predicts change in marital interaction over time? A study of alternative models. *Fam Processes* 38:143-158, 1999.

Gottman J, Silver N: *The seven principles of making marriage work*, New York, 2000, Three Rivers Press.

Groth AN: *Men who rape*, New York, 1979, Plenum Press.

Guay A: Decreased testosterone in regularly menstruating women with decreased libido: a clinical observation, *J Sex Marital Ther* 27:513-519, 2002.

Harman SM et al: Longitudinal effects of aging on serum total and free testosterone levels in healthy males, *J Clin Endocrinology and Metabolism*, 86:724, 2001.

Hillman J: *Issues in the practice of psychology: clinical perspectives on elderly sexuality*, New York, 2000, Kluwer Academic/Plenum.

Jackson G, Gillies H, Osterioh I: Past, present and future: a 7 year update on Viagra, *Int J Clinical Practice*, 59:680, 2005.

Kafka MP: Paraphilia related disorders: Common, neglected and misunderstood, *Harvard Rev Psychiatry* 2:39-42, 1994.

Kafka MP: How are drugs used in the treatment of paraphilic disorders? *Harvard Ment Health Lett* 13:8, 1997.

Kafka MP, Hennen J: A DSM-IV axis I comorbidity study of males (n = 120) with paraphilias and paraphilic related disorders, *Sex Abuse* 14:349-366, 2002.

Kaplan H: *The new sex therapy*, New York, 1974, Brunner/Mazel. (classic)

Kinsey A, Pomeroy W, Martin C: *Sexual behavior in the human male*, Philadelphia, 1948, Saunders. (classic)

Kinsey A, Pomeroy W, Martin C: *Sexual behavior in the human female*, Philadelphia, 1953, Saunders. (classic)

Klinefelter HF et al: Syndrome characterized by gynecomastia, aspermatogenesis without A-Leydigism, and increased excretion of FSH, *J Clin Endocrinol Metab* 2:615, 1942. (classic)

Koch P et al: Feeling frumpy: The relationships between body image and sexual response changes in midlife women, *J Sex Res* 42(3):215, 2005.

Laumann E, Paik A, Rosen R: Sexual dysfunction in the United States: prevalence and predictors, *JAMA* 281:537-544, 1999.

Masters W, Johnson V: *Human sexual response*, Boston, 1966, Little, Brown. (classic)

Masters W, Johnson V: *Human sexual inadequacy*, Boston, 1970, Little, Brown. (classic)

Money J: *Lovemaps*, Buffalo, NY, 1986, Prometheus Books.

Money J et al: Imprinting and the establishment of gender role, *Arch Neurol Psychiatry* 77:333, 1957.

North American Nursing Diagnosis International: *NANDA-I nursing diagnoses: definitions and classification 2007-2008*, Philadelphia, 2007, NANDA-I.

Nobre P, Pinto-Gouveia J: Dysfunctional sexual beliefs as vulnerability factors to sexual dysfunction, *J Sex Res* 43:68, 2006.

Palatin Technologies: *Bremelanotide clinical trials*. Report of presentation to the International Society for the Study of Women's Sexual Health, Lisbon, Portugal, 2006.

Proulx J, St-Yves M, McKibben A: CQSA: Computerized Questionnaire for Sexual Aggressors, Unpublished manuscript, 1994.

Rogers L: *Sexing the brain*, New York, 2001, New York University Press.

Seligman L, Hardenburg SA: Assessment and treatment of paraphilias, *J Counseling Dev* 78:107-116, 2000.

Semans R: Premature ejaculation: a new approach, *South Med J* 49:353, 1956. (classic)

Women's Sexual Health: www.womenssexualhealth.com, 2001.

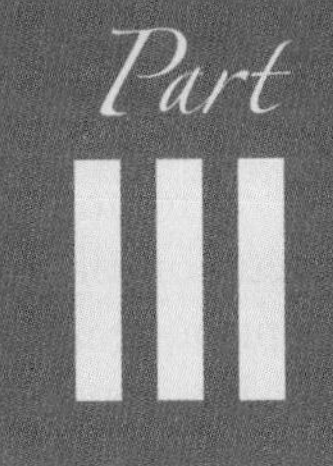

Part III: CRISIS AND AGGRESSION

Chapter 20 Crisis: Theory and Intervention

DAWN MARIE ELDERS

It holds true that man is most uniquely human when he turns obstacles into opportunities.

Eric Hoffer

OBJECTIVES

1 Describe the historical context of crisis intervention and new directions in the field.
2 Describe individual crisis triggers (external and internal).
3 Discuss the potential psychologic effects of disasters and terrorism.
4 Describe approaches to treating disaster threats and disaster victims.
5 Discuss crisis assessment "in the field" and "in the office."
6 Describe prevention strategies, planning, and intervention.
7 Describe barriers to effective crisis intervention.

KEY TERMS

bioterrorism, p. 452
coping, p. 451
coping abilities, p. 451
crisis, p. 449
crisis intervention, p. 450
crisis management debriefing, p. 454
critical incident stress management, p. 455
equilibrium, p. 450
GAF score, p. 457
homeostasis, p. 450
man-made disaster, p. 452
natural disaster, p. 452
psychiatric emergency, p. 459
terrorism, p. 452

In our present-day world, crises and disasters seem almost epidemic. The threat of mass terrorism has become an ever-increasing reality. Rape, murder, the attack on September 11, 2001, school shootings like the massacre at Virginia Polytechnic Institute, bombings, and the devastation of hurricanes and earthquakes demonstrate how vulnerable we are to crises, as individuals and communities. A crisis is not necessarily the result of a catastrophic event. Sometimes it occurs from expected, day-to-day, personal experiences that shape our lives. The word **crisis** is a dichotomy. It is defined as both a stressful event with the potential to overwhelm an individual's ability to cope effectively with a challenge or threat and as a potential crucial turning point or opportunity for growth and change (Flannery, 2000).

In a crisis, psychologic homeostasis, or a sense of balance, is disrupted, resulting in a response that is adaptive or maladaptive. With an adaptive response, the individual is able to take action and seek a solution. When the response is maladaptive, the individual experiences periods of disorganization, tension, anxiety, hopelessness, and helplessness and is less likely to take action to find a solution (Ursin, 2002). An individual's interpretation of the crisis is based on perception of the event, prior learning, memory, and prior outcomes to similar situations. Nurses use the biopsychosocial model when assessing a client in a crisis situation to determine if the response is adaptive or maladaptive. Intervention for clients with adaptive responses is supportive, but maladaptive responses frequently require additional therapy. In each case, the opportunity for growth and change exists.

Crisis intervention is a short-term strategic therapy with action-oriented interventions that focus on solving the immediate problem. The basic goals include alleviation of the acute distress, restoration of independent functioning, and prevention of psychologic trauma (Langan and James, 2005). Nurses begin interventions as soon as possible after the crisis event or the crisis response for the following reasons: (1) during a crisis individuals are more open to therapeutic interventions and (2) to avoid prolonged and further psychologic disturbances (Ursin, 2002).

Crisis intervention has primarily focused on individuals. However, when crises occur on a large scale, such as hurricanes, earthquakes, and the events of September 11, 2001, the need for group crisis interventions becomes necessary. The potential for future disasters and violence in our society has influenced the development of new strategies for planning and treating mental health disruptions that occur in large-scale disaster situations.

HISTORIC AND THEORETIC PERSPECTIVES

The Past

A variety of theorists have influenced crisis theory. Initially Claude Bernard (1813-1878), a noted French biologist, provided the theory of physiologic equilibrium (stability of the *milieu interior*). He described **equilibrium** as a natural state of balance, achieved by the interaction between an internal, biologic feedback system and the external environment that acts to maintain the body within a normal range of functioning, known as **homeostasis**. Equilibrium in both psychiatric and physiologic terms implies a steady state, resembling an optimal level of health. The term *equilibrium*, when used in psychology, refers to *that familiar state of being*. By viewing a crisis as a radical threat to or change in the norm, it is easier to understand why even a positive situation, such as the birth of a child or winning the lotto, causes a stress response *(eustress)* that a person interprets as a negative event *(distress)* (Selye, 1978). Thus, a crisis response is a mismatch between actual reality and what a person expects or desires (Ursin, 2002).

Abraham Maslow's hierarchy of human needs contributes to crisis theory in that an individual has to meet physiologic or survival needs before he or she is able to concentrate on higher needs or resolve a crisis (see Figure 2-2). Crisis intervention theory includes the assessment and treatment of needs in logical order, beginning with basic needs when formulating an action plan to assist the client in attaining a higher level of functioning.

An early proponent of crisis theory, French neurologist Jean-Martin Charcot, began with the study of "hysteria" in the late nineteenth century. From an expansive hospital complex in Paris, he studied women who had been victims of violence and exploitation. With careful observation, description, and classification of symptoms, he noted that their symptoms resembled neurologic damage but concluded that the hysteria state was psychologic because symptoms could be artificially induced and relieved through the use of hypnosis (Herman, 1997). Sigmund Freud agreed with Charcot's observation. However, he thought it was not sufficient just to observe and classify hysterics. Freud stated that it was necessary to talk with the victims as a form of therapy and catharsis. His theory of *brief therapy* (as opposed to long-term treatment) evolved from this early work. Later in his career, however, Freud insisted that long-term analysis was necessary for effective treatment. Soon after Freud's death in 1939, Alexander and French, two noted human behavior theorists, challenged the assumption that only long-term analysis was effective and promoted brief therapy once again (Budman and Gurman, 1988).

Many consider Gerald Caplan the father of crisis intervention techniques. He concluded that if an individual is able to constructively resolve a crisis, the individual will gain greater personality integration and coping abilities, whereas failure to master the situation results in disorganization. Caplan's theory states there are four phases of crisis development (Caplan, 1974):

1. The individual experiences an initial rise in tension as the stimulus continues and the individual feels more discomfort.
2. There is a lack of successful coping with the ongoing stimulus, resulting in more discomfort.
3. The individual mobilizes internal and external resources and uses emergency problem-solving skills. The problem is sometimes redefined or the goal determined unattainable.
4. If the problem continues, either resolution, avoidance, or increased tension leading to disorganization will occur.

The ability to maintain or return to a state of equilibrium in a crisis depends on the individual's ability to withstand stress and anxiety, the degree of reality recognition faced in solving problems, and the range of coping abilities (Caplan, 1964). The individual's experience in the past with similar situations also influences the state of equilibrium.

Eric Lindemann from Massachusetts General Hospital derived his theory from the treatment of relatives of 493 victims in the Coconut Grove fire in Boston in 1942. His studies of the psychologic symptoms of clients involved in the fire led him to believe that those individuals who were able to confront the crisis, turn to others for support, and

2. *Honeymoon phase.* O
after the event, feeli
high social attachme
3. *Disillusionment phase*
years after the even
anger, resentment, a
of support that were
4. *Reconstruction phase.* (
after the event, phy
ment takes place.

Individuals proceed thr
pace. Nurses providing c
stages and provide appro
Populations at special risk
ditions following a disaste
children and adolescents; t
elderly; refugees and migr
mentally or mentally disabl
As seen in Hurricane Katri
tion was the poor. They we
passes, roofs, and in the
Center without adequate
quickly overwhelmed with
ness (Rhoads, 2006). Yet, e
some individuals perceive t
saster quite differently from

Individuals tend to feel e
guilt following a disaster. It
transforms behavior from i
tion with others after the fi
belief. Individual identities a
and for a time the focus is
Hazards Observer, Novembe
ments that disaster experie
sonal growth and strength
cases (Friedman, 2005).

At present, the art and s
natural and man-made disa
tion. September 11, 2001, c
the need for police and ef
levels of government. The F
ment Agency (FEMA), thou
been dedicated to the develo
ness and crisis intervention
now recommends and requir
variety of settings including
occupational settings (Ever
twenty-first century, the N
Health (NIMH) has funded
scale research on the preventi
disorders resulting from exp
tional Institutes of Health
searchers are now investigati
will affect future roles of m
cluding the following:

- How do emergency ma
spond when many of th
victims?

express feelings were able to integrate the nightmare into their lives in a more positive way. Those who denied the importance of the event and did not seek assistance with the mourning process continued to have psychologic difficulties, especially depression. From his experience working with grief reactions, Lindemann proposed that grief is either "normal" or "morbid" (abnormal) depending on the individual's preexisting vulnerabilities and the ability to process loss and other stressful events. He believed that brief therapy was helpful to both the victims and their families in their long-term mastery of the emotional impact of a crisis.

In 1957, the Short-Doyle Act provided funds for each community to provide mental health clinics, but the emphasis was on long-term therapy. It was not until the 1970s and 1980s when the cost of health care increased dramatically that many began using brief therapy again because of its cost-effectiveness. Additionally, therapists who used cognitive-behavioral approaches were able to quantify and demonstrate significant therapeutic gains using brief therapy techniques. The general focus of these models is on identifying the client's maladaptive ways of thinking and acting, and then teaching ways to correct the maladaptive thoughts or behaviors. However, no specific cognitive-behavioral therapeutic technique among the many variations showed better results than another. Therefore, the use of a flexible selection of cognitive-behavioral techniques is preferable to adherence to one particular formula or model (Budman and Gurman, 1988).

The Present

The twenty-first century brings new ways to deliver crisis intervention. Computerized online chat capabilities now provide brief crisis therapy. This method shares similar goals and interventions as traditional crisis therapy encounters, but with a few interesting differences. Computer-based therapy usually occurs in private practice rather than in agency-based practice. On a website, professional qualifications are unregulated, but there is greater disclosure of professional interests, treatment philosophy, and resumes than agency practice usually allows. Computer services are almost always paid for by the user, and insurance seldom reimburses for this service. It is often more difficult to refer to appropriate local supporting resources associated with computer programs, as the provider on the computer is sometimes a long distance from the client and unfamiliar with local supports. Computer services do provide general information and advice on numerous mental and emotional problems, for both the clients and health care professionals.

In many states, there are in-home counseling services for families in a crisis. The focus is predominantly on children and adolescents with poor anger management, depression, anxiety, parent-child conflicts, and delinquent behavior such as truancy and gang involvement. The goal is to assist the family with coping, reduce crisis incidents, and retain the child in the home when possible.

CRISIS DEFINITIONS AND DESCRIPTION

Several definitions of crisis exist and are similar in scope. A crisis occurs "when a person faces an obstacle important to life goals that is, for a time, insurmountable through the utilization of customary problem solving skills" (Caplan, 1964). Some crises occur in the face of actual or perceived threat to an individual's physical or social integrity or occur as the result of a contradiction to some deeply held belief (Everly and Lating, 1995). Victimization also occurs when individuals witness traumatizing events happening to others and this results in a crisis.

During a crisis, psychologic homeostasis is disrupted because the individual's coping abilities fail. **Coping** is an adjustive reaction or habitual patterns of behavior that an individual uses in response to actual or imagined stress in order to maintain psychologic integrity (Aguilera, 1998). **Coping abilities** emphasize various conscious and unconscious strategies used to deal with stress and tension. Human coping abilities include flight, fight, or compromise reactions such as anxiety, hypervigilance, sleep disturbance, emotional withdrawal, and impairment in concentration and normal daily functioning (Flannery and Everly, 2000). Coping does not imply mastery over the crisis; rather it is the *process* to solve the situation.

According to criteria in the *Diagnostic and Statistical Manual of Mental Disorders* (DSM-IV-TR; American Psychiatric Association, 2000), crisis is not a distinct diagnostic category but is often associated with several psychiatric disorders. The most common disorders are depression, anxiety, adjustment disorders, and posttraumatic stress disorders (PTSD). An adjustment disorder is described as distress that is in excess of what would be expected from exposure to the stressor. In posttraumatic stress disorder (PTSD), the event is an extreme or even a catastrophic stressor that is outside the range of usual human experience according to Matthew J. Friedman, M.D., executive director of the National Center for PTSD, U.S. Department of Veterans Affairs. As seen during the Vietnam War, soldiers became profoundly demoralized when victory in battle was an impossible objective and the standard of success became the killing itself. The meaningless acts of destruction made many soldiers vulnerable to lasting psychologic damage. In one study, 30% of Vietnam veterans were symptomatic for PTSD (National Institutes of Health [NIH], 2001), and PTSD continues to be a significant problem in the war in Iraq.

The risk of PTSD for women in the general population is more than twice that for men, and there is frequent concurrent depression, anxiety, and substance abuse as well (National Institute of Mental Health [NIMH], 2001). In a longitudinal study of children who experienced Hurricane Andrew in Florida in 1992, researchers found that younger children and adolescents were at greater risk for PTSD than older adults (Rhoades et al., 2006). A study 6 weeks after the terrorist attack on the World Trade Cen-

- Psychiatric mental health nurses working in the community are especially in demand in catastrophic situations such as fires, floods, earthquakes, or acts of terrorism for those who have been traumatized by the event itself and those who have lost significant others in the tragedy. However, first responders are at the greatest risk for psychiatric problems after trauma, and plans for the care of caregivers is a priority for agencies providing crisis services to the community.

REVIEW QUESTIONS

1 A category 5 tornado hits a small Midwestern town causing major destruction of homes and buildings. Many fatalities occur. Place in sequence the psychologic stages the people of this community will experience.
1. Disillusionment phase
2. Heroic phase
3. Honeymoon phase
4. Reconstruction phase

2 A nurse on vacation comes upon a severe automobile accident. The driver emerges from the car without apparent physical injuries. Which behavior(s) would be expected from the driver immediately after this traumatic event? You may select more than one answer.
1. Urinary or fecal incontinence
2. Long-term memory loss
3. Inability to recall the spouse's phone number
4. Difficulty finding a driver's license
5. Diaphoresis and trembling

3 An adult recently diagnosed with multiple sclerosis says, "I'm worried I won't be able to support my family or send my children to college." This person begins drinking alcohol heavily and omitting prescribed medications. Select the correct analysis of the client's condition.
1. In a state of situational crisis
2. In a state of equilibrium
3. Reflecting on the situational event
4. Perceiving the event in a distorted way

4 A parent seeks counseling after the rape and murder of a child. The parent tearfully says, "I hate the man who did this. He's being tried for the murder, but I don't know what I will do if he's not found guilty." What is the nurse's highest priority response?
1. "Have you talked to a psychiatrist about taking some medication to help you cope?"
2. "Do you have enough support from your family and friends?"
3. "What resources do you need to help you cope with this situation?"
4. "Are you thinking of killing yourself or others like the man who killed your child?"

5 After a major hurricane destroys a community, which statement best indicates that an individual is likely to maintain or promptly return to a state of equilibrium?
1. "This storm wasn't so bad. It could have killed more people or destroyed the water and sewer lines."
2. "I've been through big storms before. If we pull together, we can help each other and rebuild our community."
3. "When my parent died 8 years ago, I got so depressed I was unable to care for my children or return to work."
4. "I think we'll be fine. We're getting plenty of support and assistance from other communities."

Additional self-study exercises and learning resources are available to you on the ***Companion CD*** *at the back of the book and on the* ***Evolve website*** *at* ***http://evolve.elsevier.com/Fortinash/.***

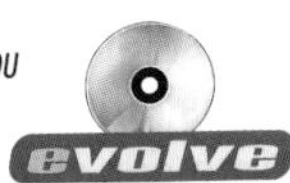

ONLINE RESOURCES

American Academy of Experts in Traumatic Stress: **www.aaets.org**

American Red Cross: **www.redcross.org**

Centers for Disease Control and Prevention: Emergency Preparedness and Response: **www.bt.cdc.gov**

National Institute of Mental Health: **www.nimh.nih.gov**

Substance Abuse and Mental Health Services Administration: **www.samhsa.gov**

U.S. Department of Energy: **www.energy.gov**

U.S. Department of Health and Human Services: **www.hhs.gov**

U.S. Environmental Protection Agency: Office of Emergency Management: **www.epa.gov/swercepp**

REFERENCES

Aguilera DC: *Crisis intervention: theory and methodology*, ed 8, St Louis, 1998, Mosby.

American Psychiatric Association: *Diagnostic and statistical manual of mental disorders*, ed 4, text revision, Washington, DC, 2000, American Psychiatric Association.

Arendt M, Elklit A: The effectiveness of psychological debriefing, *Acta Psychiatr Scand* 104:424-437, 2001.

Arron SS et al: Botulinum toxin as a biological weapon: medical and public health management [consensus statement], *JAMA* 285:1059-1070, 2001.

Beck A: *Beck anxiety inventory*, San Antonio, 1993, Psychological Corporation.

Beck A, Steer R, Brown G: *Beck depression inventory*, ed 2, San Antonio, 1996, Psychological Corporation.

Bisson J, McFarlane A, Rose S: Effective treatment for PTSD: practice guidelines from the International Society for Traumatic Stress Studies, *Psychological Debriefing*, New York, 2000, Guilford Press.

Bloom B: Focused single-session psychotherapy: a review of the clinical and research literature, *Brief Treat Crisis Interv* 1:75-86, 2001.

Breire J: *Trauma symptom inventory professional manual*, Odessa, 1995, Psychological Assessment Resources.

Budman S, Gurman S: *Theory and practice of brief therapy*, New York, 1988, Guilford Press.

Caplan, C: *Support systems and community mental health: lectures in concept development*, New York, 1974, Behavioral Publications.

Caplan G: *Principles of preventive psychiatry*, New York, 1964, Basic Books.

Everly G: Crisis management debriefing (CMB): large group crisis intervention in response to terrorism, disasters, and violence, *Int J Emerg Ment Health* 2:53-75, 2000.

Everly G, Lating J: *Psychotraumatolgy: key papers and core concepts in posttraumatic stress*, New York, 1995, Plenum.

Flannery RB, Everly GS Jr: Crisis intervention: a review, *Int J Emerg Ment Health* 2:119-125, 2000.

Friedman M: Posttraumatic stress disorder: an overview, a National Center for PTSD fact sheet, 2005; www.ncptsd.va.gov/facts/general/fs_overview.html.

Goodman D: Responding to terrorism: recovery, resilience, readiness, and readiness, *SAMHSA News*, Rockville, MD, 2000, Offices of Communication, Department of Health and Human Services.

Herman J: *Trauma and Recovery*, New York, 1997, Basic Books.

Langan J, James D: *Preparing nurses for disaster management*, Upper Saddle River, NJ, Pearson Prentice Hall, 2005.

Lerner M: An overview of acute traumatic stress management, *Trauma Response* 8:3-5, 2002.

Manning A, Henretig F: Bioterrorism, *J Spec Pediatr Nurs* 2:49-50, 84, 85, 2002.

Marshall R, Galea S: Science for the community: assessing mental health after 9/11, *J Clin Pyschiatr* 65(supp l l):37-43, 2004.

Mason T: Managing protest behavior: from coercion to compassion, *J Psychiatr Ment Health Nurs* 7:269-275, 2000.

Natural Hazards Observer, Dane S, editor: vol 26, University of Colorado at Boulder, November 2001; HAZCTR-spot.colorado.edu.

National Institutes of Health [NIH] News Release: NIMH awards new grants in response to terrorist attacks of September 11, 2001; www.nih.gov/news/pr/apr2002/nimh-18.htm.

National Institute of Mental Health [NIMH] Publication #01-4597; www.nimh.nih.gov, October 2001.

Noji E: The public health consequences of disasters, *Prehospital Disaster Med* 15:147-157, 2000.

Raphael B, Wilson J: *Psychological debriefing: theory, practice, and evidence*, Cambridge, 2000, Cambridge University Press.

Rhoades J, Mitchell F, Rick S: Posttraumatic stress disorder: after Hurricane Katrina, *JNP* 2:18-26, 2006.

Selye H: *The stress of life*, New York, 1978, McGraw Hill.

Ursin H, Eriksen H: *The cognitive activation theory of stress*, Bergen, Norway, 2002, Department of Biological and Medical Psychology, University of Bergen; hege.eriksen-psych.uib.no.

Chapter 21 Suicide: Prevention and Intervention

PAMELA E. MARCUS

The most authentic thing about us is our capacity to create, to overcome, to endure, to transform, to love, and to be greater than our suffereing.

BEN OKRI

OBJECTIVES

1 Analyze the scope of suicide by age, gender, ethnicity, socioeconomic status, and familial factors.

2 Compare and contrast biologic, psychologic, and sociologic theories regarding the etiology of suicide.

3 Distinguish among suicidal ideation, gesture, threat, attempt, and successful suicide.

4 Discuss key elements in the assessment of suicide risk.

5 Apply the nursing process for suicidal clients and their families.

6 Construct a nursing care plan for a client admitted to the psychiatric care unit with depression and suicidal ideation.

7 Describe the responsibility of mental health professionals in protecting clients from self-harm.

8 Discuss the use of emergency petition or involuntary inpatient hospitalization to prevent an imminent suicidal gesture.

9 Discuss the role of parents and guardians in observing self-destructive clues in youth and in offering guidance and assistance.

KEY TERMS

cognitive rigidity, p. 464
co-occurrence, p. 467
conscious suicidal intention, p. 471
imminence, p. 469
lethality, p. 469
perturbation, p. 464
suicidal ideation, p. 471
suicidology, p. 463
unconscious suicidal intention, p. 471

Society has become more complex and stressful for most individuals. Some people express that they feel hopeless, without any future. Individuals who feel they are unable to cope with the issues they face sometimes become depressed and suicidal. The National Center for Health Statistics ranks suicide as the eleventh cause of death in the United States. On average, one person dies from a suicidal act every 16.6 minutes. There are approximately 25 suicide attempts in the United States for every completed suicide. The statistics show that approximately 5 million individuals in the United States have attempted suicide and survived their attempts. Of these individuals, there are three women who attempt suicide for every man, but more men succeed in completing suicide than women. Approximately 4.1 men die by suicide for each female who has completed a suicidal act. Teenagers and preteens have a high risk factor, with suicide ranking as the third cause of death for people in this age-group. In 2003, 31,484 individuals completed suicide; 3988 were youth between 15 and 24 years old (American Association of Suicidology, 2006).

To prevent an individual from completing a suicidal act, it is essential that the nurse understand the person's thoughts and behavior that increases the suicidal drive. This is different for each person and depends on the individual's response to the circumstances. A thorough assessment is essential to determine the appropriate intervention and level of care necessary to prevent the person from committing suicide. Employing interventions aimed at assisting the individual to feel less hopeless is an important aspect of crisis intervention during an acute suicidal attempt, gesture, or ideation.

Suicidal thoughts, threats, and attempts often precede clients' search for mental health treatment in a variety of settings. Imminent risk for suicide is one of the leading criteria for medical care of clients admitted to mental health hospitals. Health professionals in all disciplines assist with assessing suicide risk and ensuring that clients receive prompt intervention to provide physical and psychologic safety. Nurses are in a position to contribute to these efforts because of their practice in multiple health care settings.

HISTORIC AND THEORETIC PERSPECTIVES

Throughout history, people have turned to suicide because they thought it would serve as a solution to their disappointments and obstacles. It was not until the late 1800s that pioneers such as Durkheim and Freud began to study the phenomenon from theoretic viewpoints.

Sociologic Theory

In 1897, Erik Durkheim, a sociologist, first classified the social and cultural aspects of suicide into four subtypes: anomic, egoistic, altruistic, and fatalistic (Durkheim, 1951). He defined anomic suicides as acts of self-destruction by individuals who have become alienated from important relationships in their groups, especially as this relates to their standard of living (e.g., the suicides after the 1929 stock market crash). Durkheim characterized egoistic suicides as self-inflicted deaths of individuals who turn against their own conscience (e.g., the suicide of a devout Catholic adolescent after she has had an abortion forbidden by her religion). Altruistic suicides are self-inflicted deaths based on obedience to a group's goals instead of the person's own best interests (e.g., the terrorist incidents on September 11, 2001). Durkheim defined fatalistic suicides as self-inflicted deaths resulting from excessive regulation (e.g., the suicide of a convicted prisoner who hung himself to escape a prolonged period of incarceration).

Psychoanalytic Theory

Freud viewed suicide from a psychoanalytic viewpoint. At the 1910 psychoanalytic meeting on suicide in Vienna, he described self-destruction as anger directed inward toward the internalized love object (Freud, 1920; Stekel, 1967). These early formulations ignored other critical feeling states, such as shame, hopelessness, helplessness, worthlessness, and fear. Later Freud incorporated many accompanying psychologic and sociologic clinical features, such as guilt, into his views about suicide (Litman, 1967).

Psychoanalytic theorists who followed Freud have added their own perspectives to the notion of suicide. Menninger described several sources of suicidal impulses: the wish to kill, the wish to be killed, and the wish to die. According to Jung, the suicidal person holds an unconscious wish for spiritual rebirth after feeling that life has lost its meaning. Adler identified the importance of inferiority, narcissism (self-absorption), and low self-esteem in suicidal acts. Horney believed suicide was a solution for someone experiencing extreme alienation of self as a result of a great gap between the idealized self and the perceived psychosocial self (Weiss, 1966).

Interpersonal Theory

Sullivan broadened the theoretic knowledge base of suicide by emphasizing the importance of interpersonal relationship factors. According to Sullivan, individuals are never isolated from the interactions of significant people in their lives (Sullivan, 1931). Therefore, Sullivan believed we need to view the suicidal act within the context of the perceptions of the suicidal person by his or her significant others. He viewed suicide as evidence of failure to resolve interpersonal conflicts (Sullivan, 1956).

ETIOLOGY

Suicidology is the scientific and humane study of suicide. This research began in the early 1960s with the establishment of the Center for Studies of Suicide Prevention established at the National Institute of Mental Health in 1966. The American Association of Suicidology was founded in 1967. The *Bulletin of Suicidology*, the first professional journal devoted to the study of self-destruction phenomena, began publication in 1967. Since that time, there has been an increase in the number of suicide prevention centers, and there are two national suicide prevention hotlines: 1-800-SUICIDE and 1-800-273-TALK. These hotlines provide counseling and crisis intervention for individuals throughout the United States who are suicidal. The American Association of Suicidology sponsors research and clinical competence and presents the findings during its yearly convention. The information is also available on the association's website at www.suicidology.org.

Current research is investigating steps that a clinician needs to take to prevent an individual from committing suicide. The American Psychiatric Association established the clinical practice guidelines to outline acceptable practices based on research (American Psychiatric Association [APA], 2003). The clinical practice guidelines provide the legal standard of practice for evaluation in court if a client completes suicide and the therapist or mental health staff is sued for negligence. The principles outlined in the clinical practice guidelines help nurses to provide safe and effective care. Along with these guidelines, one study cited six recurrent problems to consider when providing comprehensive care to clients who express suicidal thoughts (Hendin et al., 2006) (see the Research for Evidence-Based Practice box).

Biologic Factors

Researchers have studied the structure and chemistry of the brain in relation to affective or mood disorders (see Chapter 11). Research with adults has found irregularities in the serotonin system in suicidal clients. In 1994, Nielson and colleagues studied the major metabolite of

RESEARCH for EVIDENCE-BASED PRACTICE

Hendin H et al: Problems in psychotherapy with suicidal patients, *American Journal of Psychiatry* 163: 67-72, 2006.

This research was done to understand areas for mental health providers to improve in providing care to individuals who display imminent suicidal intent. The authors interviewed therapists for 36 patients who had completed suicide. The therapists completed comprehensive clinical case studies, reported medication the patient was taking before death, and presented the patient's treatment history in an all-day workshop. The authors identified six problem areas that were consistently evident in the therapist's clinical report of the patient's history before death:

1. Poor communication with treatment providers involved in the care of the patient
2. Allowing the patient or relatives to control the therapy
3. Avoidance of discussion of issues related to sexuality
4. Ineffective or coercive actions that resulted from the therapist's anxiety as opposed to the patient's clinical presentation
5. Inability to recognize the meaning of the patient's communication
6. Untreated or undertreated symptoms, such as anxiety or alcohol abuse

If the mental health providers assess their ability to prevent these six recurrent problem areas, there will possibly be a decrease in the completion of suicide in individuals receiving psychotherapy.

serotonin, 5-hydroxyindoleacetic acid (5-HIAA), found in cerebrospinal fluid, in conjunction with the genotype tryptophan hydroxylase (TPH). This was the first report to implicate a specific gene in the predisposition to certain antisocial and suicidal behavior regulated by serotonin (Nielson et al., 1994). Researchers have determined that there are changes in the brain's ability to manufacture and utilize serotonin. In postmortem studies, the dorsal raphe nucleus in the brain stem sent less than usual amounts of serotonin to the orbital prefrontal cortex (Ezzell, 2003). A research study using a positron emission tomography (PET) study of the serotonin function in the brain of individuals who are depressed and have a history of low-lethal (less serious) suicidal attempts, and those individuals who have high-lethal (more serious) suicidal attempts, showed biologic differences between these two groups. Individuals who are high lethal suicide attempters have less activity in the ventral, medial, and lateral prefrontal cortex. The individuals with a low lethality were often young and showed an increase in impulsiveness and more activity in the lateral prefrontal cortex. This research also demonstrates that there are alterations in the serotonin transporter binding that indicate serotonin hypofunction, particularly in the individuals with high-lethality suicide attempts (Oquendo, 2003) (Parsey et al., 2006). Currently there are no medications that specifically affect suicidal behavior. However, medications that regulate serotonin levels are effective in the treatment of mood disorders that often accompany suicidal ideation (see Chapters 11 and 24).

Another psychologic factor is the neurobiologic relationship between depression and suicide. Suicide most occurs with depression, and as depression resolves, suicide risk diminishes. The biologic changes in depression relate to alterations in specific areas of the brain (see Chapters 6 and 11):

- *Mood.* Sadness and dysphoria are associated with limbic lesions that can be moderated with dopamine.
- *Affect.* Separate motor systems of the limbic and brainstem regions of the brain influence control of the face and facial expressions and the muscular responses associated with emotional affect (e.g., crying).
- *Motivation.* Changes in the pleasure response, which is moderated by dopamine and dopamine antagonists, have an affect on motivational levels.
- *Cognitive content.* Researchers believe frontal lobe dysfunction is related to feelings of hopelessness and worthlessness, both of which are signs of suicidal thoughts.

The explosion of knowledge in psychobiology requires that nurses integrate the psychophysiologic aspects of illness with the behavioral sciences in their own nursing practice.

Psychologic Factors

Intrapsychologic and interpersonal theories continue to dominate the psychologic view of suicidal behavior. Contemporary etiologies include the following:

- Self-directed aggression or self-destruction as an act of murder directed at the love object, leading to states of isolation and loneliness
- Death as an atonement for wrongdoings
- Death as a way to recapture the lost love object
- Suicidal death as a secondary result of the major depressive processes
- Suicidal ideation and parasuicidal behavior resulting from abandonment anxiety

Most psychodynamic theorists after Freud have theorized that depression follows the loss of a significant love object and leads to feelings of helplessness, hopelessness, guilt, and diminished self-esteem. Suicide serves as a way to end those painful feeling states. This model emphasizes the functioning of the psyche and the reporting of subjective experiences.

Cognitive theory adds to the understanding of suicidal episodes by emphasizing the role of particular thought patterns: negativism, self-worthlessness, and a bleak view of the future. Some have hypothesized that **cognitive rigidity**, the inability to identify problems and solutions, is a factor in suicide when accompanied by stress (Rudd et al., 1994).

Shneidman (1985) developed the term **perturbation**, defined as a determination of an individual's level of distress and rated on a scale of 1 to 9. Perturbation refers to how upset, disturbed, or perturbed the individual is. Shneidman (1985), building on his 35 years of work as a suicidologist, lectured about the common psychologic features of suicide.

He defined suicide as a "response to an inner decision that the pain is unendurable, intolerable, and unacceptable. It is an unwillingness to endure that pain rather than the pain itself."

It is important to understand feelings of abandonment and abandonment anxiety in order to prevent a suicidal gesture in clients with interpersonal disturbances, especially in individuals with borderline personality disorder (Linehan, 1993; Masterson, 1976) (see Chapter 13).

In addition, the development of behavioral approaches based on learning theory contributed to the understanding and treatment of mental health problems. Interventions for suicidal ideation based on learning theory are directed toward decreasing unpleasant events and increasing pleasant events. Tension-reducing relaxation techniques, stress management skills, and rehearsal of problem-solving techniques are valuable adjuncts to reducing depression and suicidal behavior (Chiles and Strosahi, 2005).

Sociologic Factors

Contemporary sociologists have reinforced Durkheim's earlier work on suicide. Contemporary social scientists have supported the idea that alienation from social groups after disruption of family, community, or social relationships leads some individuals to attempt or commit suicide (Richman, 1986; Maris, 1985).

Thus, the findings of sociologic studies have provided added dimensions to the biologic and psychologic explanations of suicidal behavior. A more holistic approach is to consider a biopsychosocial model that combines all of these schools of thought in explaining such complex human concepts as suicide (Box 21-1).

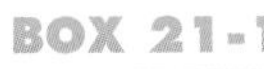

BOX 21-1

Etiologic Factors Related to Suicide

BIOLOGIC FACTORS

The neurotransmitters—principally serotonin, dopamine, norepinephrine, and γ-aminobutyric acid (GABA)—are linked to emotional responses.

Serotonin plays a major role in regulating mood and influences the occurrence of depression and suicidality.

Genetic influences are evident; researchers believe they have found a specific gene that predisposes a person to suicide.

Others have found that dimensions of depression, such as mood, affect, motivation, and cognitive content, are correlated to alterations in specific brain structure.

PSYCHOLOGIC FACTORS

Self-directed aggression
Hopelessness
Unresolved interpersonal conflicts
Negativistic thinking patterns
A reduction in positive reinforcement
Difficulty problem solving

SOCIOLOGIC FACTORS

Isolation and alienation from social groups
Biopsychosocial influences

EPIDEMIOLOGY

Prevalence

Suicide and suicidal behavior are present among persons of all ages (including young children), among both sexes, and among all ethnic groups and socioeconomic levels (Box 21-2). In 2003, 31,484 people died by suicide in the United States. This statistic places suicide as the third cause of death among 15- to 24-year-olds, the fourth cause of death among 25- to 44-year-olds, and the eighth cause of death in 45- to 64-year-olds in America. Approximately 90,000 individuals were treated in hospitals after a suicide attempt, with another 324,000 treated in an emergency room in 2002 (CDC, 2006).

Age

The two most vulnerable age-groups for suicide are older adults and youths between 15 and 24 years old.

Older Adults. Rates of suicide are highest among the older population, age 65 years and greater. Older adults have a suicide rate that is approximately 50% higher than all other reported suicidal statistics nationally. There are approximately 14 deaths per day, or 5248 completed suicides in 2003 (American Association of Suicidology, 2006). White men over the age of 85 were most at risk, with the completed suicide rate 4.8 times the current rate for men of all ages, or 10.8 per 100,000. Of all the completed suicidal acts among the elderly for 2003, 85% were enacted by males. The number of completed suicides for women peaks from ages 45 to 49 and declines after age 60 (American Association of Suicidology, 2006). The elderly most often use firearms to commit suicide. In 2003, 73% of all elderly suicide completions were by firearms. The main cause is undiagnosed or untreated depression. Many times the person completes suicide because of a recent loss, a physical illness with uncontrollable pain or a prolonged illness, loneliness and isolation, and major changes in role, such as a caretaker or recently retired (American Association of Suicidology, 2006).

Shneidman (1985) suggested that the high suicide rates among older adults represent failure to adapt to significant losses, inability to tolerate emotional pain, and negative attitudes toward the aging process related to loneliness, illness, rejection by family and society, sudden termination of meaningful work, disruption of long-standing relationships, and feelings of emptiness. As the population ages and seniors become the dominant subgroup, suicide increasingly becomes a major public health problem.

Youth. Young people ages 15 to 24 years have a suicide rate of 10 deaths out of every 100,000 young individuals, which adds up to 11 suicides daily. This means completed suicide in youth is the third leading cause of

BOX 21-2

Epidemiology of Suicide

AGE, GENDER, AND ETHNICITY

- Of the 31,383 completed suicides in the United States annually, the majority are white males of all ages.
- The two groups most at risk are youth ages 15 to 24 years (with suicides increasing at the fastest rate in African-American men ages 19 to 24 years) and white men over age 65 years (with suicides increasing at the fastest rate in men in the 85+ age-group).
- Native-American adolescent males and Hispanic females are high-risk groups among ethnic minority populations.
- Females in general attempt more suicides than males.

SOCIOECONOMIC AND FAMILIAL FACTORS

- Suicide crosses all socioeconomic levels.
- Affluent, educated overachievers are as vulnerable to suicide as people at the poverty level who are unemployed, undereducated, living in poor housing, and often the victims of crime.
- Prolonged family disruption and familial predisposition to depression and suicide, biologically or as a learned behavior from other family members, contribute to the incidence rates.
- Family turmoil, disturbed parent-child relationships, physical and sexual abuse by family members, and hostile and rejecting parental attitudes have been found to promote suicidal behavior.

CO-OCCURRENCE WITH RELATED HEALTH ISSUES

- Suicidal behavior is strongly associated with psychiatric disorders.
- Mood disorders, substance abuse, schizophrenia, borderline personality disorder, and panic disorders have a co-occurrence with high-risk suicidal behavior.
- Depression remains as the single best predictor of suicide risk in all ages.
- Suicide is the leading cause of death during the first 10 years of the course of schizophrenic illness.
- The research is mixed on the correlation of suicide with panic disorders, but it associated with suicide risk, especially when panic disorder coexists with depression, obsessive-compulsive disorder, or phobias.
- Independent of another specific psychiatric diagnosis, alcohol use and abuse are highly correlated with most suicidal acts, especially among youth. It is underdiagnosed and underreported among older adults.
- Similarly, chronic physical illness contributes to suicidal behavior. More than half of the outpatient clients who committed suicide in several studies had physical health problems, such as heart disease, hypertension, obesity, and diabetes. Older adults are particularly at risk for suicide.

death, after accidents and homicides. The 2003 statistics showed 244 individuals from the age of 10 to 14 years old completed suicide in the United States, with firearms the most common method of suicide. The rate of suicides by suffocation has increased from 1.9 in 1992 to 2.7 in 2002. As many as 16.9% of all high school students have contemplated suicide and with 16.5% who have made plans for a suicide attempt (National Center for Injury Prevention and Control, 2004).

To prevent suicide in youth, it is helpful to understand the possible causal factors. Screen adolescents for psychiatric disorders, such as drug or alcohol abuse; depression; and conduct disorders. Individuals are at high risk if they are experiencing difficulty interacting with their peers. This includes bullying, a breakup in a significant relationship, a pregnancy, issues related to sexual orientation, and feelings of isolation. Adolescents are at a higher risk if there is conflict within the family or the individual feels alienated from the family. Monitor adolescents who have experienced a peer who has been suicidal or completed suicide; this increases the possibility of a suicidal attempt (American Association of Suicidology, 2006; CDC, 2006; Carroll, 2003; McDaniel et al., 2001).

Gender and Ethnicity

National suicide rates are vague regarding the importance of gender and ethnicity in defining the scope of suicidal behavior. Suicide rates for whites are approximately twice those of nonwhites as a whole. However, it is important to note that suicide rates for African-American men have tripled since the early 1990s among the 85-plus age-group.

After older white men, African-American young adult men have the next highest rate of suicide. Males commit suicide at rates three to four times those of African-American females. Suicide is the third cause of death for male and female African-American youth. The suicide completion rate is the lowest in African-American females of all the racial and gender groups (American Association of Suicidology, 2006).

Native American individuals have a high degree of completed suicide. In 2003, 322 Native Americans completed suicide, which is approximately 10% of the Native American population (CDC, 2006). Assistance for Native American youth needs to incorporate cultural aspects of the unique tribe as well as treatment for issues such as alcoholism, family conflict, and depression.

Socioeconomic Status

Suicide crosses all socioeconomic levels. Both economic well-being and poverty create circumstances leading to the choice of suicide as a solution to stressful events.

Familial Influences

Suicidal behavior is frequently a symptom of prolonged and progressive family disruption and dysfunction. In addition, significant changes in the family, such as divorce, death of a loved one, and social isolation, contribute to high suicide rates.

The family is most influential in the lives of children and adolescents and contributes to the incidence of suicidal behavior in those age-groups. A suicidal adolescent often feels estranged from family members and sometimes experiences rejection and a loss of love. Actual physical or psychologic loss, as in death, separation, or emotional distancing from the family, is one of the most significant factors in the high incidence of adolescent suicides (American Association of Suicidology, 2006).

There is a familial predisposition to suicide in that many suicidal adolescents often have histories of suicidal behavior among their immediate and extended families. Adolescents who completed suicide usually had mothers who had previously completed suicide. Suicidal behavior becomes a learned familial adaptation to problems and stressors (Lieb et al., 2005; Qin et al., 2002, 2003).

Familial cultural values also are strong factors in suicidal behavior. For example, in Hispanic families, family honor and family centeredness and cohesiveness are factors that shield against suicidal behavior or contribute to it. Hispanic youth often experience conflict between traditional Hispanic values and the values of the dominant culture. Intergenerational tension, language barriers, and role conflicts also contribute to mental health problems. Adolescents who relate positively to the main culture and still have positive relationships with their family members who have more traditional values are often less at risk for suicide.

Co-occurrence With Related Health Issues

There is a relationship between suicidal behavior and the occurrence of psychiatric disorders and other health-related problems (see Box 21-2). Psychiatric illness, alcohol and other drug use and abuse, and medical illnesses are important indicators of suicidal events.

Suicidal ideation and completion often occur when individuals feel hopeless about their health problems. In the study by Waem et al. (2002) of older adults with health problems, the researchers rated the population depending on the severity of the illness. They discovered that serious illness or disability increased the risk for suicide completion, particularly in men. In this study sample, individuals with mood disorders as well as physical illness had a higher probability of suicide.

Psychiatric Disorders

The presence of a diagnosable mental disorder increases the risk for suicide, regardless of age. The **co-occurrence** of mood disorder and substance abuse increases the probability of suicide. The risk for completed suicide secondary to a mental disorder is higher in men than in women. Women attempt suicide twice as many times as men; but four times as many men succeed in completing suicide than women. Approximately 90% of individuals who complete suicide have a psychiatric disorder that fits DSM-IV-TR criteria. The most commonly identified mental illnesses are mood disorders, such as depression and bipolar disorder, substance abuse, schizophrenia, and borderline personality disorder (American Association of Suicidology, 2006).

Mood Disorders. The single best predictor of suicidal thinking is the presence of a mood disorder. Untreated depression is responsible for approximately 20% of completed suicidal deaths. The possibility of suicidal risk increases with recurrent episodes of depression because of the feelings of hopelessness, worthlessness, anger, social isolation, an inability to problem-solve, and cognitive rigidity. Individuals with bipolar disorder in a hypomanic or manic aspect are often impulsive, increasing the risk for suicide. Swann, Dougherty, and colleagues found that individuals with bipolar disorder were impulsive and had the most medically severe suicide attempts (Swann et al., 2005). The risk for suicidal attempts increases if the individual has had depression early in life, aggressive and impulsive behaviors, and childhood abuse (Mann et al., 2005). The suicidal risk increased with alcohol or substance abuse and depression (APA, 2003).

One aspect of treatment for major depressive disorder is the use of antidepressants. In March 2004, the U.S. Food and Drug Administration (FDA) had a black box warning regarding an increased risk of suicide with some of the newer atypical antidepressants. This warning indicates that antidepressants increase the risk of suicidal ideation and behavior in children and adolescents with major depressive disorder. Close observation of individuals placed on antidepressants is necessary to prevent a suicide attempt (APA, 2003).

Schizophrenia. Another diagnostic category linked with suicide is schizophrenia. Suicide is the leading cause of premature death in that population, with an estimated 10% incidence of suicide in the first 10 years of the illness and a 15% lifetime incidence (Thornton et al., 2001). Individuals with schizophrenia have high levels of subjective stress and feelings of hopelessness, loneliness, and dissatisfaction with social relationships because of the chronic aspect of this illness. Because the onset of schizophrenia usually occurs in late adolescence or early young adulthood, the high-risk period for suicide is in the 20- to 30-year age-group. Other risk factors associated with suicide completion in this population are active psychotic symptoms, depression, and a history of prior suicide attempts. Women have a higher completion rate after an acute exacerbation of the illness, as well as depressive symptoms and the use of alcohol. Nurses need to carefully evaluate and reevaluate this population for suicide risk, particularly during the first 10 years of the illness (APA, 2003).

Panic Disorder. When assessing the individual for suicidal potential, it is important to assess the person with a panic disorder for the possibility of suicidal ideation. There is a high comorbidity (co-occurrence) of suicidal behavior with panic disorder, major depression, and substance abuse. Evidence supports that panic disorder, in conjunction with phobias and obsessive-compulsive dis-

CLINICAL ALERT

Conflicting findings among researchers lead nurses and other clinicians to overlook the possible lethality of clients with **panic disorder, obsessive-compulsive disorder,** and **phobias.** A careful suicide assessment is necessary to ensure that health care providers consider this because clients with anxiety disorders develop depression that sometimes results in suicide ideation (see Chapters 9 and 11).

orders, is a risk factor for suicide and suicide attempts (APA, 2003).

Some individuals who complete suicide have panic disorder along with a major depressive disorder and alcohol use, as well as an Axis II disorder, such as borderline personality disorder (APA 2003).

Borderline Personality Disorder. DSM-IV-TR criteria for borderline personality disorder include "recurrent suicidal behavior, gestures, or threats, or self-mutilating behavior" (APA, 2000). Often the individual with this disorder experiences suicidal behavior when there is a loss or a perceived loss (Gunderson, 1984; Masterson, 1976). The trait of impulsivity is an important risk factor for suicide attempts with individuals with borderline personality disorder. It is therefore essential for nurses to assess the client for impulsive behavioral patterns (Oldham, 2006) (see Chapter 13).

Alcohol and Other Drugs

There is a high occurrence of alcohol and other drug use with suicidal behavior. The practice guidelines state that alcoholism increases the rate of suicide completion by six times that of the general population. Alcohol is a strong risk for suicide and is present in 25% to 50% of individuals who completed suicide (APA, 2003).

Garlow initiated a study exploring differences in patterns of cocaine and alcohol use before completion of suicide. Of the individuals who used cocaine before completed suicide, 94.6% were male, with 51.4% African American and 43.2% white. The white adolescents used alcohol, cocaine, or both before completing suicide (50% of the study population), and 41.7% used alcohol before the suicide attempt. African-American adolescents in this study did not use any substance before the suicide attempt (86.7%) (Garlow, 2002). Drugs contribute to poor, impulsive decisions that lead to high-risk, self-injurious behaviors. A high percentage of alcohol- and drug-related automobile accidents among teens are sometimes suicide attempts.

Some factors to consider when determining the risk of suicide in individuals who abuse alcohol or drugs are comorbid depression or the loss of a relationship, job, or functioning because of a medical illness. Social isolation, increased drinking, recent unemployment, and a poor social system all increase the risk of suicide. If an individual has some legal issues, he or she should be monitored for suicidal risk.

Medical Illnesses

Physical health problems are also a component of the profile for persons at risk for suicidal behaviors because of their co-occurrence with depression. The Medical Outcomes Study, one of the first major national studies to link medical illnesses and depression (Wells et al., 1989), found the physical and social dysfunctions associated with depression were greater than with most chronic medical conditions. Researchers believe depression causes as much physical and social impairment as chronic heart disease. In the study, depressed persons perceived their current health as poor and experienced greater body pain. In comparison with chronic illness, the physical functions of depressed clients were worse than those of clients with hypertension, diabetes, arthritis, and gastrointestinal and back problems. When depression and a medical condition such as advanced coronary artery disease coexisted, the client suffered nearly twice the loss of social function that occurred when either condition existed by itself. Suicide risk also increased in such coexisting conditions (Waem et al., 2002).

A complicating factor is that these clients often seek medical care for their health problems, and health care providers often miss the coexistence of a depressive disorder. It is important to assess the individual with a medical problem, particularly a chronic or potentially fatal illness, for signs and symptoms of depression.

Physical health problems often add to the emotional pain experienced by suicidal persons and sometimes contribute to their decision to end their life. Nurses play a critical role in assessing clients for depression and suicide risk in medical-surgical health care settings. Alerting the health care team to these findings will help to prevent suicide attempts and deaths.

Erroneous Beliefs About Suicide

Despite the numerous studies done on suicide, the massive efforts to educate people about suicide risk and the efforts of mental health advocacy groups, mistaken beliefs and myths still exist. Several long-standing incorrect beliefs contribute to errors in judgment when assessing for suicidal intent. These beliefs are listed in Table 21-1.

CLINICAL DESCRIPTION

The assessment of suicide risk is an important skill for the professional nurse practicing in all clinical settings. Only voicing a concern about a client's possible suicidality to other members of the health care team is not an adequate or safe response. The nurse needs to use interviewing skills to talk directly with the client and family about suicide during the initial nursing assessment and at points of reassessment in the treatment process. Being alert to the client's past medical history and the psychiatric history of suicidal behavior gives the nurse clues for identifying areas for further inquiry.

This section describes the background information needed to complement the assessment phase of the nursing process. Definitions of the five levels of suicidal behavior are listed in Box 21-3, along with risk factors. Of-

TABLE 21-1

Erroneous Beliefs and Facts About Suicide

ERRONEOUS BELIEF	FACT
People who talk about suicide do not commit suicide.	Most people communicate directly about their suicidal intent verbally, in writing, through artwork, and behaviorally through previous suicide attempts. These are all high-risk indicators of suicidal intent. Manipulation is not usually a factor. Treat all messages of intent seriously.
People who are serious about committing suicide do not give clues.	Most suicidal people give warnings of their intent by giving away possessions; wrapping up business affairs; isolating from friends; demonstrating an increased incidence of accidents; being preoccupied about death in writing, music, and art; and making self-deprecating comments related to worthlessness and hopelessness.
Young children do not commit suicide.	There were 250 suicide deaths of children between 10 and 14 years old in 2003 in the United States. Consider all threats from young children seriously. Suicidal behavior is the leading cause for the psychiatric hospitalization of young children.
An improved mood means the suicide crisis is over.	Persons who completed suicide often showed improved mood and energy before their deaths. The improved mood and energy level mean that the person's ambivalence has ended and that he or she has made the decision to commit suicide.
Only people with the diagnosis of depression kill themselves.	Although depression is the single best indicator of suicidal risk, some people who commit suicide are not diagnosed as depressed, although they often experience depressed feelings. At risk are those with schizophrenia, substance-related disorders, panic disorder, posttraumatic stress disorder, obsessive-compulsive disorder, and the manic phase of bipolar disorder. Some people do not exhibit a specific mental disorder at all (e.g., an older man who commits suicide after learning that he has terminal cancer or after his beloved wife of 60 years dies suddenly).
Individuals who self-mutilate are really suicidal.	Self-mutilation occurs when the individual has difficulty adjusting his or her affect or is feeling numb after an emotional upheaval or trauma flashback. People who are suicidal are thinking about death, as opposed to individuals who self-mutilate who are overwhelmed with unmodulated feelings.

ten the five levels of suicidal thought or action are called *suicidal behaviors*, yet it is important to be specific in naming the types of thoughts and actions in the nursing assessment with clear descriptions or examples so that others are able to judge the level of intent.

Risk Factors for Suicide

Nurses need to use the knowledge of risk factors to assist in assessing intent and lethality. Risk factors based in part on key points from the epidemiologic findings are listed in Box 21-4. Box 21-5 describes a mnemonic useful for remembering the warning signs of suicide.

Lethality Assessment Factors

In addition to the suicide risk factors, nurses need to consider the assessment of **lethality**, or the potential for causing death related to the level of danger associated with the suicide plan. **Imminence** (the likelihood that an event will occur within a specific time period), intent (the method chosen and its accessibility), and level of hopelessness often help determine the level of lethality and the extent of interventions required for safety.

Imminence Versus Nonimminence

The determination of imminence is critical. If persons are imminently in danger of killing themselves, the nurse will need to act quickly. However, determination of imminence is subjective and at best is a clinical judgment based on the professional's experience, knowledge base, and intuition. The specifics of the suicide plan often offer clues as to when the individual will be ready to act.

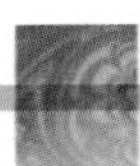

BOX 21-3

Five Levels of Suicidal Behavior

The following terms describe the five levels of suicidal thought or action:

1. **Suicidal ideation.** Direct or indirect thoughts or fantasies of suicide or self-injurious acts expressed verbally or through writing or artwork without definite intent or action expressed. Sometimes clients express this symbolically.
2. **Suicide threats.** Direct verbal or written expressions of intent to commit suicide but without action.
3. **Suicide gestures.** Self-directed actions that result in no injury or minor injury by persons who neither intended to end their lives nor expected to die as a result, but were done in such a way that others interpret the act as suicidal in purpose (e.g., taking eight tablets of valium 5 mg).
4. **Suicide attempts.** Serious self-directed actions that sometimes result in minor or major injury by persons who intend to end their lives or seriously harm themselves. Gestures and attempts that are unsuccessful and of low lethality are sometimes called *parasuicidal behavior.*
5. **Completed or successful suicides.** Deaths of persons who ended their lives by their own means with conscious intent to die. However, it is important to note that some suicides sometimes occur based on unconscious intent to die (e.g., engaging in high-risk activities).

Some mental health professionals define imminence as the likelihood that the person will engage in suicidal behavior within the next 24 hours. A specific plan, access to lethal measures, behaviors that signal a decision to die, and admission of wanting to die suggest imminent risk for

BOX 21-4

Risk Factors for Suicide

- **Age.** Persons most at risk for suicide are youth ages 15 to 24 years and older adults age 65 years and older, with those 85 years and older being the most vulnerable.
- **Sex.** Men by far have a greater incidence of completed suicides. Women have a higher rate of suicide attempts and gestures.
- **Race/ethnicity.** Suicide rates for whites are twice those of nonwhites. However, rates for African-American men over age 85 years are increasing faster than those for any other group. Second most at risk are young African-American and Native-American males.
- **Physical and emotional symptoms.** High-risk indicators are serious depression, significant changes in weight, serious sleep disturbances, extreme fatigue and loss of energy, self-deprecation, anger, feelings of hopelessness, and preoccupation with themes of death and dying. Serious depression is often a sign of suicidal behavior.
- **Suicide plan.** The presence and nature of the suicide plan are the most critical factors in assigning suicide risk. A plan clearly signals forethought and intent and often helps determine the level of lethality. Plans that are more precise, detailed, and explicit about the method indicate high risk. If the method described is highly lethal (e.g., a gunshot to the head versus an overdose of pills), and if the method is readily available, the risk is elevated even more. Add alcohol and other drugs, poor impulse control, and limited time for rescue attempts, and the risk reaches a critical level. Plans often include giving away possessions and sometimes mention of the intent to join a deceased loved one in afterlife, especially if the loved one had committed suicide.
- **History of previous attempts.** The majority of persons who complete suicides have made previous suicide attempts.
- **Social supports and resources.** The availability of a support system for a suicidal person often determines the outcome of an emotional crisis. This "life line" of caring, support, confrontation, and limit setting, as appropriate from family, friends, and community resources, assists suicidal persons in choosing other alternatives in solving their problems. Real or perceived lack of support systems or failure to use the support system that is available significantly increases the risk for suicide.
- **Recent losses.** One of the major emotional determinants of suicidal behavior is real or perceived losses, separations, or abandonment. Unresolved grief reactions lead to depression and suicidal behavior.
- **Medical problems.** Persons who suffer painful, debilitating, acute or chronic conditions or who have terminal illness are of special concern for suicide risk.
- **Alcohol and other drugs.** These substances are often lethal companions to suicidal acts. Drugs lower inhibition, heighten depression, and quicken impulsivity. According to estimates, at least 50% of adolescents are legally drunk at the time of their death by suicide. An even higher percentage has a history of recent alcohol or other drug abuse.
- **Cognition and problem-solving ability.** The inability to adequately identify problems and corresponding solutions greatly contributes to the choice of suicide as a solution to problems.

BOX 21-5

Warning Signs of Suicide: IS PATH WARM?

I Ideation
S Substance abuse

P Purposelessness
A Anxiety
T Trapped
H Hopelessness

W Withdrawal
A Anger
R Recklessness
M Mood change

A person in acute risk for suicidal behavior most often will show one or more of the following warning signs:

- Threatening to hurt or kill self or talking of wanting to hurt or kill self
- Looking for ways to kill self by seeking access to firearms, available pills, or other means
- Talking or writing about death, dying, or suicide when these actions are out of the ordinary

These might be remembered as expressed or communicated *ideation.* If observed, seek help as soon as possible by contacting a mental health professional or calling 1-800-273-TALK (8255) for a referral.

Additional warning signs:

- Increased *substance* (alcohol or drug) use
- No reason for living, no sense of *purpose* in life
- *Anxiety*, agitation, unable to sleep or sleeping all the time
- Feeling *trapped*, like there is no way out
- *Withdrawing* from friends, family, and society
- Rage, uncontrolled *anger*, seeking revenge
- Acting *reckless* or engaging in risky activities, seemingly without thinking
- Dramatic *mood* changes

If observed, seek help as soon as possible by contacting a mental health professional or calling 1-800-273-TALK (8255) for a referral.

Courtesy American Association of Suicidology, 2006, www.suicidology.com.
These warnings signs were compiled by a task force of expert clinical researchers and translated for the general public.

the client. This is especially true if combined with a sense of hopelessness, no vision of the future, or guilty thoughts. If a person has a high lethality (imminently dangerous to self) and refuses treatment, there is a legal consideration for safety called an involuntary hold-and-treat status. Each jurisdiction has rules and regulations that govern involuntary psychiatric admission. However, the client normally receives care in an inpatient setting, usually for 72 hours, depending on specific state statutes. This allows clinicians to hospitalize these individuals for an evaluation of risk and to determine appropriate treatment recommendations. These clients' rights are protected to prevent abuse. Those judged not to be imminently in danger of hurting or killing themselves sometimes choose less restrictive treatment options such as partial hospitalization programs or outpatient programs. In some states, involuntary outpatient treatment assists an individual who has demonstrated a risk over time to harm him or herself or others. This involuntary outpatient treatment usually involves an outpatient structured program and medication administration. An advance directive is generally written that gives the individual choices in care, such as where the individual wants to be hospitalized, any specified practitioner to provide care during the crisis period, and any reactions to medications the client has experienced in the past. The combination of requests outlined in the advance directive and the legal statutes mandating care provide a level of safety for the individual at risk (APA, 1999). *Any suicidal thoughts or behaviors, whether ideation, threat, gesture, or attempt, indicate an emergency situation and require prompt assessment and intervention.* Suicide risk and imminence usually decrease after health care providers answer the cry for help and establish support systems for those at risk.

Ideation vs. Intent

Suicidal ideation, or thinking about suicide without clear intent, places a person at lower risk than a person who intends or proposes to die through a suicidal act. There are two categories of intention: conscious and unconscious. **Conscious suicidal intention** has various aspects of awareness:

- Awareness of the outcomes or anticipated results of the suicidal behavior
- Awareness of others' responses to suicide threats or attempts
- Awareness of the lethality index of the chosen method
- Awareness of rescue possibilities (i.e., part of the plan includes various avenues of rescue or the plan is designed so that rescue is difficult or remote)

Unconscious suicidal intention is often more difficult to assess because it requires a higher level of skill and knowledge of psychodynamic theory. Often, there is a cluster of symptoms characteristic of the dynamics of self-destruction: depression, anxiety, guilt, hopelessness, hostility, and dependency, along with fantasies symbolic of death, hurting others, killing oneself, failure, and hopelessness. The motivation to hurt or kill oneself is outside of awareness, yet the client often expresses it by extreme risk-taking behaviors. For example, a platform parachutist who jumps from low heights off stationary objects such as buildings, towers, or cliffs has unconscious wishes to hurt himself or end his life. Others seek dangerous occupations, such as skyscraper workers, bridge builders, and high-wire artists without nets, as metaphors for suicidal wishes. Some may place themselves in dangerous, vulnerable situations that result in their deaths at the hands of others (e.g., victim-precipitated homicides). Some psychiatric clients unconsciously manipulate others through suicide threats or attempts and unconsciously arrange to be found or rescued. Unfortunately, the rescue plans sometimes fail, resulting in completed suicides.

It is important to listen to the communication of intent among suicidal persons. Often, individuals who were at higher risk and have completed suicides communicated their intent in advance only to their significant other. Individuals who are at moderate risk of suicide communicate this by threatening suicide to family members or health care providers. Nurses are able to anticipate how severe the intent is by listening to the extent of the suicidal thoughts of the individual, as well as the feelings of hopelessness and the availability of a method to carry out the suicidal plan (Box 21-6).

Nurses need to carefully observe and listen for direct and indirect communication regarding clients' suicidal intent. They need to listen not only for the words but also for the underlying themes that the words refer to or symbolize. Although a suicidal intent seems manipulative in terms of the individual's reason for this action, nurses should never ignore it. *Suicidal intent accompanied by imminence represents a high level of lethality.*

Chosen Method and Accessibility

The third determining factor of lethality is perhaps the most critical. The method and its availability determine the outcome of the suicidal behavior. People are more likely to seriously injure or kill themselves if there is an easily accessible means or method.

Persons who complete suicide tend to engage in only one high-lethality act through violent methods: using firearms, piercing of vital organs, hanging, jumping from high places, or using carbon monoxide poisoning. Men who complete suicides are more likely to select more violent means and use guns or knives or hang themselves; women are more likely to jump from high places or overdose. Nonfatal attempters tend to engage in multiple, low-lethality acts and use self-poisoning by pill ingestion (the most common method for suicide attempts), followed by wrist cutting. These methods allow time for rescue because of the slowness of their physiologic actions. Most who attempt suicide use the same method for repeated suicide attempts.

Accessibility to dangerous weapons raises the suicide risk. The increase in youth suicide rates is in proportion to the increased use of firearms. The most rapid increase in firearm

BOX 21-6

Severity Index for Suicide Risk

1. ***Suicidal ideation.*** No risk of suicide.
2. ***Mild thoughts of suicide.*** Passing thoughts of suicide. For example, "This is stupid, don't think like that; you have much to do yet, like raising your child." The client tells you that he or she is not going to make any suicide attempt. The client has support systems in his or her life and is able to identify a purpose for living.
3. ***Moderate thoughts of suicide.*** The client thinks about suicide as an option for solving his or her problems. The client describes the feeling of wanting to go to sleep and never wake up. The client has no plan for suicide. Client states that he or she does not want to die so much as escape from problems. The client has support people in his or her life but does not utilize them because the client feels that he or she is a burden to others. Religious beliefs help prevent suicidal tendencies.
4. ***Advanced thoughts of suicide.*** The client makes a suicidal gesture, not necessarily lethal (e.g., a small overdose, cutting wrists), or has more intrusive thoughts of suicide, and tells the psychotherapist or nurse that he or she is suicidal. The client does not use a support system, starts to give things away, does not buy needed items, and checks insurance policies. The client rationalizes religious beliefs. This client needs hospitalization to prevent a lethal suicide gesture.
5. ***Severe thoughts of suicide.*** The client wants to die and cannot identify any other solution but suicide. The client cuts off communication with others and isolates self from others. The client demonstrates an increase in energy after deciding on the details of suicide, including the means of death and the place and time death will occur. The client does not always tell the plan to the psychotherapist or nurse because that person will possibly intervene and prevent the suicide attempt. If the client is experiencing auditory hallucinations, he or she will not tell the psychotherapist or nurse about the commanding voices because the voices are demanding that the client not talk about the suicidal ideas. The client has begun to question and rationalize his or her relationship with God, if any, and states that he or she is not worthy in God's eyes. The client experiences intrusive thoughts of death and suicide throughout most of his or her thought process.

Data from Green E, Katz J, Marcus P: Practice guidelines for suicide/self-harm prevention. In Green E, Katz J, editors: *Clinical practice guidelines for the adult patient,* St Louis, 1995, Mosby.

suicides has been in the 15- to 24-year age range. Because of the increasing availability of firearms and other weapons, it is important for parents to be aware of the activities and peers of their children. Parents, guardians, and teachers need to investigate any clues or signs of self-destructive behavior, symptoms of mental illness such as paranoia or psychosis, or any verbalizations regarding violence toward self or others to prevent a possible tragedy, such as the shootings as Virginia Polytechnic Institution.

Suicidal clients in psychiatric hospitals or on psychiatric units in general hospitals are high suicide risks. The most vulnerable periods for attempts are within the first 24 hours after admission and as discharge approaches. Close observation is necessary as clients move from one suicide precaution level to another. Remember that *a sudden brightening of affect or lifting of depression signals that the client has resolved his or her indecision about living or dying and has made the decision to commit suicide.* Some clients have attempted or completed suicide while they were not on suicide precautions at all. Observation of all clients at least every 15 to 30 minutes, whether or not they are suicidal, is vital in detecting early clues to self-destructive behavior.

CLINICAL ALERT

Asking suicidal clients and their family members about their **access to dangerous weapons** *must* be a part of the nursing assessment. Many will verify that there are guns and other dangerous weapons in the home that are easily accessible. If the clients are experienced in firearms use (e.g., police officers, military personnel, or hunters), the risk for suicide rises sharply. Make provisions at the end of the assessment to secure the weapons, and have family and friends remove them from the home or from automobiles and trucks. Usually, a physician's order is necessary before dangerous weapons are returned to the at-risk client.

Hanging is the most prevalent suicide method used in hospital settings. Sharp objects are usually not available to clients, as part of the safety program of the unit. However, clients have used sheets, towels, belts, cords, plastic garbage bags, shoestrings, and articles of clothing to create nooses. Other clients "cheek" their psychotropic medications and use them later in overdose attempts. Some chronically suicidal clients who sneak sharp objects into the hospital are prone to cutting attempts, usually of the wrists or antecubital areas of the arms. Clients diagnosed with borderline personality disorders or dissociative disorders are especially prone to these attempts. Searching the client on admission and when returning from off-ground passes is an important safety intervention to detect razors, knives, pieces of glass, and aluminum cans.

It is not possible to prevent all suicides, even in the most secure facilities such as psychiatric hospitals and jails, but *close observation and continued reassessment of suicide risk minimize the chances of completed suicides.* Mental health professionals have an obligation to protect clients from harming themselves, just as parents and significant adults must be responsible for youth who demonstrate signs of self-destructive behavior requiring prompt intervention.

PROGNOSIS

Suicidal behavior is a treatable mental health problem. The prognosis for many suicidal clients is related to the severity of their accompanying mental disorder. Because most suicidal behavior is connected closely to major depressive disorders, effective treatment of depression reduces the risk of suicide. The majority of clients with depression who are treated with antidepressant medications demonstrate increased improvement or complete remission of their depressive symptoms (APA, 2003). Clients with schizophrenia and panic disorder who maintain therapeutic blood levels of the prescribed psychotropic

CLINICAL ALERT

A sudden **change in affect** for the better or a dramatic lifting of depression is an indication that the person has made the decision to commit suicide (is no longer ambivalent or uncertain about it). Increased energy and the ability to concentrate and plan the suicidal act facilitate the suicidal actions. *Be alert.*

medications also have a favorable response and a positive outcome related to reduction in suicide risk (see Chapter 24 for further information about medication).

DISCHARGE CRITERIA

Discharge criteria are necessary guidelines for both the client and the nursing staff and lead to a completion of treatment goals. The admission assessment establishes the groundwork for discharge criteria. An accurate, thorough, and knowledgeable assessment and appropriate treatment plan promotes effective interventions and timely discharge activities. Discharge criteria help to establish time frames to achieve goals, designate areas of responsibility and accountability through documentation, and meet specific institutional, professional, certifying, legal, or funding requirements.

Discharge criteria for the suicidal client include the following:

- Indications that the client is no longer imminently suicidal
- Determination that the client's living environment is safe for his or her return
- A consistent, available support system for the client to determine if the client has self-destructive feelings
- A commitment from the client to use psychotherapy to understand the crises that led to the suicidal ideation or attempt
- An agreement by the client to use a suicide hotline (1-800-SUICIDE or 1-800-273-TALK) or call a supportive friend or family member if suicidal ideation happens again

THE NURSING PROCESS

ASSESSMENT

The nursing assessment is a critical step toward ensuring the client's safety. Accurate assessment, continuing throughout the course of hospitalization, helps the nurse provide appropriate intervention and discharge planning. Determining an individual's risk for self-harm requires a thorough evaluation of factors that contribute to suicidality (e.g., a mental status examination and an evaluation of the client's support resources).

The initial assessment helps determine the presence of specific risk factors. Noting the presence of symptoms does not necessarily mean that a client is suicidal. However, recognizing a cluster of certain symptoms within a given time frame is necessary to accurately assess suicidal intent.

When assessing the client's risk for suicide, the nurse will observe for the following:

- *The observable behavior of the client.* A calm client may be highly suicidal, whereas an agitated client is not always in danger. Although appearances are deceiving, increased irritation (Shneidman, 1985, 1996) often signals an imminent suicide attempt, evidenced by impulsivity, restlessness, excessive motor agitation, and a brightening of affect. With some clients, however, withdrawal, apathy, irritability, and immobility intensify with suicidality. Suicides do occur in hospitals. It is important that nurses consistently monitor a suicidal client's behavior, affect, and interactions with others. Lethality levels increase during hospitalization, particularly as depression lifts and discharge is about to happen.
- *The history from the client.* Careful scrutiny sometimes reveals events that contribute to current self-destructive thoughts. It is important to determine why the client is feeling suicidal at this time. In gathering the client's history, the nurse will identify self-defeating coping patterns and past experiences that have negatively affected the client's self-esteem. Making note of significant anniversary dates will help to predict a future suicide attempt.
- *Information from friends or relatives.* Nurses obtain useful information regarding the client's history from friends or relatives. Often it is helpful to interview the client and family together and separately in case the friend or relative is hesitant to speak openly in front of the client. The nurse assesses how family members and friends feel about the client's suicidal behavior. Family members who are angry, disgusted, or frustrated with the self-destructive client will actually provoke the client to complete a plan of suicide.
- *History of suicidal gestures or attempts.* The suicide attempt is often a way of coping with painful feelings. People who have used this coping style in the past are at greater risk for using it again.
- *The mental status examination.* Disturbance in concentration, orientation, and memory suggests possible organic brain syndrome or a severe major depressive disorder, which reduces the client's impulse control and increases the potential for self-harm. Disturbance in thought processing evidenced in command hallucinations, places the client at greater risk to act destructively (refer to Chapter 3 for a discussion of mental status examination).
- *The physical examination.* Always conduct a physical examination when there are obvious signs and symptoms of substance abuse (e.g., impaired attention, irritability, euphoria, slurred speech, unsteady gait [walk], flushed face, psychomotor agitation, needle tracks), previous suicide attempts (e.g., scars on wrists), or debilitating medical conditions, including chronic pain.
- *The nurse's intuition.* The nurse's own feelings of uneasiness, anxiety, or unexplained sadness are

NURSING ASSESSMENT QUESTIONS

Suicide

1 Is the client hopeless? Does the client see no prospects for the future? Does the client express that there are no solutions to his or her problems?
2 Has the client made a recent suicide attempt? Are the client's suicide attempts severe or multiple? Does the client show impulsivity?
3 Are suicide attempts increasing in frequency or lethality? Is the client obsessing or fantasizing about suicide or death?
4 Does the client have insomnia with suicidal thoughts at night that continue into the early morning hours?
5 Is the client anxious? Are there any symptoms of panic or posttraumatic stress disorder (PTSD)?
6 Does the client have bipolar disorder, postpartum psychosis, or psychotic depression? Is the client experiencing pathologic grief, especially with command hallucinations, guilt, or other co-occurring conditions (e.g., chemical dependency, alcoholism, or personality disorder)?
7 Is there a history of suicide by a relative or close friend? Is the client isolated? Does the client lack resources and available family?
8 Does the client have detailed suicidal plans? Are lethal means available to the client for suicide, such as a gun or other weapon?
9 Did the client leave a suicide note or give away valued possessions?
10 Is the client becoming increasingly frustrated with therapy, illness, or problems? Is the client feeling powerless and unable to learn how to cope?
11 Has the client been offered electroconvulsive therapy (ECT) and demonstrated ambivalence over it? Has the client interpreted the recommendation as an admission of failure and hopelessness versus a positive solution?

A yes answer to any one of these questions suggests that the client needs careful assessment by the treatment team for possible admission to a locked facility, with suicide precautions instituted as per policy.

Developed by the Committee for Suicide Assessment, Sharp Mesa Vista Hospital, San Diego, California.

sometimes the only clues that a seemingly calm client will act on suicidal impulses. Although these feelings seem like intuition, research suggests that "intuitive feelings" tend to be based on previous experiences in similar client care situations. Nevertheless, if the nurse does not "feel right" about a client, do not ignore this important source of information (see Chapter 3 for more information on intuitive reasoning).

Use the questions in the Nursing Assessment Questions box above to determine the client's risk for suicide.

The following discussion refers to the Case Study. The nurse knew the first task of assessment was to make psychologic contact with the client. She planned to listen to how Scott viewed his situation and then communicate her understanding of his thoughts and feelings. The nurse realized that it was important to establish rapport and trust with Scott. She believed that the client-centered approach, developed by Rogers (1961), facilitated open communication and in turn assisted her in more accurately assessing Scott's risk for suicide (see Chapter 23 for more information about Carl Rogers).

The nurse used empathic listening techniques by listening for both facts and feelings (i.e., what happened and how the client felt about it). The nurse demonstrated caring and interest by using reflective statements so that Scott knew the nurse had heard what he had been saying.

When feelings were obviously present but not yet expressed, the nurse would gently comment, "I sense how upset you are by the way you are speaking. It seems like you are also angry and frustrated about what has happened."

Psychologic contact does not always happen solely through verbal communication. Sometimes, nonverbal, physical contact is quite effective. A gentle touch on the forearm or placing an arm around a shoulder will have an important calming effect and signify human concern as well.

The nurse demonstrated concern for Scott by offering him a tissue when his eyes filled with tears. The nurse not

CASE STUDY Scott, age 26 years, had been hospitalized at age 19 years after overdosing on tricyclic antidepressants. At the time, Scott's suicide attempt seemed to be linked to the end of a 3-year relationship with his girlfriend. Since the initial episode of major depression, Scott successfully graduated from college and returned home to live with his mother after his father died. Soon, however, he began to feel frustrated and inadequate when he could not find a job that suited his education and intellectual capabilities. Scott was eventually forced to accept a part-time position that paid minimum wage and lacked benefits. When his steady girlfriend suddenly relocated to another state, he felt rejected and abandoned.

Scott's mother, who noticed that he had become more withdrawn and isolative, was concerned that Scott was possibly self-destructive. After finding a loaded pistol lying on a table next to Scott's bed, his mother phoned the local mental health crisis intervention center to discuss her concerns about her son's behavior. While talking with the intake nurse, she mentioned that Scott had recently instructed her to donate his body organs to medical science "if anything should happen" to him. The nurse requested that Scott come to the center immediately for an assessment to determine his risk for suicide.

CRITICAL THINKING

1 What information did the nurse gather during the phone conversation with Scott's mother that alerted her to his need for an immediate suicide assessment? Why is this information pertinent to suicidal ideation?
2 What other factors will the nurse consider when assessing Scott's risk for suicide during the face-to-face evaluation?
3 Identify one factor noted in the assessment that will help reduce Scott's risk for self-harm.

NURSING ASSESSMENT QUESTIONS

Case Study: Scott

1. What does the client (Scott) understand about why his mother suggested he come to the center for a mental health assessment? *To determine if the client will validate his mother's concerns or deny that a problem exists*
2. What was Scott's intention in having a loaded gun lying next to his bed? Did he intend to kill himself or someone else? *Asking directly about a client's intentions will decrease anxiety and feelings of humiliation and shame.*
3. Has Scott taken antidepressants or mood-stabilizing medications in the past? Currently? Have medications used in the past been effective in improving Scott's mood and lowering his lethality level? Does he have access to other lethal means of suicide?
4. When was the last time Scott used alcohol or other drugs? When was he last intoxicated? *Clients who use alcohol and other drugs are at higher risk to complete a suicide attempt; increased impulsivity, disorientation, and confusion, which often accompany drug and alcohol use, place people at higher risk for suicide.*
5. With whom does Scott share his feelings? *To determine if Scott has a trusted and reliable support system; if so, the lethality level is lower*
6. What were the circumstances surrounding the death of Scott's father? Is there a history of depression or suicide on either side of Scott's family? *To determine the nature of Scott's father's death, family history of depression, or family style of coping, all of which increase the risk of suicide*
7. The nurse asked Scott's mother: "How do you feel about Scott's thoughts of suicide?" *To determine if Scott's mother is a support resource for him*

only recognized and acknowledged his feelings but also responded in a calm, controlled manner, resisting the tendency to become anxious, angry, or depressed because of the intensity of the client's feelings. During the assessment of Scott, the nurse included the questions in the Nursing Assessment Questions box above.

After a suicide attempt, an individual sometimes continues to be at high risk for attempting suicide again. When clients are admitted to the hospital after a suicide attempt, ongoing assessments are necessary to determine whether the person continues to be at high risk.

NURSING DIAGNOSIS

Clients who are suicidal are frequently admitted to psychiatric units, emergency departments, and intensive care units of general medical hospitals. Suicide attempts occur before or during hospitalization. Hangings, medication overdoses, and jumps from high places are frequent methods of suicide in hospitals. An accurate nursing diagnosis based on a thorough, ongoing assessment is necessary when identifying and prioritizing the client's needs for nursing interventions.

A complete nursing diagnosis is individualized and related to the client's behaviors and nursing needs. Validation of the nursing diagnosis with the client is necessary. However, some clients deny suicidal intent or the need for extra precautions. In the case of the diagnosis of risk for suicide or risk for self-directed violence, nurses must take caution in determining the level of risk. *It is best to err on the side of caution when diagnosing suicidality than to allow serious injury or death to occur.*

The primary nursing diagnoses for these clients may be the following:

- Risk for suicide
- Risk for self-directed violence

Secondary diagnoses may include the following:

- Ineffective coping
- Hopelessness
- Powerlessness
- Chronic low self-esteem
- Social isolation
- Disturbed thought processes

OUTCOME IDENTIFICATION

Outcomes come from the nursing diagnoses and are anticipated, expected client behaviors or responses achieved as a result of nursing interventions. State outcomes in clear behavioral or measurable terms, prioritizing them according to client needs, from most urgent to least urgent.

Client will:

- Remain safe and free from self-harm.
- Verbalize an absence of suicidal ideation/plan/intent.
- Verbalize a desire to live and list several reasons for wanting to live.
- Agree to inform staff immediately if suicidal feelings/thoughts recur.
- Display brightened affect with broad range of expression and spontaneity and speech that reflects a hopeful, optimistic attitude.
- Initiate social interactions with peers and staff (individually and in groups).
- Use effective coping methods to counteract feelings of hopelessness.
- Express a sense of self-worth. Meet own needs through clear, direct methods of communication.
- Verbalize realistic role expectations and goals for meeting them.
- Demonstrate absence of psychotic thinking (e.g., delusions, command hallucinations directing self-harm).
- Make plans for the future that include follow-up psychotherapy and prescribed medication compliance.
- List several friends or supportive individuals (such as a clergy member) or use a suicide hotline (1-800-SUICIDE or 1-800-273-TALK) to prevent a possible suicide attempt when experiencing increased suicidal thoughts.

- The plan of care emphasizes a reduction in the risk of self-destructive behaviors by monitoring the client's behaviors and providing a safe environment, promoting feelings of self-worth and hope, improving coping skills, limiting social isolation, and building self-esteem.
- The client is encouraged to follow the discharge plan of psychotherapy and medications, if ordered.

REVIEW QUESTIONS

1 A nurse assesses five new clients admitted to a psychiatric unit. Which client(s) would have the highest risk for suicidality? You may select more than one answer.
1. 86-year-old white male
2. 36-year-old African-American male
3. 65-year-old white female
4. 22-year-old African-American male
5. 20-year-old Native-American male

2 A nurse administers medications to a client on suicide observation. Which action by the nurse is most important?
1. Inform the client about the name, action, and side effects of the medication.
2. Verify that the client swallowed the entire dose of the medication.
3. Document the client's willingness to voluntarily take the medication.
4. Tell the client it takes several weeks for the drug to reach a therapeutic level.

3 When counseling a client with suicidal ideation, which comment by the nurse would be most therapeutic?
1. "I'm glad to see you taking ownership of your problems and trying to find solutions."
2. "When you experience negative feelings, try to focus on something more positive."
3. "Let's make a chart of all your problems and try to create solutions for each one."
4. "Let's talk about which problems are most important and which are least important."

4 A client draws a picture of dark skies shadowing a cemetery. How would a nurse document this level of suicidal behavior?
1. Ideation
2. Threat
3. Gesture
4. Attempt

5 A nurse reviews the report from a depressed client's PET scan. Which finding is most likely if the client has high-lethality suicide attempts?
1. Increased serotonin activity in the medulla, midbrain, and hypothalamus
2. Decreased serotonin activity in the ventral, medial, and lateral prefrontal cortex
3. Decreased dopamine and glutamate receptors in the parietal and temporal lobes
4. Increased norepinephrine and acetylcholine reserves in the thalamus and pons

Additional self-study exercises and learning resources are available to you on the ***Companion CD*** *at the back of the book and on the* ***Evolve website*** *at* ***http://evolve.elsevier.com/Fortinash/.***

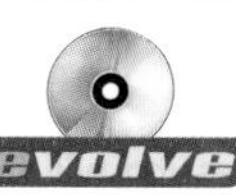

ONLINE RESOURCES

American Association of Suicidology: **www.suicidology.org**

American Foundation for Suicide Prevention: **www.afsp.org**

The Link Counseling Center: **www.thelink.org**

National Suicide Prevention Lifeline: **www.suicidepreventionlifeline.org**

Suicide Prevention Resource Center: **www.sprc.org**

Survivors of Suicide: **www.survivorsofsuicide.com**

Yellow Ribbon Suicide Prevention Program: **www.yellowribbon.org**

REFERENCES

American Association of Suicidology: African American suicide fact sheet; facts about suicide and depression; elderly suicide fact sheet; suicide in the USA based on current (2003) statistics; survivors of suicide fact sheet; and youth suicide fact sheet; retrieved Sep 3, 2006, from www.suidology.org.

American Psychiatric Association: *Resource document on mandatory outpatient treatment* Washington, DC, 1999, American Psychiatric Association.

American Psychiatric Association: *Diagnostic and statistical manual of mental disorders*, ed 4, text revision, Washington, DC, 2000, American Psychiatric Association.

American Psychiatric Association: *Practice guideline for the assessment and treatment of patients with suicidal behaviors*, Arlington, Va, 2003, American Psychiatric Association; www.psych.org.

Carroll L: Children who are bullied more often depressed and suicidal, *Reuters Health Information;* retrieved June 18, 2003, from www.medscape.com/viewarticle/457001.

Centers for Disease Control and Prevention: Self-inflicted injury/suicide; retrieved Sept 4, 2006, from www.cdc.gov/nchs/fastats/suicide.htm.

Chiles JA, Strosahi KD: *Assessment and treatment: clinical manual for assessment and treatment of suicidal patients*, Washington, DC, 2005, American Psychiatric Publishing.

Durkheim E: *Suicide*, Glencoe, Ill, 1951, The Free Press (originally published as *Le Suicide* in 1897).

Ezzell C: Why? The neuroscience of suicide: physical clues to suicide, ScientificAmerican.com, Jan 12, 2003; retrieved Oct 18, 2003 from www.sciam.com/print_version.cfm?articleID=000D8D31.

Freud S: *Mourning and melancholia*, Collected papers, London, 1920, Hogarth Press (originally published in Germany in 1917).

Garlow SJ: Age, gender, and ethnicity differences in patterns of cocaine and ethanol use preceding suicide, *Am J Psychiatry* 159:615-700, 2002.

Gunderson JG: *Borderline personality disorder*, Washington, DC, 1984, American Psychiatric Press.

Hendin H et al: Problems in psychotherapy with suicidal patients, *Am J Psychiatry* 163:67-72, 2006.

Lieb R et al: Maternal suicidality and risk of suicidality in offspring: findings from a community study, *Am J Psychiatry* 162:1665-1672, 2005.

Linehan MM: *Cognitive-behavioral treatment of borderline personality disorder*, New York, 1993, Guildford Press.

Litman R: Sigmund Freud on suicide, *Bull Suicidology*, p 11, 1967.

Mann JJ et al: Family history of suicidal behavior and mood disorders in probands with mood disorders, *Am J Psychiatry* 162:1672-1679, 2005.

Maris R: The adolescent suicide problem, *Suicide Life Threat Behav* 15:91, 1985.
Masterson JF: *Psychotherapy of the borderline adult: a developmental approach*, New York, 1976, Brunner/Mazel.
McDaniel JS, Purcell D, D'Augelli AR: The relationship between sexual orientation and risk for suicide: research findings and future directions for research and prevention, *Suicide Life Threat Behav: Am Assoc Suicidology* 31(suppl):84-105, 2001.
NANDA-I: *NANDA nursing diagnoses: definitions and classification 2007-2008*, Philadelphia, 2007, NANDA-I.
Nielsen D et al: Suicidality and 5-hydroxyindoleacetic acid concentration associated with tryptophan-hydroxylase polymorphism, *Arch Gen Psychiatry* 51:34, 1994.
Nyman A, Jonsson H: Patterns of self-destructive behavior in schizophrenia, *Acta Psychiatr Scand* 73:252, 1986.
Oldham JM: Borderline personality disorder and suicidality, *Am J Psychiatry* 163:20-26, 2006.
Parsey RV et al: Lower serotonin transporter binding potential in the human brain during major depressive episodes, *Am J Psychiatry* 163:52-58, 2006.
Qin P, Agerbo E, Mortensen PB: Suicide risk in relation to family history of completed suicide and psychiatric disorders: a nested case-control study based on longitudinal registers, *Lancet* 320:1126-1121, 2002.
Qin P, Agerbo E, Mortensen PB: Suicide risk in relation to socioeconomic, demographic, psychiatric, and familial factors: a national register-based study of all suicides in Denmark, 1981-1997, *Am J Psychiatry* 160:765-377, 2003.
Richman J: *Family therapy for suicidal people*, New York, 1986, Springer.
Rogers C, editor: *On becoming a person*, Boston, 1961, Houghton Mifflin.
Rudd D et al: Problem-solving appraisal in suicide ideators and attempters, *Am J Orthopsychiatry* 64:136, 1994.
Shneidman E: *Definition of suicide*, New York, 1985, John Wiley & Sons.
Shneidman ES: *The suicidal mind*, New York, 1996, Oxford University Press.
Stekel W: Suicide and will. In Freidman P, editor: *On suicide*, New York, 1967, International Universities Press.
Sullivan H: Socio-psychiatric research: its implications for the schizophrenia probelm and mental hygiene, *Am J Psychiatry* 10:977, 1931.
Sullivan H: The manic-depressive psychosis. In Perry H et al, editors: *Clinical studies in psychiatry*, New York, 1956, WW Norton.
Swann AC et al: Increased impulsivity associated with severity of suicide attempt history in patients with bipolar disorder, *Am J Psychiatry* 162:1680-1687, 2005.
Waem M et al: Burden of illness and suicide in elderly people: case-control study, *Br Med J* 324(7350):1355-1358, 2002.
Weiss J: The suicidal patient. In Arieti S, editor: *American handbook of psychiatry*, New York, 1966, Basic Books.
Wells K et al: The functioning and well-being of depressed patients, *JAMA* 262:914, 1989.

Chapter 22 Violence and Forensics in Clinical Practice: Abuse, Neglect, Anger, and Rape

ANN WOLBERT BURGESS and DONA PETROZZI

What is done to children they will do to society.
KARL MENNINGER

OBJECTIVES

1 Describe various theories of family violence for application to nursing practice.
2 Discuss conditions that discourage a battered person from leaving a violent situation.
3 Discuss the role of control in the etiology of domestic violence.
4 Compare the child physical offender with the child sexual offender.
5 Define child maltreatment in terms of emotional and psychologic abuse, physical abuse, and sexual abuse.
6 Construct examples of how society revictimizes women who are raped.
7 Apply the nursing process in the care of victims of family violence.
8 Describe the dynamics of sexual assault.
9 Identify the barriers in identifying elder abuse.

KEY TERMS

acquaintance rape, p. 484
battering, p. 487
child abuse, p. 492
child neglect, p. 492
domestic violence, p. 483
elder abuse, p. 500
emotional abuse, p. 493
family development phases, p. 483
family violence, p. 483
forensic evidence, p. 488
homicide, p. 485
psychologic abuse, p. 493
sexual victimization, p. 493
stalking, p. 484

Violence is a pervasive public health problem that plagues contemporary society. According to the Federal Bureau of Investigation (Bureau of Justice, 2003) someone reports a violent crime every 2 minutes in the United States, the highest incidence of any industrialized nation in the world. As a society, we have become increasingly concerned with both the physical injuries associated with violence and with the traumatic psychosocial impact it has on its victims. A traumatic event indefinitely inhibits overall functioning, altering an individual's perception of themselves, of others, and of the world. Indeed, the threat of terrorism, such as on September 11, 2001 or the school massacre at Virgina Polytechnic Institute in 2007, and biochemical warfare in the twenty-first century has impacted the nation's sense of safety and security. As survivors of violence continue to seek treatment in the clinical setting, nursing is expanding its professional practice and knowledge base to address the complex needs of victims of violence. Nurses are frontline responders and practice in a wide variety of settings. They need to be prepared to address the issues relating to the assessment, care, and protection of victims of violence, whether the abuse occurs at the hands a family member, a stranger, acquaintance, date, or caregiver. Nurses need to direct therapeutic interventions to prevent additional abuse, violence, and even death.

VIOLENCE WITHIN FAMILIES

The United States has made great progress since the 1950s. As a result of groundbreaking research, journal articles and books, and media attention, there are now more than 15,000 child abuse prevention, rape crisis, domestic violence, and elder abuse prevention programs throughout the United States. In particular, nurses have been pioneers and actively involved in providing services to victims of domestic violence and crime.

The possibility that people might be injured or that strangers have invaded their homes is a frightening thought, but hundreds of thousands of Americans face an even more devastating reality when they are harmed not by strangers, but by someone they trusted. Vicious crimes of violence occur against children, parents or grandparents, spouses, and other close relatives.

The family is still the center of society. Abuse by a partner, a parent, a trusted adult, or one's own child or to witness such abuse leaves deeply ingrained memories and other serious consequences. Victims of **domestic violence** wrestle with different emotions than do other victims of violence. They deal with mixed feelings of fear, loyalty, love, self-blame, guilt, and shame, all at the same time. Adults become torn between the desire to shield and help a loved one and their responsibility toward their own safety and the safety of others in the household. Children face the reality that those who should protect them are in fact the source of harm. For most people, home represents security; to domestic violence victims, home is a place of danger.

The problem of **family violence** has always existed. Spousal abuse has existed in almost every society in the world. The beginning of services for battered women and children dates back to 1885 when the Chicago Protective Agency for Women, established to help women who were victims of physical abuse, provided legal aid, court advocacy, and personal assistance to the women. However, by the 1940s, few shelters remained, partly because of marital separations caused by World War II.

Throughout history, there has been evidence of children suffering, from biblical times to the present. The landmark Wilson case of 1874 opened America's eyes to the difficulty of many children. Eight-year-old Mary Ellen Wilson lived with her adoptive parents in New York City. She was held there in chains, starved, and beaten. The police responded but did nothing because it was a "family matter" and parents held the "rights" (Zigler and Hall, 1989). A man named Henry Berg had founded a protective group the preceding year called the American Society for the Prevention of Cruelty to Animals. Berg was able to rescue Mary Ellen from her family torture chamber.

This section presents definitions and current statistical trends from a developmental perspective of family violence. It covers bullying behavior as a precursor to abusive dating relationships, courtship abuse, partner threat and violence, domestic violence and pregnancy, batterers' stalking patterns, and domestic homicide. It also discusses key concepts of family violence such as socialization into violence and learned socialized violence; the psychodynamics of violent behavior including altered attachment, jealousy, guilt, and revenge; and the biology of trauma.

BULLYING BEHAVIOR

Because of its connection to violent and aggressive behaviors that result in serious injury to the self and to others, bullying is now considered a major public health issue. Once viewed as a ritual of childhood and adolescence, bullying has now captured media headlines nationally and internationally (Burgess et al., 2006).

Bullying is the abuse of power by one child over another through repeated aggressive behaviors. For some bullies, power comes from physical strength and maturity, from higher status within a peer group, by knowing another child's weakness, or by recruiting support of other children. As bullies age, they rely less on physical means to intimidate their victims and turn to indirect forms that include verbal abuse and social exclusion (Olweus, 1991). Nurses are conducting research on childhood teasing and bullying. For example, the use of bibliotherapy is an innovative approach recommended to school nurses as they work to promote a healthful school environment (Gregory and Vessey, 2004).

DEVELOPMENTAL ASPECTS OF THE FAMILY AND ITS STRUCTURE

Just as there are developmental stages and tasks for the child maturing into an adult, there are also three **family developmental phases** that families progress through. The first phase begins with dating, courtship, and marriage; the middle phase includes partnership and work, with childbearing and parenting being an option; and the third phase continues a work focus, optional grandparenting, and retirement. Because violence within families has only recently surfaced as a legal matter, research into the causes and consequences is limited. As a first step, the definitions help to begin classification for the research process.

Family

Nowhere in the criminal law and its administration is the social construction of violent crime changing more rapidly than in what constitutes family violence and society's response to it (Reiss and Roth, 1993). Because of the many different statutes and regulations, there is no national legal definition of a family.

Trends in family violence, according to Reiss and Roth (1993), need to be interpreted against a decline in the percentage of households containing exclusively married couples and their biologic children. Violence between growing numbers of same-sex and opposite-sex cohabiting partners is increasingly regarded as family violence

NURSING ASSESSMENT QUESTIONS

For the Battered Woman

1 We often see women who have been hurt by their partners. Is your partner responsible for your injuries?
2 Has your partner ever hurt you?
3 Have you noticed any pattern to this behavior such as an increase in frequency and severity?
4 Does he threaten to use or has he ever used a weapon to hurt you?

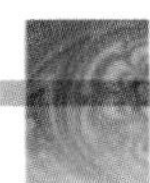

BOX 22-2

General Case History Questions for the Abused

1. Have you ever been emotionally or physically abused by your partner or someone important to you?
2. Within the past year, have you been hit, slapped, kicked, or otherwise physically hurt by someone? If yes, by whom and how many times?
3. Within the past year, has anyone forced you to have sexual activities? If yes, who and how many times?
4. Are you afraid of your partner or anyone else listed above?

the injury are cues that indicate abuse. Often, abused women seek treatment for indirect effects of their violent relationships. Complaints reflect the stress of these violent relationships or residual pain from past injuries. Often the woman appears depressed, anxious, and fatigued. Behaviors manifested in these depressed victims include soft speech, poor visual contact, hypervigilance, decreased interest in daily activities, and suicidal ideation. The battered woman typically has more chronic, pain-related, vague complaints than her nonbattered counterpart. Health history indicates frequent accidents and other traumatic injuries such as lacerations, bruises, and fractures. Spontaneous abortions, suicide attempts, and substance abuse also may be reported.

Other potential indicators of abuse are in the family history. The following potential indicators relate to the woman's partner:

- Strict disciplinarian
- Belief in physical punishment
- Child abuse
- Alcohol and drug abuse
- Extremely possessive and jealous
- History of violence in his family of origin
- Unemployed
- Seeks to isolate family members

Assessment of the battered woman begins with the nurse's critical examination of her or his own beliefs and biases about battering. For example, if the nurse believes that a woman has brought the problem on herself for not leaving the abusive relationship, then the nurse will communicate this attitude, consciously or unconsciously, to the battered woman. The nurse's attitude and resulting interactions can often revictimize the woman.

Because holistic assessments are the foundation of the nursing process, culture is an important consideration in that assessment. Culture often defines how the battered woman interprets and responds to violence she has experienced. Understanding the battered woman's culture is critical for developing a treatment plan. Culture is also an important determinant of whether the battered woman seeks assistance from community resources such as the police and shelters. Some ethnic women are isolated and unaware of community resources for abuse, are suspicious of caregivers outside of their own cultural group, and fear judgment from their cultural group if they reach out to the broader community. Most battered women's shelters make a concerted effort to reach out to women of all colors and ethnic groups. When caring for a client from a minority culture, it is the nurse's responsibility to learn about the client's culture in order to provide culturally sensitive care. Questions about the woman's culture are appropriate, but the nurse needs to present them in a sensitive, respectful way so that the woman understands that the nurse is concerned and is intent on learning more about the woman's values and customs to provide effective holistic nursing care.

An understanding of culture is as important when working with the male batterer as it is when working with the battered woman. Before planning treatment strategies for the abuser, the nurse respectfully acknowledges his cultural attitudes, values, and beliefs. No cultural beliefs and traditions, however, are acceptable or tolerable at the expense of another person's health and well-being. Because physical abuse, including rape, of women by the partners is common, it is critical to ask about physical, sexual, and emotional abuse in the histories of all women. The nurse also needs to ask if the abuser hits the children. Nurses will notify protective services if the children have been abused. Box 22-3 presents the most important physical examination indicators of wife/woman abuse.

The nurse accurately documents all statements the woman makes. Open-ended questions that reflect what the woman is disclosing will make the woman feel she is in charge of the interview. Documented information includes the name of the abuser and when and how the abuse occurred. The nurse records direct quotes from the survivor and documents with quotation marks to illustrate that the statement came from the victim. An inquiry into the safety of other persons in the home is also the responsibility of the nurse. If the nurse discovers that children, disabled, or elder persons are being abused in the home, then the appropriate protective agency or agencies are notified.

Forensic evidence is critical. Nurses document a detailed description of the woman's injuries in the narrative and use a body chart diagram to indicate the location and type of injury. In addition, the nurse collects bloodied or

BOX 22-3

Physical Indicators of Possible Abuse

GENERAL APPEARANCE
- Anxious and frightened
- Depressed and passive
- Ashamed and embarrassed
- Poor eye contact
- Weight problems
- Looks to partner for answers
- Partner does all of the talking
- Partner exhibits smothering and extremely possessive behavior

SKIN
- Contusions
- Abrasions and minor lacerations
- Scars
- Burns, particularly on breasts, arms, abdomen, chest, neck, face, and genitals

MUSCULOSKELETAL
- Fractures and sprains, especially of distal versus proximal bones (e.g., skull, facial bones, extremities)
- Dislocated shoulder
- Evidence of old fractures

GENITAL/RECTAL
- Evidence of vaginal/anal rape such as bruising, edema, and bleeding
- Evidence of direct kicks or punches

ABDOMINAL
- Internal bleeding or other injuries
- Chronic pelvic pain

NEUROLOGIC
- Acute stress disorder
- Hyperactive reflexes
- Chronic headaches and backaches
- Paresthesias from old injuries

soiled clothing and footwear and places the items in a paper bag as the items may contain vital evidence for the existence of domestic assault. All evidence is kept in a location that is accessible only with a lock and key until the police pick up the evidence.

The nurse asks the woman if she was forced into unwanted sexual acts and then examines her for anal and vaginal tears. If there is a possibility of marital rape, the nurse follows the rape protocol and uses an evidence collection kit. If a nurse suspects a sexual assault, a sexual abuse nurse examiner (SANE) will collect evidence. The nurse also assesses the woman for sexually transmitted diseases (STDs) and documents all laboratory and x-ray results. At least two photographs are taken of each injury before cleaning the areas, but the woman will first sign a consent form. The nurse places one set of photographs in the woman's record with identifying data on the back that includes the date, woman's name, hospital number, and name of photographer. Because of the possibility of future legal proceedings, the nurse requests a safe address from the woman where the second set of photographs can be mailed.

It is crucial to reassure the woman that the documentation is confidential and that her partner will not have access to it without her permission. Retaliation by the batterer is always a major concern for the abused woman. However, the woman needs to understand that she has the right to access her records and that these will be valuable to her in child custody cases or if she chooses to file charges against the abuser.

It is imperative to assess the woman's potential danger in cases of domestic violence. Information regarding the pattern of abuse and its severity and frequency is vital. Other critical signs that indicate increased danger are that the abuser has a weapon, has been violent outside the house, is a substance abuser, has been stalking the woman, and has threatened suicide/homicide. At times, some women contemplate suicide. It is well documented that the battered woman is at greatest risk of harm when she tries to leave her abuser (Walton-Moss and Campbell, 2002; Gelles, 1997). Therefore, it is imperative that the woman becomes aware of this risk, and the nurse assists her in developing a safety plan. Such a plan typically involves helping the victim create an emergency exit from the home, planning times to escape, and providing the phone numbers of nearby shelters, crisis lines, and community resources. In addition, the nurse refers the woman to the local victim's assistance program.

NURSING DIAGNOSIS

The following prioritized nursing diagnoses are examples of those that are relevant to the case study on Nina (see the Case Study on p. 490). They are based on information identified in the case study. However, all nursing diagnoses come from information obtained during the assessment phase of the nursing process. The accuracy of the diagnoses depends on a careful, in-depth assessment. Based on the provided information, the nurse identifies additional nursing diagnoses:

- Risk for injury related to present and past abuse by husband
- Pain related to injuries sustained by battering as evidenced by difficulty breathing deeply and sleeping (multiple fractures)
- Anxiety and fear related to threat of further battering
- Ineffective family coping related to abuse by husband and denial by wife

The DSM-IV-TR has not assigned a diagnosis for the battered woman. Stark and Flitcraft (1996) recommended the DSM-IV designation of "physical abuse of adult"—because it is not a formal diagnosis, it is nonstigmatizing and allows the woman access to resources. Some researchers and clinicians maintain that posttraumatic stress disorder (PTSD) is an appropriate diagnosis for many battered women who are repeatedly and severely abused (Briere, 1996; van der Kolk et al., 1996). The battered-woman syndrome is a description of what happens over time to the battered woman. This syndrome, as described by Walker (1994), has been allowed in courtrooms in all

CASE STUDY Nina's husband, to whom she has been married for 10 years, brought her to the emergency department. He was attentive to her, spoke reassuringly, and appeared concerned about Nina's condition. According to her husband, a day ago Nina slipped as she was getting out of the bathtub. When she slipped, she bumped her head on the faucet and then fell on her arm. As her husband spoke, Nina sat quietly with her head down. She cradled her right arm and appeared to be in severe pain. Her right eye was red and swollen shut, and she seemed to have some difficulty breathing. Despite protests from her husband, the nurse interviewed Nina separately from her husband in a private consultation room. Although the nurse inquired directly whether Nina's husband had beaten her, Nina denied the abuse. The physician performed a complete physical and neurologic examination and took a series of x-ray films. When Nina returned to her room, the physician told her that she had fractures of the wrist, facial bones, and several ribs. The x-ray films also indicated multiple old, healed fractures of the ribs and pelvic girdle. The nurse spent time explaining to Nina how unlikely it was for her injuries to result from a fall in the bathtub. The nurse also reassured Nina that nothing she could have done would deserve such abuse by another person. Nina finally acknowledged that her husband had abused her but insisted she had no intention of leaving him because he was a good husband. According to Nina, the only time her husband is abusive is when she fails to fulfill her domestic responsibilities and therefore provokes him into losing his temper and beating her. Nina has no children and no family nearby, except for a younger sister who is currently overwhelmed with her own family problems. Nina is psychologically and economically dependent on her husband and has no means of financial or psychologic support.

CRITICAL THINKING

1. What is the first priority for the nurse who suspects abuse when assessing a woman?
2. How should the nurse respond to the shame, guilt, and self-blame of the battered woman?
3. What should a nurse do if he or she becomes angry and rejecting with a battered woman who is in denial about being battered?
4. If you suspected that your neighbor was in an abusive situation, what signs would you look for in the relationship?

states as a defense in cases in which battered women have murdered their abusers.

OUTCOME IDENTIFICATION

The following prioritized outcome criteria come from the nursing diagnoses identified in the case study on Nina. These outcomes are the expected behaviors that Nina will demonstrate as a result of her plan of care. Stabilizing Nina's physical condition and securing her safety are the immediate short-term goals.

Client will:

- Report a decrease in her pain resulting from injuries sustained during her abuse.
- Demonstrate no difficulty breathing and verbalize feeling more relaxed.
- Demonstrate less fear and anxiety by being able to discuss her abuse and explore possible options for resolving it with the nurse.
- Verbalize an awareness of her increasingly dangerous situation because her abuse has intensified over time.
- Discuss with the nurse the implications for herself, her spouse, and other family members if she remains in the present abusive situation and explore with the nurse alternative means of family coping.
- Demonstrate an awareness of the need for safety by taking steps to protect herself in the future.
- Explore the possibility of pursuing litigation against her husband and requesting a restraining order if her husband is not jailed.
- Devise plans to secure her safety in case of future threats of abuse.
- Take advantage of community resources that increase her self-esteem and independence and become involved with an outreach group for battered women.

PLANNING

The plan of care for any survivor of violence focuses on securing the immediate safety of the victim, addressing critical physical problems, collecting appropriate evidence, examining the implications of the abuse on the woman and other family members, and discussing future plans for safety. In the case of a battered woman such as Nina, who acknowledges the abuse only when confronted by the nurse, the nurse needs to explore all possible options because she may need to use them in the future. The nurse develops the care plan with the client and recognizes that any effort to impose personal beliefs on the battered woman will ultimately fail. Instead, the battered woman needs reassurance that she is capable of making appropriate decisions for herself—even if her decision is to return to her abuser. It is only through empowerment, not threats and intimidation, that the woman is most likely to develop the strength to make independent decisions that foster growth.

IMPLEMENTATION

Once the battered woman's physical condition and safety have stabilized, it is critical to assess her future safety and collaboratively explore her fears, anxieties, and concerns. Despite the need to leave the abusive situation, the woman often strongly believes that she has no other option except to return. If the woman chooses to return to the batterer, it is important to respect this decision. Making a decision to leave the batterer is usually a gradual process. However, it is critical that the woman realize that she has options. The nurse often serves as the key factor in a beginning awareness that other options do exist.

At present, all states have laws that provide some level of protection for survivors of domestic violence, and there is a definite trend across the country to pass further legislation to ensure this protection. The reality is, however, that there is a large gap between the actual laws and their implementation by the police and criminal justice system. In some localities, police are mandated to arrest the abuser if there is evidence of probable violence. In many states the police have to provide the battered woman with

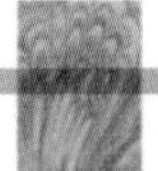

TABLE 22-1

Nursing Interventions for Battered Women

INTERVENTIONS	RATIONALE
Report abuse to police.	To provide for safety
Provide medications to relieve pain and anxiety.	To relieve her pain and reduce anxiety
Discuss validity of the woman's anxiety.	
Encourage the woman to discuss events leading to past and present abuse.	To reduce her guilt and shame
Point out the increasingly violent nature of the relationship and concern for her safety.	
Insist that no person has the right to abuse another.	
Explore effectiveness of her current coping skills and suggest additional skills.	To increase her independence and effective coping skills
Focus on strengths, endurance, and abilities.	To increase her self-esteem
Discuss destructive societal expectations of women.	
Discuss frequency of woman abuse.	
Explore family and/or friends as support possibilities.	To increase her awareness of potential support
Discuss potential for using community resources (e.g., shelters and/or hotlines and police).	
Describe current laws on domestic violence.	To increase her awareness of abuse implications
Explore implications of pressing charges against the batterer.	
Explore meaning of potential relationship loss.	
Explore various options for the future.	
Provide fact sheet on domestic violence.	To identify long-term goals
Provide referrals.	
Develop a safety plan with critical papers, money, clothing, and other essentials to be set aside for emergency exits.	
Offer to be available for further questions.	To provide continuity of care

information on local shelters, domestic violence crisis lines, and her legal rights. However, the police may not always respond appropriately, so it is important for the nurse to inform the battered woman of her legal rights.

In recent years, some women's rights advocates and criminal justice experts have debated mandatory reporting laws on domestic violence (Walton-Moss and Campbell, 2002). Women's rights advocates claim that mandatory domestic violence reporting laws discourage battered women from seeking treatment for their injuries because the women fear that health care providers will report their situation to the police and consequently place her in even greater danger with her abuser. Because some women are not ready to deal with the police, being forced to do this is nontherapeutic and disempowering and even increases their danger of abuse. If no mandatory reporting laws exist, then the nurse does not notify the police unless the woman consents. Although some professionals choose to maintain confidentiality if the battered woman requests it, the deciding factor on reporting is the degree of danger that the woman faces.

Nursing Interventions

Primary prevention for woman abuse begins with identifying families at risk and changing societal views toward wife abuse. Nurses need to educate clients on societal acceptance of violence against women as portrayed in films, television, magazines, and music. Nurses become more knowledgeable about factors such as poverty, drugs, access to guns, and unemployment, which increase the risk of domestic violence, and work with other members of the community to establish public policy and programs to address these issues.

Secondary prevention of woman battering involves early case finding and decisive prioritized intervention. Specific nursing interventions depend on the stage that the battered woman is in, because a woman in denial about the abuse requires a different strategy than one who is determined not to return to the relationship. In relationships where the abuse is just beginning and is mild, it is possible to work with the marital couple when both partners choose to do so. In these cases, the male accepts all responsibility for his abusive behavior of his partner and the counseling focuses on preventing further abuse. In many situations, an advanced practice nurse is the appropriate professional to work with the battered woman.

Tertiary prevention is necessary when the woman has been repeatedly abused, as in the case of Nina. In such instances, the focus is on helping the abused woman to overcome the physical and psychologic effects of the abuse and to prevent future abuse. Because the abuser frequently threatens and harasses the woman when she attempts to leave, it is often difficult for her to follow through. Frequently, these women seek assistance from local shelters that provide safety and counseling. Nurses are often in the position to provide support and counseling to battered women in shelters. The nursing interventions identified in Table 22-1 relate to the case study describing Nina, who requires tertiary prevention measures in an emergency department setting.

EVALUATION

Evaluation is a critical component of the nursing process. It is especially critical with the battered woman because inadequate or inappropriate nursing interventions will possibly result in more serious abuse or even death for the woman. Nurses who work in settings where battered women seek treatment need to be knowledgeable about the many different responses that occur in the battered woman. Correct evaluation of outcomes and interventions depends on this recognition. Once the nurse develops a complete nursing care plan, the evaluation is based on achievement of client goals.

CHILD MALTREATMENT

Since the beginning of time, children have been mistreated. The major types of **child abuse** are physical, psychologic, emotional, and sexual. As bruises, fractures, and lacerations are easy to observe and detect, physical abuse is the type most often reported. Sexual assault is not rare, but the victim and family often hide it. Emotional and psychologic abuse is often concealed, making it more difficult to detect and treat the victims, and is more long-lasting than physical injury.

The various types of **child neglect** (nutritional, medical, emotional, caregiver) are more subtle than abuse, but nevertheless they cause irreparable harm to the dependent child. About 10% to 15% of children who fail to thrive are nutritionally deprived, and a high incidence of such deprivation has been found in physically abused children. For religious or other reasons, parents deliberately deprive their children of essential medical care. Some parents are detached and disengaged and unable to provide the fundamentals for normal emotional development. Also, some children are not adequately supervised and therefore suffer major and repeated injuries.

No single theory explains the causation of child abuse. It is generally recognized that many complex interacting factors are involved that place children at risk for abuse. Box 22-4 summarizes the various theories of child abuse and neglect.

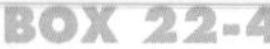

BOX 22-4

Etiologic Theories Related to Child Abuse and Neglect

BIOLOGIC THEORY

Parents who were abused as children are at risk for abusing their own children.

SOCIAL LEARNING THEORY

Family teaches and accepts violent behavior.
Violence is glorified in the media.
Violence is accepted in families, schools, and churches.

ENVIRONMENTAL THEORY

Socioeconomic level
Unemployment
Stressful life events

PHYSICAL ABUSE

Physical abuse, brought to health professionals' attention in the early 1960s by pediatrician Kempe as the "battered child syndrome," is the intentional physical infliction of injury by a parent or caretaker. The spectrum of injuries is broad, ranging from a few bruises to injuries that cause death.

Bruising is apparent through finger and palm prints on the face or buttock and through teeth or human bite marks. Loop and lash marks on the skin are easy to identify and indicative of a doubled over cord or belt. In most true accidents, bruising occurs on only one body surface, except when a fall occurs down a flight of stairs.

Burns are another source of physical abuse. A cigarette causes circular areas of similar size on the soles, palms, or abdomen. Hot-water burns are evident by a clear water level mark on the buttocks, perineum, or legs and are sometimes caused by dunking the child as a disciplinary measure for problems in toilet training. Dry contact burns to the palms of hands or the soles of feet occur from holding the child against a hot stove or radiator.

Fractures of the long bones, ribs, or skull are often apparent in abused and neglected children. Children with neurologic injury sometimes present in coma or convulsions and have suffered subdural or retinal hemorrhage.

Emily died on March 13, 2005, at the age of 9 months. She was the youngest in a family known to the Department of Children and Families for over 3 years. Emily suffered a broken leg, with no reasonable explanation, only 3 weeks before the injuries that led to her death.

A review of the Emily case revealed several points at which the extreme danger to children in this family was obvious. First, the medical staff at a local hospital failed to recognize the multiple injuries to a sibling as suggestive of abuse during sporadic clinic appointments. When the department of children's services received a report on severe medical neglect of another child, they did not understand the serious consequences of that neglect and did not seek medical information concerning the siblings (which would have revealed a pattern of possible abuse), and the case was closed. In October 2001, the police arrested the mother for risk of injury. The arrest record states that the officers found two children hanging out of an open, third-story window. There were no adults in the unheated apartment (52° F), there was animal excrement on the beds, and no food was available. The responding police officers placed the children with a relative, arrested the mother, and did not call the department of children's services until the next day. The last opportunity to avoid tragedy came in February and March of 2005, when Emily presented at a local hospital emergency room with a spiral fracture of her leg. The hospital reported this injury to the department of children's services 6 days after an emergency care physician and orthopedist initially treated the child. The counselor on this case believed the mother's explanation of an "accidental" injury. Emily remained in the home and was fatally raped and abused at the age of 9 months.

EMOTIONAL ABUSE

Often, the emotional abuse and neglect of a child is ignored until the child's formative years have been impaired by the threats and rejection that are an integral part of these families' day-to-day routines. The deprivation and misery that was a part of many neglecting parents' own childhoods often continues in their roles as parents or caregivers. They are indifferent to their children, do not wish to harm them, but have little capacity to help them. As a result, the children are more frequently withdrawn rather than aggressive.

Abusive language and verbal expressions of hostility are present in a high percentage of severely abusing families. Some parents state bluntly that they hate their children and never wanted them. Others wish their death and threaten to kill them. Frequently they yell and curse at them and call them derogatory names such as "idiot" or use other unspeakable terms. The parent will ridicule the child with comments such as "You are ugly, stupid, clumsy, hopeless, and never will amount to anything." Hopelessness, despair, and defeat are obvious in these children's attention-seeking and approval-seeking overtures for love. They trust no one and expect little except rejection.

Emotional abuse is the sustained, repetitive, inappropriate emotional response of the adult to the child's experience of emotion and behavior. Such actions do the following:

- Inflicts fear, humiliation, distress, despair
- Inhibits emotional feeling/expression
- Impairs emotional development
- Minimizes learning about emotional life
- Affects social development

PSYCHOLOGIC ABUSE

Psychologic abuse is not the same as emotional abuse. **Psychologic abuse** is the sustained, repetitive, inappropriate behavior that damages or substantially reduces the creative and developmental potential of crucially important mental faculties and mental processes of a child. These faculties and processes include intelligence, memory, recognition, perception, attention, imagination, and moral development. Psychologic abuse occurs in the following ways:

- Through domestic violence or desertion
- Unpredictability, lies, deception, exploitation by the parent/caretaker
- Various other forms of abuse (particularly sexual abuse, violence, and neglect)

Psychologic abuse impairs children's capacity to understand and manage their environment, confuses or frightens them, and renders them vulnerable (Brassard et al., 1993). Such abuse affects education, general welfare, and social life. The following also determine the consequences of psychologic abuse:

- The nature, intensity, and duration of the abuse
- The damaged mental faculties and processes
- The age and stage of development of the abused child
- The quality of life, treatment, and therapy following the abuse

SEXUAL ABUSE

A person achieves sexual contact with another person in three basic ways: (1) through consent, which involves negotiation and mutual agreement; (2) through exploitation, which involves a person's capitalizing on his position of dominance (economic, social, vocational, etc.) to take sexual advantage of a person in a lower position; and (3) through assault, which involves threat of personal injury or the use of physical force. The latter two methods constitute **sexual victimization** because a person is intimidated because of the individual's vulnerable status and, therefore, is not in a position to freely decide and determine his or her own sexual behavior. Only negotiation and consent properly achieve sexual relations. However, such consent is prohibited in sexual encounters between a child and an adult, by virtue of the adult being mature and occupying a position of authority and dominance in regard to the child. A child by definition is an immature person, and most children have not developed sufficient knowledge or wisdom or social skills to be able to negotiate such an encounter on an equal basis with an adult. Even a physically mature child is not matured enough to emotionally cope with the sexual demands from an adult. An older person or adult is able to easily take advantage of a child, and although the child agrees to and cooperates with the sexual activity, the child does so without an awareness or appreciation of the impact such activity will have on his or her subsequent psychosocial development, or personality formation, attitudes and values, and identity. In general, children are not well informed about human sexuality or adequately prepared for this important area of human behavior, and the offender exploits their innocence in self-serving ways that harm the physical, social, psychologic, and emotional development of the children.

Gaining Access to the Child

The child molester gains access to his victim through deception or by directly approaching the child. Use of the Internet by predators is a major source of this problem. In the majority of cases, the offender will use some type of psychologic pressure, such as enticement or encouragement, to persuade the child to enter into sexual activity, but in some cases the offender forces the child, either in the form of threats and intimidation or through physical strength.

Pressure Situations

The most common approach a child molester uses is to initially establish a nonsexual relationship with the victim, which has meaning to the child. The offender becomes a familiar and trusted figure in the child's life. Over time they introduce sexual intimacy into the context of this involvement. The offender deceives the child by misinterpreting social standards ("All boys and girls do this—it's okay.") or misidentifying the activity ("We're going to wrestle."), or tricking the child ("I'm going to give you a bath."), or presenting the activity in the context of game ("I've hidden some money in my clothes, and if you find it you can have it."). Then the offender rewards the child's cooperation with money, gifts, candy, or toys. Children will exchange the sexual activity for these other nonsexual rewards, and one of the most prized rewards is attention. The child molester capitalizes on the child's need for attention to lure the child into the sexual activity by making the child feel special or important.

Forced Situations

In fewer cases, the offender directly confronts the child with sexual demands in the content of verbal threats ("Do what I say and you won't get hurt."), intimidation with a weapon (e.g., brandishing a knife), or direct physical assault (e.g., grabbing the child). These tactics are to overcome any resistance on the part of the victim even though the intent is not to hurt the child. Such sexual assaults constitute child rape, in which sexuality becomes the means for expressing power and anger. The offender's method is either one of intimidation, in which the offender exploits the child's helplessness, naiveté, and awe of adults, or is one of physical aggression in which the offender attacks and overpowers the victim.

Acts of Sexual Assault

The sexual abuse of children includes a wide range of sexual acts perpetrated by persons 5 or more years older than the victim. These acts include exhibitionism, fondling or manipulation of the genitals, digital penetration, penile penetration of the vagina or rectum, or genital contact, insertion of foreign objects into the genitals or rectum, and the use of children in pornography and prostitution. Sexual abuse also includes noncontact sexual activity, such as sexually explicit language directed toward a child, obscene telephone calls, the showing of pornographic materials to a child, and voyeurism. Most sexually abused children experience multiple types of sexually abusive acts. The legal definition of sexual abuse varies by state jurisdiction, and nurses need to familiarize themselves with the laws in their district (Kelley, 1997).

Incest

Research on intrafamilial sexual abuse indicates that incest families are highly dysfunctional, although overtly they may appear normal. Studies do not find a correlation with incest and characteristics such as socioeconomic status, culture, race, and ethnicity. Incest seems to cross all boundaries.

Within incestual families, multiple forms of abuse are likely to be present including physical and other forms of psychologic/emotional abuse. Most incestual families are enmeshed, which means that they are relatively isolated from those outside the family and tend to focus most of their energies on relationships within the family. There are poorly defined boundaries within the family, and they often have excessive dependency on each other for physical, social, and psychologic needs. Role reversals often occur. One example is the abused child assuming a caregiver role for the parents and other family members. However, no single pattern accurately describes the complexity of the incestual family.

Offenders

Characteristics of offenders are primarily based on research of those cases that are examined within the criminal-justice system and therefore are more serious abuse cases. Most cases of sexual abuse are never reported, so these criminal cases are not representative of all offenders. Researchers have begun to focus on nonincarcerated offenders.

At present, experts recognize that child sexual offenders constitute a diverse population that is difficult to classify. Offenders vary in age, occupation, income, marital status, and ethnic group. Some researchers are also beginning to study the female perpetrator, because they believe that this group is more common than studies indicate (Barnett et al., 1997). Data showed that males were perpetrators in 89% of cases compared to 11% by females. Existing research on female perpetrators indicate that they are often accomplices to males or to a general pattern of abuse among all family members (Elliot, 1993).

More juveniles are being identified as offenders, and they demonstrate more violent behavior than do typical adult offenders (Prentky et al., 2000). In addition, more of these juvenile offenders are prepubescent and include growing numbers of female offenders (Schwartz et al., 2006). These juvenile offenders range in age from 5 to 19 years and represent all ethnic, racial, and socioeconomic classes; 90% are males. The majority of adult offenders report beginning their deviant sexual behavior during adolescence.

Characteristics of the Nonoffending Parent

When the abuser is the father, the mother is typically blamed for failing to satisfy her husband's psychologic and sexual needs, of being rejecting and dominating, and of expecting her daughter to assume the role of lover with the father and be caregiver to both parents. The literature has also blamed the mother for being absent when the incest occurred, even if she was working to support the family. In addition, the claims state that when the child discloses the abuse to the mother, the mother commonly denies that the abuse occurred or blames the child for initiating or encouraging it.

Although these are common themes in the literature, little or no research exists to support the claims. Many nonoffending mothers are initially shocked and unable to believe their child's claim of sexual abuse by the mother's partner. It is especially devastating to the woman if she loves and trusts her partner, because she now copes with her partner's betrayal in addition to her child being violated and traumatized. It is much simpler and less painful to believe that it did not occur. Nevertheless, many mothers who are initially in shock experience a process involving a crisis of disbelief or ambivalence followed by gradual acceptance and eventual dedication to healing the child's trauma as well as their own. It is probably most accurate to recognize that a variety of scenarios exist with regard to the nonoffending mother and that it is inappropriate to try to categorize the complexity of the nonoffending mother according to any one particular pattern or description.

Impact on Victim

The following factors demonstrate the impact on the young person who has been forced or pressured into sexual activity:

- *Relationship of secrecy and sexual activity.* Sexual activity that occurs over a period of time usually means that the offender has pressured the child into secrecy. If the offender is successful with his victim, he tries to hide the deviant behavior from others. In his attempt to achieve sexual control of the child, he will try to make the child swear to secrecy in several ways. The child is not always aware of the existence of the secret. The offender often says it is something secret between them, or in the entrapment cases he threatens to harm the child or parents if the child does tell. In most situations, the child experiences the burden to keep the secret as fear. Victims have spontaneously described the following fears, which bound them secretly: fear of punishment, fear of repercussions from telling, fear of abandonment or rejection, and communication barriers about use of correct words.
- *Conflict in feelings when the offender is a family member.* Psychologically, the child experiences the decision of siding with one of two family members as a sense of divided loyalty. When the offender is a family member, families are caught between two conflicting expectations. Should they be loyal to the child victim and treat the offender as they would treat any assailant—thinking of their duty as citizens to bring the offender before the law? Or should they be loyal to the offender, making an exception for him because he is a family member? Clearly, they cannot honor both expectations. They have to choose, and the choice is sometimes a difficult one. Careful attention to the feelings of the child is important for conflict resolution when the family knows the offender.
- *Vulnerability to physical and psychologic symptoms.* Young victims are more likely to express their distress through physical and psychologic means. School problems develop if the child is unable to concentrate and focus on studies.
- *Surveillance issue.* Children who have been pressured into secrecy over sexual activity often have been kept under surveillance by the adult authority figure. This enforced surveillance affects the victims' feelings and perceptions of themselves, especially the development of low self-esteem.
- *Sexuality.* Sexual identity is often compromised in young victims, as a result of premature introduction into adult sexuality or learning to use sex in the service of reward and approval.

LONG-TERM CONSEQUENCES: TRAUMA LEARNING

Nurses need to realize that when traumatized children become upset, it is hard for them to calm down because the behavioral inhibition of longer lasting hormones in the brain is not as effective as it is in nontraumatized children. Biologic dysregulation drives the shifts in integrative behavior. The following sections review and discuss the patterns of trauma learning, utilizing an expanded model of information processing of trauma. There is a progression of symptomology and behaviors for the victim of a traumatic event.

Integration of Trauma

The optimal response pattern from a traumatic event is that no posttraumatic stress disorder (PTSD) occurs, and there is subsequent integration of the traumatic event in to the life experience of the victim. In the integrated pattern, the patient is able to relate to the sexual abuse experience but is not required to think about it or avoid it through psychologic defenses.

Posttraumatic Stress Disorder

A classic PTSD response occurs in two phases. The victim displays intrusive or avoidant behaviors. Exposure to stimuli induces a state of hyperarousal and numbing, which causes the victim to experience highly emotional states with lower levels of thinking. The disruptions also have an impact upon sensory, perceptual/cognitive, and interpersonal performance.

Symptoms of sensory disruption include hyperactivity, headaches, stomachaches, back pain, genitourinary distress, and nightmares. Symptoms of interpersonal disruption include behaviors such as excessive fear of others and an inability to assert or protect oneself. Aggressive behaviors include agitation, aggression toward peers/family/pets, and potentially sexualized behavior toward others. Several patterns of PTSD symptoms are evident in traumatized children:

- The anxious pattern is generalized fears and anxious recollection of the abuse situation if probed or asked. Anxiety disorder, eating disorder, phobic disorder, and obsessive compulsive disorder are associated with unresolved trauma.
- The avoidant pattern is denial or recanting that the abuse has occurred. These youths often have a substance abuse history, depression and suicidal thoughts, phobic behavior, adjustment problem, or conduct disorder.
- The aggressive pattern is aggressive or sexual behavior. Minimal acknowledgment or denial of prior

abuse is typical. There is the testing and breaking of rules, impulsivity, and fighting with peers. Diagnostic labels of hyperactive, learning disabled, conduct disorder, or impulse disorder are sometimes used.
- The disorganized pattern is fragmented and sometimes bizarre behavior. Dissociative states need to be ruled out. There is often denial or amnesia for prior sexual abuse.

Delayed Posttraumatic Stress Disorder

Some victims of trauma do not initially develop PTSD but rather progress to delayed PTSD, displaying no visible connection to the event. Avoidant behaviors include low sexual involvement, passivity, substance use to reduce tension, somatic complaints and depression. Aggressive patterns include participating in high-risk behaviors and antisocial acts, substance use as a stimulant, and high sexual involvement.

THE NURSING PROCESS

ASSESSMENT

As with the assessment of other victims of violence, the nurse begins with an assessment of her own assumptions, beliefs, and attitudes about childhood sexual abuse. Nurses who believe that the child is responsible in any way for the sexual abuse find it difficult to be supportive toward the child. The nurse needs to be comfortable when speaking with the child about the abuse and avoid expressing a verbal or nonverbal attitude of discomfort to the child. Children are skilled at picking up nonverbal cues, and the child will interpret the nurse's discomfort as a sign that she should not talk about the abuse or that the nurse does not believe her or him.

As with all nursing assessments, a holistic approach is essential. Because childhood sexual abuse trauma is highly complex and multiple interacting factors affect it, the nurse needs to gain as much information as possible without subjecting the child to unnecessary and repeated questioning. Most often the nurse encounters the sexually abused child in the emergency department or outpatient clinic. Often, the mother or other caregiver brings the child to a medical facility to determine if the child has been sexually abused. Whenever there is a suspicion of childhood abuse, a complete physical examination is necessary.

The primary objective is to establish a trusting nurse-client relationship with the child so that she or he is as comfortable as possible in relating relevant events and cooperating with the physical examination. The developmental age of the child is an important factor in the ability to successfully provide data about the abuse; a young child is less able to describe events and understand the interviewer's questions. It is important to assess the relationship between the caregiver and the child to determine if the child is more comfortable with or without that person. Usually younger children do not want to be separated from their caregiver, whereas older children are often too shy to disclose in front of the caregiver for a variety of reasons, such as fear of blame from family members, disbelief, or breaking up the family. Sometimes the child retracts the disclosure in an effort to protect the abuser with whom she or he has had an ambivalent relationship.

The majority of children who have been sexually abused do not display any physical signs of abuse because the most common type of abusive activity is fondling, and it seldom leaves physical manifestations. The occurrence of oral copulation or mock intercourse is also difficult to physically document unless the examination occurs within a short time after the activity.

In addition to the lack of physical evidence, the sexually abused child does not always display signs of emotional trauma and denies, retracts, and is inconsistent when describing the abuse. Caregivers often interpret this behavior to mean that the abuse did not occur and the child is lying. The nurse needs to clearly explain to the child's caregivers that an absence of physical or emotional signs does not mean that abuse has not occurred. Conversely, multiple emotional/psychologic indicators are sometimes present; however, because many of these signs also reflect other problems, their presence alone is not a conclusive sign that sexual abuse has occurred. The diagnosis of sexual abuse is difficult and challenging because there is no single profile or set of symptoms that guarantees its presence. Many of the following signs and symptoms are only potential indicators of sexual abuse, whereas others are highly probable indicators. The American Professional Society on Abused Children (APSAC) Task Force (2002) has developed detailed psychosocial protocols and guidelines for health care professionals who interview and evaluate children for sexual abuse. Giardino et al. (2002) have published guidelines for evaluation of physical signs of sexual abuse. The indicators addressed in Boxes 22-5 and 22-6 come from these two sets of guidelines and from clinical observation.

Clearly, the nurse needs to explore the meaning of any child's acting-out behavior. Such behavior in abused children usually reflects the anger, confusion, and sense of betrayal that the child is experiencing and is unable to discuss. Although many abused children are able to act out their feelings through rebellious and delinquent behavior, others withdraw, blame themselves, become guilt ridden, and continuously try to be a "better" or "good" child. Such children function at a high level in school and are even praised and admired for what appears to be mature behavior because they often assume major responsibility for adult caregiver roles in their homes. Finally, some children with abusive histories do not exhibit signs of trauma during childhood but do exhibit them later in life, whereas others seem to escape trauma from abuse throughout their life. As previously discussed, the presence of sexual abuse trauma depends on a wide variety of complex factors, in particular, the degree to which the child receives validation, protection, and support after disclosure is crucial to the resolution of the trauma.

BOX 22-5

Physical Indicators of Possible Child Abuse and Neglect

GENERAL APPEARANCE
Excessive fearfulness and watchfulness
Disheveled and malnourished
Failure to thrive

MULTIPLE INJURIES
No history of significant trauma

SKIN
Unexplained bruises, welts, and scratches in various stages of healing (different colors)
Regular patterns of bruises and welts such as bite marks or marks from electrical cords
Untreated infected wounds
Lacerations from rope burns, especially on the neck, wrists, ankles, and torso
Bruises on buttocks, genitalia, thighs, side of the face, trunk, and upper arms

BURNS
Small round cigarette burns (infected insect bites resemble cigarette burns)
Immersion burns (even boundaries that are glovelike, socklike, or symmetric; accidental burns are asymmetric with splash marks)
Patterned burn marks (e.g., from an iron or grill)

FRACTURES
Fractures in infants younger than age 1 year
Fractures of femur, humerus, posterior ribs, skull, and long bones and any uncommon fractures

HEAD INJURIES
Skull fractures and subdural hematomas (leading cause of death among abused children)
Brain hemorrhages or contusions without external signs of injury (shaken baby syndrome)
Alopecia caused by hair pulling

ABDOMINAL INJURIES
Ruptured liver or spleen
Ruptured blood vessels
Kidney, bladder, or pancreatic injuries
Injuries to jejunum or duodenum

INJURIES TO EYES, EARS, NOSE, AND MOUTH
A wide variety of injuries including missing teeth, bruising, perforation of tympanic membrane, epistaxis and nasal fractures, retinal hemorrhage or detachment corneal abrasions, and periorbital hematomas

OTHER TYPES OF ABUSE/NEGLECT
Munchausen's syndrome by proxy
Deprivational syndromes

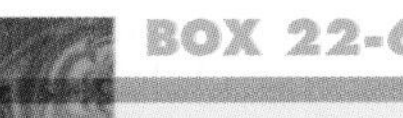

BOX 22-6

Physical, Behavioral, and Psychosocial Indicators of Possible Childhood Sexual Abuse

GENERAL APPEARANCE
Varies from normal to anxious, fearful, and depressed

PROBABLE PHYSICAL EXAMINATION INDICATORS
Bruises, lacerations, or bite marks on breasts, neck, buttocks, extremities, and oropharynx
Presence of sexually transmitted disease, including human immunodeficiency virus
Presence of adult pubic hair and semen
Edema, abrasions, petechiae, and erythema of genital area
Lacerations to vagina or anus
Alterations or enlargement of hymenal orifice
Dysuria caused by periurethral trauma
Rectal fissures, chafing and erythema, bruising, lacerations, and perianal scarring
Semen in the oropharynx or nasopharynx
Scar tissue of labia minora, hymenal membrane, and anus

HIGH-RISK FAMILY HISTORY INDICATORS
Substance abuse in caregivers
History of abuse in parents
Domestic violence
Inadequate impulse control/mental illness in caregivers
Alleged offender with sexual dysfunction or poor coping skills, poor social skills
Socially isolated family
Sexual abuse of sibling

BEHAVIORAL INDICATORS
Disclosure and spontaneous discussion of the abuse
Preoccupation with drawing genitals or anxious avoidance of anything to do with genitals/sex
Inappropriate sexual play behavior with dolls or other children, compulsive masturbation, inserting objects into vagina or anus, sexualized kissing, fondling genitals of others, and imitating intercourse
Dissociation
Avoidance of particular people
School/learning problems

POSSIBLE PSYCHOSOCIAL INDICATORS
Increased anxiety, fears, depression, low self-esteem
Multiple somatic complaints
Signs of posttraumatic stress disorder
Antisocial behavior, promiscuity, substance abuse
Running away, self-destructive behavior

NURSING ASSESSMENT QUESTIONS

For the Sexually Abused Child

1. Who do you like to play with best of all?
2. What kind of fun things do you and [name] do together?
3. What kinds of games do you and [name] play when mom isn't around?
4. Are there any games that you and [name] play that you don't like?

The assessment of child sexual abuse includes a physical examination, interviews with the child and family members, outside information from sources such as teachers and baby-sitters, and psychologic tests if needed. In general, the interview with the child needs to take place in an environment where the child feels safe and comfortable. As with all sensitive topics, questions begin with the least sensitive and most positive topics and progress to the most sensitive and direct ones. Initial questions gain the trust of the child and assist her or him to relax and become more spontaneous. The developmental age of the child is a critical factor in the type and level of question the nurse uses; therefore, nurses modify all techniques according to the child's needs. Small children have difficulty with nondirective, open-ended, or abstract questions. Interviewers need to be extremely cautious not to use leading questions such as "Daddy likes to tickle your bottom, doesn't he?"

The nurse's role is to provide comfort and safety for the child. Thus, the nurse needs to determine and address the immediate physical and psychologic needs of the child. Once the nurse has addressed these needs, it is always critical for the nurse and other health care professionals to make a determination as to whether the child will be safe if returned to her or his home.

Eventually the nurse has to ask the child directly about the possibility of sexual abuse. In a nonemergency situation, questions such as those listed in the Nursing Assessment Questions box are for a small child whose father, stepfather, or other male caregiver is suspected of the abuse.

NURSING DIAGNOSIS

The following nursing diagnoses are based on data identified in the case study on Suzy (see the Case Study). Nursing diagnoses come from the information obtained during the assessment phase of the nursing process. The accuracy of the diagnoses depends on a careful, in-depth assessment.

- Risk for injury related to sexual abuse by stepfather (increased chances of recurrence and possible prior incidents of sexual abuse by stepfather)
- Pain related to injuries sustained from abuse (physical, sexual)
- Anxiety and fear related to further abuse
- Disabled family coping related to sexual abuse by stepfather and mother's possible denial as evidenced by the mother's inability to protect her daughter

CASE STUDY Suzy is a 5-year-old girl who was brought to the emergency department by her mother and stepfather, Mr. and Mrs. Jones, because she was bleeding from the vagina. Mrs. Jones reported that while she was bathing Suzy in the tub, the phone rang, so she left Suzy for a few minutes to answer it. Mr. Jones claims that he went in to check on Suzy when he heard her crying and found her standing in the tub crying and bleeding from the vagina. Mr. and Mrs. Jones maintained that Suzy tried to get out of the tub but slipped and injured herself on the tub faucet. No other persons were in the home at the time of the accident. Suzy was obviously distressed and unable to give a history. She clung to her mother and would not allow anyone, including her stepfather, to touch her. On physical examination Suzy was found to have lacerations of the hymenal membrane and vaginal wall, trauma to surrounding perineal area, and old scarring.

CRITICAL THINKING

1. What are the possible explanations for the injury that Suzy received?
2. How would you best prepare Suzy for her physical examination?
3. What kind of questions and comments would be appropriate and helpful to Suzy?
4. How can the nurse structure the environment so that Suzy will feel safer?

DSM-IV-TR does recognize sexual abuse of the child. Many adult survivors have been identified as experiencing PTSD, but symptoms for both children and adult survivors of abuse vary greatly, and no single profile clearly describes sexual abuse survivors. However, sexual abuse is reportable under the DSM-IV-TR Axis IV, which focuses on psychosocial and environmental problems. For more information on DSM axes, see Chapter 3.

OUTCOME IDENTIFICATION

Outcome criteria for Suzy come from the nursing diagnoses identified earlier. These outcomes are the expected behaviors that Suzy and her mother will demonstrate as a result of the plan of care.

For Suzy, the first priority is addressing the physical trauma of the sexual abuse, which is the hymeneal and vaginal laceration and localized trauma to the perineal area. Presence of scar tissue indicates prior abuse. Depending on the extent of damage and bleeding, Suzy's injuries may require surgical repair. Based on her plan of care, the first outcome will focus on stabilizing her physical condition. The second priority will be to ensure that the abuse will not recur and the child will be protected in the future.

Child will:

- Report a decrease in pain and anxiety.
- Discuss her present perceptions, distortions, and fears with the nurse.
- Verbalize an awareness that she will be protected in the future and that no one will be allowed to injure her again.

TABLE 22-2

Nursing Interventions for the Sexually Abused Child

INTERVENTIONS	RATIONALE
Call police and protective services.	To provide for safety needs
Provide medication prn; reassure child that she is safe and that no one will hurt her again.	To relieve the child's pain and anxiety
Encourage her to talk about her fears and concerns.	To allow expression of feelings
Reassure her that she is not to blame and that her abuser did a bad thing to hurt her.	To reduce guilt
Verify that the appropriate agencies have been notified and will follow through.	To coordinate contact of appropriate agencies
Document the mother's responses in terms of supporting her child and being committed to protecting her child in the future.	To assess and strengthen the mother's coping abilities
Provide support and educate about potential resources (e.g., treatment centers, role of social services and criminal justice system).	
Educate the mother about the signs and symptoms of abuse that the child may exhibit and how to support her.	
Assess the mother for her ability to cope with possible feelings of grief and betrayal.	

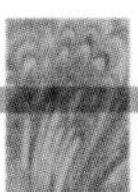

TABLE 22-3

Nursing Interventions for the Physically Abused Child

INTERVENTIONS (SECONDARY PREVENTION)	RATIONALE
Develop a trusting relationship with parents.	To provide environment for parents that facilitates their sharing the sequence of events leading to abuse
Be direct and open but supportive.	
Obtain a holistic history, including the stresses and problems the family is experiencing.	
Explore how to alter events that lead to abuse.	To problem-solve and educate on how to avoid similar scenarios in the future
Explore alternative strategies for child-care problems.	
Discuss basic child growth and development.	
Provide parents with basic materials on child growth and development.	
Have parents apply child development principles.	
Discuss need for parenting classes.	
Discuss strategies for anger control.	
Discuss reporting laws on child abuse.	To gain parental agreement to cooperate with protective services
Explain child welfare function of protective services.	
Take steps to inform protective services.	
Observe parent-child interactions unobtrusively.	To role-model providing care and support for child
Involve parents in child care during hospitalization when appropriate.	
Discuss physical impact of abuse with parents.	To have parents verbalize their understanding of abusive behavior on child
Discuss short- and long-term psychologic effects of child abuse.	
Provide referral to postdischarge public health child nursing.	To support parents in the prevention of future abuse
Coordinate services and monitor parental progress.	
Role model and assist parents to apply principles learned in parenting classes in their own lives.	To involve parents in child-care classes
Have father discuss how he will maintain anger management skills.	To demonstrate anger-control skills
Teach mother to intervene if father exhibits negative parenting.	
Help parents to develop social support systems.	To prevent isolation and expand support system
Explore community resources with family.	

Parent will:

- State the need to personally engage in the protection, safety, and nurturing support of the child.
- Follow through on referral sources for herself and her family. (Because Suzy's abuse was ongoing and severe, she will require an individual therapist.)
- Participate in individual or group therapy. (Many organizations exist that conduct groups for survivors, nonoffending parents, offenders, and siblings in families in which sexual abuse has occurred. All family members need to be assessed for the level of their therapy needs.)
- Attend parenting classes. (She will require assistance in learning how to nurture, support, and protect her daughter in the future.)

PLANNING

The plan of care for the abused child begins with stabilizing the child's physical needs, securing the child's safety, and addressing the child's psychologic needs (Table 22-2). Because the child depends on the parents for the continuation of these goals outside of the hospital, the nurse needs to address the family system as well (Table 22-3). In the case study on Suzy, the stepfather is the suspected abuser; therefore, the nurse clearly establishes that the stepfather will not have access to his stepdaughter and that the mother is capable of nurturing and protecting her child in the future. The attending staff will complete police and protective services reports.

IMPLEMENTATION

Nurses need to be educated about the signs and symptoms of childhood sexual abuse so that they are able to recognize them and take quick action in all potential cases. Because the child's safety is critical, nurses become knowledgeable about the laws in their state and the policies and procedures of their institution for caring for all survivors of abuse, especially children who are the most vulnerable. In severe cases such as Suzy's, the stepfather is removed from the home. Nurses are often the coordinators who make sure that protective services and law enforcement agencies are notified and that treatment referrals are made and are followed through. Usually the court mandates treatment after protective services and the criminal justice system make investigations.

Nursing Interventions

Types of long-term treatment depend on the child's developmental level and the mother's potential for supporting and protecting the child in the future. With a younger child, play therapy is often useful because the child often has difficulty verbalizing feelings about the abuse but is able to express them during interactive play with a skilled and empathic therapist. Group therapy with other young children is also useful because the child learns he or she is not alone in this distressing situation and is able to address common fears and misperceptions. As the child becomes able to repeatedly address these fears and misperceptions, they will gradually be resolved. Group therapy with other children is also a powerful modality for teaching self-assertive behavior and how to self-protect in the future.

A multitude of treatment modalities that have recently become available for adult survivors include antidepressant medications to treat depression, anxiety, and complex PTSD. Practice guidelines from the International Society for Traumatic Stress Studies (Foa, Keane, and Friedman, 2000) provide evidenced-based practice interventions for PTSD in both children and adults. These research guidelines indicate that cognitive behavioral therapy is effective in addressing the distorted guilt, blame, shame, and low self-esteem that survivors of childhood sexual abuse experience. Group therapy that incorporates cognitive- behavioral interventions is also a powerful modality. Somatic techniques are helpful in treating the psychobiology of the PTSD through body-mind integration exercises. These modalities include hypnotherapy, eye movement desensitization and reprocessing, imagery and deep breathing, art therapy, body-focused therapy, and thought field therapy (Wilson, Friedman, and Lindy, 2001; Phillips, 2000; Rothschild, 2000; Chu, 1998).

EVALUATION

Ongoing evaluation of the client and family outcomes reveals the efficiency of the nursing interventions and is critical to ensure that the child is protected and supported in order to recover from the trauma of the abuse. In addition, an ongoing evaluation of the caregiver is necessary to determine if this person is following through with the plan of care and to address any problems that occur. A reliable evaluation of the mother's motivation and ability to support and protect her child requires both short- and long-term assessment. Sometimes the mother becomes involved with another partner who is at high risk for abusing children. Thus, the mother has to confront her own behavior and the decisions she makes with regard to the safety of her children.

ELDER ABUSE

TYPES OF ELDER ABUSE

Elder abuse is classified as follows:

- Physical abuse of an elder is the use of physical force that results in bodily injury, physical pain, or impairment. Physical abuse includes but is not limited to acts of violence such as striking (with or without an object), hitting, beating, pushing, shoving, shaking, slapping, kicking, pinching, and burning. In addition, inappropriate use of drugs and physical restraints, force-feeding, and physical punishment of any kind also are examples of physical abuse. Nurses observe for signs and symptoms of bruises, black eyes, welts, lacerations, and rope marks; bone or skull fractures; open wounds, cuts, punctures, untreated injuries in various stages of healing; sprains, dislocations, and internal injuries/bleeding.
- Sexual abuse is nonconsensual sexual contact of any kind with an elderly person or sexual contact with a person incapable of giving consent. It includes, but is not limited to, unwanted touching; all types of sexual assault or battery, such as rape, sodomy, coerced nudity; and sexually explicit photographing. Nurses observe for bruises around the breasts or genital area; unexplained venereal disease or genital infections; unexplained vaginal or anal bleeding; and torn, stained, or bloody underclothing.
- Emotional or psychologic abuse is the infliction of anguish, pain, or distress through verbal or nonverbal acts. Emotional/psychologic abuse includes but is not limited to verbal assaults, insults, threats, intimidation, humiliation, and harassment. In addition, treating an older person like an infant; isolating an elderly person from his or her family, friends, or regular activities; giving an older person the "silent treatment"; and enforced social isolation are examples of emotional/psychologic abuse. Nurses observe for an elder who is being emotionally upset or agitated, is extremely withdrawn and noncommunicative or nonresponsive, or displays unusual

behavior usually attributed to dementia (e.g., sucking, biting, rocking).
- Neglect is the refusal or failure to fulfill any part of a person's obligations or duties to an elder. Neglect also includes failure of a person who has responsibilities to provide care for an elder (e.g., pay for necessary home care services) or the failure on the part of an in-home service provider to provide necessary care. Neglect typically means the refusal or failure to provide an elderly person with such life necessities as food, water, clothing, shelter, personal hygiene, medicine, comfort, personal safety, and other essentials included in an implied or agreed-upon responsibility to an elder. Nurses observe dehydration, malnutrition, untreated bedsores, and poor personal hygiene, as well as unattended or untreated health problems.

THEORIES ON ELDER ABUSE

Although many theories seek to explain elder abuse, no single theory is completely adequate (Box 22-7). Sengstock and Barrett (1993) identified three main elements for theories on elder abuse: abuser characteristics, situational stress, and family relationships. Pillemer (1986) identified five risk factors for elder abuse, which are within the three foci of Sengstock and Barrett: (1) psychopathology of the abuser, (2) external stress, (3) dependency, (4) social isolation, and (5) transgenerational violence.

Many frequently compare elder abuse with child abuse because in both cases neglect is common. With elder abuse, however, elders continue to have the rights of adults unless a judge declares them incompetent. Therefore, decisions cannot be legally forced on the elder as they can with children. Elders have the right to choose to remain in a particular environment, even when it is obvious that they are being abused or neglected.

> **BOX 22-7**
>
> **Etiologic Factors Related to Elder Abuse**
>
> **BIOLOGIC THEORY**
> Psychopathology of the abuser
>
> **SOCIAL LEARNING THEORY**
> Dependency (financial and relational)
> Social isolation
> Transgenerational violence
>
> **ENVIRONMENTAL THEORY**
> External stress

ELDER SEXUAL ABUSE

The incidence of elder sexual assault is difficult to estimate with any degree of confidence. The National Citizens' Coalition for Nursing Home Reform (NCCNHR) identified 1749 cases of such abuse in the institutionalized elderly in its first 3 years of keeping records starting in 1996. Furthermore, according to the National Crime Victimization Survey (2000), 261,000 rapes and sexual assaults occurred in the United States in 2000, with collateral data from the National Crime Victimization Survey of 2000 identifying 3270 of these victims as age 65 or older. Serious underreporting continues to occur, with an estimate of only 30% reported to police.

Underreporting of sexual abuse occurs in all age-groups in a significant number of cases with the extent of nondisclosure or nonreporting estimated as high as 68% (Bureau of Justice, 1990). For elders, the typically inherent nature of dependence on others (family members, caretakers, agency staff) often combined with physical frailty and/or alterations in mental status provide for increased risk of abuse with subsequently low rates of reporting. A National Institute of Justice report notes fear of the offender as the major reason for nonreporting (Tjaden and Thoenes, 1998).

From a medical standpoint, bruises are often attributed to the aging process rather than to an assault. Sometimes nursing procedures explain genital bruising (and bleeding) in institutionalized elderly as either a "botched catheterization" or "rough perineal care." Bruising to the abdominal area is attributed to tight restraints. Clearly, there are multiple reasons to believe that the known cases of elder sexual assaults are underestimates of the true number of cases.

DIFFICULTIES IN RECOGNIZING ELDER TRAUMA

There are no prevalent data on PTSD for those victimized by others in a crime or other forms of elder abuse. However, the literature suggests elder victims meet the diagnostic criteria for PTSD. Delayed onset of PTSD is an infrequently diagnosed variant of the disorder and is receiving attention among older combat veterans.

Another consideration with older adults is comorbid disorders. Many physical illnesses are attributed to elders including cardiac, respiratory, and cognitive impairment as well as psychiatric disorders including depression, substance abuse, and personality disorders.

Although the sexual assault of elders has likely been ongoing throughout time, it is clearly both a contemporary and an emergent public health issue requiring increased awareness, comprehensive and sensitive assessment, and foundational approaches for effective intervention to promote adaptive coping and mental health (Vierthaler, 2004).

Older adults residing in nursing homes are an especially vulnerable group. They often require assistance with basic activities of daily living such as bathing, dressing, and feeding because of physical and cognitive impairments. These disabilities make an individual dependent on others and an easy target for a sexual predator (Burgess et al., 2000).

There are approximately 17,000 nursing homes in the United States with 1.5 million older adults residents (United States General Account Office, 2002). In a study of 5297 nursing homes in Pennsylvania, New Jersey, and New York, a quarter of these nursing homes had serious complaints alleging situations that harmed residents or placed them at risk of death or serious injury (United States General Account Office, 2002). Concerns about the quality of care have mostly focused on malnutrition, dehydration, and other forms of neglect. However, there is growing concern about physical violence perpetrated by those who care for the elderly, particularly sexual abuse (Burgess et al., 2000).

Reasons for untimely reporting of allegations concerning the elderly residing in nursing homes include the following:

- Residents often fear retribution if they report the abuse.
- Family members are troubled with having to find a new place because the nursing home may ask the resident to leave.
- Staff do not report abuse promptly for fear of losing their jobs or recrimination from coworkers and management.
- Nursing homes want to avoid negative publicity and sanctions from the state and loss of revenue.

THE NURSING PROCESS

ASSESSMENT

It is critical to conduct the interview of the elder apart from the caregiver. In the hospital it is easy to simply state that hospital policy mandates that clients are assessed alone. If the nurse is conducting the interview at home, it is much more difficult to gain access to the elder; nurses even jeopardize their own safety by insisting on privacy. In these cases, assess suspected abusers for their potential to harm nonfamily members. This assessment needs to determine whether the abuser is a substance abuser or has a history of mental illness or violence, because these factors further compromise the nurse's safety. Sometimes it is possible to identify a family member who is trusted and is able to provide the nurse with an opportunity to visit the elder, as well as to ensure the safety of the nurse. Having another nurse present during a home visit is always an option, but at no time do nurses intentionally place themselves in dangerous home-visit situations.

It is not uncommon for both the abuser and the abused to maintain secrecy about the abuse. As with other types of family violence, abusers frequently threaten their victims with harm if they disclose the abuse. Even without threats of retaliation, however, a great deal of time often lapses before the abused elder is comfortable disclosing the mistreatment. Reluctance is usually due to shame, self-blame, or fear of abandonment, institutionalization, and serious consequences for the abuser. Box 22-8 identifies physical indicators of actual or potential elder abuse. Many of these symptoms are present with normal aging. Therefore, as with other types of family violence, the nurse needs to perform a comprehensive assessment and consider the physical symptoms within the broader context of the client's life history (see the Nursing Assessment Questions box).

Besides possible physical signs and symptoms of elder abuse and neglect, it is also necessary to assess the older adult for signs of exploitation or abandonment. Signs of exploitation include complaints by elders or evidence of misuse of their money, loss of control over their finances, material goods taken without consent or approval, and unmet financial needs that are inconsistent with their actual financial status. Signs of abandonment include reports by elders or evidence of being left alone and helpless for extended periods without adequate assistance.

BOX 22-8

Physical Indicators of Actual or Potential Elder Abuse/Neglect

GENERAL APPEARANCE
- Anxious, fearful, and passive
- Poor eye contact
- Looks to caregiver for answers
- Poor hygiene and inappropriate dress
- Underweight or malnourished
- Physically handicapped
- No glasses, false teeth, or hearing aid despite need

SKIN
- Contusions, abrasions, burns, and scars in various stages of healing
- Decubitus ulcers, urine burns
- Rope marks

ABDOMINAL/RECTAL
- Distended
- Internal bleeding
- Fecal impactions

MUSCULOSKELETAL
- Evidence of old, healed fractures
- Current fractures and sprains
- Limited range of motion
- Contractures

GENITAL/URINARY
- Vaginal lacerations, bruises, and infections
- Urinary tract infections

NEUROLOGIC
- Slurred speech
- Confusion

NURSING ASSESSMENT QUESTIONS
For the Abused Elder

1 Are you satisfied living with your [daughter, grandson]?
2 Can you tell me about your financial assets and how they are managed?
3 Whom do you turn to when you are feeling down?
4 How are family disagreements handled in your household?
5 Has anyone ever hurt you or touched you when you didn't want to be touched?

CASE STUDY Eighty-year-old Marjorie Jones is brought to the emergency department by her daughter and son-in-law and is anxiously holding her chest and gasping for breath. Marjorie is currently on medication for congestive heart failure. She is underweight, dehydrated, without dentures, and has poor hygiene. When asked about her missing dentures, she states that they have been lost for several months and that no one has been able to find them. After receiving medical treatment to stabilize her heart condition, Marjorie begins to feel much better and is able to give a brief history to the nurse in the privacy of her hospital room.

Marjorie appears depressed and withdrawn, and had difficulty making eye contact. She states that because of her inability to maintain her own apartment any longer, she moved in with her daughter and son-in-law 18 months earlier. Until that time, Marjorie had a full life with her widowed friends and had participated in social activities. She had a part-time housekeeper since her husband died 5 years before, and she was able to maintain her independence until she developed congestive heart failure.

Marjorie reports that life is very different for her now that she is no longer independent. She states that she is having difficulty adjusting to being "so dependent" and that she "misses her friends." She denies ever being hurt by anyone. After gentle questioning, Marjorie gradually admits living with her daughter and son-in-law is difficult because of their alcohol abuse. Although neither physically harmed her, they discouraged her friends from visiting her and have continually demanded exorbitant room and board payments. Recently, she noticed that some of her jewelry disappeared. Marjorie is left alone for long periods, sometimes for an entire weekend, which is frightening to her because she is physically unable to provide for her own needs and has no access to the telephone. In addition, she becomes dyspneic periodically and experiences chest pressure.

CRITICAL THINKING

1. What is the first priority for the nurse in the care of an older person who is a possible victim of abuse, neglect, or exploitation?
2. What is the best way to assist an older client like Marjorie to disclose feelings, concerns, and fears?
3. What type of mistreatment has Marjorie been experiencing from her daughter and son-in-law?
4. What characteristics require assessment in Marjorie's daughter and son-in-law?

NURSING DIAGNOSIS

The following nursing diagnoses are based on the assessment data gathered by the nurse who interviewed and examined Marjorie (see the Case Study). These diagnoses represent a few of the possibilities that are relevant for similar cases. Nursing diagnoses come from the information obtained during the assessment phase of the nursing process. The accuracy of the diagnoses depends on a careful, in-depth assessment.

- Decreased cardiac output and activity intolerance related to change in health status (congestive heart failure)
- Powerlessness related to physical illness, loss of role functioning, and lack of social support
- Moderate to severe anxiety related to change in health status and role functioning
- Ineffective family coping related to alcohol abuse by caregivers and caregiver role strain
- Disturbed personal identity related to changes in health status and role functioning

No diagnosis in the DSM-IV-TR is currently appropriate for the abused older person.

OUTCOME IDENTIFICATION

Outcome criteria for this section are based on the nursing diagnoses from the case study on Marjorie. These outcomes are the expected behaviors that someone like Marjorie will demonstrate or achieve as a result of the implementation of the plan of care and the interventions. Because Marjorie came to the emergency department with severe cardiac distress, the first priority is stabilizing her congestive heart failure so that she will regain normal cardiac output as evidenced by normal vital signs, freedom from chest pain and dyspnea, and decreased anxiety and fear. The remainder of Marjorie's nursing diagnoses relate to her psychosocial needs, including her depression. Because of her change in health status and her dependency on caregivers who are exploitative and neglectful, Marjorie also is feeling helpless, frightened, and depressed.

Client will:

- Explore options that exist in relation to her home situation. (Because Marjorie is an adult, health care providers cannot force her to leave her children's home or press charges against them. If there are mandatory reporting laws in Marjorie's state, her children's abusive behavior will have to be reported.)
- Verbalize feelings about her change in health care status, her dependency on her children, the treatment she has received from her children, and available options for dealing with these concerns.

PLANNING

As with other victims of family violence, securing health and safety are major priorities in the plan of care for abused older adults. In the case of Marjorie, stabilizing her congestive heart failure had to occur before assessing her abusive home situation and establishing a plan of care for this aspect of her life. Because most states have mandatory elder abuse reporting laws, it is critical that nurses and other health care professionals remain open to the possibility of elder abuse whenever there are potential indicators for it. As noted earlier, many times older adults will deny the existence of the abuse; therefore, it is necessary to establish a trusting relationship with older clients to facilitate disclosure. Sengstock and Barrett (1993) suggested that the establishment of trust is the most critical component in planning the care of the abused client. In particular, they warned about being critical of the abuser because older adults are most likely to strongly defend their loved ones, despite the abuse they have experienced. Because nurses have time constraints in such settings as emergency departments and clinics, it is difficult to establish the trust necessary to facilitate disclosure by older abused clients. Nevertheless, the nurse is often in the best position to assess and identify abused clients. Thus, the plan of care includes the nurse's taking time to communicate concern, compassion, and a desire to explore options and resources, which will determine whether clients disclose critical information or continue to suffer in silence.

IMPLEMENTATION

Stabilization of the client's physical health is a necessary first step in her care. As with other cases of family violence, the nurse often functions as the coordinator of care. In Marjorie's case, the nurse will work closely with the social worker to develop and implement the plan of care. Because the nurse has frequent opportunities to discuss Marjorie's problems with her, she will be a key person in helping Marjorie to identify her feelings, recognize her strengths, realistically assess the situation, and explore all possible options before making decisions. Thus, the nurse is in a position to address the total biopsychosocial, spiritual, and cultural needs of the client.

Nursing Interventions

The highest nursing priority is to balance safety and autonomy. As previously mentioned, nursing interventions focus on meeting the biopsychosocial, spiritual, and cultural needs of the client. Thus the nurse helps Marjorie to accept the limitations of her congestive heart failure while encouraging her to maximize her self-care abilities. It is also important to assist Marjorie to learn about available community resources to maximize her mental and physical health. Marjorie will require assistance with the guilt and shame she feels about being a burden to her daughter and son-in-law and the abuse. The nurse will make a plan with the family if Marjorie insists on remaining with them. This plan will clearly explain the family's obligations, Marjorie's rights, and the consequences of abusive or neglectful behavior in the future. As Marjorie's care requirements increase, the potential for greater abuse increases proportionately. Ongoing monitoring and evaluation are necessary, a role that is becoming more important for nurses as they provide ever-increasing amounts of care for older clients in their homes.

The home health care nurse is prepared to provide counseling, referrals, support, and education to older clients and their families (Table 22-4). Sometimes the caregiver is in desperate need of stress management techniques, general information on the aging process, basic nursing care principles, and community agencies that provide assistance for caring for older adults. Caregiver support groups are also valuable. Providing this support will dramatically ease the burden of caring for the older relative and prevent the occurrence of abuse and neglect.

EVALUATION

Evaluating the effectiveness of the outcomes and nursing care plan for elders who have been abused is important because the abuse often continues and even escalates if older clients choose to return to the abusive environment. In a situation like Marjorie's, the potential for escalating abuse is significant because she will probably require increasing assistance from dysfunctional caregivers who are at high risk for continuing the abuse as a result of their substance abuse. However, nurses often are not in a position to follow up with clients once they leave the hospital.

Sengstock and Barrett (1993) claimed that certain clues are helpful in determining whether the nursing interven-

TABLE 22-4

Nursing Interventions for the Abused Elderly

INTERVENTIONS	RATIONALE
Monitor the client's response to decreased cardiac output. Monitor the client's response to medications. Provide reassurance and support. Educate the client about medications and limitations.	To support return of normal cardiac output
Monitor the client for increased depression and suicide potential. Explore with the client the reasons for feelings of helplessness and grief. Discuss the client's capabilities and strengths. Explore options that provide the client with increased control. Explore ways for the client to increase self-care.	To reduce the client's sense of helplessness and grief and increase feelings of control
Explore the client's feelings related to family abuse.	To increase the client's awareness of feelings related to abuse by family
Explore the client's options for remaining with family versus alternative living arrangements. Coordinate referrals. Show respect for the client's decisions.	To increase the client's awareness of options relating to living arrangements
Evaluate the caregiver's motivation for seeking and using assistance. Evaluate family's coping skills. Evaluate possible substance abuse by caregiver. Evaluate the caregiver's willingness to acknowledge and work on family problems.	To evaluate the caregiver's motivation and ability to provide care in the future

tions will be successful. These include the willingness of the older client to acknowledge the abuse and the willingness of the older client and the abusive family members to accept outside interventions or removal of the elder from the abusive environment. Although many resources for the older client exist in most communities, no one can help the family if they deny the existence of the abuse. Like battered women, older clients often experience multiple occasions of abuse before they gradually make the decision to leave their abusive environment.

RAPE AND SEXUAL ASSAULT

Sexual violence includes attempted or completed rape, sexual coercion and harassment, sexual contact with force or threat of force, and threat of rape (Fisher, Cullen, and Turner, 2000; WHO, 1997). Over half of all victims of sexual crimes that include rape and sexual assault are women under the age of 25 years. Often this violence occurs within the context of dating or acquaintance relationships, with the female partner the likely victim of violence and the male partner the likely perpetrator.

CULTURAL VALUES AND SEXUAL ASSAULT

The way a cultural or ethnic group defines gender roles and the woman's place in society impacts how individuals will perceive rape. In the United States, multiple examples of male superiority and female subjugation exist in popular literature, media, fashion, art, and language. These cultural symbols help to form our attitudes and beliefs that become laws, court proceedings, police behavior, educational curricula, and social service programs (Dasgupta, 1998).

Ethnic-specific cultural values and norms create myths that blame victims for rape and influence broad conceptualizations of sexual assault. Cultural values are the basis of our beliefs and attitudes and help the victim, friends, family, police, and any helper to find meaning in the experience.

Research Related to Rape and Culture

Researchers have attempted to increase our understanding of the cultural definition of rape. Sexual abuse and rape by an intimate partner is not a crime in many countries around the globe, and women in many societies do not consider forced sex to be rape (Leininger, 1996). Culturally sanctioned beliefs about the rights and privileges of husbands have historically legitimized a man's domination over his wife and allowed his use of violence to control her. However, women who have been forced into sex by an intimate partner are open to the same risks and consequences as women who are sexually assaulted by a stranger. This includes sexually transmitted diseases, physical trauma, and emotional consequences.

ADOLESCENT POPULATIONS

Developmentally, an adolescent has to balance newly gained independence from parents as they master developmental milestones, such as driving a car and dating, and learn to negotiate new relationships with peers and intimate partners. As such, youth, which is associated with limited knowledge and lack of experience in interpersonal relationships, is a significant risk factor for experiencing sexual victimization (WHO, 1997). Adolescents are particularly vulnerable when they have early menarche, early dating, and early sexual activity, all of which are linked with an increased risk for experiencing victimization by an intimate (Harner, 2005).

Similar to adult victims, adolescent victims of sexual violence experience negative physical health consequences following sexual victimization. Although physical injuries do not always occur as a result of violence, victims suffer physical trauma to the genital or anal track, including vaginal or rectal bleeding, bruises, lacerations, and contusions (WHO, 1997). Trauma is often more extensive among younger females, especially those who have not yet reached menarche and thus have less elastic, more easily damaged vaginal tissue. Virginal adolescents are also at increased risk for physical trauma, including hymeneal and perineal tears. This trauma, in turn, increases the adolescent's risk of contracting sexually transmitted infections (STIs), including gonorrhea, chlamydia, herpes (HSV), and HIV. According to the Centers for Disease Control and Prevention (CDC, 2001), the risk of STI transmission following rape is between 3.6% to 30%.

Female victims are also at risk for experiencing an unplanned pregnancy. Among adult victims, almost 5% of pregnancies are the result of rape (CDC, 2001). The incidence of rape-related pregnancies among adolescent victims is likely higher as younger women are often unaware of or have limited access to postcoital contraceptives or are not using any long-term contraceptive method, such as the birth control pill, at the time of the assault (Wilson and Klein, 2002).

Risk Factors

Researchers have linked several factors with an increased risk for either experiencing or perpetrating sexual victimization during adolescence, including age and developmental level, previous victimization, drug and alcohol use, and adherence to rigid social roles dictating acceptable behaviors.

Alcohol Use

Alcohol has been cited as one of the major risk factors for both experiencing and perpetrating sexual victimization. It is important to note that while alcohol has been strongly linked to sexual assault and other violent crimes, its relationship with victimization is one of correlation and not causation. Alcohol acts as a central nervous system depressant that decreases inhibition and impairs the judgment of users.

For females, intoxication, especially binge drinking (which is four or more drinks in a row for women and five or more drinks in a row for men), decreases awareness of a partner's actions and advances as well as makes it more difficult to stop sexual advances that have gone too far. In their study of sexual victimization on college campuses, Fisher et al. (2000) noted that drinking enough alcohol to get drunk was significantly related to experiencing sexual violence.

Alcohol use and intoxication is also significantly related to the perpetration of sexual violence. Among male users, intoxication has been linked with misinterpretation of sexual cues as well as overestimation of a women's sexual interest, which sometimes ultimately results in increased aggression and forced or coerced sex. Belief in the myth that alcohol use increases sexual arousal for both parties also serves to legitimize and excuse sexually aggressive and coercive behaviors that would not otherwise be acceptable. Furthermore, despite advances in neutralizing gender-based roles and stereotypes, preservation of outdated beliefs that divide women into categories of "good" and "bad" lead possible perpetrators to view women who drink alcohol as sexually available and appropriate targets compared to their nondrinking counterparts.

A female college sophomore and her roommate took the campus bus to study at the school library. After studying for 3 hours, two male students invited the young women back to their dorm to play cards. The game required the loser of each game to drink a glass of beer. Over the new few hours, the four became intoxicated and the women missed the bus back to their dormitory. The young men said they would sleep on the couch and offered their beds to the women. Nancy fell asleep immediately but was awakened to the presence of one of the young men who removed her clothes and proceeded to force sex on her despite her protests. The next morning, the women returned to the dorm and attended classes. Nancy became increasingly anxious and distressed. She could not get the thought of the rape out of her mind. She was unable to concentrate in class, do homework assignments, continue her part-time job, or attend social functions. By the end of the semester she had failed two courses and was on academic probation. Her roommate encouraged her to report the rape to the Women's Health Center, which she did. In turn, she reported the rape to local police, but criminal charges were not filed. A civil suit was filed against the university and later settled out of court. Nancy received short-term counseling and attended group sessions at the local rape crisis center.

Drug Use

While victims are sometimes sexually assaulted after knowingly taking illegal drugs, such as marijuana, heroin, and cocaine, they are also unknowingly drugged by so-called date-rape drug (Drug Enforcement Agency, 2001). Two of the more common date-rape drugs, gamma-hydroxybutyrate (GHB) and Rohypnol, are central nervous system depressants that when dissolved in either alcoholic or nonalcoholic beverages become odorless and tasteless. Once ingested, a person becomes disoriented, confused, and is unconscious for several hours (Seymour and Rynearson, 2001). In an effort to reduce the incidence of drug-facilitated rape, pharmaceutic companies recently included a color additive to the drug Rohypnol. In addition to similar preventative measures, criminalization of drug-facilitated rape is also enforced under the Drug-Induced Rape Prevention and Punishment Act of 1996 and the Hillory J. Farias and Samantha Reid Date-Rape Prohibition Act of 2000. However, despite these efforts, sources of date-rape drugs remain plentiful both in the United States, internationally, and online. As with other substances knowingly or unknowingly taken by victims, memory impairment, a common side effect of the medication, makes it difficult to remember and identify perpetrators of the crime (Harner, 2005).

Prior Victimization

Society cannot ignore the correlation between earlier victimization and later perpetration of physically and sexually violent crimes. Researchers have postulated that males who have been exposed to early victimization, including experiencing child physical or sexual abuse as well as witnessing domestic violence within the family, are more likely to adapt to these negative experiences by using externalizing behaviors. These behaviors include increased acceptance and utilization of aggression, violence, and control within future relationships as well as other maladaptive behaviors, including lying, stealing, substance use, and truancy.

Previous victimization, including experiencing or witnessing violence in childhood, has been linked with future victimization. Past sexual victimization in childhood is a predictor of experiencing future sexual victimization. Whereas past victimization does not guarantee future victimization, previous victimization, including lack of control over one's body, sexuality, and choices, set relational norms that become acceptable in future intimate relationships. Furthermore, if previous victimization, especially in childhood, went unrecognized or unreported, especially by someone charged with their care, an adolescent will believe the victimization is unimportant and the abuse of little consequence (Harner, 2003).

Statutory Rape

There has been a growing interest in the partnering of adolescent females with older adult males, often referred to as adult-teen sex. Although most adult women do partner with slightly older males, application of this social norm to adolescent females is linked to an increased risk for victimization, including physical and sexual violence. Furthermore, imbalances in power and control, financial resources, levels of life experience, and even physical strength place younger females partnered with adult males at risk for experiencing unplanned and unprotected sex, unwanted pregnancy, and exposure to sexually transmitted infections, including HIV and AIDS. Whereas partnering with an older male is considered consensual in nature to the female, her peers, and possibly her family, sexual relationships with significantly older males sometimes meet the legal definition of statutory rape. As such, several teen advocacy and pregnancy prevention programs have called for increased utilization of existing statutory rape laws to aid in the prosecution and punishment of adult men who have sex with adolescent females (Harner et al., 2001). Nurses must also remember that underage males may be involved in underage sex with older partners and not hesitate to assess for this increasingly problematic occurrence.

DYNAMICS OF RAPE

Rape is an interactional process involving at least two persons and it involves a control issue where one person gains control over another person. It becomes clear when talking with rape victims that from their point of view, rape is an act initiated by the assailant; it is not primarily a sexual act but an act of aggression, power, and violence. One factor of great importance to the victims was how the assailant gained access and control over them (i.e., his style of attack). Two main styles of attack were the blitz rape and the confidence rape. The assailant has two goals—physical and sexual control of the victim. Some rapists gained control with a direct physical action, such as a sudden surprise attack, whereas others used verbal strategies in an attack that has the qualities of a confidence game. In both types, the rapist gains sexual control of the victim by force and without her consent.

The *blitz rape* occurs "out of the blue" and without any prior interaction between the assailant and victim. A split second later a lifestyle is shattered and that individual is a victim. As one survivor reported, "He came from behind. There was no way to get away. It happened so fast—like a shock of lightning going through you. I was so helpless at the time." From the victim's point of view, there is no ready explanation for the man's presence. He suddenly appears, his presence is inappropriate, he is uninvited, and he forces himself into the situation. Often he selects an anonymous victim and tries to remain anonymous himself. He often wears a mask or gloves or covers the victim's face as he attacks. The "mark," to use the language of the criminal world, is the person destined to become a victim of some form of illegal exploitation. The classic example of the blitz-type rape is a woman walking down the street and who, from the assailant's viewpoint, is the "right mark at the right time." He is looking for someone to capture and attack. The victim happens on the scene, and she becomes the target. Victims who have experienced a blitz attack describe being jumped upon, grabbed, pushed, or shoved when the assailant approached the victims from behind. Children and adolescents who were victims of the blitz rape were often walking home from school, walking home from a friend's house, or playing with neighborhood friends when the attack occurred.

The *confidence rape* is a more subtle setup than the blitz style. The confidence rape is an attack in which the assailant obtains sex under false pretenses by using deceit, betrayal, and often violence. There is interaction between the victim and the assailant before the assault. Sometimes he knows the victim from some other time and place and thus already has developed some kind of relationship with her. Or he establishes a relationship as a prelude to attack. Often there is quite a bit of conversation between victim and assailant. Like the confidence man, he encourages the victim to trust him, and then he betrays this trust. An analysis of rapists' talk during rape revealed a number of linguistic strategies that the attacker uses to control the victim before, during, and after the rape. One of the linguistic strategies used by the rapists is the confidence line. The rapist uses this line in various ways: offering or requesting assistance or the victim's company; promising information, material items, social activities, employment, business transactions; making reference to someone the victim knows; or trading on social pleasantries and niceties.

MOTIVATION IN RAPE

Working with identified rapists, both convicted and not convicted, it becomes apparent that sexual desire is not the dominant motive in rape, nor is sexual frustration. The majority of rapists are involved in consenting sexual relationships. If sex is not the primary motive, then what is? Clinical work with offenders and victims reveals that rape is in fact serving nonsexual needs; it is the sexual expression of power and anger. Rape is motivated more by compensatory motives than sexual ones; it is a pseudosexual act, complex and multidetermined, but addressing issues of hostility and control. The defining issue in rape is the lack of consent on the part of the victim. Sexual relations occur through physical force, threat, or intimidation. Rape, therefore, is first and foremost an aggressive act and, in any given instance of rape, multiple psychologic meanings are expressed in regard to both the sexual and the aggressive components of the act.

EFFECTS OF RAPE ON THE VICTIM

Victims suffer a significant degree of physical and emotional trauma during the rape, immediately following the assault, and over a considerable time period afterward. Victims consistently described certain symptoms over and over. A cluster of symptoms that most of the victims experienced as the rape trauma syndrome include physical, emotional, and behavioral stress reactions that result from the person facing a life-threatening event to one's life or integrity.

Stereotypically, the main reactions of women who have experienced rape are to feel ashamed and guilty. This is not the primary reaction in the majority of victims. A primary feeling expressed is that of fear of physical injury or retaliation. A common myth about rape victims is that they are hysterical and tearful following a rape, but victims described and indicated an extremely wide range of emotions. The physical and emotional impact of the incident is sometimes so intense that the victim feels shock and disbelief. As one victim said, "I remember doing some strange things after he left such as biting my arm . . . to prove I could feel . . . that I was real."

Victims show two main styles of emotion: expressed and controlled. In the *expressed style*, the victim demonstrated feelings of anger, fear, and anxiety. The victims expressed these feelings by being restless during the interview, becoming tense when certain questions were asked, crying or sobbing when describing specific acts of the assailant, and smiling in an anxious way when stating certain points. In the *controlled style*, the victim masked or hid feelings, and the interviewer could note a calm, composed, or subdued affect. It is not uncommon for victims to have a flat affect, to be stoic in demeanor or to be highly emotional.

Victims express other feelings in conjunction with fear ranging from humiliation, degradation, guilt, shame, and embarrassment to self-blame, anger, and revenge. Victims report feeling distress over reminders (or cues) of the assault. Seeing a man who looks like the assailant will evoke a strong emotional reaction. Victims become cautious with all people; in stranger rape, they expect the assailant to be everywhere.

Many symptoms develop following a rape or sexual assault. The woman will feel numb and continually tries to block the thoughts of the assault from her mind, and that reaction is evident as a flat affect or indifference. She will say she is trying to blot it from her mind, to push it from her mind, but the thought of the assault continually haunts her. There is a strong desire for the victim to try to think of how she could undo what has happened. She reports going over in her mind how she might have escaped from the assailant, how she might have handled the situation differently. However, she usually ends up saying that she would have been beaten or killed if she did not do what the assailant demanded.

Dreams and nightmares of two types are a major symptom with the rape victim. One type is a situation in which the victim dreams of being in a similar situation and is attempting to get out of the situation but fails. These dreams are similar to the actual rape itself. The second type occurs as time progresses. The dream content changes and often the victim will report mastery in the dream. Often victims see themselves committing acts of violence such as killing. Therefore they gain power in this second type of dream, and this represents mastery. However, the victim still has to deal with this violent image of herself or himself.

Trauma and the Limbic System

One way to explain the long-term effects of rape and sexual assault is to understand the neurobiology of trauma and its effect on the limbic system. The important factor is how psychologic trauma affects the brain, in particular the key regulatory processes that control memory, aggression, sexuality, attachment, emotion, sleep and appetite. The specific area of the brain is the limbic system, which is also the location of the alarm system that protects the individual in the face of danger. It is the site where all sensory information enters the human system and is encoded. When trauma occurs, the neurohormonal system releases and is regulated by epinephrine, which facilitates learning during dangerous states. However, when individuals are trapped and cannot remove themselves either through fleeing or fighting, a particular type of learning occurs, termed *trauma learning*, which interferes with a reduction of stress through adaptive means of the fight-or-flight response. Because of excesses and depletion of hormones in the brain structures responsible for interpreting and storing incoming stimuli, alterations occur in memory systems. The individual becomes immobilized, and as the level of autonomic arousal increases, there is a shift into a numbing state through the release of opiates in the brain. This numbing state accounts for disconnection of the processing and encoding of information. In a sense, when the trauma is over, the alarm system remains somewhat stuck between the accelerated fight-or-flight response and the numbing state. There is now an alteration in an adaptive capacity. This alteration occurs at a cellular level and becomes fixed in its patterning and is difficult to change or extinguish. Of particular importance are various theories of modulating effects in the brain. All can appreciate this fight-or-flight and numbing response in the face of danger: now researchers understand that trauma has a lasting effect on basic processes of adaptation and growth.

Because these neurosystems of arousal and numbing are intricately related to information processing and memory, there is a distinctive type of memory in which an individual recalls experiences as if they were happening in the present (e.g., a flashback). Thus, when external events trigger an association to the abuse itself, the person experiences this panic memory and feels subjected to a hostile environment even though nothing like that is happening. Internal events also trigger trauma-specific reactions, such as night terrors. These experiences are not like typical dreams, but inside are vivid, visceral responses as if the trauma is reoccurring.

INTERNET VIOLENCE

CYBER-STALKING

Cyber-stalking, an extension of the physical form of stalking, targets unsuspecting victims on the Internet. Stalkers use electronic media such as the Internet to pursue, harass, or contact another person in an unsolicited way. In some instances, this pursuit transforms into the physical world where interpersonal violence occurs.

The Internet has made the search for unsuspecting individuals easier than ever. With a touch of a key, individuals are able to enter a special interest chat room, such as a sadism-masochism (S&M) chat room, and have potential victims at their disposal. Most often subjects use the Internet to convince and lure individuals to actually meet in person. Once individuals step over from the imaginary world of the Internet into the real world, they are putting themselves in a highly risky situation. An August 2002 *Washington Times* article reported how one jewelry dealer, a Mr. Rick Chance, met a woman online and planned a meeting in a hotel where he would present her and an interested friend an estimated $1 million dollars worth of jewelry. He was found murdered with a bullet in his chest and the jewelry and women were gone. In this case, the woman used violence and also engaged in another criminal act with regard to the jewelry that was stolen.

INTERNET HOMICIDE

Luring a person from a chat room to an actual meeting can turn deadly. The Internet's first serial killer, John Robinson, eventually led authorities to many women around the country whom he met online. When making contact with them in chat rooms, he called himself "John" or "JT" or "JR" or "Jim Turner" and said he was a wealthy businessman. Almost every woman he encountered responded favorably to the financial condition as he presented it. To some, he hinted at an interest in sadomasochism, and this did not discourage the women. But he usually presented a wholesome image. He sent out pictures of himself dressed like a cowboy wannabe: dark western hat cocked jauntily, shiny black cowboy boots, crisply pressed blue jeans, denim shirt, and bolo tie. He wore a friendly grin and leaned against a post on farmland he owned in Linn County, Kansas. He was soon attracting women from all over. He met one named "Lauralei" from Kentucky who'd gone online looking for someone who was "over 45 and was sure of himself and secure financially." Her main concern was not becoming involved with someone she would have to support. She and "JT" flirted and did some sexual role-playing. He presented himself as divorced (which was false) and as having an open and caring heart. When Lauralei's brother died, he expressed great sympathy and began phoning her regularly. He asked to meet her in Kansas City, but she was one of the fortunate ones who declined. Several women who had come into contact with Robinson could no longer be found in cyberspace—or anywhere else.

Law enforcement began to close in on Robinson, and he was eventually arrested for several homicides of women he lured from the Internet. While John Robinson was on death row, the law enforcers continued pursuing details of three murders that they discovered across the state line. Robinson's attorneys negotiated with the prosecutor in an attempt to get Robinson to lead them to the bodies of the three women. Eventually the prosecuting team became convinced the women's remains would not be found. At that point, the prosecutor and the victims' families agreed to accept the guilty pleas in exchange for life-without-parole sentences.

In mid-October 2003, Robinson acknowledged that the prosecutor had enough evidence to convict him of capital murder for the deaths of the three women. He demanded the unusual plea agreement because an admission of guilt in Missouri might have been used against him in Kansas. The prosecutor said John Robinson, the Internet's first serial killer, was a "gamesman to the end." He gave no hint at what prompted his homicidal acts but found an aid on the Internet.

CHILD PORNOGRAPHY

Before the Internet, people who engaged in pedophilia usually had to pursue this activity alone and had to keep it extremely secret. Now the Internet offers support groups for those interested in molesting children. These sites not only encourage predators but also advise them on how to lure kids away from parents and coach them on the best techniques to seduce children without getting caught. There is an entirely new criminal realm across the face of the globe, and it has, in every sense of the word, no boundaries.

The Internet opened a vast array of communication, entertainment, and educational resources for children; however, it also opened a gateway to home and school for persons motivated to exploit children. Researchers examined a convenience sample of 225 cases published in the news media (Alexy et al., 2005). They classified the cases using law enforcement terminology to describe Internet offenders as "traders," "travelers," or "combination traders/travelers." The largest occupational category of Internet offenders was Professional (64%) and included persons in the fields of education, computers, medicine, and law. Other occupational categories included Laborer (11.2%), Unemployed (8.8%), Student (7.2%), Military (5.6%), and Clergy (3.2%). More than one fifth of the offenders lived outside the United States.

Traders are Internet offenders who trade or collect child pornography online. They are involved with any or a combination of the following: production, possession, and distribution of child pornography online. More than half of the cases in this sample involved traders (59.1%). Descriptions of the Internet online traders noted they could be charged with child pornography, be interested in a wide variety of sexual acts with children, produce Internet child pornography, distribute child pornography, collect a very large collection, or operate as partners or for profit. Travelers seek to meet a child in person after communicating through e-mail or chat room. Characteristics of travelers included offenders with a wide range of sexual interests with children including sadistic and homicidal acts.

Combination traders/travelers are individuals who participate in trading child pornography as well as traveling across state or national boundaries to engage in sexual interaction with a child. Slightly more than 19% of the analyzed cases involved offenders that engaged in a combination of trader and traveler activities.

In 1999, the FBI had opened up 1500 new cases of child pornography in the United States, and many experts maintain that this was the fastest growing criminal frontier in cyberspace. By 2000, the number of child pornography websites had grown to 23,000, and the next year it climbed to 100,000. Mainstream magazines like *Newsweek* were running cover stories on the dangers of letting youngsters explore certain corners of the Internet, and websites were providing tips and clues for parents to protect their children from online predators.

COMBATING CYBER-CRIME

As crime spread across the Internet, law enforcement began to catch up with those using the Web for illicit purposes. In 1996, the Computer Crime and Intellectual Property Section of the U.S. Department of Justice created the Infotech Training Working Group to investigate online violations of the law. This office evolved into the National Cyber-crime Training Partnership (NCTP). The NCTP worked with all levels of law enforcement to develop long-range strategies, raise public awareness, and build support to fight this problem on many different fronts. The National White Collar Crime Center (NW3C) based in Richmond, Virginia, offered operational support to the NCTP and functioned as an information clearinghouse for cyber-crime. All these agencies worked together to generate more funding to help law enforcement keep up with the ever-changing computer world.

Others joined government groups in sending out warning signals about the Internet. Two Virginia-based private organizations, the National Law Center for Children and Enough Is Enough, provided information to parents, teachers, and local, state, and federal employees about the dangers of child pornography, while supporting legislative efforts to control or get rid of it. Written material produced by Enough Is Enough described child pornography as a billion-dollar-a-year industry that was a threat to children "both morally and physically. . . . Any child with a computer can simply 'call up' and . . . 'print out' pictures that are unspeakably pornographic." The literature described in detail how child predators used the Internet to find kids before meeting them in person and molesting them.

Nursing Interventions

While law enforcement is investigating and arresting adults who commit cyber-crimes, nursing has been developing interventions to assess and treat the child and adult victims of these crimes. Nurses will implement interventions as described earlier in the chapter for health assessment and psychologic counseling with victims of cyber-stalking and child pornography. Families of homicide victims need referrals to groups that specialize in such counseling.

The Internet presents endless opportunity to improve our lives and the way we communicate and conduct business. Criminals have also seized this moment and opportunity to take advantage of unsuspecting victims. These victims go on the Internet to find a loving and understanding companion, hopeful for a better way of life and a happy ending. Although this dream comes true for a select few, it has cost others a great deal of pain and disappointment and has even cost some their lives.

CHAPTER SUMMARY

- Violence and abusive behaviors are major public health concerns.
- Because nurses assume many roles in a variety of settings, they are in prime positions to intervene and advocate for those who are victims of family violence.
- Interpersonal violence is more likely to be done by someone the victim knows.
- Battering is the most common cause of injury to women in the United States.
- Domestic violence is generally physical, psychologic, and sexual abuse primarily directed at women by men for the purpose of maintaining control and power.
- Emotional and psychologic abuse is just as devastating as direct physical abuse.
- Most child physical and sexual abuse is perpetrated by an adult the child knows.
- Actions that ensure protection and safety for the victim are the most important nursing interventions in abusive situations.
- Elder abuse is becoming a greater public concern because the number of older persons in the population is growing.
- Rape is an aggressive act and a crime. The primary motive is power and control and not for sexual satisfaction.
- Cyber-stalking is a rapidly growing activity with many victims of many ages, and often ends in crime.

ONLINE RESOURCES

General

Rape, Abuse and Incest National Network (RAINN): **www.rainn.org**

Intimate Partner Abuse

Family Violence Prevention Fund: **www.endabuse.org**

National Coalition Against Domestic Violence: **www.ncadv.org**

National Domestic Violence Hotline: **www.ndvh.org**

U.S. Department of Justice Office on Violence Against Women: **www.usdoj.gov/ovw**

Child Abuse and Neglect

American Professional Society on the Abuse of Children: **www.apsac.org**

Child Welfare Information Gateway: **www.childwelfare.gov**

Child Welfare League of America: **www.cwla.org**

Elder Abuse

American Society on Aging: **www.asaging.org**

National Center on Elder Abuse: **www.elderabusecenter.org**

National Committee for the Prevention of Elder Abuse: **www.preventelderabuse.org**

National Fraud Information Center: **www.fraud.org**

REVIEW QUESTIONS

1 A woman seeks outpatient therapy 2 weeks after being raped. She complains of insomnia, decreased appetite, depression, and anxiety when she is away from home. Select the most appropriate nursing intervention(s) for the plan of care. You may select more than one answer.

1. Refer the client to a support group for victims of rape.
2. Provide the client with information on self-defense classes.
3. Use active listening to validate the client's feelings.
4. Ask the client, "Why did you wait 2 weeks to report the rape?"
5. Teach the client relaxation techniques.

2 An emergency department nurse assesses a woman suspected of marital rape. The woman's clothes are torn and bloody. What should the nurse do with the clothing?

1. Place them in a plastic bag for return to the woman.
2. Seal the clothes in a paper bag for law enforcement.
3. No action should be taken. The clothes belong to the woman.
4. Place them in the facility's contaminated waste disposal.

3 A child is referred by a teacher for individual therapy. The child has been aggressive at school and had frequent absenteeism. The teacher recently found bruises on the child's back. Identify the best initial outcome.

1. The child will form a trusting relationship with a therapist.
2. The child will refrain from aggressive behavior.
3. The parents will attend parenting classes.
4. School attendance will become regular and timely.
5. The child will acknowledge being abused.

4 A school nurse interviews a child. Which aspect of the child's history alerts the nurse to a high risk for sexual abuse?

1. Undereducated parents
2. Low-income family
3. Multiple siblings
4. Parents were sexual abuse victims

5 A 79-year-old client is brought to the hospital by the family and diagnosed with pneumonia. The client is 5 feet 6 inches and weighs 93 pounds. The client's clothes are old, dirty, and have holes. The client also has a sacral pressure ulcer. Which question would best assess for the possibility of abuse or neglect?

1. "How long have you lived with your children?"
2. "How much money do you have in your bank account?"
3. "Describe a typical day at home. What you eat, and what you do?"
4. "Who buys your clothes and does the laundry for you?"

Additional self-study exercises and learning resources are available to you on the ***Companion CD*** *at the back of the book and on the* ***Evolve website*** *at* ***http://evolve.elsevier.com/Fortinash/.***

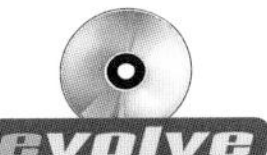

REFERENCES

Alexy EM, Burgess AW, Baker T: Internet offenders: traders, travelers and combination trader-travelers, *J Interpers Violence* 20:804-812, 2005.

American Professional Society on Abused Children Task Force: *Guidelines for psychosocial evaluation of suspected sexual abuse in young children*, Chicago, 2002, The Task Force.

Barnett OL, Miller-Perrin CL, Perrin R: *Family violence across the lifespan: an introduction*, Thousand Oaks, Calif, 1997, Sage.

Bowlby J: The nature of the child's tie to his mother, *Intl J Psychoanalysis* 39:359-373, 1958.

Brassard MR, Hart SN, Hardy DB: The psychological maltreatment rating scale, *Child Abuse Neglect* 17:715-729, 1993.

Briere J: *Therapy for adults molested as children: beyond survival*, New York, 1996, Springer.

Brownell P, Berman J, Salamone A: Mental health and criminal justice issues among perpetrators of elder abuse, *J Elder Abuse Neglect* 11:81-94, 1999.

Bureau of Justice: *Bureaus of Justice crime statistics*, 2003; retrieved Feb 23, 2003, from www.ojp.usdoj.gov/bjs/cvict_c.htm.

Bureau of Justice Statistics, U.S. Department of Justice: *Criminal victimization in the United States, 1988: a national crime survey report*, December, NCJ-122024, Washington, DC, 1990, U.S. Government Printing Office.

Burgess AW: *Advance practice in psychiatric nursing*, Stamford, Conn, 1998, Appleton-Lange.

Burgess AW, Roberts AL: Levels of stress and crisis precipitants: a stress-crisis continuum, *Crisis Intervention Time-Limited Treat* 2:31-47, 1995.

Burgess AW et al: Response patterns in children and adolescents exploited through sex rings and pornography, *Am J Psychiatry* 141:656-662, 1984.

Burgess AW, Hartman CR, Clements P: Biology of memory and childhood trauma, *J Psychosoc Nurs* 33:1-11, 1995.

Burgess AW et al: Stalking behaviors within domestic violence, *J Fam Violence* 12:389-403, 1997.

Burgess AW, Dowdell EB, Prentky RA: Sexual abuse of nursing home residents, *J Psychosoc Nurs Ment Health Serv* 38:10-18, 2000.

Burgess AW et al: Batterers stalking patterns, *J Fam Violence* 16:4, 2001.

Burgess AW, Garborino C, Carlson MI: Pathological teasing and bullying turned deadly: shooters and suicide, *Victims Offenders* 1:1-14, 2006.

Campbell JC, Humphreys J: *Nursing care of survivors of family violence*, St Louis, 1993, Mosby.

Centers for Disease Control and Prevention: Intimate partner violence fact sheet, National Center for Injury Prevention and Control home page, 2001; retrieved Dec 2, 2001, from www.cdc.gov/ncipc/factsheets/ ipvfacts.htm.

Chu JA: Rebuilding shattered lives: the responsible treatment of complex post-traumatic and dissociative disorders. New York, 1998, John Wiley.

Crowell NA, Burgess AW: *Understanding violence against women*, Washington, DC, 1996, National Academy Press.

Dasgupta SD: Women's realities: defining violence against women by immigration, race, and class. In Bergen RK, editor: *Issues in intimate violence*, Thousand Oaks, CA, 1998, Sage.

Dutton DG: *The domestic assault of women: psychological and criminal justice perspectives*, British Columbia, 1995, UBC Press.

Dwyer DC et al: Domestic violence and woman battering: theories and practice implications. In Roberts AR, editor: *Helping battered women: new perspective and remedies.* New York, 1996, Oxford University Press.

Elliot M: *Female abuse of children.* New York. 1993, Guilford.

Federal Bureau of Investigation: *Uniform crime reports for the United States: 1990*, Washington, DC, 1991, U.S. Government Printing Office.

Fischer B, Cullen FT, Turner MG: *The sexual victimization of college women.* Washington, DC, 2000, US Department of Justice, National Institute of Justice.
Foa EB, Keane TM, Friedman MJ: *Effective treatments for PTSD,* New York, 2000, Guilford Press.
Gelles RJ: *Intimate violence in families.* Thousand Oaks, Calif, 1997, Sage.
Giardino A et al: *Sexual assault: victimization across the life-span,* Maryland Heights, Mo, 2002, GW Medical.
Gidycz CA, Layman MJ: The crime of acquaintance rape. In Jackson, TL, editor: *Acquaintance rape: assessment, treatment and prevention,* pp. 23-61, Sarasota, Fla, 1996, Professional Resource Press.
Gregory KE, Vessey JA: Bibliotherapy: a strategy to help students with bullying, *J School Nurs* 20:127-133, 2004.
Harner H: Childhood sexual abuse, teenage pregnancy, and partnering with adult men: exploring the relationship, *J Psychosoc Nurs Ment Health Serv* 43:20-28, 2005.
Harner H et al: Caring for pregnant teenagers: medicolegal issues for nurses, *J Obstet Gynecol Neonatal Nurs* 30:139-147, 2001.
Kelley S: Child maltreatment. In AW Burgess, editor: *Psychiatric nursing: promoting mental health,* p. 476, Stamford, Conn, 1997, Appleton-Lange.
Leininger M: Major directions for transcultural nursing: a journey into the 21st century, *J Transcult Nurs* 7:28-31, 1996.
Males M, Chew KS: The ages of fathers in California adolescent births, 1993, *Am J Public Health* 8:565-568, 1996.
Mechanic MB, Weaver TL, Resick PA: Intimate partner violence and stalking behavior: exploration of patterns and correlates in a sample of acutely battered women, *Violence Vict* 15: 55-72, 2000.
National Crime Victimization Survey: Bureau of Justice statistics, U.S. Department of Justice, 2000; retrieved Jul 04, 2002, from www.ncpa.org/studies/s229/s229.html.
National Research Council: *Understanding child abuse and neglect,* Washington, DC, 1993, National Academy Press.
Olweus D: Bully/victim problems among school children: basic facts and effects of a school based intervention program. In Pepler D, Rubin K, editors: *The development and treatment of childhood aggression,* pp. 411-448, Hillsdale, NJ, 1991, Lawrence Erlbaum.
Parker B et al: Physical and emotional abuse in pregnancy: a comparison of adult and teenage women, *Nurs Res* 42:1783-1788, 1993.
Phillips M: *Finding the energy to heal.* New York, 2000, Norton.
Pillemer KA: Risk factors in elder abuse: results from a case-control study. In Pillemer KA, Wolf R, editors: *Elder abuse: conflict in the family.* Dover, England, 1986, Auburn House.
Prentky RA et al: An actuarial procedure for assessing risk with juvenile sex offenders, *Sex Abuse* 12:71-93, 2000.
Reiss AJ, Roth JA: *Understanding and preventing violence,* Washington, DC, 1993, National Academy Press.
Rhatifan DL, Street AE: The impact of intimate partner violence on decisions to leave dating relationships, *J Interpers Violence* 20:1580-1597, 2005.
Rothschild B: *The body remembers: the psychophysiology of trauma and trauma treatment.* New York, 2000, Norton.
Schwartyz BK et al: Descriptive study of precursors to sex offending among 813 boys and girls: antecedent life experiences, *Victims & Offenders* 1:61-77, 2006.
Sengstock MC, Barrett S: Abuse and neglect of the elderly in family settings. In Campbell JC, Humphreys J, editors: *Nursing care of survivors of family violence,* St Louis, 1993, Mosby.
Seymour A, Rynearson EK: Substance abuse and victimization. In Seymour A et al, editors: *National Victim Assistance Academy textbook.* Washington, DC, 2001, US Drug Enforcement Agency.
Stark E, Flitcraft A:Women at risk: domestic violence and women's health, Thousand Oaks, Calif, 1996, Sage.
Straus MA: Social stress and marital violence in a national sample of American families, *Ann N Y Acad Sci* 247:229-250
Tjaden P, Thoennes N: *Prevalence, incidence, and consequences of violence against women: findings from the National Violence Against Women survey,* Washington, DC, 1998, National Institute of Justice.
U.S. Department of Health and Human Services: *Child maltreatment 2004;* retrieved from www.act.hhs.gov/programs/cb/publications/CMOZ/index.html.
United States General Account Office: *Nursing homes: more can be done to protect residents from abuse* (report to Congressional Requesters), Washington, DC, 2002, United States General Accounting Office.
van der Kolk BA, Fisler R: Dissociation and the fragmentary nature of traumatic memories: overview and exploratory study, *J Trauma Stress* 8:505-525, 1995.
van der Kolk BA, McFarlane AC, Weisaeth L: *Traumatic stress: the effects of overwhelming experience on mind, body, and society,* New York, 1996, Guilford Press.
Vierthaler K: Speaking out on a silent crime: elder sexual abuse—the dynamics of problem and community based solutions, *Natl Center Elder Abuse Newslett* 6:2-3, 2004.
Walker LE: *Abused women and survivor therapy.* Washington, DC, 1994, American Psychological Association.
Walton-Moss B, Campbell J: Intimate partner violence: implications for nursing, *Online J Issues Nurs* 7:1-17, 2002.
Widom CS: Does violence beget violence? A critical examination of the literature, *Psychol Bull* 106:3-28, 1989.
Wilson JP, Friedman MJ, Lindy JD: *Treating psychological trauma &PTSD.* New York, 2001, Guilford Press.
Winpisinger KA et al: Risk factors for childhood homicides in Ohio: a birth certificate-based case-control study, *Am J Pub Health* 81:1052-1054, 1991.
World Health Organization (WHO): *Violence against women fact sheets,* Geneva, 1997, World Health Organization.
Ziegler E, Hall NW: Physical child abuse in America: past, present and future. In Cicchetti D, Carlson V, editors: *Child maltreatment,* Cambridge, 1989, Cambridge University Press.

THERAPEUTIC INTERVENTIONS

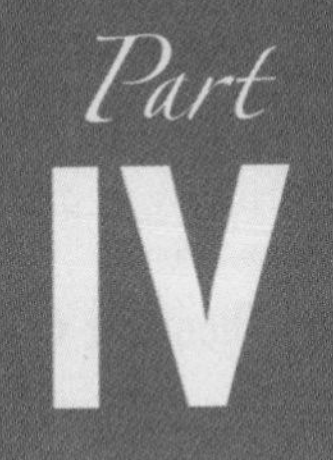

Part IV

Chapter 23 Therapies in Clinical Practice

NANCY A. COFFIN-ROMIG

You must be the change you wish to see in the world.
MOHANDAS K. GANDHI

OBJECTIVES

1 Discuss the underlying theories of the humanistic, behavioral, cognitive-behavioral, and psychodynamic therapies.
2 Describe the principles of individual, group, and family therapies and the role of the nurse.
3 Describe the role of the nurse in maintaining a therapeutic community in the psychiatric-mental health setting.
4 Compare and contrast the stages and tasks of the family life cycle.
5 Distinguish between occupational, recreational, art, music, psychodrama, and movement/dance therapies.
6 Describe the historical evolution of electroconvulsive therapy as a biologic therapy and the role of the nurse.

KEY TERMS

activity therapies, p. 533
attachment, p. 529
boundaries, p. 531
classical conditioning, p. 515
cognitive appraisal, p. 517
community meeting, p. 522
continuous reinforcement, p. 515
countertransference, p. 520
curative factors, p. 525
defense mechanisms, p. 520
ego function, p. 519
electroconvulsive therapy, p. 534
emotional triangle, p. 530
genogram, p. 531
intermittent reinforcement, p. 515
modeling, p. 515
occupational therapy, p. 534
operant conditioning, p. 515
recreational therapy, p. 534
role modeling, p. 522
therapeutic milieu, p. 520
transference, p. 520

Clinical therapies are numerous in the field of psychiatry and mental health. This chapter discusses the most common clinical therapies and underlying theories (Table 23-1) and how the nurse will use their principles in providing nursing care to clients diagnosed and suffering from a psychiatric disorder. A body of knowledge and research in the efficacy of clinical therapies is steadily growing.

Hildegard Peplau (1952, 1992), a pioneer and educator in psychiatric nursing, regarded the nurse-client relationship as the central framework for implementing therapeutic interventions. During the working phase of the nurse-client relationship, the nurse helps the client to identify difficulties, express feelings and thoughts, explore options and possibilities, and reinforce healthy coping. The nurse helps the client to change ineffective coping by

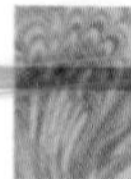

TABLE 23-1

Theoretic Components of Therapies

	PSYCHOANALYTIC	HUMANISTIC	BEHAVIORAL	RATIONAL EMOTIVE	COGNITIVE	DIALECTICAL BEHAVIORAL
Basic orientation	All behavior is meaningful; unconscious impulses and conflicts influence behavior	Human beings move toward constructive change and integration	Behavior is learned	Individuals can choose thoughts and behaviors that promote or limit self-acceptance	An individual's organization of thoughts and assumptions determines his or her affect and behavior	Behaviors result from emotional dysregulation and an invalidating environment
Concepts	Id, ego, superego; unconscious and preconscious	Interpersonal relationships are basis for health and neurosis	Conditioning; separation of client from problem	ABCs of interaction	Core beliefs; automatic thoughts; dysfunctional thinking	Emotional regulation; distress tolerance; interpersonal effectiveness; core mindfulness
Goal	Uncover unconscious conflict and increase ego consciousness	Bring aspects of self into awareness and acceptance	Modify observable behavior	Provide skills to scientifically change irrational premises and change behavior	Restructure cognitive appraisal thus changing mood and behavior	Accurately labeling emotions, monitoring behaviors, and developing a here-and-now awareness
Techniques	Dream analysis; free association	Person-centered; genuineness, unconditional positive regard, and empathetic understanding	Systemic desensitization; relaxation training	Cognitive approach; behavioral: role-playing, progressive tasks, questioning	Cognitive: questioning, reattribution; behavioral: activity schedule, cognitive rehearsal	Chain analysis; telephone support; meditation skills

providing alternative strategies in identifying and expressing underlying needs, acquiring new strategies in symptom management, adhering to medication, and role-playing interpersonal skills. (See Chapter 4 for more information about Peplau.)

THEORETIC PERSPECTIVES

Humanistic Approach

The humanistic approach emphasizes the human potential and inherent worth of human beings as unique, self-actualizing, and self-determined with the capacity to develop self-awareness. This self-awareness allows an individual to more fully make choices to enhance their quality of life in the full range of human experiences. Numerous therapies have developed since the movement began in the 1950s.

Abraham Maslow (1908-1970), considered the father of humanistic psychology, viewed human beings as motivated by basic needs. He ordered basic needs in a hierarchy, starting with survival needs such as physiologic and safety and progressing toward more self-transcendent needs such as love and belonging, esteem, and, ultimately, self-actualizing (see Figure 2-2). Maslow theorized that the coping behaviors available to an individual determine that individual's ability to meet basic needs and satisfaction in meeting those needs. The blocking or inability to meet basic needs leads to ineffective coping or in more serious cases, the development of psychopathology (Maslow, 1943). The nurse in working with clients will assist the clients to identify current needs, how those needs are met, and the effectiveness of coping behaviors.

Carl Rogers (1902-1987), a renowned humanistic psychologist, developed the "person-centered" approach and identified genuineness, unconditional positive regard, and empathetic understanding as the three essential conditions necessary in the therapeutic relationship that foster constructive personality change. The experience of these three elements by the client in a therapeutic relationship results in the client developing these characteristics in themselves (Rogers, 1957, 1980). The nurse fosters the development of trust by integrating these three essential elements into the nurse-client relationship to build a therapeutic alliance and facilitate progression through all three phases of the therapeutic relationship.

Behavioral Approach

Behavioral therapies are based on the premise that behavior is a learned response to a stimulus in the environment. The behavioral approach in combination with cognitive and pharmacologic therapies has proven to be effective in attention deficit hyperactivity disorder, anxiety disorders, and eating disorders. The purpose of behavioral therapy is to decrease or increase the probability of an identified behavior.

Classical Conditioning

Ivan Pavlov (1849-1936) was a Russian physiologist who won the Nobel Prize for his work on the digestive system, which he studied through his famous experiments with dogs. Pavlov observed that dogs salivated whenever they anticipated that food was forthcoming, and he labeled this phenomenon *psychic secretion.* He theorized that the dogs learned to associate certain events with the presence of food and therefore salivated before tasting the food (learned association). Pavlov developed his theory of **classical conditioning** (1928) when he paired a neutral stimulus (bell) with another stimulus (food which triggered salivation). Eventually, the sound of the bell alone triggered salivation in the dogs. Extinction occurred when the dogs were no longer offered food, and therefore stopped salivating at the sound of the bell (Pavlov, 1928).

Behaviorism

John B. Watson (1878-1958) was an American psychologist who developed the behaviorism school of thought. He was influenced by Pavlov's principles and stressed the importance of the social environment in shaping behavior. Watson is well known for his work with a child named Albert in which the therapist made a loud noise each time Albert reached for a white rat. Eventually, Albert became frightened of the rat and later all furry animals, even without the noise. Some have questioned Watson's ethics in conducting such an experiment with a child; yet he showed that controlling the stimulus could change or shape one's behavior.

Operant Conditioning

B.F. Skinner (1904-1990), American behavioral psychologist, coined the term **operant conditioning** as a method to modify behavior in animals and then applied his approach to people. In operant conditioning, changing a behavior involves identifying three elements: stimulus (S), response (R), and reinforcer (R) (Figure 23-1). *Stimulus* is the environmental event that immediately precedes a behavior. *Response* is the action or overt behavior occurring immediately after the stimulus. *Reinforcer* or consequence/feedback strengthens the behavior, either raising or lowering the probability of the behavior occurring again (Skinner, 1987).

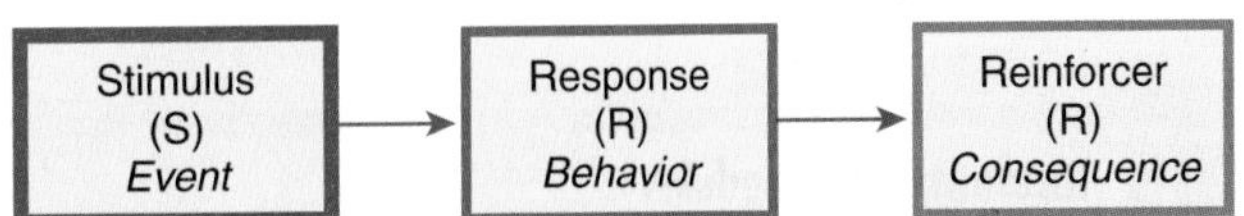

FIGURE 23-1 Operant conditioning.

Reinforcement. There are two categories of consequences used in operant conditioning designed to increase or decrease the probability of a behavior occurring in the future by changing the type of consequences over a set time interval. Reinforcement of a behavior by rewarding each behavior on the same time interval or when a correct response occurs is **continuous reinforcement. Intermittent reinforcement** is when the reinforcer is delivered on a slightly different time interval or set number of correct responses called a schedule (Table 23-2). Table 23-3 describes four types of reinforcement.

Underlying Principles of Behavioral Therapy

Modeling. The principle of **modeling** argues that behavioral change occurs through observing behaviors in others that brings positive or negative consequences (Bandura, 1969). Children, for example often imitate the behavior patterns of parents, teachers, and peers. Role-playing is another form of modeling in which clients have the opportunity to observe the modeling of new behavior and than practice the new behavior and receive feedback. An example is a nurse conducting a psychoeducational group on assertive behavior. One of the roles of the nurse on the inpatient unit is to model healthy behavior and provide guidance and feedback to clients who exhibit difficulties with verbalizing needs, speaking to the physician about medications, managing and expressing feelings such as anxiety, anger, fear, and interpersonal conflict. The nurse provides positive reinforcement with verbal praise when the client exhibits behavior on the inpatient unit that is adaptive in everyday social encounters.

Premack Principle. The Premack principle states that a frequently occurring positive behavioral response serves as a positive reinforcer for less frequent desired responses (Premack, 1959). For example, parents require their child to pick up the toy room before going out to play or going online to chat with friends after homework is completed. This principle is best employed with children and adolescents when facilitating behavioral changes to increase tolerance for delayed gratification.

Shaping. Using this principle, the nurse selects reinforcements in a *step sequence* leading to a change in a target behavior. The nurse schedules reinforcements or consequences in close approximation to the desired behavior response. For example, a child with attention deficit disorder and hyperactivity disrupts class by interrupting the teacher's lesson. First, the nurse designs a behavioral token system to reward the child for not speaking out during class each hour of the school day. The following week, the nurse adds the behavior of raising his hand to the first behavior and gives a reward. The following week, the nurse adds waiting to be called on to the two previous behaviors and gives a reward when the child performs all three behaviors in the correct sequence.

Counterconditioning. The aim of counterconditioning is to replace a negative response to a stimulus, with a positive response. This method of behavior modification

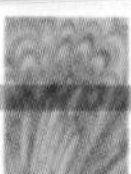

TABLE 23-2

Intermittent Schedules

CLASS	METHOD	EXAMPLE
Fixed interval	The first correct response or consequence is given within a set amount of time.	A child is rewarded with a star on a chart for sitting in his or her seat quietly within 1 minute after the bell rings for class to begin.
Variable interval	The first correct response or consequence is given after a set of time passes, but after the consequence is given, a new time period (either shorter or longer) is set. Behavior reinforced by a variable interval schedule is more difficult to change or extinguish.	Often seen with inconsistent enforcement of rules or rewards with children by parents and/or teachers.
Fixed ratio	After a specified amount of a correct behavior or response occurs, a reinforcer or consequence is given.	A child is given a token at the end of the day for washing his or her hands before every meal.
Variable ratio	A reinforcer or consequence is given with varying correct number of responses or desired behavior. This type of variable-ratio schedule is most effective for maintaining behavior.	Children on the inpatient psychiatric unit receive a reward of praise by staff when they use verbal expression of feelings instead of acting out their feelings of frustration or anger.

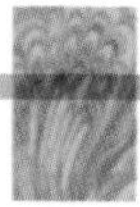

TABLE 23-3

Types of Reinforcement

TYPE	DEFINITION	EXAMPLE
Positive	A pleasant or desirable behavior occurs and a positive reinforcer or consequence is added to increase the frequency of the response.	A teacher smiling at a student during class when the student gives a correct response to a question
Negative	A behavior is used to stop or avoid a stimulus or condition that is undesirable.	Testing the temperature of the water before stepping into the shower so as not to be burned
Punishment	A negative consequence is given in response to an undesirable behavior to weaken the frequency.	Giving a time out or removing points for hitting another child
Extinction	Breaking the connection between a behavior and response by removing the reinforcer.	Ignoring or walking away when a child engages in a temper tantrum

was developed by Joseph Wolpe (1958), a South African–born American psychiatrist (1915-1997). Wolpe's method, called *reciprocal inhibition*, aims to assist the client in learning an alternative response to disturbing stimulus such as phobias, anxiety disorders, and pain. The most common technique of counterconditioning is *systematic desensitization*, which assists individuals to overcome a fear of a particular stimulus (e.g., animal, heights, elevator, public speaking, flying). The therapist, along with the client, forms a systematic hierarchy of progressive encounters with the feared stimulus. A number ranking from 1 to 10 is assigned to each encounter leading to the final direct encounter with the feared stimulus. The therapist pairs relaxation techniques with each stage of exposure and the client progresses to each stage to a direct encounter with the feared stimulus until symptoms are extinguished. Recent advances in computer technology and software development have lead to the development of virtual reality exposure therapy for treatment of the phobias of flying and height (Botella et al., 2004; Horowitz and Russell, 2004; Krihn et al., 2004). *Aversion therapy* is another type of therapy, which pairs a noxious response or unpleasant consequences to a stimulus. The most common form is the use of the drug disulfiram (Antabuse), which induces severe nausea and vomiting and headache when an individual ingests alcohol. The purpose is to remove the positive effect (consequence) with a negative response, creating an aversion to the drinking of alcohol.

Role of the Nurse

The nurse using the behavioral therapy needs to perform an assessment to first identify the problem behaviors in collaboration with the multidisciplinary team. Next, the nurse determines the schedule of reinforcement and reinforcers. Two types of behavior management programs most frequently used in a variety of mental health settings are the contingency contract and token economy. The *contingency contract* is a written agreement between the mental health providers or team and the client and family regarding the behavior change desired and the consequences for performing the desired behavior. Also, negative consequences are stated within the contract. All parties sign the contract, and the nurse places it in the chart along with a timetable for evaluation. *Token economy* is a system of behavior reinforcement using tokens. Clients earn tokens by performing predetermined desired behaviors. Tokens carry a value or points and are then tallied and exchanged for items on a predetermined list of rewards with different point values.

Rational Emotive Therapy

Albert Ellis (1973, 1993), an American psychologist (1913-2007), developed rational emotive therapy (RET). It is considered the precursor to cognitive behavioral therapy. Ellis has theorized that psychologic symptoms mainly come from disturbances in thinking leading to irrational beliefs not based on actual facts. According to RET, mental health is the ability to be flexible and open minded and to use alternative thinking. Individuals holding the irrational beliefs are largely responsible for their "emotional disturbances" either consciously or unconsciously. Healthy and unhealthy behaviors "are caused by the interactions among their innate predispositions and their external milieu, particularly their social milieu" (Ellis, 1993, p. 1). Thinking, feeling, and behavior are related in a close circular pattern. Ellis differs from other cognitive behaviorists (Meichenbaum, 1977; Beck, 1976) in that he sees irrational beliefs as the primary cause of disturbances. He theorized three core irrational beliefs regarding self, others, and the world (Ellis, 1993, p. 7):

1. "I (ego, or self) absolutely must perform well and win significant others' approval or else I am an inadequate, worthless person."
2. "You (other people) must under all conditions and at all times be nice and fair to me or else you are a rotten, horrible person."
3. "Conditions under which I live absolutely must be comfortable, safe, and advantageous or else the world is a rotten place, I can't stand it, and life is hardly worth living."

The methods of RET include active-directive engagement, questioning and challenging irrational beliefs, didactic instruction, and homework assigning.

ABC Model

The ABC model is the cornerstone of RET. The *A* represents an *activating* event, which is either an internal or external factor with an accurate description. *B* stands for *beliefs* regarding the event. These beliefs are categorized as rational (preferences and wishes) or irrational beliefs (dogmatic musts and imperative demands). Individuals choose from these two categories, which leads them to *C*, to create or construct cognitive, emotional, and behavioral *consequences* about the event *(A)*. These consequences are feelings of anxiety, depression, and rage, as well as behaviors of suicide, withdrawal, compulsions, and procrastination, among others. Therapy is highly structured and the therapist is highly active in the session. The client learns the ABC model and begins by identifying and agreeing on a target problem. The first phase of work involves working on identifying the *C* or the response or consequence—thinking, feelings, and behaviors to the event *(A)*. The client learns to identify the irrational or rational beliefs *(B)* to the response or consequence. Once the client makes the connection between *A* and *C*, he or she learns to dispute irrational beliefs and adopt or strengthen rational beliefs. In his later work, Ellis expanded RET to include a behavioral component, which then became rational emotive behavioral therapy (REBT).

Cognitive Behavioral Therapy

Aaron T. Beck, an American psychiatrist born in 1921, developed cognitive therapy at the University of Pennsylvania in the early 1960s. Cognitive therapy is based on the premise that distorted or dysfunctional thinking cause psychologic disturbances in mood and behavior. A large body of research exists proving the efficacy of cognitive therapy in depression and anxiety disorder (Beck, 1995). The therapist works with the client to identify and correct dysfunctional thinking patterns, which in turn alleviate symptoms of depression and anxiety.

The cognitive model proposes that perceptions, or the interpretation of events through a process called **cognitive appraisal**, influence emotions and behaviors. How the person thinks about a situation or event governs an individual's emotional response and behavior. Individuals beginning at childhood develop certain *core beliefs* about themselves, which tend to be global, rigid, and overgeneralized.

Core beliefs for individuals who are depressed usually involve self-worth or self-esteem and are often statements such as "I am worthless," "I am incompetent," "I will never amount to anything," "I am a terrible person," and so on. These core beliefs lead to attitudes, rules, and assumptions that influence the way an individual perceives a situation/event. *Intermediate beliefs* or attitudes, rules, and assumptions become a way to manage or deal with core beliefs. The core belief of "I am not smart" has for an intermediate belief "I must get an A," or "No matter how much I study I will never get an A." These intermediate beliefs go on to generate *automatic thoughts* when a situation occurs regarding studying. In this instance, the individual says, "I don't understand the reading material." The person feels anxious and frustrated *(emotion)* and closes the book *(behavior)* (Figure 23-2).

The goal of cognitive therapy is to assist the client in beginning to identify automatic thoughts and their connection to feelings. Clients have homework in the form of a diary or log for tracking feelings, thoughts, and behaviors; reading assignments, and exercises. During sessions with the therapist, the client and therapist review logs and explore situations generating difficulties. The therapist employs Socratic questioning as a method to discover, with the client, the situation or event that generated distress or difficulty. Then the therapist asks such questions as "What was going through your mind at that time?" "What did you think when he told you the news?" "How did you feel after hearing your grade?" "What did you do then?" Through the process of questioning, the validity of automatic thoughts, the therapist challenges intermediate and core beliefs and helps the client to generate alternative responses.

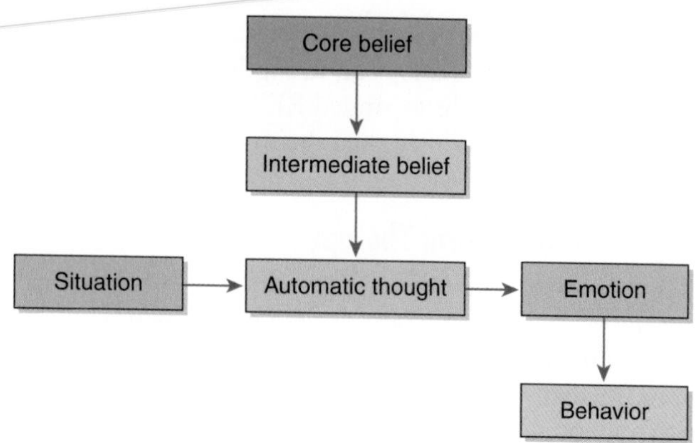

FIGURE 23-2 Cognitive behavioral model.

Beck, Rush, and Shaw (1979) listed the most common types of automatic thoughts or cognitive errors among depressed clients as follows:

- *Overgeneralization.* General conclusions reached based on a single event and excludes any other facts, often negative, and leading to feelings of helplessness or hopelessness.
- *Mental filtering.* Filtering out certain facts, often positive, to fit a core belief or assumptions regarding an event.
- *Catastrophizing.* Focusing on the negative aspects of a situation or event and predicting an outcome of failure to the exclusion of other possible outcomes.
- *Minimization.* Discounting positive results of accomplishments, which reinforces negative self-appraisal; this often leads to an overemphasis and reinforcement of negative outcomes from the past.
- *Magnification.* Focusing only on the negative facts of a situation and excluding other facts.
- *Dichotomization.* Sorting or dividing events into judgment categories of good or bad, all or nothing, leading to narrow definitions of success and failure.
- *Arbitrary inference or fortune telling.* Individual draws automatic conclusions regarding the outcome of a situation without considering the actual facts in the situation and alternative solutions available.
- *Personalization.* Interpreting the outcome of an event as reflective only of one's actions and excluding responsibility of others or other facts that have influenced the situation.

Dialectical Behavioral Therapy

Traditional treatment in cognitive behavioral therapy focuses on changing thoughts, feelings, and behaviors. Marsha M. Linehan, an American psychologist, initially developed dialectical behavioral therapy (DBT) in 1993 for clients diagnosed with borderline personality disorder (BPD) who often exhibit self-harm behaviors. This includes self-cutting or burning, chronic pattern of suicide attempts, impulsivity, and intense emotional displays alternating with episodes of anxiety, shame, and depression. Several studies of DBT have found the therapeutic techniques developed by Linehan successful with clients suffering from BPD (Bohus et al., 2004; Linehan et al., 1991, 1999, 2002; Turner, 2000) and more recently with other disorders such as eating disorders (Tech et al., 2001), chronically depressed older adults (Lynch et al., 2003), and substance abuse (Linehan et al., 2002).

Linehan (1993) broadens her definition of behavior from other cognitive behaviorists by redefining the role and impact of emotions in cognitive processes and behavioral responses. Linehan (1993) postulates that emotional dysregulation or difficulties in regulating emotions are due to an inborn temperament leading to an inability to regulate emotions or an *emotional vulnerability*, which includes high sensitivity to emotional stimuli, emotional intensity, and difficulty in returning to a more neutral emotional baseline. The other central factor is the presence of an *invalidating environment*. Characteristics of an invalidating psychologic environment include dismissal of an individual's interpretation of feelings, thoughts, or behaviors, informing the individual that his or her description and analysis of the individual's experience is "wrong" and the individual's experiences are socially unacceptable or undesirable personality traits. In addition, an invalidating environment does not permit or ignores attempts at communicating private inner experiences of thoughts and feelings, experiences of others, and resulting self-appraisal and interpretation of the social environment. Clients who have experienced physical, emotional, and sexual abuse; clients with borderline personality disorder or eating disorders such as bulimia, anorexia, and obesity; and clients with depression and substance abuse often describe experiencing an invalidating environment. The consequences of invalidating environment and emotional vulnerability lead to an inability to accurately describe or label inner experiences and emotional states, difficulty in tolerating distressing states, difficulty forming realistic goals and expectations, and the inability to trust one's own thoughts, emotions, and interpretations of outer events and individuals (Linehan, 1993).

Clients engaged in dialectical behavioral therapy receive three treatment modalities of individual therapy, group therapy, and telephone support. The goal of treatment is to assist the clients to increase their ability to tolerate and regulate emotions and learn to adopt more effective behavioral responses in a validating environment provided by the therapist and group.

Individual Therapy

Therapists identify behavioral targets and rank them from life-threatening, therapy-interfering, and quality of life interfering behaviors. The client self-monitors the behaviors via weekly diary cards, and the therapist highlights the highest priority behaviors. Sessions focus on a particular problematic behavior in detail through a *chain analysis* of events leading to the problem, and they explore all emotional responses leading to the problematic or target behavior. During this process, the therapist provides validation and simultaneously provides the client with alternative behavioral responses to emotions experienced.

Telephone consultation is available between sessions to help the client implement new behavioral responses.

Group Skills Training

This second phase of treatment consists of four modules:

1. *Core mindfulness skills.* The therapist teaches mediation skills to assist the client in developing a here-and-now awareness through observing, describing, and participating fully in one's actions and experiences without judgment.
2. *Interpersonal effectiveness skills.* The therapist teaches effective ways of achieving objectives with other people by learning and practicing assertiveness skills, managing conflict, and maintaining relationships and self-esteem.
3. *Emotion modulation skills.* The therapist helps the client to evaluate and manage emotional responses through exposure, blocking ineffective behavioral responses, and substituting effective responses.
4. *Distress tolerance skills.* The therapist teaches learning techniques for tolerating emotional distress and unmet needs through finding meaning and acceptance.

Researchers are still studying the applicability and effectiveness of DBT in the inpatient psychiatric setting. In a controlled study, Bohus et al. (2004) found that clients who participated in a 3-month inpatient DBT treatment program based on Linehan's program demonstrated statistically significant improvement in symptoms of depression, anxiety, interpersonal functioning, social adjustment, global psychopathology, and self-harm compared to patients on a waiting list who received usual community treatment.

Dialectical behavioral therapy provides nurses with an opportunity to develop nursing interventions for assisting clients to develop skills in managing emotional dysregulation and ineffective behavioral responses such as self-harm and chronic suicide attempts.

Psychoanalytic and Psychodynamic Approach

Gallop and O'Brien (2003) have emphasized the value of psychodynamic theory in psychiatric mental health nursing practice. The psychodynamic approach provides a deeper understanding of how early childhood relationships and experiences heavily influence the client's present symptoms and interpersonal difficulties.

Sigmund Freud (1856-1939), an Austrian, is the founder of psychoanalytic theory. A variety of schools of thought regarding personality structure and development have evolved over the past century from Freud's original theory, in an attempt to more fully explore the relationship between the ego and the unconscious (Jung, 1966), ego formation or object relations (Mahler et al., 1975; Winnicott, 1965), and self-psychology (Stern, 1985; Kohut, 1977) from Freud's original theory. The initial focus of psychoanalytic psychotherapy was on the psychic or psychologic structure of the personality. Freud (1960) proposed the structure of id, ego, and superego:

- The *id* is the primitive undifferentiated level of the personality and consists of drives, instincts, needs, and reflexes. It is irrational by nature and operates on the pleasure principle.
- The *ego* develops or emerges during the first 6 months of life and develops with the purpose of mediating between the outside world and the irrational id impulses. The ego operates on the reality principle.
- The *superego* is the last stage of personality structure development and represents the moral aspect of the personality. The superego consists of the internalized rules of conduct learned from parents and other authority figures regarding morality and strives for the ideal in personality development.

BOX 23-1

Ego Competency Model

- **Impulse control:** Effectiveness with which impulses are adaptively controlled
- **Mood:** Ability to sustain a normal range of moods that vary appropriately with external occurrences
- **Judgment:** Ability to anticipate the consequences of one's behaviors
- **Reality testing:** Accuracy of perception of external events
- **Self-perception:** Ability to regulate appropriate feeling of self-esteem
- **Object relations:** Degree and quality of relatedness to others
- **Thought processes:** Characteristic mode of thinking and language expression
- **Activities of daily living:** Ability to use existing ego strengths to achieve self-maintenance
- **Stimulus barrier:** Degree to which sensory stimuli are adaptively "screened"

From Kerr NJ: The ego competency model of psychiatric nursing: theoretical overview and clinical application, *Perspect Psychiatr Care,* 26:13-24, 1990.

The psychosexual phases of personality development of oral, anal, phallic, and genital represent the stages of personality of development. These four phases occur from birth to 15-plus years. Subsequent followers of psychoanalytic theory have focused on expanding a more interpersonal model of ego development, called object relations theory, which outlines descriptions of **ego function.** Kerr (1990) proposed the ego competency model for psychiatric nursing practice based on object relations theory involving the assessment of ego functioning in terms of ego strengths and deficits. Clients receive mental health treatment because of deficits or weakness in ego functioning in coping with common stressors of everyday living, difficulties in social and personal relationships, and impairment in self-identity. The number of ego functions affected and the severity of deficits govern the client's level of overall functioning and treatment goals. An assessment of ego functioning (Box 23-1) provides the nurse with important data in developing a care plan designed to help clients to increase ego functioning and enhance their quality of life.

The common thread in the contemporary psychoanalytic psychodynamic approach is the existence of the unconscious as a component of the individual's personality structure. The unconscious is a reservoir of repressed memories from childhood; in particular they are traumatic memories, which are the source of psychopathology. Present day difficulties in relationships or overwhelming feelings of depression or anxiety originate in early childhood relationships and traumatic experiences. Unconscious repressed unmet childhood needs or traumas influence conscious behavior. The goal of psychoanalytic/psychodynamic therapy is to bring repressed memories into conscious awareness with the help of a psychotherapist or analyst. The psychodynamic therapist helps the client to develop a conscious awareness of defenses employed by the ego to ward off intrapsychic conflict.

Defense Mechanisms

Anna Freud (1895-1982), in *The Ego and the Mechanisms of Defense* (1937), developed the concept of the ego as the mediator between the id and the superego and the use of **defense mechanisms** when conflicts occur between the ego and the id or the superego. The defense mechanisms protect the ego by channeling overwhelming anxiety generated by the conflict. Defense mechanisms operate unconsciously or consciously and are sometimes adaptive or become unhealthy when they prevent an individual from confronting reality or impair psychologic growth (see Chapter 9 for more information about defense mechanisms). Symptoms of psychopathology are largely reflective of an ineffective use of defense mechanisms.

Transference/Countertransference

Sigmund Freud (1912) is credited with the discovery of the phenomenon of transference. **Transference** refers to the unconscious projection of feelings, thoughts, or unsatisfied or repressed wishes, which are transferred on to the therapist or nurse in the therapeutic relationship. Transference is marked by strong feelings from the client toward the therapist or nurse and is positive or negative. For example, a client sends letters to a nurse requesting additional contact after discharge from the hospital. The phenomenon of transference can occur in any relationship. These feelings often evoke a response in the therapist or nurse of empathy, nurturing, approval, sexual attraction, self-importance, anger, irritability, rejection, or caretaking. These feelings or thoughts toward a client from the therapist or nurse are called **countertransference**. An example of countertransference is a strong dislike or attraction to a client that affects the ability of the nurse to provide care. They are conscious or unconscious feelings, signaled by an overly strong emotional reaction to the client that is either positive or negative. Just as in the client, the therapist or nurse is projecting or displacing feelings toward people in the past on to the client, which represents unsatisfied or repressed needs. Recognition of transference and countertransference reactions by the therapist or nurse remains vital in maintaining the boundaries of the therapeutic relationship. A lack of awareness or consciousness leads to boundary violations and prevents progress in assisting the client to meet treatment goals (Stiles, 2004; Peternelj-Taylor and Yonge, 2003).

Therapeutic Techniques

Psychodynamic-oriented psychotherapists primarily work with the transference and countertransference within the therapeutic relationship as a source of unconscious material. By developing a strong foundation of trust with the client, the therapist forms a therapeutic alliance, which facilitates the formation of the transference leading to the exploration of projected wishes and needs. Together they identify defense mechanisms and carefully challenge them, allowing a gradual release of repressed memories. The psychotherapist helps the client to explore emerging memories and associated feelings and thoughts and integrate them into consciousness by gaining a deeper understanding of the effect of childhood memories on present symptoms. In contrast, psychoanalysts use primarily the techniques of word association (Jung, 1966) and dream analysis (Jung 1969; Freud, 1961) in working with clients. For this technique, dreams are an objective source of material reflecting symbolically the intrapsychic conflict that causes the client's symptoms. Clients record dreams and interpret them with the therapist. Through personal associations to symbols, images, or individuals appearing in the dreams, unconscious feelings and memories emerge. The analyst helps the client to integrate repressed material, eventually leading to a reduction or absence of symptoms.

THERAPEUTIC MILIEU

The **therapeutic milieu** is an environment specifically created and maintained to restore and promote optimal psychologic health and wellness. Since its early days, the nursing profession has always recognized the importance of the therapeutic milieu to healing. Florence Nightingale (1820-1910), a British-born nurse considered the founder of modern nursing, defined her work as organizing the environment to allow the body to heal. The same principle holds true in psychiatric mental health nursing.

The psychiatric unit is a social system in its own right, with clients at various points of length of stay. Each client has his or her own agenda and interacts within the milieu to meet his or her unique personal and social needs. As such, the milieu is both a large work group with the definitive task of healing and a community with all the tasks of communal living. The psychiatric mental health nurse is a constant in this system, interacting with clients and staff in a variety of ways. These interactions are significant for a number of reasons, which include (1) the promotion of the healing process and (2) the creation of the atmosphere or culture that is unique to each particular psychiatric milieu. Many authorities believe that the atmosphere or culture of a psychiatric milieu has a significant influence on the healing process.

Historical Development

Maxwell Jones, a social psychiatrist, developed the concept of the therapeutic community in the 1950s. His goal was the development of a structure in psychiatric settings that builds a therapeutic environment (Jones, 1968). He held that the therapeutic community was an extremely important factor in determining successful treatment outcomes. He based his writings largely on his experiences and observations of long-term state psychiatric hospitals. His writings were an effort to establish hospital or community mental health treatment environments that optimize treatment outcomes for clients with a psychiatric disorder. Jones (1968) identified three factors as determining the therapeutic effectiveness of the social environment:

1. Presence of two-way communication between clients and members of the multidisciplinary team
2. An effective decision-making process among all levels of treatment and between staff and clients
3. Opportunities for social learning around interpersonal problem areas

Jones (1968) saw the psychiatric setting as providing a living laboratory situation for experimenting or learning new ways of problem-solving conflicts and crisis. The psychiatric setting in essence becomes a social microcosm of the larger society. The various roles of the nurse in promoting a therapeutic milieu include the following:

- Observing behaviors and providing opportunities for the client to receive feedback and develop new skills in coping with everyday interpersonal relationships
- Problem-solving in order to meet basic needs
- Identifying feelings, thoughts, and behaviors in response to stressors
- Managing psychiatric symptoms and improving communication skills

Goals of Milieu Therapy

Maintaining and supporting the therapeutic milieu is the primary responsibility of nursing in collaboration with the clients and the multidisciplinary team. The most common goals of the therapeutic milieu in the psychiatric setting are as follows:

- Providing a physically and psychologically safe environment
- Maximizing the highest level of psychologic functioning
- Identifying acute or chronic physical illnesses that are affecting psychiatric symptoms
- Promoting healthy coping behavioral strategies and symptom management
- Helping to promote independent activities of daily living
- Educating clients and their families about medications and other therapeutic modalities
- Establishing collaborative discharge planning between the client or family and the multidisciplinary team

Structure in the Psychiatric Milieu

The goals of the therapeutic milieu are structured by the boundaries, roles, and functions of the client and members of the multidisciplinary team. Clients are responsible for being active participants in the treatment plan by doing the following:

- Attending scheduled activities
- Participating in treatment planning and goal setting
- Meeting regularly with members of the interdisciplinary team
- Acquiring effective problem-solving skills and emotional coping strategies
- Performing self-care activities
- Adhering to the medication regimen

Nurses are largely responsible for managing the structure of the psychiatric unit by maintaining the unit schedule of client activities, which include the following:

- Completing hygiene and grooming
- Participating in mealtimes
- Taking medications at the prescribed times
- Participating in unit assignments (e.g., watering plants, keeping dayroom organized, running community meeting, attending planned activity therapies)
- Meeting with multidisciplinary team members

Clients have free time for patio breaks, social interactions, and individual meetings with staff.

Boundaries

The nurse maintains boundaries in the psychiatric setting by clearly outlining the roles of the staff and the client, meeting responsibilities for achieving treatment goals, and maintaining the integrity of the therapeutic milieu.

Safety

To promote and maintain a safe environment in the psychiatric setting, the roles and responsibilities of the nurse include enforcing the following basic rules:

- Clients will not have access to harmful items such as sharps, belts, and shoelaces.
- Clients will not have the means to harm themselves or others on the unit.
- Methods for managing clients at high risk for aggressive behavior are available to the staff.
- Strong communication skills, staff training, and collaborative relationships among staff are essential for ensuring clients that the environment is safe.

Therapeutic Interactions

The responsibility of the nurse is to maintain a therapeutic relationship built on trust, rapport, mutual respect, and interactions that focus on the client and his or her treatment goals.

Communication

Open communication by the nurse and other team members regarding observations of client behaviors, interactions with peers, adherence to unit activities, and one-on-

one interactions helps to develop flexible boundaries for communication among treatment team members. Evaluating the client's treatment plan and goals is an ongoing process requiring periodic modification. Nurses provide 24-hour care and play a key role in the evaluation process (see Chapters 3 and 4).

Role Modeling

The nurse who role models effective interpersonal skills, such as respect, caring, genuineness, assertiveness, and conflict resolution, promotes an atmosphere of trust and emotional safety for clients in the therapeutic environment. The nurse is responsible for modeling nurse-client interactions that demonstrate and reinforce healthy boundaries between the nursing staff and clients or between clients and their peers. **Role modeling** provides significant opportunities for clients to learn mature, effective interpersonal interactions with staff and with each other (see Chapter 4).

Yurkovich (1989) described three phases through which clients progress during their hospitalization as they adapt to the therapeutic milieu. The role of the nurse changes to accommodate the length of time and familiarity the client has with the treatment setting. The nurse's function is to respond in ways that consistently promote these goals. The three phases and the different roles of the nurse are presented in Table 23-4.

Community Meeting

Most mental health units conduct some type of group meeting designed to review staff and client roles and responsibilities in the milieu and to address issues that inevitably occur in communal living. The mental health **community meeting** is part of the structure of the unit. It is made up of staff and clients and generally occurs during the morning shift, with a brief review sometimes held in the afternoon. The goals of the meeting include the following:

- Introduce new clients to staff, milieu, and other clients.
- Orient all clients to scheduled unit activities/groups of the day, and explain functions.
- Introduce clients to their primary contact person for each shift and medication nurse.
- Ask each client to state at least one goal he or she has for the day. A goal may be as simple as taking a shower. Sometimes it is more complex, such as preparing for discharge. All goals are accepted, as they reflect the client's place on the health-illness continuum.
- Review old business that clients want to bring up (e.g., "The smoking rules are way too strict." "My shower still has cold water." "What did we decide about telephone use?").
- Discuss new business that clients have (e.g., "I suggest we have some new videos. How do other people feel?" "I don't think the client assignments are fair.").
- Assign each client (with client's consent) to a unit activity in accordance with the client's capability and length of time spent on the unit. Typical assignments include kitchen and day-room organization, taking meeting minutes, and presenting unit rules for smoking, laundry, telephone, visiting hours, and so on.

In summary, a community meeting provides an opportunity for clients to orient to the unit, meet other clients and their primary contact person, voice concerns, ask questions, state the goal of the day, discuss old and new business, and problem-solve issues related to communal living. Because appropriate task completion is essential to mental health, the nurse carefully explains the functions and tasks of the various groups and activities offered on the unit.

TABLE 23-4

Client and Nurse Roles in the Therapeutic Community

PHASES	CLIENT ROLES	NURSE ROLES
Newcomer	Follower Seeks information Observes group	Gives information Provides introductions Supports socialization
Member	Gives information Gives opinions Encourager Activator Compromiser	Encourages risk-taking Provides opportunity for contributions Plans for behavioral change
Leader	Initiator/contributor Coordinator Orientor Evaluator/critic Standard setter Gatekeeper	Gives feedback to client from therapeutic community Provides positive feedback Shares evaluation of client roles in the therapeutic community with client

From Yurkovich E: Patient and nurse roles in the therapeutic community, *Perspect Psychiatr Care* 25:18-22, 1989.

This promotes the opportunity for each group or activity to be used as effectively as possible for each client.

Table 23-5 illustrates an example of an effective therapeutic community meeting. The nurse leader in this community meeting facilitated movement toward the stated goals of introductions, orientation, and organization. The nurse took the opportunity to assess the general tone of the milieu and make observations regarding individual clients. For example, Patty seemed somewhat bewildered and Lynette appeared angry. The nurse will share this information with staff in context to the situation, and it will be extremely useful as staff interact with the clients throughout the course of the day. In effect, the structured meeting assists the nurse in becoming oriented to the tone of the unit and the status of the clients. This information will also help the nurse to organize the day while considering client needs, keeping in mind that needs could change as the day goes on. In summary, the therapeutic milieu is structured to provide nursing interventions that clearly define expectations of the client "through a mutually collaborative process in order to augment and enhance ego functions and to promote a positive sense of self" (Sebastian et al., 1990, p. 26).

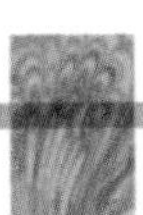

TABLE 23-5

Therapeutic Community Meeting

PURPOSE	DIALOGUE
Leader defines purpose of meeting.	***Leader:*** Good morning. It's Tuesday, June 14, and this is our community meeting. This is the meeting where we get ourselves organized for the day and take care of any business that comes up. This is important, because there are many people living in this community.
Leader provides structure for task.	***Leader:*** Let's do first things first and introduce ourselves and discuss what we all do here.
Leader defines tasks and explains how clients can use her in this role.	***Leader:*** I'm Tracy, and I'm one of the nurses. I'll be passing out the medications today, so if any of you have questions about your medications, please see me. I'll also be leading the process group, and I'll tell you more about that later.
Leader provides structure.	***Leader:*** [To each client] Would you please introduce yourself to everybody and say something about yourself?
	Client: Well, I think everybody knows me. I'm Sara. I've been here since Friday. I'll probably go home Wednesday or Thursday.
	Client: I'm Cory. I don't know if I'll ever go home.
	Client: I'm Mark. I'm Cory's roommate, and he snores! So loud!
Leader focuses on task.	***Leader:*** Mark, please say something about yourself.
	Client: I'm tired. I'm not sleeping well.
	Leader: Thanks.
	Client: I'm Patty. I just came in yesterday, and I've met a few of you. This is a real nice place.
	Client: I'm Lynette. I've got nothing to say.
	Client: I'm Claire. Uh, I don't like to talk in front of people.
Leader models acceptance.	***Leader:*** I appreciate your effort.
	Staff: I'm Jana. I'm the occupational therapist. I'll be leading the 9 AM and 2 PM groups today in the activity room. I also want to meet with you, Patty, to get to know you and make some plans with you about how you can best use occupational therapy. Could you meet with me after the meeting to set up a time?
	Patty: Sure.
Leader acknowledges effort.	***Leader:*** Thanks for your introductions.
Leader defines role and how to use contact person to promote task accomplishment.	***Leader:*** Each one of the staff acts as a contact person for each of you. A contact is the person who is working with you for the day. You can talk to your contact about anything that concerns you. I'll be the contact person for Sara, Mark, and Claire. Jana will be the contact person for Cory, Patty, and Lynette. Any questions so far?
Leader promotes self-responsibility by telling clients how to meet their own needs.	***Leader:*** Let me introduce today's schedule to you. It's posted on the bulletin board if you forget the times. We mostly want to tell you about the activities and groups.
	Jana: From 9 to 10 AM is Roles Group. This group helps you look at the different parts you play in your various relationships. It's a good place to look for patterns that recur in your life. I will be the group leader.
Leader defines purpose and structure of groups and activities.	***Leader:*** You have free time until 10:30 AM. From 10:30 to 11:30 AM is Process Group. In this group, we pay attention to how we communicate with each other. It's a good place to look at any problems you may be having communicating with other people. I will be group leader. Lunch is at 11:45 AM, and at 1 PM you have a choice of taking a walk (if you have privilege to do so), or playing a game like bingo here on the unit. From 2 to 3 PM is the activity group that Jana leads. This is where you can make something. It's a good opportunity to look at how you approach doing a task. At 3:30 PM we go home, and the evening staff will meet with you to go over the evening schedule and staffing. Any questions?
Client uses information and responds to cooperative style modeled by leaders.	***Cory:*** Do we have to play bingo? I hate that game.
	Leader: No, that was just what came to mind. Actually, as a group you can choose any game you'd like at that time.

Continued

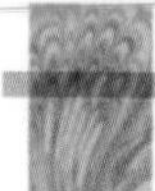

TABLE 23-5

Therapeutic Community Meeting—cont'd

PURPOSE	DIALOGUE
Leader supports client initiative, clarifies the situation, and models acceptance of question asking.	***Leader:*** Thanks for asking. It helps us to make ourselves clear and share understanding of what happens here on the unit.
Leader reiterates ways to be self-responsible.	***Leader:*** Any other questions about the schedule? [Pause] It's a lot to remember. If any questions come up during the day, check the schedule on the bulletin board or see your contact person.
Leader continues providing structure.	***Leader:*** I think we can move to the last piece of business for this meeting, and that's to deal with any issues that come up whenever so many people live together. Anything you want to bring up? ***Lynette:*** I still don't have any hot water.
Leader promotes interaction.	***Leader:*** I heard about that from night staff again. It's been a while, hasn't it? ***Lynette:*** Three days, and nothing has happened yet.
Leader clarifies information.	***Leader:*** Well, actually, something is happening. Engineering found that the valve is broken, and they're waiting for a replacement.
Group follows up on problem solving (probably based on leader's earlier modeled acceptance and encouragement to be self-responsible).	***Lynette:*** [Sarcastically] Great! They're waiting, and I still don't have any hot water. ***Sara:*** No hot water at all? ***Lynette:*** Well, my shower works, but I don't have any hot water in my sink to wash up. I don't want to take a whole shower just to wash my face. ***Mark:*** Why don't you just wet your washcloth in the shower? ***Lynette:*** That's what I've been doing, but I get soaked and my clothes get soaked. ***Sara:*** Well, I don't mind if you want to use my sink for washing up, as long as you give me notice.
Clients have clarified their action appropriate to their role.	***Lynette:*** Really? Thanks. I'll do that.

GROUP THERAPY

Human beings are social by nature, and Maslow identified *belonging* as one of the basic needs. The meeting of needs occurs primarily in groups, beginning with the family where physical and psychologic needs are met and are essential for healthy growth and development of family members. The need for belonging and social development progresses through the life span and moves to larger social groups such as school, church, recreation, work, local community, society, and the cultural or international community. A basic understanding of how groups function and the therapeutic role of groups helps the nurse to more effectively participate as a member and leader in professional and clinical settings. Northouse and Northouse (1998) defined a group as a "set of three or more individuals whose relationships make them in some way *interdependent*" (p. 196). Groups in the health care settings fall somewhere in the range between *content oriented* to *process oriented* (Figure 23-3), and the designation depends on the purpose of the group. *Content* refers to the tasks or activities to accomplish the goal(s) of the group. *Process* refers to the interpersonal relationships between members of the group and the leader. All groups contain both elements and vary according to the goal of the group (Northouse and Northouse, 1998). A *therapeutic group* is a specific type of group where the goal is psychologic change and growth. Therapeutic groups generally fall in the process-oriented range of the continuum and are largely dependent on the level of change members are seeking. Therapeutic groups range from a behavior focus to a psychoanalytic approach involving personality change.

Types of Groups

Task groups focus primarily on tasks or activities and procedures and the quality of work necessary to meet the goal. There is generally some processing going on among members. Examples of task groups are committees formed to develop or revise a policy or procedure, monitor quality improvement, or plan a client outing or unit activity. Task groups are made up of nurses, therapists, and clients or are mutually exclusive.

Midrange groups are groups that combine the functions of task and process. *Support* and *self-help groups* are examples of groups that provide an opportunity for individuals and families to come together to process experiences by sharing feelings and thoughts with others who have found ways to cope with similar experiences over time. Members further along in the process of coping (sharing information) with loss, disability, sobriety, addiction, illness, rehabilitation, and other challenges help other members by giving (altruism) their knowledge to newer members. Some self-help or support groups are led by a mental health professional or an experienced member volunteer who is elected by group members. Another type of midrange group is the *psychoeducational group*, which is the most common type of group facilitated by nurses in inpatient, outpatient, and community settings. This type of group has a more formal structure and goals. These goals generally include gaining new knowledge in

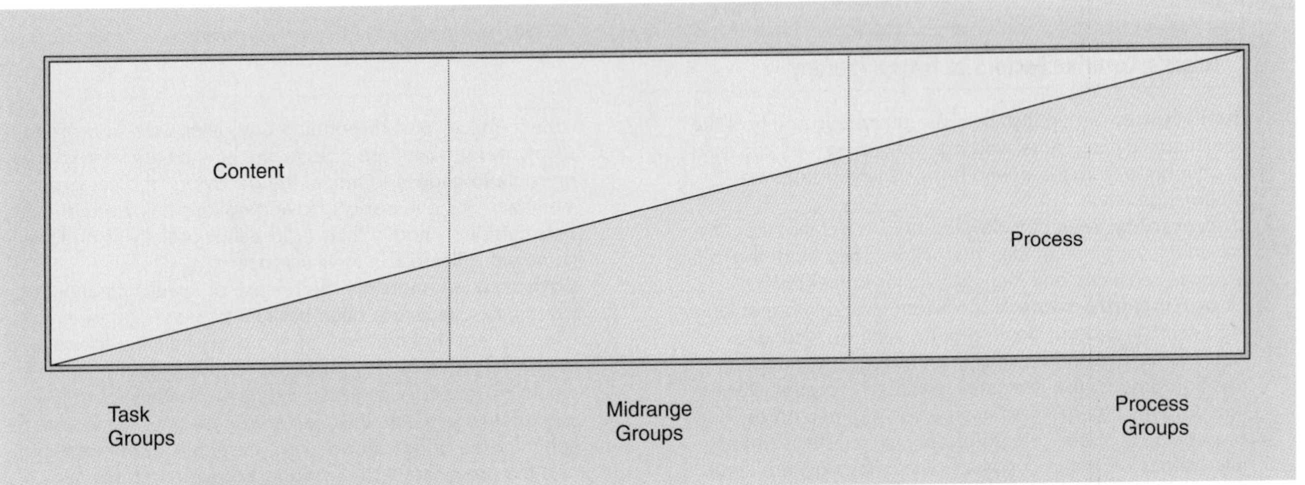

FIGURE 23-3 The emphasis on content and process in different types of groups. Psychiatric mental health nurses are most involved with process group therapy. (Modified from Loomis M: *Group process for nurses*, St Louis, 1979, Mosby.)

understanding and managing a psychiatric disorder, learning activities for increasing self-awareness, and developing strategies that promote effective coping skills.

Process groups focus on interpersonal relationships among members and their communication styles or patterns. A type of process group is psychodynamic group therapy. A key assumption of this type of therapeutic group is that psychopathology has its source in disordered relationships (Yalom, 2005). The goal of group psychotherapy is to help individuals develop more functional and satisfying relationships. Because the dysfunction in each group member will eventually manifest in the group, the task of the group therapist is to monitor and support the development of the **curative factors** (Box 23-2), which facilitate change by assisting members to understand their patterns of interacting within the group. Therapists hope that this greater understanding will help members transfer their new insights to the larger society outside the confines of the group. Irvin Yalom (2005), an American psychiatrist and innovator of group inpatient therapy, advocated the following steps to help group members accomplish this task:

- Get feedback on how they present themselves to others.
- Assess whether their fixed patterns are realistic or effective in the current situation.
- Discover previously unknown parts of themselves (strengths, skills, abilities, desires).
- Gradually try new behaviors within the safety of the group.
- Accept ultimate responsibility for the way they live their lives.

Group Dynamics

Once the nurse establishes the goal and formation of a group, a number of factors or dynamics influence the success of the group in meeting its goal. It is essential for the nurse to understand the importance of leadership, norms, cohesiveness, and roles in developing the necessary skills to practice successful nursing interventions in a group format.

Leadership

The leader's role and leadership style largely depend on the goals of the group. The leader plays an important role in guiding the group to meet its goals, developing group norms, and facilitating communication among members. Leadership is the "process in which one person attempts to influence others in order to attain some mutually agreed-upon goal" (Northouse and Northouse, 1998, p. 202). The leader's ability to influence the group largely depends on communication skills that are positive, open, assertive, flexible, tactfully honest, and receptive, while acknowledging others as the group moves forward to meet the stated goal. According to Lieberman, Yalom, and Miles (1973), characteristics of an effective therapeutic group leader are as follows:

- *Emotional stimulation.* Occurs when a leader actively encourages members to express their feelings, helps them confront and reflect ideas and values in a safe setting, and role models effective communication strategies that move the group closer to its stated goal.
- *Caring.* Is demonstrated when a leader expresses sincerity, openness, warmth, and kindness to the members.
- *Meaning attribution.* Refers to a leader who helps members develop insight into the underlying meaning of their behavior and a deeper understanding and acceptance of feelings that emerge from everyone involved in the group process.
- *Executive functioning.* Refers to the leader's ability to monitor group norms, set limits, and attend to group rules and procedures.

BOX 23-2

Yalom's Curative Factors of Group Therapy

1. **Instill hope.** Group members are at various points of the health continuum. Those who are not coping well are able to gain hope from those who have benefited from the group experience.
2. **Universality.** Members develop awareness that they are not unique or alone in their discomfort. They learn that others have reactions and thoughts similar to their own.
3. **Imparting information.** Both formal and informal learning occurs in groups. Some groups, such as Alcoholics Anonymous (AA) and medication-education or symptom-recognition groups, are designed specifically to give information. Groups that focus on interpersonal relationships, however, help members gain insight about the effects of their interactions on group dynamics, which they generalize to the larger society.
4. **Altruism.** By and large, members of groups give credit to the other group members for their support and insight. Members view their improvement as related to the work done by all group members. The knowledge that they are useful to others helps members experience an improved sense of self-value.
5. **Corrective recapitulation of the family group.** As noted earlier, people act as they were taught to act in their families. As is often the case with psychiatric clients, these patterns are dysfunctional and the client continues to repeat these dysfunctional patterns in all interactions. Group therapy provides the opportunity for clients to identify, evaluate, and change these patterns.
6. **Development of social techniques.** By interacting with others, members are able to improve their social skills. Members will often give other members feedback on their reactions to each other's interpersonal style. This enriches member recognition of the various effects of their style on others and gives them opportunities to choose and practice styles that are more in keeping with their goals.
7. **Imitative behavior.** Group members are often "caught" or trapped in a specific style of interacting because they cannot conceive of responding any other way. In a group situation, members are able to see how others interact and are able to choose to model the behaviors of other group members or the therapist. Having options helps group members curtail or modify their rigid behavioral styles and become more flexible in their interactions.
8. **Catharsis.** Catharsis is the release of intense emotions. Psychiatric clients are often hesitant to express these emotions for fear that they will be too overwhelming for anyone to handle and that the consequence of expressing them would be grievous. In group therapy, members learn how to express these emotions and experience the immediate relief catharsis brings. In addition, members learn that they and the group have survived the expression of emotions without calamity.
9. **Existential factors.** Human beings must inevitably deal with the fact that we all exist alone in the universe, in spite of the presence of others. Psychiatric clients (and others) tend to be unrealistic in their expectations of human relationships, thinking that with the perfect mate, friend, or family, all feelings of aloneness would vanish. In group therapy, members learn that human companionship can decrease feelings of loneliness, but this does not ever completely eliminate it. By not reaching for what is unattainable, members are able to enjoy what is attainable.
10. **Cohesiveness.** This is one of the most powerful benefits of an effective group. Many members experience extreme isolation in their daily lives and consequently feel disconnected from others even when they are not alone. Being part of a cohesive group that achieves its stated goals allows members to experience a sense of belonging and a feeling of being part of a whole that is greater than any one individual.
11. **Interpersonal learning.** In groups designed to examine interpersonal relationships, the members learn to identify, clarify, and modify maladaptive behaviors.

From Yalom ID: *The theory and practice of group psychotherapy*, ed 3, New York, 2005, Basic Books.

Norms

Norms are the rules of behavior established by the leader and group members. They represent the shared expectations of appropriate behaviors (Sampson and Marthas, 1990) and serve to maintain the function and work of the group. The norms emerge out of interactions among members and the leader and ultimately have an effect on the development of cohesion and other curative factors. Norms are either *enabling* (those that assist the group in accomplishing its work) or *restrictive* (those that hinder movement toward accomplishment of the group's goal).

Norms are overt or covert (Northouse and Northouse, 1998). *Overt norms* are the rules explicitly known and agreed upon by all members. For example, an overt norm is the time of group sessions, when they begin and end. The group usually agrees upon this norm during the forming phase of the group. If the normal times of the group change, the leader and group members discuss the effects these changes will have on the group and the group goal. *Covert norms* are the unspoken or implied rules among group members. For example, actively listening without interruption when another member is talking is a covert norm. Nonverbal glances of disapproval or stopping of dialogue usually signal the violation of this norm.

Norms tend to develop early in groups and are difficult to change later in the course of the group's development. The leader or group therapist and the members are all responsible for monitoring the norms and their effectiveness in meeting individual and group goals. Nurses on the inpatient psychiatric unit are responsible for promoting norms that meet the goal of a therapeutic environment or milieu when conducting community meetings and leading psychoeducational groups.

Cohesiveness

Cohesion or *cohesiveness* is the extent to which group members work together to accomplish stated goals. This is the sense of "we-ness" that a group experiences. Cohesion acts as a bond between group members and has been associated with positive group outcomes such as increased

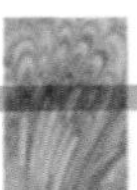

TABLE 23-6

Factors That Influence Group Cohesiveness

CHARACTERISTIC	CONSIDERATIONS
Group goals	Clear goals, based on similar member values and interests, motivate members to seek/maintain group membership.
Similarity among members	Members are frequently attracted to other members who share similar values and beliefs. There are some instances, however, in which people are attracted to those who are dissimilar in values and attitudes.
Type of interdependence among members	Groups that function in a cooperative versus competitive manner tend to have higher cohesion among members.
Leader behavior	For the most part, democratic styles of leadership are associated with higher group cohesiveness than are other styles of leadership (e.g., autocratic).
Communication structures	Decentralized communication structures, characterized by increased member interaction, are associated with higher morale and increased satisfaction among members.
Group activities	Members who are asked to perform group activities they believe are beyond their capabilities will feel less attracted toward the group, whereas members who believe group activities are within their capabilities will feel more attracted toward the group.
Group atmosphere	Members are frequently attracted to groups that help them feel valued and accepted.
Group size	Group size should match the number of members needed to complete the task. Larger groups can compromise group cohesiveness if there are too many members for the task.

From Cartwright D: The nature of group cohesiveness. In Cartwright D, Zander A, editors: *Group dynamics: research and theory,* ed 3, New York, 1968, Harper & Row.

interactions, norm conformity, goal-directed behaviors, and member satisfaction (Northouse and Northouse, 1998). Table 23-6 summarizes factors that influence group cohesiveness.

Roles

The behavior of individual members toward each other has a significant impact on the functioning of the group and the group's ability to accomplish the goal. Member behavior is categorized by roles assumed by group members. These roles often reflect the characteristics and roles adopted in early family life. Three broad categories of roles assumed by group members are group tasks roles, group-building and maintenance roles, and individual roles. Members of a group often have more than one role.

Task roles are members' behaviors that contribute to the group's ability to perform its function toward meeting the group goals. The primary concern of task roles is to obtain and share information in order to solve problems. *Group building and maintenance roles* enhance the development of member relationships, supporting the ability of the group to work together and build group cohesiveness. *Individual roles* are the roles a member adopts to meet individual needs, and sometimes these adversely affect group cohesion, function, and tasks when the leader or group do not confront them. Examples of the three categories of member roles are presented in Box 23-3.

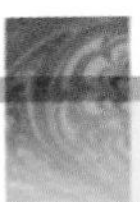

BOX 23-3

Role Functions Within a Group

TASK FUNCTIONS

Initiator: Proposes new ideas, directions, tasks, and methods
Elaborator: Expands on existing suggestions; further develops the group's plans
Evaluator: Critically evaluates ideas, proposals, plans, and procedures; examines their practicality and effectiveness
Coordinator: Helps pull together ideas and themes to clarify members' suggestions; assists various subgroups to work more effectively toward their common goal

GROUP MAINTENANCE FUNCTIONS

Encourager: Offers praise to members when warranted; communicates acceptance of others and their ideas; is open to differences within the group
Harmonizer: Mediates conflicts and disagreements that emerge in an effort to relieve or reduce tension within the group
Compromiser: Assumes a position between contending sides; seeks a compromise that all parties can accept

INDIVIDUAL FUNCTIONS

Aggressor: Acts hostile and negative toward other members; criticizes others' contributions; attacks the group and its members
Recognition-seeker: Calls attention to own activities; boasts; redirects things toward self
Help-seeker or *confessor:* Uses the group as a vehicle either to gain sympathy or to achieve personal insight and self-satisfaction without consideration for others or the group as a whole
Dominator: Asserts authority and seeks to manipulate others so as to be in control of everything that happens

Phases of Group Development•

All groups progress through the phases of development governed by the group dynamics previously outlined. Northouse and Northouse (1998) developed a model based on small group research findings. The model consists of five phases: orientation, conflict, cohesion, working, and termination. Understanding the phases of group development and common characteristics of group behavior for each phase, gives the nurse a framework for recognizing and assisting the group through each phase.

Orientation Phase

Individuals in this beginning phase of group development are evaluating the leader and other members regarding trustworthiness, compatibility between individual goals and group goals, type of requirements (i.e., time, tasks, and roles), level of self-disclosure, and establishment of norms. The role of the leader is to help group members to feel like part of the group and to achieve a sense of privacy, trust, and independence. The establishment of structure, group guidelines, and shaping of group norms is the primary responsibility of the leader.

Conflict Phase

Conflicts occur when group members compete with each other and the leader for control, influence, and authority regarding group decisions. The conflict over control is common in groups and possibly comes from resistance to forming a new group because of fear about entering into a new set of interpersonal relationships. It is the leader's responsibility to guide members through the conflict by helping them negotiate issues of influence and control while accepting the conflict as a normal phase of group dynamics.

Cohesion Phase

Cohesion begins when group members have worked through conflicts and are more aware of individual differences. A greater understanding and acceptance of differences are evident, and members begin to feel more positive toward each other. Trust begins to build, self-disclosure increases, and a greater expression of feelings, thoughts, and behaviors begins to emerge. As members continue to work as a cohesive group, the leader's role is one of minimal guidance and direction.

Working Phase

The hallmark of the working phase is the group's greater depth of self-disclosure and expression of both positive and negative emotions and thoughts. It sometimes takes up to 2 months for the working phase to fully develop, depending on such factors as group size, whether it is a short- or long-term group, or member commitment. Members of short-term task groups generally exhibit positive feelings toward each other in the form of praise, joking, a high spirit of camaraderie, and work productivity. The leader's role is minimal in task-oriented groups during this phase, unless otherwise indicated. The role of the leader in any therapeutic group varies according to the issues being worked on in the group.

Termination Phase

A group disbands when the goals of the group are fulfilled or the allotted time has finished. The termination phase in long-term therapeutic groups is sometimes a time of grief and loss for group members and the therapist. Feelings of abandonment, guilt, fear, anger, gratitude, positive affection, or frustration sometimes emerge during this phase. Members recognize that the uniqueness of their group can never be recreated or duplicated. Each individual member will confront this phase according to previous personal experiences of loss and separation. The leader during this phase summarizes the group accomplishments and helps members to confront their feelings regarding individual group members, the leader, and the ending of the group as a whole.

FAMILY THERAPY

A family is a primary social group of individuals who are related by biologic lines, legal bonds of marriage, or adoption and are emotionally related or interdependent. The developmental stage of each family member and the family's phase in the family life cycle influence the function or tasks of the family. Carter and McGoldrick (2005) outlined six stages of the family life cycle (Table 23-7). The authors defined the key emotional processes necessary at each stage for successful transition to the next stage of the family life cycle. As the family moves through the life cycle stages, there is an ongoing redefinition of roles, entry and exit of members, changes in emotional/attachment needs, and realignment of boundaries. The hallmarks of healthy family functioning include the following:

- Open communication patterns among family members in negotiating individual needs/tasks
- Secure attachment or emotional bonds between family members
- Flexibility and adaptability to change
- Ability to express and distinguish emotions and thoughts
- Ability to effectively manage social and economic stressors

Several schools of family therapy have emerged from the treatment models of individual and group therapies since the 1960s (Table 23-8).

Family Systems Theory

The common underlying theory in all forms of family therapy is the family systems theory that views the family as the primary emotional system that shapes and determines the outcome and course of one's life. A healthy emotional and psychologic environment is created by family interactions and relationships that help individual members to meet developmental tasks while allowing the family as a whole to move through the stages of the family life cycle. Relationships and functioning among family members "are interdependent, and a change in one part of the system is followed by compensatory changes in other parts of the system" (Carter and McGoldrick, 2005, p. 436). The family system strives to maintain a psychologic *homeostasis* or balance through emotional interactions or relationships among family members. The couple or marital dyad, siblings, and parent-child are the common *subsystems* or relationships within the family. A relationship

TABLE 23-7

Stages of the Family Life Cycle

FAMILY LIFE CYCLE STAGE	EMOTIONAL PROCESS OF TRANSITION: KEY PRINCIPLES	SECOND-ORDER CHANGES IN FAMILY STATUS REQUIRED TO PROCEED DEVELOPMENTALLY
Leaving home: single young adults	Accepting emotional and financial responsibility for self	Differentiating self in relation to family of origin Developing intimate peer relationships Establishing self in respect to work and financial independence
The joining of families through marriage: the new couple	Commitment to new system	Forming a marital system Realigning relationships with extended families to include spouse
Families with young children	Accepting new members into the system	Adjusting marital system to make space for children Joining in child-rearing, financial, and household tasks Realigning relationships with extended family to include parenting and grandparenting roles
Families with adolescents	Increasing flexibility of family boundaries to permit children's independence and grandparents' frailties	Shifting of parent-child relationships to permit adolescent to move into and out of system Refocusing on midlife marital and career issues Beginning to shift toward caring for older generation
Launching children and moving on	Accepting a multitude of exits from and entries into the family system	Renegotiating marital system as a dyad between grown children and their parents Developing adult-to-adult relationships between grown children and their parents Realigning relationships to include in-laws and grandchildren Dealing with disabilities and death of parents (grandparents)
Families in later life	Accepting the shifting generational roles	Maintaining own or couple functioning and interests in face of physiologic decline: exploration of new familial and social role options Supporting the more central role of middle generation Making room in the system for the wisdom and experience of the elderly, supporting the older generation without overfunctioning for them Dealing with loss of spouse, siblings, and other peers and preparation for death

From Carter B, McGoldrick M: Overview: the expanded family life cycle: individual, family and social perspectives. In Carter B, McGoldrick M, editors: *The expanded life cycle: individual, family and social perspectives,* ed 3, Boston, 2005, Allyn & Bacon.

between two or more individuals constitutes a subsystem. Extended family members also interact to form other subsystems affecting the overall family functioning. Some of the following brief descriptions of key concepts of family systems therapy are the components of the assessment process that enable the family therapist to identify areas of intervention.

Attachment

Attachment refers to the emotional bond between couples, parents, and children. Seeking and maintaining an emotional bond with significant others is an innate, primary, and motivating need in human beings across the life span (Johnson, 2003). Positive attachment is built on a strong sense of trust that someone is available to provide a sense of safety and security, and it serves as a buffer against the effects of stress, thus allowing psychologic development to proceed. A secure, positive emotional attachment for a child with a parent provides a safe psychologic environment for the child through the stages of individual development and maturity, leading to psychologic autonomy within a network of emotional bonds between immediate and extended family members. Some forms of attachment, such as avoidant and insecure attachment, result from traumas such as physical or sexual abuse, emotional abuse, loss of a parent, mental illness in a parent (e.g., depression leading to emotional abandonment), severe illness, or trauma by war, famine, or catastrophe impacting one or more members in a family. The developmental stage of the infant, child, or adolescent governs the extent of attachment impairment. An extensive body of research has shown that how a caregiver responds to a child's needs and expectations and how a child's needs are met lead to three distinct attachment patterns: secure, avoidant, and anxious-ambivalent attachment. Observing attachment styles in children, researchers concur that being responsive, attentive, and approving leads to a securely attached child that exhibits less inhibited and more explorative behavior. Being inconsistent in responding and in giving attention leads to an anxiously, ambivalently attached child that tends to try to reestablish contact, clings to the caregiver, and constantly checks to see that the caregiver is nearby. Constantly ignoring or deflecting the needs and the attention of the child leads to an avoidant attachment style in which the child attempts to maintain proximity but avoids close contact with the caregiver (Siegel, 1999). Adults that have a secure attachment style have reported positive early family relationships and trusting attitudes toward others. These individuals have also shown to have

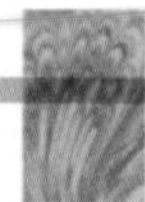

TABLE 23-8

A Comparison of Family Therapy Models

MODEL	DESCRIPTION	GOALS
Psychodynamic	Regards family pathology as resulting from internal intrapsychic forces manifested in intimate interactions. Symptoms result from family projection processes stemming from unresolved conflicts and losses in the family of origin (Boszormenyi-Nagy & Spark, 1973).	To bring about reconstructive personality change achieved by a working through of unconscious transference distortions among family members and with the therapist. Over an extended period, clients explore the connection between past relationships and current problems (Bentovin & Kinston, 1991).
Bowen	Regards family pathology as resulting from lack of differentiation and high anxiety. Those who lack differentiation are emotionally reactive, anxious, and dysfunctional (Bowen, 1976a).	To promote differentiation and less reactivity. Therapy focuses on the family of origin within a multigenerational context. The therapist coaches family members to resolve undifferentiated relationships with the family of origin (Kerr & Bowen, 1988).
Structural	Regards family pathology as resulting from stressors on a family that cannot nurture its members owing to faulty social organization and structure as well as dysfunctional interactions among members (Minuchin, 1974).	To transform family structural patterns by challenging the family's idea of where the problem lies and how to solve it. The therapist joins the family to challenge the system from within, transforming the structure, patterns, and behavior (Colapinto, 1991).
Strategic	Focuses on the social context of human dilemmas and habits, avoiding the use of psychiatric labels. Instead problems are seen as solvable by the use of directives to change how family members relate to one another (Lankton & Lankton, 1983).	To organize family members to take charge of problems, to facilitate the ability of family members to love and be loved, to promote the family's ability to reframe the distribution of power and responsibility, to promote shifts between hierarchy and equality, and to address personal gain and altruism that contribute to maintaining or resolving family problems (Madanes, 1991).
Behavioral	Problems are overt behavioral acts rather than emotional states or cognitions. Combines training strategies with individuals and conjoint problem-solving among members (Falloon, 1991).	To change reinforcements so family members receive rewards for desired behavior instead of maladaptive behavior. This occurs through education, training, conditioning, and management strategies (Patterson, 1975).
Feminist	Problems result from the unique problems women face as a result of socialization. Enacts a political, institutional, gender-sensitive viewpoint aimed at gender equality in defining and changing family structure and function (Goodrich, 1991).	To equalize access to influence, control, choice, resources, opportunity, and status. Uses role modeling, education, rebalancing of relationship power and authority, reframing authority, and reinforcing of new beliefs (Avis, 1991).

From Haber J: Family therapy. In Lego S, editor: *Psychiatric nursing: a comprehensive reference*, ed 3, p 62, Philadelphia, 1966, Lippincott-Raven.

higher levels of self-esteem compared to individuals with insecure attachment styles. Adults with an avoidant attachment style tend to view relationships as less satisfying and intimate compared to securely attached individuals. They are also less trusting of others and tend to avoid getting close to others. Adults with an anxious-ambivalent attachment style view others in a relationship as unreliable and unable to commit themselves. They also see their relationships as having less interdependence, trust, and satisfaction when compared to securely attached individuals. Parents or adults with avoidant or insecure attachment styles have difficulty forming healthy or secure attachment with their infants and children, leading to difficulties in meeting the developmental needs of infants and children as they mature to adolescence and young adulthood.

Symptom Development

The development of symptoms in a family depends on the amount of anxiety and stress being generated in the family and how much it disrupts the family system. The degree of symptoms in one or more family members and the level of anxiety present in relationships reflect the level of psychologic development and coping skills available in managing internal and external stressors. For example, few symptoms appear in families with strong emotional bonds and healthy coping skills under high levels of stress, whereas other families under similar conditions exhibit symptoms that indicate high levels of anxiety that result from ineffective family coping skills caused by poor communication patterns and high levels of interpersonal conflict. Symptom development is generally based on the emergence of various types of stressors as the family moves through time and available psychologic and social support resources (Carter and McGoldrick, 2005). (See examples of stressor types in the Role of the Family Therapist section.)

Emotional Triangles

An **emotional triangle** is a situation occurring in a family that tends to redirect anxiety and avoid actual or potential conflict between two people by introducing a third person

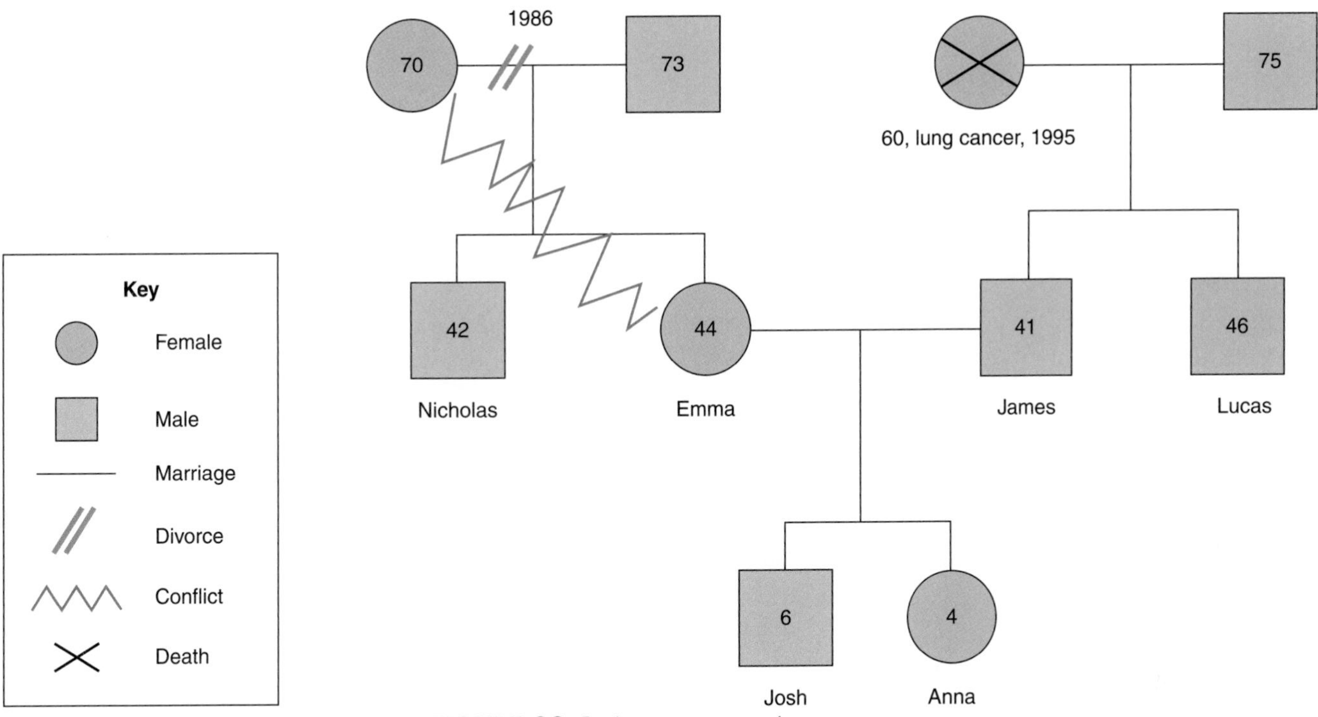

FIGURE 23-4 Three-generational genogram.

or third issue into the mix. Although triangles decrease anxiety, they also keep the two individuals from addressing the source of the conflict that has produced the anxiety. A triangle temporarily diffuses a problem relationship, but if it becomes fixed and the original conflict is not resolved, then symptoms begin to appear in one of the members of the triangle. Identifying triangles in the family and their role in the psychologic symptoms of its members is essential in planning interventions that help families more effectively manage anxiety-producing stressors within and outside the family.

Boundaries

Boundaries are rules in the family that regulate interpersonal, emotional contact between individual family members and subsystems within the family. Boundaries or rules that become rigid and do not allow contact with outside subsystems result in isolation and limit emotional support or *disengagement*. An extreme amount of stress needs to occur before an individual family member or the family as a whole seeks assistance. In contrast, *enmeshment* refers to limitless contact and support that intrude on the development of independent emotional competence. The development of boundaries or interactions between subsystems allowing emotional independence is necessary (Nichols and Schwartz, 2001).

Genogram

A **genogram** is a two- to three-generational diagram designed to track family processes over time. These processes include conflicts, types of boundaries, enmeshment, disengagement, and family triangles (Figure 23-4).

Role of the Family Therapist

The goal of the family therapist using the systems approach is to effect change by helping family members work out their differences and concerns by communicating and relating directly with each other. The family therapist works as a coach by observing and providing feedback regarding the family's patterns of interaction and communication and evaluating the family's responses, strengths, and weaknesses. The therapist introduces new strategies for the family to use that will result in more positive interactions (Carter and McGoldrick, 2005). The family therapist conducts an extensive assessment of all family members and the family as a whole by using a genogram to identify relationship patterns, communication styles, and the level of communication skills between the couple dyad, the parent-child dyad, the child-child dyad, and any other extended family relationships.

Family therapists look at symptoms related to the overall family system that is exhibiting difficulty in one or more subsystems such as the couple or parent dyad, mother-son dyad, father-daughter dyad, or mother-daughter dyad, in contrast to individual therapy where the focus is on a single individual.

Families generally seek therapy when they experience some difficulty in performing or completing one or more of the developmental family life cycle tasks or when an individual member or subsystem is encountering difficulty in moving through a developmental task. Identifying stressors within and outside the family system and assessing how family members are coping or reacting are critical priorities for the family therapist. Symptoms of psychologic distress in one family member affect other family

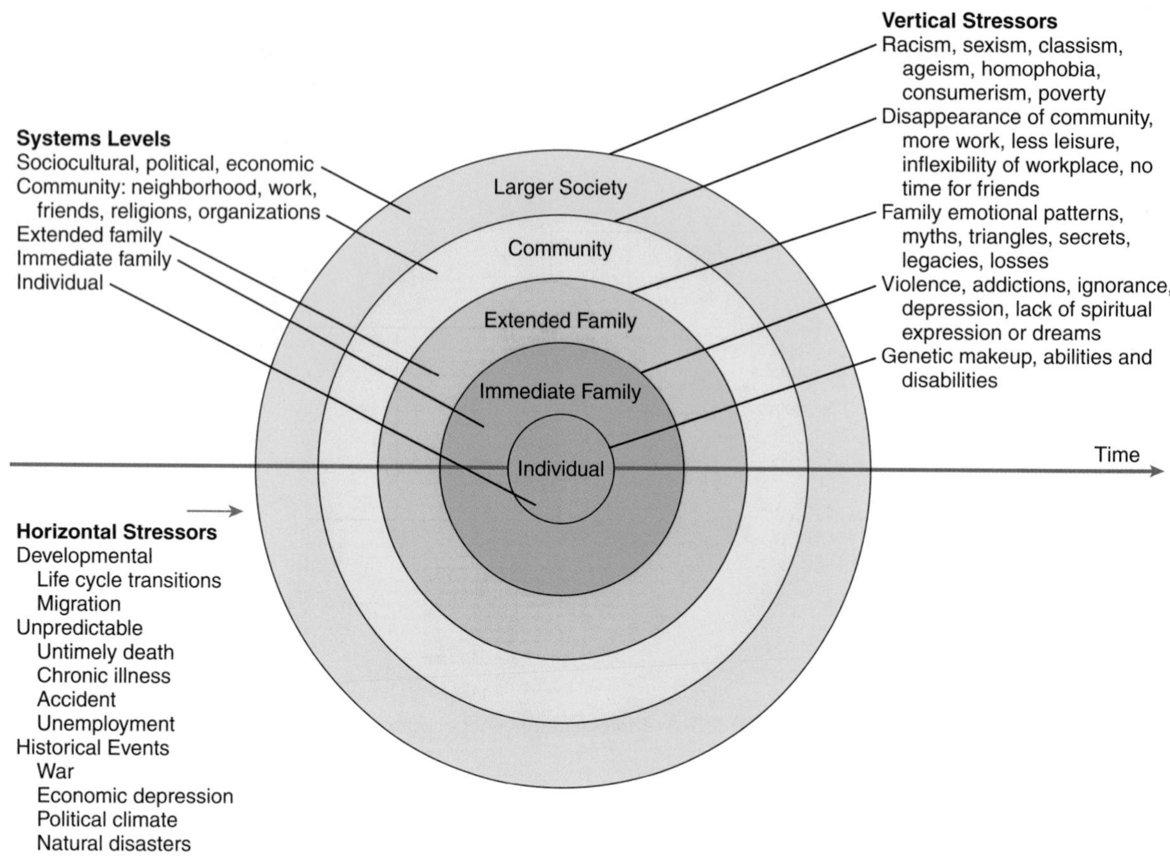

FIGURE 23-5 Flow of stress through the family. (From Carter B, McGoldrick M: Overview: the expanded family life cycle: individual, family and social perspectives. In Carter B, McGoldrick M, editors: *The expanded life cycle: individual, family and social perspectives,* ed 3, p 6, Boston, 2005, Allyn & Bacon.)

members and also create secondary stressors. Carter and McGoldrick (2005) identified stressors as flowing in both vertical and horizontal lines within the life cycle of the family over time (Figure 23-5). Social factors inherent in the family's society or culture progresses downward toward the community, extended family, immediate family, and finally to the individual.

Vertical stressors include societal attitudes and values regarding race, gender, work, and leisure time, as well as individual family factors such as the generational transmission of family history, family emotional patterns, attitudes, family secrets, taboos, and cultural beliefs. *Horizontal stressors* are predictable developmental stressors that arise during the normal stages of family development, such as marriage, childbirth, and entering college.

In addition to the vertical and horizontal stressors, unpredictable events such as untimely death, chronic illness, or accidents also occur, which further disrupt the family life cycle. At the sociocultural level, war, famine, health epidemics, natural disasters, social policy, and political climate also negatively impact families (Carter and McGoldrick, 2005).

Difficulties arise most often for families during a transition or movement to the next stage of the family life cycle. Carter and McGoldrick (2005) cited research indicating that the highest points of stress occur during times of loss or when there is an addition to the family. These transitions require families to redefine their relationships as they form new emotional attachments and lose other attachments. Families enter into crisis when they do not have the psychologic resources to manage the stressors. Some families seek help or enter the mental health care system during a developmental crisis or situational crisis. Referral to a family therapist occurs when the parents, school system, or juvenile court identifies a child or adolescent as not exhibiting or adhering to age-appropriate behaviors set by social or cultural standards. Examples of inappropriate behaviors include aggression, difficulty concentrating, significant change in school performance (such as poor grades), an unusual or abrupt change in behavior (such as withdrawal in a normally outgoing child or adolescent), difficulties with peer relationships, substance use/abuse, extreme difficulty with separation, inappropriate fears, fire setting, or cruelty to animals. Some families also require additional support with the onset of an acute physical or psychiatric illness of a family member.

Role of the Nurse

The nurse plays a vital role in assessing symptoms of distress in family members and in helping the family to identify and mobilize available resources that facilitate emotional support and functioning in the family as a whole. Tapp (2000)

RESEARCH for EVIDENCE-BASED PRACTICE

Johnson ED: Differences among families coping with serious mental illness: a qualitative analysis, *American Journal of Orthopsychiatry* 70:126-134, 2000.

Researchers interviewed families of 180 people diagnosed with a serious mental illness about their understanding of their family member's illness, coping with problems caused by the illness, and sources of support. They also asked families about the effects of medication and substance abuse and dealing with mental health professionals. Results demonstrated that different members interpret the illness in different ways. Fathers had more difficulty accepting mental illness in their sons, mothers were often the primary caregiver, and siblings were more sympathetic if they understood the illness as biologic and more distant or rejecting if behavioral symptoms were understood as "manipulative, stubborn, lazy." Interpretations varied among family members. The majority of families among all ethnic and socioeconomic groups reported feeling disregarded or dismissed as irrelevant by mental health professionals and not heard when seeking help when the early stage of decompensation began to occur in their family member. The majority of the families felt family members benefited from the use of medication for remission of symptoms, but also voiced concern over concurrent substance use and its effect on the client's level of functioning, need for hospitalization, or incarceration. Families identified faith or religious beliefs, other family members, connection with self-help groups, and helping the ill family member obtain treatment as ways of coping.

Recognize that individual family members often differ in their understanding of the client's illness and therefore require education. Also, nurses can provide families with valuable information on medication response and early signs of relapse and can help families to identify self-help groups as sources of support to increase their sense of competence.

emphasized the nurse's responsibility to acknowledge the reciprocal influence between illness in a client and other family members. The nurse is able to employ a brief 15-minute assessment using a genogram by asking the following three important assessment questions:

- *Which family members are most involved with the client?* This involves making a genogram to illustrate family structure (see Figure 23-4).
- *How does the illness affect the family?* The nurse explores, with family members, the amount of distress and anxiety being experienced and acknowledges their concerns and fears by answering questions and promoting communication and support from other family members (see the Research for Evidence-Based Practice box).
- *How does the family affect the illness?* The nurse engages in therapeutic conversations to help the family reveal its method of managing the demands of caregiving. This gives the nurse the opportunity to provide feedback for effective coping and to suggest additional resources for the family to use while negotiating the crisis. Referrals to community resources provide additional support to families as they cope with the stressors. Numerous support groups are available to help family members learn how to cope and manage family stressors, such as the loss of a child, parenting concerns, a chronic psychiatric illness, developmental disabilities, addictions, a chronic physical illness, widowhood, single parenting, and divorce.

ACTIVITY THERAPIES

Health care providers have practiced **activity therapies**—also known as *therapeutic activities, expressive therapies, experimental therapies,* or *adjunct therapies*—in psychiatric mental health settings since the 1980s. With the onset of managed care and cost containment, the use of these activities has diminished, and in many instances, nurses pair up with recreational therapists to conduct these activities in inpatient, outpatient, and community settings.

Types of therapeutic activities include recreational, occupational, art, music, movement/dance, and psychodrama. These activities provide service to children, adolescents, adults, and older adults of all functional levels and diagnostic categories. The primary intent of these activities is to increase the client's awareness of feelings, behaviors, thoughts, and sensations through the medium of art, music, or dance and to use that medium to minimize pathology and promote mental and emotional health. Activities also allow clients to express themselves on multiple levels, to be creative, and to demonstrate conflicts, strengths, and limitations in a safe, nonthreatening environment, which will help prepare them for life outside the hospital. Activity therapists and nurses generally collaborate to recommend activity therapies to the client's primary physician.

Historical Perspectives

Activity therapies date back to 2000 BC when exercise and the arts were found to be healing, especially for melancholia, known today as depression. In the eighteenth and nineteenth centuries, the moral treatment of persons with mental illness increased, and nurses were among the first to recognize the therapeutic value of these activities. Two nurses, Susan E. Tracy and Florence Nightingale, contributed greatly to the birth of recreational therapy and occupational therapy. As the activities evolved and became more complex in theory and practice, activity therapy eventually became recognized as its own specialty with professional, ethical, and educational standards.

Role of the Nurse

The nurse's role in activity therapies is extremely valuable for the following reasons:

- Involvement of nurses provides more availability for client activities.
- The nurse is an additional trained professional observer who represents safety and comfort, which reduces the client's anxiety and inhibitions.
- The collaboration of the nurse and the therapist, along with the physician, allows multiple disciplines to view client problems from different perspectives, which increases the opportunity for more effective outcomes.

Occupational Therapy

Occupational therapy focuses on assessment of task performance, cognitive functioning, psychosocial development, recognizing strengths, ameliorating weaknesses, and adapting to change. The nurse's role in occupational therapy includes daily contact with clients to provide encouragement, support, role modeling, teaching, discussion, and reality testing of prescribed tasks. The nurse's assessment of overall client functioning provides valuable information for occupational therapists. For example, a client who is experiencing cognitive decline based on the nurse's mental status assessment will benefit from the occupational therapist's evaluation and perspective of cognitive functioning. Also, nurses observe a client's frustration tolerance and problem-solving skills as the client performs activities of daily living or attempts other simple tasks. Nurses and occupational therapists work together and with the physician to provide the best possible outcomes for the client by promoting client strengths based on the specialized roles of each discipline.

Recreational Therapy

Recreational therapy, also known as *therapeutic recreation*, is sometimes called the art of work, love, and play. The nurse's role in recreational therapy includes promoting activities and interactions that foster independence, responsibility, problem-solving skills, leisure activities, and interactive skills. Table 23-9 describes the various types of recreational therapy and the nurse's role in each type.

ELECTROCONVULSIVE THERAPY

Many healing methods focus on affecting changes on the physical parts of the body that result in positive effects on the individual's mental or emotional state. Psychiatry has a unique form of biologic treatment known as **electroconvulsive therapy** (ECT), which stipulates that a brief, controlled electrical stimulus applied to the brain produces a change in brain chemistry that results in an improved mood state, even though the precise mechanism of action is unknown. In this instance, the individual's physical state also improves once the depression has lifted. Unlike nutritional therapy, ECT was not always favorably viewed, and even today this mainstream biologic-based treatment has its share of skeptics.

Historical Perspectives

ECT, sometimes known as *electroshock therapy*, is not a new discovery. It was first used as a treatment in 1934 to "cure" psychotic disorders by inducing convulsions. Paracelsus, a sixteenth-century Swiss physician, gave camphor to induce convulsions as a method of treating "lunacy." Von Auenbrugger in 1764 used the same intervention to treat symptoms of mania. In 1934, Meduna administered an injection of camphor oil to a patient with schizophrenia who had been in a catatonic stupor for 4 years. After a series of these treatments, the patient made a remarkable recovery. Meduna administered this same treatment to 26 patients, 13 of whom showed significant improvement. Reports of the success of this new form of therapy spread, and others soon explored additional methods to induce convulsions. By 1938, two Italian scientists, Cerletti and

TABLE 23-9

Recreational Therapy and the Nurse's Role

THERAPY	DESCRIPTION	NURSE'S ROLE
Art therapy	The use of art to help resolve conflicts and promote self-awareness through nonverbal media	Observing client's use of art, encouraging verbal responses to artwork, and noting content of artwork and how it relates to client's specific issues. NOTE: Do not comment on the quality of the artwork or the client's artistic talents, as this is not an art contest but simply each client's self-expression.
Music therapy	The use of music in a defined structure to bring about change and promote self-organization, social connection, and expression	Observing whether the client is active or passive during the experience and noting any verbal and nonverbal feelings expressed by the client. NOTE: The client's taste in music is not the focus of this activity.
Movement/dance therapy	The use of movement (kinesics) to express emotions, work out tensions, develop improved body image, and achieve body awareness and social interactions through rhythmic exercises and responses to music	Participating in the activity, observing and encouraging all clients to participate, and promoting discussion when possible. NOTE: The client's dancing talents are not the focus of this activity.
Psychodrama/sociodrama	The use of spontaneous expression and dramatic technique to act out emotional problems to promote health through the development of new perceptions, behaviors, and connection with others; a method of group psychotherapy developed by Jacob Moreno (1889-1974), a Viennese physician.	Observing the client's reactions and encouraging the client to relate these reactions to the client's own issues. NOTE: A client's acting talent is not the focus of this activity. Psychodrama is not a mainstream activity in most psychiatric mental health facilities. However, it is sometimes used in a simpler form, such as role-playing, in which individuals act out conflicts with significant others in a safe setting. Role-playing is often used to help children and adolescents reenact conflicts with a trusted nurse or therapist.

Bini, administered 11 separate transcerebral treatments using an electrical stimulus to induce a seizure in a client with schizophrenia. The client fully recovered from his illness, and Cerletti and Bini received worldwide acclaim for their efforts (Abrams, 1988). It is doubtful that this client would be diagnosed with schizophrenia by today's standards, but the relative safety and efficacy of this procedure opened up a whole new treatment technique in psychiatry.

Modern Electroconvulsive Therapy

ECT is currently considered a safe and effective treatment for major depression. Despite advances in the pharmacologic treatment of major depression, approximately 15% of depressed people do not respond to medications and continue to experience depression. Of this 15%, however, approximately 90% find relief from depression through ECT, making it an effective treatment for clients who are resistant to pharmacotherapy.

ECT involves sending an electrical current through the brain of an anesthetized client to induce a grand mal seizure. The exact mechanism of action is not known. Because of this lack of understanding, as well as issues surrounding clients' rights, ECT has had a poor reputation in the publics mind based on media portrayal of this treatment. The most appropriate candidates are those experiencing a major mood disorder. Clients with melancholic, delusional, and psychotic depression also tend to respond well to ECT.

Other indications for ECT include previous positive results from ECT, clients who cannot tolerate side effects of antidepressant medications, clients with acute suicidal thoughts and behaviors, and clients in danger of fluid and electrolyte imbalance as a result of an inability to eat or drink because of severe depression. ECT has also been used in the treatment of mania, severe catatonia, and schizophrenia that is unresponsive to antipsychotic medications.

ECT is used for clients with a mental disorder who are in the first trimester of pregnancy when pharmacotherapy is contraindicated. It is also an effective treatment for older adult clients experiencing mental illness, who cannot tolerate the effects of pharmacotherapy.

Absolute contraindications of ECT include clients with space-occupying lesions in the brain with increased intracranial pressure. Risk factors are recent myocardial infarction, aneurysms, acute respiratory infection, cardiac arrhythmias, organic syndromes, thrombophlebitis, and narrow-angle glaucoma.

ECT is not used for clients with the following diagnoses: drug dependence, personality disorders, reactive depression, and paranoid schizophrenia. Physicians generally administer ECT treatments three times a week, with an average series of 8 to 12 treatments.

Informed Consent

Informed consent authorizes the physician to perform ECT. The client gives consent before treatment, and the health care provider obtains it only after thoroughly educating the client about the procedure and preparing the client for any possible effects. The nurse is often a witness to informed consent (see Chapter 8).

Preparation

Basic preliminary tests before ECT include a complete blood count, a comprehensive metabolic profile, a urine analysis, an electrocardiogram, and a physical examination. ECT currently is performed on an inpatient or outpatient basis depending on the physician's assessment of the client's condition and support system. Clients scheduled for ECT must fast overnight and are prepared as if they were undergoing a routine operative procedure (i.e., they empty the bladder and remove any jewelry, dental work, or nail polish).

Approximately 30 minutes before ECT, the client receives an intramuscular injection of atropine, typically 0.5 mg. This drug reduces secretions and protects against vagal bradycardia, which can occur with application of the electrical stimulus.

Procedure

In the ECT treatment room, blood pressure, cardiac, and electroencephalogram monitors assess the client's vital functions. Emergency equipment such as oxygen, suction, and a cardiac arrest cart (crash cart) are also available. The minimum staff in attendance includes the treating psychiatrist, an anesthesiologist, and a nurse.

The anesthesiologist gives a short-acting anesthetic and a muscle relaxant intravenously, as muscle paralysis prevents increased movement, which reduces the risk of fracture or injury. A mouth guard and 100% oxygen are administered. After obtaining anesthesia and paralysis, the ECT electrodes are placed. For bilateral ECT, electrodes are placed on the right and left anterior portion of the client's temples. For unilateral ECT, the electrode is placed on the anterior side of the client's nondominant temple. For example, if the client is right-handed, the electrode is placed on the right temple.

Once the electrodes are placed, a brief electrical stimulus (generally no more than 2 seconds in total duration) is applied. The body does not move because of the paralyzing agent, and the seizure is confirmed by EEG monitoring. The client wakes in a few minutes, and oxygen is discontinued accordingly. The client is monitored for any respiratory distress or excess secretions that need to be suctioned.

Postprocedure

After ECT, the client remains in the recovery room for about 1 to 3 hours until vital signs are stable and the client is alert, oriented, and able to walk without assistance. The client is now able to eat and resume normal activity. Some clients feel sleepy and return to bed for a while. Side effects most associated with ECT are headache and memory loss.

Clients experiencing headaches sometimes receive a mild analgesia and are instructed to rest. Memory impairment tends to be more pronounced with bilateral ECT. It can be quite severe during the course of treatment but generally improves significantly after completion of a series of treatments.

Role of the Nurse

Nurses play an integral role in ECT treatment by providing accurate education to the client and family to reduce fear and prevent distortions and myths regarding the use of ECT. Nurses need to fully understand the indications, contraindications, procedures, and side effects of ECT in order to educate, prepare, monitor, and support the client and family.

The nurse also witnesses the informed consent procedure and ensures that the client's rights regarding treatment are understood by the client and accurately documented. Before and after the procedure, the nurse calms the client's fears, anxieties, and concerns; administers vital signs; and performs other necessary nursing interventions. The nurse also supports, comforts, and reassures clients experiencing headache or memory loss and recognizes the need for repetitive teaching for clients with memory loss throughout the course of treatment. This is often challenging, as the depression itself sometimes impairs memory and concentration. Nurses need to be aware that there is still some controversy about whether mild cognitive deficits remain after ECT (Blazer and Cassel, 1994). Nurses work closely with the client, family, physician, and anesthesiologist to provide a safe, effective ECT procedure and to prepare the client for transition to another unit or discharge home.

CHAPTER SUMMARY

- The humanistic approach emphasizes the human potential and inherent worth of human beings as unique, self-actualizing, and self-determined individuals with the capacity to develop self-awareness.
- Behavioral therapies are based on the premise that behavior is a learned response to a stimulus in the environment.
- Cognitive therapy is based on the theory that distorted or dysfunctional thinking causes psychologic disturbances in mood and behavior.
- Group therapy allows the client to define her or himself through human interaction and task accomplishment.
- Family therapy promotes the health and functioning of the entire family system as it helps to define the member's roles and tasks during times of stress and transition.
- The goal of activity therapy is to increase the client's awareness of sensations, feelings, perceptions, thoughts, and behaviors.
- Activity therapy includes occupational, recreational, art, music, movement/dance, and psychodrama/sociodrama.
- Occupational therapy focuses on assessment of task performance, cognitive functioning, and psychosocial development.
- Recreational therapy focuses on assessing the individual's capacity to incorporate the curative elements of play and leisure into his or her lifestyle.
- The nurse's role in therapeutic activities is that of a professional observer and participant who works with the therapist to enhance the client's capabilities and functioning within the parameters of the assigned activity.
- Electroconvulsive therapy (ECT) is a safe, effective biologic treatment for major depression and other select diagnoses despite residual consumer perceptions.
- Nurses play an integral role in preparing and educating clients and families about ECT.

REVIEW QUESTIONS

1 A nurse interacts with a woman recently widowed when her husband was killed in a plane crash. While supporting and comforting this client, the nurse experiences distressing personal feelings associated with the death of a parent 5 years earlier. What is the nurse's best action?

1. Acknowledge the transference evident in this relationship and discuss the phenomenon with the client.
2. Carefully select the words the nurse uses in interactions with this client to avoid influencing the client.
3. Disregard the nurse's personal feelings and proceed with helping this client resolve the grief.
4. Recognize development of countertransference and introspectively explore ways to cope with it.

2 A client says to the nurse, "The treatment team wants me to attend individual therapy sessions to help me with my problems, but I'm not going. I've seen psychoanalysis in movies, and it's not for me." Select the nurse's most therapeutic response.

1. "Psychoanalysis is an effective short-term approach to solving problems. You should follow the recommendation."
2. "Psychoanalysis is just one type of individual therapy. You and your therapist can decide which type is best for you."
3. "It is your right to decide whether or not to participate in any type of therapy, regardless of the team's recommendation."
4. "It doesn't sound like you like this plan. Perhaps you should consider changing to a new psychiatrist."

3 A nurse talks with a client engaged in an arts and crafts activity. The client says, "I've never been artistic. I shouldn't even come to these silly groups." The client also attends cognitive behavioral therapy (CBT) sessions two times a week. Which comment by the nurse would be supportive of the CBT?

1. "I noticed that you made interesting color combinations and encouraged others."
2. "What activities do you think you would enjoy more than arts and crafts?"
3. "You should try harder to finish projects that you start. You give up too easily."
4. "These are simply recreational activities. Talk to your therapist about your reactions."

4 These comments are made by members of a group. Which comment best contributes to the group's cohesiveness?
1. "I need to talk about how my problems developed and get some ideas for solving them."
2. "We aren't making progress because our group leader has as many problems as we do."
3. "No one in this group wants to hear anything else about failed romantic relationships."
4. "We started out talking about losses, but we have strayed from that subject."

5 The leader opens the discussion at the first meeting of a new group. Which comment would be appropriate for this phase?
1. "Let's start by asking each person here to define his or her problems."
2. "Let's begin by establishing the ground rules for our group."
3. "I would like each person to explain why you are attending this group."
4. "Bringing family members to our group will help us achieve our goals."

Additional self-study exercises and learning resources are available to you on the ***Companion CD*** *at the back of the book and on the* ***Evolve website*** *at* ***http://evolve.elsevier.com/Fortinash/.***

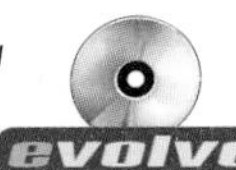

ONLINE RESOURCES

Albert Ellis Institute: **www.albertellisinstitute.org**

American Art Therapy Association: **www.arttherapy.org**

American Dance Therapy Association: **www.adta.org**

American Music Therapy Association: **www.musictherapy.org**

American Occupational Therapy Association: **www.aota.org**

American Society of Group Psychotherapy and Psychodrama: **www.asgpp.org**

American Therapeutic Recreation Association: **www.atra-tr.org**

Beck Institute for Cognitive Therapy and Research: **www.beckinstitute.org**

Behavior Tech: Dialectical Behavior Therapy: **www.behavioraltech.com**

REFERENCES

Abrams R: *Electroconvulsive therapy*, New York, 1988, Oxford University Press.

Avis, JM: Power and politics in therapy with women. In Goodrich TJ (Ed.): *Women and power: perspectives for family therapy*, New York, 1991, Norton & Company, pp. 183-200.

Bandura A: *Principles of behavior modification*, New York, 1969, Holt, Rinehart & Winston.

Beck AT: *Cognitive therapy and the emotional disorders*, New York, 1976, International Universities Press.

Beck AT, Rush AH, Shaw BF: *Cognitive therapy of personality disorders*, New York, 1979, Plenum.

Beck JS: *Cognitive therapy: basics and beyond*, New York, 1995, Guilford Press.

Bentovin A, Kinston W: Focal family therapy: joining systems theory with psychodynamic understanding. In Gurman AS, Kiskern DP, editors: *Handbook of family therapy*, vol 2, New York, 1991, Brunner/Mazel.

Blazer DG, Cassel CE: Depression in the elderly, *Hosp Pract* 29:37-41, 1994.

Bohus M et al: Effectiveness of inpatient dialectical behavior therapy for borderline personality disorder: a controlled trial, *Behav Res Ther* 42:487-499, 2004.

Botella C et al: Treatment of flying phobia using virtual reality: data from a 1 year follow-up using a multiple baseline design, *Clin Psychol Psychother* 11:311-323, 2004.

Boszormeyni-Nagy I, Spark G: *Invisible loyalties: reciprocity in intergenerational family therapy*, New York, 1973, Harper & Row.

Bowen M: Theory in the practice of psychotherapy. In Guerin P, editor: *Family therapy: theory and practice*, New York, 1976, Gardner Press, pp. 42-90.

Carter B, McGoldrick M: Overview: the expanded family life cycle: individual, family and social perspectives. In Carter B, McGoldrick M, editors: *The expanded life cycle: individual, family and social perspectives*, ed 3, vols 1-26, Boston, 2005, Allyn & Bacon.

Colapinto J: Structural family therapy. In Gurman AS, Kniskem DP: *Handbook of family therapy*, vol 2, New York, 1991, Brunner/Mazel, pp. 417-443.

Ellis A: *Humanistic psychotherapy: the rational-emotive approach*, New York, 1973, McGraw-Hill.

Ellis A: Fundamentals of rational-emotive therapy for the 1990s. In Dryden W, Hill LK, editors: *Innovations in rational-emotive therapy*, pp 1-32, Newbury Park, Calif, 1993, Sage.

Falloon IRH: Behavioral family therapy. In Gurman AS, Kniskem DP: *Handbook of family therapy*, vol 2, New York, 1991, Brunner/Mazel, pp. 65-95.

Freud A: *The ego and the mechanisms of defense*, London, 1937, Hogarth Press and Institute of Psychoanalysis.

Freud S: The dynamics of transference. In *Collected papers*, vol 2, New York, 1959, Basic Books, pp. 312-322.

Freud S: *The ego and the id*, New York, 1960, W.W. Norton (edited and translated by J Strachey).

Freud S: *The interpretation of dreams*, New York, 1961, Scientific Editions (edited and translated by J Strachey).

Gallop R, O'Brien L: Re-establishing psychodynamic theory as foundational knowledge for psychiatric/mental health nursing, *Issues Ment Health Nurs* 24 213-227, 2003.

Goodrich TJ: Women, power, and family therapy: what's wrong with this picture? In Goodrich TJ, editor: *Women and power: perspectives for family therapy*, New York, 1991, WW Norton & Company, pp. 3-35.

Horowitz ER: Virtual graded exposure therapy treatment for phobias: a program design. Diss Abst Int: *Sci Engineer* 64:4040, 2004.

Johnson SM: Introduction to attachment: a therapist's guide to primary relationships and their renewal. In Johnson SM, Whiffen VE, editors: *Attachment processes in couple and family therapy*, pp 3-17, New York, 2003, Guiford Press.

Jones M: *Beyond the therapeutic community*, New York, 1968, Basic Books. (classic)

Jung CG: *Two essays on analytical psychology*, ed 2, vol 7, collected works, New York, 1966, Princeton University Press. (classic)

Jung CG: *The structure and dynamics of the psyche*, ed 2, vol 8, collected works, New York, 1969, Princeton University Press. (classic)

Kerr ME, Bowen M: *Family evaluation: an approach based on Bowen theory*, New York, 1988, WW Norton & Company.

Kerr NJ: The ego competency model of psychiatric nursing: theoretical overview and clinical application, *Perspect Psychiatr Care* 26:13-24, 1990.

Kohut H: *The restoration of the self*, New York, 1977, International Universities Press.

Krihn M et al: Virtual reality exposure therapy of anxiety disorders: a review, *Clin Psychol Rev* 24:259-281, 2004.

Lankton SR, Lankton CH: *The answer within: a clinical framework of Ericksonian hypnotherapy*, New York, 1983, Brunner/Mazel.

Lieberman MA, Yalom ID, Miles MB: *Encounter groups: first facts*, New York, 1973, Basic Books.

Linehan MM et al: Cognitive-behavioral treatment of chronically parasuicidal borderline patients, *Arch Gen Psychiatr* 48: 1060-1064, 1991.

Linehan MM: *Cognitive-behavioral treatment of borderline personality disorder*, New York, 1993, Guilford Press.

Linehan M et al: Dialectical behavior therapy for patients with borderline personality disorder and drug-dependence, *Am J Addictions* 8, 279-292, 1999.

Linehan MM et al: Dialectical behavior therapy versus comprehensive validation therapy plus 12-step for the treatment of opioid dependent women meeting criteria for borderline personality disorder, *Drug Alcohol Depend* 67:13-26, 2002.

Lynch TR et al: Dialectical behavior therapy for depressed older adults: a randomized pilot study, *Am J Geriatr Psychiatry* 11: 33-45, 2003.

Madanes C: Strategic family therapy. In Gurman AS, Kniskem DP: *Handbook of family therapy*, vol 2, New York, 1991, Brunner/Mazel, pp. 396-416.

Mahler MS, Pine F, Bergman A: *The psychological birth of the human infant: symbiosis and individuation*, New York, 1975, Basic Books.

Maslow AH: A theory of human motivation, *Psychol Rev* 50: 370-396, 1943.

Meichenbaum D: *Cognitive-behavior modification*, New York, 1977, Plenum.

Minuchin S: *Families and family therapy*, Cambridge, 1974, Harvard University Press.

Nichols MP, Schwartz RC: *The essentials of family therapy*, Boston, 2001, Allyn & Bacon.

Northouse P, Northouse L: *Health communication: strategies for health professionals*, Norwalk, Conn, 1998, Appleton & Lange.

Patterson G: *Families: applications of social learning to family life*, Champaign Ill, 1975, Research Press.

Pavlov I: *Lectures on conditioned reflexes*, New York, 1928, International Publishers (edited and translated by WH Grant).

Peplau HE: *Interpersonal relations in nursing*, New York, 1952, GP Putnam's Sons. (classic)

Peplau, HE: Interpersonal relations: a theoretical framework for application in nursing practice, *Nurs Sci Q* 5:13-18, 1992.

Peternelj-Taylor CA, Young O: Exploring boundaries in the nurse-client relationship: professional roles and responsibilities, *Perspect Psychiatr Care* 39:55-66, 2003.

Premack D: Toward empirical behavioral laws: I. Positive reinforcement, *Psychol Rev* 66:219-233, 1959.

Rogers CP: The necessary and sufficient conditions of therapeutic personality change, *J Consult Psychol* 21:95-103, 1957.

Rogers CP: *A way of being*, Boston, 1980, Houghton-Mifflin. (classic)

Sampson E, Marthas M: *Group process for the health professions*, New York, 1990, Delmar.

Sebastian L, Kuntz G, Shocks D: Whose structure is it anyway? *Perspectives in Psychiatr Care* 26:25-7, 1990.

Siegel DJ: *The developing mind: how relationships and the brain interact to shape who we are*, New York, 1999, Guilford Press.

Skinner BF: Whatever happened to psychology as the science of behavior? *Am Psychol* 42:780-786, 1987.

Stern DN: *The interpersonal world of the infant*, New York, 1985, Basic Books.

Stiles AS: Personal versus relational boundaries: concept clarification and therapeutic interventions, *J Theory Construction Testing* 8:72-78, 2004.

Tapp DM: Therapeutic conversations that count, *Canadian Nurse* 96:29-32, 2000.

Tech CF, Agras WS, Linehan M: Dialectical behavior therapy for binge eating disorder, *J Consult Clin Psychol* 69:1061-1065, 2001.

Turner R: Naturalistic evaluation of dialectical behavior therapy-oriented treatment for borderline personality disorder, *Cogn Behav Pract* 7:413-419, 2000.

Winnicott DW: *The maturational processes and the facilitating environment: studies in the theory of emotional development*, New York, 1965, International Universities Press.

Wolpe J: *Psychotherapy by reciprocal inhibition*, Stanford, Calif, 1958, Stanford University Press.

Yalom ID: *The theory and practice of group psychotherapy*, ed 3, New York, 2005, Basic Books. (classic)

Yurkovich E: Patient and nurse roles in the therapeutic community, *Perspect Psychiatr Care* 25:18-22, 1989.

Chapter 24

Psychopharmacology

PAULINE CHAN

Better to use medicines at the onset than at the last moment.

PUBLILIUS SYRUS

OBJECTIVES

1 Describe and discuss the client considerations and nursing responsibilities related to antipsychotic medication therapy.

2 Describe and discuss the client considerations and nursing responsibilities related to antidepressant medication therapy.

3 Describe and discuss the client considerations and nursing responsibilities related to mood stabilization therapy.

4 Describe and discuss the client considerations and nursing responsibilities related to anxiolytic and hypnotic medication therapy.

5 Describe and discuss the client considerations and nursing responsibilities related to stimulant medication therapy.

KEY TERMS

agranulocytosis, p. 548
akathisia, p. 543
atypical antipsychotics, p. 541
conventional antipsychotics, p. 541
extrapyramidal side effects, p. 543
hypertensive crisis, p. 556
metabolite, p. 540
neuroleptic malignant syndrome, p. 544
neuroleptics, p. 541
photosensitivity, p. 545
psychotropic, p. 540
refractory, p. 541
serotonin syndrome, p. 553
serum level monitoring, p. 543
side effects, p. 540
tardive dyskinesia, p. 543
titration, p. 554

The National Institute of Mental Health estimates that 26.2% of Americans 18 years and older—about one in four adults—suffer from a diagnosable mental disorder in a given year. When applied to the 2004 U.S. census residential population estimate, this figure translates to 57.7 million people. According to Substance Abuse and Mental Health Services Administration (SAMHSA), about half (46.6%) of all Americans will have a mental illness during their lifetimes, and for most, the symptoms will manifest during the teen years. About 20% of Americans will experience mood disorders, and 28.8% will experience anxiety disorders. Nearly a quarter (24.8%) will experience an impulse control disorder; 14.6% will experience a substance abuse disorder.

Until the discovery of chlorpromazine (Thorazine) and other psychoactive medications, clients with mental illness had few options and often were left untreated. Edward Shorter (1998), in his book *History of Psychiatry*, summarized the discovery of chlorpromazine for psychiatry as important as the discovery of penicillin for general medicine. The significant discovery that chlorpromazine reduces agitation, hallucinations, and psychotic symptoms marked the beginning of the era of psychopharmacology. In the years following this discovery, researchers developed additional antipsychotic medications. Initially these included more phenothiazines, as represented by chlorpromazine, and then other structurally different chemical compounds such as the butyrophenone class, as represented by haloperidol (Haldol). In the 1960s, researchers studied these drugs to establish clinical efficacy using the double blind, placebo-controlled study method, which greatly increased our knowledge of the mechanism of actions of these drugs. The studies also provided evidence that the various antipsychotic drugs are also effective, although their potency varies. New medications continually emerge as the result of ongoing research in an effort to alleviate debilitating psychiatric symptoms and also to reduce many of the adverse side effects that occur during psychopharmacotherapy.

MODE AND MECHANISM OF DRUG ACTION

The *mode of action* of a drug describes what it does to the body. The *mechanism of action* describes how the drug works to affect the symptoms, cure the disease, or cause side effects.

Neurotransmitters

To understand the modes of action of psychotropic medications, it is important to understand the neurotransmitter systems in the brain that are affected during psychopharmacotherapy (Kramer, 2002). The classic neurotransmitters include the following: acetylcholine, histamine, serotonin, dopamine, norepinephrine, epinephrine, aspartic acid, γ-aminobutyric acid (GABA), glutamic acid, glycine, homocysteine, and taurine. A thorough discussion of the brain's neurotransmitter systems appears in Chapter 6.

The four neurotransmitters that are *most* important in the study of psychotropic medications are as follows:

1. Acetylcholine
2. Dopamine
3. Serotonin (also called 5-hydroxytryptamine or 5-HT)
4. Glutamate (glutamic acid)

Acetylcholine

Numerous receptors exist for acetylcholine. The major subdivisions are the nicotinic and muscarinic cholinergic receptors. There are numerous muscarinic receptors; the M1 postsynaptic receptor is the most important because of its mediating effect in the memory function linked to cholinergic neurotransmission. It is also related to the side effects of anticholinergic drugs such as dry mouth, blurred vision, urinary retention, and constipation. Dopamine and acetylcholine have a reciprocal relationship. Dopamine suppresses cholinergic activities in the nigrostriatal dopamine pathway.

Dopamine

Dopamine is produced in dopaminergic neurons from the precursor tyrosine. Receptors for dopamine regulate dopaminergic neurotransmission. There are four dopamine receptor pathways in the brain:

1. Nigrostriatal dopamine pathway controls movements.
2. Mesolimbic dopamine pathway is involved in behaviors such as pleasurable sensation, euphoria resulting from drugs of abuse, and delusions and hallucinations resulting from psychosis.
3. Mesocortical dopamine pathway mediates positive and negative psychotic symptoms, as well as cognitive side effects of antipsychotic medications.
4. Tuberoinfundibular (endocrine) dopamine pathway controls the release of prolactin.

Serotonin

Serotonin is produced when the enzyme tryptophan hydroxylase converts tryptophan, after being transported into the serotonin neuron. It is first converted to 5-hydroxytryptophan (5HTP) and then further converted to 5-HT by the enzyme aromatic amino acid decarboxylase. Serotonin is an inhibitory catecholamine that is stored in the vesicles until released by neuronal impulses. The enzyme monoamine oxidase type A destroys serotonin, forming an inactive metabolite. There are numerous subtypes of serotonin receptors. The key receptor, $5HT_{1D}$, is a presynaptic receptor, and other key postsynaptic receptors are $5HT_{1A}$, $5HT_{2A}$, $5HT_3$, and $5HT_4$. At least five serotonin pathways exist in the central nervous system (CNS). Serotonin mediates cognitive effects, emotions, panic, memory, anxiety, violence and aggression, sexual function, and sleep-wake cycles through the various serotonin pathways. Serotonin also interacts with many dopamine pathways and has the ability to inhibit dopamine release.

Glutamate

Glutamate, or glutamic acid, is an amino acid that is synthesized in the brain and functions as a major excitatory neurotransmitter. Glutamate is identified in an increasing number of neurologic and psychologic disorders. The psychoactive drug phencyclidine (PCP) has the ability to block the *N*-methyl-D-aspartate receptor channel. Because glutamate is the neurotransmitter of cortical and hippocampal pyramidal neurons, researchers hypothesize that the effects of PCP reflect interference with glutamatergic neurotransmission in these brain regions.

PSYCHOTROPIC PHARMACOTHERAPY ASSESSMENT

Before starting pharmacotherapy treatment, a thorough assessment of the client is necessary. Many drugs cause psychiatric symptoms ("Drugs That May Cause Psychiatric Symptoms," 2002), and it is important to evaluate the client carefully. Treatment focuses on stabilization of the illness with the goal of achieving remission, defined as complete return to baseline level of functioning and absence of symptoms. Following remission, the client enters the maintenance phase where the goal is to optimize protection against recurrence of illness. Equally important is consideration of treatment that maximizes client functioning and minimizes subthreshold symptoms and adverse effects of treatment with medications.

Variables Affecting Drug Therapy

Sherr advocated that when assessing clients before or during pharmacotherapy, it is necessary to incorporate information from both drug-related and client-related vari-

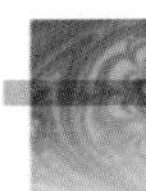

BOX 24-1

Variables Affecting Drug Therapy

DRUG-RELATED VARIABLES
- Mode/mechanism of action
- Available dosage form: oral (solid, liquid, sublingual), parenteral
- Bioavailability of various formulations
- Onset, peak, and duration of action
- Serum half-life
- Method of elimination from the body (hepatic or renal)
- Side effects/toxicities (both predictable and idiosyncratic)
- Cost (drug price, administration, and monitoring costs)

CLIENT-RELATED VARIABLES
- Diagnosis
- Other disease states (cardiovascular, liver, renal disease)
- Other medications
- Age and weight
- Previous responses and history of side effects (client and family)
- Willingness, ability to comply/insight into illness
- Financial and/or health insurance
- Support systems

BOX 24-2

Symptoms of Psychosis

POSITIVE SYMPTOMS
- Delusions
- Hallucinations
- Disorganized speech
- Disorganized behavior
- Catatonia
- Agitation

NEGATIVE SYMPTOMS
- Blunted affect
- Passiveness
- Social apathy and withdrawal
- Alogia (inability to speak)
- Avolition (inability to decide)
- Anhedonia (lack of pleasure)
- Lack of attention or spontaneity

COGNITIVE FUNCTION IMPAIRMENT
- Thought disorder
- Incoherence
- Loose association
- Difficulty processing information

AGGRESSIVE/HOSTILE SYMPTOMS
- Verbal abuse
- Assault
- Sexual acting out
- Poor impulse control

DEPRESSIVE/ANXIOUS SYMPTOMS
- Worry
- Guilt
- Anxiety
- Irritability
- Depression

ables before initiation of therapy. Box 24-1 describes common drug- and client-related variables.

PSYCHOSIS

In the past, the medical community thought psychosis was due to overactivity of dopamine neurons (referred to as the *dopamine hypothesis of psychosis*). Psychosis is traditionally described as having positive and negative symptoms, which research has concluded is not an adequate description. Instead, researchers now describe psychosis with five symptom dimensions: positive symptoms, negative symptoms, cognitive, aggressive/hostile, and anxious/depressed (Box 24-2).

Many think that positive symptoms occur as a result of the overactivity of the dopamine neurons in the mesolimbic dopamine pathway (increased brain activity), whereas negative symptoms occur as a result of cortical dopamine deficiency in the mesocortical pathway of the brain (decreased brain activity).

Antipsychotic Medications

Antipsychotic medications, previously known as *major tranquilizers* or **neuroleptics**, have been the mainstay of treatment for schizophrenia and other psychotic disorders since the introduction of chlorpromazine in 1952. These medications are effective and were directly and indirectly responsible for deinstitutionalization of clients diagnosed with schizophrenia during the 1950s and 1960s. Antipsychotic medications are generally divided into two broad categories, the *conventional* or *typical* antipsychotics and the *atypical* or *unconventional* antipsychotics. The **conventional antipsychotics** are similar in mode of action and efficacy but differ in side effects and potency. These medications block D_2 receptors in the limbic region of the brain. The **atypical antipsychotics**, also referred to as *second-generation* medications, differ in mode of action, side effects, and potency. When compared to conventional antipsychotics, the atypical antipsychotic agents generally have lower potential for extrapyramidal effects and greater efficacy in negative symptoms, cognitive symptoms, and **refractory** (treatment-resistant) illness. They also lower potential to cause prolactin elevations and have greater serotonin/dopamine D_2 effects.

Indications

Antipsychotics are for the treatment of psychosis (American Psychiatric Association [APA], 2000), which includes a wide spectrum of illnesses such as schizophrenia, schizoaffective disorders, and delusional disorders. Atypical antipsychotics are used as an adjunctive or monotherapy for bipolar disorders (Schatzberg and Nemeroff, 2001). Clients with psychosis from secondary causes, such as electrolyte or hormonal imbalances, drug abuse, brain tumors, mania, or depression with psychotic features, also benefit from short-term antipsychotic medications while the underlying illness is being treated. Table 24-1 lists the various types of antipsychotic medications and their dosages.

Goals of Therapy

Typical (conventional) antipsychotic medications are effective in reducing or alleviating the positive symptoms of psychosis. Atypical antipsychotics are more effective in alleviating negative symptoms and other symptoms associated with psychosis. It is important to observe clients for signs and symptoms and to assess clients regularly, docu-

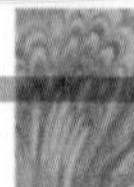

TABLE 24-1

Antipsychotic Medications

GENERIC NAME (TRADE NAME)	POTENCY	RECOMMENDED DOSAGE RANGE (MG/DAY)*	CHLORPROMAZINE EQUIVALENTS (mg/DAY)†
FIRST-GENERATION ANTIPSYCHOTICS			
Phenothiazines			
Chlorpromazine (Thorazine)	Low	300-1000	100
Fluphenazine (Prolixin)	Very high	5-20	2
Fluphenazine decanoate (Prolixin Decanoate)	Very high	6.25-75 mg/3 weeks	—
Perphenazine (Trilafon)	High	16-64	10
Thioridazine (Mellaril)	Low	300-800	100
Trifluoperazine (Stelazine)	High	15-50	5
Butyrophenone			
Haloperidol (Haldol)	Very high	5-20	2
Haloperidol decanoate (Haldol Decanoate)	Very high	100-450 mg/month	—
Others			
Loxapine (Loxitane)	High	30-100	10
Molindone (Moban)	High	30-100	10
Thiothixene (Navane)	High	15-50	5
SECOND-GENERATION ANTIPSYCHOTICS			
Aripirazole (Abilify)	—	10-30	—
Clozapine (Clozaril)	—	150-600	—
Olanzapine (Zyprexa)	—	10-30	—
Quetiapine (Seroquel)	—	300-800	—
Risperidone (Risperdal)	—	2-8	—
Ziprasidone (Geodon)	—	120-200	—

*Dosage range recommendations are adapted from the 2003 Schizophrenia Patient Outcome Research Team Recommendations.
†Chlorpromazine equivalents represent the approximate equivalent to 100 mg of chlorpromazine (relative potency); this applies to first-generation antipsychotics only.

menting specific behavior changes. The overall goal is to enable the client to return to normal daily functions and to be able to provide self-care. Another important goal is to minimize side effects, using the optimal dose with the least possible side effects, and to help clients manage these side effects so that they will continue to comply with their treatment plan on a long-term basis. Clients frequently stop taking their medications if side effects are too difficult to tolerate.

Absorption, Distribution, Metabolism, and Excretion

Sometimes the presence of food, antacids, anticholinergics, and smoking influences the absorption of drugs. Cigarette smoking tends to activate hepatic enzymes, which metabolizes drugs faster, thus smokers sometimes require higher doses. The distribution of the drug depends on the route of administration, with intramuscular injections generally having greater bioavailability than oral preparations. All drugs are metabolized in the liver and excreted through the kidneys.

Clinical Use and Efficacy

Although antipsychotics are important and effective medications, they are also the most toxic drugs used in psychiatry. A major principle for nurses and other health care providers is to use the lowest possible effective dose for the shortest amount of time.

Target symptom response varies with time. Positive symptoms are the most responsive, and symptoms such as combativeness, hostility, psychomotor agitation, and irritability often are relieved within hours. Affective symptoms, anxiety, tension, depression, inappropriate affect, reduced attention span, and social withdrawal often take 2 to 4 weeks to respond. Cognitive and perceptual symptoms such as hallucinations, delusions, and thought broadcasting usually take 2 to 8 weeks to respond. The most negative symptoms—poor social skills, unrealistic planning, poor judgment and insight—are the least responsive and slowest. Many clients have fixed hallucinations and delusions that respond minimally to medications. Given the varied time course of different symptoms, keep in mind that increases in medication dose will not hasten the relief of slow-responding symptoms.

Antipsychotic therapy usually begins with divided doses three or four times a day. This regimen is useful in determining a client's ability to tolerate a medication and to minimize the initial impact of side effects. Once an effective total daily dose is established and the client has had time to develop tolerance to side effects, the medication is often reduced to once or twice a day. Reduced frequency of administration increases the likelihood of compliance with the regimen.

Drug Level Monitoring. In general, the gastrointestinal (GI) tract absorbs antipsychotics well and the liver extensively metabolizes them. The half-life varies widely among individuals but is usually between 20 and 40 hours in adults, with the client reaching the steady state in 4 to 7 days. Serum level monitoring (i.e., obtaining blood samples to determine drug concentration) is not routinely useful. Serum level monitoring is useful in specific situations, including lack of response to normal doses after 6 weeks, severe or unusual adverse reactions, in clients who are taking multiple medications, in the physically ill, in the elderly or young children, and as a check for compliance. The side-effect profile and specific needs of each client largely determine the choice and dosage of medication.

Treatment Therapy for Acute Episodes. Atypical antipsychotics such as olanzapine (Zyprexa) 10 to 20 mg daily, risperidone (Risperdal) 3 to 6 mg daily, quetiapine (Seroquel) 300 to 800 mg daily in divided doses, ziprasidone (Geodon) 120 to 180 mg daily, and aripiprazole (Abilify) 10 to 30 mg daily are currently first-line treatments for acute episodes. Clozapine (Clozaril) is *not* a first-line treatment and is usually for refractory illness because of the risk of the serious adverse effect of agranulocytosis.

Adverse Effects of Antipsychotics: Nursing Management

The conventional antipsychotics block the D_2 receptors and the extrapyramidal motor system. Therefore, even though effective in treating psychosis, the medications also induce troublesome extrapyramidal side effects (EPS) (movement disorders). In addition, antipsychotics also block noradrenergic, cholinergic, and histamine receptors to varying degrees, resulting in a unique side-effect profile for each drug. Box 24-3 lists side effects associated with receptor blockade.

BOX 24-3

Side Effects Associated With Receptor Blockade

DOPAMINE$_2$
- Extrapyramidal side effects
- Prolactin

HISTAMINE$_1$
- Sedation
- Weight gain

CHOLINERGIC
- Dry mouth
- Blurred vision
- Sinus tachycardia
- Constipation
- Impaired memory/cognition

ALPHA$_1$
- Orthostatic hypotension
- Reflex tachycardia

SEROTONIN$_2$
- Weight gain
- Gastrointestinal upset
- Sexual dysfunction

Extrapyramidal Side Effects. The use of *high-potency conventional* antipsychotic medications poses a higher risk for EPS. High-potency conventional antipsychotic medications include fluphenazine (Prolixin), perphenazine (Trilafon), trifluoperazine (Stelazine), and haloperidol (Haldol). Four EPS symptoms are described next. Table 24-2 lists adjunctive medications used to treat EPS.

Dystonia. Dystonia reactions include spasms of the eye (oculogyric crisis), neck (torticollis), back (retrocollis), tongue (glossospasm), or other muscles, which are often frightening to the client. Fortunately these symptoms are readily reversed with intramuscular injection of 50 mg of diphenhydramine (Benadryl) or 1 or 2 mg intramuscularly of benztropine (Cogentin), followed by oral agents to prevent recurrence.

Dystonia reactions usually occurs during the early stages of treatment and are common after intramuscular injections of antipsychotics. They seldom occur after 3 months of treatment. Risk factors include administration of high-potency agents, large doses, and parenteral injections.

Pseudoparkinsonism. Symptoms include decreased movements (bradykinesia, akinesia), muscle rigidity (cogwheel and lead pipe), resting hand tremor, drooling, mask like face, and shuffling gait. This EPS is often misdiagnosed, untreated, or unrecognized. Some clients have a behavioral form of akinesia, characterized by lack of motivation, blunted affect, decreased speech, and apathy, making it difficult to distinguish this symptom from negative symptoms of their illness. Physicians need to be on the alert for this symptom complex for proper diagnosis, and nurses are alert in recognizing medication-related symptoms versus illness-generated symptoms.

Treatments include reduction of the antipsychotic medication dose, change of antipsychotic medications to one with less potential for EPS, and use of an oral anti-Parkinson agent such as benztropine (Cogentin), trihexyphenidyl (Artane), diphenhydramine (Benadryl), or amantadine (Symmetrel). EPS are not treated prophylactically.

Akathisia. Symptoms of akathisia include restlessness, pacing, rocking, or inability to sit still. These symptoms are often dose related. Akathisia is sometimes confused with anxiety and agitation. To differentiate the diagnoses of akathisia and anxiety/agitation, careful observation of the client is warranted. Akathisia improves with decreasing antipsychotic dose, whereas anxiety/agitation worsens. Akathisia is also difficult to control over a period of time, whereas anxiety/agitation is not. Propranolol (Inderal) with daily dose of 80 to 120 mg (divided dose) is usually an effective treatment. It is advisable to monitor the client's blood pressure when using this agent. A benzodiazepine such as lorazepam (Ativan) 1 mg orally is often helpful.

Tardive Dyskinesia. Tardive dyskinesia manifests as abnormal movements of any voluntary muscle groups after a prolonged period of dopamine blockade. Most commonly affected muscles are those of the face, mouth, tongue, and digits resulting in grimacing, lip smacking, tongue poking, and writing movements of the fingers and toes. These movements are often severe and disabling. Risk factors include longer lengths of time of antipsychotic use and exposure, high doses, high-potency drugs, and use of conventional antipsychotics. There is no effective treatment for tardive dyskinesia; the use of vitamin E has shown some benefit. Atypical antipsychotics have much lesser risk of causing tardive dyskinesia (less than 1% with risperidone and olanzapine) and clozapine carries no risk of causing tardive dyskinesia. Conversion to atypical antipsychotics is an ideal choice whenever possi-

TABLE 24-2

Adjunctive Medications Used to Treat Extrapyramidal Side Effects

GENERIC NAME (TRADE NAME)	EQUIVALENT DOSE (mg)	DOSE RANGE (mg)	DOSAGE FORMS*
ANTICHOLINERGIC			
Benztropine (Cogentin)	1	1-8	Injectable, capsule
Trihexyphenidyl (Artane)	2	2-15	Capsule—extended release, elixir
ANTIHISTAMINE			
Diphenhydramine (Benadryl)	50	50-400	Capsules, liquid, injectable
DOPAMINE AGONIST			
Amantadine (Symmetrel)	N/A	100-400	Capsule and liquid only

*All available as tablets unless noted.

CLINICAL ALERT

Tardive dyskinesia (TD) occurs as a result of up-regulation of dopamine receptors (i.e., prolonged blockade results in the increase in the number of receptors). **Extrapyramidal side effects** (EPS), on the other hand, occur as a result of temporary blockade of these same receptors. Therefore, when TD occurs, decreasing the dose temporarily worsens TD but improves EPS; increasing the dose temporarily improves TD but worsens EPS. A long-term solution is to decrease the dose and change to an atypical antipsychotic medication.

Recognition of TD during its early stage is crucial. Clients need to be examined using the Abnormal Involuntary Movement Scale (AIMS) or Dyskinesia Identification System: Condensed User Scale (DISCUS).

ble. Note that clozapine carries the risk of producing agranulocytosis.

Drowsiness. Drowsiness is most common during the first days of treatment and usually disappears in 1 to 2 weeks. Sedation is particularly significant with the *low-potency conventional* antipsychotics such as chlorpromazine and thioridazine (Mellaril). Clients need to avoid alcohol, medications such as antihistamines (common in some cough and cold preparations), and sleeping aids. Some clients take the daily dose at bedtime instead of during the daytime to avoid interference with daily activities.

Anticholinergic Side Effects. The use of *low-potency conventional* antipsychotics such as chlorpromazine and thioridazine presents a greater risk of anticholinergic side effects. Tolerance sometimes develops over the first 4 to 8 weeks. Anticholinergic side effects are mostly annoying but not serious and include dry mouth, blurred vision, constipation, urinary retention, nasal congestion, and ejaculatory inhibition. The following interventions are often useful suggestions for the client:

- *For dry mouth:* Use ice chips, lemon swabs, sugarless gums or candies.
- *For blurred vision:* Read in well-lighted areas, read for short periods, and vary the distance of the reading materials.
- *For constipation:* Exercise (including walking) regularly, drink plenty of fluids, eat plenty of fruits and vegetables, and use a stool softener such as docusate sodium (Colace).
- *For urinary retention:* Medical attention is often necessary. Oxybutynin (Ditropan) is successful in some cases.
- *For nasal congestion:* Use nasal decongestants to relieve symptoms.
- *For ejaculatory inhibition:* This is more prominent in men using thioridazine. Refer the client to a physician for further interventions or medication change.

Cardiovascular Side Effects

Postural Hypotension. Postural hypotension is dizziness associated with sudden changes in position such as lying down and getting up. The use of *low-potency antipsychotics* such as chlorpromazine and thioridazine presents a greater risk for postural hypotension as a result of α-adrenergic receptor blockade. Advise clients to rise from bed or chair slowly and to avoid the risk of falling. This is especially important with older adults.

Arrhythmias, Palpitations (Changes in the Heart Rhythm). Arrhythmias or palpitations sometimes occur with higher doses or in clients with preexisting heart disease, as well as in combination with certain drugs such as thioridazine and ziprasidone (Geodon).

Changes in QT Intervals. Do a baseline electrocardiogram (ECG) and repeat at maximum dose **titration**. Carefully monitor for changes in ECG. Some clients will need to use an alternative medication (Taylor, 2002).

Neuroleptic Malignant Syndrome. Neuroleptic malignant syndrome (NMS) is a medical emergency (Berkow, 1992). A client with NMS has symptoms that include decreased level of consciousness, greatly increased muscle tone (rigidity), and autonomic dysfunction (hyperpyrexia, labile hypertension, tachycardia, tachypnea, diaphoresis, and drooling). Muscle necrosis, or rhabdomyolysis, is sometimes so severe that it causes myoglobinuric renal failure, as large amounts of myoglobin are released from the muscle tissue and excreted in the urine causing myoglobinuria.

NMS is potentially fatal with a mortality rate of about 10%, and it occurs in approximately 1% of clients using antipsychotics. Major risk factors identified for the development of NMS include past history of NMS, adjunctive and polypsychotropic medications, rapid dose titration, use of high-potency antipsychotics at high dose, or use of parenteral antipsychotics. Young male clients are more frequently affected. Most of the time NMS occurs during the early stages of treatment with antipsychotics, but it may at times occur even after years of treatment.

Laboratory findings are an important diagnostic aid with this diagnosis. Typically, laboratory abnormalities include leukocytosis (15,000 to 30,000 cells/mm^3), greatly elevated creatine phosphokinase levels (over 3000 IU/ml), and myoglobinuria (Hermesh et al., 2002).

Treatments include the following:

- Immediate discontinuation of all antipsychotic medications
- Hydration of client, including administration of intravenous infusion of fluids
- Administration of acetaminophen (Tylenol) along with cooling blankets for hyperthermia
- Consideration of intravenous heparin infusion to reduce the risk of pulmonary emboli
- Management of arrhythmias
- Intravenous infusion of dantrolene (Dantrium), a direct muscle relaxant, to reduce muscle rigidity and to treat hyperthermia resulting from breakdown of muscle tissues
- Consideration of use of dopaminergic drugs such as bromocriptine (Parlodel), amantadine, or anticholinergic drugs

Most clients recover from NMS. Once the client has recovered, it is advisable to wait for 1 to 2 weeks before restarting the antipsychotic medication. Carefully evaluate clients for the need for antipsychotics. Consider possible alternatives such as lithium, carbamazepine (Tegretol), and divalproex sodium (Depakote). If the practitioner determines that the client should continue with an antipsychotic medication, another antipsychotic medication with a different chemical structure will be prescribed and doses will be slowly titrated. Note any history of NMS in the client's medical record, and the client should not receive depot antipsychotic drugs (haloperidol or fluphenazine) because of their long half-lives.

Recently, clients with a history of NMS are prescribed the atypical antipsychotics clozapine and risperidone. It is important to note that NMS has also occurred with the use of these agents. The most important rule is careful monitoring for recurrence and relapse. Monitor clients for additional signs and symptoms such as psychomotor excitement, refusal of food, anuria, and weight loss.

Weight Gain. Clozapine and olanzapine have higher weight gain potential (Box 24-4). Carefully monitor the client's blood glucose levels and screen for adult onset diabetes. Weight gain is especially significant when the client is taking other drugs, such as lithium, divalproex sodium (Depakote), or mirtazapine (Remeron) that also cause weight gain.

Counsel clients about weight gain and obesity before initiating antipsychotic therapy. Record the client's weight as a baseline, and monitor it weekly. Excessive weight gain will possibly indicate the need for a change of antipsychotics. Preventive education includes dietary counseling, including calorie counts, portion size, choice of low-fat/low-calorie foods, and exercise. Excessive weight gain, along with high blood glucose level, high blood pressure, and high cholesterol and triglycerides level, increase the risk factors contributing to metabolic syndrome, leading to diabetes and other chronic illness.

CLINICAL ALERT

Neuroleptic malignant syndrome (NMS) is a medical emergency that may be fatal if untreated. Nurses will observe excessive muscle rigidity, fever, rapid heart beat, diaphoreses, and client drooling. Immediate discontinuation of antipsychotic medications is necessary, followed by treatment of other adverse symptoms.

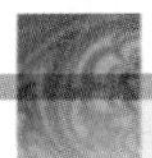

BOX 24-4

Antipsychotics Associated With Weight Gain*

- Clozapine
- Olanzapine
- Low-potency conventional antipsychotics (e.g., chlorpromazine)
- Quetiapine
- Risperidone
- High-potency conventional antipsychotics (e.g., haloperidol)
- Ziprasidone and molindone

*Ranked from greatest to least potential.

Photosensitivity and Skin Changes. Phenothiazines such as chlorpromazine induce photosensitivity reactions. Haloperidol sometimes causes photosensitivity, but this is rare. The word **photosensitivity** is a general term used to describe either the common phototoxic response or the uncommon photoallergenic reaction. Phototoxic response is nonimmunologic resembling sunburn and occurs immediately after exposure to sunlight, usually within hours. Clinical signs and symptoms include erythema, pain, and edema. Photoallergenic reactions are immunologic, require previous exposure to the photosensitizing agent, and are commonly delayed reactions (i.e., usually in 1 day to 2 weeks after exposure to sunlight). Clinical signs and symptoms include papulovesicular eruption, pruritus, and eczematous dermatitis. Treatment of sunburn includes topical burn cream and antihistamines, whereas steroids are often indicated for photoallergenic reactions. Advise clients to wear protective clothing and to use a good sunscreen during outdoor activities. Titanium dioxide is the least likely sunscreen product to cause photosensitivity disorders (Reid, 1996). Skin discoloration such as gray-blue skin is associated with antipsychotic use. Low-potency conventional antipsychotics such as chlorpromazine and thioridazine are associated with skin pigmentation. Management of these side effects requires switching to another antipsychotic.

Poikilothermia. The loss of ability to regulate internal body temperature with environment temperature change occurs and is often problematic with older adults. Closely monitor older clients using antipsychotics in the outdoors during hot weather.

Galactorrhea and Gynecomastia. These conditions are due to dopamine blockade, which results in hyperprolactinemia. Management of these side effects includes client counseling and may require medication change.

Injectable and Oral Antipsychotics

Three depot conventional antipsychotic medications are marketed in the United States: fluphenazine decanoate (Prolixin), risperidone, and haloperidol decanoate. Long-acting antipsychotics in the decanoate form are effective for clients who are unable to maintain more frequent dosage regimens because of their symptoms. The manufacturer has discontinued fluphenazine enanthate. In addition, risperidone (Risperdal Consta), a depot long-acting atypical antipsychotic medication, is available in United States.

Clinical Use and Dosage Regimen. In general, the nurse administers antipsychotics in divided doses to minimize side effects and to determine the client's ability to tolerate the medication. Once an effective dose is established, simplify the dosage regimen to once-a-day dosing. Studies show that client medication compliance improves with daily dosing or less frequent dosing.

In general, the GI tract absorbs antipsychotic medications well. To improve compliance, liquid doses are available, and both olanzapine and risperidone are available in an orally disintegrating tablet form, which readily dissolves on the tongue. It is generally not necessary to obtain serum blood samples to determine the drug concentration in the blood. The nurse obtains serum levels in specific situations such as lack of response to normal dose after an adequate trial period (6 weeks), severe or abrupt adverse drug reactions, or when a client is seriously ill.

Fluphenazine Decanoate Injection. Once the provider determines that a depot injection is necessary and the client is able to tolerate the adverse effects, the client will probably receive an initial dose of 12.5 to 25 mg (0.5 to 1 ml). Fluphenazine decanoate is administered intramuscularly or subcutaneously. The onset of action is about 24 to 72 hours. Normally the client will see the effects of the drug within 48 to 96 hours. The client receives subsequent dosages in intervals according to his or her response. Maintenance therapy dosage is usually established in 4 weeks.

A controlled multicenter study showed that fluphenazine hydrochloride 20 mg daily (orally) is equivalent to 25 mg of fluphenazine decanoate every 3 weeks. This represents a conversion of every 10 mg daily dose to be equivalent of 12.5 mg (0.5 ml) of fluphenazine decanoate every 3 weeks.

Haloperidol Decanoate Injection. Haloperidol decanoate can be given only as a deep intramuscular injection. The maximum dose should not exceed 100 mg. If an additional dose is necessary, the initial injection does not exceed 100 mg, with the balance of the dose given in 3 to 7 days as a separate injection. Clients receive haloperidol decanoate usually every 4 weeks or monthly.

The initial conversion of an oral haloperidol daily dose to decanoate injection occurs by administering 10 to 20 times the daily oral dose; for older clients, use a conversion factor of 10 to 15. For clients who previously received higher doses of antipsychotics for whom a low-dose approach risks recurrence of psychiatric decompensation, and for clients whose long-term use of haloperidol has resulted in a tolerance to the drug, 20 times the previous daily dose in oral haloperidol equivalents should be considered for initial titration, with downward titration on succeeding injections. Maintenance dosage is usually 10 to 15 times the previous daily oral dose.

Table 24-3 compares haloperidol decanoate and fluphenazine decanoate in onset, peak time, half-life, and therapeutic range. The pharmacokinetic response after intramuscular injections varies among clients.

Long-Acting Risperidone Injection. The initial dose of long acting risperidone is 25 mg by deep intramuscular injection. Do not administer it until after the initial oral dose to ensure there are no significant adverse effects. Increase the IM dose every 2 weeks up to 37.5 mg. A maximum dose is 50 mg every 2 weeks. Beyond that dosage, side effects increase with no increase in clinical benefit.

Atypical Antipsychotics

Clozapine is the first atypical antipsychotic that demonstrated efficacy in the treatment of both positive and negative symptoms in schizophrenia. Subsequently, risperidone,

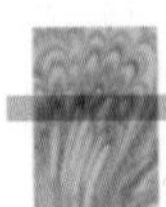

TABLE 24-3

Pharmacokinetics Comparison of Depot Antipsychotics

	HALOPERIDOL DECANOATE	FLUPHENAZINE DECANOATE
Onset	Slow onset	1-3 days
Time to peak	6 days	2-4 days
Half-life	21 days (3 weeks)	14-26 days (2-3 weeks)
Therapeutic range	100-450 mg/month	12.5-75 mg/3 weeks

olanzapine, quetiapine, ziprasidone, and aripiprazole were approved for use in the United States. EPS occur much less frequently with use of atypicals, and there is much less risk for developing tardive dyskinesia compared to high dose of high-potency typical antipsychotics. Olanzapine, risperidone, quetiapine, and aripiprazole are first-line treatment of schizophrenia because of their effectiveness and favorable side-effect profiles. Ziprasidone is also considered first-line treatment, but it has greater capacity to prolong the QT/QTc interval in the heart compared to other antipsychotics, and clients should use it with caution. Clozapine is not a first-line therapy because of the risk of agranulocytosis. It is used for refractory illness. The most recent study (CATIE) advocates the use of low to moderate doses of mild potency first-generation antipsychotics for first line therapy, along with the atypical antipsychotics.

Inappropriate uses of atypical antipsychotics include the following:

- Combination with another atypical antipsychotics or with other atypical antipsychotics
- High doses (increase side effects and is more expensive)
- Subtherapeutic doses (too low) (often ineffective and lead to treatment with combination therapy resulting in polypharmacy, especially with the elderly)

Clozapine. Clozapine is a dibenzodiazepine. It was the first atypical antipsychotic introduced for use in the United States.

Mechanism of Action. Clozapine has high receptor affinity for the D_4, 5-HT_2, α-1 adrenergic, muscarinic, and histamine H_1 brain cell receptors, and it has relatively weak receptor affinity for the D_1, D_2, and D_3 receptors. Researchers believe the high-receptor affinity for D_4 and 5 HT_2 is responsible for the many advantages of clozapine over the typical antipsychotics. Positron emission tomography scan techniques have demonstrated the dramatic difference between the atypical antipsychotic clozapine and the conventional antipsychotic haloperidol (Figure 24-1).

Clinical Use. Clozapine is for refractory illness. The dose is usually titrated slowly to avoid side effects such as sedation and orthostatic hypotension. The initial dose is 12.5 mg daily on the first day, which is then quickly titrated to 12.5 mg twice a day. The dose may be increased in 25-mg increments every other day until reaching an optimal dosage of 300 to 500 mg/day. To avoid oversedation, clients take the larger dose in the evening. Serum therapeutic level monitoring is not necessary, but a serum level of 350 μg/ml or greater is necessary for optimal response. The typical trial period of clozapine is 6 months,

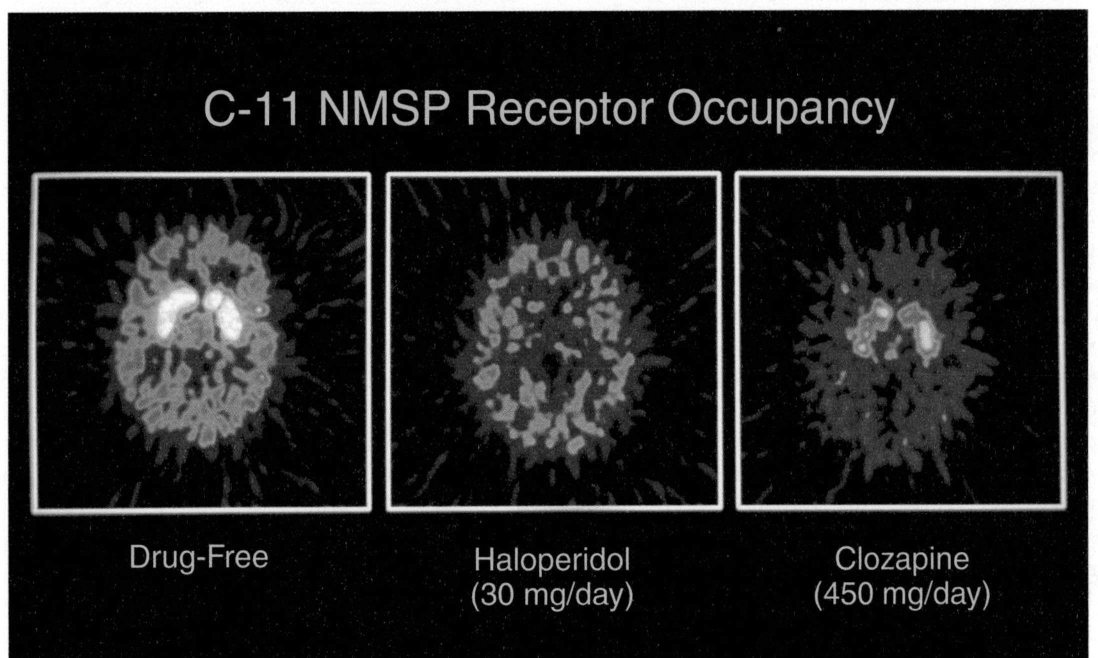

FIGURE 24-1 A transaxial positron emission tomography (PET) scan image at the level of the basal ganglia. Carbon-11 *N*-methylspiperone (NMSP) is a radioactive tag that binds and thus highlights dopamine type 2 (D_2) receptors. The three panels are from the same 36-year-old man with schizophrenia. In the first panel, the man is drug free, and the D_2-rich basal ganglia are highlighted by the NMSP. Note the absence of NMSP in the next panel, 6 weeks later, when the client was taking haloperidol, 30 mg/day, with 85% of his basal ganglia D_2-receptors occupied with haloperidol. Finally, with the man taking clozapine, 450 mg/day, only 37% of the D_2-receptors are occupied by drug. Although the psychosis was responsive to both medications, motor side effects were considerable with haloperidol and absent with clozapine. (Data from Tamminga CA et al., Maryland Psychiatric Research Center, University of Maryland at Baltimore, unpublished research.)

and if the client does not respond, providers often consider a higher dose.

Risks. Agranulocytosis occurs in 1% to 3% of clients. In the United States, clients on clozapine (Clozaril) are required to register with the Clozaril National Registry. The physician registers the client by filling out a Clozaril Client Safety Assurance Form at the initiation of therapy and also applies for a rechallenge clearance authorization from the national registry. To limit "rechallenge" of clients at risk, the physician submits weekly white blood cell (WBC) counts and evaluation (normal and abnormal) to the pharmacy that is dispensing the medication for submission to the National Registry within 7 days of collection. The physician also agrees to notify the National Registry promptly of all clients who have discontinued therapy and submit to the National Registry the results of the four required weekly blood tests after discontinuation of therapy.

A weekly WBC is drawn for the first 6 months of therapy and every other week thereafter. If the weekly WBC count is between 3000 and 3500/mm^3, these counts need to be obtained more frequently, such as twice a week. If total WBC falls between 2000 and 3000/mm^3, and the absolute neutrophil count is between 1000 and 1500/mm^3, carefully monitor the client, and check WBC with differentials daily. Discontinue clozapine permanently if the total WBC count falls below 2000/mm^3, or absolute neutrophil count falls below 1000 mm^3. Do not restart the client on clozapine. Update allergy history to include clozapine to prevent readministration. If no WBC is available from the client, discontinue the therapy. Administration of granulocyte colony-stimulating factor is necessary to reduce the risk of prolonged agranulocytosis and subsequent infections.

Clients who are at risk of agranulocytosis, such as immunocompromised clients (e.g., clients with AIDS or active tuberculosis), are not good candidates for clozapine therapy. Also the client should not receive other medications, such as carbamazepine, that carry the risk of agranulocytosis.

Side Effects. Side effects related to use of clozapine include the following:

- *Sedation.* Sedation is the most common side effect of clozapine, especially during initiation of therapy. Dose reduction is necessary in some situations. Giving a larger dose at bedtime and a smaller dose during the day is helpful.
- *Anticholinergic side effects.* Dry month, blurred vision, GI upset, urinary retention, and constipation are common.
- *Extrapyramidal side effects.* EPS are uncommon with clozapine, even with higher doses. However, akathisia is common.
- *Neuroleptic malignant syndrome.* Clozapine is not risk free for NMS.
- *Cardiovascular effects.* Tachycardia sometimes occurs. Orthostatic hypotension is often significant. Advise clients to rise slowly to prevent falls.
- *Weight gain.* Weight gain is often significant and clients need nutritional counseling before initiation of therapy. Some clients are at risk for diabetes mellitus (Wang et al., 2002) and metabolic syndrome.
- *Hypersalivation.* Hypersalivation is common, and an anticholinergic medication often alleviates symptoms.
- *Fever.* Transient rise of temperature occurs in clients treated with clozapine, especially during initiation of therapy. Monitor clients with fever and evaluate for possible infection, agranulocytosis, or NMS.
- *Seizures.* Seizures associated with clozapine are dose related. The vast majority of clozapine-induced seizures are tonic-clonic type seizures. Clients who take dosages higher than 600 mg/day have a 5% greater risk of seizures. Because of this risk, dosage greater than 600 mg/day is not recommended unless the client has failed to respond to a lower dose. Use sound judgment to discontinue or continue clozapine if the client has a seizure. Consider an anticonvulsant, but avoid carbamazepine because of increased risk of agranulocytosis. Avoid drugs that increase risk of seizures, such as bupropion (Wellbutrin).

Risperidone. Risperidone is a benzisoxazole derivative. It blocks dopamine (D_2) receptors and 5-HT receptors. Risperidone also blocks D_1, D_4, α-1, α-2 and H_1 histamine receptors and is effective in treating both positive and negative symptoms of psychosis.

Clinical Use. The usual dosage range for risperidone is 4 to 8 mg/day in two divided doses. Higher doses increase the chance of EPS and other side effects. Titrate it slowly, starting with 1 mg daily in divided doses. In the older adult, the dose is usually lower, usually starting at 25% to 50% of usual adult dose. When titration is complete, administer a once-a-day dose at bedtime. For older clients, the bedtime dose is not always appropriate because of the risk for falls. Bedtime doses are also not appropriate for clients who experience agitation and insomnia. Compared to other atypical antipsychotics, risperidone has fewer anticholinergic side effects and is often preferred for older clients (Ranier et al., 2001). Risperidone long-acting injection (Risperdal Consta) is available. The initial dose is 25 mg deep intramuscular injection every 3 weeks. The dose is sometimes increased to 37.5 mg every 2 weeks up to a maximum dose of 50 mg every 2 weeks. Before administering long-acting injections, give clients risperidone orally to ensure there are no serious adverse side effects.

Side Effects. Common side effects are insomnia, hypotension, agitation, and headache. Hyperthermia sometimes occurs, especially in older clients. Additional side effects include the following:

- *Extrapyramidal side effects.* Risperidone has a lower incidence of EPS compared with conventional antipsychotics. Administering an anticholinergic drug such as benztropine is helpful.

- *Tardive dyskinesia.* The incidence of risperidone-associated tardive dyskinesia is less than with conventional antipsychotics, but this does occur. Monitor clients closely for this.
- *Cardiovascular effects.* Hypotension occurs from α-adrenergic blockade. Caution older clients to prevent falls.
- *Weight gain.* Weight gain is associated with risperidone, but is not as significant as with clozapine or olanzapine.
- *Hyperprolactinemia.* Risperidone is associated with a rise in prolactin levels.

Olanzapine. Olanzapine is a thienobenzodiazapine. It is an atypical antipsychotic with greater D_2 and weaker D_4 and α-adrenergic blockade. Structurally, olanzapine is similar to clozapine but does not have the risk of agranulocytosis. Olanzapine is effective in treating positive and negative symptoms of schizophrenia. It is also approved for use as monotherapy for bipolar disorder in manic episodes. It is effective in the treatment of schizoaffective disorders.

Clinical Use. The recommended starting dose is 5 to 10 mg daily at bedtime and is often titrated to 20 mg/day. The rapidly disintegrating olanzapine tablet is particularly useful in clients who prefer a rapid disintegrating tablet without the need to swallow the entire tablet. Olanzapine is available in intramuscular injection and it treats agitation (overexcited, hostile, or threatening behavior) in clients with schizophrenia or bipolar disorder. Elderly clients with dementia-related psychosis who are treated with atypical antipsychotic drugs, like olanzapine, are at an increased risk of death compared to placebo. Risperidone is not for the treatment of clients with dementia-related psychosis.

Side Effects. Side effects related to use of olanzapine include the following:

- *Sedation and anticholinergic side effects.* Sedation is common because of the drug's H_1-blocking properties. Clients commonly take doses at bedtime. Anticholinergic side effects are not as significant. The most common side effect is dry mouth.
- *Weight gain and metabolic syndrome.* Weight gain is a significant side effect of many atypical antipsychotics, including olanzapine. Weight gain, increases in cholesterol and triglycerides levels, and hyperglycemia have been associated with olanzapine use (Meyer, 2001), as have adult-onset diabetes mellitus and diabetic ketoacidosis. Adult-onset diabetes mellitus has occurred between 5 weeks and 17 months after initiation of olanzapine therapy. Discontinuation of olanzapine is sometimes necessary (Zobor et al., 2002). When this cluster of conditions called *metabolic syndrome* occur together, there is increased risk for heart disease, stroke, and diabetes.
- *Seizures.* Risk of seizure with use of olanzapine is approximately 0.9%. Avoid clomipramine (Anafranil) and other drugs such as bupropion and clozapine, which induce seizures.
- *Hyperprolactinemia.* High prolactin levels are associated with higher doses of olanzapine.

Quetiapine. Quetiapine is a dibenzothiazepine derivative with weak affinity for serotonin 5-HT_{1A}, 5-HT, dopamine D_1, D_2, histamine H_1, adrenergic α-1, and α-2 receptors. Quetiapine has no appreciable affinity for cholinergic muscarinic and benzodiazepine receptors.

Clinical Use. The recommended initial dose of quetiapine is 25 mg twice a day, with increases in increments of 25 to 50 mg twice or three times a day on the second or third day, as tolerated, to a target range of 300 to 400 mg daily on the third or fourth day. Subsequent titration generally occurs in no less than 2 days with 50-mg increments. The usual dosage range for treatment of schizophrenia is 150 mg to 750 mg/day. Doses greater than 800 mg/day are not recommended. The U.S. Food and Drug Administration (FDA) has recently approved a new once-a-day dosing formulation. The advantage of a once-a-day dose is ease of administration, which directly helps to improve client adherence to the medication regimen.

Side Effects. Side effects related to use of olanzapine include the following:

- *Sedation.* Sedation is due to the H_1-antagonistic effect. Sedation and psychomotor slowing are dose dependent, and clients become more tolerant to this side effect with time.
- *Cardiovascular effects.* Because of the α-1 adrenergic antagonism, the symptoms of orthostatic hypotension with dizziness, tachycardia, and syncope are common. Hypotension sometimes occurs especially during the initiation of quetiapine. Avoid quetiapine in clients with cardiovascular diseases or other illnesses predisposed to hypotension. Postural hypotension is common during the initial titration period and can be minimized by a slower titration of 25 mg twice a day, smaller dosage increments, or a return to the previous dose titration. Nurses need to carefully monitor older clients to prevent falls.
- *Weight gain.* Weight gain is not as significant with quetiapine as with olanzapine.
- *Cholesterol and triglycerides elevations.* Elevated cholesterol and triglyceride levels have been associated with quetiapine and occur with and without weight gain. Nurses need to monitor cholesterol and triglyceride levels regularly with these clients.

Ziprasidone. Ziprasidone is a benzisothiazol piperazine derivative and a serotonin $(5HT)\text{-}2_A$/dopamine D_2 antagonist. It is also a 5HT-$_{1A}$ agonist and therefore has greater protection against adverse EPS. Ziprasidone also inhibits norepinephrine reuptake.

Clinical Use. The recommended starting dose of ziprasidone oral capsule is 20 mg twice a day and needs to be taken with food. It is usually titrated with increments of 20 mg every 2 days up to 80 mg twice a day. An increase in dose over 80 mg twice a day is not recommended.

Ziprasidone for injection is indicated for the treatment of acute agitation for clients with schizophrenia when the use of ziprasidone is appropriate and when a rapid control of agitation is necessary. The DSM-IV-TR defines *psychomotor agitation* as "excessive motor activity associated with a feeling of inner tension" (APA, 2000). Clients with a diagnosis of schizophrenia who experience agitation frequently manifest behaviors that interfere with their care (e.g., threatening behaviors, escalating or urgently distressing behavior, or self-exhausting behavior). Be aware that elderly clients with dementia-related psychosis who are treated with atypical antipsychotic drugs like ziprasidone are at an increased risk of death compared to placebo.

Risks and Contraindications. Because of ziprasidone's dose-related prolongation of the QT interval and the known association with fatal heart arrhythmias with QT prolongation by some other drugs, it is contraindicated in clients with a known history of QT prolongation (including congenital QT syndrome), recent acute myocardial infarction, or uncompensated heart failure (Glassman and Thomas Bigger, 2001).

Ziprasidone should be avoided in combination with other drugs that prolong the QT interval. Certain circumstances increase the risk of occurrence of torsades de pointes (unstable ventricular tachycardia) or sudden death in association with the use of drugs that prolong the QT interval and includes (1) bradycardia; (2) hypokalemia or hypomagnesemia; (3) concomitant use of other drugs that prolong QT interval, including quinidine, sotalol, other class Ia and III antiarrhythmics, thioridazine, chlorpromazine, pimozide, pentamidine, tacrolimus, and others; and (4) presence of congenital prolongation of the QT interval (see the Research for Evidence-Based Practice box).

Side Effects. The most common side effects of ziprasidone use are GI discomfort, including nausea, dyspepsia, constipation, diarrhea, and dry mouth. CNS side effects include drowsiness, akathisia, dizziness, EPS, dystonia, and hypertonia. Cardiovascular side effects include tachycardia and postural hypotension. Dermatologic side effects include rash and fungal dermatitis. Other side effects include abnormal vision and upper respiratory infections. Side effects associated with intramuscular injections include pain at the injection site, headache, postural hypotension, bradycardia, nausea, constipation, dizziness, drowsiness, and sweating.

Summary

In general, providers should initially administer antipsychotic medications in divided doses to minimize side effects and to determine the client's ability to tolerate the medication. Once an effective dose has been established, simplify the dosage regimen to once-a-day dosing. Studies have shown that client medication adherence and compliance improve with daily dosing or less frequent dosing. Nurses continually observe for major side effects that may occur. This is especially important with clients whose psychosis may prevent them from telling the nurse when they experience side effects.

RESEARCH for EVIDENCE-BASED PRACTICE

FDA Alert: Increased Mortality in Patients With Dementia-Related Psychosis, April 11, 2005.

This alert, issued by the Food and Drug Administration (FDA), reported that patients with dementia-related psychosis treated with atypical (second-generation) antipsychotic medications are at an increased risk of death compared to placebo. Based on currently available data, the FDA has requested that the package insert for all atypical antipsychotics include a black box warning describing this risk and noting that the drug is not approved for this condition (indication). The decision was made after the FDA reviewed reports of analyses of 17 placebo-controlled trials that enrolled 5106 elderly patients with dementia-related behavioral disorders revealing a risk of death in the drug-treated patients of between 1.6 to 1.7 times that seen in placebo-treated patients. Researchers performed clinical trials with Zyprexa (olanzapine), Abilify (aripiprazole), Risperdal (risperidone), and Seroquel (quetiapine). Over the course of these trials, averaging about 10 weeks in duration, the rate of death in drug-treated patients was about 4.5%, compared to a rate of about 2.6% in the placebo group. Although the causes of death varied, most of the deaths appeared to be either cardiovascular (e.g., heart failure, sudden death) or infectious (e.g., pneumonia) in nature.

The GI tract generally absorbs antipsychotic medications well. To improve adherence and compliance, liquid doses are available. Olanzapine and risperidone are available in an oral, rapidly disintegrating tablet form, which readily dissolves on the tongue. Olanzapine and ziprasidone injections are available for acute agitation in people with schizophrenia or bipolar disorder. In addition, risperidone is available in depot long-acting intramuscular injection that can be administered every two weeks with added convenience. It is usually not necessary to obtain blood samples to determine the drug concentration in the blood. However, serum levels are necessary in specific situations, such as lack of response despite titration to a normal dose range after an adequate trial period (6 weeks) and severe or abrupt adverse drug reactions when client is seriously ill.

MAJOR DEPRESSION

Antidepressants

The first modern antidepressant medication, imipramine, was marketed in 1958. This tricyclic compound is a modification of the structure of the antipsychotic chlorpromazine. The reason imipramine and similar drugs are called tricyclics is due to the compound's three-ring chemical structure (Figure 24-2). Dr. Roland Kuhn, a Swiss psychiatrist, originally administered imipramine to clients with schizophrenia and found no clinical efficacy. Astute observation and the persistence of Dr. Kuhn, who studied imipramine in clients with depression, quickly led to proving imipramine's efficacy in the treatment of depression. This success served as the catalyst in the search for additional antidepressant medications exhibiting improved efficacy and reduced side effects. At the same time, advances in the understanding of the role of serotonin in

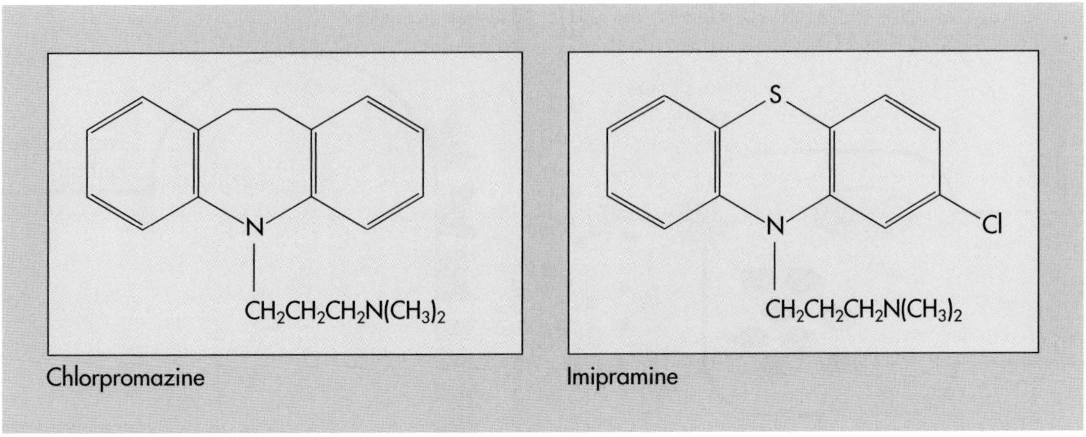

FIGURE 24-2 Chlorpromazine and imipramine are referred to as tricyclics because of their three-ring chemical structure.

depression pointed toward a new class of antidepressants, the selective serotonin reuptake inhibitors (SSRIs).

Indications

The antidepressants have many therapeutic uses, but the primary approved use is to treat major depression as defined by DSM-IV (Katon and Sullivan, 1990). Antidepressants are also effective in the treatment of a number of other conditions including the following:

- Anxiety
- Obsessive-compulsive disorders
- Panic disorders
- Bulimia
- Anorexia nervosa
- Posttraumatic stress disorder
- Bipolar depression
- Social phobia
- Irritable bowel syndrome
- Enuresis
- Neuropathic pain
- Migraine headache
- Attention deficit/hyperactivity disorder
- Smoking cessation
- Autism

Biologic Theory

The biologic theory states that depression occurs because of a decreased amount or inadequate function of the catecholamine neurotransmitters norepinephrine or serotonin. Antidepressant drugs affect the responses of these neurotransmitters. Presynaptic neurons synthesize these neurotransmitters, which are incorporated into vesicles. The action of the various antidepressants causes the vesicles to release their contents into the synapse. After they are released, neurotransmitters cross the synapse and impact receptors on the postsynaptic neuron. Most of the neurotransmitters are taken back into the presynaptic neuron to conserve this valuable resource. Then they reenter the synthesis process and are incorporated into the vesicles for future use. The cyclic antidepressants partially block reuptake of norepinephrine and serotonin. Initially, this results in increased amounts of neurotransmitter in the synapse, which reduces the number of receptors on the postsynaptic membrane. This change in receptor density, called *down-regulation*, takes several weeks to occur and is temporarily associated with the antidepressant response (Figure 24-3).

According to the biologic theory, a client who fails to respond therapeutically to one antidepressant will respond more favorably to a different antidepressant. It makes sense to switch to an antidepressant that more specifically affects the neurotransmitter that is associated with that individual client's depressed state. Even with the strength of the biologic hypothesis, a single theory does not fully explain the etiology of depression. The efficacy of medications and the ability to measure the complex effects of neurons offer important clues toward better understanding of the causes of depression.

Major Classes of Antidepressants

Selective Serotonin Reuptake Inhibitors. SSRIs remain first-line drug therapy for the treatment of depression (Celexa, 2000) because of their safety and favorable adverse effect profile. Unlike the tricyclic antidepressants (TCAs), there has been no fatality associated with an overdose of an SSRI. Escitalopram oxalate (Lexapro) is the newest SSRI approved by the FDA (Lexapro, 2002).

SSRIs work by inhibiting the reuptake of 5-HT, which results in an increase of 5-HT concentrations in the synapse. There are six SSRIs approved by the FDA, including the newest escitalopram (Table 24-4); more are being studied. Except for fluvoxamine, which is approved for use in anxiety, all the SSRIs are approved for the treatment of major depression disorder. All SSRIs are effective in the treatment of panic disorders, obsessive-compulsive disorders, bulimia nervosa, social phobia, and posttraumatic stress disorders.

Efficacy. The efficacy among SSRIs is similar. Choosing a particular antidepressant depends on the client's acceptance and tolerance to the adverse effects and, to a

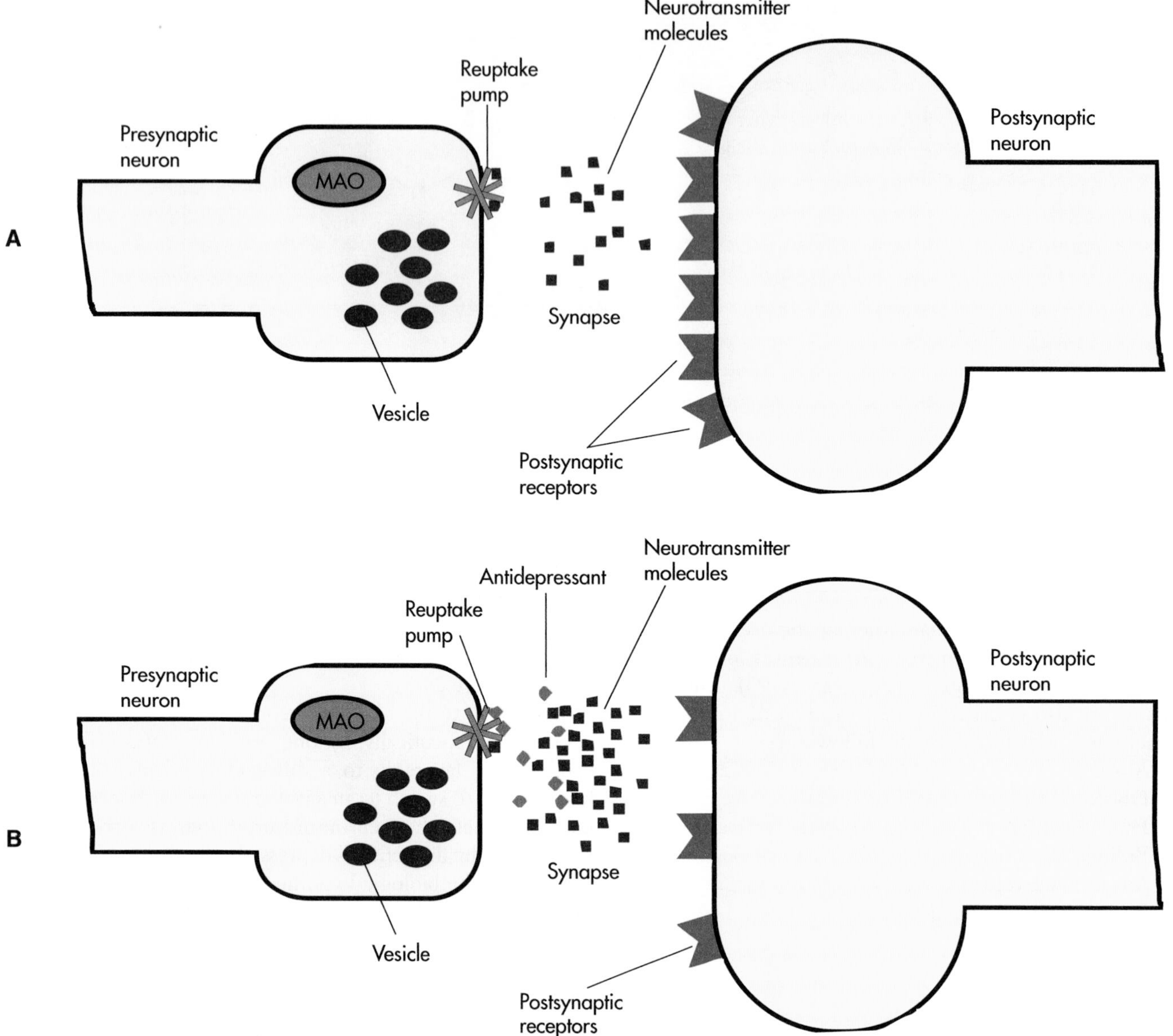

FIGURE 24-3 Neurotransmitter responses to antidepressant therapy. **A,** In the depressed state, sparse amounts of neurotransmitter are available in the synapse of a depressed person. **B,** With treatment, the reuptake of neurotransmitter is blocked by the antidepressant drug (in red). The result is increased amounts of neurotransmitter in the synapse, and, finally, after several weeks the postsynaptic receptors have decreased (i.e., downregulated), which is associated with resolving depression. For the sake of clarity, this drawing omits numerous receptors and postsynaptic intracellular mechanisms that may ultimately prove to be important components of the pathophysiologic substrate of depression and antidepressant response.

lesser extent, cost. Adverse effects differ among the SSRIs mainly because of their differing affinities for the 5-HT receptor subtypes, including 5-HT_{2A}, 5HT_{2C}, 5-HT_3, and 5-HT_4. Some clients tolerate one antidepressant better than another, so it is important to assess the client thoroughly before choosing a particular drug. To maximize client acceptance and compliance with these medications, monitoring side effects is important and needs to continue for the duration of therapy.

Half-Lives. The half-lives of SSRIs differ; this difference is considered when choosing a particular dosing schedule. For example, fluoxetine has the longest half-life and an active metabolite, norfluoxetine, which prolongs the drug effect. This enabled the development of a **sustained release** fluoxetine formulation that allows the client to take the drug once a week (Claxton et al., 2000). This is a convenient dosing schedule and normally improves client compliance.

Cost. The cost of SSRIs is taken into consideration. Fluoxetine is now available in generic formulation, although Prozac is the only fluoxetine that is available in a sustained-release formulation suitable to be taken once a week. Parox-

TABLE 24-4

Antidepressant Dosing

GENERIC (TRADE NAME)*	STARTING DOSE (mg/DAY)	MAINTENANCE DOSE (mg/DAY)	
CYCLIC ANTIDEPRESSANTS			
Tricyclics			
Amitriptyline (Elavil, Endep)	25-50	100-300	
Clomipramine (Anafranil)	25	100-250	
Desipramine (Norpramin)	25-50	100-300	
Doxepin (Sinequan)	25-50	100-300	
Imipramine (Tofranil)	25-50	100-300	
Nortriptyline (Aventyl)	25-50	100-300	
Maprotiline (Ludiomil)	50	100-225	
Tricyclic Dibenzoxazepine			
Amoxapine (Asendin)	50	100-400	
Triazolopyridines			
Nefazodone (Serzone)	200	300-600	
Trazodone (Desyrel)	50	150-500	
Piperazinoazepine			
Mirtazapine (Remeron)	15	15-45	
Monoamine Oxidase Inhibitors			
Phenelzine (Nardil)	15	15-90	
Tranylcypromine (Parnate)	10	10-40	
Selegiline (EMSAM) (transdermal patch)	6	6-12	
Serotonin-Selective Reuptake Inhibitors			**FDA Indications in Addition to Depression**
Citalopram (Celexa)	20	20-40	Depression only
Fluvoxamine (Luvox)	50	100-300	Obsessive-compulsive disorder
Fluoxetine (Prozac)	5-20	20-80	Obsessive-compulsive disorder, bulimia nervosa
Paroxetine (Paxil)	10-20	20-50	Obsessive-compulsive disorder, panic
Sertraline (Zoloft)	50-100	50-200	Obsessive-compulsive disorder, panic
Indolamine			
Bupropion (Wellbutrin)	200	300-450	
Phenylethlyamine			
Venlafaxine (Effexor)	75	150-350	

*Use about half the dose for the elderly.

etine is available in a sustained-release formulation, Paxil CR, but still requires a once-a-day dose. There is a slight advantage in using Paxil CR, as the slow-release formulation helps to reduce GI upset. There appears to be no advantage compared to the regular Paxil formulation in the clinical setting because Paxil CR cannot be cut or split in half to save cost. *Pill splitting* or *cutting* reduces the overall cost of some of the SSRIs. For example, paroxetine 20-, 40-, or 60-mg tablets are priced comparably regardless of the dose. By splitting or cutting in half the higher dose tablet, such as using half tablet of 40 mg for a 20-mg dose, the client is able to substantially reduce the cost of the medication.

Serotonin Syndrome. SSRIs are subject to a variety of drug interactions, some very serious, due to complex metabolism process. The potential drug interactions of SSRIs with other drugs that also affect serotonin lead to the **serotonin syndrome**, which is life threatening. Interacting drugs include monoamine oxidase inhibitors (MAOIs), dextromethorphan, meperidine, and sympathomimetics. The clinical signs of serotonin syndrome include confusion, hypomania, restlessness, myoclonus, hyperreflexia, diaphoresis, shivering, tremor, and diarrhea.

Serotonin syndrome is treated in an acute care hospital setting by the following:

- Discontinuation of medications causing the increase in serotonin
- Supportive measures such as cooling blanket for hyperthermia, benzodiazepines (e.g., clonazepam) for myoclonus (sudden twitching of muscle or muscle parts without any rhythm or pattern), anticonvulsants for seizures, and antihypertensives for increased blood pressure

Side Effects. The most common side effects are mild. They are often more severe at the initiation of treatment

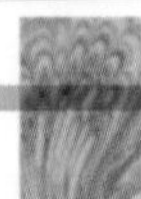

TABLE 24-5

Side Effects of Antidepressants with Nursing Interventions

SIDE EFFECT	NURSING INTERVENTIONS
ANTICHOLINERGIC EFFECTS	
Dry mouth	Offer sugarless gum and candy, artificial saliva. For persistent problems, treat with pilocarpine 1% rinse and spit (4 drops of 4% pilocarpine and 12 drops water) or bethanechol (Duvoid, Urecholine) 5 mg sublingual or 10-30 mg once daily or twice daily.
Blurred vision: disturbance of presbyopia (near vision), far vision usually preserved	Ask if vision prescription is current; try pilocarpine 1% eye drops or bethanechol 10-30 mg tid.
Urinary retention	When not caused by benign prostatic hypertrophy (BPH) may be treated with bethanechol 10-30 mg tid.
Constipation	Prevention: encourage fluids (medication givers may offer), fruits and vegetables, mild physical exercise (walks). Treat with bulk-forming laxatives (e.g., Metamucil 1-2 tablespoons qAM or docusate 100 mg daily or twice daily). Avoid stimulant laxatives when possible; if needed, limit duration to avoid laxative dependence. Or treat with bethanechol 10-30 mg daily or twice daily.
Anticholinergic delirium (also known as atropine psychosis)	Monitor for agitation restlessness, psychotic signs and symptoms, myoclonic jerking. Sometimes occurs with or without peripheral anticholinergic signs. Hold anticholinergic drugs. Physostigmine 5 mg IV rapidly reverses but requires life-support backup and cardiac monitoring.
α-BLOCKADE	
Orthostatic hypotension	Consider other contributing factors such as low-salt diets, restricted fluid intake, dehydration. Antihypertensive medications exacerbate. Advise client to change positions slowly, dangle feet 1 minute in sitting position when rising from prone; sit immediately when lightheaded. Offer support hose, exercise to strengthen calf muscles to improve venous return.
SEXUAL DYSFUNCTION*	
Decreased libido	Neostigmine 7.5-15 mg 30 minutes before anticipated intercourse.
Impaired erection	Often an anticholinergic problem; change to less anticholinergic drug or try bethanechol.
Priapism	Rare disorder associated with trazodone. Prolonged painful, nonsexual erection. Medical urgency treated with epinephrine injections to the corpus cavernosa. Requires surgical intervention leading to permanent impotence.
Impaired ejaculation	Requires switching drug. Try Neostigmine 7.5-15 mg 30 minutes before anticipated intercourse.
Inhibition of orgasm	Less serotonergic drug. Try cyproheptadine 4 mg daily. Note that cyproheptadine, a serotonin antagonist, has caused loss of antidepressant efficacy in some clients. The addition of bupropion has been successful.
HEMATOLOGIC	
Agranulocytosis	Exceedingly rare allergic reaction usually occurring in the first 3 months of treatment. Monitor for fever, sore throat, mucosal ulceration, weakness. Discontinue drug; change to different chemical class.
Petechia, ecchymosis, easy bruising, bleeding	Associated with selective serotonin reuptake inhibitor (SSRI) effect on platelet. Often occurs with normal or decreased platelet counts. Discontinue drug. Monitor CBC, dizziness, lightheadedness.
OTHER	
Weight gain	Associated with cyclic antidepressants and monoamine oxidase inhibitors. Recommend diet and exercise. Treat with diuretics (e.g., hydrochlorothiazide for edema).
Weight loss	Associated with SSRI; rarely clinically significant.
Tremor	Caffeine exacerbates tremors. Determine degree of interference with daily activities. Propranolol 10-20 mg tid-qid is often useful.
Antidepressant withdrawal	Anticholinergic rebound results in GI upset, cramps, diarrhea. Educate client on potential withdrawal symptoms. When discontinuing, taper slowly over several weeks. SSRI withdrawal symptoms include nausea, lightheadedness, dizziness, faintness, fatigue, paresthesias, flulike syndrome. Taper slowly.

*Obtain a clear history that the complaint does not predate the depression or medication use.
From Andrews JM, Nemeroff CB: Contemporary management of depression, *Am J Med* 97:24S, 1994; modified from Pollack MH, Rosenbaum JF: Management of antidepressant-induced side effects: a practical guide for the clinician, *J Clin Psychiatry* 48:3, 1987.

but lessen or become more tolerable with time and use. Side effects include GI upset, insomnia, restlessness, irritability, headache, and sexual dysfunction (Fava and Rankin, 2002). If sexual dysfunction is significant, consider switching to an antidepressant not associated with sexual dysfunction, such as bupropion or nefazodone. SSRIs are associated with EPS including akathisia, dystonia, and bradykinesia. The SSRIs are not lethal in overdose, which is an advantage over other antidepressants such as the TCAs, especially for clients with suicidal risk. Table 24-5 lists side effects of all antidepressants and nursing interventions.

Discontinuation of Therapy. A withdrawal syndrome can occur, making it important to gradually taper (**titration**) the SSRIs over 2 to 4 weeks. Symptoms of the withdrawal syndrome include severe headache, GI upset, dizziness, impaired concentration, flulike symptoms, insomnia, and anxiety.

Tricyclic Antidepressants. The tricyclics (TCAs) (see Table 24-4) were the first widely used antidepressants to treat depression; however, they have an unfavorable adverse effects profile. With the emergence of the SSRIs, the TCAs have become second-line therapy. This class of antidepressants acts by blocking the reuptake of 5-HT and norepinephrine.

The tertiary amines are frequently metabolized to secondary amines, and the secondary amines are more potent in blocking the reuptake of norepinephrine. This is why the use of tertiary amine TCAs also produces norepinephrine response even though they are primarily active in blocking serotonin reuptake.

TCAs also act on other receptors. These actions contribute to the adverse effects, including antihistaminic, anticholinergic, and effects on cardiac conduction.

Anticholinergic Side Effects. All TCAs have substantial anticholinergic side effects, such as dry mouth, blurred vision, GI upset, constipation, urinary retention, and confusion. Among the TCAs, desipramine and nortriptyline have the least intense anticholinergic side effects. All tricyclics are very sedating, and clients usually take them at bedtime. Because they cause cardiotoxicity, an ECG is recommended before the initiation of therapy and is repeated periodically. TCAs cause orthostatic hypotension. Instruct clients, especially the elderly, to rise slowly to prevent falls. Another disadvantage of TCAs is the risk of fatality with an overdose, particularly in clients with suicidal risk.

Monitoring Parameters. Therapeutic blood level monitoring is useful to confirm that the administered dose is maintaining serum drug concentration within the effective range and to prevent toxicity and serious adverse effects. Avoid tricyclic antidepressants in elderly clients because of anticholinergic side effects, orthostatic hypotension, sedation and cardiac arrhythmias. SSRI are preferred for elderly clients.

Discontinuation of Therapy. TCAs should be tapered for discontinuation. Abrupt withdrawal leads to a withdrawal syndrome with GI complaints, dizziness, insomnia, and irritability. Reduce the dose by 25 to 50 mg/week to minimize withdrawal symptoms. Box 24-5 explains the time course of response to antidepressants.

BOX 24-5

Time Course of Response to Antidepressants

FIRST WEEK
Decreased anxiety
Improved sleep
Client often unaware of these changes

1 TO 3 WEEKS
Increased activity, sex drive, self-care
Improved concentration, memory
Psychomotor retardation resolves

2 TO 4 WEEKS
Relief of depressed mood
Less hopelessness
Suicidal ideation subsides

Monoamine Oxidase Inhibitors. Iproniazid, a drug used to combat tuberculosis in the 1950s, was an MAOI. Some clients receiving iproniazid became euphoric. This observation ultimately led to the use of MAOIs as antidepressant agents. The use of MAOIs is now limited as a result of the potentially dangerous side affects and necessary strict dietary modifications with its use, as described next. Thus, investigation for new antidepressant agents continued.

Mode of Action. The neurotransmitters norepinephrine, serotonin, and dopamine are monoamines. In the CNS, these molecules are synthesized inside the presynaptic neuron. Maintenance of cellular homeostasis requires a mechanism to degrade monoamines. Monoamine oxidase is an enzyme found in the mitochondria of cells that participate in the normal process of degradation of these amines; MAOIs inhibit this enzyme initially resulting in increased availability of these neurotransmitters. As with other antidepressants, these initial neurotransmitter increases result in postsynaptic receptor down-regulation that is temporally related to the antidepressant response.

Clinical Use and Efficacy. MAOIs are used in the treatment of atypical (novel) depression, major depression without melancholia, or depressive disorders resistant to TCAs. Hypersomnia, hyperphagia, anxiety, and the absence of vegetative symptoms characterize atypical depression. In addition, MAOIs have been used with variable success in the treatment of other disorders such as certain anxiety disorders, eating disorders, and some pain syndromes (e.g., migraines).

MAOIs are rapidly absorbed, metabolized in the liver, and have average half-lives of approximately 24 hours. A majority of individuals metabolize MAOIs relatively slowly. This metabolic difference among individuals results in wide variation with respect to required doses for efficacy and sensitivity to side effects at a given dose. There is no clinically available test for this metabolic rate. Thus, many clinicians begin MAOI therapy with a 10- or 15-mg test dose. Monitor vital signs and complaints of side effects closely before beginning titration.

Contraindications to the use of MAOIs include cerebrovascular defects, major cardiovascular disease, and pheochromocytoma (tumor of the adrenal medulla). Older clients do not tolerate MAOIs well, so use is uncommon in individuals over 65 years old. MAOIs sometimes worsen symptoms of Parkinson's disease, induce manic states in bipolar clients, and exacerbate psychotic symptoms in clients with schizophrenia. Clients with diabetes require adjustment of their hypoglycemic medication. MAOIs are contraindicated in pregnancy.

The use of MAOIs requires additional considerations. As with cyclic antidepressants, titrate initial dosing to give clients time to tolerate side effects. Table 24-4 lists initial and maintenance dosing ranges. Clients taking MAOIs need to comply with a tyramine-restricted diet (Box 24-6)

BOX 24-6

Dietary Restrictions for Clients Taking Monoamine Oxidase Inhibitors

PROHIBITED

- Aged cheeses
- Ripe avocados
- Ripe figs
- Anchovies
- Bean curd/fermented beans
- Broad beans (fava/Italian)
- Yeast extracts and yeast-derived vitamin supplements
- Liver
- Delicatessen meats (especially sausage)
- Pickled herring
- Meat extracts (Marmite, Bovril)
- Fermented foods
- Chianti and sherry

ALLOWED WITH MODERATION

- Beer and ale (tyramine content varies with brand and can be especially high in imported beers and some nonalcoholic beers)
- White wine/distilled spirits
- Cottage cheese, cream cheese
- Coffee (2 cups/day)
- Chocolate
- Soy sauce (tyramine content varies with brand)
- Yogurt and sour cream
- Spinach, raisins, tomatoes, eggplant, plums

CLINICAL ALERT

It is extremely important for nurses to teach clients to avoid certain foods and other drugs when taking monoamine oxidase inhibitors (MAOIs) to avoid a **hypertensive crisis.** Nurses need to teach and discuss these with the clients, give them lists of potentially dangerous foods and drugs as reminders, and especially document the nursing actions and nurse-client interactions.

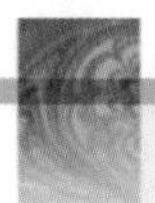

BOX 24-7

Drugs to Avoid When Taking Monoamine Oxidase Inhibitors

- Antiasthmatics: theophylline and inhalers containing epinephrine or β-agonists (e.g., albuterol [Proventil, Ventolin])
- Antihypertensives: methyldopa (Aldomet), guanethidine (Ismelin), reserpine
- Anesthetics with epinephrine
- Allergy, hay fever, cough and cold products, decongestants, diet pills (many combination over-the-counter products; look for inclusion of phenylpropanolamine, ephedrine, phenylephrine, dextromethorphan)
- Buspirone (BuSpar)
- Meperidine (Demerol)
- Serotonin selective reuptake inhibitors: fluoxetine (Prozac), sertraline (Zoloft), paroxetine (Paxil), fluvoxamine (Luvox), nefazodone (Serzone)
- Yohimbine (Yocon)

and avoid stimulant medications to prevent the risk of a potentially fatal **hypertensive crisis.** Thus, the client's ability to comply with dietary and medication restrictions is an important consideration before initiating therapy. Response to therapy takes 3 to 6 weeks. Except in emergencies, discontinuations should be tapered.

Drug-Drug and Drug-Food Interactions. Dietary tyramine is a precursor in the synthesis of norepinephrine. In the presence of an MAOI, foods high in tyramine (an amino acid by-product formed by the bacterial breakdown of tyrosine in fermented foods) lead to a sharp increase in available norepinephrine and potentially fatal hypertensive crisis. Tyramine is not the only factor in food that interacts with MAOIs. For instance, fava beans contain dopamine, which affect blood pressure in the presence of MAOIs. Previously, dietary restrictions for MAOIs were extensive and made compliance unlikely. Estimates of compliance with an MAOI diet have been as low as 40%. Yet, for several reasons, there are not an overwhelming number of MAOI hypertensive reactions. Foods, different brands of prepared foods, and a client's susceptibility to this interaction all vary widely. For instance, although a cup of coffee elevates blood pressure and causes headaches, some clients who take MAOIs benefit from a cup of coffee as an adjunct to treat hypotension on awakening. Thus, client education consists of simple, clear, written and verbal instructions to absolutely avoid certain foods. Nurses need to review warnings of other foods that cause problems in some clients or when taken in large quantity. Clients need to maintain dietary restrictions for 2 weeks after discontinuing MAOIs. All clients need to know the warning signs of hypertensive crisis, which include headache, stiff neck, sweating, nausea, and vomiting. Clients with such symptoms need to seek medical attention immediately.

Many drugs also interact with MAOIs and lead to a hypertensive crisis or dangerous hypotension (Box 24-7). Many over-the-counter medications are dangerous when taken with MAOIs, including diet pills, nasal decongestants, asthma medications (including inhalers), and cough suppressants (dextromethorphan). Literally hundreds of over-the-counter and prescription combination products under many different brand names contain sympathomimetics that are unsafe to use with MAOIs. Therefore, nurses need to educate every client taking an MAOI and to consult a physician, dentist, nurse, or pharmacist before taking any additional medication. Although hypertensive events are generally more dangerous and more common, the response to a sympathomimetic medication or dietary indiscretion is sometimes hypotension rather than hypertension. Whether a hypotensive or hypertensive reaction ensues is a function of the overall adrenergic tone of the client and is not predictable.

Treatment for hypertensive crisis usually begins with nifedipine (Procardia, Adalat) 10 mg. Absorption from oral administration is extremely rapid, and the client's blood pressure often lowers in a matter of minutes. Monitor vital signs every 10 to 15 minutes until the client is stable. Other therapies include the α-adrenergic blockers phentolamine (Regitine) 5 mg intravenous and chlorpromazine 50 mg PO.

Clients who fail to respond to a non-MAOI antidepressant usually wait at least 2 weeks before starting an MAOI. An important exception to this is fluoxetine. Because of the long half-life of fluoxetine and its active metabolite norfluoxetine (approximately 7 to 10 days), clients discontinuing fluoxetine need to wait at least 5 weeks before starting an MAOI. In general, this class of medication is not suitable for clients with suicidal risk or cognitive inability or unwillingness to follow the rigid regimen of dietary and drug restrictions.

Client Education and Documentation. Careful and thorough client education and monitoring are required with use of MAOIs. Instruct clients to avoid foods high in tyramine (Hedberg et al., 1966) and to be extremely cautious in taking other medications, especially over-the-counter cold and cough medications. Be diligent about providing each client with lists of potentially harmful foods and drugs that cannot be taken with the MAOI medications. Nurses also carefully document the client teaching and monitoring activities while responsible for the client's care.

Other Side Effects. Orthostatic hypotension is a common initial and sometimes persistent side effect of MAOIs. Dangling feet on rising, changing positions slowly, wearing support stockings, and increasing fluid and salt intake are often effective treatments. A caffeinated drink in the morning is useful as long as the nurse has monitored vital signs initially. Edema, sexual dysfunction, and weight gain are also common and often lead to drug discontinuation. Complaints of insomnia occur with all MAOIs. Moving the last dose of the day to an earlier time is helpful. Complaints of confusion or feeling drunk indicate an excessive dose. Although these drugs do not have direct effects on cholinergic receptors, anticholinergic-type side effects (e.g., dry mouth, urinary hesitancy, constipation) are common. Sometimes MAOI-induced pyridoxine (vitamin B_6) deficiency causes paresthesias (numbness, prickling, tingling feelings). This is treated with oral pyridoxine.

Abrupt discontinuation of MAOIs may produce *monoamine oxidase inhibitor withdrawal syndrome* and so should be avoided. Symptoms include nausea, sweating, palpitation, nightmares, hallucinations, delirium, and paranoid psychosis.

Other Antidepressants

Duloxetine. Duloxetine is a selective serotonin and norepinephrine reuptake inhibitor (SNRI). The FDA has approved it for the treatment of major depression in adults and diabetic neuropathy as well. Venlafaxine is the only other SNRI approved for use in United States. Duloxetine inhibits serotonin, norepinephrine, and weakly inhibits dopamine reuptake in the neuronal synapse.

Formulations and Dosage. Duloxetine is available in 20-, 30- and 60-mg enteric-coated delayed-release capsules. The initial recommended dose is 20 mg twice a day and is sometimes increased to 30 mg twice a day or 60 mg once a day.

Absorption, Metabolism, and Elimination. Duloxetine is well absorbed orally. Clients reach the peak plasma level at 6 hours if administered without food and 10 hours with food. It has an elimination half-life of 12 hours. The enzymes CYP1A2 and CYO2D6 metabolize duloxetine in the liver, and it is excreted in urine (70%) and feces (20%).

Drug Interactions. Inhibitors of 1A2, such as fluvoxamine and ciprofloxacin increase duloxetine serum concentrations and lead to possible toxicity. 2D6 inhibitors such as paroxetine, fluoxetine and quinidine also have the same possible affect. Duloxetine is a moderate inhibitor of CYP 2D6, which increases serum concentration of tricyclic antidepressants, type 1C antiarrhythmics (flecainide), and phenothiazines. Do not co-administer with thioridazine.

Venlafaxine. Venlafaxine is a serotonin norepinephrine reuptake inhibitor (SNRI). Unlike TCAs, it does not affect other receptors that cause the undesirable adverse effects such as anticholinergic and antihistaminic side effects.

Because venlafaxine affects both serotonin and norepinephrine, clients with less than optimal response to an SSRI use it (Thase et al., 2001). It is also used to treat anxiety disorders (Gelenberg et al., 2000).

Formulations and Dosage. Venlafaxine is available in regular and sustained-release formulations (Product Information for Effexor, 2002). Clients take regular tablets two or three times a day. Clients take venlafaxine XR, the sustained-release formulation, once a day. If the client cannot tolerate a single sustained-release dose, the dose is divided to reduce side effects such as GI upset. The initial dose of regular release venlafaxine is 50 to 75 mg/day, administered in two or three divided doses with food. The dose is increased by 75-mg increments every 4 days. Doses beyond 225 mg do not usually demonstrate increased efficacy; however, severely depressed clients often need up to 350 mg/day. The maximum recommended dose is 375 mg/day (Product Information for Effexor, 2002).

For the sustained-release formulation, the initial recommended dose for venlafaxine XR is 37.5 mg/day administered with food. The maximum recommended dose 225 mg/day (Product Information for Effexor, 2002).

Side Effects. The most common adverse effect is GI upset, which is more significant in older clients. Venlafaxine causes increases in blood pressure and clients with uncontrolled hypertension need to use it with caution. The increase in blood pressure is dose related. Other side effects are similar to those associated with the SSRIs, including insomnia, restlessness, headache, and irritability.

Trazodone. Trazodone is an SSRI, and it also blocks serotonin ($5HT_{2A}$) receptors. Because of its sedative effects, trazodone is used as an agent to counteract insomnia.

Formulations and Dosage. The therapeutic dosage range is 50 to 600 mg/day. Most clients respond to a dosage of 100 to 300 mg/day in single or divided daily doses (Rawls, 1982). The manufacturer recommends that therapy be initiated at a dose of 150 mg/day in divided doses and increased gradually, as needed, every 3 to 4 days in increments of 50 mg. Outpatient doses should not exceed 400 mg/day in divided doses. Inpatients receive up to 600 mg/day in divided doses, but do not exceed this dosage. Clients should take the lowest effective dose (Product Information for Trazodone, 1998).

Side Effects. Sedation is a frequent and often intense side effect. Therefore, trazodone is currently used as a hypnotic and an antidepressant adjunctive therapy to SSRI to counteract insomnia. The most frequent cardiovascular side effect during therapy is postural hypotension, which is often accompanied by syncope, especially in clients taking concomitant antihypertensive therapy (Spivak et al., 1987). Adjustment of antihypertensive medication is necessary if administered concurrently (Product Information for trazodone, 1998).

A rare but serious side effect is priapism. *Priapism* is painful, persistent, abnormal penile erection, unaccompanied by sexual stimulation. This is an emergency and requires prompt medical attention.

Client Education. Discuss sedation and the risk of fall, as well as orthostatic hypotension with the client. Warn male clients of the potential serious side effect of priapism.

CLINICAL ALERT

Antidepressants sometimes increase the risk of **suicidal thinking and behavior** in adults, as well as children and adolescents, with depression and other psychiatric disorders. Families or caregivers need to watch children and adolescents for any signs of suicidal thinking and behavior. It is important to notify the physician or nurse before having the client stop taking an antidepressant. Stopping an antidepressant suddenly may cause other symptoms.

Bupropion. Bupropion has inhibitory effects on dopamine and norepinephrine reuptake, and it has a lesser effect on serotonin reuptake. It is commonly referred to as a norepinephrine-dopamine reuptake inhibitor (NDRI). The exact mechanism is unknown.

Half-Life and Dosing Schedule. Bupropion has a short half-life, and clients take doses three times a day. An extended-release product is available for once-a-day dosing. The recommended initial dose of bupropion is 200 mg/day, administered as 100-mg doses once in the morning and once in the evening (Product Information for Wellbutrin, 2001). The recommended initial dose of bupropion-sustained release is 150 mg given as a single daily dose in the morning. If the client tolerates the initial dose, an increase to 150 mg twice a day is recommended as early as day 4 (Product Information for Wellbutrin SR, 2001). To prevent the risk of seizure and adverse effects such as dystonia, the maximum single dose of bupropion SR is limited to 150 mg/dose and 450 mg/day, and the non-SR is 100 mg/dose. Minimum interval of dosage is 8 hours for SR formulation and 4 hours for non-SR formulation (Product Information for Wellbutrin, 2001).

Side Effects. Common side effects include nervousness, headache, and insomnia. Seizure is a significant risk; titrate the dose and follow the dosing schedule closely. Another common side effect is dystonia.

Other Therapeutic Uses. The drug is helpful with reducing cigarette and alcohol and drug craving (Chengappa et al., 2001). Zyban is the brand name of bupropion as labeled for use as an adjunct therapy for cigarette smoking cessation (Bupropion, 1997). Bupropion is an antidepressant often used in association with alcohol and drug detoxification and rehabilitation.

Mirtazapine. Mirtazapine increases both norepinephrine and serotonin in the synapse. It also blocks serotonin receptors (Davis and Wilde, 1996).

Dosage. The recommended starting dose is 15 mg/day as a single dose. It is preferable to give the dose in the evening before sleep. The effective dose range appears to be 15 to 45 mg/day. Do not make dosage changes in less than 1- to 2-week intervals (Product Information for Remeron, 2000).

Side Effects. The major side effects are sedation and weight gain (Gorman, 1999). Interestingly, sedation is more prominent with a lower dose. Weight gain is significant and is sometimes desirable in older clients. Other side effects include constipation. Serious but rare side effects include neutropenia, agranulocytosis, and hepatotoxicity. Regular monitoring parameters include complete blood count and liver function tests.

Other Therapeutic Uses. Mirtazepine, 15 mg orally, is often administered the night before surgery to reduce insomnia and to minimize presurgical anxiety.

Augmentation Therapy for Major Depression

Psychostimulants

Psychostimulants such as dextroamphetamine and methylphenidate are not FDA approved for treatment of depression. Researchers have determined the efficacy for adult treatment because of a lack of controlled studies. Dextroamphetamine is an effective in the treatment of depression with low energy in AIDS clients (DSM-III-R). In another study, dextroamphetamine was effective for treatment of poststroke depression. Researchers retrospectively evaluated 17 clients with poststroke depression treated with either dextroamphetamine or methylphenidate during a 5-year period (Masand et al., 1991). A total of 82% of clients improved on psychostimulants; 47% of clients demonstrated a marked or moderate improvement in depressive symptoms. No significant difference in efficacy existed between the two agents. Clients improved quickly within the first 2 days. Only three clients discontinued the psychostimulant treatment because of side effects. In another study, dextroamphetamine was used successfully to improve depression and low energy in 24 clients with AIDS (Wagner et al., 1997).

Methylphenidate or dextroamphetamine may be used occasionally as antidepressants; both have been effective for treating depression in some older clients. The dose range is 5 to 40 mg/day for methylphenidate and 10 to 30 mg/day for dextroamphetamine.

Not all clients are suitable for treatment with these drugs, especially clients with potential for drug abuse. Avoid these drugs in clients already nervous, anxious, or psychotic.

Lithium

Lithium is sometimes prescribed for refractory (treatment-resistant) depression. Therapeutic blood level monitoring is an imperative requirement. Use lithium with caution in older clients and in clients with renal impairment.

Thyroid Therapy

Clients with low thyroid function often exhibit symptoms of depression. Levothyroxine (T_4) is used, and some clients require combination therapy that includes antidepressants. Clients need monitoring and periodic thyroid function tests.

Herbal Supplements

Saint John's wort is a mild herbal antidepressant commonly used in Europe and has gained considerable popularity in the United States. Caution clients that Saint John's wort should be avoided in combination with other antidepressants.

BIPOLAR DISORDERS

Mood Stabilizers

This section describes the role of mood stabilizers in the treatment of bipolar disorder, which include lithium, valproate, carbamazepine, and other anticonvulsant mood stabilizers. Many of the anticonvulsant mood stabilizers have risks of adverse drug reactions and drug interactions (Frances et al., 1996). Atypical (second-generation) antipsychotic drugs have received FDA approval for treatment of acute mania or mixed episodes of mania and depression. In addition, the FDA has approved olanzapine and aripiprazole for maintenance treatment of bipolar disorder. The FDA has also approved the fixed-dose combination of olanzapine and fluoxetine (Symbyax) for the treatment of depressive phase of bipolar disorder. The available dosages are 6 mg olanzapine/25 mg fluoxetine, 6/50, 12/25, and 12/50. Many clients prefer taking the combination once daily in the evening as olanzapine is sedating.

Lithium. Lithium, a single ion, was medicinally used for more than a century for several ailments, but its use for mania was discovered by accident. Physicians have used lithium in the treatment of bipolar mania for more than 50 years. It has antimanic, antipsychotic, and antidepressant activity, but it is most effective in the treatment of pure mania and less effective in the treatment of a mixed state mood disorder ("Bipolar Disorder," 1999).

Therapeutic Dosage Regimen. Close monitoring by the nurse of client's laboratory reports of blood serum lithium levels is imperative. The therapeutic index, or the range between therapeutic and toxic levels of lithium, is narrow. The diligent nurse is therefore instrumental in helping clients avoid potentially severe adverse reactions to this medication. The therapeutic index varies slightly among facilities, and the nurse's responsibility is to follow current procedures.

Clients usually begin lithium in low divided doses to minimize side effects. The dose is titrated according to response and the appearance of side effects, until serum lithium concentration is within the range of 0.5 to 1.2 mEq/L (Tohen and Grundy, 1999). A typical starting dose is 300 to 400 mg three times a day depending on the client's age and weight.

On a given dose regimen, lithium levels achieve a steady state after 5 days. Because of its narrow therapeutic index, check lithium levels periodically at steady state and after each dose increase. It is appropriate to check lithium levels more frequently when rapid titration is necessary, such as in the treatment of acute mania, or when the nurse suspects toxicity. As levels reach the upper limits of the therapeutic range, check them more frequently to minimize the risk of toxicity. Older clients are more at risk for lithium toxicity, and need the dose adjusted with the upper end of the therapeutic range of approximately 0.6 mEq/L.

In addition to monitoring serum lithium levels, other baseline and periodic monitoring includes the following: renal function, thyroid function, urinalysis, complete blood count with differentials, serum electrolytes, ECG, and weight. It is advisable to perform a pregnancy test for women of childbearing age before initiating lithium therapy. Order renal function and thyroid function tests periodically, and carefully monitor them.

Pharmacokinetics. Absorption of oral lithium is rapid, with peak serum concentrations occurring in 30 minutes to 1 hour. The elimination half-life is about 24 hours and is prolonged in older clients and in clients with renal impairment. In all, 90% to 98% of a dose is excreted as unchanged drug in the urine. Box 24-8 describes lithium baseline monitoring.

Clinical Use

Acute Treatment. Lithium is effective for acute and prophylactic treatment of both manic and depressive episodes in clients with bipolar disorders. The first-line treatment is to combine lithium or valproate with an antipsychotic. For less ill clients, monotherapy with lithium and valproate or an antipsychotic (atypical antipsychotic such as olanzapine or risperidone) is used. Benzodiazepines are often helpful as a short-term adjunctive treatment.

For clients who have rapid cycling bipolar disorder (with four or more mood disorder episodes within 12 months), valproate plus an antipsychotic is sometimes preferred over lithium. Carbamazepine or oxcarbazepine may

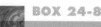

BOX 24-8

Lithium Baseline Monitoring

- Vital signs
- Weight
- Blood chemistry (electrolytes)
- Blood urea nitrogen/creatinine
- Complete blood count with differentials
- Urinalysis
- Thyroid function test
- Electrocardiogram
- Pregnancy test (for women of childbearing age)

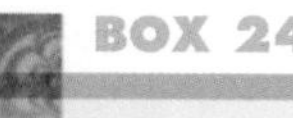

BOX 24-9

Lithium Side Effects

TRANSIENT EFFECTS AND MILD TOXICITY
- Fine tremor
- Gastrointestinal upset
- Mild polyuria, polydipsia
- Muscle weakness, lethargy

PERSISTENT EFFECTS
- Fine tremor
- Mild polyuria, polydipsia
- Increased white blood cell count
- Nontoxic goiter, hypothyroidism
- Exacerbation of psoriasis
- Acne
- Alopecia
- Weight gain
- *Effective acute treatment and prophylaxis: 0.5-1.2 mEq/L*

MODERATE TOXICITY
- *Lithium level >1.5 mEq/L*
- Coarsening of tremor
- Reappearance of gastrointestinal symptoms
- Confusion
- Sedation, lethargy
- *As levels increase:*
  - Ataxia
  - Dysarthria
  - Mental status deterioration

SEVERE TOXICITY
- *Lithium level >2.5 mEq/L*
- Seizures
- Coma
- Death
- Cardiovascular collapse

be used instead of lithium or valproate. Antidepressants should be tapered or discontinued. Psychosocial therapy should be used in combination with pharmacotherapy.

Other Uses of Lithium. Lithium is also prescribed for acute treatment of major depressive disorder, prevention of recurrent major depression, and for the treatment of cluster headaches.

Side Effects and Toxicity. As many as 75% of clients treated with lithium experience some side effects. Lithium toxicity is closely related to serum lithium levels but also occurs when levels approach the upper end of the therapeutic range. Some side effects are minor, and lowering the dose can reduce them. Side effects that are correlated to peak serum levels, such as tremors, may be reduced by changing to a slow-release formulation or by changing to a single bedtime dose. Box 24-9 shows potential side effects of lithium therapy in relation to blood serum concentration levels.

Mild to Moderate Effects. Some of the strategies used to manage persistent side effects include use of beta-blockers to treat tremor, diuretics for polydipsia, polyuria or edema, topical antibiotics, or another acne preparation for acne. Manage GI upset by changing the dose to a slow-release formulation or controlled-released formulation, or by giving lithium with meals. If the client uses a diuretic, reduce lithium dose (sometimes up to 50%) because of increased intrarenal reabsorption induced by the diuretics. In addition, it is advisable to monitor electrolyte balance, particularly sodium and potassium. A starting dose of 5 mg twice a day of amiloride, a potassium-sparing diuretic that does not alter the lithium level, is recommended. Lithium sometimes induces hypothyroidism. Perform thyroid function tests and prescribe levothyroxine for these clients as appropriate. Treat exacerbation of psoriasis with dermatologic preparations. However, in some cases discontinuation of lithium is necessary.

Severe Toxicity and Lithium Overdose. As the serum level increases to greater than 2.5 mEq/L, the risk of permanent neurologic impairment is significant. It is important therefore to reduce the serum level rapidly. Hemodialysis is the only reliable method to rapidly reduce the serum level, especially in acute poisoning or when a client deteriorates rapidly and is showing clinical signs of intoxication such as coma, convulsions, cardiovascular collapse, or respiratory failure. Nurses continuously monitor clients, especially in the case of an overdose of sustained-release lithium, as manifestation of symptoms may be delayed.

Client Education. During client education, nurses address potential side effects of lithium, as well as potential drug interactions. Counsel clients to monitor fluid intake according to activity and exercise levels and to avoid a salt-restricting diet; also advise clients about potential drug interactions with thiazide diuretics, angiotensin-converting enzyme inhibitors, nonsteroidal antiinflammatory drugs, and cyclooxygenase-2 inhibitors. Childbearing age female clients need to discuss use of lithium and other psychotropic medication if client should become pregnant. Follow-up appointments and monitoring are important for all clients.

Valproate. Valproate, an anticonvulsant medication, is for the treatment of manic episodes and is the first-line treatment for rapid cycling of bipolar disorder. It is more effective than lithium in treating bipolar disorder with prominent depressive symptoms. It is also effective in adjunctive treatment of schizoaffective disorder (Bogan et al., 2000). Divalproex, valproate, and valproic acid formulations are available in several dosage forms as different salts of valproate. Valproate is a common compound in the plasma.

Absorption, Distribution, Metabolism, and Excretion. The body rapidly absorbs valproate orally, with peak serum concentrations occurring within 4 hours. Therapeutic serum concentrations are monitored. Valproate is highly protein bound (i.e., approximately 90%). The cerebrospinal fluid levels are about 10% of corresponding serum levels. The elimination half-life is 6 to 17 hours. Valproate is metabolized extensively in the liver and excreted in the urine.

Dosage and Titration Regimen. It is generally advisable to start with a dose of 20 to 30 mg/kg per day in hospitalized clients. This usually occurs on a divided dose regimen, until desired serum level is reached.

In the outpatient setting or in older clients, doses are titrated until serum level is stabilized. Once the client is stable, it is advisable to simplify the dose to once or twice a day to enhance client compliance. Extended-release divalproex (Depakote ER) is available for once-a-day dosing. The bioavailability is 15% lower, so the dose often needs a small adjustment upward. Clients usually tolerate the extended release form better.

Side Effects. The main reasons for using valproate for bipolar disorders are its relative safety and more rapid symptom abatement when compared with lithium. Minor side effects include sedation and GI distress. These occur early in treatment and typically resolve with continued treatment or dose adjustment. Divalproex has a wider therapeutic range than lithium. Inadvertent overdose is uncommon, and accidental or intentional poisoning is less likely to be lethal than with lithium, making it a preferred choice over lithium for older clients. In rare incidences, however, valproate causes serious adverse effects.

Common dose-related side effects include (1) sedation; (2) GI distress, nausea, vomiting, diarrhea, dyspepsia, and anorexia; (3) benign transaminase elevation; (4) osteoporosis; and (5) tremor. These side effects are often transient. Other side effects that are persistent include hair loss, increased appetite, and weight gain. Mild, asymptomatic leukopenia and thrombocytopenia sometimes occur, but usually return to normal when client discontinues therapy.

Hepatotoxicity. Clients with a history of hepatic disease are at higher risk for hepatotoxicity. Hepatic failure has occurred mostly in children 2 years old or younger receiving multiple drug therapy. Life-threatening pancreatitis has occurred in both children and adults shortly after initial use and after several years of use. Baseline liver function tests are necessary before initiation of valproate therapy. Monitor clinical signs of hepatotoxicity and laboratory levels of liver enzymes.

Transient and mild elevation of liver enzymes, up to three times the upper limits of normal, do not require discontinuation of valproate. Transient elevated levels of ammonia are also common with valproate therapy. The dose of valproate is sometimes reduced, and the nurse needs to monitor the client carefully.

Persistent GI Distress. Indigestion, heartburn, and nausea are common side effects of valproate therapy. Taking the dose with food, or using enteric-coated tablets, or change of formulation to divalproex instead of using valproic acid is generally helpful. Administration of a histamine-2 antagonist such as famotidine (Pepcid) is sometimes helpful. If the client vomits and has severe abdominal pain, monitor the client's serum amylase level and carefully evaluate the client for pancreatitis.

Tremor. Essential tremor is a common side effect of valproate. Dose reduction or administration of a beta-blocker such as propranolol (40 to 160 mg in divided doses) reduces this effect.

Sedation. This is a common side effect and is more prominent at the initiation of therapy. A more gradual titration is often necessary. The once-a-day bedtime dose using an extended-release valproate is also useful.

Hematologic Effects. Mild leukopenia (total WBC count $>3000/mm^3$) is usually reversible on dose reduction or discontinuation. Discontinuation reverses mild cases of thrombocytopenia, but more serious cases have occurred. For clients receiving anticoagulation therapy, monitor an appropriate test of clotting function closely.

Serious Adverse Effects. Rare, idiosyncratic, but potentially fatal adverse effects with divalproex include fatal hepatic failure, pancreatitis, and thrombocytopenia. Monitoring parameters include hepatic function and complete blood count on a regular basis, usually every 6 months.

Potential Drug-Drug Interactions. Valproate displaces highly protein-bound drugs from their binding sites, resulting in the increased blood levels of the drugs displaced. An example is the drug interaction of valproate with lamotrigine. Valproate interferes with the metabolism of lamotrigine by competing with the glucuronidation enzyme sites in the liver. As a result, the use of valproate increases lamotrigine blood level twofold.

Client Education. Client education includes management of minor side effects as well as the signs and symptoms of hepatic and hematologic side effects. Advise clients to report these potentially serious side effects promptly.

Other Uses. Valproate is an anticonvulsant and is effective in the treatment of grand mal, petit mal, myoclonic, and temporal lobe seizures. The drug is much less effective for focal or complex partial seizures. It is also indicated for prophylaxis of migraine headache and as an adjunctive therapy for pain management.

Carbamazepine. Carbamazepine and oxcarbazepine (Trileptal) are also anticonvulsants and are an alternative treatment for acute bipolar mania in place of lithium or divalproex.

Mechanism of Action. Carbamazepine is structurally related to imipramine, a TCA. It enhances GABA activity in the brain and inhibits glutamate and aspartate activity. Carbamazepine has psychotropic effects and is less sedating than most anticonvulsants. The drug elevates mood in some depressed clients and is a second-line treatment for bipolar disorder. Although effective in psychiatric disorders, carbamazepine does not have a neurochemical profile resembling that of classic antipsychotics. However, data suggest that carbamazepine decreases dopamine turnover without directly blocking dopamine receptors.

Absorption, Distribution, Metabolism, and Excretion. Carbamazepine has a unique pharmacokinetic profile. Metabolism occurs via cytochrome P450 3A4 enzyme. Initially it has a half-life of approximately 36 hours. However, carbamazepine induces its own metabolism during treatment; this is complete within 3 to 5 weeks. After this period the half-life is about 24 hours. For this reason, the client does not reach the steady state until about 4 weeks after initial therapy. Also, with increasing carbamazepine doses in children, a dose-dependent auto-induction process occurs.

Extended-release capsules taken every 12 hours provide steady-state plasma levels comparable to immediate-release tablets taken every 6 hours at the same milligram dose. Food increases bioavailability; therefore, providers recommend giving carbamazepine with food. Total protein binding is 76%. Unbound drug decreases with increasing total concentrations.

Dosage Regimen and Monitoring Parameters. Carbamazepine dose ranges from 200 to 800 mg/day. The dose is usually started at the lower end of the range and titrated upward according to response and side effect tolerance. In clients over 12 years old, carbamazepine is usually initiated at 200 to 600 mg/day in divided doses. Usual titration increases the dose by 200 mg/day. In hospitalized clients with acute mania, the dose is initially titrated faster. Rapid titration causes an increase in side effects such as drowsiness, dizziness, ataxia, and diplopia. Serum levels are determined 5 days after a dose change, or sooner if the nurse suspects toxicity. The maintenance dose range is 1000 to 1600 mg/day. Doses greater than 1600 mg/day are not recommended.

Baseline laboratory orders include a complete blood count (CBC) with differential and platelet count; a hepatic panel with lactate dehydrogenase, serum glutamic-oxaloacetic transaminase, serum glutamate-pyruvate transaminase, bilirubin, and alkaline phosphatase; and renal function test. A pregnancy test is necessary for women of childbearing age.

Side Effects and Toxicity. Overdoses or undetected excessive accumulation of carbamazepine can be *fatal.* Signs of carbamazepine toxicity include dizziness, ataxia, sedation, and diplopia. Acute toxicity results in stupor or coma. Treatment includes gastric lavage and management of symptoms.

Rare, idiosyncratic, but potentially fatal side effects include agranulocytosis, aplastic anemia, thrombocytopenia, hepatic failure, exfoliative dermatitis (e.g., Stevens-Johnson syndrome), and pancreatitis. Other serious side effects include cardiac conduction disturbances.

A CBC with differential and platelet count as well as liver function tests are recommended every 2 weeks during the first 2 months of therapy. If the results of the tests are normal, the tests can be done every 3 months thereafter. However, whenever there are signs or symptoms of hepatic, hematologic, or dermatologic reactions, the client should have laboratory tests preformed more frequently.

Manage minor side effects, such as nausea, by taking carbamazepine immediately before or after meals, by dividing the doses throughout the day, by changing to a sustained-release form, or by using a histamine-2 antagonist such as famotidine. Cimetidine (Tagamet) is not recommended because of potential drug-drug interactions. Manage sedation and dizziness by decreasing the dose or shifting the dose to bedtime.

Client Education. It is important for nurses to counsel clients to monitor for signs and symptoms of hematologic and hepatic abnormalities so that clients report them promptly. Instruct the client to notify the physician immediately if a rash occurs.

Potential Drug-Drug Interactions. Carbamazepine induces the metabolism of many drugs, including its own, through induction of cytochrome P450 oxidation and conjugation. Erythromycin, calcium channel blockers, and SSRIs increase carbamazepine levels, whereas carbamazepine decrease the levels of many other drugs including antipsychotics, some steroids, oral contraceptives, thyroid hormones, benzodiazepines, TCAs, and anticonvulsants.

Concomitant use of clozapine increases the risk of aplastic anemia and clients need to avoid this. Concomitant use of lithium sometimes causes an acute state of confusion.

Oxcarbazepine. Oxcarbazepine is as effective as carbamazepine in the treatment of bipolar disorder, and clients usually tolerate it better. This is often an alternative for clients unable to tolerate carbamazepine.

Mechanism of Action. Oxcarbazepine is the 10-keto (10, 11-dihydro-co-oxo-carbamazepine) analog of carbamazepine.

Risks. Hyponatremia is a *major* concern with oxcarbazepine therapy, and some limit its use as an anticonvulsant and antineuralgic. The mechanism is thought to be due to an antidiuretic hormone-like action on the kidney. Most cases of hyponatremia are asymptomatic, although confusion and an increase in seizure frequency have occurred in some clients. Hyponatremia with oxcarbazepine occurs most commonly in older clients and during administration of high doses of the drug (Van Amelsvoort et al., 1994; Steinhoff et al., 1992; Kloster et al., 1998; Pendlebury et al., 1989; Zakrzewska and Patsalos, 1989; Nielson et al., 1988; Houtkooper et al., 1987; Johannessen and Nielsen, 1987).

Side Effects. Headache, drowsiness, dizziness, ataxia, tremor, abnormal gait, fatigue, sedation, encephalopathy, and oculogyric crises have occurred with administration of oxcarbazepine. Sedation, difficulty in concentration, and memory impairment are also associated with its use.

Hyperlipidemia, antidiuretic hormone effects, and altered reproductive hormones, as well as weight gain and effects on thyroid function, have also occurred with the administration of oxcarbazepine. Use of oxcarbazepine is associated with decreases in T_4 hormone, but not in T_3 or thyroid-stimulating hormone (MICROMEDEX, 2003).

Lamotrigine. Researchers have studied lamotrigine in bipolar depression and in rapid cycling bipolar disorders. It has been effective for both types of bipolar disorder (Botts and Raskind, 1999).

Dosage Titration and Risk. The initial dose of lamotrigine is 25 mg once a day and is increased in 25-mg increments every other week. When the client is taking valproate in addition to lamotrigine, reduce the dose of lamotrigine by half because of drug interaction. Lamotrigine requires a slow titration; the titration schedule must be followed to minimize the risk of skin rash. Approximately 5% of clients develop a maculopapular rash, and approximately 0.1% develop Stevens-Johnson syndrome, which is often *fatal.*

Side Effects. Common side effects include headache, dizziness, GI distress, and blurred or double vision.

Drug Interactions. Significant drug interactions occur with valproate.

Topiramate. Topiramate is a sulfamate-substituted monosaccharide used for treatment of epilepsy. Topiramate is an anticonvulsant and is an adjunctive therapy for partial seizures and generalized tonic-clonic seizures. It is not used as monotherapy for bipolar disorder but is sometimes useful as an adjunctive therapy. Topiramate is also for the treatment of binge eating, bulimia, cluster headache, trigeminal neuralgia, and Tourette's syndrome.

Absorption, Distribution, Metabolism, and Excretion. Topiramate is well absorbed after oral doses; peak serum concentration occurs in 2 to 4 hours. Food alters the rate of absorption, but not significantly. Topiramate is minimally bound to protein. The drug is not metabolized and is excreted unchanged in the urine.

Dosage. Titrate topiramate dosage slowly, with an initial dose of 50 mg/day for the first week and increased in 50-mg increments per week until the client reaches a dose of 400 mg/day (in two divided doses). Slower titration is necessary to minimize side effects, primarily impaired cognitive function (Martin et al., 1999). Slow titration also minimizes other side effects such as dizziness and drowsiness.

The dosage of topiramate is 11 to 35 mg/kg/day for children 5 years or younger and 5.5 to 16.5 mg/kg/day for children 6 to 12 years old. The clearance of topiramate is 50% greater in children, which results in a shorter half-life. In children topiramate has a faster elimination rate, which results in a 30% lower plasma concentration as compared to adults. Topiramate has significant drug interactions with enzyme-inducing anticonvulsants. These result in an increased clearance rate and shorter half-life.

The dose needs to be adjusted in clients with renal impairment. In clients with creatinine clearance of less than 70 ml/min, 50% of the usual dose is adequate. The clearance of topiramate decreases by 42% with creatinine clearance of 30 to 69 ml/min and by 54% with creatinine clearance of less than 30 ml/min.

Risks. Use topiramate with caution in clients with renal impairment, and adjust the dose (Bialer, 1993). Topiramate may cause acute myopia and secondary close-angle glaucoma and should be avoided by clients with glaucoma. Slowly taper topiramate to avoid the risk of precipitating seizures.

Side Effects. Anemia has occurred with topiramate use. Cardiovascular effects include hypertension, postural hypotension, vasodilation, arrhythmias, palpitations, atrioventricular block, and bundle block.

The most common side effects of topiramate include drowsiness, dizziness, ataxia, speech disorders and related speech problems, psychomotor slowing, nystagmus, fatigue, confusion, language problems, anxiety, and cognitive problems. Auditory hallucination has occurred as well.

New Anticonvulsants

Several newer anticonvulsants are only indicated and approved by FDA for treatment of seizures. These include tiagabine, zonisamide, and levetiracetam. The newer anticonvulsants listed are not FDA approved for the treatment of bipolar disorders at this time.

Treatment of Mania

The first step in treating mania includes the use of a mood stabilizer such as lithium or valproate. The FDA has approved atypical antipsychotics in treating mania, and they have been effective.

For clients with agitation associated with mania, a benzodiazepine is often added to the initial treatment regimen until the client stabilizes. High-potency benzodiazepines such as lorazepam and clonazepam are sometimes used. Alprazolam is not used because its antidepressant effect precipitates mania.

Atypical Antipsychotics for Mania

The atypical antipsychotics have effectively treated mania and include olanzapine, clozapine, quetiapine, risperidone, and ziprasidone. The atypical antipsychotics are replacing haloperidol and conventional or typical antipsychotics. When clients receive haloperidol, a mid range dose is often adequate for treatment. A typical dose of haloperidol is 10 to 15 mg/day.

Combination of Mood Stabilizers

Lithium is sometimes combined with valproate for effective treatment of bipolar disorder in the manic phase. Use of valproate in combination with carbamazepine is generally best avoided because of drug interactions. If there are no other alternatives and the client is using a combination of valproate and carbamazepine, the dose of valproate needs be increased and the dose of carbamazepine needs to be lowered because of their mutual drug interactions.

Treatment of Bipolar Depression

Treating bipolar depression is different from treating unipolar or major depression. The first attempt is optimization of the mood stabilizer. Monitor thyroid function tests. Clinical signs of hypothyroidism include depression, which is usually treated with thyroid hormone replacement therapy. If the client will be using an antidepressant, carefully monitor the client, as this predisposes the client to mania. In general, SSRIs and bupropion are safer. Avoid TCAs.

Maintenance Therapy and Lifelong Intervention

Because clients with bipolar disorder face the prospect of requiring lifelong medication therapy, the noncompliance rate is high, which results in multiple recurrent episodes of mood disorders. Clients frequently discontinue their medications when symptoms subside. The goal of maintenance therapy is to prevent recurrences, and there is a fine balance between optimal therapy and client acceptance. The risk of relapse is high on discontinuation of a mood stabilizer, and clients often become refractory to treatment, even when they resume use of the same drug. Therefore, it is important to educate clients to avoid stopping their medication when they feel better and to emphasize the need for prophylactic treatment despite the lack of symptoms. In addition, to avoid noncompliance with medication, clients need to know that they must tolerate an acceptable level of side effects. For example, a lithium dose between 0.8 and 1.0 mEq/L is an optimal level for maintenance therapy but usually causes side effects. There are attempts to maintain a level of 0.4 to 0.6 mEq/L to reduce the side effects and correspondingly improve client compliance.

ANXIETY DISORDERS

Twenty million people in the United States suffer from anxiety disorders. They are the most prevalent of all psychiatric conditions and among the leading causes of disability in the United States and worldwide, costing billions of dollars in lost wages and for treatment. There is also a strong association between alcohol and drug abuse and anxiety disorders worldwide (Kushner et al., 1990).

Generalized Anxiety Disorder

Excessive worry, poor concentration and insomnia, and an unidentifiable cause characterize anxiety disorder. Symptoms last more than 6 months, and the client is not always able to function in daily life. Treatment options include antidepressants, benzodiazepines, and buspirone.

Treatment Medications

Antidepressants. Several antidepressants have proven effective in the treatment of anxiety disorders, particularly the second-generation antidepressants. Venlafaxine is an FDA-approved antidepressant drug for generalized anxiety disorder (GAD). Clients commonly use the sustained-release formulation, venlafaxine XR, because of better compliance with the less frequent dosing schedule. It has a somewhat more rapid onset than other antidepressants. Other first-line drugs include SSRIs such as paroxetine, the TCA imipramine, nefazodone, and mirtazapine. Bupropion, an antidepressant with insignificant serotonin activity, is ineffective. The onset of action of these drugs is typically within 4 weeks.

The advantage of antidepressants over benzodiazepines is that these drugs are also effective for clients with co-occurring disorders such as major depression or other anxiety disorders. Other advantages include lower potential for drug dependence and abuse that occurs with many antianxiety medications. The disadvantage compared to benzodiazepines includes longer onset of peak action (4 weeks versus 1 week or less) and less efficacy for physical or somatic symptoms of anxiety.

Antidepressant doses for GAD are similar to those for major depression. Gradual titration minimizes side effects and increases client compliance. Adverse effects of SSRIs and venlafaxine include GI upset, insomnia, irritability, headache, and sexual dysfunction. Imipramine has the side effects of TCAs, that is, anticholinergic effects, drowsiness, and dizziness. Nefazodone causes drowsiness and liver toxicity.

Benzodiazepines. Clonazepam, lorazepam, and alprazolam are all FDA approved for use in GAD. The longer-acting benzodiazepine, clonazepam, is desirable because of its ease of dosing. Clients usually take it once or twice a day. The advantage of benzodiazepine is its rapid onset (1 week or less). Disadvantages include cognitive impairment, decreased coordination, potential drug abuse, and withdrawal symptoms. In general, shorter-acting benzodiazepines are more difficult to taper and potentially cause more problems with withdrawal.

Buspirone. Buspirone is a 5-HT_{1A} receptor partial agonist requiring two or three times a day dosing. It is effective in generalized anxiety disorder, but it does not appear to be effective in panic disorder.

The major disadvantage of buspirone is its longer onset, usually 2 to 4 weeks. Initial therapy includes the addition of benzodiazepines until the client sees the effect of buspirone. Table 24-6 describes the therapeutic indications of hypnotic and anxiolytic agents.

Obsessive-Compulsive Disorder

Obsessive-compulsive disorder (OCD) is characterized by persistent and recurrent thoughts, images, impulses, and behaviors that are distressing to the individual and impair daily function.

Treatment Medications

Antidepressants. SSRIs and clomipramine are effective in treating OCD. Physicians prefer SSRIs because of their more advantageous adverse effect profile and better client

TABLE 24-6

Hypnotic and Anxiolytic Agents

GENERIC NAME (TRADE NAME)	APPROVED INDICATION	APPROXIMATELY BENZODIAZEPINE EQUIVALENCY (mg)	ACTIVE METABOLITE	USUAL DOSAGE RANGE (mg/DAY)	HALF-LIFE HOURS
BENZODIAZEPINES					
Alprazolam (Xanax)	A, AD, P	0.5	No	0.75-4 (A) 4-10 (P)	12-15
Chlordiazepoxide (Librium)	A, AW, PS	10	Yes	25-200	5-30
Clonazepam (Klonopin)	LGS	2.5	No	1-6*	20-50
Clorazepate (Tranxene)	A	7.5	Yes	7.5-90	20-80
Diazepam (Valium)	A, PS, SE	5	Yes	2-40	20-80
Estazolam (ProSom)	Hypnotic	2	No	1-2	10-15
Flurazepam (Dalmane)	Hypnotic	15	Yes	15-30	8-40
Halazepam (Paxipam)	A	20	Yes	20-160	10-20
Lorazepam (Lorazepam)	A, PS	1	No	0.5-10	10-20
Oxazepam (Serax)	A, AD, AW	15	No	30-120	5-20
Prazepam (Centrax)	A	10	Yes	20-60	20-80
Quazepam (Doral)	Hypnotic	2	Yes	30-50	30-50
Temazepam (Restoril)	Hypnotic	15	No	15-30	10-20
Triazolam (Halcion)	Hypnotic	0.25	No	0.125-0.25	1.5-5
NONBARBITURATE, NONBENZODIAZEPINE					
Buspirone (BuSPAR)	A	—	—	10-60	2-4
Chloral hydrate (Noctec)	Hypnotic	—	—	500-2000	8-11
Diphenhydramine (Benadryl)	Hypnotic	—	—	25-100	3-9
Diphenhydramine (Unisom)	Hypnotic	—	—	25-100	8-12
Ethchlorvynol (Placydyl)	Hypnotic	—	—	500-1000	18-20
Eszopiclone (Lunesta)	Hypnotic	—	—	2-3	
Rozerem (Ramelteon)	Hypnotic	—	—	8	2-5
Zaleplon (Sonata)	Hypnotic	—	—	10-20	—
Zolpidem (Ambien)	Hypnotic	—	—	5-10	1.5-4
Zolpidem CR (Ambien CR)	Hypnotic	—	—	6.25-12.5	—

A, Anxiety; *AD*, anxiety associated with depression; *AW*, alcohol withdrawal; *LGS*, Lennox-Gastaut syndrome (seizures); *P*, panic disorders; *PS*, psychotic disorders; *SE*, status epilepticus.
*Dosed up to 20 mg/day for seizure.

compliance. Fluvoxamine, fluoxetine, paroxetine, and sertraline are all effective. The choice of a particular SSRI depends on side effects, client tolerance, and potential drug interactions.

Drug Interactions. Fluvoxamine is the only SSRI that has potent inhibitory effects on the CYP_{1A2} enzyme. Significant drug interactions occur with clozapine, TCAs, and theophylline; dose reduction of these drugs is recommended. Fluvoxamine also inhibits CYP 2C19 and CYP 3A4 enzymes, and dose reduction of several drugs, including alprazolam, is necessary.

Tricyclic Antidepressants. Clomipramine is effective for the treatment for OCD, whereas other TCAs, such as desipramine and imipramine, are not. Clomipramine has the usual side-effect profile of the TCAs including sedation, anticholinergic side effects, orthostatic hypotension, sexual dysfunction, and seizure risk. TCAs are second-line therapy.

Augmentation Therapy

Cognitive behavioral therapy is an important nonpharmacologic intervention for OCD. Other augmentation therapies includes the use of (1) dopamine blocking agents, (2) buspirone, (3) lithium, and (4) clonazepam.

Dopamine Blocking Agents. Haloperidol has been effective as an adjunct to fluvoxamine for OCD associated with tics. Researchers are currently studying olanzapine for use in OCD.

Buspirone. Researchers have studied buspirone, 10 mg three times a day, as an adjunct. Lithium and clonazepam have been prescribed and further studies are necessary with this agent.

Posttraumatic Stress Disorder

Posttraumatic stress disorder (PTSD) is recurrent anxiety symptoms in response to very serious life event (i.e., war combat, child abuse, rape). Symptoms interfere with daily function and with relationships.

Treatment Medications

Antidepressants. SSRIs are effective treatment as a class for PTSD (Foa et al., 1999b). Drug selection is based on client preference, side-effect profile, and client tolerance. Nefazodone and bupropion are also effective. TCAs and MAOIs are effective but generally not used because of their side-effect profile and drug and food interactions. The use of a combination of different drug classes is often necessary.

Benzodiazepines. Benzodiazepines are an effective treatment for PTSD. Clonazepam is effective to reduce flashbacks and nightmares. The major problems with the use of benzodiazepines are tolerance and dependence. There is also risk for the client with alcohol abuse because of additive depressant effects.

Mood Stabilizers. Lithium, divalproex, and carbamazepine are an adjunct therapy for explosiveness, irritability, and other symptoms associated with PTSD.

Social Phobia

Social phobia is the most common anxiety disorder. Strong and persistent anxiety resulting from fear of scrutiny by others, or embarrassment, or humiliation characterize this disorder. This response is disproportionate and unrealistic to the situation. A high incidence of alcohol abuse and depression is associated with social phobia, as clients are often isolated in their avoidance.

Treatment Medications

Antidepressants. The SSRIs, including paroxetine, fluoxetine, fluvoxamine, sertraline, and citalopram, are first-line treatments for social phobia. Dosing is similar to that for major depressive disorder. Slow titration increases client compliance and tolerability. The onset of therapeutic effect is about 4 weeks, with optimal effects in 8 to 12 weeks.

Nefazodone is an option if sexual dysfunction is a significant side effect. Nefazodone is contraindicated in clients with hepatic impairment.

Benzodiazepines. Clonazepam and alprazolam are effective.

Gabapentin. The effective dose is 900 to 3600 mg/day. Side effects are sedation, dizziness, and dry mouth.

Herbal Therapy for Anxiety

Kava

Kava *(Piper methysticum)* is an herb that has anxiolytic and sedative properties. It is available as a root extract in capsule form. The recommended dose for treating anxiety is 100 to 125 mg dried kava root extract, taken three times a day. It is also available in tablet form as a purified kavalactone, and the dose is 50 to 70 mg three times a day. As a tincture, the usual dose is 30 drops with water three times a day.

Side Effects. Kava was thought to be relatively mild and safe. Recently literature has warned of kava-associated hepatitis, cirrhosis, and liver failure. Other side effects include altered judgment, altered motor reflexes, GI upset, skin rash, and visual disturbances.

Herb-Drug Interactions. Kava is associated with interactions with several drugs including barbiturates, benzodiazepines, dopamine agonists, alcohol, and MAOIs. There is added risk with combinations of other hepatotoxic drugs.

Valerian

Valerian *(Valeriana officinalis)* has anxiolytic and hypnotic properties. It is for treatment of mild to moderate insomnia and restlessness and tension. Valerian is available as a capsule, extract, tincture, and tea. The dose for anxiety relief is 220-mg valerian extract three times a day.

Side Effects. Some clients have had hepatotoxicity with long-term use of valarian. Side effects include sedation and withdrawal symptoms similar to those associated with benzodiazepines.

Client Education

Important teaching points for clients with an anxiety disorder and their families include the following:

- Educate the client that anxiety disorder is a treatable illness and is not a personal weakness or failure.
- Educate the client regarding the different types of medications that are effective, the side-effect profiles, precautions, and contraindications.
- Encourage clients to participate in the decision-making process when choosing therapy.
- Medications generally take several weeks to achieve maximal effects. Encourage the clients to continue the medications even though they do not see an immediate effect.
- Encourage nonpharmacologic interventions, when appropriate.
- Advise the client of potential drug-drug and drug-herb interactions. Advise clients to report any medications they are taking to their physician or health care professional. This includes herbal remedies, prescription drugs and over-the-counter drugs.
- As with all herbal preparations, caution clients to use only those products where unit dose is clearly defined on the label.
- Counsel the client regarding the risk of mixing alcohol with these medications, especially benzodiazepines.
- Counsel the client to avoid driving or operating machinery, as many of these drugs cause drowsiness and sedation.

Summary

Pharmacotherapy for anxiety disorders is moving away from benzodiazepines toward the serotonergic antidepressants, particularly the SSRIs and venlafaxine. SSRIs and venlafaxine have better safety profiles and do not have the risk of substance abuse, tolerance, and dependence associated with the benzodiazepines. The disadvantage is their slow onset of action. Benzodiazepines are still widely prescribed because of their rapid onset of action and the lack of sexual dysfunction.

INSOMNIA

Hypnotics

Benzodiazepines

Triazolam. Triazolam (Halcion) has a short half-life and a fast onset of action. It is for use with the client who has difficulty falling asleep.

Temazepam. Temazepam (Restoril) has an intermediate half-life with a slow onset of action. It is for the client who awakes early and cannot stay asleep.

Flurazepam. Flurazepam (Dalmane) has a long half-life with a fast onset of action. It is good for clients who have difficulty both falling asleep and staying asleep. The disadvantage is rebound insomnia.

Nonbenzodiazepine Hypnotics

Zolpidem (Ambien), zaleplon (Sonata), eszopiclone (Lunesta), and ramelteon (Rozerem) are the nonbenzodiazepine receptor agonists (NBRAs). They are structurally unrelated to benzodiazepines and do not appear to have abuse potential. They possess minimal muscle relaxant, anticonvulsant, or anxiolytic properties. Advantages over benzodiazepines include lack of rebound insomnia, lack of development of dependence, and lack of adverse withdrawal effects. The main disadvantage of zolpidem and zaleplon is their high cost compared to the benzodiazepines hypnotics.

Zolpidem. Zolpidem is an oral imidazopyridine sedative-hypnotic agent.

Pharmacokinetics. Onset is within 30 minutes, and the duration is 3 to 5 hours. It is rapidly absorbed. The half-life of the drug is 2.5 to 5 hours. It is metabolized to inactive compounds (Greenblatt et al., 1998).

Dose. The usual dose is 10 mg immediately before bedtime; the dose for older adults is 5 mg. Repeating the dose is not recommended. Limit the therapy to 7 to 10 days, and reevaluate the client if a longer duration is necessary.

Ambien CR is a dual-layer tablet that works in two distinct ways:

- The first layer dissolves quickly to help clients get to sleep fast.
- The second layer dissolves slowly to help clients stay asleep.

Ambien CR is available in 6.25 mg and 12.5 mg tablets. It is a controlled release formulation, but there are no comparative sleep studies between the regular formulation and the sustained release formulation.

Side Effects. Clients have reported dizziness, headache, GI upset, nausea, and mild anterograde amnesia. For doses over 10 mg/day, there is risk of hallucinations.

Drug Interactions. Zolpidem is highly protein bound. Food decreases absorption. Avoid the use of other CNS depressants, including alcohol.

Zaleplon. Zaleplon is a nonbenzodiazepine hypnotic agent.

Pharmacokinetics. Zaleplon is a short-acting pyrazolopyrimidine hypnotic with a rapid onset of action. Onset is within 30 minutes and the duration is 2 hours. The half-life is 1.1 hours. Because of its short onset and short half-life, zaleplon is useful for treating insomnia that occurs in the middle of the night and early morning (Elie et al., 1999).

Dose. The recommended dose for the treatment of insomnia is 10 mg before bedtime. A 5-mg dose is sufficient for a small or low-weight client or for an older adult. The dose may be repeated once.

Side Effects. Dizziness and headache are common.

Eszopiclone. Eszopiclone is the newest of the three nonbenzodiazepine benzodiazepine receptor agonists (NBRAs) available in the United States and also has the longest half-life. It has a rapid onset of action (15 to 30 minutes) and is available in 1, 2, and 3 mg tablets. The usual dose is 2 to 3 mg for adult. Older adult clients need to receive lower doses (usually 50% of the usual adult dose).

Rozerem. Rozerem (Ramelteon) is short acting and has a half life of 2to 5 hours (similar to triazolam). The usual dose is 8 mg; 16 mg to 32 mg has been administered with no apparent additional side effects but higher doses did not provide added benefits.

New Drugs Pending Approval

Gaboxadol and indiplon are hypnotics currently in development and not yet FDA-approved. Gaboxadol may have advantages over current hypnotics available on the market. Indiplon is an indirect GABA agonist.

Other Agents Used for Sleep

Trazodone

Mechanism of Action. Trazodone is a serotonin reuptake inhibitor that blocks serotonin receptors. The dose as a hypnotic is 50 to 200 mg at bedtime.

Pharmacokinetics. There is delayed onset, with a long half-life of 6 hours and longer for older adults and obese clients. Side effects are sedation and orthostatic hypotension. Priapism, which is a rare but serious adverse effect, sometimes occurs. Trazodone is preferred over benzodiazepines for clients on drug or alcohol detoxification programs or when clients need to avoid benzodiazepines.

Chloral Hydrate

Mechanism of Action. The mechanism of action of chloral hydrate (Noctoc) is unknown. The active metabolite is trichloroethanol, which possesses hypnotic effect and is responsible for cross-tolerance.

Pharmacokinetics. Rapid onset is 30 minutes. The half-life is 8 to 11 hours. The duration of effect is 4 to 8 hours.

Dose. The recommended dose is 500 to 1000 mg at bedtime, with a maximum dose of 2 g.

Side Effects. Side effects include GI upset, nausea, vomiting, ataxia, confusion, headache, hallucinations, and rash. All clients using this drug need to avoid alcohol. This is recommended for short-term treatment (a few nights) for transient insomnia. It is not for initial treatment as doses exceeding 4 grams can be fatal, and there are many safer drugs such as the nonbenzodiazepine hypnotics that are available.

Diphenhydramine. Diphenhydramine is available over the counter. Many over-the-counter sleep remedies contain diphenhydramine, including Nytol, Sominex, and Unisom. It is an antihistamine and an H_1-receptor antagonist.

Pharmacokinetics. Diphenhydramine is metabolized in the liver.

Dose. The recommended dose is 25 to 50 mg at bedtime. Maximum dosage is 300 mg/day.

Side Effects. Tolerance sometimes develops after 2 weeks. Avoid this drug in older adults because of its anticholinergic side effects.

Barbiturates. The use of barbiturates has dramatically decreased because of the many safer and better hypnotics now available. Table 24-6 lists their dosages and half-lives.

Melatonin. Melatonin (Micromedex, 2003) is an *N*-acetyl-5-methoxytryptamine. It is a naturally occurring hormone secreted by the pineal gland and is a by-product of serotonin metabolism. The dose is 0.3 to 5 mg at bedtime. It is often used to counteract jet lag.

Melatonin is not an herbal product; however, it is commercially available in combination with other herbal remedies. Side effects include drowsiness and daytime fatigue. Avoid other CNS drugs when taking melatonin.

Herbal Products for Sleep

Kava. The dose used as a hypnotic is 60 to 120 mg dried extract (Micromedex, 2003).

Valerian. The dose being used as a hypnotic is 400 to 900 mg at bedtime. Because of its slower onset, clients need to take valerian 1 hour before bedtime (Micromedex, 2003).

AGGRESSIVE AND VIOLENT BEHAVIORS

Aggressive and violent behaviors are frequent in clients with a wide spectrum of underlying disorders. Brain injury, brain trauma, dementia, mental retardation, and seizure disorders are some of the underlying disorders that lead to aggressive and violent behaviors. CNS infections and drug abuse may also lead to aggressive behaviors. Clients with schizophrenia and personality disorders often display these behaviors.

Careful diagnosis always precedes treatment to avoid overuse and misuse of medications. Although the FDA has not approved any medications specifically for aggression, many medications are being used, primarily for the following two purposes:

- To sedate and calm the client and prevent self harm or harm to others
- To treat chronic aggressive behaviors

Factors most important in the selection of an initial emergency medication include availability of an intramuscular injection, liquid formulation, speed of onset, and previous history of response (Allen et al., 2001b).

Acute Agitation and Aggression

Sedating medications are commonly used to treat the acutely aggressive or violent situation. It is important to select a sedating medication that is limited in duration to avoid oversedation and potential adverse effects. Antipsychotics or benzodiazepines are commonly used. Treatment does not exceed 4 weeks. When a client requires more than 4 weeks of treatment, change the approach toward chronic treatment.

Antipsychotics

Antipsychotics are commonly used to treat acute aggressive and violent behaviors. Often it is the sedating property of the antipsychotics that produces the calming effect for the client. An important point to remember is that antipsychotics cause side effects such as akathisia (increased psychomotor restlessness), which nurses often mistake for increased irritability and agitation. It is an error to administer an extra PRN dose of the antipsychotic medication in this instance and worsen the client's symptoms.

The atypical antipsychotics are becoming more commonplace in the treatment of aggressive behavior and have fewer side effects. The disadvantage of using atypical antipsychotics is that only ziprasidone is available in intramuscular injection, and it is expensive. All of the atypical antipsychotics are effective, and the choice depends on the client's condition and the side-effects profile of each drug. For example, clients with diabetes and with weight gain need to avoid the use of olanzapine. Instead, quetiapine is preferred for clients with a history of EPS, and risperidone is preferred for older clients and clients who are delirious because this drug produces fewer anticholinergic side effects (Allen et al., 2001a).

Haloperidol. In clients with brain injury and acute aggression, low-dose haloperidol is preferred. The recommended dose is 1 mg orally or 0.5 mg intramuscularly, with repeated injections every hour until aggression is controlled. Once a client shows no aggression for 48 hours, the dose of haloperidol is gradually tapered, with a decreasing daily dose schedule of 25% until achieving the discontinuation goal.

In clients with dementia and schizophrenia, risperidone is often used (Ranier et al., 2001). Low-dose risperidone of

0.5 to 1 mg is preferred, and the doses should be smaller for older adults with dementia. Trazodone, a sedating antidepressant, has been used to treat older adult clients with sundowning syndrome and aggressive behaviors. Some providers prescribe a low dose of 50 to 100 mg.

Benzodiazepines

The sedating properties of benzodiazepines are helpful in the management of acute agitation and aggressive and violent behavior. Another advantage of the benzodiazepines is their rapid onset of action. There have been reports of paradoxical reactions where benzodiazepines cause violent and aggressive behaviors, but these are rare.

Lorazepam is the most common benzodiazepine in use. Nurses administer it orally or by injection. It is commonly used in combination with antipsychotic medication such as haloperidol. Other nonbenzodiazepine sedating agents used include valproate, chloral hydrate, and diphenhydramine.

Chronic Aggression

When a client continues to exhibit aggressive behavior for more than several weeks, the choice of medication to counteract aggression is guided by the client's underlying condition. For example, when aggression is related to schizophrenia, antipsychotic medications are sometimes used. When aggression is related to mania, lithium or valproate is used. When aggression is related to seizure disorder, carbamazepine or valproate is used.

Antipsychotics

Do not use antipsychotics solely for treatment of aggressive behavior but rather to treat the underlying condition.

Buspirone

Buspirone, an antianxiety agent, has been effective in treating aggressive behavior. The initial dose is 5 mg twice a day, which is increased by 5-mg increments every 3 to 5 days. The client usually does not see the full effect for several weeks, and the effective dose may be as high as 45 to 60 mg/day.

Anticonvulsants

Carbamazepine and valproate treat bipolar disorders and associated aggressive behavior because of their important antikindling properties as described in Chapter 11. Carbamazepine has been effective in reducing aggressive behavior associated with dementia. Lithium is also useful in treating aggression associated with mania.

Antidepressants

Trazodone has been prescribed for the treatment of aggression associated with organic mental disorders. Other antidepressants such as the SSRIs have also been used. The dose range of the antidepressants used to treat aggression is the same as that used for treatment of depression.

Antihypertensive Medications

The beta-blocker propranolol has been effective in treating aggression related to organic brain syndrome. Major side effects of propranolol include lowering of blood pressure and heart rate. Remember that beta-blockers may cause depression.

Special Considerations for Children

If antipsychotic medication is necessary for the treatment of aggression in children, a low-dose atypical antipsychotic such as olanzapine or risperidone is preferred (Allen et al., 2001c).

CHAPTER SUMMARY

- Atypical antispychotic medications have improved efficacy over conventional antipsychotics in the treatment of negative symptoms, but both are effective in treating psychosis.
- Response to antipsychotic medication is heterogeneous and varies among clients.
- In general, the sequence of symptom response is as follows: positive symptoms, affective symptoms, cognitive/perceptual symptoms, and negative symptoms.
- Neuroleptic malignant syndrome (NMS) may be a fatal response to any antipsychotic medication, but it is most frequently associated with conventional antipsychotics. It is important to recognize NMS and to treat it early. Careful diagnosis is necessary.
- A great majority of clients respond favorably to pharmacologic treatment. Failure rates are often caused by inadequate dosing or length of trial, particularly with antidepressants.
- Antidepressants usually cause change in energy levels, and increased energy may result in a client's suicide attempt.
- Suicidal ideation often persists, so clients are at the highest risk to act on suicidal impulses during the early stage of treatment. Protect clients, and counsel them about the delay of desired effects with use of antidepressants.
- Pharmacotherapy for depression has risk. Therefore, knowledge of toxicity and efficacy is important for optimal therapeutic response.
- Adjunctive therapy such as antipsychotics is often used with lithium for bipolar disorder.
- Antianxiety medications such as benzodiazepines are an adjunct to therapy for short-term use. They are often an additive in the long term.
- Selective serotonin reuptake inhibitors (SSRIs) are first-line treatment for depression and many anxiety disorders.
- Anticonvulsants are useful in treating bipolar disorders and as adjunctive therapy for pain and other uses.
- Herbal therapy is common. Caution clients about drug-drug and drug-herb interactions and instruct them to consult the physician. Clients should only use products with specifically labeled unit doses.

REVIEW QUESTIONS

1 A client has been taking citalopram (Celexa) for 2 years for depression. The client's outcomes have been achieved and the client wants to discontinue the medication. Which information should the nurse provide?
1. "It's important for you to gradually stop taking this drug over 2 to 4 weeks."
2. "Citalopram is an antidepressant medication that is usually taken for life."
3. "Because your depression is alleviated, you may discontinue the medication."
4. "Stopping this medication all of a sudden can cause serotonin syndrome."

2 A client with schizophrenia was changed to a new antipsychotic medication 3 weeks ago. The client calls the clinic nurse complaining of sore throat, fever, and malaise. Which laboratory test would be most helpful in determining the cause of these findings?
1. Serum lithium level
2. Complete blood count
3. Liver panel
4. Urinalysis

3 A client hospitalized for major depression has been taking (sertraline) Zoloft for the past week and has verbalized increased energy and improved sleep. What is the highest priority question the nurse should ask?
1. "Have you experienced any side effects from this drug?"
2. "How has your appetite changed since starting this drug?"
3. "Do you think your depression is less severe?"
4. "Are you having any thoughts of harming yourself?"

4 A client with bipolar disorder takes lithium. After playing soccer on a hot summer day, the client complains of nausea, vomiting, diarrhea, and thirst. The client's hands begin to tremble and the gait becomes unsteady. Select the priority nursing intervention(s). You may select more than one answer.
1. Complete an AIMS evaluation on this client immediately.
2. Instruct the client not to take any more lithium until directed the physician.
3. Collaborate with the physician about drawing a serum lithium level immediately.
4. Administer an antiemetic medication to the client.
5. Collaborate with the physician regarding increasing the daily lithium dose.

5 Quetiapine (Seroquel) is prescribed for a client who smokes two packs of cigarettes per day. Which effect would be expected?
1. Quetiapine will have a longer half-life for the client, so fewer doses per day are needed.
2. The doses of quetiapine will be lower than usual because of slowed metabolism.
3. This client has a higher risk of developing tardive dyskinesia.
4. Higher doses of quetiapine will likely be needed to achieve therapeutic effects.

Additional self-study exercises and learning resources are available to you on the ***Companion CD*** *at the back of the book and on the* ***Evolve website*** *at* ***http://evolve.elsevier.com/Fortinash/.***

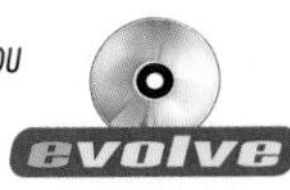

REFERENCES

Allen MH et al: Guidelines 10: initial medication strategies for a violent and unmanageable child: treatment of behavioral emergencies, Expert Consensus Guideline Series: a postgraduate medicine special report, White Plains, NY, 2001a, Expert Knowledge System; www.psychguides.com.

Allen MH et al: Guidelines 12: Choice of oral atypical antipsychotic for an agitated, aggressive client with a complicating medical condition: treatment of behavioral emergencies, Expert Consensus Guideline Series: a postgraduate medicine special report, White Plains, NY, 2001b, Expert Knowledge System; www.psychguides.com.

Allen MH et al: Treatment of behavioral emergencies, Expert Consensus Guideline Series: a postgraduate medicine special report, White Plains, NY, 2001c, Expert Knowledge System; www.psychguides.com.

American Psychiatric Association: *Diagnostic and statistical manual of mental disorders*, ed 4, text revision, Washington, DC, 2000, American Psychiatric Association.

Berkow R, editor: *The Merck manual of diagnosis and therapy*, ed 16, Whitehouse Station, NJ, 1992, Merck and Co.

Bialer M: Comparative pharmacokinetics of the newer antiepileptic drugs, *Clin Pharmacokinet* 24:441-452, 1993.

Bipolar disorder: management of acute mania in adults. In Manolakis PG: *Guide to drug treatment protocols: a resource for creating and using disease-specific pathways*, Washington, DC, 1999, American Pharmaceutical Association.

Bogan AM, Brown ES, Suppes T: Efficacy of divalproex therapy for schizoaffective disorder, *J Clin Psychopharmacol* 20:520-522, 2000.

Botts SR, Raskind J: Gabapentin and lamotrigine in bipolar disorder, *Am J Health Syst Pharm* 56:1939-1944, 1999.

Bupropion (Zyban) for smoking cessation, *Med Lett Drugs Ther* 39:77-78, 1997.

Celexa, citalopram product information, St Louis, 2000, Forest Pharmaceuticals.

Chengappa KNR et al: Bupropion sustained release as a smoking cessation treatment in remitted depressed clients maintained on treatment with selective serotonin reuptake inhibitor antidepressants, *J Clin Psychiatry* 62:503-508, 2001.

Claxton A et al: Client compliance to a new enteric-coated weekly formulation of fluoxetine during continuation treatment of major depressive disorder, *J Clin Psychiatry* 61:928-932, 2000.

Davis R, Wilde MI: Mirtazapine: a review of its pharmacology and therapeutic potential in the management of major depression, *CNS Drugs* 5:389-402, 1996.

Drugs that may cause psychiatric symptoms, *Med Lett* 44:59-62, 2002.

Effexor XR, venlafaxine product information, Wyeth-Ayerst Laboratories, Philadelphia (PI revised Sep 2000), reviewed Jan 2001.

Elie R et al: Sleep latency is shortened during 4 weeks of treatment with zaleplon, a novel nonebnzodiazepine hypnotic, *J Clin Psychiatry* 60:536-544, 1999.

Fava M, Rankin MA: Sexual functioning and SSRIs, *J Clin Psychiatry* 63(suppl 5):13-16, 2002.

Foa EB, Davidson JRT, Frances A: *Treatment of posttraumatic stress disorder*, Preferred medications for guideline 3: selecting a specific medication strategy, Expert Consensus Guideline Series, White Plains, NY, 1999b, Expert Knowledge System; www.psychguides.com.

Frances A, Docherty JP, Kahn DA, editors: The expert consensus guideline series: treatment of bipolar disorder, *J Clin Psychiatry* 57(suppl 12A):1-88, 1996.

Gelenberg AJ et al: Efficacy of venlafaxine extended release capsules in nondepressed outclients with generalized anxiety disorder: a 6-month randomized controlled trial, *JAMA* 283: 3082-3088, 2000.

Glassman AH, Thomas Bigger JT: Antipsychotic drugs: prolonged QTc interval, torsades de pointes, and sudden death, *Am J Psychiatry* 158:1774-1782, 2001.

Gorman JM: Mirtazapine: clinical overview, *J Clin Psychiatry* 60(suppl 17):9-13, 1999.

Greenblatt D et al: Comparative kinetics and dynamics of zaleplon, zolpidem and placebo, *Clin Pharmacol Ther* 64:553-561, 1998.

Hedberg DL, Gordon MW, Glueck BC: Six cases of hypertensive crisis in clients on tranylcypromine after eating chicken livers, *Am J Psychiatry* 122:933-937, 1966.

Hermesh H et al: High serum creatinine kinase level: possible risk factor for neuroleptic malignant syndrome, *J Clin Psychopharm* 22:252-256, 2002.

Houtkooper MA et al: Oxcarbazepine (GP 47.680): a possible alternative to carbamazepine? *Epilepsia* 28(6):693-698, 1987.

Johannessen AC, Nielsen OA: Hyponatremia induced by oxcarbazepine, *Epilepsy Res* 1(2):155-156, 1987.

Johne A et al: Decreased plasma levels of amitriptyline and its metabolites on comedication with an extract from St. John's wort, *J Clin Psychopharmacol* 22:46-54, 2002.

Katon W, Sullivan MD: Depression and chronic medical illness, *J Clin Psychiatry* 51(suppl):3-11, 1990.

Kloster B, Borresen HC, Hoff-Olsen P: *Sudden death in two patients with epilepsy and the syndrome of inappropriate antidiuretic hormone secretion (SIADH)*, Sandvika, Norway, The National Center for Epilepsy.

Kramer TA: Dopamine system stabilizers, *Medscape Psychiatry Mental Health eJournal* 7, 2002.

Kushner MG, Sher KJ, Beitman BD: The relation between alcohol problems and the anxiety disorders, *Am J Psychiatry* 147: 685-695, 1990.

Lexapro (Escitalopram) product information, St Louis, 2002, Forest Pharmaceuticals.

Martin R et al: Cognitive effects of topiramate, gabapentin, and lamotrigine in healthy young adults, *Neurology* 52:321-327, 1999.

Masand P, Murray GB, Pickett P: Psychostimulants in post-stroke depression, *J Neuropsychiatry Clin Neurosci* 3:23-27, 1991.

Meyer JM: Novel antipsychotics and severe hyperlipidemia, *J Clin Psychopharmacol* 21:369-374, 2001.

MICROMEDEX Healthcare Series, vol 115, 1974-2003, Greenwood Village, Colo, Thomson MICROMEDEX.

Murray CJL, Lopez AD: *The global burden of disease*, Cambridge, Mass, 2000, Harvard University School of Public Health & World Health Organization.

Neurontin, gabapentin product information, Morris Plains, NJ, 1999, Parke-Davis.

Nielson CP et al: Polymorphonuclear leukocyte inhibition by therapeutic concentrations of theophylline is mediated by cyclic-3,5-adenosine monophosphate, *Am Rev Respir Dis* 137:25-30, 1988.

Pendlebury SC, Moses DK, Eadie MJ: Hyponatremia during oxcarbazepine therapy, *Hum Toxicol* 8:337-344, 1989.

Ramsay RE: Clinical efficacy and safety of gabapentin, *Neurology* 44(suppl 5):S23-S30, 1994.

Ranier MK et al: Effect of risperidone on behavioral and psychological symptoms and cognitive function in dementia, *J Clin Psychiatry* 62:894-900, 2001.

Rawls WN: TrazodoneB, *Intell Clin Pharmacol* 16:7-13, 1982.

Reid CD: Chemical photosensitivity: another reason to be careful in the sun, *FDA Consumer Magazine*, 1996.

Schatzberg AF, Nemeroff CB: *The American Psychiatric Press textbook of psychopharmacology*, ed 2, Washington, DC, 2001, American Psychiatric Publishing.

Shorter E: *A history of psychiatry: from the era of the asylum to the age of Prozac*, Hoboken, NJ, 1998, John Wiley & Sons.

Spivak B, Radvan M, Shine M: Postural hypotension with syncope possibly precipitated by trazodone, *Am J Psychiatry* 144:11, 1987.

Steinhoff BJ et al: Hyponatremic coma under oxcarbazepine therapy, *Epilepsy Res* 11:67-70, 1992.

Tandon R: Introduction (Ziprasidone), *Br J Clin Pharmacol* 49(suppl 1):1S-3S, 2000.

Taylor DM: Prolongation of QTc interval and antipsychotics, *Am J Psychiatry* 159:1062; discussion 1064, 2002.

Thase ME, Entsuah AR, Rudolph RL: Remission rates during treatment with venlafaxine or selective serotonin reuptake inhibitors, *Br J Psychiatry* 178:234-241, 2001.

Tohen M, Grundy S: Management of acute mania, *J Clin Psychiatry* 60(suppl 5):31-34, 1999.

Van Amelsvoort TH et al: Hyponatremia associated with carbamazepine and oxcarbazepine therapy: a review, *Epilepsia* 35: 181-188, 1994.

Wagner GJ, Rabkin JG, Rabkin R: Dextroamphetamine as a treatment for depression and low energy in AIDS patients: a pilot study, *J Psychosom Res* 42:407-411, 1997.

Wang PS et al: Clozapine use and risk of diabetes mellitus, *J Clin Psychopharmacol* 22:236-243, 2002.

Zakrzewska JM, Patsalos PN: Oxcarbazepine: a new drug in the management of intractable trigeminal neuralgia, *J Neurol Neurosurg Psychiatry* 52:472-476, 1989.

Zobor P et al: Antipsychotic-induced weight gain and therapeutic response: a differential association, *J Clin Psychopharmacol* 22:244-251, 2002.

Chapter 25 Complementary and Alternative Therapies

RUTH N. GRENDELL

The part can never be well unless the whole is well.

PLATO

OBJECTIVES

1. Describe the philosophic differences between complementary/alternative medicine (CAM) and traditional (allopathic) therapies.
2. Discuss the use of various CAM therapies, including mind-body interventions, pharmacologic and biologic treatments, herbal medications, diets, and dietary supplements, and alternative systems of medical practice.
3. Describe the nurse's role in providing holistic nursing care.
4. Discuss the impact of integrating complementary/alternative therapies into nursing practice, education, and research.
5. Outline a client education program that focuses on the concurrent use of alternative therapies and traditional (allopathic) therapies.

KEY TERMS

allopathic (traditional) medicine, p. 573
complementary and alternative medicine, p. 573
disease, p. 572
health, p. 573
holistic, p. 573
illness, p. 572
stress response, p. 575

People have used herbal mixtures and teas, poultices and homemade salves, acupuncture and massage, as well as meditation and prayer for centuries to treat a variety of diseases. There is a resurgence of interest in the use of these self-treatment alternatives. Consumers take megadoses of vitamin C and newly marketed over-the-counter (OTC) products as preventive and treatment measures during the cold and flu season. Many pharmacies and health food stores stock products to prevent or alleviate physical and mental health problems. Many promote certain foods, beverages, and vitamins for their specific benefits and suggest changes in lifestyle to provide a healthy life. The renewed focus on treating the whole person has strongly influenced the interest in these products and practices.

Consumers also continue to use some of the alternative therapies along with the prescribed therapies without informing their health care providers. In some instances, combining herbal and OTC medications with prescribed medications is potentially very harmful. Therefore, it is important that health care professionals are knowledgeable about the numerous alternative therapies available to the public (Cosentino, 2006).

The biomedical model is based primarily on the following assumptions: (1) the scientific method identifies causes of **disease**, a pathologic condition, and providers implement curative treatments to correct abnormal physiology; (2) the germ theory defines infections; (3) prevention of disease is based on proper hygiene, public sanitation, and personal lifestyle choices; (4) disease is usually tangible and measurable. The terms *disease* and *illness* are often used simultaneously; however, **illness** is a highly individual and personal response, exhibited as pain, suffering, or distress (Venes, 2005). Biomedicine utilizes an *opposing approach* to eliminate or correcting an underlying problem, such as prescribing a laxative for constipation or a decongestant for nasal congestion.

In contrast, the focus of the **holistic** or alternative care model is on strengthening one's inner resistance to disease and healing from within, or enhancing the body's innate healing powers (Snyder and Lindquist, 2001; Chen, 2000; Kreitzer and Jensen, 2000). Although biomedical practices have strongly influenced the nursing discipline, it also has deep roots in the holistic perspective that considers the impact of all intrapersonal, interpersonal, and environmental interactions as contributing factors to a person's well-being or illness (American Holistic Nursing Association [AHNA], 2006).

Some alternative medical practices have been integrated into **allopathic (traditional) medicine,** particularly in pain management and the treatment of chronic illness, anxiety, depression, and disease prevention. This chapter describes the contrast in philosophies and treatment modalities between biomedical and holistic models of care and selected alternative therapies and their significance to the practice of nursing.

ALTERNATIVE THERAPY FIELDS

Complementary and alternative medicine (CAM) covers a broad range of healing philosophies, approaches, and therapies and their accompanying theories and beliefs. There are more than 1800 approaches to healing (Snyder and Lindquist, 2001). Some therapies are based on physiologic principles of modern medicine, whereas others come from concepts that are in contrast to the accepted medical practices. In 1992, Congress established the Office of Alternative Medicine (OAM) under the direction of the National Institutes of Health (NIH) to evaluate the effectiveness of alternative therapies. In 1998, OAM became the National Center for Complementary and Alternative Medicine (NCCAM). There are regional centers for objective, evidenced-based research on alternative therapies throughout the nation (NCCAM, 2002). The NCCAM has classified complementary and alternative therapies into seven broad categories: (1) alternative medicine systems; (2) mind-body interventions; (3) pharmacologic- and biologic-based therapies; (4) herbal medications; (5) diet, nutrition and supplements, and lifestyle changes; (6) manipulative and body-based methods; and (7) energy therapies. More than 600 CAM therapies are within this continually evolving taxonomy (Pelletier, 2000). The list of CAM practices is constantly revised as a result of the gradual acceptance of some CAM modalities that are based on research findings (Cosentino, 2006). Box 25-1 lists selected CAM therapies.

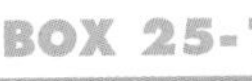

BOX 25-1

Complementary and Alternative Therapy Fields and Selected Examples

ALTERNATIVE SYSTEMS OF MEDICAL PRACTICE
Traditional Chinese medicine (TCM) including acupuncture
Ayurvedic medicine
Homeopathic medicine
Naturopathy
Environmental medicine
Culture-based community medicine (folk medicine)

MIND-BODY INTERVENTIONS
Meditation
Mindfulness-based therapy
Prayer
Yoga
The arts: music, dance, drama, art, literature
Humor
Exercise
Animal-assisted therapy
Psychotherapy
Hypnosis

PHARMACOLOGIC AND BIOLOGIC TREATMENTS
Vaccines and medicines not yet approved by mainstream medicine—animal cartilage, chelating chemicals

HERBAL MEDICINE
Chinese herbals
European herbals
American herbals

DIET, NUTRITION, SUPPLEMENTS, AND LIFESTYLE CHANGES
Vitamins, minerals, and supplements
Designer diets—macrobiotic, cancer, weight reduction
Food elimination diets—allergy detection
Vegetarian
Ethnic-based diets

MANUAL HEALING METHODS
Osteopathy
Chiropractic
Massage
Acupressure
Foot and hand reflexology
Therapeutic touch

ENERGY THERAPIES
Biofeedback
Bioelectromagnetics
Light therapy
Bone growth stimulation
Magnet therapy

HISTORICAL OVERVIEW

Ancient Cultural Beliefs

In ancient times, many often believed illness was punishment for sin or at the whim of the gods—a matter of fate. Healing came through purification of the body through the use of herbs, fasting, purgatives, incantations, and ceremonies. Individuals believed evil spirits caused diseases and adverse events; good spirits intervened on the behalf of an individual or group. People made animal sacrifices to appease the gods, and calling on spirits became part of healing rituals. Some countries, however, passed laws to regulate the practices of hygiene, sanitation, and preservation of food to protect people from disease.

Hippocrates (400-377 BC), known as the father of modern medicine, introduced beliefs that the gods did not control **health,** the state when all functions of the body and mind are normally active. Instead, health was dependent on the harmony, or balance, between the body, the mind, and the environment. He used a patient-centered approach to treat the whole person. The dominant beliefs in most Asian countries considered that individuals attained this balance between human beings and nature by finding inner peace and spiritual contentment and by understanding and practicing the interactive powers of the mind and body and spirit. In many cultures, healers were priest-physicians referred to as holy men, or shamans, and the care they provided was shamanistic medicine (Ellis and Hartley, 2003; Weil, 2000).

Biomedicine Model Concepts

Western biomedicine (allopathic medicine) is based on a worldview strongly influenced by Cartesian dualism (separation of mind and body) and Newtonian physics of the seventeenth and eighteenth centuries. "Disease occurs when the parts break down" (The New Medicine Video [KPBS], 2006; Snyder and Lindquist, 2001). Science and technology revolutionized the practice of medicine and facilitated a greater understanding of human biology and methods of intervention in disease and illness. In Western biomedicine, practitioners have standardized treatments and care regimens that match the client with a disease category of defined signs and symptoms. These technically oriented interventions aim for rapid results in reversing the deteriorative physiologic disease process and to prolong life (Parkman and Ullrich, 2000). In turning to technology, however, Western medicine lost touch with its own historical roots of treating the whole person (Weil, 2000). Weil stated that allopathic medicine is also *physician centered*, granting the caregiver the authority for making decisions and placing the client in a passive, somewhat powerless position that limits the client's responsibility in the recovery process.

Holistic Model Concepts

In contrast, the holistic perspective focuses on the healing of the total person rather than the cure of a specific disease. Each person is uniquely separate from another human being and is *more* than the sum of the individual parts—what affects one aspect affects all (Topham, 2004; Parkman and Ullrich, 2000). In addition to examining physical symptoms, the clinician considers the influence of cultural and genetic factors, past and current experiences, family structure, and role functions on the person's perception of health and illness and the use of coping mechanisms. Many therapies are *preventive* measures rather than treatments for disease symptoms. Research indicates that many of the CAM therapies, such as diet, exercise, and psychologic stress-reduction therapies, are particularly effective in preventing and managing chronic disease processes (Snyder and Lindquist, 2001; Pelletier, 2000). CAM therapies encourage individuals to take active responsibility for their own health and participate in the recovery process when diseases do occur. A change in attitude and lifestyle, a sense of control and peace, and decreased anxiety indicate healing, even though the particular disease is not cured. Multiple methods are sometimes incorporated into the individualized plan of care. Many alternative therapies are based on Oriental and Far Eastern beliefs and practices. Some unifying themes among the several alternative therapies include a person's inherent recuperative ability, the importance of self-esteem, and the influence of spiritual and emotional beliefs on health. Treatment methods are based on maintaining or restoring a balance within all aspects of the individual. Box 25-2 presents a detailed listing of themes.

BOX 25-2

Common Themes of Integrative Therapies

- Humans have recuperative powers.
- Religious and spiritual values are important to the state of health.
- Self-esteem and purpose of life are positive influences in the healing process.
- Thoughts, feelings, emotions, values, and perceived meanings affect physical function.
- Most therapies rely on diet, exercise, relaxation techniques, lifestyle, and attitude changes.
- Focus is on the total person—one's physical, emotional, mental, and psychosocial health.
- Illness is an imbalance; interventions are directed toward restoring balance.
- Energy is the force needed to achieve balance and harmony.

Rise in Dominance of the Biomedical Model

Before the 1800s, biomedicine and alternative medicine coexisted and competed on a somewhat equal basis. During the latter part of that century, however, many considered the biomedical model superior because of the scientific discovery of microbes as the cause of many infectious diseases and the development of methods to eliminate those causes. Disease cure rates rose, and favorable surgical outcomes soon followed through the use of proper aseptic techniques and new anesthesia discoveries. Another significant event that legitimized biomedicine was the research report by Abraham Flexner in 1910. It indicated the need for standards in education and licensing of physicians. Philanthropic funding of medical education institutions quickly stopped any financial assistance to the schools with nonmedical, nonscientific curricula.

As a result of the rising dominance of the biomedical model, many questioned the credibility of alternative therapies. These practices were soon relegated to the fringes of health care and were often referred to as quackery. Although chiropractic and osteopathic practices continued, others such as homeopathy and naturopathy were almost forgotten (Tedesco and Cicchetti, 2001). Yet today more than 40% of Americans have reported using alternative therapies; worldwide, more than 90% of people use them (Cosentino, 2006; Parkman and Ullrich, 2000). Although Europe and other countries have largely accepted

CAM therapies, most U.S. health care professionals sometimes ignore the fact that people use many alternative methods to manage their diseases and chronic illnesses.

Merging Philosophies

Renewed interest in mind-body interactions grew in the mid-twentieth century. The discovery that some people exposed to pathogens did not become ill led researchers to challenge the existing biologic theory and to explore other possible influencing causes. Subsequent epidemiologic studies revealed that diet, smoking, and environmental pollution were strongly associated with increased incidences of lung cancer. They also found that widowed persons had higher death rates than married persons in the same age group; socioeconomic factors had impact on disease; and certain religious groups had fewer reports of illness and death from specific diseases. The technologies of modern biomedicine did not provide explanations. The strong possibility of a cause-effect relationship between the environment and the mind, spirit, and body in health and illness encouraged further investigation. These findings indicated that many chronic conditions are the result of common lifestyle risks (smoking, diet, sedentary lifestyle, stress). These are not treatable by means of the one-dimensional solutions prescribed by conventional (allopathic) medicine.

Psychoneuroimmunology (PNI), a relatively new field, is the study of a person's psychobiologic factors and their interaction with the **stress response** and influence on health outcomes. Arousal of the hypothalamic-pituitary-adrenal axis affects the nervous, endocrine, and immune systems. Prolonged exposure to stress and high anxiety levels are linked to lowered immunity, whereas a greater resistance to illness is associated with lower stress and anxiety. The PNI model provides a framework for screening risk factors of health problems including stress stimuli, sociodemographic factors, lifestyle behaviors, and health history (Anderson, 2004a). PNI is also possibly the framework for conducting future studies on the efficacy of mind-body therapies because of its emphasis on the relationships between stress, increased cortisol levels, and impairment of the immune system (Maes, 2001).

Scientists have explored the age-old mind-body healing modalities of other societies, particularly Oriental medicine. As a result, mainstream health care has integrated acupuncture, meditation, relaxation techniques, massage, and other related interventions into care plans. Some medical schools have included courses in CAM in the curriculum. Additional researchers are conducting studies, and several practitioners have published articles (Anderson, 2004b; Pelletier, 2000). However, progress in integrating CAM into mainstream medicine will be slowed because of regulatory and reimbursement measures, values, and misconceptions still held by many allopathic (biomedicine) practitioners and the lack of large-scale clinical trials to demonstrate the effectiveness of CAM (Box 25-3).

BOX 25-3

Examples of Completed and Ongoing Research Funded by the National Center of Complementary and Alternative Medicine (NCCAM) and Safety Warnings

NOTE: Many of the studies are longitudinal and require several months or years to produce results. Large-scale, long-term, randomized clinical trials are the gold standard of biomedical research (NCCAM, 2006; Pelletier, 2000). Preliminary findings have been reported on some of the studies. After evidence-based studies, the Agency for Healthcare Research and Quality has issued several safety alerts. Some herbals are harmful as a result of certain health problems and their interactive effects with other herbals and medications. Consider the following examples:

- *Ephedra (Ma huang)* is used for weight loss, to increase energy, and to enhance athletic ability. The amphetamine-like effects are harmful for persons with hypertension, hyperthyroid, cardiovascular problems, glaucoma, depression, diabetes mellitus, prostate hypertrophy, and retention.
- *Kava (Piper methysticum)* is a member of the pepper family and is used for insomnia, stress, and anxiety reduction. It is linked with hepatitis and cirrhosis.
- *Garlic* is popular for use in reducing cholesterol levels. It is harmful when combined with drugs for treatment of AIDS. It reduces saquinavir by 50%.
- *St John's wort* should not be used with protease inhibitors such as indinavir.
- *Bioterrorism protection herbals* have been advocated by some as protection against virulent infections spread by biologic weapons. The Centers for Disease Control and Prevention states there is no scientific basis for this practice. Anthrax and smallpox progress too rapidly for the immune system to counteract them via the use of any complementary and alternative medicine dietary supplement.

Modified from the NCCAM website: www.nccam.nih.gov.

CURRENT ISSUES

The Changing Complexion of Health Care

Modern medicine has become so expensive that it is straining the economy of the United States and many other developed nations, putting itself beyond the reach of much of the world's population, particularly for long-term regimens. Chronic and degenerative illnesses, including cardiovascular disease, cancer, diabetes, arthritis, and depression, are reaching epidemic proportions (Bodenheimer and Fernandez, 2005; Pelletier, 2000). Nearly 70% of the U.S. health care budget is spent on the treatment of persons with chronic diseases, and costs will escalate as the baby-boomer generation grows older. The United States spent more than $1.7 trillion, or 15.3% of the U.S. gross domestic product (GDP), on health care in 2003. (Researchers predict this will increase to $4 trillion by 2015, or 20% of the GDP.) These costs are straining all systems that finance health care (Gutierrez and Ranji, 2005).

Many traditional medicine physicians think they are not receiving adequate payment for services because of the managed care model that dominates health care. Concierge medicine—also known as boutique medicine or platinum medicine—is a relatively new practice method for physicians who choose to limit their practice to clients who are able to privately pay an annual fee for extra and special services from the physician (Kalogredis, 2004). There is a wide range of services offered that depend on the individual physician's imagination and choices. Annual fees range from $1000 to $20,000 and include house calls, priority days of service, preventive care, spa care, and other services. This type of service is obviously in the minority in the United States, but the American Medical Association and other legal governing organizations consider this legal and ethical. The obvious disadvantage is that it eliminates those who are not privileged and wealthy from participating.

Unfortunately, biomedical treatments and advanced technology also have negative consequences. Microbes have become resistant to medications. Some chronic diseases that still defy scientific interventions have replaced infectious diseases as the major cripplers and killers. Side effects of many of the new wonder drugs sometimes have dangerous psychologic and physiologic effects.

Consumer confidence in conventional treatment methods has deteriorated, and citizens are turning to legislators to change the health care system. The reasons for the growing dissatisfaction include the increasing costs and restrictions imposed by managed care and health maintenance organizations. Consumers also want to have more control in health care decisions. Health care reform requires a focus on disease prevention and health promotion rather than on disease treatment (Topham, 2004; Ellis and Hartley, 2003). Exposure to the various alternative therapies through the combination of cultures and abundant information provided by the media has a strong influence on the public's acceptance and use of alternative therapies. The media covers information on health care almost daily, and it is easily accessible on the Internet. Articles frequently appear in popular magazines, and many bookstores have substantial sections for self-help books that have become bestsellers. Convenience and fewer side effects from natural substances, less invasive techniques, the possibility of an overall decrease in cost, and the ability to choose are appealing alternatives to traditional medicine (Topham, 2004; Snyder and Lindquist, 2001; Parkman and Ullrich, 2000).

In May 2004, the NCCAM released the most comprehensive findings regarding the use of CAM by Americans. The report was based on data from the 2002 National Health Interview Survey of 31,044 Americans aged 18 years or older who answered questions about their health practices and status and their use of 27 types of CAM. The therapies included acupuncture, hypnosis, chiropractic care, and others, in addition to self-administered therapies such as meditation, prayer, and herbal supplements. The survey revealed that 75% of the respondents used CAM at some point in their lives; 62% had used CAM within the previous 6 months. When researchers eliminated the use of prayer specifically for healing purposes from the data, the amount dropped to 50%, and 36% had used some form of CAM during the previous 12 months (Cosentino, 2006). Eisenberg et al. found similar results in a landmark national study in 1993. According to a 1997 update of this study, there was an almost 10% increase in the use of these therapies and an expenditure of more than $22 billion (Eisenberg et al., 1998).

Barriers to Acceptance of Alternative Therapies

Although alternative practices have been in style for centuries in Europe, Asia, and the Far East, therapeutic results were primarily reported through subjective reports, so the medical community questioned the validity of the research methods. The Western medical world continues to call for clinical studies conducted within strict, controlled limits. The U.S. Food and Drug Administration (FDA) also expressed great concern over the lack of guidelines to ensure purity and dosage accuracy of herbal remedies and supplements (NCCAM, 2002; Silva and Ludwick, 2001). Currently these substances are exempt from FDA approval. There is also a concern over claims that one substance is a cure-all for many health problems. The FDA continues to argue for the right to regulate these products. Another great concern is the validity of media reports, the credentials of the report writers, and the fact that no effective control exists for the more than 15,000 health care information sites on the Internet (Box 25-4).

Many advocates of alternative therapies cannot afford the tremendous costs of investigation, thus many methods will not be tested. Additional barriers are society's heavy reliance on high-technology treatments by society, the dependence on pharmaceuticals, and state laws that limit the practice of medicine or the healing arts to those with professional medical licensure. Political lobbying and the advertising influence of drug manufacturers are other major barriers, although most pharmaceutical companies produce OTC compounds that are attractive substitutes to costly prescriptive medications.

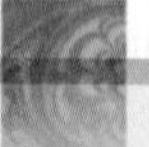

BOX 25-4

Evaluation Strategies of Medical Resources on the Web

- Who establishes and maintains the site?
- Who finances the site?
- What is the purpose of the site?
- Where does the information come from?
- What is the basis for the information? Is it research based? Are references listed?
- How is the information selected?
- Is the information current? When was the site last updated?
- Are there links to other sites? How were these sites chosen?
- What information does the site collect from you? Why?
- How does the site interact with visitors to the site?

Modified from the NCCAM website: www.nccam.nih.gov.

The many barriers are typical for innovative proposals that challenge any current traditional practices. Additional concerns focus on the dangers of self-diagnosis, potential and critical delay in seeking appropriate medical care, the potential interactions during the concurrent use of herbal and other drugs with prescribed medications, and the detrimental effects of not informing health care providers about the use of CAM products. The scientific research projects at NCCAM have produced a notable shift in thinking by mainstream medical practitioners. Because the use of CAM is continuing to increase, the medical community and consumers deserve to know which therapies have demonstrated effectiveness and which have not (Pelletier, 2000).

Pelletier, a past director of NCCAM, cautions that some advocates of CAM view it as a religion and tend to believe that all CAM therapies are superior to any form of conventional medicine. CAM has limitations and is harmful if used improperly. He stated that Western medicine also includes some practices that research has not yet validated. Pelletier (2000) advocated that the same stringent standards of evidence-based medicine be employed in all therapeutic interventions, thereby helping to prevent double standards.

Impact of the *Healthy People 2000* Report

As early as the 1970s, the rising costs of medical care led several physicians and educators to see the need for integrating technical sophistication with humanistic values. The debate over quality-of-life issues required a focus on changes in educating the public and the profession. Alternative strategies evolved, such as permitting family members to assist in patient care in intensive care units, creating a homelike atmosphere during labor and delivery, presenting health education programs, and establishing self-help support groups. Health care agencies made health appraisal questionnaires available in health care facilities, and illnesses were creative opportunities for instruction on self-care. Some practitioners introduced a limited number of alternative therapies, including acupuncture and stress-reduction measures, into the system (Leonard and Plotnikoff, 2001; Snyder and Lindquist, 2001).

Health care reform became a major issue in the 1980s, and as a result, researchers conducted several nationwide studies. The *Healthy People 2000* report published by the U.S. Public Health Department in 1990 contained three major goals: (1) to increase healthy life span for all Americans, (2) to reduce the discrepancies in care provided among Americans, and (3) to provide access to preventive services for all. Primary, secondary, and tertiary levels of illness/disease prevention were referred to as healthy lifestyle practices, early screening and treatment, and rehabilitation measures to inhibit complications. These protective and preventive measures required active participation by both individuals and health care providers. The report also targeted the specific needs of several high-risk groups, including infants, children, ethnic and low-income groups, and older adults. The amount of progress in meeting these goals was included in the *Healthy People 2010* report. Ongoing research will monitor the incidence of health and illness. Statistical indicators of a healthy population include evidence of physical activity, a reduction in obesity, a decline in tobacco and substance abuse, responsible sexual behavior, improved mental health, a decrease injury and violence, enhanced environmental quality, and a more widespread application of immunizations. (The nurse plays a primary role in health promotion and education. Consider these indicators as you learn about human responses to health and illness.)

EXPLORING EFFECTIVENESS OF ALTERNATIVE THERAPIES

The Informed Client

As mentioned earlier, physicians have less control over disease information as consumers become more active in decisions about their methods of treatment. Many people are turning to therapies that address them as whole beings. Self-help and discussion groups often use the Internet for the exchange of information. The Internet has provided a collection of current expertise about a variety of health problems that often goes beyond current information known by the practicing health care provider. However, the public needs to evaluate the validity of information. Box 25-4 describes how to evaluate Internet sources. Broadcasts of documentary films and programs in health education and fitness have also enhanced public awareness of developments in health care and alternative therapies, as well as self-care options.

The Nurse's Role

The health of individuals, families, and communities is a major focus of nursing, with consideration for the effect of the individual's health status, health beliefs, and interactions with self, others, and the environment. Several practice models help to guide the nurse in carrying out these practices. All of the new integrative therapy (CAM) models are designed around a holistic view of the client, giving consideration to the ability for adapting and coping with life events, the impact of social and cultural values on health/illness beliefs, and personal responsibility for healthy outcomes (The New Medicine Video, 2006; Topham, 2004; Kreitzer and Disch, 2003).

People from every culture have a different perspective of the Western health care model and will respond in different ways. They often view the system as cold and abrupt—even rude. They often turn away unless health care providers understand them. Knowing this, it is important to keep people of all cultures connected to the system, particularly related to public health concerns. It is important for the nurse to respect people's dignity and the integrity and belief systems, to negotiate a situation that allows for as much independence in the care as possible, and to create an environment that promotes partnership with clients in all phases of the nursing process. The Joint Commission

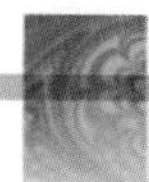

BOX 25-5

Summary of AHNA Standards of Holistic Nursing Practice

1. The standards are based on the philosophy and theory of holism (emphasizing the whole and the interdependence of the parts) and ethical practice.
2. The nurse will obtain and maintain current knowledge and competency in the practice of holistic nursing. The practice will be consistent with research findings.
3. The nurse will practice holistic self-care to permit personal development and facilitate in the healing process of others.
4. The nurse will communicate within the holistic framework; consider the environment within and surrounding the individual client; and consider the client's cultural background, health beliefs and practices, sexual orientation, values, and preferences.
5. The holistic caring process will consist of the following:
   a. Assessment that honors the uniqueness of the individual
   b. Prioritization of actual/potential problems and needs
   c. Developing outcomes that correlate with the identified problems and needs
   d. Care plans focusing on health promotion, recovery and restoration or peaceful dying; plans support the independence of the individual as much as possible
   e. Nursing interventions conducive with the plan of care
   f. Evaluation recognizing each person's response to the care provided

Modified from the American Holistic Nursing Association website: www.ahna.org/about/standards.html, retrieved 2006.

(TJC) also requires documentation of the ways in which nurses meet clients' cultural needs (Williams, 2006; Frisch, 2001a).

The AHNA has published standards for holistic practice (Box 25-5), and resources are available through the several nursing specialty groups (Frisch, 2001b; Snyder and Lindquist, 2001). Nurses often integrate CAM techniques with the traditional medical practices such as teaching breathing and visualization strategies in managing pain and reducing stress. Serving as teacher and facilitator empowers the client (Parkman and Ullrich, 2000).

APPLICATION OF SELECTED ALTERNATIVE THERAPIES

Since the mid-1970s, there has been a major effort to identify strategies to assist individuals in coping with acute diagnoses and chronic psychologic and physiologic health problems, as well as managing sudden and long-term life changes. The greatest benefits of CAM therapies lie in promoting healthy lifestyles and managing chronic illnesses and diseases (Kreitzer and Disch, 2003: Snyder and Lindquist, 2001; Pelletier, 2000).

Mind-Body Interventions

Meditation

The relaxation response to meditation consists of a wide range of beneficial physiologic and psychologic effects, including lowered heart and blood pressure rates, decreased serum levels of adrenal corticosteroids, increased immunity to disease, a sense of calmness and peace, and mental alertness. Meditation therapies include biofeedback, visual imagery, and other stress-reduction measures, including yoga and progressive relaxation techniques. Originally, meditation was a religious practice (i.e., saying prayers, reciting scripture, saying the rosary, or concentrating on a religious symbol). Nurses can teach meditative techniques, and there are a number of audiotapes that facilitate mastery of concentration. Guidelines for meditating include a routine of selecting a special time and place, assuming a comfortable position, using deep breathing and progressive relaxation exercises, and focusing attention on a chosen mental image (Topham, 2004; Kreitzer and Jensen, 2000; Parkman and Ullrich, 2000).

Prayer

Prayer differs from meditation in that it involves communication with God, or a superior being, who answers the prayer. "There are as many different types of prayer as there are different religions or cultures" (Ameling, 2000, p. 43). Prayer for healing purposes is an individual or group action or an intercessory prayer (distant prayer) conducted by other people with or without the knowledge of the individual for whom the prayers are said. An ancient form of intercessory prayer is the laying on of hands and anointing the ill person with oil.

Prayer is silent or spoken, conversational or formal, or a recitation of a favorite psalm. Illness sometimes interferes with an individual's ability to pray because of feelings of isolation, guilt, grief, or anxiety (Maier-Lorentz, 2004). Prayer is one of the therapeutic tools nurses use when providing spiritual care to calm a client's worried feelings. Many hospitals have chaplains to support clients and their families of all faiths. "Each of these threads—religion, ethnicity, and culture—is woven into the fabric of a person's particular response to treatment and healing" (Spector, 2003, p. 123). Numerous studies—some poorly constructed and others with a strong scientific base—have demonstrated significant positive associations between religion (faith) and health; therefore, do not ignore the role that beliefs play in a person's coping (Koenig, 2006).

Mindfulness-Based Therapy

Jon Kabat-Zinn is the founder of the Mindfulness-Based Stress Reduction (MBSR) Clinic at the University of Massachusetts Medical School. The program is based on Zen consciousness—paying attention to one's own inner experience by quieting the mind and investigating the mind through personal experiences, asking questions such as, "Who am I?" Individuals learn how to balance physical, mental, and spiritual health by using all the senses. They learn how to develop a deeper knowing of self from silence and stillness and to perceive thoughts more clearly because of embodied wakefullness. Many use MBSR for a variety of health problems including anxiety, eating disorders and addictions. In an interview, Kabat-Zinn stated, "Humans are miraculous beings, and we have infinitely more capacity and dimensions associated with our brains and our nervous system and with our deep intelligences, *and I emphasize the plural*, that we usually simply ignore" (Gazella, 2005, p. 59). MBSR therapy has also proved effective for persons with prostate cancer, for those receiving bone marrow transplant, for prison inmates and staff, and for persons in multicultural settings as well as corporate and work environments.

The goal of the meditation process is not to change thoughts but to allow an awareness to emerge through, paying attention only to the present moment and being nonjudgmental about the thoughts that pass through the mind. Although the meditation is based on Buddhist beliefs, the spiritual aspects are de-emphasized for a Western audience. Hatha yoga and controlled breathing eliminate distractions and permit the participant to be more objective about inner thoughts. The person also learns to scan the body systematically, as part of a desensitization process to inhibit the automatic learned responses to unhealthy thoughts (Telner, 2005; Laidlaw and Dwivedi, 2004). Kabat-Zinn's (1990) book *Catastrophe Living: Using the Wisdom of Your Body and Mind to Face Stress, Pain and Illness*, which outlines the practices at the MBSR clinic, is a major resource for mindfulness-based cognitive therapy (MBCT) programs that also includes principles of cognitive therapy (Segal et al., 2002).

MCBT is a promising new approach for preventing recurring episodes of depression. Sad moods reactivate thinking styles associated with previous sad moods, and as a sad mood becomes more negative, thoughts and behaviors become repetitive, ruminative (focusing on a thought for an extended period of time), and self-perpetuating (a self-fulfilling prophecy). The therapy uses the *decentering*, or disengagement, concept to help the individual visualize passing events in the mind that are neither necessarily valid reflections of reality nor central aspects of the self. Culture and upbringing strongly influence the meaning of an event and an individual's response. Reframing, or cognitive restructuring (cognitive optimizing), is a strategy that encourages the individual to monitor and evaluate the negative thoughts and replace them with positive ones, therefore changing the meaning of an experience. This strategy often helps the individual to gain control over the unpleasant experience. For example, "I can cope. I had pain before and I was able to handle it. I can manage this too." The major principles of cognitive behavioral therapy (CBT) are as follows (National Association of Cognitive-Behavioral Therapists [NACBT], 2006):

- Our thoughts strongly influence our feelings and actions; external factors or events do not cause feelings and actions.
- We can learn to identify which thoughts cause unwanted feelings and behaviors and how to replace them with thoughts that lead to more desirable responses.

Cognitive therapy is based on the education model. It involves teaching rational self-correcting skills, and is a collaborative effort between the client and the therapist.

RESEARCH for EVIDENCE-BASED PRACTICE

Meadows G, Mitchell P (principal investigators): *Randomized controlled trial of MBCT and maintenance of adherance therapy (MAT) for the prevention of relapse and recurrence of depression in primary care*, Mental Health Australia and Monash University, 2005.

Researchers are conducting a randomized controlled 3-year clinical trial to evalaute the effectiveness of mindfulness-based cognitive therapy (MBCT) and medication adherance therapy (MAT) for the prevention of depressive relapse. The ultimate goal is to develop a service model involving collaboration between primary care providers and mental health specialty professionals. A literature review indicated that both treatment protocols have been effective; however, a combination of the therapies is even more effective for the long-term care of clients in outpatient settings. The project includes developing training manuals, educating the primary and mental health care providers, establishing protocol for recruiting participants, and establishing a time frame as well as the selection of measurement tools. A follow-up report in December, 2005, stated that these strategies have been accomplished. The first treatment group will begin early in 2006. A second follow-up report will be given in 1 year. Projected outcomes for the adherance therapy include the following: adherence to the prescribed psychotherapeutic medications for at least 1 year, preferably for 2 years; for the MBCT, participants will develop an individualized depression relapse prevention plan, follow the stress-reduction strategies learned in the therapy program, keep bimonthly appointments with the health care provider, respond to the telephone contacts regarding adherance to medications and utilizing the learned strategies to recognize warning signs of potential depressive relapse, and seek professional help if needed.

The Socratic questioning method tests the perceptions and hypotheses thoughts create (e.g., How do I know that people are criticizing me? How do I know that I am a failure?). Homework is a central feature of CBT. CBT requires a relatively short duration of time compared with other psychotherapies.

The MBCT classes consist of a series of 8 to 12 group meetings and 4 follow-up sessions. Each week the therapist introduces a new strategy followed by instructions for daily homework assignments. Subsequent classes build on the previous content. Daily homework assignments consist of viewing videos, practicing meditation, keeping a diary, visualizing how the body responds to healthy and unhealthy thoughts, and planning an individualized strategy to use when a future depressive mood occurs. During the sixth week, in some programs, the participants attend an all-day silent retreat. MBCT is particularly helpful for persons who have had three or more depression episodes and who experienced depression early in life (Kabat-Zinn, 2002) (see the Research for Evidence-Based Practice box).

Psychotherapists are also looking at *Johrei*, a Japanese strategy that is a nontouch method of sending subtle energy toward another person, which includes not only paying close attention to the recipient but also being open hearted and feeling goodwill toward the recipient. The Johrei method uses Zen meditation principles. In Asian languages, mindfulness means being affectionate and having kind-hearted characteristics when the person is attending to the here and now. Some have used this method in conjunction with hypnosis. Studies have shown lower immune system responses in an experimental group of students who have been exposed to the Johrei experience than the control group when taking exams. Current studies are investigating the changes in EEG patterns in the practitioner and the recipient (Laidlaw and Dwivedi, 2004).

Yoga

Living a balanced life is central to yoga principles. The individual achieves the use of specific body postures *(asanas)*, gentle movements and stretches, breath control, and minimizing stimulation of the senses, leading a simple life, and directed meditation through daily practices. Concentration on purity of body and mind, self-restraint and contentment with life, studying relevant literature, and daily dedication to a higher being are the means to attain that balance. Originally practiced in India, yoga has become a popular practice as a part of health enhancement and as a therapy for stress reduction and for people with chronic diseases. Hatha yoga, also called Hatha *vidya*, is the most familiar form of yoga. Its many forms focus on purification of the physical body, thus leading to purification of the mind and renewal of vital energy. Outside of India, Hatha yoga is mainly practiced for mental and physical health. Conversely, the focus of Raja yoga is on purifying the mind and spirit, then, purification comes to the body via body postures and the breath (Hatha Yoga: Wikipedia, 2006; Ameling, 2000; Pelletier, 2000).

Use of the Arts

The use of music, dance, drama, literature, humor, and art is part of environmental therapy for clients and health care providers. Quiet background music provides a soothing atmosphere and is distracting medium during times of stress and pain. Music is often used in intensive care units, in birthing rooms, during dental procedures, and even as a stimulus for people with lowered levels of consciousness. Mood music allows the listener to express emotions and feelings through dancing, singing, and creative thinking. Music is also beneficial in reducing agitation in persons with dementia (Goodal and Etters, 2005; Gaskill, 2004; McCaffrey and Locsin, 2002; Young-Mason, 2002).

Dance is an expression of joy and celebration throughout the world. Many have used it as a means to increase self-esteem and body image; lessen depression, fear, and isolation; and express emotions. Art has often been used to help children and adults express their feelings about stressful situations and unconscious concerns about their illnesses. Art expression has been a psychotherapy tool in geriatric centers, with children and adolescents, in hospices, in alcohol treatment programs, and in prisons. Books, poetry, and religious writings are often inspirational and cause a person to become immersed for long periods in reading. Journals and diaries are also forms of expressing one's emotions and are called *process meditation* and a conversation with the self. Duran (2000) discussed the use of drama, quilting, and story telling as therapeutic tools used by women for centuries. Helpful distractions such as handheld video games and virtual reality glasses have been used during painful procedures for children; other distractions include suggesting that the client visualize a medication flowing through the circulation to bring pain relief or to perform its intended purpose and intentional conversations with clients about their interests and their lives (Gaskill, 2004).

Humor

Humor and laughter are also helpful for expressing emotions, relieving tensions and anxiety, and coping with painful or unpleasant situations. Laughter often has a positive effect on cognitive ability, respiratory and heart rates, blood pressure, and muscle tension (Kreitzer and Jensen, 2000). In some places, humor rooms supplied with videocassettes and audiotapes, books, cartoons, and artwork are available for clients, families, and agency staff; all are encouraged to use humorous artwork on bulletin boards in patient rooms and staff work areas. Minden (2002) conducted a qualitative study of humor as a focal point of therapy for hospitalized male forensic (criminal) psychiatric patients. Under supervision, student nurses held humor groups over a 16-week clinical rotation with a total of 10 rotation time frames. Interview findings indicated enhanced physical, psychologic, and social health. More than half of the men felt an increased sense of spiritual well-being. In his classic book *Anatomy of an Illness as Perceived by the Patient* (1979), Norman Cousins, a famous journalist, wrote about the value of humor in relieving the severe pain he experienced from ankylosing spondylitis by stating that a good belly laugh when watching *Candid Camera* episodes and the Marx Brothers films allowed him to be pain free for at least 2 hours at a time. Cousins wrote that humor healed him (Anderson, 2004).

Exercise

The benefits of physical exercise are well known. Exercise brings a general sense of health and vitality, increases respiratory and cardiovascular efficiency, and promotes a longer life. People who exercise often sleep better and have improved appetites; society now considers exercise a major factor in self-care (Pelletier, 2000). People with disabilities are able to perform even simple exercises. Special Olympics events for wheelchair athletes are excellent examples of using exercise to enhance the self-image and general health. (*Tai chi* exercise is included with traditional Chinese medicine.)

Animal-Assisted Therapy

This discussion of mind-body interventions is not complete without mentioning the use of companion animals to induce the relaxation response and enhance emotional and physiologic well-being. Animal-assisted therapy (AAT) is a goal-directed intervention designed to improve human physical, social, emotional, and cognitive function in a variety of settings. It is for groups or individuals. AAT is frequently used in conjunction with occupational and physical therapies for refining fine-motor skills, assisting with maintaining balance and walking tolerance, and increasing attention and self-esteem. Studies show a reduction in a person's hypertension, heart rate, and social isolation when pets are a treatment modality. Studies have also shown the benefits to the morale of staff and caregivers. Individuals who are blind, deaf, or paralyzed use companion animals to assist them in accomplishing activities of daily living. Some acute and long-term health care agency policies now allow pets into intensive care units, pediatric wards, hospices, rehabilitation units, and geriatric and other areas. Nurses are active supporters of animal-assisted therapy (Animal Assisted Therapy, 2006; Cole and Gavlinski, 2000).

Psychotherapy and Hypnosis

A variety of social support and self-help groups have implemented many of the psychologic methods such as multiple therapy approaches and cognitive, behavior, and body-oriented therapies to bring about beneficial effects for the participants. Groups are common in adjunct therapy for substance abuse control, weight loss, cancer, grief counseling, and caregiver support.

Hypnosis has been in use since the eighteenth century as a deep relaxation technique and is a useful tool in the treatment of substance addiction, smoking cessation, pain control, fears, and phobias. It is also successful before anesthesia induction, as a means for reducing hypertension, for relieving pain and muscle spasms for persons with cerebral palsy, for relaxing children during invasive procedures, and for dietary management. Hypnosis involves the use of mental images, concentration, the use of repetitive words or sounds, and total relaxation. Hypnosis produces an altered state of consciousness that permits the person to concentrate with minimal distraction. Self-therapy at home consists of education in self-hypnosis through the aid of guided audiotapes designed to meet the individual's specific problem. Hypnosis relies heavily on the person's openness to suggestion (The New Medicine Video, 2006; Pelletier, 2000). There is a concern that selective serotonin-reuptake inhibitor (SSRI) medications are a contributing factor to the increase in the suicide rate for people with depression. A systematic meta-analysis of several clinical studies indicated that minimal benefits come from SSRI medications compared to placebo effects. The research recommended that the use of hypnosis in psychotherapy was a better choice (Kirsch, 2005).

Energy Therapies

Biofeedback

Biofeedback is a technique that initially uses electrical equipment to assist persons in gaining conscious control over body processes that are normally beyond voluntary command. Biofeedback training (BFT) is often combined with controlled breathing techniques or meditation to provide individuals with increased awareness about their bodies. Electrodes that are attached to the affected area send information into a monitoring device, which emits a signal to alert the person to changes in a particular body function (e.g., an increase or decrease in muscle tension). Transcutaneous electrical nerve stimulation (TENS) is one example. It is most often used for clients with chronic pain and muscle spasm (Keck and Baker, 2001).

Several other electrical biofeedback devices have been used to assist clients to gain self-control of body functions. By watching their responses on the device, clients learn to use mental processes to control that particular body action. A therapist instructs the client in the mental exercises during a series of sessions. Eventually the client is able to practice the exercises without the aid of the machine. Biofeedback has been used in the treatment of multiple physical, cognitive, and behavioral symptoms. Among these are hypertension, temperature control, gastrointestinal activity, substance abuse, stress, sleep disorders, migraine headaches, and other vascular disorders (Saito and Saito, 2004; Pelletier, 2000).

Bioelectromagnetics

Concepts of magnetic field therapy relate to the electrical currents that exist within and external to the body, the influence of external currents on the body, and the result of physical and behavioral changes. Examples are the electromagnetic energies produced by x-rays, television, microwaves, and light rays. Prolonged exposure to such fields produces hazardous effects. However, scientists also discovered that lower-level energy frequencies are beneficial in designing diagnostic and treatment tools.

Health care providers use nonthermal electromagnetic fields—which do not cause heating of tissues—for bone repair, nerve stimulation, and wound healing; as electrostimulation via acupuncture needles for stimulation of the immune system; and for neuroendocrine modulations. Unipolor magnets are for pain relief, particularly from arthritis. Magnets are taped to various areas of the body, inserted inside shoes, and placed in mattress covers. Anecdotal accounts yield favorable responses (Kreitzer and Jensen, 2000). A new clinical trial by NCCAM (2002) is examining the effectiveness of electrostimulated acupuncture on minimizing delayed nausea after cancer chemotherapy that occurs 24 hours to 5 days posttreatment.

Alternative Systems of Medical Practice

Alternative systems of medical practice include traditional Oriental medicine; acupuncture; Ayurvedic, homeopathic, naturopathic, and environmental medicines; and anthroposophically extended medicine (which builds on naturopathy, homeopathy, and modern scientific medicine).

Traditional Chinese Medicine

Traditional Chinese medicine (TCM) uses a variety of therapies, including acupuncture and acupressure, massage, herbal medicine, *qigong*, and *tai chi*. *Tai chi*, a Chinese exercise program with roots in the ancient martial arts, has gained popular appeal for people of all ages in the West. It consists of slow, gentle rhythmic movements, controlled breathing and creating an "inner stillness." Individuals have used tai chi to prevent and remedy of a variety of muscular and joint problems and to reduce stress. It is an excellent exercise for persons with osteoarthritis; other benefits are pain relief, a reduction of joint soreness and stiffness, and balance maintenance. There are many different styles of tai chi exercises, and choosing an instructor is important, as some of the movements need to be modified. Individuals need to consult their health care provider before beginning an exercise program (Horstman, 2000).

Variations of TCM are practiced in Japan, Korea, and Vietnam. Oriental medicine centers on the diagnosis of disturbances of *qi* (pronounced "chee"), or the vital energy, and the balance between *yin* and *yang* (female and male, cold and hot, dark and light) forces. TCM diagnostic procedures consist of observing facial expressions and body movements, careful listening and questioning, and palpating body pulses. The relationship of physical and emotional behaviors is used to plan a range of traditional therapies. The most frequent methods used in the United States are acupuncture and massage.

Acupuncture. Acupuncture is a process in which the practitioner inserts small needles at selected energy points of the body that correspond to energy pathways, or meridians, that traverse from the body surface to inner organs. Its purpose is to activate the *qi* and achieve a balance when imbalance exists. The needles are sometimes heated and attached to a mild electrical current or are twirled by hand to cause vibrations. Numerous studies reveal the positive effects of acupuncture on a wide range of disorders, including gynecologic, mental, and neurologic problems and substance dependence. Its effectiveness in pain control and anesthesia is attributed to the release of endogenous opioids (endorphins) produced within the central nervous system. Acupuncture is one of the most thoroughly researched and documented alternative medical practices (Eshkevari and Heath, 2005; Parkman and Ullrich, 2000; Pelletier, 2000).

Ayurveda/Ayurvedic Medicine

Ayurvedic (science of life) medicine originated in India and dates back thousands of years. This method uses a combination of therapies including meditation, yoga, massage, herbs, aromatherapy, and biofeedback. In ayurvedic medicine, the body is a pharmacy that can make its own natural drugs to heal itself.

The human body is also a microcosm of the universe, with principles, or *doshas*, that interact in maintaining balance. The basic nature *(prakriti)*, or genetic code, and the relationship among the *doshas* remain unaltered throughout a person's life. Each *dosha* has a principal location in the body, with emphasis on the interdependence of health and the quality of the person's sociocultural life. When any imbalance occurs, an individual achieves a restoration of balance of the internal environment through proper diet and lifestyle. A study funded by the NIH Alternative Medicine Branch demonstrated the positive effects of Ayurvedic practices with healthy adults (Pelletier, 2000).

Homeopathic Medicine

Homeopathic medicine is based on the belief that substances that produce certain disease symptoms in a healthy person provide a cure for a sick person experiencing the same symptoms. Diluted substances are used to elicit a cure (e.g., a very dilute solution containing poison ivy compound is used for a skin rash). The medication has to be shaken vigorously or "potentized" for the greatest effectiveness as the solution picks up energy from the dissolved substance. These products are often for acute and chronic health problems, as well as for health promotion.

The homeopathic drug market has become a multimillion-dollar industry. The FDA currently regulates the remedies, and drugs manufactured by reputable pharmaceutical companies are in the *Homeopathic Pharmacopoeia of the United States.* Some are sold as OTC drugs, but products used for serious conditions must be dispensed by a licensed practitioner (Tedesco and Cicchetti, 2001).

Naturopathy

A small group of physicians practice naturopathy. These physicians have been educated in the sciences and have received specialized training in the disciplines of alternative medicine. They use an eclectic selection of herbs, homeopathy, nutrition, TCM, hydrotherapy, and manipulative therapy in conjunction with modern scientific medical diagnostic methods and standards. Naturopathy focuses on self-healing, and practitioners individualize health care to meet the individual's needs. The basic principles include the following (Pelletier, 2000):

- Use of therapies that do no harm
- The physician's primary role as teacher
- Establishing and maintaining an optimal health and balance
- Treatment of the whole person
- Prevention of disease through a healthy lifestyle
- Therapeutic use of nutrition

Many of the therapies occur in treatment spas where practitioners using sunlight, fresh air, and water therapies. Fasting, natural food diets, colonic enemas, acupuncture, massage, and Chinese medicine are also used. Allopathic practitioners view naturopathy with skepticism (Barrett, 2006).

Environmental Medicine

Allergy treatment was the original impetus for the development of environmental medicine in the 1940s. Scientists noted that the sensitivity and allergy symptoms of some individuals improved after eliminating certain foods or chemicals, molds, dust, pollens, and other substances. Emotional stress was also a source of immune system dysfunction. The person's environmental history became an important component in the diagnostic process by providing a chronologic account of etiologic circumstances leading to the health problem. The elimination of health hazards from the environment has become a major health issue. Examples include the removal of asbestos building insulation materials, the instillation of devices that recapture gasoline fumes and smog emissions on automobiles, the removal of certain pesticides from the market, and the elimination of preservatives and color additives from foods, medicines, and nutrition supplements.

Culture-Based Community Medicines

The many culture-based practices, or folk medicine, follow naturalistic methods; and a spiritual healer or shaman usually provides religious rituals, which are a major component. Symbols such as prayer wheels, sand paintings, meditation, amulets, group singing, chanting, and dancing ceremonies are part of the healing rituals. On the Navajo reservation, modern hospitals and the shaman's healing room are under the same roof. Some people believe that spells cast by the witch doctor have sometimes proved to be more powerful than Western medicines (Grendell, personal observation; Leonard and Plotnikoff, 2001; Parkman and Ullrich, 2000).

Manual Healing Methods

Included in manual healing methods are osteopathic and chiropractic medicines, massage, reflexology, and techniques that use pressure points and other various touch therapies.

Osteopathy and Chiropractic Medicines

These practices involve manipulation of soft tissues and joints. Both require specialized education and licensure to practice. Much of the public considers osteopathic practices to be mainstream medicine, and the practitioner often is the primary health care provider. Chiropractic practitioners study the relationship between pressure, strain, or tension on the spinal cord and the ability of the neuromusculoskeletal system to act efficiently. Manual adjustments of the spine to correct alignment are a mainstay of treatment. Some insurance carriers have approved chiropractic medicine, and NCCAM has recently established a center to study its effects (NIH, 2002).

Massage

Touch, which is the basic medium of massage therapy, is a form of communication and caring (Kreitzer and Jensen, 2000). There are more than 80 different forms of massage therapy. These forms vary from gentle stroking to deep kneading, rubbing, and percussion. Most massage is done with the hands; however, forearms, elbows, and feet are sometimes used. The primary purposes of massage therapy are to produce muscle and total-body relaxation and to increase circulation. In the past, massage techniques were in fundamental nursing courses.

Acupressure

The same meridian points used in acupuncture are manipulated in pressure-point therapies. The therapists use their fingertips to apply pressure to more than 600 designated points in soft tissues. Acupressure is both a diagnostic tool and a treatment. The sessions sometimes last up to an hour, with the recipient spending equal time lying in the prone and dorsal positions for a total body treatment. The therapist also places a strong emphasis on mind-spirit-body balance in counseling the client. *Shiatsu*, a Japanese form, is similar to acupressure, with the therapist applying pressure with the palm of the hand as well as the fingers.

Hand and Foot Reflexology

Reflexology, which originated in Egypt, is also referred to as zone therapy. This technique is based on the premise that the feet (and hands) are mirrors of the body, with reflex points that correspond to glands, organs, and other structures in the body. (The feet are more responsive to massage than the hands.) Massage of a reflex point (without the use of oil, cream, or lotion) stimulates the corresponding organ in that zone. The main goal is to provide relaxation by removing tension in a zone area (Shirley, 2004).

Therapeutic Touch

Healing through touch can be traced back to early civilizations. Nurses have practiced various forms of therapeutic touch for many years. Benefits of contact touch such as massage have been recently identified as providing a sense of spiritual balance, relieving mental and emotional tension and anxiety, improving blood flow, easing pain, and stimulating the immune system.

Therapeutic touch also refers to a noncontact technique that comes from the laying on of hands associated with Far Eastern, European, and religious philosophies. This method is based on a theory that the release of excess energy from the healer assists the ill person in the healing process. Individuals can learn the basic principles, and workshops are available throughout the country and the world. Healing touch is a similar technique and became a certificate program of the American Holistic Nurses Association in 1993 (Kreitzer and Jensen, 2000; Zerwekh, 2000).

Pharmacologic and Biologic Treatments

Pharmacologic and biologic alternative therapies consist of a variety of drugs and vaccines that are not yet included in mainstream medicine. Some stimulate the immune system to ward off diseases and consist of older herbal remedies. All are considered nontoxic. One example is shark and other animal cartilage used to treat acquired immunodeficiency syndrome (AIDS), cancer, and arthritis. Cartilage possibly inhibits tumor growth by cutting off the blood supply to the tumor, suppressing autoimmune reactions, and promoting wound healing. Ethylene diamine tetraacetic acid (EDTA) is a chemical that binds with metallic ions and is used as a treatment (chelation) for poisoning from lead and other toxic metals. It is now being proposed as treatment for ridding the body of free radicals and thus removing fat deposits from artery walls and improving cardiovascular circulation. A total of 70 studies yielded

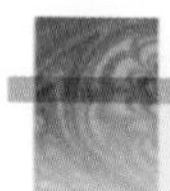

BOX 25-6

Examples of Herbs and Food Herbals Used as Alternative Therapies and as the Basis for Allopathic Medicines

Most of the herbs come from tropical rain forests; others come from the sea, and still others come from countries around the world. Flowers, seeds, leaves, woods and barks, vines, tubers, roots, and even grasses have been the basis of alternative and traditional allopathic medicine therapy. (More than one fourth of allopathic medicines are based on plant properties.) Different portions of a plant or tree often have different properties and different concentrations and are also used for different purposes. These products are used as inhalants, taken internally, added to bathwater, or applied externally. The following is a small list of examples:

- *Analgesics:* Meadowsweet, poplar (balm of Gilead) tree, willow tree (aspirin), wintergreen, oil of clove (used in dentistry), feverfew, nutmeg (for migraine), marijuana (nausea and pain for cancer patients and people with AIDS)
- *Narcotics:* Belladonna, celandine, nightshade, opium poppy
- *Aromatics.* Allspice, angelica, anise, avicena, camomile, ginger, juniper, lavender, mint, nutmeg, pennyroyal, rosemary, wormwood, pine and balsam woods, cinnamon (as incense); used as relaxants, for bronchodilator effects, and so on
- *Stimulants:* Marijuana, nutmeg, peyote, Scotch broom for euphorics and hallucinogens; ginseng (American and Asian) for mental and physical energizer—ginseng is also considered a panacea for its variety of healing properties; belladonna for atropine effects on the central nervous system; dronabinol (Marinol), a synthetic derivative of marijuana components, is used as an antiemetic, especially for nausea and vomiting in persons on chemotherapy for cancer and as an appetite stimulant for persons with AIDS
- *Sedatives:* Celery, feverweed, hops, Indian pipe, lavender, monkshood, wild black cherry, mountain laurel, passion flower, peach tree, peony, periwinkle, heliotrope (valerian)
- *Antidepressant/antianxiety agents:* Borage, St. John's wort, lobelia (in correct dosage), rosemary, pasqueflower, aromatics
- *Antiaging agents: Ginkgo biloba* (increases circulation, dilates blood vessels; has been used with clients diagnosed with Alzheimer's and dementia)
- *Antiseptics:* Garlic (also used to reduce cholesterol), onion, wintergreen, camphor
- *Diaphoretics:* Seneca snakeroot
- *Antioxidants:* Ginger, spices (Indian)
- *Cardiotonics:* Foxglove (digitalis), lily of the valley, *Strophanthus* (ouabain)
- *Ophthalmic agents:* Calabar bean (physostigmine); used for glaucoma
- *Antihypertensives:* Parsley, skullcap, garlic, hawthorn, wild black cherry, seneca snakeroot (rauwolfia)
- *Contraceptive agents:* Mexican yam—diosgenin that can be converted to progesterone (Syntex)
- *Muscle paralyzing agents: Strychnos toxifera* produces a powerful poison—curare (used to create intercostal muscle paralysis during surgery)
- *Antineoplastic agents:* Yew tree bark (paclitaxel), rosy periwinkle (vincristine, vinblastine); used for childhood leukemias and Hodgkin's disease
- *Gastrointestinal agents:* Papaya for dyspepsia, liquorice flower (carbenoxolone) as treatment for peptic ulcer
- *Antidiarrheal agents:* Opium poppy (paregoric)
- *Cathartics: Ricinus communis* (castor oil)
- *Dermatologic agents:* Aloe vera, wintergreen (ointment)
- *Antibiotic agents:* Fungi (penicillin), iris versicolor (antisyphilitic), lobelia (antisyphilitic)
- *Antimalarials:* Chinchona bark or Peruvian bark (quinine); also used as antiarrhythmic
- *Antiviral agents:* May apple (used for venereal warts and AIDS)

positive results. However, the American Heart Association and other organizations do not endorse its use (American Heart Association, 2006; Turner, 2001).

Herbal Medicine

The use of herbal and plant medicine is an ancient practice worldwide. Tree barks, plant roots, berries, leaves, resins, seeds, and flowers have all been ground into powders, mixed with solutions, brewed in teas, and used singly or in combination as the treatment for ailments (Box 25-6). One third of adult Americans (an estimated 60 million people) use herbal remedies. In all, 64% of the world's population relies on herbal remedies. More than 1500 herbs are marketed in the United States (Parkman and Ullrich, 2000; Pelletier, 2000).

Records of herbal medicines appeared in the Bible and in Egypt extending back to 2000 BC, in Greece and Rome at the time of Aristotle, in the Muslim world, in India, and in the Orient. Each culture compiled a *materia medica*—a listing of drugs and their uses. The American Indians contributed a vast array of herbals to the Colonial American medicine formulary, and herbals continued to be a mainstay of medical practices for many years. Today herbal products are marketed only as food supplements, and the FDA and other regulatory agencies consider some of these potentially dangerous. There are not any safety guidelines for these products. Nevertheless, the public is purchasing alternative medicines at a greater rate than ever before and adopting many remedies from other cultures.

> **CLINICAL ALERT**
>
> It is important to inquire and document whether the client is taking any **herbal preparations** or using **food supplements.** Natural substances may cause toxic adverse effects, severe allergic reactions, and adverse drug reactions. They may also interfere with laboratory test results (see Boxes 25-7 and 25-8).

The formulas of Chinese medicine are based on the correct ratio or balance of a variety of *food herbs* that are harvested and prepared at an appropriate time to enhance their effects. Food herbs are composed of plants (85%), animals (12%), and minerals (3%). The various herbal ingredients are mixed according to the diseases caused by imbalance of yin and yang rather than the chemistry makeup of the herb. Yin and yang characteristics and their

BOX 25-7

Potential Interactions Between Medications and Herbals, Food Supplements, and Allopathic Medications

- *Ginkgo biloba* may intensify the anticlotting effects of warfarin (Coumadin) and other anticoagulant drugs, including aspirin.
- Garlic and ginseng have similar effects on the anticoagulant drugs.
- Many of the fortified foods have high concentrations of calcium and other minerals (calcium fortified orange juice, breakfast cereals) that bind with antibiotics (ciprofloxacin, gatifloxacin, levoflosacin, and tetracycline) and prevent drugs from being absorbed. Tetracycline also binds with aluminum, magnesium, and other minerals.
- Calcium carbonate antacid preparations interferes with the absorption of levothyroxine (thyroid hormone).
- Echinacea interferes with efficacy of birth-control pills.
- Alfalfa (used for hot flashes) interferes with effects of immunosuppressant drugs.
- Grapefruit juice increases the bioavailability of many drugs such as antihypertensive drugs, cholesterol-lowering drugs, benzodiazepine and nonbenzodiazepine sedatives, carbamazepine (an anticonvulsant), sertraline (antidepressant), cyclosporine (anti rejection drug), and amiodarone (antiarrhythmic).
- St. John's wort reduces blood concentrations of indinavir (a protease-inhibitor used to treat HIV infection) and cyclosporine.
- Caffeine (coffee, tea, cocoa, and guarana) increases blood levels of theophylline. Mixed together, these foods also increase caffeine side effects including nervousness, tremor, and sleeplessness.
- Fiber delays absorption of drugs and nutrients including vitamins and minerals. Clients need to take bulk-forming laxatives at least 2 hours before or after taking medications to prevent these problems. Persons taking digoxin need to avoid taking their medications with bran fiber and bulk-forming laxatives and food that contains pectin (apples and pears).
- Foods that acidify urine include cheese, eggs, and meat, thus extending acidity; foods that alkalinize urine include citrus and vegetables that decrease acidity. A high-salt diet increases urinary excretion of lithium and limits drug effects (treatment for bipolar disorder).

Modified from Spencer, J: New red flags raised on mixing medications, herbal remedies, *San Diego Union Tribune*, pp A-1, A-14, June 23, 2004; and Leigh E: Nutrient-drug interactions, *The Natural Foods Naturalizer*, pp 42-44, Feb 1, 2005.

related properties of cold and heat are used to categorize diseases and medicines. These mixtures are supplements to a well-balanced diet and are often prescribed along with daily exercise and positive thinking, in the belief that a balanced body is a result of a balanced life. Many Chinese herbal stores have captured a large share of the U.S. alternative medicine market.

Examples of commonly used herbs worldwide are *Ginkgo biloba*, Echinacea, saw palmetto, *Prunus africanum*, ginseng, and St. John's wort. Both European and Oriental varieties of *Ginkgo biloba* increase circulation and bring oxygen to the brain and to retard the effects of aging. European studies have shown its effectiveness for improvement in mental alertness, increased circulation to the extremities, lowered cholesterol, and improved blood flow to the retina. Echinacea, or purple coneflower, is prized for its antiseptic properties and ability to stimulate the immune system, particularly against infections such as flu, colds, and wound healing. Saw palmetto berries and *P. africanum* have become popular treatments for benign prostatic hypertrophy. Ginseng root has been used as a tonic in China for more than 3000 years. Many have used it as an antistress agent and to alter circadian rhythms and amounts of circulating corticosterone. *Hypericum*, the principal ingredient of St. John's wort, has been termed "nature's Prozac" because of its popular use as an antidepressant (Eberhardie, 2005: Parkman and Ullrich, 2000; Pelletier, 2000). Examples of natural herbal remedies new to the U.S. market include black cohosh for menopausal symptoms; mental acuity formula, a combination of vitamins and herbs for mild memory problems; probiotic pearls, a dietary supplement with acidophilus and *B. longum* to promote healthy intestinal flora; and pantetheine plus, a triple action combination formula to enhance the breakdown of fat and cholesterol (Rite-Care Pharmacy, online, September 2002). Additional herbal remedies appear in Box 25-6. Box 25-7 describes potential interactions between herbal medicines, food supplements, and allopathic medicines.

CLINICAL ALERT

Concerns regarding **safety of herbal medications** include the following (Eberhardie, 2005):

- Some herbal medications have been mixed with synthetic chemicals including heavy metals.
- Safe dosage of food supplements and herbal medications may not have been established.
- Concentrations of an active ingredient are not always consistent in the liquid or pill.
- Chemical and microbiologic contamination may occur.
- Packages, labeling, and advertising policies need to be more rigorous with regard to ingredients, purpose, and effectiveness.
- Some dangers are associated with self-medication and mixing different medicinal approaches for a health problem. This is concern is particularly important when interacting with clients from multicultural backgrounds.

Aromatherapy was initially used in Egypt to relieve pain. Today individuals use it for relaxation or as an adjunct to stress-reduction measures. More than 300 essential plant oils are currently in use as inhalants, for massage and compresses or as additions to bathwater, and for use in candles. In ancient times, people used the burning of aromatic woods to purify the air. Some still use incense as part of healing ceremonies. Other examples include the use of birch oil as an antiinflammatory agent, lavender for its calming effect and headache relief, rosemary added to vaporizers for relief of congestion, citrus as an energizing agent, and peppermint for nausea relief and as an antipyretic and respiratory stimulant. Aromatherapy is included in Ayurvedic therapy (Parkman and Ullrich, 2000).

Diet and Nutrition

Diet and nutritional needs are integral to both traditional and alternative therapies. Today's affluent diet, which is high in animal fats, refined carbohydrates, and partially hydrogenated vegetable oils, contributes to many of the current health problems in the United States. Educational information provides alternative healthy diets and a change in lifestyle to prevent or correct obesity, cardiovascular disease, diabetes, and other chronic health problems. Vitamins and other food supplements are frequently added to the health maintenance plan. Studies include research on the value of the antioxidant vitamins A and E as antioxidants and β-carotene in the prevention of cataracts and cancer, and on the effects of vitamin C and nicotinic acid as replacement therapy for psychiatric clients receiving electroconvulsive and tranquilizer therapy. Megadoses of niacin have helped to reduce serum cholesterol. Some providers have given nutritional supplements to offset the effects of medicines prescribed for people with AIDS (Parkman and Ullrich, 2000; Pelletier, 2000). Health food stores and the Internet are promoting popular new foods and juices. Pomegranate juice and blueberries are being promoted because of their antioxidant properties, and juice from the Acai, a native berry from Brazil, is a "superfood," rich in antioxidants and omega fatty acids. Noni juice, a plant found mainly in the South Pacific, is supposedly a cure for a range of health problems from high blood pressure to poor digestion. Guarana, a South American berry that has chemical properties similar to caffeine, is an ingredient added to "energy" food bars and drinks. Mangosteen, a Southeast Asia fruit, has been used as an antioxidant and for a variety of health problems as well.

Several diets have been developed as specific treatments for diseases. Macrobiotic cancer diets are based on Oriental beliefs of creating a balance of yin and yang. Research by environmental medicine scientists has helped to identify potential food antigens such as chemical additives and natural food substances. Food-elimination diets reduce sensitivity to certain substances and hasten recovery from allergic responses. These diets have also been used to treat children with attention deficit/hyperactivity disorder (Pelletier, 2000). Health care providers need to be sensitive to ethnic and cultural diets when planning health care activities. Some of these diets pose health risks because of a lack of essential ingredients or because they interact with prescribed medications (Box 25-8). Incorporating familiar foods into the diet also facilitates a person's recovery, and substances in the diet actually facilitate healing.

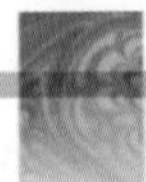

BOX 25-8

Potential Nutrient/Drug Interactions

- Fish oils are commonly used for rheumatoid arthritis, psoriasis, inflammatory bowel disease (IBS), and to improve immunity; however, they increase the anticoagulant action of aspirin and dipyridamole and produce increased bleeding if taken with vitamin E.
- Iron compounds reduce the absorption of carbidopa-levodopa (Sinemet) and levodopa. Antacids reduce the uptake of iron, and there is a reduced absorption of methyldopa.
- Broccoli, brussels sprouts, kale, parsley and spinach, coffee, green tea, and liver are rich in vitamin K; these foods neutralize the effects of anticoagulant drugs.
- A hypertensive crisis may occur between foods rich in tyramine (aged cheese, fava beans, salami/pepperoni, pickled fish, red wines, and some beers) and monoamine oxidase inhibitor (MAOI) drugs (antidepressants). The newer SSRI drugs have mostly replaced the older MAOI drugs; however, MAOIs are still available.
- Certain foods alter the rate of drug excretion. Acidic foods (eggs, cheese, meat) lengthen the half-life of drugs; alkaline foods (citrus and vegetables) decrease the half-life of drugs. A high-salt diet hastens the urinary output of lithium, a drug therapy for bipolar disorder.
- Many drugs need to be taken with food to prevent the drug-related gastrointestinal irritation; however, some drugs need to be taken on an empty stomach, such as erythromycin, levodopa, most penicillins, and tetracycline. Drug absorption is often delayed or enhanced because of the presence of food. Fatty foods delay gastric emptying, thereby delaying the time for a drug to reach the desired peak level. High-carbohydrate meals enhance the absorption of some drugs.

Modified from Leigh E: Nutrient-drug interactions, *Nutr Sci News*, pp 42-44, Feb 1, 2005.

CHAPTER SUMMARY

- A historical overview reveals that contrasting perspectives exist regarding the nature of human beings (1) as individuals and as whole persons with mind-body-spirit interactions to (2) adopting a dualistic view that separates the functions of the body from the functions of the mind and spirit.
- Allopathic medicine has traditionally been a dualistic model with an emphasis on curative methods of biologic diseases based on empirical evidence outcome criteria. In contrast, the focus of the holistic or alternative care model is on strengthening one's inner resistance to disease and "healing from within" or enhancing the body's innate healing powers.
- There is still a stigma attached to alternative methods. The scientific community often labels alternative methods as a hoax, witchcraft, or magicoreligious practices and attributes results to placebo effects. Nevertheless, nurses need to become knowledgeable about the many CAM methods used by clients from diverse cultural and ethnic backgrounds to manage their lives. Nurses must be nonjudgmental about these practices.

- The public must become educated regarding the potential harmful effects of the concurrent use of alternative and prescription medicines, and the need to inform health care providers when taking alternative medicines is essential. People also need to understand the consequences of self-diagnosis, self-treatment, and delay in seeking help.
- Several factors have influenced the use of CAM interventions, including the spiraling costs of today's health care, restrictions imposed by third-party payers, the influence of media coverage, the introduction of ancient cultural therapies, and an increase in consumer interest in self-control, especially for promoting health and for managing chronic health problems.
- The traditional allopathic system has included some CAM interventions, especially stress-reduction therapies; however, barriers still exist for herbal medicines, dietary supplements (because of the lack of significant empirical evidence of their effectiveness), and safety control issues.
- The American Holistic Nurses Association (AHNA) suggests that alternative and traditional therapies complement each other in providing holistic care, and it recommends that nurses become familiar with the alternative methods and incorporate them into the plan of care whenever possible. Use of the term "integrative therapies" has become a common practice.
- Nurses educate clients about the potential harmful effects of concurrent use of alternative and prescription medicines and emphasize the need to inform their health care providers about what therapies they are using.
- The concepts of caring and healing, as well as commitment to global health, are integral components of nursing.
- The nurse attends to a wide range of human experiences and responses to health and disease, and in the provision of a caring relationship the nurse promotes healing and health maintenance.
- The goal of holistic nursing is to enhance the healing of all aspects of the whole person. The nursing profession performs independent and interdependent actions that are largely technical, such as teaching, administration, and research. It is dynamic and evolutionary, humanistic, and a discipline that is fundamentally based on scientific and theoretic knowledge and founded on moral, ethical, and spiritual values.
- Concepts of health, illness, and disease are deeply embedded. Cultural competency requires an awareness of one's own values and those of the health care system. Nurses frequently have to support decisions that differ from their own cultural norms and values. Culturally incompetent care challenges the belief system of clients and their families, causes undue stress, and inhibits the healing process. Efficient and effective clinical care in cross-cultural circumstances is a new competency for all nurses.

REVIEW QUESTIONS

1 A nurse assesses a newly admitted client. The client says, "I've been taking feverfew for my migraine headaches. It has really helped a lot." The nurse knows there are no hazardous interactions between feverfew and the client's current medications. Select the nurse's best response.

1. "I'm glad feverfew helps your headaches. I'll make a note in your chart that you take it."
2. "You should never take any medications unless you have a physician's prescription."
3. "I also take feverfew for my own migraine headaches. It has really helped me too."
4. "Feverfew is not backed by reliable research for treatment of migraine headaches."

2 A client with chronic psoriasis takes various fish oils and vitamin E to improve immunity and skin condition. This physician instructs the client to take aspirin daily to reduce the risk of heart disease and stroke. When the nurse assesses this client 3 weeks later, which observation indicates a dangerous drug interaction?

1. The client's psoriatic skin lesions are dry and crusty.
2. There a numerous bruises on the client's extremities.
3. The client reports that movement occurs with less pain.
4. Scales are being shed from the client's psoriatic skin lesions.

3 When used in combination with an anticoagulant medication, ingestion of large quantities of which food(s) would be likely to reduce medication effectiveness? You may select more than one answer.

1. Broccoli
2. Green tea
3. Pickled herring
4. Aged cheese
5. Scrambled eggs

4 A nurse interviews for new employment at four facilities. This nurse values holism, including the healing powers of complementary and alternative therapies. Which observation(s) would suggest to this nurse that the facility has similar values? You may select more than one answer.

1. The facility advertises the purchase of a new SPECT diagnostic device.
2. The facility sponsors weekly articles in a local newspaper about new cures for disease.
3. The interview includes a tour of the facility's high-tech biomedical laboratory.
4. The interview concludes with a tour of the facility's massage therapy suites.
5. Each client at the facility has input into his or her plan of care and then signs the plan.

5 The nurse cares for a client who uses alternative vitamin therapies to manage a chronic disease. The nurse believes the vitamins are not therapeutic. Select the nurse's best initial action.

1. Report the situation to the ethics committee
2. Ask the client to discontinue taking the vitamins
3. Determine whether the vitamins pose any danger
4. Teach the client about more effective strategies

ONLINE RESOURCES

American Association of Oriental Medicine: **www.aaom.org**

American Holistic Nurses Association: **www.ahna.org**

National Center for Complementary and Alternative Medicine: **www.nccam.nih.gov**

Additional self-study exercises and learning resources are available to you on the ***Companion CD*** *at the back of the book and on the* ***Evolve website*** *at* ***http://evolve.elsevier.com/Fortinash/.***

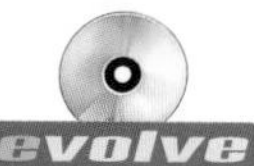

REFERENCES

Ameling A: Prayer: an ancient healing practice becomes new again, *Holistic Nurs Pract* 14:40-48, 2000.

American Heart Association: Questions and answers about chelation therapy; retrieved 4/24/06 from www.americanheart.org.

American Holistic Nursing Association: Mission statement and standards, 2006; retrieved from www.ahna.org.

Anderson RA: The immune system and mind function, *Townsend Letter for Doctors and Patients*, issues 265-266:102-106, 2004a; retrieved from EBSCOhost.com.

Anderson RA: Psychoneuroimmunoendocrinology review and commentary, *Townsend Lett Doctors Patients*, issue 269:126-129, 2004b; retrieved from EBSCOhost.com.

Animal Assisted Therapy (AAT): Delta Society; retrieved Apr 3, 2006, from www.deltasociety.org/AnimalsAAAAbout.htm.

Barclay L, Vega C: Intercessory prayer may not decrease complications from CABG, Apr 4, 2006; retrieved from www.medscape.com/viewarticle/529043.

Barrett S: Naturopathy, Apr 4, 2006; retrieved from www.quackwatch.org/01QuackeryRelatedTopics/Naturopathy/naturopathy.html.

Bodenheimer T, Fernandez A: High and rising health care costs: can costs be controlled while preserving quality? IV. *Ann Intern Med* 143:26-32.

Cearley A: Three Tijuana alternative clinics shut down as part of probe, *San Diego Union Tribune*, p B-3, Feb 2, 2006a.

Cearley A: U.S. man dies at alternative detox clinic in Tijuana, *San Diego Union Tribune*, p B-3, Feb 2, 2006b.

Chen K: The focus of the discipline of nursing: caring in the human health experience, *Grad Res* 2, 2000; retrieved from www.graduateresearch.com/Archives.htm#GRM11.

Cole K, Gavlinski A: Animal-assisted therapy: the human-animal bond, *AACN Clin Issues Adv Pract Acute Crit Care* 11:139-149, 2000.

Cosentino BW: Complementary and alternative medicine in the mainstream, *Pathways to Professional Development: Nursing Spectrum Nurseweek*, pp 120-122, 2006.

Cousins N: *Anatomy of an illness as perceived by the patient*, New York, 1979, WW Norton.

Duran D: Integrated women health holistic approaches for comprehensive care (review), *AORN J* 74:683-689, 2000.

Eberhardie C: Food supplements and herbal medicines, *Nurs Standard* 20:52-56.

Eisenberg DM et al: Unconventional medicine in the United States—prevalence, costs, and patterns of use, *N Engl J Med* 328:246-252, 1993.

Eisenberg DM et al: Trends in alternative medicine use in the United States, 1990-1997, *JAMA* 280:1569-1575, 1998.

Ellis K, Hartley C: *Nursing in today's world: Challenges, issues and trends*, Philadelphia, 2003, Lippincott.

Eshkevari L, Heath J: Use of acupuncture for chronic pain, *Holist Nurs Pract* 19:217-221, 2005.

Frisch N: Nursing as a context for alternative/complementary modalities, *Online J Issues in Nurs* 6, 2001a; retrieved from www.nursingworld.org/ojin/topic15/50c15_2.htm.

Frisch N: Standards for holistic nursing practice: a way to think about our care that includes complementary and alternative modalities, *Online J Issues in Nurs* 6, 2001b; retrieved from www.nursingworld.org/ojin/topic15/50c15_2.htm.

Gaskill M: Forces of nature (complementary/alternative therapies), *Nurseweek*, pp 11-13, July 26, 2004.

Gazella K: Bringing mindfulness to medicine: an interview with Jon Kabat-Zinn, *Altern Therap* 11:56-64, 2005.

Goodall D, Etters L: The therapeutic use of music on agitated behavior in those with dementia, *Holist Nurs Pract* 19:258-262, 2005.

Gutierrez C, Ranji U: U.S. health care costs, Kaiser Family Foundation, 2005; retrieved Apr 3, 2006, from www.kaiseredu.org/topics.im.asp?=1&parentID=61&id=358.

Horstman J: Tai chi, *Arthritis Today Online Edition*, 2000; retrieved Apr 3, 2006, from www.arthritis.org/resources/arthritistoday/2000.archives/2000_07_08_Taichi.asp.

Kabat-Zinn J: *Catastrophe living: using the wisdom of your body and mind to face stress, pain and illness*, New York, 1990, Guilford Press.

Kabat-Zinn J: Commentary on Majumdar et al: Mindfulness meditation for health, *J Altern Complement Med* 8:731-735, 2002.

Kalogredis V: Should you consider concierge medicine? *Physicians News Digest, Delaware Valley Edition* 17:8, 10, 2004.

Keck J, Baker S: Clients with pain: Promoting positive outcomes. In J Black et al, editors: *Medical-surgical nursing: clinical management for positive outcomes*, Philadelphia, 2001, Saunders.

Kirsch I: Medication and suggestion in the treatment of depression, *Contemporary Hypnosis* 22:59-66, 2005.

Koenig H: Separating fact from fiction, *Science & Theology News Online edition;* retrieved Apr 3, 2006, from www.stnews.org/Commentary-2758.htm.

Kreitzer M, Disch J: Leading the way: the Gillette nursing summit on integrated health and healing, *Altern Therapies in Health Med* 9:3A-10A, 2003.

Kreitzer M, Jensen D: Healing practices: trends, challenges, and opportunities for nurses in acute and critical care, *AACN Clin Issues* 11:7-16, 2000.

Laidlaw T, Dwivedi P: Combining cognitve, emotional, behaviora, and dare we say it, the spiritual: review of mindfulness-based cognitive therapy for depression: a new approach to preventing relapse. *Contemp Hypnosis* 21:205-209, 2004.

Lawson W: Taking humor therapy seriously, *Positive Health* 89: 18-21, 2003.

Leigh E: Nutrient-drug interactions, *The Natural Foods Merchandiser*, pp 42-44, 2005.

Leonard B, Plotnikoff G: Awareness: the heart of cultural competence, *AACN Clin Issues* 11:51-59, 2001.

Maes S: Nurses explore relationships among mind, body, spirit, *Oncol Nurse Society News* 16:1-3, 2001.

Maier-Lorentz M: The importance of prayer for mind/body healing, *Nurs Forum* 39:23-33, 2004.

McCaffrey R, Locsin R: Music listening as a nursing intervention: a symphony of practice, *Holist Nurs Pract* 16:70-77, 2002.

Meadows G, Mitchell P: Randomized controlled trial of MBCT and adherence therapy (MAT) for the prevention of relapse and recurrence of depression in primary care: the Southern Health Adult Psychiatry Research Training and Evaluation Center & Monash University, 2005; retrieved Apr 1, 2006, from www.mindfulbasedcbtblogspot.com/2005/12/midfulnes-based.cognitive-behavior.html.

Minden P: Humor as focal point of therapy for forensic psychiatric patients, *Holist Nurs Pract* 16:775-786, 2002.

Myers D: Commentary on Harvard prayer study results, *Science & Theology News Online edition*; retrieved Apr 3, 2006, from http://davidmyers.ort/Brix?pageID=122.

National Association of Cognitive-Behavioral Therapists: What is cognitive-behavioral therapy? 2006; retrieved Mar 28, 2006, from www.nacbt.org/whatiscbt.htm.

National Center for Complementary and Alternative Medicine: Examples of completed and ongoing research related to use of complementary alternative medicine, 2006; retrieved from www.altmed.od.nih.gov/nccam.

National Institutes of Health: Manipulative and body-based practices: an overview; retrieved 4/30/06 from www.health.nih.gov.

Parkman C, Ullrich S: *Keeping current on age-old practices: a complementary and alternative medicine guide for nurses,* Sunnyvale, Calif, 2000, Nurseweek.

Pelletier K: *The best alternative medicine,* New York, 2000, Simon & Schuster.

Rite-Care Pharmacy: Homeopathic medicine, 2002; retrieved from www.LookSmartWorld.com.

Saito I, Saito Y: Biofeedback training in clinical settings, *Biogenic Amines* 18:463-476, 2004.

Segal Z et al: The mindfulness-based cognitive therapy adherence scale: inter-rater reliability adherence to protocol and treatment distinctiveness, *J Clin Psychol Psychother* 9:131-138, 2002.

Silva M, Ludwick R: Ethical issues in complementary/alternative medicine therapy, *Online Journals in Nursing,* 2001; retrieved from www.nursingworld.org/ojin/topic.

Snyder M, Lindquist R: Issues in complementary therapies: how we got to where we are, *Online J Issues in Nur,* 6, 2001; retrieved from www.nursingworld.org/ojin/topic15/50c15_1.htm.

Spector R: *Cultural diversity in health and illness,* Upper Saddle River, NJ, 2003, Prentice Hall.

Spencer J: New red flags raised on mixing medications, herbal remedies, *San Diego Tribune,* pp A-1, A-14, June 23, 2004.

Tedesco P, Cicchetti J: Like cures like: homeopathy, *Am J Nurs* 101:43-50, 2001.

Telner J: A review of text: mindfulness-based cognitive therapy for depression: a new approach to prevent relapse. In Segal Z et al, *Canadian J Psychiatry* 50:432, 2005.

The new medicine (video), KPBS, San Diego State University, San Diego, Calif, 2006.

Topham D: Alternative and complementary therapies. In Daniels R, editor: *Nursing fundamentals: caring and clinical decision making,* New York, 2004, Delmar Learning.

Turner J: Chelation therapy, *Gale encyclopedia of alternative medicine,* 2001; retrieved from www.LookSmartWorld.com.

Venes D (editor): *Taber's cyclopedic medical dictionary,* Philadelphia, 2005, F.A. Davis.

Weil A: Introduction. In Pelletier K: *The best alternative medicine,* New York, 2000, Simon & Schuster.

Wikipedia: Mindfulness-based therapy, 2006; retrieved from www.en.wikipedia.org/wiki/mindfulness.

Williams S: Beyond belief: transcultural nurses provide culturally competent care, *Nurseweek,* pp 54-55, 58, May 8, 2006.

Young-Mason J: Music therapy: a healing art, *Clin Nurse Spec* 16:153-154, 2002.

Zerwekh J: Contemporary health care delivery: trends and economics. In Zerwekh J, Claborn J, editors: *Nursing today: transitions and trends,* ed 3, Philadelphia, 2000, Saunders.

Part V

SPECIAL POPULATIONS

Chapter 26

Grief and Loss

KATHERINE M. FORTINASH

A heavier task could not have been imposed/than I to speak my griefs unspeakable.
WILLIAM SHAKESPEARE

OBJECTIVES

1 Describe three components of the normal grief process.
2 Differentiate between grief, bereavement, and mourning.
3 Discuss the four major categories for symptoms of grief.
4 Distinguish between symptoms/behaviors of grief and those of depression.
5 Analyze the risk for dysfunctional grief reactions in high-risk clients.
6 Examine the major goals for intervention in acute grief.
7 Evaluate effective interventions in various stages of grief.
8 Compare and contrast chronic sorrow with other types of grief.
9 Identify persons at risk for chronic sorrow.
10 Explain how posttraumatic stress disorder is sometimes a feature of dysfunctional grief.
11 Discuss the profound effects of grief and loss on individuals across the life span.
12 Apply the nursing process in managing clients who are experiencing grief.

KEY TERMS

Grief is a natural and normal reaction to loss. It is a multifaceted response with painful psychologic, physiologic, cognitive, and behavioral responses that vary among individuals. Although it is most commonly associated with the death of a loved one, grief occurs when there is any significant loss, including loss of self-esteem, identity, dignity, or sense of worth. Grief descends on everyone, regardless of age or status. The following persons might be vulnerable to grief:

- The client newly admitted to a psychiatric hospital
- The parents of an infant with birth defects
- The victim of violence (e.g., abuse, war, natural disaster)
- The child who changes schools, leaving friends behind
- The wife caring for a husband with Alzheimer's disease
- The nurse working with terminally ill clients
- The betrayed lover
- The elderly widow who loses a pet
- The person whose time has come to retire

Although we know that grief is part of life, many of us are unprepared for the long journey of grieving which is often devastating, frightening, and lonely. In grief, many think, say, and do things that are normally uncharacteristic. There seems to be no relief, no end to the intense feelings that we experience, and there is no right way of coping with death (National Institutes of Health [NIH], 2006). Grief has been compared to a raw, open wound. With great care, it eventually will heal, but there will always be a scar. Most nurses are in daily contact with grief—other people's and their own.

The terms *grief*, *bereavement*, and *mourning*, listed below, are often used in place of each other, but they have different meanings (Tomita and Kitamura, 2002):

- **Grief** is the normal process of reacting to loss that is sometimes felt in response to physical losses (for example, a death) or in response to symbolic or social losses (for example, divorce or job loss). Each type of loss means the person has had something taken away. As a family goes through a catastrophic illness such as cancer, each member experiences many losses, and each loss triggers its own grief reaction.
- **Bereavement** is the period following a loss during which grief is experienced and mourning occurs. The time spent in a period of bereavement depends on how attached the survivor was to the person and how much time was spent anticipating the loss. The greater the bonding was to the deceased, the more profound the loss.
- **Mourning** is the process by which people adapt to a loss. Cultural customs, rituals, and society's rules for coping with loss also influence grief (NIH, 2006).

Although grief is painful, it is important to understand that grief and its pain are normal and inevitable life experiences (American Psychiatric Association [APA], 2000; Freud, 1917). In some cases, a grieving person benefits from psychosocial or pharmacologic intervention, and in other cases, grief becomes pathologic.

RESPONSES

Responses to bereavement (loss) may be examined as a range of physical, cognitive, relating, and affective (emotional) manifestations of pain—the intensity of which is often a surprise to the mourner. Lindemann's classic study of grief (1944) and other more current studies (Tomita and Kitamura, 2002; Parkes, 2001; Stroebe et al., 2000) identified many of the manifestations of grief, including physical distress, preoccupation with the image of the deceased, guilt, hostile reactions, and disruptions in normal patterns of conduct. These and other physical and psychologic manifestations of grief are summarized as follows.

Physical Manifestations

Physical responses of grief include weakness, anorexia, feelings of choking, shortness of breath, tightness in the chest, dry mouth, and gastrointestinal disturbances. Fatigue, exhaustion, insomnia, and episodes of sobbing are common. Bereaved persons frequently seek medical attention for vague symptoms such as chest discomfort or gastrointestinal problems, some of which seem to have no physiologic basis. In addition, although grief is seldom a direct cause of illness or death (except for suicide), there is a clear link between grief and increased vulnerability to physical and mental illness, especially myocardial infarction, hypertension, rheumatoid arthritis, depression, alcohol and other drug abuse, and malnutrition (Tomita and Kitamura, 2002; Charlton et al., 2001; Ringdal et al., 2001).

Cognitive Manifestations

Cognitive manifestations center on preoccupation with the deceased person. The involuntary nature and intensity of the preoccupation are surprising and distressing to some. It is common for the preoccupation to take the form of conversations with the deceased (in normal grief, with the recognition that the deceased person is not actually present). Especially with older adults, these conversations sometimes continue for the rest of the survivor's life. Over time, preoccupation usually diminishes, although some individuals maintain links with the deceased for many years, and for some people, this continues until death. These links are sometimes in the form of remembrances such as treasured things or renegotiated relationships with the deceased. Many now recognize the drive to maintain links between the living and the dead as normal behavior (Reisman, 2001; Silverman and Worden, 1992). In some cultures (e.g., Chinese and Vietnamese), the failure to maintain formal links with deceased ancestors is pathologic (Kemp and Chang, 2002). Another common symptom is difficulty concentrating, such as complete lapses of focus or even orientation to time and place. Seeking and longing for the lost person or object are universally experienced. Some grieving persons experience hallucinations. Individuals most often describe these as momentary glimpses of the person who died or brief (two or three words) auditory messages perceived to be spoken by the deceased. In most cases hallucinations diminish within a month or two after the loss and thus are considered as part of the normal grieving process. In a few cases hallucinations persist, increase in number or intensity, or become derogatory or threatening, such as beckoning the survivor to join the deceased. They are then considered negative hallucinations (pathologic grief), and therapeutic interventions, including hospitalization or antipsychotic medications, are indicated (APA, 2000).

Behavioral and Relating Manifestations

Grief and bereavement figure prominently in the DSM Axis IV dimension of psychosocial and environmental stressors. Among the Axis IV problems directly or indirectly related to grief and bereavement (APA, 2000) are the following:

- Death of a family member
- Health problems in a family
- Inadequate social support
- Adjustment to life-cycle transition
- Inadequate finances
- Marital difficulties

Behavioral and relating manifestations of grief include disruptions in patterns of conduct ranging from an inability to perform even basic activities of daily living; to dragging through daily activities; to a restless, disorganized behavior that includes "searching" for that which is lost and obsessive reflection and reminiscence; and overall, an intense sense of isolation (Hentz, 2002; Lindemann, 1944). The old life and patterns lose meaning and satisfaction without the lost object or person, and there does not seem to be a new life or patterns to which the bereaved individual can turn. This loss of relating and meaning is a major etiology of despair or hopelessness.

Affective Manifestations

Affective manifestations of grief are often overwhelming, with sadness, guilt, loneliness, hopelessness, and anger being the most common. Sadness, loneliness, and hopelessness tend to predominate and sometimes, along with other symptoms, meet the criteria for diagnosis of an affective (mood) disorder (e.g., major depression or dysthymic disorder). The most common differences between symptoms of bereavement and major depression or dysthymic disorder are that psychomotor retardation, morbid guilt, and suicidal ideation are less common in bereavement and that affective disorders are of longer duration than bereavement (Hentz, 2002; APA, 2000; Nuss and Zubenko, 1992). Dysfunctional or unresolved grief, however, will possibly result in major depression.

Guilt is a pervasive theme in grief, even in children as young as 2 years (Jacob, 1996; Gibbons, 1992). Many survivors search for their failures or omissions in the relationship, and when they do not find significant mistakes, some proceed to magnify whatever small errors they have done (Lindemann, 1944). Many people are tortured by "if onlys" and "what ifs" (e.g., "If only I had called"; "If only we hadn't let her take the car that night"; "If only I had taken time to listen and visit more often."). Guilt is especially troublesome for those whose relationships with the deceased were ambivalent (uncertain about feelings toward the person) and characterized by unresolved or unexpressed feelings. Survivor guilt is common among people who go through an intense experience (e.g., war) and survive when others do not. Individuals experience a similar guilt when survivors believe that they should have died instead of the loved one. Grief accompanied by "guilt about things other than actions taken or not taken by the survivor at the time of death" (APA, 2000), sustained loss of self-esteem, and ambivalence about living is an indication that an individual is at increased risk for suicide and needs help. All we can do with the guilt is to learn from it for the other people in our lives. When the death is by suicide, it is especially important to remember we cannot control the behavior of another person, even as we search for answers (Hsu, 2002).

Anger is common and is sometimes directed toward the person who died, toward family members, toward the health care staff, or toward God. Some turn it inward to the self. Anger is generally a response to the anxiety that comes from the powerlessness and vulnerability resulting from the death of a loved one and other losses. For example, some express anger toward the deceased in statements such as "How could she do this to me? It's not fair!" or "How does he expect me to take care of things alone?" Many survivors believe it is wrong to feel anger toward a deceased loved one and thus turn the anger inward. Anger turned inward also reflects a survivor's inability to release the lost person or object. To those who have spent a lifetime suppressing anger, these overwhelming and "wrong" or ego-dystonic feelings (unnatural or uncomfortable feelings) are distressing and indicate to some individuals that they are "going crazy." Some need permission to express anger. For others, if the death itself is not enough to create anger, for some tending to the business death requires, such as funeral preparations and legal matters, results in anger. For some morticians, lawyers, and others, death is just another way to make a profit. Even if their motives are exemplary, the normally cool, detached attitude they display toward their vulnerable clients evokes anger and even hostility. Talking about anger also helps survivors to define, understand, and learn how to handle it. Suppressing anger will possibly lead to deeper than normal depression or bitterness. The impulse to use drugs, including prescription drugs and alcohol, occurs for some. Bereaved persons with a history of any sort of drug misuse or mental illness are at risk for recurrence or exacerbation of these problems.

STAGES AND PROCESS OF GRIEF

Stages

Grief is often described in terms of stages. Although there is variation among the different conceptions, many stage-oriented theories have three basic stages: avoidance (numbing and blunting), confrontation (disorganization and despair), and reestablishment (reorganization and recovery) (Kemp, 2006). *Avoidance* includes both the initial denial and subsequent brief periods of time when the survivor "forgets," then "remembers" with shock and pain, the losses and the grief. *Confrontation* is the often lengthy period of active mourning and includes the previously discussed most acute physical, cognitive, behavioral and relating, and affective manifestations of grief. *Reestablishment* occurs, not as a distinct stage but as the *gradual* decrease of symptoms and adjustment to life without that which was lost. The problem with stages is that they tend to be neater in theory than they are in reality. Thus, sometimes these stages mislead some individuals into thinking that grief is a matter of progressing in an orderly manner through definitive stages, and then grief is over. In reality, no two people grieve the same way, even in the same family. Like a snowflake or a fingerprint, each person's grief has characteristics and a timetable all its own.

Process

Characteristics

It is more helpful to think in terms of a process of common and dynamic responses to grief than to think of grief as occurring in well-defined stages. Some initially respond to the death of a loved one with shock and disbelief, followed by protest and despair. Others go through a period of emotionless cognitive activity (planning the funeral, etc.) mixed with waves of despair, then experience yearning, despair, and disorganization (sobbing, confusion, wandering). Most gradually begin the long, painful, and varied process of rebuilding a life without the person who died. An essential feature of this process is its dynamic, changing nature (Kemp, 2006). For example, some experience periods of normal functioning interspersed with periods of psychologic distress or symptoms (almost indistinguishable from those of major depression). Countless people say, "It seems like I'm doing fine, and then, for no reason at all, I start crying" (as if some external or practical reason was needed).

The grief process sometimes includes all of the aforementioned responses, phases, or symptoms, or only some of them. There is not always a "stage of avoidance" or a period of organized cognitive activity; or there may be very little in the way of resolution, reorganization, or adjustment to the environment in the absence of the deceased. Moreover, when death is expected, the grief process begins before the person dies. Grief occurring before the death or other loss is called anticipatory grief, and this chapter discusses the concept later. Box 26-1 summarizes grief theories.

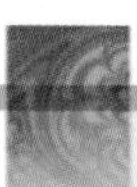

BOX 26-1

Summary of Grief Theories

LINDEMANN

Grief is manifested by predictable psychologic and somatic symptomatology. Somatic distress, preoccupation with the deceased person's image, guilt, hostile reactions, and loss of patterns of conduct all characterize acute mourning. Dysfunctional or "morbid" grief reactions are distortions of some aspect of "normal grief." The duration of grief and development of dysfunctional grief are largely dependent on the success with which the mourner *works* through the grief.

KÜBLER-ROSS

Elisabeth Kübler-Ross's stages of dying (denial, anger, bargaining, depression, and acceptance) are often applied to grief. The initial response to loss often includes denial, anger, and bargaining. Denial is characterized by refusal to accept the loss. Individuals initially direct anger at the health care staff and then, later in the process, at the person who died. Bargaining and denial are often mixed in a futile attempt to "reverse reality." Depression tends to be the lengthiest phase, and in dysfunctional grief it becomes chronic and meets DSM-IV-TR criteria for major depression. Acceptance of the loss is a gradual process that includes aspects of previous stages. As the grief work progresses, acceptance increases.

BOWLBY

Grief and loss are characterized first by numbness in which the loss is recognized but not necessarily felt as real. Numbness is followed by yearning and searching, in which the loss is still not fully realized. In the third phase, disorganization and despair, the loss is real, and intense emotional pain and cognitive disorganization occur. Reorganization is the final phase and is characterized by a gradual adjustment to life without the deceased.

ENGEL

The initial response to loss is shock and disbelief. Awareness of the loss and the meaning of the loss develop during the first year of mourning. Eventually, the relationship is resolved and put into perspective.

SHNEIDMAN

Conceptualizing less structure or stages than other theorists in regard to grief, Shneidman views the expression of grief as being dependent primarily on an individual's personality or style of living. An individual who goes through life feeling depressed and guilty is likely to grieve similarly. One who avoids emotional investments with others will also tend to try to avoid grief as well.

THEORY SYNTHESIS

Grief tends to occur in several phases. The initial response to loss is shock, numbness, denial, or other attempts to defend against the reality and pain of loss. This initial phase is followed by painful psychologic and physical disequilibrium—which, in the case of chronic grief, lasts indefinitely. The third phase of resolution or recovery is a gradual process in which "the good days begin to outnumber the bad." Ultimately, although not forgotten, the relationship with the deceased is resolved and placed into perspective.

Grief Work

Named first by Lindemann (1944), **grief work** is the means by which people move through the stages and processes of grief (Carpenito, 2002). Grief work is both a struggle to not give in to despair and a willingness to confront the reality of despair. Within the grief process, the bereaved person must continue to move forward with the business of life. This includes paying the bills, making decisions, and, at the same time, being able to separate him or herself from the person who died and readjust to a world without the deceased. In grief work, the mourner begins the difficult task of turning to others for emotional satisfaction and redirecting energy that was once given to the person who died. The survivor continues to express the deep, painful emotions of grieving, which also includes grieving for the self as well as the deceased and all the plans and dreams that will never be fulfilled. The process is exhausting as it requires physical and mental energy, yet it is a necessary journey both for closure and new beginnings (NIH, 2006).

Tasks in Grief

Accomplishing the following **tasks in grief** helps to resolve issues that otherwise obstruct the grief process (Carpenito, 2002; Kemp, 2006):

- Telling the "death story" or describing (in detail) events surrounding the death or loss
- Expressing and accepting the sadness of grief
- Expressing and accepting guilt, anger, and other feelings perceived as negative
- Reviewing the relationship with the deceased
- Exploring possibilities in life after the loss (e.g., new relationships, activities, sources of support)
- Understanding common processes and problems in grief
- Being understood or accepted by others

Complicating Factors

Several factors complicate grief work. First, it is extremely painful. Many people are surprised at the intensity and depth of the pain and often make an attempt to avoid the distress by throwing themselves back into a busy schedule or taking a vacation. Second, the work is inherently contradictory. The pain demands expression, but many often fear that they will lose control over their feelings if they express the pain, saying, "I know that if I start crying, I will never stop." Third, individuals need both emotion-based coping (such as expressing deep, powerful feelings) and problem-solving coping (such as developing strategies for going on with life) to successfully complete the work. Finally, in most of the Western world, cultural values support avoiding the expression of grief. For example, Western cultures value self-control highly, especially in men. There is a tendency to try to rush through grief and get back to work or get on with one's life (as said *ad nauseam,* "Let the healing begin"). Rituals that formerly helped in individual and community expressions of grief are now often brief "celebrations" of the deceased's life or other upbeat and usually brief events. Memorial services have replaced the ritual of the funeral mass. The viewing of the body, a customary ritual by some ethnic groups, has been cut back to one or two days instead of 4 or 5 days. The expression of grief, therefore, is limited to what the public considers appropriate or what is convenient for today's busy lifestyle. After the burial or cremation, the survivors are left alone with the pain and a long journey of healing ahead.

TYPES OF GRIEF

Types of grief include anticipatory, acute, and dysfunctional, as well as chronic sorrow. There is disagreement about definitions, especially in terms of the time required for resolution of a particular form of grief.

Anticipatory Grief

Anticipatory grief, or *premourning,* is grief associated with anticipation of a predicted death or developing loss (Ackley, 2002; Heffner and Byock, 2002; Shneidman, 1980). Anticipatory grief sometimes begins with a catastrophic diagnosis, characterized by a sharp sense of vulnerability. The old and comfortable illusion of immortality that we all have when life is good suddenly dies, and grief for that life begins at the time of diagnosis. Here, as in other situations, the grief is often complex. For example, in a family in which a loved one develops dementia, grief is possibly acute (related to the current condition), ongoing (as the family continuously loses aspects of the loved one), and anticipatory (as the long-term reality of the disorder becomes clearer).

Early in the development of the anticipatory grief model, anticipatory grief was viewed as an adaptive process that helped resolve relationships and prepare survivors for the anticipated loss. Ideally the realization that loss was approaching gave the people involved an opportunity to work on interpersonal and spiritual reconciliation and provide support for one another (Parkes, 1998). More recently, some clinicians and researchers have seen an association between anticipatory grief and a high incidence of depression or family withdrawal from the client. There is general agreement that (1) grief begins when a serious physical or mental illness occurs; (2) this grief is sometimes anticipatory and involves pain, as do other forms of grief; and (3) a lack of emotional response to serious illness or other loss is an indication that dysfunction or dysfunctional grief is likely (Ackley, 2002; Carpenito, 2002). Thus, the nurse needs to view anticipatory grief as normative, and persons experiencing it will possibly benefit from intervention.

Acute Grief

Acute grief, usually simply referred to as grief, is the prototype of a painful experience after a loss. Its symptoms and process are described earlier in the chapter. Although there is agreement that acute grief is time limited, there is no agreement on how long acute (or normal) grief lasts. An early theory is that acute grief lasts approximately 1 year (Shneidman, 1980). More recently, researchers have integrated the time span for acute grief with the severity of symptoms, severity of trauma or loss, nature of the relationship, and cultural values (Kemp, 2006; APA, 2000; Stroebe et al., 2000). Acute grief does not have a clear ending; gradually the sadness lessens, the pain diminishes, and eventually the mourner moves forward with his or her life—even though complete recovery may never occur (Hentz, 2002). In some traditional cultures (e.g., East Indian) and among some individuals in certain religions (e.g., Jewish and Hindu), grief is ongoing and not limited by time (Kemp, 1998; Goodman et al., 1991).

Within the process of healing and moving on, there are times of acute exacerbation, when some situation or event brings back the pain, and the mourner again feels overwhelmed with grief. Holidays, birthdays, and other significant milestones are obvious events with the potential to revive the grief. Other precipitants are less obvious, and thus the mourner is unable to prepare for them. For example, a song, an image, or a smell occurs in an unguarded moment and the sadness returns as powerful as it was in the beginning. These moments of exacerbation also decrease over time.

Dysfunctional Grief

Early theorists have described **dysfunctional grief** in multiple ways, and many of these definitions are still true today. Lindemann (1944) and a host of contemporary writers and researchers (APA, 2000; Stroebe et al., 2000; Parkes, 1998; Cowles and Rodgers, 1991; Bowlby, 1980) have emphasized normative and dysfunctional aspects of grief. In other words, up to some point, grief is *normal*, and beyond that point, grief is variously considered *dysfunctional*, *pathologic*, *complicated*, and more recently, *traumatic* (Jacobs et al., 2000; Stroebe et al., 2000; Horowitz et al., 1997). Posttraumatic stress disorder (PTSD) is sometimes a feature of dysfunctional grief (Melhem et al., 2001). PTSD is a disorder in which individuals reexperience past traumatic events with extreme symptoms of anxiety (Fortinash and Holoday Worret, 2007). Many people who witnessed the death and devastation of September 11, the Iraq War, Hurricane Katrina, and the violence at Virginia Polytechnic Institute and State University will develop PTSD (see Chapter 9). If depression is the predominant feature of bereavement and is incapacitating 2 months after the loss, the client may be diagnosed as having a major depressive disorder (APA, 2000) (see Chapter 11).

Although there is considerable debate about the details of exactly what constitutes dysfunctional grief, all sources agree that dysfunctional grief lasts longer than other types of grief and is characterized by greater disability or other dysfunctional patterns than usual, as defined by cultural values. In addition, studies (e.g., Piper et al., 2001) have identified levels of severity of dysfunctional grief.

Types of dysfunctional grief include the following (APA, 2000; Kemp, 2006; Silverman et al., 2001):

- *Traumatic grief.* Occurs when there is traumatic loss such as a spouse murdered, a child dying suddenly and unexpectedly, rape, or multiple deaths. PTSD is often a concurrent or complicating factor, sometimes characterized by psychic numbing, intrusive thoughts, avoidance of stimuli, increased arousal, and other aspects of PTSD (Fortinash and Holoday Worret, 2007; Melhem et al., 2001). For some there is distortion or exaggeration of one or more normative components of grief, with anger and guilt being most common. As noted previously, the term *traumatic grief* is used by some (e.g., Jacobs et al., 2000) to refer to pathologic, dysfunctional, or complicated grief.
- *Absent or inhibited grief.* Characterized by minimal emotional expression of grief and is sometimes related to trauma as noted previously. Absent grief sometimes converts to **delayed grief**, and the individual experiences it years after the loss. Precipitating factors for conversion to delayed grief often are powerful experiences such as psychotherapy or religious conversion.
- *Conflicted grief.* Occurs when the relationship with the deceased or lost object is characterized by ambivalence or conflict. Initial responses to the loss are often minimal and then intensify rather than diminish over time, and the survivor feels "haunted" by the deceased. An adult survivor of childhood sexual abuse whose abusing parent dies is an example of a person at risk for conflicted grief.
- *Chronic grief.* Unending grief after a loss. Chronic grief is sometimes related to the survivor and the deceased having a highly codependent relationship. In other cases, chronic grief is a result of (1) severe loss and (2) lack of resources or support to deal with the loss. Chronic grief is especially common in some cultural groups such as Cambodian refugees or Native Americans.

Dysfunctional grief is generally associated with one or more of the following (Ackley, 2002; Parkes, 2001):

- Unresolved issues in the relationship with the person who died
- Inhibited expression of grief
- Lack of social support
- The "deritualization" of Western culture (e.g., reduced mourning periods of 1 or 2 days)
- Uncertain loss (e.g., prisoners of war, kidnapping)
- Traumatic loss (e.g., by murder, accident)
- Multiple losses (e.g., war, natural disaster, mass murders)
- Loss that is seldom discussed (e.g., rape, abortion)
- Undervalued loss such as that felt by some experiencing miscarriage or other losses that may not be recognized by others as significant
- The accumulated effects of current grief on past unresolved grief

Chronic Sorrow

Chronic sorrow is a form of grief that often includes characteristics of other forms of grief but differs in several essential aspects. First, chronic sorrow is a response to

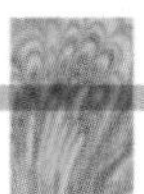

TABLE 26-1

Comparison of Grief, Depression, and Posttraumatic Stress Disorder

	GRIEF	DEPRESSION	POSTTRAUMATIC STRESS DISORDER
Process	Related to loss	Relatively static or cyclic affective disorder not necessarily related to loss	Relatively static anxiety disorder related to trauma; precipitating event is outside the range of usual human experience
Manifestation of symptoms	Usually appear shortly after the loss	Sometimes associated with an identified loss	Often appear years after the trauma
Depressive symptoms	Dysphoric mood of sadness, hopelessness, and despair; anger is common, as are periods of agitation	Similar to but more intense than grief, except that the individual seldom expresses anger; psychomotor retardation, morbid guilt, and suicidal ideation are more common	Common; other symptoms include persistent reexperiencing of the trauma (versus preoccupation with the image of the deceased, as in grief); increased arousal is common
Physical symptoms	Cover a wide spectrum; physical symptoms sometimes include heart disease and other chronic illness	Primarily neurovegetative	Sleep disturbances often resemble those of grief or depression; hypervigilance is common
Spiritual beliefs	Sometimes provide meaning or context	Seldom provide context or meaning	Seldom any relation

CLINICAL ALERT

The following increase a client's risk for developing **dysfunctional grief:**

- Premorbid psychiatric history or history of psychosocial trauma
- Social isolation
- Relationship with the deceased that was characterized by unresolved conflict or ambivalence (e.g., "love-hate")
- Relationship with the deceased that was characterized by enmeshment and a high level of introjection, hence difficulty "letting go"
- Tendency to suppress grief
- Young age

ongoing loss such as the chronic illness of a loved one. Second, persons experiencing chronic sorrow seldom experience disability such as major depression and typically function at a higher level in activities of daily living than those experiencing other forms of grief (Burke et al., 1992). Persons at risk for chronic sorrow include parents with children who have mental retardation, schizophrenia, or other chronic illness; spouses of persons with long-term chronic illnesses such as multiple sclerosis, alcoholism, or Alzheimer's disease; and persons with similar disorders (Lichtenstein et al., 2002; Pejlert, 2001). There is no documentation on the effects on the grief process when the etiology of chronic sorrow is removed (i.e., when the disabled person dies).

Grief and Depression

Grief and depression are often compared with one another. Grief, especially dysfunctional grief, also shares characteristics with PTSD, particularly in that both invariably involve loss (Table 26-1).

BEREAVEMENT CARE

Before Loss

Grief is a universal experience that comes with or without warning and occurs many times and with varying intensity throughout life. The major psychosocial determinants of pathology in grief are a psychiatric history before the loss and inadequate social support (Silverman et al., 2001). It follows, then, the first and primary promotion of mental health, such as family involvement in community and faith activities, improved parenting, and other such efforts to promote mental and spiritual health, are best to address grief.

When Loss Is Impending

A second point for the nurse to consider health promotion or disability prevention is in the case of terminal illness or other anticipated loss. Interventions in these situations include assisting individuals and families in working toward personal, interpersonal, and spiritual reconciliation—and not necessarily anticipatory grief. Even in the best of relationships, there are sometimes unresolved issues or areas in which growth is possible, and promoting health in this stage of life includes promoting participation of the *client and family* in care. Clearly, effective participation in care has a positive effect on the grief process after death (although long-term effects are not known for caregivers in Alzheimer's disease, schizophrenia, and other similar chronic illnesses). A variety of means exist for intervention at this point, including individual informal or formal counseling in acute care settings, family support groups, hospice care, and spiritual support. Nurses and other health care professionals need to address the health needs of family members, as well as those of clients.

Health care providers offer preventive grief therapy to survivors in several circumstances. For example, hospice and palliative care programs typically offer bereavement calls or visits at specified intervals to survivors. Many hospice programs also periodically hold seminars and other events or activities for bereaved adults or children. Churches and synagogues hold grief workshops for members and others in the community. These are generally weekend or time-limited groups similar to self-help groups such as I Can Cope and others. Religiously oriented grief activities are also held in some cases in association with significant religious holidays related to death or remembrance.

After the Loss

The third intervention point is after the loss occurs (**postvention**). Intervention at this point is often preventive and directed toward addressing existing problems that are interpersonal in nature or related to normative or dysfunctional grief. The tasks in grief (see the earlier discussion) provide a framework for intervention after loss.

SPIRITUALITY AND GRIEF

The grief experience can threaten all basic spiritual needs or issues: meaning, hope, relatedness, forgiveness, and transcendence sometimes fall away and leave the mourner in a spiritual vacuum. The nature of God and previously held beliefs, including any easy answers to life's problems (e.g., that faith protects one from pain), are called into question and do not always support the reality of the current feelings. Grief is then a test of faith, and the awareness or acknowledgment of anger or other negative feelings is interpreted as a personal spiritual failure (a source of more guilt).

Although dreams and visions are significant spiritual events in some cultures, in the context of Western cultures they are discounted as either immaterial or pathologic. There is often reluctance by the grieving individual to discuss these experiences and feelings with family, friends, or clergy. As mourners struggle to find a context for the doubt and confusion that accompanies these experiences, it is important for the nurse to listen with openness, determining how these experiences either confirm or challenge the mourner's spiritual and religious beliefs. Some individuals are confirmed in their traditional beliefs; others see the dissolution of their faith; some find or rediscover a deeper faith (see Chapter 7).

Grief has the potential to transform those who experience it, for better or worse. Grief is an "invitation to a new life" in which the individual can take the discontinuity of death/loss and grief to a "higher continuity" (Carse, 1980). For others, grief is a context for retreat into an impoverished life. Interventions in grief are most effective when used to promote health, offer comfort and hope, and prevent dysfunction. Interventions are less effective in the postvention period and least effective in treating dysfunctional or complicated grief.

THE NURSING PROCESS

ASSESSMENT

Nursing assessment of a person who is bereaved is based on knowledge of normative and pathologic aspects of the grief process, influences on the grief process, and the person's resources. Assessment encompasses (1) the grief experience of the mourner; (2) factors that inhibit or promote working through the grief process, including cultural and religious norms; and (3) the mourner's ability to mobilize cognitive, behavioral, and emotion-based coping strategies. The nurse assesses the client's current level of functioning with the understanding that up to a point impaired functioning is to be expected (see the Nursing Assessment Questions box).

Physical Disturbances

Physical disturbances in acute grief include weakness, anorexia, shortness of breath, tightness of the chest, dry mouth, and gastrointestinal disturbances such as constipation or diarrhea, abdominal pain, gas, and nausea and vomiting. Cardiovascular and gastrointestinal problems predominate in chronic grief. Vague physical complaints such as unfocused abdominal pain or shortness of breath are especially common in all stages and types of grief.

Cognitive Disturbances

Cognitive disturbances are often focused on preoccupation with images and thoughts of the deceased. This preoccupation is sometimes so pervasive that the bereaved person is unable to carry on with some activities of daily living. The inability to control thoughts is distressing to many mourners. In acute grief, these obsessive thoughts are normal; they are simply part of the process. Preoccupation that results in significant disturbance of daily life (e.g., work) is widely considered pathologic after about 1 year past the date of death when the person who died was an adult and 2 or more years past the date of death when the deceased was a child.

NURSING ASSESSMENT QUESTIONS

Grief

1. Describe how it has been for you since [your husband] died.
2. How have you reacted to other major losses in your life?
3. Whom do you depend on when you are having a hard time, like now? Talk about how it is when you ask for help.
4. Let's go over all the prescription and other medicine and vitamins you are taking.
5. How often do you have alcoholic drinks (or other drugs)? When you drink (take drugs), how much do you take, and how does it make you feel?

A question *not* to ask is, "How are you doing?" Cultural norms are to respond to such questions with "pretty good," "okay," or "fine." These answers are essentially meaningless.

Behavioral and Relating Disturbances

Behavioral and relating disturbances often result from the depressive aspects of grief. Some people who are bereaved describe themselves as "stopped" and thus unable to participate in relationships (see the Case Study). There is a tendency in survivors to reflect on the death and the relationship with the deceased. In at least the earlier phases of the process, talk of the deceased tends to focus only on his or her "good" qualities and ignore the multifaceted nature of the individual. Many people who are bereaved cry with little apparent provocation, which often results in discomfort for the mourner and others. In chronic grief, the talk of the death and the relationship tends to be repetitive and superficial rather than progressive and insightful.

Affective Disturbances

Affective disturbances are primarily those of sadness or depression, anger, and guilt. Cultural norms of "carrying on" inhibit expression of these feelings. People who are bereaved soon learn that "nobody wants to hear your sad story." Sadness and even feelings of depression are not considered pathologic unless they persist a year or 2 past the death or include suicidal ideation.

NURSING DIAGNOSIS

In diagnosing grief or problems occurring in grief, nurses need to be mindful that the typical approach in diagnosing is to identify problems of a physical or psychologic nature and then try to alleviate the discomfort. Because grief normally includes discomfort, attempts to avoid or eliminate the discomfort, no matter how well intentioned, will impede the grieving process. On the other hand, extreme discomfort will possibly require pharmacologic intervention. The point at which discomfort is classified as extreme or abnormal versus normal has not been defined. An insightful diagnosis therefore focuses on the *expression* of normal feelings (e.g., anger, guilt, sadness) as much as on what feelings exist. Nursing diagnoses are prioritized according to client needs and safety issues.

Acute Grief

- Disturbed personal identity related to change in role and relationships, as evidenced by the inability to establish new patterns of relating to others and the environment after the death of a spouse or loved one
- Situational low self-esteem related to pervasive feelings of guilt and cognitive distortions secondary to guilt, as evidenced by thinking about inadequacies in the relationship with the deceased and blaming self for all problems in the relationship
- Impaired social interaction related to altered role performance and disruptions in usual patterns of conduct/interactions, as evidenced by difficulty in adapting to life changes and developing relationships according to the current situation

Dysfunctional Grief

- Risk for self-directed violence; risk factors: feelings of hopelessness and anger and reports and observed incidents of rage over perceived inability to live without the deceased
- Complicated grieving (unexpressed) related to fear of catastrophe if grief is expressed, as evidenced by absence of expression of feelings related to the grief process
- Complicated grieving related to unresolved guilt, as evidenced by frequent references to personal failings in the relationship with the deceased

Chronic Sorrow

- Chronic sorrow related to effects of the death of a loved one or experiences of chronic physical or mental illness or disability (e.g., Alzheimer's disease, schizophrenia, mental retardation, cancer), as evidenced by recurring feelings of sadness and grief that vary in intensity over time and interfere with the person's ability to reach the highest level of personal and social well-being
- Caregiver role strain related to chronic sorrow, as evidenced by caregiver withdrawal from community life to care for a loved one with chronic schizophrenia

Other Nursing Diagnoses

- Risk for other-directed violence
- Risk-prone health behavior
- Disabled family coping
- Ineffective coping

CASE STUDY

Mrs. Downs is 72 years old and lives alone in the apartment she shared with her husband for the past 19 years, since retirement. Her husband died the previous month, after a 2-year struggle with prostate cancer. Since her husband's death, Mrs. Downs has felt sad and depressed. She wants to spend time with others but says, "They are happy, and I'm sad, and it's no good for anyone." For the past week, except for "forcing" herself to take her daily walk around the block, Mrs. Downs has spent most of her time alone in her apartment. She has a poor appetite, difficulty sleeping, and feels guilty about "all the things I could have done to help my husband." Most of the other residents in the complex are similar in age to Mrs. Downs, and she is close to several of them. Her only daughter lives in another state and has invited her mother to move into her home.

CRITICAL THINKING

1. According to your assessment, what type of grief is Mrs. Downs experiencing?
2. From your knowledge of the grieving process, what are three important needs of Mrs. Downs?
3. What personal resources are likely to be most helpful to Mrs. Downs at the present time?
4. What questions would you ask Mrs. Downs at this stage in her grief?

- Ineffective denial
- Interrupted family processes
- Fatigue
- Grieving
- Hopelessness
- Posttrauma syndrome
- Powerlessness
- Insomnia
- Social isolation
- Disturbed thought processes
- Spiritual distress
- Ineffective sexuality pattern

OUTCOME IDENTIFICATION

Outcome criteria focus on enhancement of emotional coping skills or methods (e.g., greater expression of feelings of grief) and cognitive and behavioral coping abilities (e.g., strategies to develop more functional patterns of living, appropriate to changed life circumstances). Outcomes are prioritized according to client needs and safety issues.

Client will:

- Verbalize absence of suicidal ideations.
- Express guilty or angry feelings related to the death and grief versus suppression of grief.
- Express both positive and negative feelings about the deceased versus idealizing the qualities of the deceased.
- Explore the relationship with the deceased in a multifaceted way that includes both positive and negative aspects.
- Formulate and implement reasonable plans for adapting life and the identified role to present circumstances.
- Participate in at least one social or community activity each week.

CASE STUDY Mr. and Mrs. Casey have a 24-year-old son, Sean, who has chronic undifferentiated schizophrenia. Sean lives at home most of the year, except when he is admitted to the county hospital (two or three times a year). Sean has never worked, has no friends, is withdrawn most of the time, has violent episodes about once a month, and is noncompliant with medications. The Caseys have tried different hospitals until they ran out of insurance coverage for Sean. Sean has experienced a variety of antipsychotic medications, different therapists, alternative therapies, and spiritual counseling, but nothing has changed the course of his illness. Mr. Casey works long hours at an auto parts store, and Mrs. Casey stays home with Sean. Mr. and Mrs. Casey have begun seeing the clinical nurse specialist from the county hospital community outreach program. Their chief complaints as a couple and individually are overwhelming feelings of hopelessness and physical and mental exhaustion. The clinical nurse specialist has diagnosed their problem as caregiver role strain related to chronic sorrow, as evidenced by the caregivers' withdrawal from community life to care for their son with chronic schizophrenia. The nurse has implemented a plan of care that includes (1) weekly couples' counseling, (2) joining a regular family support group in a community facility, and (3) biweekly home visits by an outreach staff member to assist Sean with medication compliance.

CRITICAL THINKING

1. What is your opinion about whether Sean will experience significant improvement in his disorder?
2. Part of the care is directed to the parents. Why are they also receiving care instead of Sean alone, as he is the one who is mentally ill? What might happen to Sean if his parents are no longer able to cope?
3. Discuss potential success in relation to this plan. Are the Caseys likely to achieve happiness or even contentment as a result of receiving care?
4. Discuss each of the following feelings that family members with relatives with chronic mental illness sometimes experience: anger, sorrow, love, disgust, and despair.

PLANNING

The plan of care for a person with acute grief consists primarily of (1) supporting mobilization of the person's personal and community resources, (2) providing normative data about the grief process, and (3) supporting the person in her or his grief work (see the Case Study). The next section discusses each of these steps.

Assistance is sometimes necessary in mobilizing resources (e.g., family, friends, and spiritual supports), because individuals often are reluctant to ask for help and resources often do not know how to provide help. In addition, some of the symptoms of grief (e.g., fatigue, sadness, and anger) promote isolation rather than relating to others. Frequently, if either the bereaved person or his or her support systems are able to initiate contact, the other will respond appropriately. Too often, however, the mourner and his or her resources exist in isolation, each wishing they knew how to make contact with the other.

Nurses can provide normative data on grief (i.e., explanation of physical, emotional, social, and spiritual difficulties inherent in the grief process) to both the bereaved and his or her support systems. In a culture in many ways lacking in ritual and tradition, grief sometimes seems mysterious or pathologic even to those one might expect to be helpful (e.g., clergy). The nurse teaches survivors and others (such as family members) what they might experience in the grief process. Bereavement (survivor) groups are an excellent forum for such teaching.

Supporting the mourner in his or her grief work includes facilitating the telling of how the deceased died and related events and exploring both positive and negative aspects of the relationship with the deceased, positive and negative aspects of the deceased, and cognitive and behavioral coping strategies. Assistance with mobilizing resources and providing normative data is also part of support.

The plan of care for a person with dysfunctional grieving focuses on the specific pathologic condition of the client. The nurse also addresses normative aspects of grief.

The nurse can also direct plans toward the community. In community-focused planning, the nurse helps churches, synagogues, community centers, hospitals, and other organizations develop self-help groups for bereaved persons. Nurses also serve as facilitators for such groups.

IMPLEMENTATION

The first priority in planning care for a person with dysfunctional grief is to assess the risk for violence toward self or others. The client's physical health is also a major concern. The plan includes efforts to work toward resolving the grief through emotional, cognitive, and behavioral means. Chemical dependency presents a major barrier to the individual's goal attainment, and the nurse needs to address it. Dependence on anxiolytic medications is common. In many cases, the approach can be growth oriented rather than directed only to treatment of symptoms.

Nursing Interventions

Bereavement care ideally takes place in the community before the client deteriorates to the extent that hospitalization is required. Nursing interventions are prioritized according to client needs and safety issues.

1. Assess the client for intent to kill self or harm or kill others *to ensure safety and prevent violence.*
2. Promote a therapeutic alliance between the client and the nurse. *Developing a working relationship is sometimes difficult because of the client's suppressed feelings. Death and other major losses are often experienced as complete destruction of the certainty and order around which people structure their lives. It is therefore necessary for the nurse to be certain and orderly with respect to following through on all obligations such as schedules and appointments.*
3. Facilitate the client's expression of feelings related to the loss, and validate the feelings already expressed by the client. Also, begin to introduce the possibility of other feelings related to the loss, such as ambivalence. Help the client take an increasingly active role in exploring and understanding the full response to the grief. *Ambivalent feelings are especially difficult for many clients to acknowledge. Many clients are prone to merely repeat feelings and thoughts rather than explore, expand, and understand them. Although some repetition of feelings, concerns, and experiences is unavoidable and somewhat helpful, it is important for the client to understand the full grief response to begin the healing process.*
4. Help the client understand the relationship between self and the lost person or object and to express and understand the grief and attendant feelings. Facilitate a review of the client's relationship with the deceased, and help the client to discuss and understand meanings within the relationship, hopes fulfilled, disappointments, and strengths and weaknesses of the relationship. *It is essential for the client to move beyond the grief that is related to the death or loss and begin to understand the full meaning of the relationship, both good and bad.*
5. Facilitate the full expression of grief by assisting the client in linking together the full spectrum of feelings, both positive and negative, regarding the loss and the relationship with the deceased. *It is necessary for the client to remember the deceased as a real human being with both positive and negative qualities, to "let go" of the idealistic image of the person, and begin to move forward without guilt and remorse. Some survivors are more successful at this than others.*
6. Promote interactions with others and offer limited and specific options for the client to increase **social support,** both individually and in the community. Encourage the client to continue engaging in social relationships—even when, as some mourners say, it feels as if "it's just going through the motions." *It is important for the client to begin to move forward and "join the living," even if it means "going through the motions" at first. With encouragement from family and friends, the client will eventually develop a healthy social life while experiencing (in a healthy sense) both good and bad memories of the deceased.*

Collaborative Interventions

A multidisciplinary approach by a team consisting of nurse, psychiatrist, psychologist, social worker, occupational therapist, and other health care providers is not usually necessary, although community resources are an important part of care. Because of the frequency and vagueness of physical complaints, the most important discipline other than nursing is the client's nurse practitioner or physician or other source of primary care.

Problem-Oriented Grief Therapy

Health care providers offer grief therapy when a problem—not necessarily dysfunctional grief—exists or is anticipated. Like other of life's unavoidable processes, the difficult and painful transitions in normative grief usually respond to understanding and support. Grief therapy often focuses on emotional responses to the loss and problem solving related to moving forward in life (i.e., undoing bonds of attachment) (Parkes, 2001; Worden, 1982; Bowlby, 1980) or finding reconstructing meaning in the loss or relationship (Neimeyer, 2001).

Emotional issues center around the telling and retelling of the details of the story (of the death and surrounding issues) and the history of the relationship, with emphasis on the experience and expression of the feelings, particularly sadness, anger, guilt, or other troubling feelings (Carpenito, 2002). In earlier phases of the process, the bereaved person recalls only the positive qualities of the deceased. As the mourner progresses through the grief work, and the scar begins to heal, both positive and negative qualities of the deceased and the relationship emerge. Problem-focused strategies address questions of developing support, relationships, and other issues inherent in "the new life" or life after a loved one dies. Family-oriented therapy focuses on improving communications, increasing cohesiveness, and enhancing problem solving.

The death of a spouse is especially important. Researchers have rated it highest among all losses, although experts cite loss of a child as being the most risky. Death of a spouse presents the surviving mate with a host of new responsibilities previously performed by the deceased (e.g., paying the bills, doing the weekly shopping). Widowhood is difficult at any age. For older adults who are unable to manage their home alone, the loss of home and community compounds the grief. For parents with young children, the trauma of being both mother and father is a daunting task. Also, the loneliness experienced in suddenly living without the emotional support of a partner is profound at any age (Mabry, 2006).

Loss occurring during childhood predisposes a child to many physical, emotional, and behavioral problems. There is an increased risk for suicide in the adolescent period, as preteen and teenage children have a more mature understanding of death as being permanent rather than transitory. It is useful to listen to children and adolescents express their thoughts of death and dying and to respond in accordance with their understanding and developmental stage. Adolescents who are given some control over their lives may feel more empowered and less helpless when dealing with grief (Cerel et al., 2006).

In response to frequent overuse of medications to mask grief, some practitioners discourage the use of anxiolytic or antidepressant medications for bereaved persons. Even in cases of normal grief, however, some mourners require short-term use of these medications at certain stages of the grief process. Selective serotonin reuptake inhibitors are the mainstay of therapy in most settings and for most problems of grief, including dysfunctional grief (Fortinash and Holoday Worret, 2007; Casarett et al., 2001).

Reassurance is an essential component in grief therapy. The absence of cultural norms for expressing or otherwise dealing with grief results in some people feeling as if their grief is the beginning of insanity. They say things like, "I'm going crazy," or "I think I'm losing my mind." Although some will not initially believe it, they need to hear from the nurse that their experience is grief and is normal and not mental illness. The tasks in grief, described earlier, provide a framework for therapy.

Interventions in Dysfunctional Grief

In dysfunctional grief there is often unresolved grief from the past or a preexisting psychologic condition that the nurse needs to address as part of the grief therapy. Therapy thus includes the issues noted previously and other interpersonal issues. Often, a central issue in dysfunctional grief is the promotion of the client's ability to express the pain of the grief rather than only the anger or guilt (Ackley, 2002; Carpenito, 2002). It is common for bereaved persons to have ill-defined fantasies of catastrophe if their pain is expressed: "If I ever start crying, I will never stop." Clients with dysfunctional grief are at increased risk for suicide or, to a lesser extent, for hurting others. Some also experience physical and mental disorders as previously discussed (see the Research for Evidence-Based Practice box).

Intervention studies are looking at the validity of the constructs of dysfunctional grief (Bonanno, 2006). New research offers a cognitive-behavioral model that suggests that clients use narrative strategies that have special meaning for them to cope with devastating loss. The cognitive-behavioral model focuses on the client's struggle to integrate the loss into autobiographical memory (Boelen et al., 2006; Neimeyer, 2006).

The client's primary physician, nurse practitioner, or other source of primary health care needs to be involved or at least kept aware of treatment for several specific reasons. First, it is common for such clients to frequently seek medical care, often for vague or difficult-to-evaluate complaints that are actually somatic expressions of grief. Awareness of dysfunctional grief and ongoing therapy will help health care providers avoid unnecessary tests and treatment. Second, there is significant risk of suicide in dysfunctional grief, and an informed health care provider needs to be alert to suicidal hints, gestures, and attempts to obtain lethal amounts of medications. All health care professionals involved in the care of a person with dysfunctional grief need to be alert to the possibility of the client's seeking help from multiple sources and the potential for lethal medication admixture.

CLINICAL ALERT

The likelihood of **suicide** attempts and completion increases in grief, especially dysfunctional grief. The loss of psychosocial support systems is especially significant for men. Sustained loss of self-esteem, blaming self for the death, and ambivalence about living indicate that suicide risk is markedly increased.

RESEARCH for EVIDENCE-BASED PRACTICE

Piper WE et al: Prevalence of loss and dysfunctional grief among psychiatric outpatients, *Psychiatric Services* 52:1069, 2001.

The purpose of the clinical investigation was to examine the prevalence of significant loss through the death of another person as well as complicated (or dysfunctional) grief among psychiatric outpatients. Of 729 clients questioned about losses, 55% had suffered the loss of one or more loved one in their lifetimes. Of this 55%, 235, or about 33%, met the criteria for moderate or severe complicated grief. Criteria included intrusion or avoidance of loss stimuli, pathologic grief, grief anxiety, and general symptomatic distress. Compared with other psychiatric outpatients, including those who had suffered the loss of loved ones, those with severe complicated grief had significantly higher levels of depression, anxiety, and general symptomatic distress; 33% positive findings in any physical or mental pathology or symptomatology is highly significant. Questions about loss are uncommon in psychiatric interviews, as are client complaints about loss. Implications of this study include the need for loss and grief assessment among psychiatric clients, cost-effective means of treating complicated grief, and preventive measures among bereaved persons.

EVALUATION

The nurse evaluates the client's increasing ability to express feelings and to develop effective coping strategies such as increasing social interactions. It is important for the client to express the full spectrum of feelings that are (1) associated with the loss and (2) related to the relation-

NURSING CARE PLAN

Mr. Grey and his wife had been married for 40 years when she suddenly died 17 months ago from a cerebral aneurysm. Since his wife's death, Mr. Grey has become increasingly seclusive. He expresses extreme anger toward the physicians and nurses who were in the emergency room when his wife died. Mr. Grey keeps his home exactly as it was when his wife was alive. He has not disposed of any of her belongings and has renewed subscriptions to magazines that only Mrs. Grey read. Both Mr. and Mrs. Grey drank heavily but denied alcoholism. They had no children, and their relationship was characterized by frequent verbal and occasional physical abuse. Mr. Grey continues to drink daily. He complains of heart problems and is angry with his physician, who insists that Mr. Grey has only mild hypertension that should respond to dietary changes and a cessation of alcohol consumption. Mr. Grey has begun keeping his curtains drawn, ignoring his neighbors and friends, and denies the need for interpersonal relationships.

DSM-IV-TR DIAGNOSES

Axis I	Major depression; alcoholism
Axis II	None known
Axis III	Hypertension
Axis IV	Loss of primary support group (death of spouse) Problem related to the social environment (living alone, isolating self)
Axis V	GAF = 40 (current); GAF = 45 (past year)

Nursing Diagnosis *Complicated grieving (chronic distorted) related to inability to appropriately express the full spectrum of feelings associated with wife's death, as evidenced by social isolation, projected anger, daily alcohol use, and somatic complaints*

NOC Coping, Motivation, Psychosocial Adjustment: Life Change, Personal Health Status, Role Performance, Depression Self-Control, Communication, Grief Resolution

NIC Grief Work Facilitation, Coping Enhancement, Anger Control Assistance, Guilt Work Facilitation, Support System Enhancement, Emotional Support, Counseling

CLIENT OUTCOMES	NURSING INTERVENTIONS	EVALUATION
Mr. Grey will engage in a therapeutic alliance with the home health nurse.	Visit Mr. Grey's home at a regular time on the same day once each week. *Constancy and dependability are essential in developing productive relationships.*	Mr. Grey reluctantly agrees to visits by the nurse.
Mr. Grey will cease intake of alcohol at least 4 hours before and during visits with nurse.	Develop a contract with Mr. Grey in which he agrees to sobriety during visits. *Sobriety is essential to therapeutic relationships and personal growth.*	Mr. Grey maintains sobriety during visits.
	Institute chemical dependency care plan (see Chapter 14).	Mr. Grey enters and continues in a 12-step or other program intended to promote sobriety.
Mr. Grey will express anger, sadness, and other feelings appropriately related to his wife's death.	Gradually present Mr. Grey with aspects of his grief experience that will help him uncover his sadness and ambivalence. *Feelings of sadness and ambivalence are threatening to Mr. Grey. Do not introduce these too rapidly in the interventions.*	Mr. Grey is able to appropriately express sadness, confusion, ambivalence, and other feelings in addition to anger.
	Recognize the legitimacy of Mr. Grey's anger. Demonstrate acceptance and understanding of the ambivalence and other feelings such as sadness and confusion. *Anger is the means by which Mr. Grey is expressing other feelings not yet in his awareness. Facilitating other feelings helps to better manage anger and promote resolution of grief.*	Mr. Grey begins to accept the validity of anger and feelings other than anger that are hidden behind the expression of anger and rage.
Mr. Grey will discuss his hopes (fulfilled and unfulfilled) and his disappointments about his relationship with his wife.	Assist Mr. Grey in reviewing his relationship with his wife and the hopes each one held, including those fulfilled and those that led to disappointments. *Although Mr. Grey's problems are attributed to his wife's death, they are also, to a great extent, attributable to his relationship with his wife and his difficulty coping with the loss of his wife.*	Mr. Grey discusses his relationship with his wife in realistic terms (neither idealized nor all negative) and expresses both positive and negative feelings about their relationship.
Mr. Grey will grieve in a functional manner for his wife, for their relationship, and for himself.	Facilitate Mr. Grey's linking together all of his feelings and responses related to his relationship with his wife, to his life, and to his current dysfunctional behavior. *This is the full expression of grief.*	Mr. Grey fully expresses his grief.

Continued

NURSING CARE PLAN—cont'd

Nursing Diagnosis *Social isolation related to seclusive behavior patterns secondary to unresolved grief, as evidenced by refusal to engage in interpersonal relationships*

NOC Loneliness Severity, Depression Level, Self-Esteem, Communication, Social Support, Social Involvement, Personal Well-Being

NIC Visitation Facilitation, Grief Work Facilitation, Socialization Enhancement, Hope Instillation, Self-Awareness Enhancement, Support System Enhancement

CLIENT OUTCOMES	NURSING INTERVENTIONS	EVALUATION
Mr. Grey will agree to regular visits in his home with the nurse.	Adhere to 30-minute limit for visits; be prompt according to schedule. *Structure in care increases order, understanding, and predictability and will help promote Mr. Grey's developing cognitive coping strategies, such as making realistic plans for the future.*	Mr. Grey tolerates visits and eventually remarks that he looks forward to them.
Mr. Grey participates in one social activity weekly. (Alcohol should not be served or available.)	Give Mr. Grey choices of time-limited social activities that are likely to be enjoyable and convenient for him. *Activities that are enjoyable and sociable are more likely to be repeated; too many choices are likely to be overwhelming; time limits will reduce anxiety.*	Mr. Grey follows through and attends activities, and he expresses a favorable response.
Mr. Grey participates in the termination phase of the relationship by increasing his social activities and continuing in his recovery from alcoholism.	Include Mr. Grey in plans for termination by working *with* him to make plans for increased social activity as the relationship is terminated. Together, the nurse and Mr. Grey write a schedule for termination that decreases the frequency of visits and ultimately ends the visits. *The therapeutic alliance progresses from collaboration between the nurse and client to the client's achieving independence.*	Mr. Grey (1) participates in planning for termination, (2) initiates additional social activities, and (3) continues in his recovery.

CLIENT and FAMILY TEACHING GUIDELINES

Grief

There is little tradition related to grief in this contemporary technologic society. It is therefore extremely helpful to provide persons who are bereaved with normative data about grief. This includes common physical, cognitive, behavioral, and affective responses to grief. It is helpful to write a list of grief reactions (in lay person's terms) and review the list with the person who is bereaved. The power or intensity of feelings in response to loss is especially important to discuss with the bereaved person.

ship with the deceased. Expressing feelings only about the loss itself is not sufficient for successful progress in grief work (see the Client and Family Teaching Guidelines box). Remember that grief is a normal response to loss and that the feelings associated with grief are necessarily painful. The key to successful grief work depends on the individual's understanding of the relationship with the deceased. When that occurs, the client is able to continue the work of investing in new relationships.

CHAPTER SUMMARY

- Grief encompasses all spheres of being. Symptoms include physical, cognitive, behavioral, and affective reactions.
- Although grief is commonly presented in stages, it is more effective to conceptualize grief in terms of a dynamic process in which certain tasks are usually accomplished.
- Grief is classified as acute, anticipatory, dysfunctional or pathologic, and as chronic sorrow. Types of dysfunctional grief include traumatic grief, absent or inhibited grief, conflicted grief, and chronic grief.
- The potential for dysfunctional grief decreases in situations where clients have a healthy family life, provide care for the person who is dying, participate in community-oriented bereavement programs, and receive therapy if they are at risk.
- Therapy for persons experiencing dysfunctional grief includes facilitating expression of suppressed feelings, mobilizing cognitive and behavioral coping skills, dealing with unresolved aspects of the relationship, and encouraging reentry into socialization and meaning of life.
- Children and adolescents need to express their own thoughts and feelings about death and dying. Adolescents need to be monitored during grief as they can be at risk for suicide.
- Researchers are still studying a cognitive-behavioral approach model focusing on survivors' struggles to integrate loss into autobiographical memory for those experiencing complicated grief.

REVIEW QUESTIONS

1 A client who continues to be tearful and has difficulty verbalizing feelings of sadness regarding a parent who died 11 years ago is experiencing which type of grief?

1. Traumatic grief
2. Conflicted grief
3. Inhibited grief
4. Chronic grief

2 A client with a new diagnosis of liver cancer says, "I can't believe this is happening to me. My mother died of cancer. I can't go through that." Select the highest priority nursing diagnosis.
1. Grieving
2. Ineffective coping
3. Ineffective denial
4. Risk for self-directed violence

3 A child dies after being hit by a car. The physician tells the parents, "Your child's injuries were so severe that there was nothing we could do." What is the initial nursing intervention?
1. Bring the parents to a room to be alone.
2. Explain all the medical interventions attempted.
3. Stay with the parents until a support person arrives.
4. Give the parents a referral for a grief-counseling group.

4 A man was killed during a robbery attempt 10 days ago. His widow, who has a long history of major depression, cries spontaneously when talking to the nurse about her loss. Select the nurse's best response.
1. "The sudden death of your husband is hard to accept. I'm glad you're able to tell me how you're feeling."
2. "This loss is harder to accept because you have a severe mental illness. Try to focus on other activities."
3. "Your tears let me know you are not coping appropriately with your loss. Let's make an appointment with your physician."
4. "I'm concerned that you're crying so much. Your grief over your husband's death has gone on too long."

5 Four teenagers are killed in an automobile accident. Three days later, which behavior indicates that one of the teenagers' parents is coping effectively with their loss?
1. Returns immediately to his or her employment
2. Forbids other teens in the household to drive a car
3. Isolates him or herself at home and refuses visitors
4. Marks the site of the accident with flowers

Additional self-study exercises and learning resources are available to you on the ***Companion CD*** *at the back of the book and on the* ***Evolve website*** *at* ***http://evolve.elsevier.com/Fortinash/.***

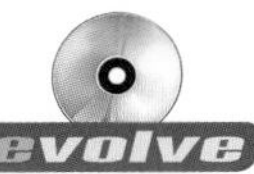

REFERENCES

Ackley BJ: Anticipatory grieving. In Ackley BJ, Ladwig GB, editors: *Nursing diagnosis handbook*, ed 5, St Louis, 2002, Mosby.

American Psychiatric Association: *Diagnostic and statistical manual of mental disorders*, ed 4, text revision, Washington, DC, 2000, American Psychiatric Association.

Boelen PA, van den Hour MA, van den Bout J: A cognitive behavioral conceptualization of complicated grief, *Clin Psychol* 13:141, 2006.

Bonanno GA: Is complicated grief a valid construct? *Clin Psychol* 13:129, 2006.

Bowlby J: *Loss: sadness and depression*, vol 3, *Attachment and loss*, New York, 1980, Basic Books.

Burke ML et al: Current knowledge and research on chronic sorrow: a foundation for inquiry, *Death Studies* 16:231, 1992.

Carpenito LJ: *Nursing diagnosis: application to clinical practice*, Philadelphia, 2002, Lippincott.

Carse JB: *Death and existence*, New York, 1980, John Wiley & Sons.

Casarett D, Kutner JS, Abrahm J: Life after death: a practical approach to grief and bereavement, *Ann Intern Med* 134:208, 2001.

Cerel, J et al: Childhood Bereavement: Psychopathology in the 2 years postprental death, *J Am Acad Child Adolesc Psychiatry* 45:681-690, 2006.

Charlton R et al: Spousal bereavement: implications for health, *Fam Pract* 18:614, 2001.

Cowles KV, Rodgers BL: The concept of grief: a foundation for nursing research and practice, *Res Nurs Health* 14:119, 1991.

Engel G: Grief and grieving, *Am J Nurs* 64:93, 1964.

Fortinash KM, Holody Worret PA: *Psychiatric nursing care plans*, ed 5, St Louis, 2007, Mosby.

Freud S: Mourning and melancholia. In Strachey J, editor: *The standard edition of the complete psychological works of Sigmund Freud*, vol 14, London, 1917, Hogarth Press.

Gibbons MB: A child dies, a child survives: the impact of sibling loss, *J Pediatr Health Care* 6:65, 1992.

Goodman M et al: Cultural differences among elderly women in coping with the death of an adult child, *J Gerontol* 46:321, 1991.

Heffner JE, Byock IR: Palliative and end-of-life pearls, Philadelphia, 2002, Hanley & Belfus.

Hentz P: The body remembers: grieving and a circle of time, *Qual Health Res* 12:161, 2002.

Horowitz MJ et al: Diagnostic criteria for dysfunctional grief disorder, *Am J Psychiatry* 154:904, 1997.

Hsu AY: *Grieving a suicide: a loved one's search for comfort, answers and hope*, Downers Grove, Ill, 2002, Intervarsity Press.

Jacob SR: The grief experience of older women whose husbands had hospice care, *J Adv Nurs* 24:280, 1996.

Jacobs S, Mazure C, Prigerson H: Diagnostic criteria for traumatic grief, *Death Stud* 24:185, 2000.

Kemp C: Refugee mental health issues, *Refugee health*, 1998; www.baylor.edu/Charles_Kemp/refugee_health.htm.

Kemp C: Spiritual care in terminal illness. In Ferrel B, Coyle N, editors: *Oxford textbook of palliative nursing*, ed 2, pp 595-604, Oxford, 2006, Oxford University Press.

Kemp C, Chang B-J: Culture and the end of life: Chinese, *J Hospice Palliative Nurs* 4:1, 2002.

Lichtenstein B, Laska MK, Clair JM: Chronic sorrow in the HIV-positive patient: issues of race, gender, and social support, *AIDS Patient Care STDS* 16:27, 2002.

Lindemann E: Symptomatology and management of acute grief, *Am J Psychiatry* 101:141, 1944.

Mabry R: *The tender scar: life after the death of a spouse*, Grand Rapids, Mich, 2006, Kregel.

Melhem NM et al: Comorbidity of Axis I disorders in patients with traumatic grief, *J Clin Psychiatry* 62:884, 2001.

National Institutes of Health (NIH): Loss, grief and beveavement (PDQ); www.cancer.gov, update June 19, 2006.

Neimeyer RA: Reauthoring life narratives: grief therapy as meaning reconstruction, *Isr J Psychiatry Relat Sci* 38:171, 2001.

Nuss WS, Zubenko GS: Correlates of persistent depressive symptoms in widows, *Am J Psychiatry* 149:346, 1992.

Parkes CM: Bereavement. In Doyle D, Hanks GWC, MacDonald N, editors: *Oxford textbook of palliative medicine*, ed 2, Oxford, 1998, Oxford University Press.

Parkes CM: Bereavement dissected: a re-examination of the basic components influencing the reaction to loss, *Isr J Psychiatry Relat Sci* 38:150, 2001.

Pejlert A: Being a parent of an adult son or daughter with severe mental illness receiving professional care: parents' narratives, *Health Soc Care Community* 9:194, 2001.

Piper WE et al: Prevalence of loss and dysfunctional grief among psychiatric outpatients, *Psychiatr Serv* 52:1069, 2001.

Reisman AS: Death of a spouse: illusory basic assumptions and continuation of bonds, *Death Studies* 23:445, 2001.

Ringdal GI et al: Factors affecting grief reactions in close family members to individuals who have died from cancer, *J Pain Symptom Manage* 22:1016, 2001.

Shneidman ES, *Voices of death*, New York, 1980, Harper & Row.

Silverman GK, Johnson JG, Prigerson HG: Preliminary of the effects of prior trauma and loss on risk for psychiatric disorders in recently widowed people, *Isr J Psychiatry Relat Sci* 38:202, 2001.

Silverman PR, Worden JW: Children's reactions in the early months after the death of a parent, *Am J Orthopsychiatry* 62:93, 1992.

Stroebe M et al: On the classification and diagnosis of pathological grief, *Clin Psychol Rev* 20:57, 2000.

Tomita T, Kitamura T: Clinical and research measures of grief: a reconsideration, *Compr Psychiatry* 43:95, 2002.

Worden J: *Grief counseling and grief therapy: a handbook for the mental health practitioner*, New York, 1982, Springer.

Chapter 27

Mental and Emotional Responses to Medical Illness

RUTH N. GRENDELL

Mental outlook has an impact on physical health. Health is improved by optimism and acceptance, and is diminished by anger, pessimism, and unrelenting chronic stress.

KENNETH PELLETIER

OBJECTIVES

1 Discuss the historical and theoretic perspectives related to stress.

2 Define the major physiologic and psychosocial stressors and their impact on health status.

3 Describe the potential negative impact that stress has on multiple body systems.

4 Summarize the biologic and psychologic responses to stress.

5 Discuss adaptation to stress (cognitive appraisal, autonomic nervous system responses, and use of coping mechanisms).

6 Discuss the prevalence of HIV/AIDS, particularly in vulnerable populations.

7 Distinguish between adjustment disorders and Axis I mood disorders in persons with HIV/AIDS using the criteria of severity of symptoms, treatment, and prognosis.

8 Examine potential interactions between behavioral characteristics of persons coping with HIV/AIDS and treatment adherence management.

9 Discuss the significance for nurses who provide holistic health care to vulnerable groups.

10 Describe the independent and collaborative interventions nurses and other health care professionals use for clients experiencing stress-related health problems.

11 Apply the nursing process for persons with HIV/AIDS.

12 Explain the concepts of empowerment and self-care.

13 Identify factors influencing the current and future trends in self-care.

KEY TERMS

acquired immunodeficiency syndrome, p. 611
acute illness, p. 610
acute stress disorder, p. 610
AIDS dementia complex, p. 614
CD4 count, p. 615
cognitive appraisal, p. 609
coping, p. 610
daily hassles, p. 609
distress, p. 608
eustress, p. 608
general adaptation syndrome, p. 609
general inhibition syndrome, p. 609
homeostasis, p. 608
human immunodeficiency virus, p. 611
psychologic stress, p. 608
psychoneuroimmunoendocrinology, p. 610
secondary appraisal, p. 609
stress, p. 608
viral load, p. 615

tations. Initial symptoms are usually memory impairment and concentration difficulties. These symptoms are often overlooked and frequently confused with symptoms associated with depression. However, some clients complain of forgetfulness, "slowed thinking," and difficulty concentrating when engaged in conversations, watching TV programs, or reading. In some cases, poor balance and coordination occur early on. As this syndrome progresses, with no chance of reversal, clients become dependent on others for completion of activities of daily living. Many clients and their caregivers fear the development of dementia. Some have observed friends whose lives were significantly compromised by AIDS dementia in all areas—cognitive, motor, and behavior. In addition, AIDS dementia is not easy to identify, and symptoms increase and decline, causing a great deal of uncertainty and anxiety. For this reason, early thorough assessment and instruction of the client and caregivers about signs and symptoms are extremely important interventions.

With the arrival of new therapies, researchers are hopeful that AIDS dementia will decline and that some clients with dementia will regain their lost abilities. Whether these symptoms are reversible and what level of cognitive improvement will result are the subjects of ongoing study.

Nurses working with clients diagnosed with AIDS, who also have dementia, participate in the neuropsychiatric assessment of their clients by recording problems related to memory, attention span, concentration, and motor deficits. They provide support to the client, family, and friends who are assuming client care. Caregivers or partners sometimes welcome respite care or home care, depending on the client's functional status and needs. It is important to help clients and their families remember treatment and medication schedules. This includes the use of checklists, bulletin boards, pill boxes, alarms, and other strategies to promote self-care management and ease the burden of care for significant others.

Additional Treatment Modalities

Nursing interventions contribute significantly to the client's ability to cope effectively with HIV disease. It is important to keep in mind, however, that other disciplines and therapies also play a critical role in the client's ability to deal with psychologic distress related to HIV. Currently accepted treatments of adjustment problems in clients with HIV/AIDS parallel those for other populations with adjustment disorders, but this section addresses important key differences related to the following: pharmacologic intervention, the preferred format for individual counseling, psychosocial support networks specific to persons living with HIV/AIDS and their significant others, and the use of other methods to decrease stress and promote clients' highest level of functioning.

Three studies reported similar results between coping and levels of depression in HIV-positive men and women. Group interaction and social support provided avenues for the individuals to express their concerns, to relieve their depression, and to acquire a sense of self-worth and acceptance (Ashton et al., 2005; Blaney et al., 2004; Sikkema et al., 2004).

Pharmacologic Intervention

Medical. Formerly the first line of treatment for HIV was prescription of a reverse transcriptase inhibitor (e.g., AZT). This was called monotherapy because only one agent was involved. With advances in antiretroviral therapies, more complex courses of therapy have replaced monotherapy approaches. Combination antiretroviral therapies include HAART and mega-HAART. These treatment plans include reverse transcriptase inhibitors and protease inhibitors. These classifications of drugs work together to interrupt production of new viruses. Combination therapies are the most effective treatment available, but some cause disabling side effects.

Psychopharmacology. Psychotropic medications are useful in the treatment of clients with HIV disease. There are no medical reasons to avoid their use. The most common psychotropic medications HIV/AIDS clients experiencing moderate to severe distress are antidepressants and anxiolytics. The best outcome results from the use of medications with combined cognitive behavioral counseling approaches. Counseling and psychotherapy are generally the standard of care for clients with significant, persistent depression or anxiety. Still, in the case of demoralization syndromes (adjustment disorders), some clients respond well to unstructured support with a caring provider who is not technically trained (Angelino and Treisman, 2001).

Antidepressant medication is sometimes prescribed if the client manifests a significant depressed or anxious condition. Sometimes an antidepressant is given as a preventative measure in anticipation of new uncontrollable stressors. Anxiolytics are prescribed in daily dosages or as needed to reduce the client's anxiety. The choice of antidepressant or anxiolytic and dose of medication often depends on the client's neurovegetative symptoms and underlying physical illness. For example, for an agitated client with gastroenteritis who is also having difficulties with diarrhea because of the disease or complications from treatment, an antidepressant medication with more anticholinergic action are sometimes the best choice. This medication reduces diarrhea and provides mild sedation and thus works to the client's advantage. In addition to the individual's overall health status and specific emotional distress, the age of the client is important. For example, older adults and adolescents are generally treated with lower doses of psychotropic medications. The first step in antidepressant treatment is to assist the client to consistently take the medication and to use an adequate therapeutic dose (Angelino and Treisman, 2001). Generally physicians begin with low doses of the chosen medication and slowly increase the level to minimize medication side effects. Remember that in addition to the potential side effects clients experience while on antidepressants, they are also experiencing to varying degrees side effects from their antiretroviral medications. Once the client is on a dose of medication for at least 2 weeks, reassess the client for improvements in mood and the presence of any continuing distressing side effects. With this assessment, nurses are able to make decisions about modifying or keeping the medications as prescribed.

Integrative Therapies

In the absence of a definitive cure, many clients with HIV have chosen to supplement their treatment programs with complementary/integrative therapies or treatments. Ordinarily, medical physicians do not provide these complementary therapies; but these thrapies can be combined with the client's medical treatment. Complementary therapies in HIV/AIDS include mind-body remedies or herbal supplements aimed at reducing the individuals' symptoms or treatment side effects, enhancing immune status, or improving their sense of well-being. Examples of these therapies include, acupuncture, massage, herbs, vitamins, meditation, and stress reduction. With few exceptions, these approaches are helpful and not harmful. Exceptions are the use of Saint-John's wort, which reduces the blood plasma concentration of indinavir, a protease inhibitor, and garlic supplements, which interact with saquinavir, another protease inhibitor. Caution clients to discuss the use of an herbal or dietary supplement with their health care provider to prevent any adverse effects resulting from interactions with their antiviral treatment therapy (see Chapter 25).

The stress of HIV infection is chronic and usually continues over long periods with acute exacerbations. Nurses need to recommended alternative methods of managing stress. Along these lines, there are well-documented techniques (e.g., stress reduction, meditation, relaxation techniques) that are extremely useful to many persons at various stages of HIV/AIDS. For example, nurses are able to teach stress management strategies and progressive relaxation exercises to clients. Stress management manuals and self-help books, as well as brief workshops in the community, are available to help clients learn these techniques. Some of these instructional aids are also on videotape.

Nurses also need to recognize, discuss, and support the individual's desire to control psychologic distress through alternative methods, including spiritual practices. Spirituality as treatment is receiving increased attention, as a growing body of literature suggests that there is an important connection between how a person interprets the meaning of his or her illness and the ability to cope with illness and loss. Taking spirituality and prayer into account when assessing an individual's needs and resources and in developing intervention strategies requires a shift in perspective.

Nurses monitor clients' self-management strategies for other reasons as well. Nurses must caution clients that bodies infected with HIV are different from disease-free systems. Weight loss generated by diet changes and physical exercise is usually more of a problem than a desired goal. Unnecessary dieting and strenuous exercise resulting in a reduction of calories need to be minimized. The recommendation for exercise focuses on moderation, with the major goal of exercise being strength building and resistance training. Adding muscle mass is a good thing; burning calories is not.

EVALUATION

When nursing interventions are successful, the client will usually show significant signs of improvement in coping ability. If coping ability improves, changes in client mood, behavior, and functional abilities will also improve. Increases in clients' understanding of their illness and treatment will also be evident. A large part of the treatment of persons with HIV/AIDS is individualized teaching to help them regain and maintain a sense of control over their lives, symptoms, and disease.

Effective coping is evident in the outcome criteria addressed in the treatment plan—that is, clients will demonstrate an ability to manage and contain uncomfortable feelings of fear, anxiety, guilt, grief, and depression. As their ability to manage symptoms improves, the client's self-esteem and perception of self-worth will also improve. Relationships with others, especially those in caregiver roles, will be stronger because of the added instruction and support from the nurse. The client will demonstrate a realistic level of hope as a result of the nurse's efforts to help him or her find meaning in life and set small, realistic goals. Although clients do not consistently experience a strong sense of well-being, they should experience improved quality of life based on increased feelings of cognitive, behavioral, and decisional control. Helping clients achieve control minimizes their fear, anxiety, and depression associated with HIV/AIDS while maximizing their ability to cope with illness and multiple losses. They will more likely follow their antiretroviral therapy regimen when they can make choices.

NURSING CARE PLAN

Steve, a 32-year-old white man, formerly a travel agent, has been retired for 2 years because of complications from AIDS. He has had a history of depression since his early 20s and has received outpatient counseling for it. He sees his physician regularly; currently he has esophageal candidiasis and wasting syndrome. He came to the clinic appointment expressing a great deal of hopelessness about his future. He stated that he did not want to live anymore and that he was tired of fighting AIDS. When asked if he had thought about suicide or had a suicide plan, he hesitated when stating that he thought about a quick death by jumping out of a window.

DSM-IV-TR DIAGNOSES

Axis I	Major depression, recurrent
Axis II	Deferred
Axis III	Acquired immunodeficiency syndrome (AIDS) with candidiasis and wasting syndrome
Axis IV	Moderate: financial difficulties
Axis V	GAF = 50 (current); GAF = 60 (past year)

Nursing Diagnosis *Powerlessness related to responses to treatment of HIV disease and symptoms, as evidenced by verbalization of suicidal thoughts and plans, inability to forecast a positive future, verbalization of powerlessness as a result of physical decline, decreased functioning, and lack of progress in treatment regimen*

NOC Hope, Self-Esteem, Health Beliefs: Perceived Control, Depression Self-Control, Stress Level, Participation in Health Care Decisions, Health Beliefs: Perceived Resources

NIC Self-Esteem Enhancement, Self-Responsibility Facilitation, Patient Contracting, Health System Guidance, Mutual Goal Setting, Decision-Making Support, Support Group

CLIENT OUTCOMES	NURSING INTERVENTIONS	EVALUATION
Steve will verbalize absence of suicidal ideation and plans.	Assist Steve to (1) identify his needs and short-term achievable goals, (2) relate these goals to his life tasks, and (3) contract to avoid acting out with suicidal gestures or attempts *to facilitate the client's adaptive coping responses and decrease feelings of loss of control; to support Steve's goal.*	Steve progressively states optimism about achieving goals within his anticipated life span.
Steve will verbalize increased feelings of personal competence and efficiency in managing his symptoms.	Assist Steve to identify options for controlling his emotional and physical distress (e.g., stress management strategies and ways to cope with fatigue and diarrhea) *to counteract feelings of powerlessness and helplessness that, if not stopped, result in hopelessness.*	Steve identifies and begins to implement new strategies for coping with his symptoms. He verbalizes feelings of competence, as identified in the main outcome.
Steve will develop a therapeutic alliance with staff.	Engage Steve in an active problem-solving approach addressing each stressor and discussing appropriate coping options/strategies *to evaluate Steve's coping options/methods.*	Steve regards the nurse as a facilitator and supportive resource. He initiates discussion of stressors and options to reduce stress.
Steve will initiate social interactions with others with HIV to gain information and support.	Refer Steve to support groups and particularly voluntary home care services *to help Steve gain information and support.*	Steve attends support group of his choice or identifies at least one other person with HIV/AIDS who he is able to talk to on a weekly basis.
Steve will identify barriers or problems associated with exacerbation of his anxiety/depression.	Assist Steve in reviewing what events or thoughts increase his anxiety/depression *to avoid such events, when possible, through increased awareness.*	Steve expresses awareness of recurring stressors that worsen his anxiety and depression.
Steve will verbalize goal-directed plans that are both achievable and solution focused.	Assist Steve in formulating goals that are realistic and achievable. Direct these goals toward improving the quality of life and reducing stressors in day-to-day living *to decrease frustration and increase success through goal attainment.*	Steve states two or three short-term goals he can realistically commit to in his present condition.

CHAPTER SUMMARY

- Historically, the scientific community considered the body, mind, and spirit as separate entities. Physical health and illness were major concerns, and few paid attention to the mental and emotional responses to physiologic problems.
- Multicausal and psychologic theories provide a framework for understanding the person's response to stress and its relationship to physiologic and psychologic interactions.
- Common psychosocial responses to stress and illness are fear, anxiety, feelings of powerlessness and helplessness, hostility, and anger. Depression often prohibits effective coping and adaptation.
- Coping is the use of resourcefulness and ability to manage the stress of daily circumstances such as the challenges posed by pain, disability, acute, or chronic disease. Coping mechanisms are conscious or unconscious, adaptive or maladaptive.

- Adaptation is a complex and a continuous demanding process, particularly in accepting loss of independence and valued roles.
- HIV disease is a major public health problem worldwide. Some persons infected with HIV are asymptomatic for long periods of time. AIDS is the advanced stage of HIV disease.
- HIV/AIDs is a chronic disease that affects multiple body systems including the brain and the central nervous system. Many individuals experience significant psychologic stress related to the awareness of their diagnosis and the subsequent need for adaptation to the consequences of this life-threatening chronic illness.
- Dramatic shifts in the numbers of persons living with AIDS have occurred as a result of the development of effective antiretroviral medication therapy. Consequently, more people are living longer with HIV and will ideally learn to cope effectively with the ongoing impact of their disease and treatment.
- Certain disadvantaged minorities have a disproportionate number of AIDS cases. These populations traditionally have experienced problems in accessing health care services. Shifts in rates of HIV infection suggest that adolescent girls and women are increasingly vulnerable for HIV/AIDS.
- One principal DSM-IV-TR diagnosis among persons with HIV/AIDS is adjustment disorder. This diagnosis is differentiated from other mood disorders (e.g., major depression).
- Nurses conduct assessments and interventions in collaboration with the client and, in some cases, family or significant others.
- Psychotropic medications are helpful for some clients experiencing more severe depression or anxiety, especially when coupled with structured or unstructured supportive counseling.
- The psychosocial needs of those infected and affected by HIV are numerous and present significant challenges to quality of life and the management of treatment adherence in these individuals and their families or significant others.
- Complementary therapies, such as stress reduction, relaxation, and spirituality or prayer, are useful to many clients in various stages of HIV disease.
- The current Western health care model includes a greater emphasis on health promotion across the life span, self-care management, and a holistic approach in managing acute and chronic psychosocial and physiologic health problems.
- The nurse has an essential role in helping clients recognize the impact of stress and assisting them in selecting appropriate coping mechanisms and promoting the best possible quality of life.

REVIEW QUESTIONS

1 Over the past 2 years, an individual's parent dies, rheumatoid arthritis is diagnosed, employment is terminated, and the person's spouse begins divorce proceedings. Which complaint(s) would the nurse expect? You may select more than one answer.

1. "I'm having trouble remembering to pay my bills every month."
2. "All this stress has helped me focus on what I really need to accomplish."
3. "It seems like I catch every little virus that goes through our community."
4. "I'm beginning to feel like I am losing control of my life."
5. "My energy levels have increased in response to these stressful events."

2 A nurse wants to research interactions between the neurologic, endocrine, and immune systems in response to psychosocial stressors. Which search term would yield the desired information?

1. Multicausal theories of disease
2. Psychoneuroimmunoendocrinology
3. General adaptation syndrome
4. Epidemiology

3 An adult is hospitalized with pneumonia and dehydration secondary to advanced AIDS. The client is confused and delusional. Which nursing diagnosis should be included in the plan of care?

1. Disturbed thought processes
2. Hopelessness
3. Powerlessness
4. Risk-prone health behavior

4 A young adult is informed of a positive laboratory test for HIV. The client tells the nurse, "Well, I know what I need to do now." What is the nurse's next action?

1. Give information on local support groups.
2. Assess the client's suicidality.
3. Discuss results of the newest medication research.
4. Arrange a consultation with the social worker.

5 Which individual would have the highest risk for clinical depression?

1. An individual with AIDS and whose CD4 count decreased over the past week
2. An individual who believes there is a risk for HIV infection but has not had testing
3. An individual with AIDS and a recent sudden onset of Kaposi's sarcoma
4. An individual with AIDS and whose viral load increased over the past month

*Additional self-study exercises and learning resources are available to you on the **Companion CD** at the back of the book and on the **Evolve website** at **http://evolve.elsevier.com/Fortinash/**.*

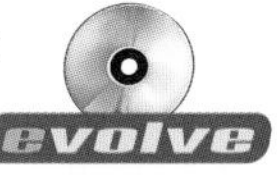

REFERENCES

American Psychiatric Association: *Diagnostic and statistical manual of mental disorders*, ed 4, text revision, Washington, DC, 2000, American Psychiatric Association.

Anderson R: Psychoneuroimmunoendocrinology review and commentary, *Townsend Letter for Doctors & Patients* 265/266: 102-106, 2003.

Angelino AF, Treisman GJ: Management of psychiatric disorders in patients with human immunodeficiency virus, *HIV/AIDS CID* 33:847-856, 2001.

Ashton E et al: Social support and maladaptive coping as predictors of the change in physical health symptoms among persons living with AIDS, *AIDS Patient Care STDs* 19:57-598, 2005.

Bing EG et al: Psychiatric disorders and drug use among human immunodeficiency virus-infected adults in the United States, *Arch Gen Psychiatry* 58:721-728, 2001.

Blaney N et al: Psychosocial and behavioral correlates of depression among HIV-infected pregnant women, *J Aids Patient Care STDs* 18:405-415, 2004.

Bottonari K et al: Life stress and adherence to antiretroviral therapy among HIV positive individuals: a preliminary investigation, *Aids Patient Care STDs* 19:719-727, 2005.

Carpenito L: *Nursing diagnosis: application to clinical practice*, ed 10, Philadelphia, 2003, Lippincott.

Centers for Disease Control and Prevention: *HIV surveillance report, June 2001*, Atlanta, 2006 U.S. Department of Health and Human Services.

Cook J, Tyor W: The pathogenesis of HIV-associated dementia: Recent advances using a SCID mouse model of HIV encephalitis, *Einstein Q J Biol Med* 22:32-40, 2006.

Cooperman N, Simoni J: Suicidal ideation and attempted suicide among women living with HIV/AIDS, *J Behav Med* 28 149-156, 2005.

Cote J, Pepler C: Cognitive coping intervention for acutely ill HIV positive men, *J Clin Nurs* 14, 321-326.

Cumbie S, Conley V, Berman M: Advanced practice nursing model for comprehensive care with chronic illness: model for promoting process engagement, *Adv Nurs Sci* 27:70-80, 2004.

Hellman E: Theories of health promotion and illness management. In Black J et al, editors: *Medical-surgical nursing: clinical management for positive outcomes*, ed 6, Philadelphia, 2001, Saunders.

Holmes T, Rahe R: The social readjustment rating scale, *J Psychosom Med* 11:213-218, 1967.

Lazarus R: Theory-based stress management, *Psychol Inq* 1:3-13, 1990.

Lazarus R, Folkman S: *Stress, appraisal and coping*, New York, 1987, Springer.

Liewer S: Hospital adding wing for combat casualties, *San Diego Union-Tribune*, pp A-1, 8, June 15, 2006.

Lenz R: Army changes tack in treating combat stress, *San Diego Union-Tribune* (Associated Press), p A-21, June 4, 2006.

Marelich W, Murphy D: Effects of empowerment among HIV+ women on the patient-provider relationship, *AIDS Care* 25:475-482, 2003.

Neurnberger P: *Freedom from stress: a holistic approach*, Honesdale, Pa, 1981, Himalayan International Institute of Yoga Science and Philosophy. (classic)

Neville K: Uncertainty in illness: an integrative review, *Orthop Nurs* 22:206-214, 2003.

Neyland T: Hans Selye and the field of stress research, *J Neuropsychiatry Clin Nuerosci* 10:230, 1988.

North American Nursing Diagnosis Association International: *NANDA-I nursing diagnoses: definitions and classification 2007-2008*, Philadelphia, 2007, NANDA-I.

Pender N, Murdaugh C, Parsons M: *Health promotion in nursing practice*, ed 4, New York, 2001, Pearson Education.

Plattner I, Meiring N: Living with HIV: the psychological relevance of meaning making, *AIDS Care* 18:241-245, 2006.

Porth C: *Pathophysiology: concepts of altered health states*, ed 5, Philadelphia, 2004, Lippincott.

Russell C, White M, White C: Why Me? Why now? Why multiple sclerosis?: Mmaking meaning and perceived quality of life in a Midwestern sample of patients with multiple sclerosis, *Fam Syst Health* 13:65-81, 2006.

Selye H: *The stress of life*. New York, 1956, McGraw-Hill. (classic)

Shea K: Reframing: a fresh outlook helps patients envision positive outcomes, *Pathways to Professional Development*, pp 56-59, 2006. (*Nurseweek* publication)

Sikkema K et al: Outcomes from a randomized controlled trial of a group intervention for HIV-positive men and women coping with AIDS related loss and bereavement, *Death Stud* 28: 187-209, 2004.

Springer L: Human immunodeficiency virus infection. In Lewis S et al, editors: *Medical-surgical nursing: assessment and management of clinical problems*, St Louis, 2004, Mosby.

State Legislatures Report: State Legislatures, 34, one page, Apr 2004.

Stuart G: *Principles and practice of psychiatric nursing*, ed 7, St Louis, 2004, Mosby.

UNAIDS Press Release: World leaders chart way to reverse AIDS epidemic: AIDS from obscurity to global emergency, Mar 31, 2006; retrieved from www.aegis.com/news/unaids/2006/UN060508.html.

U.S. Department of Health and Human Services, CDC: Update: trends in AIDS incidence—United States, 1996, *MMWR Morbid Mortal Wkly Rep* 46:861, 2006.

Williams K, Kurina L: The social structure, stress, and women's health, *Clinical Obstet Gynecol* 45:1099-1118, 2002.

Witek-Janusek L: *Stress in medical-surgical nursing: assessment and management of clinical problems*, ed 6, Lewis M et al, editors, St Louis, 2004, Mosby.

World Health Organization (WHO): Retrieved June 17, 2006, from www.who.int/health_topics/chronic_disease/en.

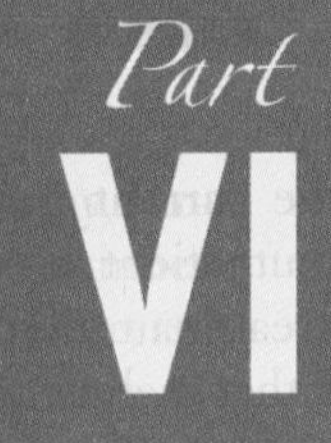

COMMUNITY PSYCHIATRIC NURSING

Chapter 28

Caring for Clients in the Community

ALWILDA SCHOLLER-JAQUISH

If there is any great secret of success in life, it lies in the ability to put yourself in the other person's place and see things from his point of view as well as your own.

Henry Ford

OBJECTIVES

1. Discuss the factors that influenced the deinstitutionalization movement.
2. Describe the components of community mental health nursing.
3. List outpatient treatment options commonly available in community settings.
4. Discuss the legal influences affecting health care for severely and persistently mentally ill persons.
5. Compare and contrast therapy and rehabilitation.
6. Discuss the components of case management.
7. Describe ways in which you will play an integral role in symptom management and medication compliance.
8. Explore ways that you will provide health promotion and early intervention for mentally ill persons at risk for HIV/AIDS.
9. Discuss the complications of obesity in persons with severe and persistent mental illness.
10. Analyze the impact of substance abuse, including smoking, on persons with severe and persistent mental illness.
11. Explain the impact of managed care on community psychiatric rehabilitation.
12. Analyze the key elements of psychiatric home health care.
13. Identify factors that contribute to the homelessness of people with severe and persistent mental illness.
14. Describe the cultural needs of community residents with severe and persistent mental illness.
15. Explore the factors contributing to the incarceration of mentally ill persons.
16. Identify the predictors of violence in the mentally ill.
17. Apply the nursing process to clients in the community and in the home.

KEY TERMS

adult family home, p. 634
adult residential treatment program, p. 633
capitation, p. 629
case management, p. 632
Clubhouse Model, p. 631
community mental health center, p. 628
congregate care facility, p. 634
deinstitutionalization, p. 626
least restrictive, p. 627
psychosocial rehabilitation/skills training program, p. 631

mentally ill persons are gay or lesbian and as such require appropriate nursing interventions (Hellman, 1996).

Pregnancy

There are legal and ethical concerns related to pregnancy and the potential effects of psychotropic medications. Antipsychotic medications affect the fetus; however, withholding medications from a pregnant woman will exacerbate psychotic behavior. Discuss concerns about the expectant mother and unborn infant in collaboration with the mother, psychiatrist, and obstetrician (Jaffe, 2002). If possible, the expectant mother needs to avoid medications that affect the fetus. An alternative to psychotropic medications is electroconvulsive therapy, which is safe to use throughout pregnancy (Lentz, 1996). Depending on the expectant mother's support system, it is advisable to include social workers and a legal advocate to protect the best interests of the fetus and the mother.

Psychiatric nurses working with mentally ill pregnant women need to be aware that pregnancy is a time of unstable behavior under the best of circumstances (Munroe, 2002). Providing for the safe care of the mother and fetus is challenging for all concerned. Pregnant mentally ill women present a complex set of obstetric, psychiatric, social, family, and legal concerns ("Gold Award," 1996; Miller and Finnerty, 1996).

One study suggested that postpartum exacerbations may be clustered in families, which may indicate a genetic connection. Nurses caring for pregnant mentally ill women need to conduct a careful family history as part of a comprehensive plan of care (Jones and Craddock, 2001).

Violent and Criminal Behavior

Persons with severe and persistent mental illness commit a disproportionate number of violent or criminal acts, which reveals lack of judgment and self-control. These persons respond with violence to perceived threats (Green, 1997). Violence by a person with severe and persistent mental illness is dangerous for family members or care providers. Children are sometimes the targets of verbal and physical aggression. Violent behavior often makes community living difficult if not impossible. There is an even greater risk for violence in persons with a dual diagnosis (e.g., when drug and alcohol abuse coexist).

Many persons with severe and persistent mental illness have had extensive contact with the criminal justice system. People with mental illness commit crimes for a variety of reasons, as poor impulse control and acting-out behaviors result in disorderly conduct, disturbing the peace, and trespassing. Some of these individuals commit more serious crimes, such as shoplifting, petty theft, and prostitution, as a means of survival (Lamb and Weinberger, 1998; Teplin et al., 1996).

Some persons with severe and persistent mental illness commit violent crimes that pose a threat to public safety, such as residential burglary, assault, rape, and robbery. Young persons with severe and persistent mental illness who have had little mental health treatment are more likely to commit criminal acts of violence, such as the recent shootings at Virginia Tech. The three primary predictors of violence are a history of past violence, drug and alcohol abuse, and failure to take medication. As many as 1000 people in the United States are murdered each year by persons with severe and persistent mental illness (Torrey, 1996). Unfortunately, murder has become the leading occupational hazard as persons with severe and persistent mental illness act out their anger and delusions against their supervisors and coworkers (Schmitt, 1999).

Many mass murders have been committed by people who experienced hallucinations or delusions coupled with poor impulse control and substance abuse. With the restricted policies for hospitalization, many violent persons are treated for a brief period and then released. Persons with severe and persistent mental illness who commit violent crimes are often delusional. These persons commit crimes because of command hallucinations. They believe voices tell them to perform certain acts. Others commit violent crimes because they are unable to control their impulsive urges (Sadock and Sadock, 2006; Silva et al., 1997; Torrey, 1997).

Persons with severe and persistent mental illness who commit criminal acts of violence are more likely go to prison than to a psychiatric institution. Even in prison, persons with psychosis are legally allowed to choose whether they will take their medication. The rights of the individual and the goal of freedom of choice often conflict with the rights of family members to live without fear of harm to themselves or others.

CLINICAL ALERT

Women with **severe and persistent mental illness** are at great risk for victimization (Center for Mental Health Services [CMHS], 2000), and children of mentally ill parents are at risk for mental and physical problems (Gopfert et al., 1996).

CLINICAL ALERT

A client who commits a **violent act** toward an individual just before admission to a hospital is likely to attack that same person within 2 weeks after discharge. Hospital personnel need to make an attempt to warn the potential victim, per hospital and regulatory protocols, if the client voices threats before discharge (Tardiff et al., 1997) (see Chapter 8).

PERSONS WITH SEVERE AND PERSISTENT MENTAL ILLNESS WHO HAVE SPECIAL PROBLEMS

Within the population of people with severe and persistent mental illness there are subgroups with unique problems that affect their ability to respond to psychiatric interventions.

Mentally Retarded Persons

Essential features of mental retardation are an IQ below 70 and impairments in adaptive functioning that began before the person was 18 years old. Behavioral patterns include cognitive deficits revealed in concreteness of thinking and neurologic dysfunction. Persons with mild to moderate retardation are more susceptible to mental illness. The conflict between the person's expectations and actual abilities are a source of lifelong stress. In addition to a variety of personality disorders, the person with mental retardation and mental illness sometimes experiences affective, as well as psychotic disorders. There are indications that at least 40% of individuals with mental retardation meet the criteria for at least one psychiatric disorder (Sadock and Sadock, 2006). Depression and psychotic disorders are underreported in persons with mental retardation (Gorman, 1997). A breakdown of central nervous system processing is a common feature in persons with a diagnosis of mental retardation and mental illness. Researchers have associated self-stimulating and self-injurious behaviors with underlying neurologic dysfunction (Gorman, 1997). Treatment for this special population requires an interdisciplinary approach. Psychopharmacology is an important modality used in conjunction with other therapies such as counseling, cognitive therapy, behavior management, social skills training, and activity therapy (Reiss, 1993).

Persons With Sensory and Communication Impairments

Individuals with sensory deprivations experience many difficulties communicating with others, which their mental illness further exacerbates. Persons with severe and persistent mental illness and sensory impairment are often hospitalized much longer and receive less treatment (Fitzgerald and Parkes, 1998). Some have reported cases in which hearing-impaired clients were institutionalized for many years before it became known that the individual's social deficits were not a result of mental illness. Any person with symptoms of severe and persistent mental illness needs to receive a careful medical evaluation before a final diagnosis is made.

Older Adults

Older adults with severe and persistent mental illness include those who have had mental illness for decades, as well as those whose mental disorder was diagnosed after age 50 years. Older adults who develop severe and persistent mental illness often have a severe onset that family members and care providers do not immediately recognize. Depression is a serious problem in older adults and requires appropriate intervention to reduce the risk of suicide. Schizophrenia usually presents during the early years of a person's life, and there are many people who have grown old with this condition (Harvey et al., 1997). Nevertheless, schizophrenia also manifests after age 45 years. Family members of older adults with severe and persistent mental illness find themselves becoming a primary caregiver in a most difficult situation at a difficult time in their lives (Eliopoulos, 2000).

Alzheimer's disease and other dementias are the most common causes of mental illness in older adults. As many as 20% of older adults over the age of 80 years suffer some form of dementia. The onset of dementia is threatening and requires careful evaluation and diagnosis (Sadock and Sadock, 2006; Pace-Murphy et al., 2002). The behavioral changes in older adults with severe and persistent mental illness are disturbing to spouses and adult children. Family members have concerns about the person's safety, as well as his or her memory loss and disorientation. Some older persons become so agitated that they require intensive treatment (Mintzer et al., 1997). As persons with senile dementia continue to lose cognitive ability, they sometimes strike out in fear at family members, who they no longer recognize. The mental deterioration of the older person sometimes precipitates emotional disturbances in the spouse or adult children. Partial hospitalization provides an effective method of treatment for individuals with agitated dementia (Shoemaker, 2000).

According to estimates, the exploding population of people over age 65 years will reach 35 million by the year 2000 and will be more than 64 million by the year 2030. There will possibly be 16 million mentally ill older adults by the year 2030. The combined effect of increased costs for extended care facilities and the limitations placed on services by insurance programs result in limited care for the aged with severe and persistent mental illness. This places an increasingly large burden on the adult children. Adult children, especially daughters, are fulfilling most dependence needs of older parents. Not only is the burden of care difficult, but it is often psychologically difficult for the caregiver who is now responsible for the dependent parent. The awareness of the stress and psychologic strain for caregivers has resulted in a variety of educational programs designed to assist them in coping with unexpected life situations (Pruchno et al., 1997; Seltzer and Li, 1996).

The stress and strain of providing care for a dependent parent affects the entire family system. Male in-laws are more likely to report marital problems than female in-laws. The presence of strong family support and the avoidance of conflict reduce the stress for caregiving family members. Emotional distance and family demands on the caregiver increase the risks for stress and strain for the caregiver, the older person, and the extended family (Lieberman and Fisher, 1999).

Research associates abuse of persons with dementia by their caregivers with the premorbid existence of family violence. Spouse abuse continues in the form of maltreatment by care providers (Buttell, 1999). Nurses working with clients with Alzheimer's disease and their families need to explore the nature of spouse and family relationships before the onset of dementia (see Chapter 15).

Substance Abuse

Persons with severe and persistent mental illness who are also dependent on one or more substances are among the most difficult to treat in either psychiatric or substance abuse treatment programs. Persons with a **dual diagnosis** mental illness from gaining access to appropriate psychiatric care. General hospital units have become locked wards to house people with severe and persistent mental illness who were a threat to the safety of others. The restriction of mental health benefits by third-party payers has significantly reduced the amount of time a client receives care (Sharfstein et al., 1998) (see Chapter 8).

Aftercare

Aftercare programs include a variety of community programs and services from partial hospitalization to sheltered living. The types of programs available in a specific community depend on the size and nature of the community, as well as the community's financial constraints. Outpatient clinics are often associated with acute care hospitals. The size of the outpatient programs and the extent of their services depend on the availability of reimbursement for services (Fenton et al., 1998; Gater et al., 1997). Insurance companies limit the number of days of therapy that they will pay for specific disorders.

Some have developed a variety of community programs in more recent years. Some include partial care services with day care provided in an acute care hospital and a return to the individual's place of residence at night. Partial care programs place their emphasis on improving the capabilities of persons with severe and persistent mental illness. Other living arrangements include lodgings for four or more people. In some situations, a manager visits the residence once a day or at other periodic intervals. Some programs provide for a live-in manager who helps the residents resolve interpersonal or household issues. People living in assertive community programs have lower rates of rehospitalization in some cases (Getty et al., 1998; Gater et al., 1997; "Gold Award," 1997; Klinkenberg and Calsyn, 1996). Community service programs such as mobile outreach and crisis interventions provide access to care for difficult-to-reach persons ("Gold Award," 1997).

Homeless Shelters

Other types of community programs that provide services to persons with severe and persistent mental illness include homeless shelters, soup kitchens, and substance abuse treatment programs. These individuals consistently use the same program or go from place to place. Most service providers for the homeless have restrictions on serving individuals who are actively hallucinating, intoxicated, or displaying threatening acting-out behaviors. Persons who are noncompliant with the provider's rules are often refused admission or forced to leave the facility. Thus, some of the most incoherent persons are turned away from the only places that remain available to them. Persons with severe and persistent mental illness who become homeless do not have contact with family, health care services, and providers therefore often suffer the full ravages of untreated mental disorders. Shelters provide an evening meal, a change of clothes, and a place to take a shower. However, they have no staff or facilities to deal with the psychotic or violent behavior homeless people with severe and persistent mental illness experience (Scholler-Jaquish, 2000a).

Foster Care

Foster care is a temporary or permanent way of removing the child, adolescent, or adult with severe and persistent mental illness from an unsafe environment. Children with severe and persistent mental illness are sometimes at risk for abusive behavior from parents or siblings. Therapeutic foster care must be carefully selected to ensure that the child is in a safe environment. Adults at risk in their own homes are sometimes removed to foster care to receive appropriate physical care and engage in healthy interpersonal relationships.

Prisons and Jails

Current reports suggest that from 6% to 15% of persons in city and county jails are those with severe and persistent mental illness and that up to 15% of those in the prison population have severe mental disorders. Many of these offenders have a history of mental illness and are unable to function well in society. A large number of prisoners with severe and persistent mental illness are also homeless (Lamb and Weinberger, 1998; Jordan et al., 1996; Teplin et al., 1996). Incarceration of persons with severe and persistent mental illness poses serious problems for these individuals, as well as for the prison system.

Some individuals are arrested for minor offenses and are held in the local jail. Mentally ill persons are sometimes arrested because no facilities are available. They are often arrested for minor offenses such as vagrancy, trespassing, disorderly conduct, or failure to pay for a meal. Jails are inadequately prepared to care for the severely mentally ill offender who is able to refuse to take psychotropic medications. The suicide rate among mentally ill offenders is higher than for any other group of offenders (Open Society Institute, 2002).

Family members often find it necessary to have a relative with severe and persistent mental illness arrested for violent or threatening behavior. In some situations, emergency involuntary admissions require that the person making the arrest or signing the commitment orders has to also witness the violent behavior. If that does not happen, the individual is jailed for his or her mental illness rather than admitted to a psychiatric facility. Many persons with severe mental illness serve long-term prison sentences with a minimal amount of psychiatric treatment. There is a concern that prison facilities are becoming like the asylums of the past.

Family

The majority of people with severe and persistent mental illness live with their families. Family members are key players in providing community mental health services. They assume responsibility for the client with little if any support, few resources, and no appreciation. The behaviors associated with severe and persistent mental illness

CLIENT and FAMILY TEACHING GUIDELINES

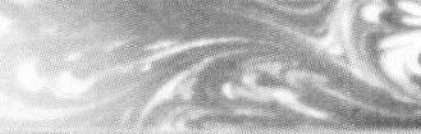

Tips for Managing a Crisis

- It is important to attempt to reverse any escalation in psychotic symptoms and provide immediate protection and support for the person with severe and persistent mental illness and for family members.
- Warning signs of a crisis include sleeplessness, ritualistic behaviors, increased suspiciousness, and unpredictable outbursts.
- Remember that things always go better if you speak softly and in simple sentences. It is uncommon for a person to lose total control of thoughts, feelings, and behaviors.
- Accept the fact that this individual is in an altered state of reality and will sometimes act out in response to hallucinations.
- It is important to stay calm. Trust your feelings; if you are frightened, take immediate action to protect yourself, according to learned techniques (if you have been instructed in self-protection). Do nothing, however, to aggravate the situation. If you are alone, call for someone to stay with you while professional help is on the way. If it is necessary to call the police, explain that your relative is mentally ill and that you need help during this crisis. (If police know that this is a psychiatric crisis, they are more likely to respond with strategies than if they think that criminal activity is in progress.)
- Some simple tips include the following:
  - *Don't threaten.* This increases fear or increases the risk of violent behavior.
  - *Don't shout.* If the person isn't listening to you, he or she is probably listening to other "voices" (hallucinations).
  - *Don't criticize.* It will only make things worse.
  - *Don't argue with other family members.* This is not the time to fix blame or prove a point.
  - *Don't bait the person.* This leads to the person acting on his or her wild threats, and the consequences could be tragic.
  - *Don't stand over the mentally ill person.* If the person is seated, seat yourself, as safety permits, because standing may pose a threat.
  - *Avoid continuous eye contact or touching.* This intimidates the person, especially if paranoia exists.
  - *Comply with requests that are not dangerous.* This gives the individual a sense of control and increases cooperation.
  - *Don't block the doorway.* However, place yourself between the client and an exit, in the event that you may need to leave the area.
  - *Evacuate.* All family members should be evacuated in the event that the person appears to be out of control and there is risk for injury. Seek immediate help.

intrude on the lives of the family members and make extraordinary demands of them. The stressors experienced by family members depend on the family's physical endurance and emotional health, as well as on the nature and intensity of the individual's illness.

It is important to know that the family structure provides the greatest support for adults with severe and persistent mental illness; however, it is a position of great responsibility for all concerned. Family providers need referrals to self-help groups or for counseling to maintain their emotional stability. The Client and Family Teaching Guidelines box details information a nurse needs to provide to the client and family.

Under any circumstance, it is difficult to live with a family member who has a severe and persistent mental illness, whether he or she is hospitalized, acting out, or in an interval between psychiatric symptoms (remission). Nurses working with persons with severe and persistent mental illness need to be aware of the needs and concerns of family members.

HEALTH PROMOTION ACTIVITIES

Health promotion activities include many forms of education programs and are often described in terms of illness prevention and a means of maintaining wellness. Health promotion activities for persons with severe and persistent mental illness reduce the frequency of exacerbations, increase the individual's ability to live independently, and improve medication compliance. These activities also improve care practices, increase recognition of signs and symptoms indicating the need for interventions, and help families function more effectively. The next sections describe examples of health promotion activities.

Activities of Daily Living

These activities are individually designed charts or plans developed with the family and client, or goals established with the individual and caregiver. A schedule of telephone contacts provides support and encouragement for persons with severe and persistent mental illness. These activities remind the individual about his or her medications and assess the person's level of functioning.

Medication Education

Nurses need to provide and reinforce education about medications, frequency, side effects, and the need for compliance. Individuals with these disorders need to know about the potential side effects of medications and the appropriate action to take when they begin to be troubled by side effects or begin to think about discontinuing their medication (see Chapter 24).

Family Education

Family education includes the nature of severe and persistent mental illness and the changes associated with long-term health problems. These educational programs include signs and symptoms of exacerbation (return of symptoms), as well as strategies about how to respond to positive and negative symptoms. Families need instruction on developing methods for coping with individuals who demonstrate psychotic or violent behaviors (see Chapter 22).

Sex Education

Sex education is an essential nursing intervention that includes appropriate sexual behaviors and personal hygiene, as well as the importance of regular gynecologic examinations and recognition of abnormal signs and symptoms. The nurse needs to teach sexually active men about the use of condoms and avoiding unsafe sexual behaviors. Women need to know about the risks involved in pregnancy and how to protect themselves from unwanted pregnancy, sexually transmitted diseases, and the potential for violence (see Chapter 19).

Family Support

Support, encouragement, and assistance in coping with daily life events are essential for families with persons who have severe and persistent mental illness. Spouses play a significant role in the quality of life for their partners. Exacerbations place additional strains on what is already a difficult life situation. Children of parents with severe and persistent mental illness need assurance that they are not responsible for their parents' illness. They also need assistance in finding healthy adult role models.

Promotion Programs for the Community

These programs consider the importance of reintegrating persons with severe and persistent mental illness into the community. School programs need to stress recognition of signs and symptoms of mental illness in children and adolescents. Nurses need to develop strategies for dealing with children and adolescents who talk about suicide, or committing destructive acts against themselves or others (see Chapter 21).

Physicians and nurses providing medical care for clients with severe and persistent mental illness need to learn about the person's normal response to pain and discomfort. It is important that persons with severe and persistent mental illness receive appropriate care when they become ill.

PUBLIC POLICY ISSUES

Nurses have opportunities to make an impact on public policies at the local, state, and national levels. National policies relating to persons with severe and persistent mental illness need to address the need for programs that are more flexible, comprehensive, and easier to access. There is a critical need for coordinated services with consistent financing at the city and state levels. Treatment programs in general and psychiatric hospitals in particular have to be more creative in their approaches to treating clients with severe and persistent mental illness. Individuals who are clearly unable to care for themselves must not be left to live on the streets without treatment and without access to psychiatric care. Persons who pose a threat to society because of their violent behavior require treatment in appropriate mental health facilities rather than criminal intervention that will worsen their condition.

One of the most acute problems facing persons with severe and persistent mental illness is housing, because they vary in their need for supervised living arrangements. Provisions for housing in a variety of settings need to be available, including adult foster care and residential treatment programs. Adequate low-income housing could be made available for persons with severe and persistent mental illness who have low-paying jobs or for those who subsist on entitlements alone. The lack of adequate housing is as severe a problem as the unavailability of adequate care.

Access to care is an increasingly important concern. The individual's ability to access the mental health system depends on his or her ability to seek assistance, as well as knowledge. Nurses play an important role in advocating for increased resources for mental health care. In addition, nurses educate self-help groups and other community groups about the nature and impact of severe and persistent mental illness. The quality of the available mental health care is also a concern for nurses. Short-term, episodic care is not sufficient to provide adequate care for persons with severe and persistent mental illness. Walk-in mental health clinics need to be available for these clients and their families. The clinics could monitor medication compliance, as well as provide individual or group psychotherapy. Psychopharmacology alone is not sufficient treatment for persons with severe and persistent mental illness. These individuals also need access to psychotherapy to assist them with the complexity of their lives and their feelings.

Models for providing mental health services to persons with severe and persistent mental illness vary according to regions of the country and resources available. Mental health professionals have advocated a comprehensive health team approach to address the variety of problems these individuals experience. A treatment team of professionals will provide more and better-coordinated services than mental health specialists working independently of one another.

Special programs need to be in place for the care and treatment of homeless persons with severe and persistent mental illness. There are strong indications that available programs such as homeless shelters or soup kitchens are effective means to reach homeless persons with severe and persistent mental illness. Nurse-managed clinics in shelters and soup kitchens allow for easy access to health care professionals (Scholler-Jaquish, 2000a). These clinics could also distribute psychotropic medications to help homeless persons with severe and persistent mental illness increase their compliance with treatment and improve their ability to function in the world.

THE NURSING PROCESS

ASSESSMENT

When conducting an initial assessment interview with a person with severe and persistent mental illness, it is important to be sensitive to the client's concerns. Establishing a therapeutic relationship begins with the development of a sense of trust between the nurse and the client. The nurse needs to explain the nature and purpose of the interview and tell the client where the interview will take place and approximately how long it will last. The nurse allows for as much privacy as possible while using appropriate precautions during the interview, as these clients may have a history of poor impulse control or violent outbursts. It is critical to review client history if available (see Chapter 3).

Effective assessment provides the nurse with information about the nature of the client's problems (Box 29-1). Clients with severe and persistent mental illness often

Text continued on p. 657

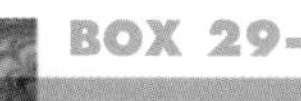

BOX 29-1

Assessment of Clients With Severe and Persistent Mental Illness

PHYSIOLOGIC DISTURBANCES

Physical Integrity

The nurse will examine the client to determine if there is evidence of impaired skin integrity, such as abrasions, bruises, lacerations, scars, and needle puncture sites. Abrasions and bruises indicate that the client had a self-inflicted injury or trauma before admission. It is important to determine if the injuries are recent or almost healed, as well as the nature and source of the injuries. When examining abrasions and bruises, it is always important to determine if infection or inflammation is present. If there is a history suggestive of trauma or violence, it is important to carefully inspect the client's body surface for additional injuries.

Hormonal/Metabolic Patterns

Children with severe mental illness often have inborn errors of metabolism. The nurse obtains this information through the client's history or from observing the child's physical characteristics. Does the client have a history of diabetes mellitus or kidney disease? Assess female clients for their menstrual patterns. In each of these areas of concern, the nurse needs to know if the client is taking any medications for metabolic or hormonal disturbances.

Circulation

The nurse will assess the client's medical record for indications of neurologic changes and cardiac status.

Nutrition

Assessment of the client's nutritional history and present status is important, as many of these individuals live a disorganized and confused lifestyle, which often alters their nutritional intake significantly.

Physical Regulation

Assessment of physical regulation includes the client's temperature and the potential for infection. The medication history for persons with severe mental illness is important. It is necessary to know the nature and type of medications that the client has been prescribed, as well as his or her compliance in taking the medications. Also, evaluate disturbances of the immune system at this time.

Oxygenation

Assessment of the client's respiratory system includes evidence of dyspnea, cough, or labored breathing. Determine if the client smokes, how long he or she has been smoking, and the number of cigarettes smoked each day.

Elimination

It is essential to know if the client has normal elimination habits. The nurse will want to know if the client has difficulties in handling urine or stool, or ritualistic behaviors associated with elimination. Screening the client's urine for nonprescription drugs and psychotropic medications is also sometimes necessary.

MOBILITY DISTURBANCES

Activity

The nature and extent of the client's activity patterns provide important information for the nurse. The presence of any physical disability such as paralysis or fractures affects the development of the nursing care plan. The nurse needs to know if there are problems walking, tremors, or ritualistic behavior associated with moving from place to place. The client with severe mental illness sometimes demonstrates lethargic movements or is hyperactive and moves rapidly from place to place. Lethargy is related to major depression or catatonic features of schizophrenia. Hyperactivity is related to agitation associated with anxiety, hallucinations, paranoid delusions, mania, or other mental or neurologic disorders.

Rest

The person with severe and persistent mental illness often has sleeping patterns that differ from the norm. Some clients exhibit sleep reversal (sleeping during the daytime and being awake during the night). Assess the person's ability to fall asleep and remain asleep. Individuals who have difficulty falling asleep sometimes have symptoms of depression or psychomotor agitation. Some obsess about suicide while awake and require a more thorough assessment and medications to help them sleep.

Recreation

Individuals with severe and persistent mental illness have a significant deficit in diversional activities. The person is often so preoccupied with the symptoms of the mental disorder, or the effort it takes to get through the day, that he or she leads a dull and uninteresting existence. Too much free time on a client's hands leads to thought disorders and suicidal ideation if there is underlying depression. The client needs support in planning activities throughout the day.

Environmental Maintenance

The nurse's assessment of the client's ability to manage his or her living arrangement provides important cues about the treatment plan, as well as for discharge planning. If the person lives in a group situation, the nurse needs to know the extent to which the client participates in maintaining individual and shared living space.

Safety

The most important component of this section and a nursing priority, includes assessing the individual's risk for injury, violence, and the possession of weapons. Persons with severe and persistent mental illness are at risk for harming themselves or others. Suicide rates are high in these individuals, so thoroughly assess for suicidal ideations, gestures, or attempts. In assessing suicidal ideations or attempts, the nurse needs to know what method the individual has used in the past (if there is a history). It is also critical to determine the availability of weapons and firearms and the person's access to them (see Chapter 21).

Self-Care

Persons with severe and persistent mental illness often have an impaired ability to perform activities of daily living, such as personal hygiene and grooming. When these individuals have significant self-care deficits, they may not be able to bathe or clean themselves appropriately.

COMMUNICATION DISTURBANCES

Verbal Communication

In times of illness and stress, bilingual individuals often resort to their native language or speak in a combined dialect that seems disordered and confused. The presence of speech impairments related to physical defects provides the nurse with important cues. Verbal symptoms of psychiatric disorders include perseveration, circumstantiality, punning, rhyming, echolalia, mutism, word salad, cryptic language, symbolic references, neologisms, poverty of content, confabulation, and logorrhea (see Chapters 12 and 15).

Continued

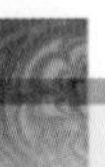

BOX 29-1

Assessment of Clients With Severe and Persistent Mental Illness—cont'd

Nonverbal Communication
Nonverbal disturbances include posture, manner of dress, and gestures. Persons with chronic mental illness may crouch on the floor, pace back and forth, or retreat from others. Their ability to make and hold eye contact provides the nurse with important cues. Gestures include ritualistic movements, striking themselves, or striking out at others. Inappropriate sexual behaviors are also important to note, as these individuals often have trouble expressing sexuality appropriately as a result of the pathology of their illness.

COGNITIVE DISTURBANCES
Orientation
Assessment of the individual's orientation to time, place, person, and situation provides essential data for the plan of care. The person with severe mental illness will possibly be aware of all issues or only a few. For example, the person knows his or her identity and whereabouts but does not know the month or the year. The client is sometimes confused about the diagnosis or does not know why he or she is hospitalized or being questioned. Mental confusion is usually related to the individual's psychiatric disorder, side effects of medications, dual diagnosis (alcoholism or substance abuse), or physical disorders (see Chapter 15).

Memory
The nurse needs to assess the individual's memory to determine if he or she has intact recent and remote memory. The individual's ability to demonstrate abstract or concrete thinking affects his or her ability to understand and communicate effectively. Problems with recent or short-term memory signify early dementia or other amnestic or cognitive disorders. Further investigation is necessary, as many things affect memory (see Chapter 15).

Perception
Also assess the person's understanding of the purpose and nature of treatment. Some persons with severe mental illness do not understand why they have been admitted to an inpatient unit, and a more thorough explanation by the nurse, done in a clear and concise way, is required. Repetition is sometimes necessary.

Thought Processes
Some with severe and persistent mental illness exhibit one or more thinking disturbances. These include dereistic and autistic thinking, delusions, thought withdrawal, thought insertion, thought blocking, thought broadcasting, magical thinking, looseness of association, ideas of reference, flight of ideas, ideas of influence, and tangentiality.

Persons with severe mental illness often have well-defined delusions such as paranoid delusions in which they believe that a force is attempting to control their minds or cause them harm. Obsessional thought patterns take the form of ritualistic behaviors or the person has an obsessive desire to control or possess another person. The nurse needs to demonstrate patience with these clients and provide a safe environment (see Chapter 12).

PERCEPTUAL DISTURBANCES
Sensory Perception
The senses include vision, hearing, taste, touch, and smell. Physical and mental disorders can impair any of these senses. Persons with severe and persistent mental illness often have hallucinations involving one or more of the senses. The more common hallucinations in schizophrenia are auditory and involve the client hearing sounds or voices. The nurse needs to acknowledge the client's hallucinations while presenting a nonthreatening reality (see Chapter 12).

Attention
The nurse assesses the client's ability to follow directions, as well as follow verbal and visual cues. Evidence of psychiatric disturbance includes distractibility, hyperalertness, inattention, or selective inattention. The individual who demonstrates extreme anxiety or manic behaviors is easily distractible and needs immediate help with focusing.

Self-Concept
The person with severe and persistent mental illness, almost by definition, has significant disturbances in self-image, self-esteem, and personal identity. Assessment for these disturbances includes statements of negative self-concept and negative self-worth. Cognitive therapy, group therapy, and activity therapy help these clients gain a sense of self-worth (see Chapter 23).

Meaningfulness
Persons with severe and persistent mental illness often have difficulty finding meaning in a life that seems purposeless and hopeless. These individuals sometimes express hopelessness (feelings and thoughts that their lives will never get better). In addition, they also express powerlessness (belief that they are unable to effect any change in their life situations). When a person expresses feelings of hopelessness and powerlessness, it is important to immediately assess for suicidal ideations (see Chapter 21).

RELATING DISTURBANCES
Role
Each person has certain role expectations that fit with societal norms. The assessment of the person's marital status and relationship with parents, siblings, spouse, children, and others provides significant information about the individual's ability to function in society.

Sexuality
Sexual relationships are often difficult for the individual to maintain. There are wide variations in sexual expression among persons with severe and persistent mental illness. Some individuals exhibit little interest, whereas others have difficulty controlling their sexual behaviors. Still others express sexuality in an inappropriate way, given the nature of their mental illness. These clients sometimes develop a sexual relationship with other clients that is not always a positive experience, as both parties are often unable to handle the responsibility of a mature sexual relationship. Education about human sexuality is useful for some clients (see Chapter 19).

Socialization
Persons with severe mental illness often have difficulties in maintaining social relationships with others. Their ability to develop a meaningful relationship with people outside their immediate family is often significantly impaired. The age of onset of the mental disorder affects the individual's ability to socialize with others.

FEELING DISTURBANCES
Comfort/Pain
The person's physical condition and the presence of any injuries before hospitalization affect the individual's awareness of pain or discomfort. Some individuals with severe mental illness are not able to describe their sense of pain or discomfort and rely on the nurse or others to be aware of changes that affect their comfort level. The Joint Commission (TJC) and the Board of Registered Nurses (BRN) currently consider pain to be the fifth vital sign for all clients and is a nursing priority.

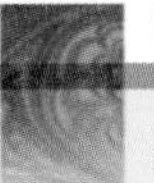

BOX 29-1

Assessment of Clients With Severe and Persistent Mental Illness—cont'd

Emotional States
Persons with severe and persistent mental illness often exhibit signs of mood disturbance such as major depression, anxiety, mania, agitation, and fear. The emotional disturbances are related to the individual's mental disorder(s). Assessing the way the individual is coping with his or her emotional disturbance is important in the plan of care. Clients sometimes express anger and aggression through sarcasm, fault finding, domineering behavior, and the threat or use of violence, in which case immediate interventions are necessary (see Chapter 11).

PROBLEM-SOLVING DISTURBANCES

Coping
Coping mechanisms of persons with severe and persistent mental illness are often inadequate or inappropriate for the situation. Defense mechanisms include rationalization, conversion, displacement, regression, introjection, projection, denial, dissociation, symbolization, fantasy, or splitting. It is important to note that some defense mechanisms are necessary for the client's emotional survival at key points in his or her illness (see Chapter 9).

Participation
The individual's ability or willingness to participate in treatment is assessed on admission and on an ongoing basis throughout the hospitalization. Persons with a history of noncompliance sometimes exhibit compliance in a controlled environment. Nurses assess the degree of compliance with the therapeutic plan through nursing observations and frequent communication with the treatment team. At some point, gentle but firm confrontation is necessary.

Judgment/Insight
Disturbances in judgment and insight are common among persons with severe mental illness. Thought disorders and disorganized living experiences seriously affect the individual's decision-making ability. These individuals exhibit indecisiveness or make poor judgments about themselves and others. The severity of the illness affects the degree of difficulty the person experiences. These individuals often need help with decisions for a period of time.

NURSING ASSESSMENT QUESTIONS

Severe and Persistent Mental Illness

1. When did you first have trouble managing your own life? *To determine duration of the illness*
2. Did your family have religious preferences? *To determine basic values in the home*
3. What is the place like where you live? *To determine the person's current living situation*
4. Is there a family member who helps you out? *To determine relationship with family members*
5. Are there times when you hear voices talking to you? *To determine presence of auditory hallucinations*
6. *(If yes)* What do the voices that you hear tell you? *To determine if voices are troubling or threatening, such as command hallucinations*
7. Have there been times when you were so excited you could hardly contain yourself? *To determine the presence of mania or hypomania*
8. Have there been times when you have thought of hurting someone else? *To determine any patterns of violence toward others*
9. Have there been times when you felt life isn't worth living? *To determine the presence of hopelessness or depression*
10. *(If yes)* Have you ever thought about ending your life? *To determine suicidal intent*
11. *(If yes)* Are you thinking about that now? *To determine if client is in imminent danger*
12. *(If yes)* Assure the client that the nurse/staff will protect him or her; proceed with usual suicide precautions *to provide safety and comfort* (see Chapter 21).

NOTE: Suicide and violence are priority nursing assessments.

have unidentified medical problems that have been neglected as a result of the individual's dysfunctional lifestyle. It is therefore important to conduct a thorough assessment of these clients, as each person presents a unique set of nursing challenges (see the Nursing Assessment Questions box).

NURSING DIAGNOSIS

Nursing diagnoses are problems formulated from the data collected during the assessment phase. Nursing diagnoses are statements that describe an individual's health state or change in life processes. They are prioritized according to the client's needs and safety risks.

Safety or Health Risks

- Risk for self-directed violence
- Risk for other-directed violence
- Risk for self-mutilation
- Risk for injury
- Imbalanced nutrition: less than body requirements
- Ineffective health maintenance
- Bathing/hygiene self-care deficit
- Dressing/grooming self-care deficit

Perceptual/Cognitive Disturbances

- Anxiety
- Fear

- Hopelessness
- Disturbed personal identity
- Powerlessness
- Chronic low self-esteem
- Disturbed sensory perception (hallucinations)
- Disturbed thought processes (delusions, impaired problem solving)

Problems Communicating and Relating to Others

- Impaired verbal communication
- Delayed growth and development
- Ineffective sexuality pattern
- Impaired social interaction
- Social isolation

Disturbances in Coping (Client or Family)

- Defensive coping
- Compromised family coping
- Disabled family coping
- Ineffective coping
- Ineffective denial

Client and Family Teaching Needs

- Deficient knowledge (medication, treatment, symptoms)
- Noncompliance (medication, therapy, aftercare)
- Ineffective role performance

OUTCOME IDENTIFICATION

Outcome criteria for persons with severe and persistent mental illness include short- and long-term client behaviors and responses to treatment. Outcomes will be stated in clear, measurable, and behavioral terms; will be identified as expected or anticipated; will be prioritized according to client needs and safety risks; and whenever possible will include a time frame in which the client is expected to achieve them. Clients with severe and persistent mental illness vary significantly in the extent and nature of their disorders. The following outcomes are not all inclusive for clients with chronic mental illness.

Client will:

- Refrain from harming self or others.
- Verbalize absence of suicidal ideation or plan.
- Demonstrate absence of violent or aggressive behaviors.
- Verbalize pain or discomfort if present
- Demonstrate absence of verbal intentions to harm self or others.
- Display control of angry, impulsive emotions.
- List several reasons for wanting to live.
- Seek staff when hallucinations begin.
- Stop talking to self.
- Demonstrate reality-based thinking in verbal and nonverbal behavior.
- Demonstrate absence of delusions.
- Sit through meals or other activities without agitation or restlessness.
- Demonstrate orientation to time, place, and person.
- Demonstrate absence of overt confusion.
- Distinguish boundaries between self and others and the environment.
- Demonstrate socially appropriate behavior.
- Initiate conversation with staff.
- Verbalize feeling in control of self and situations.
- Communicate with others using appropriate language, tone, and speech pattern.
- Participate in individual milieu and group activities without disruptions
- Engage in positive relationships with significant others or identified support persons.
- Express sense of self-worth.
- Use coping strategies in a functional, adaptive manner.
- Display consistent, optimistic attitude.
- Eat adequate amounts of different food groups.
- Demonstrate self-care appropriate for the client's age.
- Demonstrate effective problem-solving skills.
- Adhere to prescribed facility regimen.
- Make choices regarding management of care.

PLANNING

The nurse's knowledge and understanding of the complexities of providing care to persons with severe and persistent mental illness are essential in the development of a comprehensive plan of care for the individual client. Each person has his or her own history of mental disorders, previous treatment, coexisting medical illness, and current symptoms. Nursing care addresses the short- and long-term needs of the individual and family members when appropriate.

It is important to remember that the individual's disturbed disorganized thought process or mental deterioration limits how much he or she participates in the development of a plan of care. Many persons with severe and persistent mental illness have been alienated from their families and live alone or live a homeless existence (see the Case Study). For those persons, it is necessary to include community mental health care providers in the development of the nursing care plan.

IMPLEMENTATION

The plan of care for clients with severe and persistent mental illness varies depending on the nature of the person's mental disorder, age, and physical health status. Although the individual's mental disorder is long term, he or she will be admitted episodically for treatment of the disease process. General hospitals provide short-term care, whereas state psychiatric institutions provide longer term care. Nursing interventions occur in either setting; however, achievement of the goals often takes much longer for persons with severe and persistent mental illness.

These individuals experience impairment in their physical health, mental status, emotional responses, social status, and spirituality. The nurse providing care for the person with severe and persistent mental illness will be challenged to prioritize a plan that addresses the client's

CASE STUDY A psychiatric nurse who provides consultation for a local homeless shelter brought Josh (age 23) to the hospital for evaluation and possible admission. The shelter staff asked the nurse to see Josh, who was rocking back and forth on his bed, mumbling incoherently to himself. When the nurse spoke to Josh, he stated his name and date of birth. He said he had been homeless since he was 14 or 15 years old, adding, "My family thought I was strange, and they sent me away. I found a place to stay in a junkyard. The old man who owned the junkyard found me living in an old car and let me stay in an abandoned shed behind his office. He brought me food and gave me a cot to sleep on. I stayed there until last month, when the old man died. I don't have anywhere to go now. I can't stand the noise of the radio that keeps playing in my head all the time. I just wish it would stop."

CRITICAL THINKING

1 What are Josh's most immediate problems?
2 What might the hallucinations be saying to Josh?
3 What nursing diagnoses would be relevant for Josh?
4 What outcome criteria, based on the nursing diagnoses, might be established with Josh?
5 What are three appropriate nursing interventions critical to Josh's situation?

most important needs (see the Research for Evidence-Based Practice box). In addition to the manifestations of the disease process, these individuals need assistance with social interactions, self-esteem, knowledge of the disease process, compliance with the treatment regimen, and discharge planning. It is important to consider the individual's priorities when planning care away from the hospital. If the person's concerns are not addressed, this will affect his or her ability or willingness to remain compliant with the treatment plan. Involving family members or community mental health care providers in the discharge planning process will help the client maintain the highest level of functioning over a period of time.

Nursing Interventions

Nursing interventions are prioritized according to client needs and safety risks.

1. Monitor the risk of danger to client and others *to ensure safety and prevent violence.*
2. Encourage the client to alert the staff when self-destructive thoughts occur *to help client manage destructive thoughts before acting on them.*
3. Familiarize the client to the setting and modify the environment *to reduce situations that provoke anxiety.*
4. Provide positive feedback when the client demonstrates self-control *to ensure repetition of functional behaviors.*
5. Isolate the client during periods of high risk for harming self and others *to provide a safe environment.*
6. Educate family members about symptoms of noncompliance with psychotropic medications or exacerbation of the mental disorder *to promote knowledge, which enhances compliance.*
7. Educate the family in self-protective responses in relation to the client *to ensure family safety.*

RESEARCH for EVIDENCE-BASED PRACTICE

George TB: Care meanings, expressions, and experiences of those with chronic mental illness, *Archives of Psychiatric Nursing* 16:25, 2002.

The purpose of this study was to examine the care meanings, expressions, and experiences of one group of chronically mentally ill persons living in the community. Understanding their ideas about care enables nurses to provide care in a way that enhances the health and well-being of these people, reduces the frequency and length of hospital stays, and leads to more positive interactions in the community. The study included questions about the shared norms, lifeways, environment, experiences, and care meanings and how this group of people interpreted these concepts. A total of 15 clients, 9 family members, and 15 staff members participated in the study. Researchers collected data through open-ended interviews and observations over an 11-month period. They analyzed data from 54 interviews.

The meaning of care was described as listening, doing for others, spending time with others, doing things together, and sensitivity to the feelings of others. An analysis of the data related to values, norms, and lifeways revealed that the group valued respect, genuineness, honesty, and friendliness. A job was seen as a way to become independent. Many of these individuals spent time alone and often borrowed money and cigarettes. Watching television was the most frequent source of entertainment. Participants accepted waiting in line as being normal. The small amount of money they earned was spent on soft drinks, coffee, and cigarettes.

Data related to cultural and social structure factors revealed that money was a constant concern. Experiences with emergency commitments and hospitalization left the participants fearful of the police and fearful of hospitalization. Several of the participants had graduated from high school and others had taken college courses. One person was working on a baccalaureate degree. Some of the participants took part in religious services, and others thought the services were a way to make one feel comfortable. Religion was also part of the symptomatology of a few of the clients. Eleven of the 15 key informants reported that they had little if any contact with their families. Staff members stated that caring for a mentally ill relative for 20 to 30 years had sometimes resulted in families becoming "burned out." Most of the participants had never been married. Differences between themselves and the dominant culture were apparent to the participants.

The chronically mentally ill who live in the community have identifiable values, norms, and lifeways that set them apart from the dominant culture. Nurses can use this information to design and provide culturally sensitive care to those with severe and persistent mental illness.

8. Provide nonthreatening reality orientation *to decrease the risk of upsetting the client and initiating harmful reactions.*
9. Instruct the client in recognizing harmful or inappropriate behaviors *to increase the client's self-awareness.*
10. Assess the client for delusions and hallucinations *to determine the level of psychosis.*
11. Interpret the meaning of the hallucination or delusion for the client *to determine the intent.*
12. Instruct the client to alert the staff when hallucinations begin *so that the staff is able to intervene and minimize their impact.*

13. Teach techniques to stop or reduce hallucinations, such as whistling, hand clapping, and loudly telling the "voices" to stop, *to offer the client strategies to manage hallucinations.*
14. Praise efforts at controlling hallucinations *to reinforce the client's functional behavior.*
15. Work with clients to manage hygiene, grooming, and activities of daily living *to increase self-esteem by improving appearance and giving the client the satisfaction of self-help.*
16. Assist in selecting appropriate clothing *to reduce the incidence of ridicule by other clients.*
17. Monitor elimination and bathing patterns and establish a routine *to encourage proper hygiene and prevent pain or injury to the bowel and bladder. Clients with psychosis often have trouble attending to activities of daily living.*
18. Set a regular eating schedule *to remind the client when it is time to eat. Clients with psychosis often forget or refuse to eat and could become physically ill.*
19. Supervise food preparation as necessary. *Persons with psychosis are often careless in food preparation and could cut or burn themselves.*
20. Assist with regulation of sleep-wake patterns *to promote healthy sleep patterns because clients with chronic mental illness experience irregular sleep-wake patterns that could disrupt their daily routine.*
    a. Provide activities to keep the client awake during the day.
    b. Encourage dressing before breakfast and staying awake all day.
    c. Promote relaxation at night by reducing stimulation and activities.
21. Listen actively to the client's verbal and nonverbal communication *to elicit the client's style of communication and to better understand and anticipate the client's needs* (see Chapter 4).
22. Engage the client in conversations with others *to promote socialization and decrease isolation.*
23. Teach clients anxiety-reducing techniques when they are experiencing impaired communication *to reduce anxiety when clients are having difficulty expressing themselves* (see Chapters 9 and 23).
24. Praise attempts to speak clearly and effectively *to encourage repetition of the client's clear, expressive behaviors.*
25. Enhance social skills, such as proper communication, eating/table manners, and social activities *to promote the client's acceptability by others and increase self-esteem.*
26. Act as a role model for effective social interaction *to teach the client effective social skills.*
27. Praise successful social interactions or attempts *to reinforce positive social behavior.*
28. Teach the client and family about the disorder and symptom management *to promote knowledge, which may enhance compliance and reduce guilt.*
29. Arrange private meetings so that the family is able to express special concerns regarding the client *to clarify confusion about the illness and provide opportunities for expression of feelings.*
30. Teach the family to recognize early behavioral signs and symptoms of the client's failure to take medication *to be able to seek early intervention, promote medication compliance, and reduce recidivism.*

Additional Treatment Modalities

Nurses working with persons with severe and persistent mental illness are involved in collaborative interventions with a variety of mental health specialists and disciplines. These clients require an interdisciplinary approach during hospitalization, for discharge planning, and for follow-up care after discharge.

Psychotropic Medications

Psychotropic medications reduce the client's psychotic behavior and help control anxiety. The most common medications used for clients with chronic mental illness are the antipsychotic drugs.

Medications such as haloperidol (Haldol) and loxapine (Loxitane) are for both acute episodes of psychosis and long-term management of the client with severe and persistent mental illness. There is a high rate of extrapyramidal reactions (movement disorders) with haloperidol. Note any evidence of these side effects and report them immediately to the physician. Newer or atypical antipsychotic medications such as ziprasidone (Geodon), which is currently available in both oral and intramuscular forms, and risperidone (Risperdal) are sometimes effective alternatives to the older or typical antipsychotics. These drugs demonstrate less serious side effects and reduced incidence of troubling symptoms in general. Antianxiety and antidepressant medications are also used for clients with severe and persistent mental illness (see Chapter 24).

Group, Occupational, and Other Therapies

The client with severe and persistent mental illness will benefit from group therapy in that it offers the client opportunities to enhance communication skills and to express feelings in a nonthreatening setting. The group also provides an acceptable forum for the client to interact with others in a safe environment. Nurses and other therapists serve as role models for social interactions and guide the group dynamics in a fair and meaningful way.

Occupational therapy helps the client with severe and persistent mental illness to coordinate movements and express inner feelings through a variety of art forms. The client can also learn new dressing, grooming, and homemaking skills. The occupational therapist is an important adjunct to the psychiatric mental health nurse, as both the therapist and nurse work together to assess the client's level of functioning from different perspectives. Therapeutic recreation, which includes movement, dance, and other recreational activities, is also a valuable adjunct to nursing in working with these clients, as the activities help clients to get in touch with their feelings and attitudes toward themselves, others, and the world around them in a nonthreatening way (see Chapter 23).

NURSING CARE PLAN

Bradley, a 32-year-old man with a history of psychosis, was brought to the emergency department by the police for violent behavior. He was admitted to the behavioral health unit in the hospital for psychiatric care. He had been treated in the same hospital in the past and also had been committed to a state psychiatric hospital three times in the past 10 years.

Bradley was the third of six children and appeared to behave normally until he had an onset of psychosis at age 17 with episodes of hallucinations and aggression and intermittent periods of mutism (not speaking) for long periods of time. He was placed on antipsychotic medication and continued to live at home until age 27 when his parents thought he would do better in a residential supervised treatment facility so his medications could be administered on a regular basis. In the past 5 years, Bradley lived in several different treatment facilities and continued to have problems with medication compliance.

When Bradley ran out of his antipsychotic medication 4 weeks ago, he became aggressive and threatened another resident, accusing him of stealing his money. When the resident manager tried to intervene, Bradley became upset and ran away. His family was unable to find him until they were notified that he was in the emergency department.

Bradley had been living on the street and in missions for the homeless since he ran away. The police had been called to a soup kitchen because of Bradley's paranoid and aggressive behavior. He was uncooperative and aggressive to the staff and others and became violent when approached. Bradley also fought with the police until they were able to restrain him and take him to the hospital. He had been without antipsychotic drugs for almost 1 month.

On admission to the unit, Bradley was actively hallucinating and talking to an unseen presence. His affect was flat and his movements were slow. When approached by the staff or other clients, Bradley either ignored them or spoke in a rude tone of voice. He has no history of drug or alcohol abuse. He was unkempt, and his clothing was dirty.

DSM-IV-TR Diagnoses

Axis I	Schizophrenia, undifferentiated, chronic, with acute exacerbation
Axis II	Deferred
Axis III	Deferred
Axis IV	Severity of psychologic stress: chronic as a result of severe mental illness, noncompliance with medications, unable to maintain stable living environment
Axis V	GAF = 30 (current); GAF = 50 (past year)

Nursing Diagnosis *Risk for other-directed violence. Risk factors: client's paranoid, aggressive and belligerent behavior; auditory hallucinations that could be command type (telling client to harm others); stopping antipsychotic medications for 1 month; history of psychosis (unreality); unable to get along with family/caregivers*

NOC Aggression Self-Control, Stress Level, Impulse Self-Control, Risk Detection, Community Risk Control: Violence, Distorted Thought Self-Control

NIC Anger Control Assistance, Anxiety Reduction, Environmental Management: Violence Prevention, Distraction, Reality Orientation, Medication Management

CLIENT OUTCOMES	NURSING INTERVENTIONS	EVALUATION
Bradley will not act out in aggressive or violent behavior toward others in the unit.	Prevent Bradley from acting out in an aggressive or violent manner by: 1. Close observation by staff 2. Therapeutic communication that builds trust and reduces anxiety 3. Administration of prescribed medication *To maintain safety of everyone on the unit, which is the first nursing priority.*	Bradley has not demonstrated violence or aggression toward others on the unit. He is open to communication strategies and accepts staff direction and prescribed medication.
Bradley will seek staff when feeling anxious or when hallucinations begin.	Make Bradley continuously familiar with the nursing unit and to the events and activities that are going on *to present reality in a nonthreatening way.*	Bradley tells staff when he is feeling anxious or when hallucinations begin.
Bradley will understand the staff's communication and will ask them to explain words that are not clear to him.	Use clear, concrete statements and avoid abstract concepts when speaking *to help Bradley understand the message, since persons with schizophrenia lose the ability to understand concepts.*	Bradley is trying his best to understand the nursing staff and asks them to explain words that are not clear to him.
Bradley will feel safe and worthwhile in the mental health environment.	Reassure Bradley that he is safe and will not be harmed *to help him begin to trust the staff and the environment and to increase his self-esteem.*	Bradley states to the nurses that he feels safe and wanted on the unit and he is sure no one will harm him.
Bradley is aware of the behavior brought on by the hallucinations, versus the behavior following treatment including antipsychotic medication.	Help Bradley see the differences between his hallucinatory behavior and his behavior following treatment, including antipsychotic medication *to help him see the importance of medication and other treatments in managing his hallucinations.*	Bradley says he has noticed an improvement in his behavior when he follows the treatment program. He joins in the activities and takes his medication every day.
Bradley will be able to hold most conversations with staff, clients, and family without interference from hallucinations.	Help Bradley to focus on real events or activities *to reinforce reality and divert Bradley's attention from his hallucinations.*	Bradley holds several conversations with staff, clients, and family without evidence of hallucinations.

Continued

NURSING CARE PLAN—cont'd

CLIENT OUTCOMES	NURSING INTERVENTIONS	EVALUATION
Bradley will name the stressors that trigger the hallucinations and will try to avoid or reduce them.	Help Bradley to identify stressors that trigger the hallucinations *to teach Bradley, his family, and residential supervisors how to avoid or reduce his hallucinations.*	Bradley lists two stressors that provoke his hallucinations: (1) stopping his medication and (2) too much stimulation, especially loud noises.
Bradley will state that he feels calmer knowing he is accepted as a person with real feelings and not just someone who is "hearing voices."	Encourage Bradley to discuss his feelings as well as his hallucinations *to show understanding and acceptance of him as a person and to reduce anxiety, which will help reduce the hallucinations.*	Bradley is able to identify three feelings: anxiety, frustration, and anger. He says he feels calmer when he expresses his feelings to the nursing staff.
Bradley shows a reduction in anxiety and hallucinations after using techniques and strategies recommended by the nursing team and his physician.	Teach Bradley anxiety-reducing techniques and strategies such as exercising, joining an activity, listening to music, watching a favorite video, clapping or whistling when the hallucinations are too intrusive, or telling the voices to "go away" *to help reduce anxiety and hallucinations and to join in more positive, rewarding activities.*	Bradley shows effective use of techniques, activities, and strategies to manage feelings of anxiety and hallucinations before discharge.
Bradley will demonstrate trust in the staff and the treatment program and will continue to take his medication as an outpatient. He will return to his residential treatment facility and visit his parents.	Provide a consistent, structured setting that encourages the client to join activities and continue medication and other treatments in a safe, accepting setting *to promote the client's trust, safety, a sense of well-being, and the desire to continue treatment after discharge.*	Bradley expresses relief that his "voices" were significantly reduced and nearly eliminated at times and credits the staff's treatment of him as a human being with real feelings, as well as the structured treatment program and medication.
Bradley will continue to attend groups and activities as an outpatient and will continue to take medication. He will notify support persons at the first sign of returning symptoms.	Have the nurse case manager help Bradley make the transition to outpatient care and continue his treatment and medication *to reduce the risk of returning symptoms.*	Bradley is making a successful transition to outpatient care; he continues to attend groups and activities of daily living classes and takes his medication every day with supervision. He says he will call support persons at the first sign of hallucinations.

Nursing Diagnosis *Social isolation related to negative experiences of aloneness, auditory hallucinations, withdrawal from the community, and defensive behaviors, as evidenced by living apart from family; running away from residential facility, care providers, and the environment; talking to "internal voices;" noncommunicative, belligerent behaviors; flat affect; and minimal or absent eye contact*

NOC Loneliness Severity, Aggression Self-Control, Social Support, Social Involvement, Family Social Climate, Communication, Leisure Participation, Social Interaction Skills

NIC Socialization Enhancement, Support System Enhancement, Activity Therapy, Family Therapy, Environmental Management, Self-Esteem Enhancement

CLIENT OUTCOMES	NURSING INTERVENTIONS	EVALUATION
Bradley will interact socially with nursing staff, therapists and other clients.	Engage Bradley in meaningful, nonthreatening individual and group interactions every day *to let client know that participation is expected and that he is a worthwhile member of the community.*	Bradley says he is willing to participate in social interactions on the unit.
Bradley will demonstrate appropriate social behaviors in one-to-one and group interactions.	Role model for Bradley, individual and group social behaviors *to help Bradley learn appropriate social skills.*	Bradley has successfully interacted socially in individual and group settings.
Bradley will participate in social activities with family and other clients such as meals and games, as well as therapeutic activities, such as exercise, arts, and crafts.	Help Bradley to socialize with trusted family members and to seek out other clients who have similar interests *to promote more comfortable and enjoyable socialization and therapeutic activities.*	Bradley participates in social and therapeutic activities on the unit and has social contact with his family.
Bradley will continue to seek out others to socialize with who have similar interests as he does.	Praise Bradley for attempts to seek out others with similar interests *to promote continued positive socialization.*	Bradley continuously seeks out other clients with similar interests for social interactions and unit activities.
Bradley's family will have more contact with him.	Encourage Bradley's family to call him on the telephone and visit him on the unit. *A strong family network will increase Bradley's social contacts and promote self-esteem.*	Bradley's family calls and visits him frequently.

CLIENT OUTCOMES	NURSING INTERVENTIONS	EVALUATION
Bradley will express pleasure from social conversations with other clients, staff, and family.	Provide Bradley with social activities according to his level of tolerance *to gradually expose him to more complex social interactions.*	Bradley expresses pleasure in participating in social activities before discharge.
Bradley will attend unit outings with other clients.	Provide opportunities for Bradley to go on outings *to encourage a variety of more complex social experiences.*	Bradley engages in social conversations and activities during outings with other clients.
Bradley will participate in social activities within his overall capabilities.	Activate Bradley to engage in social activities that are within his physical/mental capabilities *to provide him with successful social experiences.*	Bradley participates in social activities that he is able to effectively accomplish and enjoy.

Nursing Diagnosis *Impaired verbal communication related to disturbed thought processes (paranoia), disturbed sensory perceptions (hallucinations), and inability to process and use language effectively when interacting with others (all secondary to chronic schizophrenia), as evidenced by speaking minimally or not speaking for long periods of time, defensive communications, flat affect, and lack of eye contact*

NOC Distorted Thought Self-Control, Sensory Function Status, Cognitive Orientation, Information Processing, Communication, Client Satisfaction: Communication

NIC Anxiety Reduction, Active Listening, Communication Enhancement: Speech Deficit, Art Therapy, Learning Facilitation, Support System Enhancement

CLIENT OUTCOMES	NURSING INTERVENTIONS	EVALUATION
Bradley will communicate his thoughts in a coherent, goal-directed manner with reduced anxiety.	Demonstrate a calm, quiet appearance rather than attempting to force Bradley to speak *to show acceptance and reduce anxiety.*	Bradley communicates his thoughts and feelings in a goal-directed, calm manner.
Bradley will respond positively to the nursing staff's active listening and close attention to his communication style.	Actively listen and observe Bradley's verbal and nonverbal cues during the communication process *to show interest in meeting his needs and to indicate his self-worth.*	Bradley tries hard to use effective verbal and nonverbal methods to express his needs to the staff. He states, "I feel good that they care enough to try to understand me."
Bradley will express satisfaction in having his needs met, even if he has difficulty communicating them.	Anticipate Bradley's needs until he is able to communicate them effectively *to provide for Bradley's safety and comfort.*	Bradley is verbalizing satisfaction that staff members are able to meet his needs of safety and comfort.
Bradley will demonstrate reality-based thoughts in brief 3- to 5-minute verbal conversations with others, beginning with his peers.	Teach Bradley to approach other clients for conversations about basic subjects they all have in common, such as how their day is going or what activities they like *to allow Bradley to practice simple, realistic communication skills with his own peers, in a safe setting.*	Bradley is able to maintain reality-based verbal conversations with his peers for 5 minutes.
Bradley will actively listen and give realistic responses to staff and other clients in individual and group activities.	Instruct Bradley to listen and respond to the specific topics of discussion with staff and other clients in individual and group activities *to encourage Bradley to respond to reality rather than listen to his own autistic thoughts.*	Bradley is able to listen and respond realistically to topics of discussion with staff and other clients in individual and group activities.
Bradley will use strategies to decrease anxiety to help him focus on realistic thoughts and meaningful verbal communication.	Teach Bradley anxiety-reducing strategies, such as (1) deep breathing, (2) replacing irrational or negative thoughts with realistic ones (cognitive therapy), and (3) seeking out a supportive person to help guide him when first experiencing impaired verbal communication *to decrease anxiety, which will promote more functional speech patterns.*	Bradley is able to identify and use effective strategies to control his anxiety. He uses effective verbal communication skills without signs of autistic thinking before discharge.
Bradley will continue to engage in realistic, meaningful conversations with others.	Praise Bradley for his realistic, meaningful conversations with others *to increase self-esteem and promote continued functional speech patterns.*	Bradley continues to use meaningful and logical speech in conversations with others. He says, "Positive feedback makes me feel proud."

Continued

NURSING CARE PLAN—cont'd

Nursing Diagnosis *Self-care deficit (bathing/hygiene, dressing/grooming) related to disturbed sensory perception and disturbed thought processes (secondary to schizophrenia), as evidenced by withdrawal from reality (hallucinations, isolation, paranoia), and impaired ability to perform functions of hygiene, dressing, or grooming (appears unbathed and disheveled)*

NOC Self Care: Bathing, Self-Care: Hygiene, Self-Care: Dressing, Anxiety Self-Control, Cognition, Self-Direction of Care, Comfort Level, Client Satisfaction: Physical Care

NIC Self-Care Assistance: Bathing/Hygiene, Self-Care Assistance: Dressing/Grooming, Teaching: Individual, Self-Responsibility Facilitation, Body Image Enhancement

CLIENT OUTCOMES	NURSING INTERVENTIONS	EVALUATION
Bradley will consistently perform adequate personal hygiene and grooming and dressing functions.	Assist Bradley with personal hygiene, grooming, dressing, and other activities of daily living skills until he can function independently *to preserve Bradley's dignity and self-esteem and avoid negative responses of other clients.*	Bradley performs all self-care activities of hygiene, dressing and grooming in an appropriate manner before discharge.
Bradley will perform daily routines for self-care, beginning with simple tasks and progressing to more complex functions.	Establish daily routines for Bradley's self-care functions, adding more complex tasks as his condition improves *to help Bradley organize his chaotic world and promote successful self-care.*	Bradley is able to complete all self-care functions before discharge.
Bradley will be able to verbalize positive feelings resulting from his self-care task performance.	Praise Bradley for attempts at self-care and each completed task *to increase feelings of self-worth and promote continued self-care.*	Bradley expresses feelings of pride and self-respect for successfully performing self-care tasks. He states, "I feel like a worthwhile person now that I can do my own personal care."

EVALUATION

The nurse evaluates changes in client behaviors and responses to treatment and interventions. The nurse needs to list outcomes so that there is a specified time in which the desired behavior will be evaluated. At the time of evaluation, it is important to determine if the client has satisfactorily met the desired outcome or made progress toward achieving the outcome. The nurse notes the date that the client achieves the outcome (and that outcome identification is no longer active). During evaluation, sometimes the original outcome identification is no longer applicable because of changes in the client's condition.

CHAPTER SUMMARY

- Severe and persistent mental illness manifests by acute exacerbations and remissions.
- Persons experiencing severe and persistent mental illness may have one or more mental disorders, which affects every aspect of life.
- These individuals may have difficulty managing their medication, as well as problems organizing their lives on a daily basis.
- Persons do not die from their mental disorder and often have the same life span as any other adult, yet they are at risk for injury or harm as a result of environmental and personal stressors.
- Many of these disorders are first evident during adolescence. Young adults with mental illness are more likely to live chaotic lifestyles associated with undertreated mental disorders and substance abuse.
- Family members of persons with these disorders experience a significant amount of acute and chronic stress.
- Many of these individuals live in poverty with little or no support from family or friends who have given up on them.
- Persons with severe and persistent mental illness have normal sexual drives and interests, although they may act them out in inappropriate ways.
- There is a high rate of suicide among these individuals.
- Many people with severe and persistent mental illness are able to control hallucinations and delusions through an effective medication regimen and steady support system.
- Family members who receive their own support from health care personnel and community groups are able to learn how to intervene in the client's sensory/perceptual disturbances and prevent violence.
- Cultural values and beliefs affect the individual's perception of a mental illness, presenting symptoms, and response to treatment.
- Mentally ill pregnant women need careful management by a comprehensive health care team.

REVIEW QUESTIONS

1 A nurse at the mental health center finds that a client with severe and persistent mental illness is having difficulty taking prescribed medications. The client lives alone and says, "This drug really works for me but I can't always remember whether or not I've taken it." Which strategy should the nurse use first to assist this client?

1. Obtain a daily pill minder and instruct the client on how to fill and use it.
2. Suggest that the client ask a neighbor for help with managing the medication.

3. Arrange for the client to come to the clinic every day for medication administration.
4. Collaborate with the psychiatrist about changing the client's medication to depot injections.

2 A client with a 4-year history of paranoid schizophrenia lives in the community. The client complains of feelings of increasing depression and states, "I will never live a normal life like my friends." The nurse at the clinic notes that the client exhibits a withdrawn affect and has gained 12 pounds in the past month. Select the highest priority nursing intervention.
1. Direct that the client to attend community support groups.
2. Question the client about the client for suicidal ideation and intent.
3. Reinforce to the client the importance of antipsychotic medication.
4. Monitor the client's recent daily intake of food and fluids.

3 A client with severe and persistent mental illness tells the nurse, "I'm ready to get a job. I think employment would be good for me." Select the nurse's best action.
1. Talk to the client about the chronic nature of mental illness.
2. Remind the client that employment could jeopardize disability benefits.
3. Assist the client with preparing a resume and obtaining references.
4. Talk with the client about a referral to vocational rehabilitation.

4 A client with undifferentiated schizophrenia is found wandering the streets, barely clothed, and yelling obscenities. A psychiatric nurse assesses the client in the emergency department. Which behavior meets involuntary hospitalization criteria?
1. The client stopped taking medications 1 month earlier.
2. The client is currently homeless.
3. The client says, "The voices tell me to kill little people."
4. The client admits to drinking alcohol excessively.

5 An adult with bipolar disorder becomes agitated and threatens to harm a staff person. What is the best nursing intervention?
1. Address the client with simple directions and a calming voice.
2. Tell the client, "If you do not calm down, restraints will be needed."
3. Confront the client on how inappropriate this behavior is.
4. Maintain the client's attention by patting the client's shoulders.

*Additional self-study exercises and learning resources are available to you on the **Companion CD** at the back of the book and on the **Evolve website** at **http://evolve.elsevier.com/Fortinash/**.*

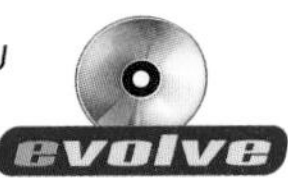

REFERENCES

Ahmed SH: Development of mental care in Pakistan past, present and future, 2000; retrieved Sep 18, 2002, from www.euro.who.int/MNH/WHD/TechPres_Pakistan1.pdf.

Alderete E et al: Lifetime prevalence of and risk factors for psychiatric disorders among Mexican migrant farmworkers in California, *Am J Public Health* 90:608, 2000.

Al-Issa I, Tousignant M, editors: *Ethnicity, immigration, and psychopathology*, New York, 1997, Plenum Press.

American Psychiatric Association: *Diagnostic and statistical manual of mental disorders*, ed 4, text revision, Washington, DC, 2000, American Psychiatric Association.

Angold A et al: Perceived burden and service use for child and adolescent psychiatric disorders, *Am J Public Health* 88:75-80, 1998.

Aponte JF, Johnson LR: The impact of culture on the intervention and treatment of ethnic populations. In Aponte JF, Johnson LR, editors: *Intervention and cultural diversity*, ed 2, Needham Heights, Mass, 2000, Allyn & Bacon.

Australian-Afghan Consulate: Afghan-Australian relations, June 20, 2000; retrieved Sep 20, 2002, from www.afghanconsulate.net/message_from_baird.htm.

Bachrach LL: The chronic patient: patient's quality of life: a continuing concern in the literature, *Psychiatr Serv* 47:1305, 1996.

Baker JA: Bipolar disorders: an overview of current literature, *J Psychiatry Ment Health Nurs* 8:473, 2001.

Beard JJ, Gillespie P: *Nothing to hide: mental illness in the family*, Boston, 2001, The New Press.

Bellack AS, Mueser KT: A comprehensive treatment program for schizophrenia and chronic mental illness, *Commun Mental Health J* 22:174, 1986.

Bernheim KF, Lehman AF: *Working with families of the mentally ill*, New York, 1985, WW Norton.

Bhui K, Puffet A, Strathdee G: Sexual relationship problems amongst patients with severe chronic psychoses, *Soc Psychiatry Psychiatr Epidemiol* 32:459, 1997.

Bond GR et al: An update on supported employment for people with severe mental illness, *Psychiatr Serv* 48:335, 1997.

Borrows JA: The Chippewa experience with the therapy process: stepping stones to healing, UMI, vol 61, 2001.

Brown C, Hamera E, Long C: The daily activities check list: a functional assessment for consumers with mental illness living in the community, *Occup Ther Care* 10:33, 1996.

Buist A: Mentally ill families: when are the children safe? *Issues Mental Health Nurs* 27:261, 1998.

Buttell FP: The relationship between spouse abuse and the maltreatment of dementia sufferers of their caregivers, *J Alzheimers Dis* 14:230, 1999.

Carey MP et al: Behavioral risk for HIV infection among adults with a severe and persistent mental illness: patterns and psychological antecedents, *Community Ment Health J* 33:133, 1997.

Castillo RLL: *Culture and mental illness*, Pacific Grove, Calif, 1996, Brooks/Cole.

Castle LN: Beyond medication: what else does the patient with schizophrenia need to reintegrate into the community? *J Psychosoc Nurs Mental Health Serv* 35:18, 1997.

Center for Mental Health Services [CMHS]: Critical issues for parents with mental illness and their families, 1999; retrieved Sep 23, 2002, from www.mental.org/publications/allpubs/KEN-01-0109/ch2.asp.

Cogan MB: Diagnosis and treatment of bipolar disorder in children and adolescents, *Psychiatr Times* 13, 1996.

Cook JA, Sliegman P: Experiences of parents with mental illness and their service needs, *J NAMI Calif* 11:21, 2000.

Dembling B: Datapoints: mental disorders as contributing cause of death in the United States in 1992, *Psychiatr Serv* 48:45, 1997.

Donnelly PL: Korean American family experiences of caregiving for their mentally ill adult children: an interpretive inquiry, *J Transcultural Nurs* 12:292, 2001.

Doornbas MM: The problems and coping methods of caregivers of young adults with mental illness, *J Psychol Nurs Ment Health Serv* 35:41, 1997.

Eliopoulos C: Cognitive disorders. In Carson VB, editor: *Mental health nursing: the nurse-patient journey*, ed 2, Philadelphia, 2000, Saunders.

Felker B, Yazel JJ, Short D: Mortality and medical comorbidity amongst psychiatric patients: a review, *Psychiatr Serv* 47:1356, 1996.

Fenton WS et al: Randomized trial of general hospital and residential alternative care for patients with severe and persistent mental illness, *Am J Psychiatry* 155:516, 1998.

Fitzgerald RG, Parkes CM: Blindness and loss of other sensory and cognitive functions, *BMJ* 316:1160, 1998.

Flaskerud JH: Ethnicity, culture, and neuropsychiatry, *Issues Ment Health Nurs* 21:5, 2000.

Fortinash KM, Holoday Worret PA: *Psychiatric nursing care plans*, ed 4, St Louis, 2007, Mosby.

Ganache G: Grandparents caring for grandchildren when parents have mental illness, *J NAMI Calif* 11:32, 2000.

Gater R et al: The care of patients with chronic schizophrenia: a comparison between two services, *Psychol Med* 27:1325, 1997.

Getty C, Perese E, Knab S: Capacity for self-care of persons with mental illnesses living in community residences and the ability of their surrogate families to perform care functions, *Issues Ment Health Nurs* 19:53, 1998.

Gold award: comprehensive prenatal and postpartum psychiatric care for women with severe mental illness, *Psychiatr Serv* 47:1108, 1996.

Gold award: linking mentally ill persons with services through crisis intervention, mobile outreach, and community education, *Psychiatr Serv* 48:1450, 1997.

Gopfert M, Webster J, Seeman MV, editors: *Parental psychiatric disorder: distressed parents and their families*, Cambridge, 1996, Cambridge University Press.

Gorman PA: Sensory dysfunction in dual diagnosis: mental retardation/mental illness and autism, *Occup Ther Ment Health* 13:3, 1997.

Gray GE: Providing mental health services to the African American community, *J Calif Alliance for Mentally Ill* 10:24, 1999.

Green SA: Silence and violence, *Psychiatr Serv* 48:175, 1997.

Grinfeld MJ: Mental consequences of conflict neglected, *Psychiatric Times* 19; retrieved Sep 25, 2002, from www.psychistrictimes.com/p020401a.html.

Harvey PD et al: Cognitive impairment in geriatric chronic schizophrenic patients: a cross-national study in New York and London, *Int Geriatr Psychiatry* 12:1001, 1997.

Hatfield AB, Lefley HP, Strauss JS: *Surviving mental illness*, New York, 1993, Guilford Press.

Hellman RE: Issues in the treatment of lesbian women and gay men with severe and persistent mental illness, *Psychiatr Serv* 47:1093, 1996.

Herrick C, Brown HN: Mental disorders and syndromes found among Asians residing in the United States, *Issues Ment Health Nurs* 20:275, 1999.

Hindle D: Growing up with a parent who has a chronic mental illness: one's child's perspective, *Child Family Social Work* 3:259, 1998.

Hodgman CH: Adolescent psychiatric conditions, *Compr Ther* 22:796, 1996.

Hornung WP et al: Psychoeducational training for schizophrenic patients: background, procedure and empirical findings, *Patient Educ Counsel* 29:257, 1996.

Howard PB: The experience of fathers of adult children with schizophrenia, *Issues Ment Health Nurs* 19:399, 1998.

Howe J, Howe C: When mentally ill children have children, *J NAMI Calif* 11:21, 2000.

Israel Mental Association: 1999; retrieved Sep 25, 2002, from www.members.tripod.com/Goldin_Yarik/about_amuta_e.htm.

Jaffe DF: Pregnancy pointers for women with NBD; retrieved Sep 18, 2002, from www.schizophrenia.com/schizoph/NBDpreg.html.

Johnson JT: *Hidden victims-hidden healers: an eight stage healing process for family and friends of the mentally ill*, New York, 1994, PEMA.

Jones I, Craddock N: Familiarity of the puerperal trigger in bipolar disorder: results of a family study, *Am J Psychiatry* 158:913, 2001.

Jordan BK et al: Prevalence of psychiatric disorders among incarcerated women: convicted felons entering prison, *Arch Gen Psychiatry* 53:513, 1996.

Keyes EF: Mental health status in refugees: an integration of current research, *Issues Ment Health Nurs* 21:397, 2000.

King SV: "God won't put more on you than you can bear": faith as a coping strategy among older African American caregiving parents of adult children with disabilities, *J Religion Disabilities* 4:7, 2001.

Klinkenberg WD, Calsyn RJ: Predictors of receipt of aftercare and recidivism among persons with severe and persistent mental illness: a review, *Psychiatr Serv* 47:487, 1996.

Kouzis AC, Eaton WW: Psychopathology and the development of disability, *Soc Psychiatry Psychiatr Epidemiol* 32:379, 1997.

Lamb HR, Weinberger LE: Persons with severe mental illness in jails and prisons: a review, *Psychiatr Serv* 49:483, 1998.

Lawrence C: *Looking for Mary Gabriel*, New York, 2002, Dunne Books.

Lechner S: The adolescent. In Carson VB, editor: *Mental health nursing: the nurse-patient journey*, ed 2, Philadelphia, 2000a, Saunders.

Lechner S: The child. In Carson VB, editor: *Mental health nursing: the nurse-patient journey*, ed 2, Philadelphia, 2000b, Saunders.

Lechner S: Travelers from many lands. In Carson VB, editor: *Mental health nursing: the nurse-patient journey*, ed 2, Philadelphia, 2000c, Saunders.

Lentz SK: Electroconvulsive therapy during pregnancy, 1996; retrieved from Sep 18, 2002, from www.ect.org/resources/pregnancy.html.

Lieberman MA, Fisher L: The impact of dementia on adult offspring and their spouses: the contribution of family characteristics, *J Mental Health Aging* 5:207, 1999.

Lloyd C, Bassett J: Life is for living: a pre-vocational program for young people with psychosis, *Aust Occup Ther J* 44:82, 1997.

Lyden J: *Daughter of the Queen of Sheba: a memoir*, New York, 1998, Penguin.

Marcus PE: Suicide. In Carson VB, editor: *Mental health nursing: the nurse-patient journey*, ed 2, Philadelphia, 2000, Saunders.

Miller LJ, Finnerty M: Sexuality, pregnancy, and childrearing among women with schizophrenia—spectrum disorders, *Psychiatr Serv* 47:502, 1996.

Mintzer JE et al: The effectiveness of a continuum of care using brief and partial hospitalization for agitated dementia patients, *Psychiatr Serv* 48:1435, 1997.

Mohr WK: Bipolar disorder in children, *J Psychosocial Nurs Mental Health Serv* 39:12, 48, 2001.

Moorman M: *My sister's keeper: learning to cope with a sibling's mental illness*, New York, 2002, WW Norton.

Mueser KT et al: Family burden of schizophrenia and bipolar disorder: perceptions of relatives and professionals, *Psychiatr Serv* 47:507, 1996.

Munroe H: The impact of schizophrenia on women: a voyage of turbulence, *Women's health matters*, Jan 2002; retrieved Sep 18, 2002, from www.womensmatters.ca/facts/quick_show_d.cfm?number=333.

North American Nursing Diagnosis Association International: *NANDA-I nursing diagnoses: definitions and classification 2007-2008*, Philadelphia, 2007, NANDA-I.

National Institute of Mental Health [NIMH]: Mental disorders in America; retrieved Sep 18, 2002, from www.nimh.nih.gov/publicat/numbers.cfm.

Neufeld J: *Lisa, bright and dark: a novel*, New York, 1999, Puffin.

News in mental nursing: sex in the state hospital a continuing headache, *J Psychosoc Nurs* 35:6, 1997.

Open Society Institute: Mental illness in US jails; retrieved Sep 17, 2002, from www.soros.org/crime/research_brief_1.html.

Pace-Murphy K, Dyer CB, Gleason MS: Delirium, dementia, and other amnestic disorders, Palestinian Counseling Center; retrieved Sep 25, 2002, from www.pcc-jer.or/affiliations.htm.

Pejlert A: Being a parent of an adult son or daughter with severe mental illness receiving professional care: parents' narratives, *Social Care Community* 9:194, 2001.

Piazza LA et al: Sexual functioning in chronically depressed patients treated with SSRI antidepressants: a pilot study, *Am J Psychiatry* 154:1757, 1997.

Pickens JM: Living with serious illness: the desire for normalcy, *Nurs Sci Q* 12:233, 1999.

Potash JB et al: Attempted suicide and alcoholism in bipolar disorder: clinical and family relationships, *Am J Psychiatry* 157:2048, 2000.

Powell J: First person account: paranoid schizophrenia—a daughter's story, *Schizophr Bull* 24:175, 1998.

Pruchno RA, Burant CJ, Peters ND: Understanding the well-being of caregivers, *Gerontologist* 37:102, 1997.

Reiss S: Mental illness in persons with mental retardation, 1993; retrieved Sep 19, 2002, from www.thearc.org/faqs/mimrqa.html.

Riggin OZ, Redding BA: Substance related disorders. In Fortinash KM, Holoday Worret PA, editors: *Psychiatric mental health nursing*, ed 2, St Louis, 2000, Mosby.

Ritsher JEB, Coursey RD, Ferrell EW: A survey on issues in the lives of women with severe mental illness, *Psychiatr Serv* 48:1273, 1997.

Ruscher SM, de Wit R, Mazmanian D: Psychiatric patients' attitudes about medication and factors affecting noncompliance, *Psychiatr Serv* 48:82, 1997.

Sachs GS et al: Comorbidity of attention deficit hyperactivity disorder with early and late-onset bipolar disorder, *Am J Psychiatry* 157:466, 2000.

Sadock BJ, Sadock VA: *Kaplan & Sadock's synopsis of psychiatry, behavioral sciences/clinical psychiatry*, ed 9, Baltimore, 2006, Lippincott, Williams & Wilkins.

Saunders J: Walking a mile in their shoes . . . symbolic interaction for families living with severe mental illness, *J Psychosoc Nurs Ment Serv* 35:45, 1997.

Schmitt SM: Criminalizing the mentally ill, *CTOnline*,1999; retrieved Sep 18, 2002, from www.counseling.org/ctonline/criminalization.htm.

Scholler-Jaquish A: Homelessness in America. In Smith C, Maurer F, editors: *Community nursing: theory and practice*, ed 2, Philadelphia, 2000a, Saunders.

Scholler-Jaquish A: Persons with chronic mental illness. In Fortinash KM, Holoday Worret PA, editors: *Psychiatric mental health nursing*, ed 2, St Louis, 2000b, Mosby.

Scott CM: Mood disorders. In Carson VB, editor: *Mental nursing: the nurse-patient journey*, ed 2, Philadelphia, 2000, Saunders.

Seltzer MM, Li LW: The transitions of caregiving: subjective and objective definitions, *Gerontologist* 36:614, 1996.

Shaner et al: Monetary reinforcement of abstinence from cocaine among mentally ill patients with cocaine dependence, *Psychiatr Serv* 48:807, 1997.

Sharfstein SS, Webb WL, Stoline AM: *Schizophrenia: questions and answers*, National Institute of Mental Health (online), 1998.

Shoemaker N: The continuum of care. In Carson VB, editor: *Mental health nursing: the nurse-patient journey*, ed 2, Philadelphia, 2000, Saunders.

Silva JA, Leong GB, Weinstock R: Violent behaviors associated with the antichrist delusion, *J Forensic Sci* 42:1058, 1997.

So YP, Toglia J, Donohue MV: A study of memory functioning in chronic schizophrenic patients, *Occup Ther Ment* 13:1, 1997.

Strasser JA: Urban transient women, *Am J Nurs* 78:2076, 1978.

Tardiff K et al: Violence by patients admitted to a private psychiatric hospital, *Am J Psychiatry* 154:88-93, 1997.

Tempier R: Long-term psychiatric patients' knowledge about their medication, *Psychiatr Serv* 47:1385, 1996.

Teplin LA, Abram KM, McClelland GM: Prevalence of psychiatric disorders among incarcerated women. I. Pretrial jail detainees, *Arch Gen Psychiatry* 53:505, 1996.

Torrey EF: *Nowhere to go: the tragic odyssey of the homeless mentally ill*, New York, 1988, Harper.

Torrey EF: *Surviving schizophrenia*, ed 3, New York, 1995, Harper Perennial.

Torrey EF: *Out of the shadows: confronting America's mental illness*, New York, 1996, John Wiley & Sons.

Torrey EF: Stop the madness, *New York Times*, July 18, 1997; retrieved Sep 18, 2002, from www.psych-.com/madness1.htm.

Treatment Advocacy Center: Many Americans with untreated psychiatric illnesses have nowhere to go: homelessness—tragic side effect of non-treatment; retrieved Sep 18, 2002, from www.psychlaws.org/GeneralResources/fact11.htm.

Tseng WF: *Handbook of cultural psychiatry*, San Diego, 2001, Academic Press.

Uba L: *Asian Americans: personality patterns, identity, and mental health*, New York, 1994, Guilford Press.

Ware NC, Goldfinger SM: Poverty and rehabilitation in severe psychiatric disorders, *Psychiatr Rehabilitation J* 21:3-9, 1997.

Webster MM: Interactive therapies and methods of implementation. In Fortinash KM, Holoday Worret PA, editors: *Psychiatric mental health nursing*, ed 2, St Louis, 2000, Mosby.

Williams DR: African American mental health: persisting question and paradoxical findings, 1995; retrieved Sep 18, 2002, from www.rcgd.isr.umich.edu/prba/perspectives/spring1995/dwilliams.pdf.

Wise TN, Mann LS: Utilization of pain medication in hospitalized psychiatric patients, *Gen Hosp Psychiatry* 18:422, 1996.

Yap EL: Neurobiological influences. In Carson VB, editor: *Mental health nursing: the nurse-patient journey*, ed 2, Philadelphia, 2000, Saunders.

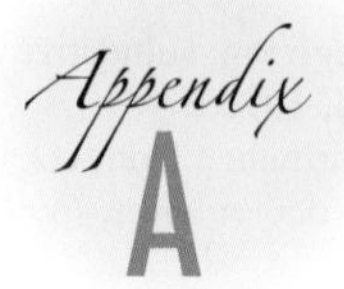

Appendix A American Nurses Association Standards of Psychiatric-Mental Health Nursing Practice

STANDARDS OF CARE

STANDARD I. ASSESSMENT

The psychiatric-mental health nurse collects patient health data.

STANDARD II. DIAGNOSIS

The psychiatric-mental health nurse analyzes the assessment data in determining diagnoses.

STANDARD III. OUTCOME IDENTIFICATION

The psychiatric-mental health nurse identifies expected outcomes individualized to the patient.

STANDARD IV. PLANNING

The psychiatric-mental health nurse develops a plan of care that is negotiated among the patient, nurse, family, and health care team and prescribes evidence-based interventions to attain expected outcomes.

STANDARD V. IMPLEMENTATION

The psychiatric-mental health nurse implements the interventions identified in the plan of care.

Standard Va. Counseling

The psychiatric-mental health nurse uses counseling interventions to assist patients in improving or regaining their previous coping abilities, fostering mental health, and preventing mental illness and disability.

Standard Vb. Milieu Therapy

The psychiatric-mental health nurse provides, structures, and maintains a therapeutic environment in collaboration with the patient and other health care clinicians.

Standard Vc. Promotion of Self-Care Activities

The psychiatric-mental health nurse structures interventions around the patient's activities of daily living to foster self-care and mental and physical well-being.

Standard Vd. Psychobiologic Interventions

The psychiatric-mental health nurse uses knowledge of psychobiologic interventions and applies clinical skills to restore the patient's health and prevent further disability.

Standard Ve. Health Teaching

The psychiatric-mental health nurse, through health teaching, assists patients in achieving satisfying, productive, and healthy patterns of living.

Standard Vf. Case Management

The psychiatric-mental health nurse provides case management to coordinate comprehensive health services and to ensure continuity of care.

Standard Vg. Health Promotion and Health Maintenance

The psychiatric-mental health nurse uses strategies and interventions to promote and maintain health and prevent mental illness.

The following interventions (Vh-Vj) may be performed only by the APRN-PMH.

Standard Vh. Psychotherapy

The APRN-PMH uses individual, group, and family psychotherapy and other therapeutic treatments to assist patients in preventing mental illness and disability, treating mental health disorders, and improving mental health status and functional abilities.

Standard Vi. Prescriptive Authority and Treatment

The APRN-PMH uses prescriptive authority, procedures, and treatments in accordance with state and federal laws and regulations to treat symptoms of psychiatric illness and improve functional health status.

Standard Vj. Consultation

The APRN-PMH provides consultation to enhance the abilities of other clinicians to provide services for patients and effect change in the system.

STANDARD VI. EVALUATION

The psychiatric-mental health nurse evaluates the patient's progress in attaining expected outcomes.

STANDARDS OF PROFESSIONAL PERFORMANCE

STANDARD I. QUALITY OF CARE

The psychiatric-mental health nurse systematically evaluates the quality of care and effectiveness of psychiatric-mental health nursing practice.

STANDARD II. PERFORMANCE APPRAISAL

The psychiatric-mental health nurse evaluates one's own psychiatric-mental health nursing practice in relation to professional practice standards and relevant statuses and regulations.

STANDARD III. EDUCATION

The psychiatric-mental health nurse acquires and maintains current knowledge in nursing practice.

STANDARD IV. COLLEGIALITY

The psychiatric-mental health nurse interacts with and contributes to the professional development of peers, health care clinicians, and others as colleagues.

STANDARD V. ETHICS

The psychiatric-mental health nurse's assessments, actions, and recommendations on behalf of patients are determined and implemented in an ethical manner.

STANDARD VI. COLLABORATION

The psychiatric-mental health nurse collaborates with the patient, significant others, and health care clinicians in providing care.

STANDARD VII. RESEARCH

The psychiatric-mental health nurse contributes to nursing and mental health through the use of research methods and findings.

STANDARD VIII. RESOURCE UTILIZATION

The psychiatric-mental health nurse considers factors related to safety, effectiveness, and cost in planning and delivering patient care.

Appendix B DSM-IV-TR Classification

NOS = Not Otherwise Specified.

An *x* appearing in a diagnostic code indicates that a specific code number is required.

An ellipsis (. . .) is used in the names of certain disorders to indicate that the name of a specific mental disorder or general medical condition should be inserted when recording the name (e.g., 293.0 Delirium Due to Hypothyroidism).

If criteria are currently met, one of the following severity specifiers may be noted after the diagnosis:

Mild
Moderate
Severe

If criteria are no longer met, one of the following specifiers may be noted:

In Partial Remission
In Full Remission
Prior History

DISORDERS USUALLY FIRST DIAGNOSED IN INFANCY, CHILDHOOD, OR ADOLESCENCE

Mental Retardation

NOTE: These are coded on Axis II.

317 Mild Mental Retardation
318.0 Moderate Mental Retardation
318.1 Severe Mental Retardation
318.2 Profound Mental Retardation
319 Mental Retardation, Severity Unspecified

Learning Disorders

315.00 Reading Disorder
315.1 Mathematics Disorder
315.2 Disorder of Written Expression
315.9 Learning Disorder NOS

Motor Skills Disorder

315.4 Developmental Coordination Disorder

Communication Disorders

315.31 Expressive Language Disorder
315.32 Mixed Receptive-Expressive Language Disorder
315.39 Phonologic Disorder
307.0 Stuttering
307.9 Communication Disorder NOS

Pervasive Developmental Disorders

299.00 Autistic Disorder
299.80 Rett's Disorder
299.10 Childhood Disintegrative Disorder
299.80 Asperger's Disorder
299.80 Pervasive Developmental Disorder NOS

Attention-Deficit and Disruptive Behavior Disorders

314.xx Attention-Deficit/Hyperactivity Disorder
.01 Combined Type
.00 Predominantly Inattentive Type
.01 Predominantly Hyperactive-Impulsive Type
314.9 Attention-Deficit/Hyperactivity Disorder NOS
312.xx Conduct Disorder
.81 Childhood-Onset Type
.82 Adolescent-Onset Type
.89 Unspecified Onset
313.81 Oppositional Defiant Disorder
312.9 Disruptive Behavior Disorder NOS

Feeding and Eating Disorders of Infancy or Early Childhood

307.52 Pica
307.53 Rumination Disorder
307.59 Feeding Disorder of Infancy or Early Childhood

Tic Disorders

307.23 Tourette's Disorder
307.22 Chronic Motor or Vocal Tic Disorder
307.21 Transient Tic Disorder
Specify if: Single Episode/Recurrent
307.20 Tic Disorder NOS

Elimination Disorders

___.__ Encopresis
787.6 With Constipation and Overflow Incontinence
307.7 Without Constipation and Overflow Incontinence
307.6 Enuresis (Not Due to a General Medical Condition)
Specify type: Nocturnal Only/Diurnal Only/Nocturnal and Diurnal

From American Psychiatric Association: *Diagnostic and statistical manual of mental disorders*, ed 4, text revision, Washington, DC, 2000, American Psychiatric Association.

Other Disorders of Infancy, Childhood, or Adolescence

309.21 Separation Anxiety Disorder
Specify if: Early Onset
313.23 Selective Mutism
313.89 Reactive Attachment Disorder of Infancy or Early Childhood
Specify type: Inhibited Type/Disinhibited Type
307.3 Stereotypic Movement Disorder
Specify if: With Self-Injurious Behavior
313.9 Disorder of Infancy, Childhood, or Adolescence NOS

DELIRIUM, DEMENTIA, AND AMNESTIC AND OTHER COGNITIVE DISORDERS

Delirium

293.0 Delirium Due to . . . *[Indicate the General Medical Condition]*
___.__ Substance Intoxication Delirium *(refer to Substance-Related Disorders for substance-specific codes)*
___.__ Substance Withdrawal Delirium *(refer to Substance-Related Disorders for substance-specific codes)*
___.__ Delirium Due to Multiple Etiologies *(code each of the specific etiologies)*
780.09 Delirium NOS

Dementia

294.xx Dementia of the Alzheimer's Type, With Early Onset *(also code 331.0 Alzheimer's disease on Axis III)*
.10 Without Behavioral Disturbance
.11 With Behavioral Disturbance
294.xx Dementia of the Alzheimer's Type, With Late Onset *(also code 331.0 Alzheimer's disease on Axis III)*
.10 Without Behavioral Disturbance
.11 With Behavioral Disturbance
290.xx Vascular Dementia
.40 Uncomplicated
.41 With Delirium
.42 With Delusions
.43 With Depressed Mood
Specify if: With Behavioral Disturbance

Code presence or absence of a behavioral disturbance in the fifth digit for Dementia Due to a General Medical Condition:
0 = Without Behavioral Disturbance
1 = With Behavioral Disturbance

294.1x Dementia Due to HIV Disease *(also code 042 HIV on Axis III)*
294.1x Dementia Due to Head Trauma *(also code 854.00 head injury on Axis III)*
294.1x Dementia Due to Parkinson's Disease *(also code 332.0 Parkinson's disease on Axis III)*
294.1x Dementia Due to Huntington's Disease *(also code 333.4 Huntington's disease on Axis III)*
294.1x Dementia Due to Pick's Disease *(also code 331.1 Pick's disease on Axis III)*
294.1x Dementia Due to Creutzfeldt-Jakob Disease *(also code 046.1 Creutzfeldt-Jakob disease on Axis III)*
294.1x Dementia Due to . . . *[Indicate the General Medical Condition not listed above] (also code the general medical condition on Axis III)*
___.__ Substance-Induced Persisting Dementia *(refer to Substance-Related Disorders for substance-specific codes)*
___.__ Dementia Due to Multiple Etiologies *(code each of the specific etiologies)*
294.8 Dementia NOS

Amnestic Disorders

294.0 Amnestic Disorder Due to . . . *[Indicate the General Medical Condition]*
Specify if: Transient/Chronic
___.__ Substance-Induced Persisting Amnestic Disorder *(refer to Substance-Related Disorders for substance-specific codes)*
294.8 Amnestic Disorder NOS

Other Cognitive Disorders

294.9 Cognitive Disorder NOS

MENTAL DISORDERS DUE TO A GENERAL MEDICAL CONDITION NOT ELSEWHERE CLASSIFIED

293.89 Catatonic Disorder Due to . . . *[Indicate the General Medical Condition]*
310.1 Personality Change Due to . . . *[Indicate the General Medical Condition]*
Specify type: Labile Type/Disinhibited Type/Aggressive Type/Apathetic Type/Paranoid Type/Other Type/Combined Type/Unspecified Type
293.9 Mental Disorder NOS Due to . . . *[Indicate the General Medical Condition]*

SUBSTANCE-RELATED DISORDERS

The following specifiers may be applied to Substance Dependence as noted:

[a]With Physiologic Dependence/Without Physiologic Dependence
[b]Early Full Remission/Early Partial Remission/Sustained Full Remission/Sustained Partial Remission
[c]In a Controlled Environment
[d]On Agonist Therapy

The following specifiers apply to substance-induced disorders as noted:

[I]With Onset During Intoxication/[W]With Onset During Withdrawal

Alcohol-Related Disorders

Alcohol Use Disorders

303.90 Alcohol Dependence[a,b,c]
305.00 Alcohol Abuse

Alcohol-Induced Disorders

303.00 Alcohol Intoxication
291.81 Alcohol Withdrawal
Specify if: With Perceptual Disturbances
291.0 Alcohol Intoxication Delirium
291.0 Alcohol Withdrawal Delirium
291.2 Alcohol-Induced Persisting Dementia
291.1 Alcohol-Induced Persisting Amnestic Disorder
291.x Alcohol-Induced Psychotic Disorder
.5 With Delusions[I,W]
.3 With Hallucinations[I,W]
291.89 Alcohol-Induced Mood Disorder[I,W]
291.89 Alcohol-Induced Anxiety Disorder[I,W]
291.89 Alcohol-Induced Sexual Dysfunction[I]
291.89 Alcohol-Induced Sleep Disorder[I,W]
291.9 Alcohol-Related Disorder NOS

Amphetamine (or Amphetamine-Like)–Related Disorders

Amphetamine Use Disorders

304.40 Amphetamine Dependence[a,b,c]
305.70 Amphetamine Abuse

Amphetamine-Induced Disorders

292.89 Amphetamine Intoxication
Specify if: With Perceptual Disturbances
292.0 Amphetamine Withdrawal
292.81 Amphetamine Intoxication Delirium
292.xx Amphetamine-Induced Psychotic Disorder
.11 With Delusions[I]
.12 With Hallucinations[I]
292.84 Amphetamine-Induced Mood Disorder[I,W]
292.89 Amphetamine-Induced Anxiety Disorder[I]
292.89 Amphetamine-Induced Sexual Dysfunction[I]
292.89 Amphetamine-Induced Sleep Disorder[I,W]
292.9 Amphetamine-Related Disorder NOS

Caffeine-Related Disorders

Caffeine-Induced Disorders

305.90 Caffeine Intoxication
292.89 Caffeine-Induced Anxiety Disorder[I]
292.89 Caffeine-Induced Sleep Disorder[I]
292.9 Caffeine-Related Disorder NOS

Cannabis-Related Disorders

Cannabis Use Disorders

304.30 Cannabis Dependence[a,b,c]
305.20 Cannabis Abuse

Cannabis-Induced Disorders

292.89 Cannabis Intoxication
Specify if: With Perceptual Disturbances
292.81 Cannabis Intoxication Delirium
292.xx Cannabis-Induced Psychotic Disorder
.11 With Delusions[I]
.12 With Hallucinations[I]
292.89 Cannabis-Induced Anxiety Disorder[I]
292.9 Cannabis-Related Disorder NOS

Cocaine-Related Disorders

Cocaine Use Disorders

304.20 Cocaine Dependence[a,b,c]
305.60 Cocaine Abuse

Cocaine-Induced Disorders

292.89 Cocaine Intoxication
Specify if: With Perceptual Disturbances
292.0 Cocaine Withdrawal
292.81 Cocaine Intoxication Delirium
292.xx Cocaine-Induced Psychotic Disorder
.11 With Delusions[I]
.12 With Hallucinations[I]
292.84 Cocaine-Induced Mood Disorder[I,W]
292.89 Cocaine-Induced Anxiety Disorder[I,W]
292.89 Cocaine-Induced Sexual Dysfunction[I]
292.89 Cocaine-Induced Sleep Disorder[I,W]
292.9 Cocaine-Related Disorder NOS

Hallucinogen-Related Disorders

Hallucinogen Use Disorders

304.50 Hallucinogen Dependence[b,c]
305.30 Hallucinogen Abuse

Hallucinogen-Induced Disorders

292.89 Hallucinogen Intoxication
292.89 Hallucinogen Persisting Perception Disorder (Flashbacks)
292.81 Hallucinogen Intoxication Delirium
292.xx Hallucinogen-Induced Psychotic Disorder
.11 With Delusions[I]
.12 With Hallucinations[I]
292.84 Hallucinogen-Induced Mood Disorder[I]
292.89 Hallucinogen-Induced Anxiety Disorder[I]
292.9 Hallucinogen-Related Disorder NOS

Inhalant-Related Disorders

Inhalant Use Disorders

304.60 Inhalant Dependence[b,c]
305.90 Inhalant Abuse

Inhalant-Induced Disorders

292.89 Inhalant Intoxication
292.81 Inhalant Intoxication Delirium
292.82 Inhalant-Induced Persisting Dementia
292.xx Inhalant-Induced Psychotic Disorder
.11 With Delusions[I]
.12 With Hallucinations[I]

292.84 Inhalant-Induced Mood Disorder[I]
292.89 Inhalant-Induced Anxiety Disorder[I]
292.9 Inhalant-Related Disorder NOS

Nicotine-Related Disorders

Nicotine Use Disorder

305.1 Nicotine Dependence[a,b]

Nicotine-Induced Disorder

292.0 Nicotine Withdrawal
292.9 Nicotine-Related Disorder NOS

Opioid-Related Disorders

Opioid Use Disorders

304.00 Opioid Dependence[a,b,c,d]
305.50 Opioid Abuse

Opioid-Induced Disorders

292.89 Opioid Intoxication
Specify if: With Perceptual Disturbances
292.0 Opioid Withdrawal
292.81 Opioid Intoxication Delirium
292.xx Opioid-Induced Psychotic Disorder
.11 With Delusions[I]
.12 With Hallucinations[I]
292.84 Opioid-Induced Mood Disorder[I]
292.89 Opioid-Induced Sexual Dysfunction[I]
292.89 Opioid-Induced Sleep Disorder[I,W]
292.9 Opioid-Related Disorder NOS

Phencyclidine (or Phencyclidine-Like)–Related Disorders

Phencyclidine Use Disorders

304.60 Phencyclidine Dependence[b,c]
305.90 Phencyclidine Abuse

Phencyclidine-Induced Disorders

292.89 Phencyclidine Intoxication
Specify if: With Perceptual Disturbances
292.81 Phencyclidine Intoxication Delirium
292.xx Phencyclidine-Induced Psychotic Disorder
.11 With Delusions[I]
.12 With Hallucinations[I]
292.84 Phencyclidine-Induced Mood Disorder[I]
292.89 Phencyclidine-Induced Anxiety Disorder[I]
292.9 Phencyclidine-Related Disorder NOS

Sedative-, Hypnotic-, or Anxiolytic-Related Disorders

Sedative, Hypnotic, or Anxiolytic Use Disorders

304.10 Sedative, Hypnotic, or Anxiolytic Dependence[a,b,c]
305.40 Sedative, Hypnotic, or Anxiolytic Abuse

Sedative-, Hypnotic-, or Anxiolytic-Induced Disorders

292.89 Sedative, Hypnotic, or Anxiolytic Intoxication
292.0 Sedative, Hypnotic, or Anxiolytic Withdrawal
Specify if: With Perceptual Disturbances
292.81 Sedative, Hypnotic, or Anxiolytic Intoxication Delirium
292.81 Sedative, Hypnotic, or Anxiolytic Withdrawal Delirium
292.82 Sedative-, Hypnotic-, or Anxiolytic-Induced Persisting Dementia
292.83 Sedative-, Hypnotic-, or Anxiolytic-Induced Persisting Amnestic Disorder
292.xx Sedative-, Hypnotic-, or Anxiolytic-Induced Psychotic Disorder
.11 With Delusions[I,W]
.12 With Hallucinations[I,W]
292.84 Sedative-, Hypnotic-, or Anxiolytic-Induced Mood Disorder[I,W]
292.89 Sedative-, Hypnotic-, or Anxiolytic-Induced Anxiety Disorder[W]
292.89 Sedative-, Hypnotic-, or Anxiolytic-Induced Sexual Dysfunction[I]
292.89 Sedative-, Hypnotic-, or Anxiolytic-Induced Sleep Disorder[I,W]
292.9 Sedative-, Hypnotic-, or Anxiolytic-Related Disorder NOS

Polysubstance-Related Disorder

304.80 Polysubstance Dependence[a,b,c,d]

Other (or Unknown) Substance-Related Disorders

Other (or Unknown) Substance Use Disorders

304.90 Other (or Unknown) Substance Dependence[a,b,c,d]
305.90 Other (or Unknown) Substance Abuse

Other (or Unknown) Substance-Induced Disorders

292.89 Other (or Unknown) Substance Intoxication
Specify if: With Perceptual Disturbances
292.0 Other (or Unknown) Substance Withdrawal
Specify if: With Perceptual Disturbances
292.81 Other (or Unknown) Substance–Induced Delirium
292.82 Other (or Unknown) Substance–Induced Persisting Dementia
292.83 Other (or Unknown) Substance–Induced Persisting Amnestic Disorder
292.xx Other (or Unknown) Substance–Induced Psychotic Disorder
.11 With Delusions[I,W]
.12 With Hallucinations[I,W]
292.84 Other (or Unknown) Substance–Induced Mood Disorder[I,W]
292.89 Other (or Unknown) Substance–Induced Anxiety Disorder[I,W]
292.89 Other (or Unknown) Substance–Induced Sexual Dysfunction[I]

292.89 Other (or Unknown) Substance–Induced Sleep Disorder[I,W]
292.9 Other (or Unknown) Substance–Related Disorder NOS

SCHIZOPHRENIA AND OTHER PSYCHOTIC DISORDERS

295.xx Schizophrenia

The following Classification of Longitudinal Course applies to all subtypes of Schizophrenia:

Episodic With Interepisode Residual Symptoms (*specify if:* With Prominent Negative Symptoms)/Episodic With No Interepisode Residual Symptoms

Continuous (*specify if:* With Prominent Negative Symptoms)

Single Episode in Partial Remission (*specify if:* With Prominent Negative Symptoms)/Single Episode In Full Remission

Other or Unspecified Pattern

.30 Paranoid Type
.10 Disorganized Type
.20 Catatonic Type
.90 Undifferentiated Type
.60 Residual Type

295.40 Schizophreniform Disorder
Specify if: Without Good Prognostic Features/ With Good Prognostic Features
295.70 Schizoaffective Disorder
Specify type: Bipolar Type/Depressive Type
297.1 Delusional Disorder
Specify type: Erotomanic Type/Grandiose Type/ Jealous Type/Persecutory Type/Somatic Type/ Mixed Type/Unspecified Type
298.8 Brief Psychotic Disorder
Specify if: With Marked Stressor(s)/Without Marked Stressor(s)/With Postpartum Onset
297.3 Shared Psychotic Disorder
293.xx Psychotic Disorder Due to . . . *[Indicate the General Medical Condition]*
.81 With Delusions
.82 With Hallucinations
___.___ Substance-Induced Psychotic Disorder (*refer to Substance-Related Disorders for substance-specific codes)*
Specify if: With Onset During Intoxication/ With Onset During Withdrawal
298.9 Psychotic Disorder NOS

MOOD DISORDERS

Code current state of Major Depressive Disorder or Bipolar I Disorder in fifth digit:

1 = Mild
2 = Moderate
3 = Severe Without Psychotic Features
4 = Severe With Psychotic Features
Specify: Mood-Congruent Psychotic Features/ Mood-Incongruent Psychotic Features

5= In Partial Remission
6 = In Full Remission
0 = Unspecified

The following specifiers apply (for current or most recent episode) to Mood Disorders as noted:
[a]Severity/Psychotic/Remission Specifiers/[b]Chronic/ [c]With Catatonic Features/[d]With Melancholic Features/ [e]With Atypical Features/[f]With Postpartum Onset

The following specifiers apply to mood disorders as noted:
[g]With or Without Full Interepisode Recovery/[h]With Seasonal Pattern/[i]With Rapid Cycling

Depressive Disorders

296.xx Major Depressive Disorder
.2x Single Episode[a,b,c,d,e,f]
.3x Recurrent[a,b,c,d,e,f,g,h]
300.4 Dysthymic Disorder
Specify if: Early Onset/Late Onset
Specify: With Atypical Features
311 Depressive Disorder NOS

Bipolar Disorders

296.xx Bipolar I Disorder
.0x Single Manic Episode[a,c,f]
Specify if: Mixed
.40 Most Recent Episode Hypomanic[g,h,i]
.4x Most Recent Episode Manic[a,c,f,g,h,i]
.6x Most Recent Episode Mixed[a,c,f,g,h,i]
.5x Most Recent Episode Depressed[a,b,c,d,e,f,g,h,i]
.7 Most Recent Episode Unspecified[g,h,i]
296.89 Bipolar II Disorder[a,b,c,d,e,f,g,h,i]
Specify (current or most recent episode): Hypomanic/Depressed
301.13 Cyclothymic Disorder
296.80 Bipolar Disorder NOS
293.83 Mood Disorder Due to . . . *[Indicate the General Medical Condition]*
Specify type: With Depressive Features/With Major Depressive-Like Episode/With Manic Features/With Mixed Features
___.___ Substance-Induced Mood Disorder (*refer to Substance-Related Disorders for substance-specific codes)*
Specify type: With Depressive Features/With Manic Features/With Mixed Features
Specify if: With Onset During Intoxication/ With Onset During Withdrawal
296.90 Mood Disorder NOS

ANXIETY DISORDERS

300.01 Panic Disorder Without Agoraphobia
300.21 Panic Disorder With Agoraphobia
300.22 Agoraphobia Without History of Panic Disorder
300.29 Specific Phobia
Specify type: Animal Type/Natural Environment Type/Blood-Injection-Injury Type/Situational Type/Other Type
300.23 Social Phobia
Specify if: Generalized
300.3 Obsessive-Compulsive Disorder
Specify if: With Poor Insight
309.81 Posttraumatic Stress Disorder
Specify if: Acute/Chronic
Specify if: With Delayed Onset
308.3 Acute Stress Disorder
300.02 Generalized Anxiety Disorder
293.84 Anxiety Disorder Due to . . . *[Indicate the General Medical Condition]*
Specify if: With Generalized Anxiety/With Panic Attacks/With Obsessive-Compulsive Symptoms
___.__ Substance-Induced Anxiety Disorder *(refer to Substance-Related Disorders for substance-specific codes)*
Specify if: With Generalized Anxiety/With Panic Attacks/With Obsessive-Compulsive Symptoms/With Phobic Symptoms
Specify if: With Onset During Intoxication/With Onset During Withdrawal
300.00 Anxiety Disorder NOS

SOMATOFORM DISORDERS

300.81 Somatization Disorder
300.82 Undifferentiated Somatoform Disorder
300.11 Conversion Disorder
Specify type: With Motor Symptom or Deficit/With Sensory Symptom or Deficit/With Seizures or Convulsions/With Mixed Presentation
307.xx Pain Disorder
.80 Associated With Psychologic Factors
.89 Associated With Both Psychologic Factors and a General Medical Condition
Specify if: Acute/Chronic
300.7 Hypochondriasis
Specify if: With Poor Insight
300.7 Body Dysmorphic Disorder
300.82 Somatoform Disorder NOS

FACTITIOUS DISORDERS

300.xx Factitious Disorder
.16 With Predominantly Psychologic Signs and Symptoms
.19 With Predominantly Physical Signs and Symptoms
.19 With Combined Psychologic and Physical Signs and Symptoms
300.19 Factitious Disorder NOS

DISSOCIATIVE DISORDERS

300.12 Dissociative Amnesia
300.13 Dissociative Fugue
300.14 Dissociative Identity Disorder
300.6 Depersonalization Disorder
300.15 Dissociative Disorder NOS

SEXUAL AND GENDER IDENTITY DISORDERS

Sexual Dysfunctions

The following specifiers apply to all primary sexual dysfunctions:
Lifelong Type/Acquired Type
Generalized Type/Situational Type
Due to Psychologic Factors/Due to Combined Factors

Sexual Desire Disorders

302.71 Hypoactive Sexual Desire Disorder
302.79 Sexual Aversion Disorder

Sexual Arousal Disorders

302.72 Female Sexual Arousal Disorder
302.72 Male Erectile Disorder

Orgasmic Disorders

302.73 Female Orgasmic Disorder
302.74 Male Orgasmic Disorder
302.75 Premature Ejaculation

Sexual Pain Disorders

302.76 Dyspareunia (Not Due to a General Medical Condition)
306.51 Vaginismus (Not Due to a General Medical Condition)

Sexual Dysfunction Due to a General Medical Condition

625.8 Female Hypoactive Sexual Desire Disorder Due to . . . *[Indicate the General Medical Condition]*
608.89 Male Hypoactive Sexual Desire Disorder Due to . . . *[Indicate the General Medical Condition]*
607.84 Male Erectile Disorder Due to . . . *[Indicate the General Medical Condition]*
625.0 Female Dyspareunia Due to . . . *[Indicate the General Medical Condition]*
608.89 Male Dyspareunia Due to . . . *[Indicate the General Medical Condition]*
625.8 Other Female Sexual Dysfunction Due to . . . *[Indicate the General Medical Condition]*
608.89 Other Male Sexual Dysfunction Due to . . . *[Indicate the General Medical Condition]*

___.__ Substance-Induced Sexual Dysfunction *(refer to Substance-Related Disorders for substance-specific codes)*
Specify if: With Impaired Desire/With Impaired Arousal/With Impaired Orgasm/With Sexual Pain
Specify if: With Onset During Intoxication
302.70 Sexual Dysfunction NOS

Paraphilias

302.4 Exhibitionism
302.81 Fetishism
302.89 Frotteurism
302.2 Pedophilia
Specify if: Sexually Attracted to Males/Sexually Attracted to Females/Sexually Attracted to Both
Specify if: Limited to Incest
Specify type: Exclusive Type/Nonexclusive Type
302.83 Sexual Masochism
302.84 Sexual Sadism
302.3 Transvestic Fetishism
Specify if: With Gender Dysphoria
302.82 Voyeurism
302.9 Paraphilia NOS

Gender Identity Disorders

302.xx Gender Identity Disorder
.6 In Children
.85 In Adolescents or Adults
Specify if: Sexually Attracted to Males/Sexually Attracted to Females/Sexually Attracted to Both/Sexually Attracted to Neither
302.6 Gender Identity Disorder NOS
302.9 Sexual Disorder NOS

EATING DISORDERS

307.1 Anorexia Nervosa
Specify type: Restricting Type; Binge-Eating/Purging Type
307.51 Bulimia Nervosa
Specify type: Purging Type/Nonpurging Type
307.50 Eating Disorder NOS

SLEEP DISORDERS

Primary Sleep Disorders

Dyssomnias

307.42 Primary Insomnia
307.44 Primary Hypersomnia
Specify if: Recurrent
347 Narcolepsy
780.59 Breathing-Related Sleep Disorder
307.45 Circadian Rhythm Sleep Disorder
Specify type: Delayed Sleep Phase Type/Jet Lag Type/Shift Work Type/Unspecified Type
307.47 Dyssomnia NOS

Parasomnias

307.47 Nightmare Disorder
307.46 Sleep Terror Disorder
307.46 Sleepwalking Disorder
307.47 Parasomnia NOS

Sleep Disorders Related to Another Mental Disorder

307.42 Insomnia Related to . . . *[Indicate the Axis I or Axis II Disorder]*
307.44 Hypersomnia Related to . . . *[Indicate the Axis I or Axis II Disorder]*

Other Sleep Disorders

780.xx Sleep Disorder Due to . . . *[Indicate the General Medical Condition]*
.52 Insomnia Type
.54 Hypersomnia Type
.59 Parasomnia Type
.59 Mixed Type
___.__ Substance-Induced Sleep Disorder *(refer to Substance-Related Disorders for substance-specific codes)*
Specify type: Insomnia Type/Hypersomnia Type/Parasomnia Type/Mixed Type
Specify if: With Onset During Intoxication/With Onset During Withdrawal

IMPULSE-CONTROL DISORDERS NOT ELSEWHERE CLASSIFIED

312.34 Intermittent Explosive Disorder
312.32 Kleptomania
312.33 Pyromania
312.31 Pathologic Gambling
312.39 Trichotillomania
312.30 Impulse-Control Disorder NOS

ADJUSTMENT DISORDERS

309.xx Adjustment Disorder
.0 With Depressed Mood
.24 With Anxiety
.28 With Mixed Anxiety and Depressed Mood
.3 With Disturbance of Conduct
.4 With Mixed Disturbance of Emotions and Conduct
.9 Unspecified
Specify if: Acute/Chronic

PERSONALITY DISORDERS

NOTE: These are coded on Axis II.
301.0 Paranoid Personality Disorder
301.20 Schizoid Personality Disorder
301.22 Schizotypal Personality Disorder
301.7 Antisocial Personality Disorder
301.83 Borderline Personality Disorder
301.50 Histrionic Personality Disorder
301.81 Narcissistic Personality Disorder
301.82 Avoidant Personality Disorder

301.6 Dependent Personality Disorder
301.4 Obsessive-Compulsive Personality Disorder
301.9 Personality Disorder NOS

OTHER CONDITIONS THAT MAY BE A FOCUS OF CLINICAL ATTENTION

Psychologic Factors Affecting Medical Condition

316 . . . *[Specified Psychologic Factor] Affecting . . . [Indicate the General Medical Condition]*

Choose name based on nature of factors:
Mental Disorder Affecting Medical Condition
Psychologic Symptoms Affecting Medical Condition
Personality Traits or Coping Style Affecting Medical Condition
Maladaptive Health Behaviors Affecting Medical Condition
Stress-Related Physiologic Response Affecting Medical Condition
Other or Unspecified Psychologic Factors Affecting Medical Condition

Medication-Induced Movement Disorders

332.1 Neuroleptic-Induced Parkinsonism
333.92 Neuroleptic Malignant Syndrome
333.7 Neuroleptic-Induced Acute Dystonia
333.99 Neuroleptic-Induced Acute Akathisia
333.82 Neuroleptic-Induced Tardive Dyskinesia
333.1 Medication-Induced Postural Tremor
333.90 Medication-Induced Movement Disorder NOS

Other Medication-Induced Disorder

995.2 Adverse Effects of Medication NOS

Relational Problems

V61.9 Relational Problem Related to a Mental Disorder or General Medical Condition
V61.20 Parent-Child Relational Problem
V61.10 Partner Relational Problem
V61.8 Sibling Relational Problem
V62.81 Relational Problem NOS

Problems Related to Abuse or Neglect

V61.21 Physical Abuse of Child *(code 995.5 if focus of attention is on victim)*
V61.21 Sexual Abuse of Child *(code 995.5 if focus of attention is on victim)*
V61.21 Neglect of Child *(code 995.5 if focus of attention is on victim)*
___.__ Physical Abuse of Adult
V61.12 (if by partner)
V62.83 (if by person other than partner) *(code 995.81 if focus of attention is on victim)*
___.__ Sexual Abuse of Adult
V61.12 (if by partner)
V62.83 (if by person other than partner) *(code 995.83 if focus of attention is on victim)*

Additional Conditions That May Be a Focus of Clinical Attention

V15.81 Noncompliance With Treatment
V65.2 Malingering
V71.01 Adult Antisocial Behavior
V71.02 Child or Adolescent Antisocial Behavior
V62.89 Borderline Intellectual Functioning
Note: This is coded on Axis II.
780.9 Age-Related Cognitive Decline
V62.82 Bereavement
V62.3 Academic Problem
V62.2 Occupational Problem
313.82 Identity Problem
V62.89 Religious or Spiritual Problem
V62.4 Acculturation Problem
V62.89 Phase of Life Problem

ADDITIONAL CODES

300.9 Unspecified Mental Disorder (nonpsychotic)
V71.09 No Diagnosis or Condition on Axis I
799.9 Diagnosis or Condition Deferred on Axis I
V71.09 No Diagnosis on Axis II
799.9 Diagnosis Deferred on Axis II

MULTIAXIAL SYSTEM

Axis I Clinical Disorder
Other Conditions That May Be a Focus of Clinical Attention
Axis II Personality Disorders
Mental Retardation
Axis III General Medical Conditions
Axis IV Psychosocial and Environmental Problems
Axis V Global Assessment of Functioning

Appendix C

Axis V: Global Assessment of Functioning (GAF) Scale

Consider psychologic, social, and occupational functioning on a hypothetic continuum of mental health–illness. Do not include impairment in functioning due to physical (or environmental) limitations. (NOTE: Use intermediate codes when appropriate, e.g., 45, 68, 72.)

CODE

100–91	Superior functioning in a wide range of activities, life's problems never seem to get out of hand, is sought out by others because of his many positive qualities. No symptoms.
90–81	Absent or minimal symptoms (e.g., mild anxiety before an exam), good functioning in all areas, interested and involved in a wide range of activities, socially effective, generally satisfied with life, no more than everyday problems or concerns (e.g., an occasional argument with family members).
80–71	If symptoms are present, they are transient and expectable reactions to psychosocial stressors (e.g., difficulty concentrating after family argument); no more than slight impairment in social, occupational, or school functioning (e.g., temporarily falling behind in schoolwork).
70–61	Some mild symptoms (e.g., depressed mood and mild insomnia) OR some difficulty in social, occupational, or school functioning (e.g., occasional truancy, or theft within the household), but generally functioning pretty well, has some meaningful interpersonal relationships.
60–51	Moderate symptoms (e.g., flat affect and circumstantial speech, occasional panic attacks) OR moderate difficulty in social, occupational, or school functioning (e.g., few friends, conflicts with peers or coworkers).
50–41	Serious symptoms (e.g., suicidal ideation, severe obsessional rituals, frequent shoplifting) OR any serious impairment in social, occupational, or school functioning (e.g., no friends, unable to keep a job).
40–31	Some impairment in reality testing or communication (e.g., speech is at times illogical, obscure, or irrelevant) OR major impairment in several areas, such as work or school, family relations, judgment, thinking, or mood (e.g., depressed man avoids friends, neglects family, and is unable to work; child frequently beats up younger children, is defiant at home, and is failing at school).
30–21	Behavior is considerably influenced by delusions or hallucinations OR serious impairment in communication or judgment (e.g., sometimes incoherent, acts grossly inappropriately, suicidal preoccupation) OR inability to function in almost all areas (e.g., stays in bed all day; no job, home, or friends).
20–11	Some danger of hurting self or others (e.g., suicide attempts without clear expectation of death, frequently violent, manic excitement) OR occasionally fails to maintain minimal personal hygiene (e.g., smears feces) OR gross impairment in communication (e.g., largely incoherent or mute).
10–1	Persistent danger of severely hurting self or others (e.g., recurrent violence) OR persistent inability to maintain personal hygiene OR serious suicidal act with clear expectation of death.
	Inadequate information.

The rating of overall psychologic functioning on a scale of 0-100 was operationalized by Luborsky in the Health-Sickness Rating Scale (Luborsky L: Clinicians' judgments of mental health, *Arch Gen Psychiatry* 7:407-417, 1962). Spitzer and colleagues developed a revision of the Health-Sickness Rating Scale called the Global Assessment Scale (GAS) (Endicott J, Spitzer RL, Fleiss JL, Cohen J: The global assessment scale: a procedure for measuring overall severity of psychiatric disturbance, *Arch Gen Psychiatry* 33:766-771, 1976). A modified version of the GAS was included in *DSM-III-R* as the Global Assessment of Functioning (GAF) Scale.

Appendix D Answers to Review Questions

Chapter 1: Principles of Psychiatric Nursing: Theory and Practice
1. 3
2. 1
3. 2, 3, 5
4. 1, 3, 5
5. 1, 5
6. 1

Chapter 2: Clinical Practice: Rewards, Challenges, and Solutions
1. 4, 5
2. 4, 1, 2, 3
3. 3
4. 2
5. 1

Chapter 3: The Nursing Process
1. 1
2. 4
3. 4
4. 3
5. 3

Chapter 4: Therapeutic Communication
1. 4
2. 4
3. 4
4. 1
5. 2

Chapter 5: Growth and Development Across the Life Span
1. 4
2. 1
3. 3
4. 1, 3, 4
5. 1, 2, 4

Chapter 6: Neurobiology in Mental Health and Disorder
1. 1
2. 4
3. 1, 3, 5
4. 4
5. 1

Chapter 7: Cultural, Ethnic, and Spiritual Considerations
1. 1, 2
2. 4
3. 4
4. 1
5. 1

Chapter 8: Legal and Ethical Aspects in Clinical Practice
1. 4
2. 1
3. 2
4. 1
5. 1, 2, 5
6. 2

Chapter 9: Anxiety and Anxiety Disorders
1. 1
2. 2
3. 2
4. 4, 1, 3, 2
5. 3

Chapter 10: Somatoform, Factitious, and Dissociative Disorders
1. 2, 4, 5, 6
2. 1
3. 3
4. 4
5. 1

Chapter 11: Mood Disorders and Adjustment Disorders
1. 4
2. 3
3. 1
4. 2, 3, 5
5. 2
6. 3, 1, 2

Chapter 12: Schizophrenia and Other Psychotic Disorders
1. 2
2. 1
3. 4
4. 1
5. 1
6. 4

Chapter 13: Personality Disorders
1. 3
2. 4
3. 1
4. 4
5. 1, 2, 5

Chapter 14: Substance-Related Disorders
1. 4
2. 1, 5
3. 1, 5
4. 2
5. 1

Chapter 15: Cognitive Disorders: Delirium, Dementia, and Amnestic Disorders

1. 1
2. 2, 3, 1
3. 2
4. 1, 3, 4
5. 4

Chapter 16: Disorders of Infancy, Childhood, and Adolescence

1. 3
2. 2, 4, 5
3. 1
4. 2
5. 4

Chapter 17: Eating Disorders

1. 1, 2, 5
2. 1
3. 2, 3, 4, 5
4. 4, 1, 2, 3
5. 4

Chapter 18: Sleep Disorders

1. 1
2. 2, 4
3. 2
4. 1, 5
5. 2

Chapter 19: Sexual Disorders

1. 4
2. 2
3. 3
4. 1
5. 1, 4, 5

Chapter 20: Crisis: Theory and Intervention

1. 2, 3, 1, 4
2. 3, 4, 5
3. 1
4. 4
5. 2

Chapter 21: Suicide: Prevention and Intervention

1. 1, 4, 5
2. 2
3. 4
4. 1
5. 2

Chapter 22: Violence and Forensics in Clinical Practice: Abuse, Neglect, Anger, and Rape

1. 1, 2, 3, 5
2. 2
3. 1
4. 4
5. 3

Chapter 23: Therapies in Clinical Practice

1. 4
2. 2
3. 1
4. 4
5. 2

Chapter 24: Psychopharmacology

1. 1
2. 2
3. 4
4. 2, 3
5. 4

Chapter 25: Complementary and Alternative Therapies

1. 1
2. 2
3. 1, 2
4. 4, 5
5. 3

Chapter 26: Grief and Loss

1. 4
2. 4
3. 3
4. 1
5. 4

Chapter 27: Mental and Emotional Responses to Medical Illness

1. 1, 3, 4
2. 2
3. 1
4. 2
5. 3

Chapter 28: Caring for Clients in the Community

1. 2
2. 1
3. 4
4. 1, 4
5. 4

Chapter 29: Caring for Persons With Severe and Persistent Mental Illness

1. 1
2. 2
3. 4
4. 3
5. 1

Glossary

A

abstinence Voluntary refraining from a behavior or the use of a substance that has caused problems in psychosocial, physical, cognitive/perceptual, or spiritual/belief dimensions of life (e.g., alcohol/drug use, food, gambling, spending, sex).

abuse (1) A maladaptive pattern of substance use leading to problems in psychosocial, biologic, cognitive/perceptual, or spiritual/belief dimensions of life. (2) Any harm or injury to a child, adult, elder (e.g., physical, psychologic, emotional, sexual).

acculturation Adapting or modifying cultural values and beliefs to accommodate living in a new culture.

acquired immunodeficiency syndrome (AIDS) A late-stage infection with HIV viruses (HIV-1 and 2).

acting-out The expression of internal affective states through external activities and behaviors, which are often destructive or maladaptive.

activities of daily living (ADLs) The set of activities used in routine daily lives, such as personal hygiene, grooming, eating, and recreation.

adaptive The ability to adapt to change in internal or external circumstances or conditions.

addiction A maladaptive, compulsive dependence on a substance (e.g., alcohol, other drugs) or a behavior (e.g., gambling, spending).

adverse drug reaction An unintended effect of a medication resulting in severe, unwanted symptoms or consequences.

affect Outward, bodily expression of emotions, ranging through joy, sorrow, anger, and so on. *Blunted affect:* Restricted expression of emotions. *Flat affect:* Lack of outward expression of emotions. *Inappropriate affect:* Affect that is not congruent with the emotion being felt (e.g., laughing when sad). *Labile affect:* Rapid changes in emotional expression.

agnosia The loss of comprehension of auditory, visual, or other sensations, although the senses are intact.

agraphia The loss of the ability to write.

akathisia Literally, *not sitting.* A syndrome caused by dopamine-blocking drugs characterized by both motor restlessness and a subjective feeling of inner restlessness.

alcoholic blackout An episode of forgetting all or part of what occurred during or following alcohol intake.

alcoholism A chronic, progressive, and potentially fatal biogenic and psychosocial disease characterized by impaired control over drinking. Eventual tolerance and physical dependence leads to loss of control, distorted thinking, and other physical and social consequences.

alexia Inability to read because of central nervous system lesion or dysfunction.

alexithymia A condition in which individuals have difficulty recognizing and describing their emotions. The term literally means *no words for feelings.* Individuals with eating disorders often have a restricted emotional life.

allele Small defects or variations in genes.

allopathic The health beliefs and practices that are derived from the scientific models of the present time and involve the use of technology and other modalities of present-day health care, such as immunization, proper nutrition, and resuscitation.

altruism The principle or practice of unselfish concern for others' welfare.

Alzheimer's disease A neurodegenerative disease characterized by progressive, irreversible, and lethal structural damage to the brain resulting from the presence of beta-amyloid proteins and leading to loss of cognitive functions and symptoms of progressive dementia.

ambivalence Simultaneously holding two different attitudes, emotions, thoughts, or feelings about a person, object, or situation.

amnestic disorders Impairments of memory without the delirium and dementia.

amyloid plaques Formed of amyloid proteins and surround affected neuronal cells. The amount of plaques is related to the degree of mental deterioration. Amyloid plaques interfere with cell-to-cell communication, resulting in decreased availability of acetylcholine. Also called *senile plaques* or *neuritic plaques.*

anger A common feeling in grief, often directed toward the deceased, family members, health care givers, or higher power. Anger is inappropriate when intent is to harm or injure others and is discussed in several chapters throughout the text.

anhedonia The loss of pleasure and interest in activities previously enjoyed or in life itself.

anticipatory grief Grief experienced before death or loss occurs (e.g., when a loved one has a terminal illness).

anxiety A vague, nonspecific feeling of uneasiness, tension, apprehension, and sometimes dread or pending doom. Anxiety occurs as a result of a threat to one's biologic, physiologic, or social integrity arising from external influences. It is a universal experience and an integral part of human existence.

aphasia *Expressive aphasia:* The inability to speak or write. *Receptive aphasia:* The inability to comprehend what is being said or written. May progress to babbling or mutism.

apraxia The loss of the ability to carry out purposeful, complex movements and to use objects properly.

assent To agree, concur, or yield.

autism A pervasive developmental disorder characterized by marked impairment of social and cognitive abilities.

autistic thinking Disturbances in thought that result from the intrusion of a private fantasy world that is internally stimulated, resulting in abnormal responses to people and events in the real world.

autodiagnosis Self-examination of one's own thoughts, feelings, perceptions, and attitudes about a particular client.

B

basal ganglia (nuclei) An area of the central nervous system made up of cell bodies and that is responsible for motor functions and association.

battering Physical, sexual, or mental abuse of women by intimate partners or those with whom they have been intimate.

behavior modification Type of therapy that focuses on modifying observable behavior by manipulating the environment, the behavior, or the consequences of a behavior.

bereavement The objective state following loss, especially of a loved one; the state of grieving.

binge eating disorder (BED) A pattern of binge eating without the purging characteristic of bulimia nervosa. BED is commonly known as compulsive overeating. It is included in DSM-IV-TR as a proposed diagnosis for further study.

blackout Loss of memory of events that occur after the onset of the causative agent or condition such as the ingestion of alcohol or drugs.

boundary Distinguishing and separating the self from others by clarifying the limits and extent of the nurse's responsibilities and duties in relationship to the client and others.

breach of duty Failure to perform by act of commission or omission within scope of practice and adhere to defined standard of care.

bulimarexia An obsession with thinness, dieting, and a compulsive cycle of bingeing and purging. This syndrome is now labeled bulimia nervosa.

C

case management Clinical coordination of inpatient and outpatient care designed to support the client's highest level of functioning. Services include crisis intervention, supportive counseling, consultation/collaboration with multidisciplinary treatment providers, medication, and mental status monitoring.

cataplexy Sudden loss of muscle tone and voluntary muscle movement.

catastrophic reaction A sudden or gradual negative change in the behavior of clients with dementia caused by their inability to understand and cope with stimuli in the environment.

central nervous system A division of the human nervous system containing the brain and spinal cord.

challenge An actual or potential task or undertaking that by its very nature may be difficult yet stimulating.

chemical restraint The use of psychotropic drugs and sedatives to reduce or eliminate psychiatric symptoms. Symptom management through medication as part of the client's standard treatment plan is another way to describe chemical restraint and is the currently accepted description.

chronic mental illness A psychiatric disorder that persists over time with remissions and recurrence of severe, disabling symptoms.

chronic sorrow Grief in response to an ongoing loss, such as a long chronic illness in a loved one.

circadian rhythm The cycle of sleep and wakefulness and fluctuation of various physiologic and behavioral parameters over a 24-hour cycle including change in body temperature, hormone secretion, and neurotransmitter secretion such as norepinephrine and serotonin, which are both believed to be involved in mood and affect states.

classical conditioning Theory developed by Ivan Pavlov involving the pairing of a neutral stimulus with another stimulus.

clinical pathway A standardized format used to provide and monitor client care and progress by way of the case management, interdisciplinary health care delivery system. Also known as critical pathway, care path, or care map.

Clubhouse Model A place where persons with severe and persistent mental illness go to rebuild their lives. The participants are viewed as members rather than patients, and the emphasis is on the members' strengths rather than their weaknesses.

codependence A relationship in which the actions of a member of the family or close friend or colleague of an alcohol- or drug-dependent person tend to perpetuate the person's dependence and thereby retard the process of recovery. The term is also now used figuratively to describe the way in which the community or society acts as an enabler of alcohol or drug dependence, or other areas of dysfunction (e.g., family, gambling, spending).

cognition Awareness and subjective meaning of an event.

commitment Court-ordered evaluation certifying that an individual is to be confined to a mental health facility for treatment.

communication A reciprocal process of sending and receiving messages between two or more people and their environment; the vehicle for establishing a therapeutic relationship.

community-linked health care Care provided by public or private partnerships using grant and government funds.

community mental health center An outpatient facility that provides multiple mental health treatments and programs for people in a specified area.

competency to stand trial The ability of an individual to understand the charges and their consequences, to understand the nature and object of the legal proceedings, and to advise an attorney to assist in the defense.

complementary/alternative medicine (CAM) CAM covers a broad range of healing philosophies, approaches, and therapies. It generally is defined as those treatments and health care practices not taught widely in medical schools, not generally used in hospitals, and not usually reimbursed by medical insurance companies (National Center for Complementary and Alternative Medicine, NCCAM). Additional terms include *holistic therapies* and *integrative medicine*.

compulsion An unremitting, repetitive impulse to perform a behavior, such as hand washing, checking, cleaning, or putting things in order; or mental acts, such as praying, counting, or repeating words silently. The goal of the behavior is to prevent or reduce anxiety or distress, not to provide pleasure or gratification. Compulsive acts often occur to reduce the distress that accompanies an obsession or to prevent some dreaded event or situation.

concept map A critical problem-solving plan that promotes the student's understanding of the relationships between ideas, concepts, or topics.

concierge medicine The practice of medicine or other health care limited to clients who can afford to privately pay for extra or special services. Also referred to as *boutique medicine* or *platinum medicine*.

confidentiality The right of the psychiatric client to keep information from people outside the health care team.

congruence Consistency of agreement between verbal and nonverbal behavior.

contraband Any objects that are prohibited by law, or the rules of a facility. On an acute care psychiatric unit, this includes illegal drugs, dangerous objects such as knives, guns, or anything that may prove harmful to clients on that unit.

conventional/traditional medicine The primary medicine practiced in the United States. The major focus is on the biologic mechanisms of disease, ruling out potential causes, then forming a diagnosis and treatment of a specific disease. Also *Western medicine, mainstream medicine, orthodox medicine, allopathic medicine, biomedicine.*

co-occurrence More than one psychiatric diagnosis occurring at the same time in the same individual. Also *comorbid* or *coexisting.*

cope To adapt to a threat to integrity using a variety of tools, including adaptive (useful) or maladaptive (ineffective) maneuvers. One can cope internally via changes in thinking or psychologic defense mechanisms, or externally, via actions.

countertransference The nurse's feelings and responses to a client that are associated with a significant person in the nurse's life. Although countertransference may be a natural part of therapy, the nurse needs to be aware of it and manage it to avoid behaving inappropriately toward the client.

crisis (1) An event that threatens well-being such as sudden death in the family or an earthquake. A response to an event, where the person interprets the event as a threat to well-being or to one's normal state of being. The interpretation of a threat leads to attempts to cope with the threat. Failed attempts to meet a threat, resulting in an assumption that the threat cannot be remedied—that is, the crisis begins when coping efforts fail.

crisis intervention Therapeutic techniques for helping individuals experiencing a crisis.

critical thinking An intellectual, disciplined process of actively and skillfully conceptualizing, applying, analyzing, synthesizing, and evaluating information through observation, experience, reasoning, and communication, as a guide to belief or action.

cultural competence Standard of practice that ensures the caregiver accepts and recognizes multiple aspects of cultural diversity among individuals and helps them receive information that they understand.

culture The collective process of acquiring shared beliefs, dominant patterns of behavior, values, and attitudes learned through socialization.

curative factors Eleven factors, as determined by Irvin Yalom, that make up the dynamic of every group and facilitate change by assisting members to understand their patterns of interacting within the group.

D

defense A means or method of protecting oneself; an unconscious mental activity or mental structure (e.g., a defense mechanism) that protects the ego from anxiety.

defense mechanisms Also known as ego defenses. Automatic and semiautomatic mental processes to protect the ego (person) against anxiety resulting from feelings and impulses that threaten psychologic harm, conflict, or exposure, for example, denial and repression.

deinstitutionalization Discharge from the psychiatric institution or hospital into the community. Specifically refers to the discharge of severely mentally ill clients with long-term hospitalizations into less-structured care during the 1960s.

delirium A disturbance of consciousness and a change in cognition that develop over a short period of time and tends to fluctuate during the course of the day, characterized by disorientation to time and place; reduced ability to focus, sustain, or shift attention; incoherent speech; and continual aimless physical activity.

delusions False beliefs that are fixed and resistant to reasoning.

dementia A global impairment of intellectual (cognitive) functions (e.g., thinking, remembering, reasoning) that usually is progressive and of sufficient severity to interfere with a person's normal social and occupational functioning.

denial Avoidance of reality that threatens an individual's self-concept. Denial is demonstrated by ignoring or deemphasizing the importance of an event, observation, or feeling. At times, denial helps one survive life stressors.

depersonalization Feelings of unreality or alienation. Individuals experiencing depersonalization have difficulty distinguishing themselves from others. Depersonalization may occur in extreme anxiety.

depression A dysphoric or depressed mood state. The relatively normal symptom of feeling somewhat depressed, sad, or blue must be distinguished from the diagnosis of major depression that is more severe; in addition to depressed mood, it includes several other symptoms (changes in appetite, weight, sleep, activity, libido, energy; thoughts of death or suicide, and more).

derealization The feeling that the surrounding world is not real or is distorted.

dereism A loss of connection with reality and logic that occurs just before autistic thinking noted in schizophrenia. Thoughts become private and idiosyncratic.

designer drugs Illegal drugs used at all-night parties, called raves or trances. Designer drugs include GHB (gamma-hydroxy butyrate), ketamine, ecstasy, rohypnol, and others.

detoxification The removal of toxins or poisons from a person. Treatment that assists the individual in withdrawing from the physical effects of substances.

devaluation A method of coping whereby a person deals with emotional conflict or stressors by attributing exaggerated negative qualities to oneself or others.

disease A term used to describe altered body functions and a condition that places limitations on daily activities with the presence of recognizable disease symptoms. It is a result of the inability to adapt to certain stressors. Formerly it was believed that a specific disease had one particular cause. Today, it is known that the individual's physical and psychologic responses are affected by multiple stimuli and interactions with their environments.

disorientation A loss of familiarity with place, time, and person, and situation.

dissociation The separation of an overwhelming event from one's conscious awareness; a prominent defense mechanism in dissociative identity disorder (formerly known as *multiple personality disorder*).

distress A subjective response to internal or external stimuli that are threatening or perceived as threatening to the self.

diurnal variation Feeling worse or more depressed in the morning and better in the evening.

domestic violence Learned behaviors used by one or more persons in an intimate or family relationship for the purpose of controlling the behavior of others. Violence may take the form of physical, psychologic, sexual, or emotional abuse; intimidation; threats; isolation; economic control; or stalking.

double-bind A situation in which contradictory messages are given to one person by another, demanding a response or choice between two opposing alternatives.

dual diagnosis A term used when the individual has two identified primary psychiatric diagnoses, most commonly used when one diagnosis is drug or alcohol related. For example, the person may have both a substance-related disorder and a mood disorder.

duty to warn The legal obligation of a mental health professional to warn an intended victim of potential harm from a client with mental illness.

dynamic Refers to an active and energetic state; the capacity or ability to change, as opposed to being static, fixed, or stationary.

dysarthria Difficulty in articulating words; this is especially frustrating because the client knows what words to use but has trouble forming them (more commonly found in vascular dementias and strokes).

dysfunctional grief Grief expressed to a significantly greater or lesser intensity over a significantly longer or shorter time than is culturally expected. It may manifest itself in serious physical or emotional disabilities (also termed *pathologic, complicated,* or *traumatic grief*).

dysphoria Depressed, sad mood.

dysthymia Chronic, low-level depression lasting more than 2 years that may lead to more severe depression if untreated.

dystonic Abnormal muscle tonicity and spasms of face, head, neck, and back (side effect of antipsychotic medication).

E

echolalia Involuntary repetition of words spoken by another person.

echopraxia Spontaneous imitation of movements made by another person.

eclectic approach Selecting or choosing from various sources and not following any one system. In therapy, refers to use of several different modalities together, when treating clients.

ego Freud's word for the self, whose major role is to find safe and appropriate ways for needs (instincts) to be met (gratified) in the external world. Lies mostly in the conscious.

ego defenses Automatic psychologic processes that keep out the threat of internal and external stressors and dangers or deny awareness to protect the self. Also known as *defense mechanisms* or *mental mechanisms.*

electroconvulsive therapy (ECT) A type of biologic therapy performed with the client under general anesthesia, most often used to treat major depression, in which a brief electrical stimulus is applied to the brain, producing a seizure.

empathy Projecting sensitivity and understanding of another's feelings and communicating the understanding in a way that the client comprehends.

enabler One who supports someone to continue on a path of substance abuse by providing excuses for or helping the affected individual avoid the consequences of his or her behavior.

encopresis The repeated passage of feces into inappropriate places (e.g., clothing or floor), whether involuntary or intentional.

enmeshed A pattern seen frequently in dysfunctional families, where members have diffuse rather than clear boundaries, lack clear role definitions, and are excessively involved in each other's lives. This makes it difficult to individuate and separate, which is a necessity for healthy functioning.

enuresis The repeated voiding of urine into bed or clothing, whether involuntary or intentional.

ethnicity A specific cultural group's sense of identification associated with its common social and cultural heritage.

ethnocentrism The tendency of members of one cultural group to view the members of other cultural groups in terms of the standards of behavior, attitudes, and values of their own group; belief in the superiority of one's own group.

ethnomethodology The study of people in context, through inductive, qualitative methods.

eustress A nonspecific stress response associated with desirable events such as marriage, birth of a child, or job promotion; from the Greek word *eu,* meaning "good."

euthymia A mood that is normal and level.

evaluative responses Responses that place a determined or conclusive value on a person, object, situation, or event, for example, "good" or "bad," "nice" or "mean," "pretty" or "ugly."

evidence-based practice Nursing practice that is proven effective by virtue of having undergone research versus being accepted merely on opinions or because of a history of having been done a certain way for a long time.

extrapyramidal symptoms (EPS) The collective term used to describe the motor side effects of dopamine-blocking medications. EPS includes acute dystonia, akathisia, parkinsonism, and tardive dyskinesia.

F

faith Belief, confidence, or trust in anything, which is not necessarily based on proof, or substantiated by actual fact. May refer to a religion, or spiritual belief.

feedback The measure by which the effectiveness of the message is gauged.

fetal alcohol syndrome (FAS) A set of congenital psychologic, behavioral, and physical abnormalities that occur in infants whose mothers consumed high amounts of alcohol during pregnancy.

flight of ideas The shifting from one idea to another without completing the previous idea, or an abrupt change of topics, expressed in a rapid flow of speech. Although most commonly seen in the manic phase of bipolar disorder, it may be noted in schizophrenia and is often confused with the looseness of associations (LOA) most often manifested in schizophrenia, in which thoughts are more fragmented.

forensic nursing A branch of nursing that focuses on the clinical observation and treatment of individuals who have mental health problems and who are charged with or convicted of crimes.

functional disabilities Difficulties with normal, day-to-day activities resulting from a mental or physical deficit.

G

gateway drugs Substances implicated as forerunners to polysubstance use or drug dependence (e.g., tobacco, alcohol, marijuana).

general adaptation syndrome (GAS) The syndrome described by Hans Selye as the body's response to stress; occurs in three stages: (1) alarm (fight or flight stage), (2) adaptation, and (3) exhaustion.

generativity In Erikson's personality theory, the positive outcome of one of the stages of adult personality development; the ability to do creative work or to contribute to the raising of one's children. The opposite of stagnation.

genuineness A quality of an effective nurse that encompasses openness, honesty, and sincerity.

gerontology The scientific study of the aging process involving multiple disciplines and settings.

Global Assessment of Functioning (GAF) score The fifth axis (assessment category) in the DSM-IV-TR that describes a person's overall functioning in society. A measure of precrisis and current level of functioning.

grief The dynamic natural response to loss. Grief affects physical, cognitive, behavioral, emotional, social, and spiritual aspects of the individual.

grief work The intense psychologic effort to (1) fully express the feelings associated with grief, (2) understand the relationship with the deceased, and, paradoxically, (3) carry on with essential activities of daily living.

guilt A pervasive theme in grief for individuals of all ages; especially troublesome for survivors who experienced difficult or ambivalent relationships with the deceased. Overwhelming guilt can be self-destructive and is discussed in several chapters throughout the text.

H

hallucination A perceptual disturbance of one or more of the five senses in the absence of external stimuli.

health The absence of disease; a state of total well-being. The various definitions imply that health is dynamic, with the focus on a healthy lifestyle. Health has been referred to as a condition of adjustment, or adaptation, to physical, psychologic, social, and environmental changes.

holistic Of or pertaining to holism, a philosophy that states that in nature, individuals function as complete units that cannot be reduced to the sum of their parts. Holistic medicine refers to the comprehensive and total care of each client, in which all needs (physical, emotional, social, spiritual, economic) are considered and treated.

homeopathic Health beliefs and practices derived from traditional cultural knowledge to maintain health, prevent changes in health status, and restore health.

homeostasis The way the body, using feedback mechanisms, maintains a stable internal environment, despite changes in the external environment.

human genome All of the genes carried on human chromosomes.

hypertensive crisis Any severe elevation of blood pressure that is a medical emergency. May occur as a result of food or drug admixtures with some psychotropic medications.

hypochondriasis A long-standing dependency. A preoccupation with the "sick role." A fear or belief that one has a serious illness in spite of medical reassurances to the contrary.

hypomania The mood of elation with higher-than-usual activity and social interaction; not as expansive as full mania.

I

id The basic level of the personality that lies in the unconscious and consists of primitive drives and instincts aimed at self-preservation.

idealization The tendency of a person with borderline personality disorder to idealize persons or groups beyond their capabilities when they are meeting that person's needs.

ideas of reference Incorrect interpretations of incidents and external events as having a particular or special meaning specific to the person.

identified client In family therapy, the member of the family (or group) whose behavior is seen as causing the problem for the family (or group).

illness Sickness, disease, or ailment. Illness has been labeled as an unexpected stressful event in individuals' lives that can interrupt them from fulfilling their usual tasks or roles. Illness is often perceived to be a crisis event. The terms *illness* and *disease* are often used synonymously; however, the disease process may be present without the person feeling ill, such as a lump in the breast that has not yet been detected. *Chronic illness* is a health problem with symptoms or disabilities requiring long-term management that affect persons across the life span.

incest Sexual intercourse between blood relatives.

incidence The frequency of occurrences of a specific disorder within a designated time period; number of new cases.

independent activities of daily living (IADLs) Activities an individual requires to function in the community (e.g., shopping, preparing meals, transportation).

indifference Refers to the nurse's disconnected or aloof lack of concern. A separation from the client's needs or situation.

inference The interpretation of behavior, assumption of motive, and formation of a conclusion before having all the information.

insight The ability to perceive oneself realistically and to understand oneself and the motives behind one's behavior.

institutionalization Placing or confining persons with mental disorders in state-run facilities, such as residential treatment programs designed to treat such disorders.

intermittent reinforcement When the reinforcer is delivered on a slightly different time interval or set number of correct responses called a schedule.

interpersonal communication Communication between two or more persons containing both verbal and nonverbal messages.

intoxication The physiologic state of being poisoned by a drug or other toxic substance.

intrapersonal communication Communication occurring within oneself that can be functional or dysfunctional.

intrapsychic Pertaining to the mind or mental process.

intuition Insight into a situation without the benefit of critical analysis. Also known as *intuitive reasoning*.

isolation A feeling of aloneness with perceived social rejection or lack of support from others during a crisis.

J

judgment An opinion or a conclusion that may affect or influence another person's life circumstances or situations. Also, the ability to make logical decisions.

K

kindling The creation of electrophysiologic sensitivity in the brain from stress that results in alteration of neural functioning.

L

label A word or phrase that describes a person or group. Usually has a negative connotation for clients with psychiatric disorders and signifies a stereotype that is detrimental for the individual.

learned helplessness The perception that events are uncontrollable, leading to apathy, helplessness, powerlessness, and depression.

least restrictive A therapeutic intervention or treatment that is applied when all other less intrusive methods have been tried and were unsuccessful; for example, initiating seclusion and restraint because talking to the client or reducing environmental stimulus did not prevent the client's behavior from escalating to a point of self-harm or harm to others.

least restrictive alternative Providing the least restrictive treatment in the least restrictive setting for a mental health client.

legal duty Something that an individual is required to do by law.

lethality The potential for causing death related to the level of danger associated with the suicidal plan along a continuum from low to high probability (e.g., a cut on both wrists versus a gunshot wound to the head).

libido The energy of the instincts held in the id. Sexual drive.

life stages The framework for several theories of adult development that divide life span into a series of sequential transitions.

locus of control An aspect of personality that deals with the degree of control one perceives over one's own destiny. *Internal locus of control* refers to the ability to actively control one's own destiny. *External locus of control* refers to the inability to control one's own destiny.

looseness of associations (LOA) Thought disturbance in which the speaker rapidly shifts expression of ideas from one subject to another in an unrelated, fragmented manner. Most commonly noted in schizophrenia.

loss A process characterized by a series of overlapping stages that include common psychologic and behavioral manifestations of recognition, adjustment, and resolution.

M

maladaptive The opposite of adaptive. Signifies a response that may result in unfavorable circumstances, situations, or conditions for an individual who is unable or unwilling to adapt to meet standards that are accepted by the medical or social communities.

mania An elevated, expansive, or irritable mood accompanied by hyperactivity, grandiosity, and loss of reality. Most commonly noted in bipolar disorder.

mental status examination An organized collection of data reflecting an individual's functioning at the time of interview. Mood, affect, thoughts and perceptions are a few components that make up the exam. Also includes psychosocial criteria such as coping.

mild cognitive impairment Cognitive functioning that is below the functioning associated with normal aging, while not meeting the criteria for dementia.

milieu therapy Re-creates a community atmosphere on an inpatient hospital unit, a partial hospitalization unit, or a day treatment setting to facilitate interaction between client peers to identify and problem-solve issues that occur while relating to others.

mirroring A technique in psychodrama and movement/dance therapy in which one individual imitates the behavior patterns of another to show the person how other people perceive and react to him or her.

modeling Principle arguing that behavioral change occurs through observing behaviors in others that brings positive or negative consequences.

mood A feeling state reported by the client that can vary with external and internal changes.

moral development Encompasses moral judgment or reasoning processes and involves making decisions about right or wrong actions in a particular situation.

mourning The social expression of grief.

N

NANDA diagnoses The North American Nursing Diagnosis Association International (NANDA-I) defines a nursing diagnosis as "a clinical judgment about an individual, family or community response to actual or potential health problems/life processes which provide the basis for definitive therapy toward achievement of outcomes for which the nurse is accountable."

negative symptoms A syndrome that includes flat affect, poverty of speech, poor grooming, withdrawal, and disturbance in volition.

neglect Intentional avoidance of attending to, or caring for, the physical or emotional or psychologic needs of another (usually child or elder).

neologisms Invented words to which meanings are attached.

neuritic plaques Insoluble deposits of protein and cellular material outside the neuron. Associated with Alzheimer's disease.

neurofibrillary tangle Insoluble twisted filaments that accumulate inside the neuron. Associated with Alzheimer's disease.

neuroleptic Literally, *to clasp the neuron;* the term used to describe antipsychotic medications.

neuroleptic malignant syndrome (NMS) A rare but potentially lethal toxic reaction to dopamine-blocking drugs that presents with a constellation of symptoms, including fever, autonomic instability, increased muscular rigidity, and altered mental status.

neurotransmitter A chemical substance released by presynaptic cells when stimulated that functions to activate postsynaptic cells and thus cause them to act as messengers in the central nervous system. Common neurotransmitters are acetylcholine, dopamine, norepinephrine, serotonin, and gamma-aminobutyric acid (GABA).

nihilism Belief that existence is senseless and useless.

nonverbal communication Nonverbal behaviors displayed by individuals during the process of an interaction.

norms The standards of behavior, attitudes, and perceptions that a group has for its members. Norms represent the shared expectations of appropriate behavior.

nuclear family A family made up of the parental dyad and the individual's siblings.

nurse-client relationship A professional, not a social, relationship with specific objectives to facilitate the client's process of achieving a state of well-being.

nursing Nursing has many definitions. The American Nurses Association (ANA) Social Policy Statement (1995) defines nursing as the diagnosis and treatment of human responses to actual and potential health problems. The statement emphasizes the nurse's role in addressing a wide range of human experiences and responses to health and disease and the provision of a caring relationship that promotes healing and health maintenance. It is the application of nursing science and theory and the integration of the art of nursing that create environments that facilitate healing. The goal of holistic nursing is nursing practice that enhances healing the whole person from birth to death.

Nursing Interventions Classification (NIC) The first comprehensive standardized classification of treatments performed by nurses; developed in 1987 by members of the Iowa Intervention Project research team.

Nursing Outcomes Classification (NOC) The first comprehensive standardized classification used to describe patient outcomes that are influenced by nursing; developed in 1991 by the Iowa Outcomes Project research team. Outcomes include indicators such as patient states, behaviors, and self-reported perceptions.

O

object constancy The ability to maintain a relationship regardless of frustration and changes in the relationship.

object relations The stability and depth of an individual's relations with significant others as manifested by warmth, dedication, concern, and tactfulness.

objectivity The state of remaining free from bias, prejudice, and personal identification in an interaction with another person.

obsessions Persistent ideas, thoughts, impulses, or images about death, sexual matters, religion, or any themes that lead to the person's efforts to resist them. They result in marked anxiety or distress.

operant conditioning A term coined by B.F. Skinner to describe his method of modifying behavior in animals, an approach he later applied to humans.

P

pain A subjective feeling of discomfort as indicated by the client, generally on a scale of 1 to 10 (1 to 3 = mild) (4 to 6 = moderate) (7 to 10 = severe). Pain is considered a fifth vital sign by the accrediting bodies of The Joint Commission (TJC) and the Board of Registered Nursing (BRN).

panic A circumscribed period of extreme anxiety. During panic, one's perceptions are distorted and the ability to integrate and separate environmental stimuli is impaired.

paradigm A side-by-side example to show a clear pattern.

paranoia A mental disorder characterized by persecutory thoughts or delusions.

paraphilias Sexual deviations/disorders presenting with inappropriate sexual fantasies involving deviant sexual acts, inappropriate sexual urges, and acting-out of these fantasies and urges.

perseveration A disturbance in thought association that is manifested by repetitive verbalizations or motions, or persistent repetition of the same idea in response to different questions. Perseveration is commonly seen in clients with schizophrenia or dementia.

personality traits Behaviors and enduring patterns of perceiving, relating to, and thinking about the environment and oneself that are exhibited in a wide range of social and personal contexts.

pervasive developmental disorders A collection of disorders in which the child experiences deficits in a broad range of developmental areas.

pheromones Airborne odorous chemicals (that are often unconscious) that may influence bonding and sexual attraction.

phobias A group of disorders primarily characterized by avoidance of a specific situation or escape, if that situation is unexpectedly encountered.

physical dependence A physiologic state of adaptation to a drug or alcohol, usually characterized by the development of tolerance to drug effects.

pleasure principle The goal of experiencing pleasure while avoiding pain. This principle represents the id's goal in the personality to satisfy a person's innate needs and instincts.

positive affirmation A self-supporting message that reinforces confidence and enhances performance.

positive cognitive set The belief that success is possible and that one can achieve what one believes.

positive regard Acceptance of and respect for a client.

positive symptoms A syndrome that includes hallucinations, increased speech production with loose associations, and bizarre behavior.

poverty of thought A psychopathologic thought disturbance in schizophrenia. The client's inability to think logically and sequentially is reflected in *poverty of content speech,* which is vague, repetitious, and disconnected.

premorbid The period just preceding the onset of a mental illness. Characteristics of the personality may indicate the type of disorder that may occur.

pressured speech Rapid speech with an urgent quality.

prevalence The number of cases of a specific disorder in a normal population at a given point in time; the number of existing cases.

primary prevention Prevention efforts that focus on reduction of the incidence of mental disorders within the community. It is directed toward occurrence of mental health problems with emphasis on health promotion and prevention of disorders.

primary process thinking Prelogical thought that aims for wish fulfillment. It is associated with the pleasure principle characteristic of the id portion of the personality.

privileged communication Communication between a professional and a client that is confidential and protected from forced disclosure in court unless authorized by the client. The privilege is delegated by statutes in the various states.

problem solving The process involved in discovering the correct sequence of alternatives leading to a goal or to an ideational solution.

prodromal symptoms Early symptoms, such as a deterioration in functioning, that may mark the onset of a mental illness.

projection The process whereby a person deals with his or her emotional conflicts or stressors, both internal and external, by unconsciously and falsely attributing to another person his or her own unacceptable feelings, impulses, or thoughts.

projective identification Projecting one's emotional conflicts and stressors to another who does not fully disavow what is projected. The individual remains aware of his or her own affects or impulses but misattributes them as justifiable reactions to the other person.

protective factors Factors that help an individual guard against risks. May be internal (capacity to tolerate stress) or external (a caring responsive teacher). Also see *risk factors*.

psychologic dependence The compulsive use of substances, leading to a state of craving a drug or alcohol for its positive effect or to avoid negative effects associated with its absence.

psychomotor agitation Agitated motor activity.

psychomotor retardation The slowing of physiologic processes, resulting in slow movement, speech, and reaction time.

psychosis Inability to recognize reality, bizarre behaviors, or inability to deal with life's demands.

psychosocial theory Erikson's eight stages in a person's social development. Each stage is marked by a particular type of crisis resulting from the ego's attempt to meet the demands of social reality.

psychosomatic illness Pertaining to a physical disorder that is notably influenced or caused by emotional or mental factors involving the mind and the body.

psychotropic Literally, *mind nutrition*. The term used to describe drugs that affect the central nervous system.

purging The use of self-induced vomiting or the abuse of laxatives, diuretics, syrup of ipecac, diet pills, or enemas to avoid weight gain following a binge. One or more of these behaviors, as well as periods of fasting and excessive exercise during an episode of bulimia nervosa, may be used.

R

rape The act of physically forcing sexual intercourse.

rapid eye movement (REM) sleep An active cerebral state. During this stage of sleep, there is an increase in cerebral metabolism with brain waves paralleling those of an awake state.

rave Raves and trance events are generally nightlong dances, often held in warehouses. Club drugs, sometimes referred to as designer drugs, are often used by teens and young adults who participate in nightclub, bar, rave, or trance scenes.

reality principle The goal of postponing immediate gratification until a suitable object for this satisfaction is found. The ego is ruled by this principle.

receptors Protein molecules located in the cell walls of tissues that receive chemical stimulation resulting in stimulation or inhibition of activity of the target cell.

refractory A term used when an individual is not responsive to medication or other types of treatment, generally requiring new or different therapeutic measures.

reframing A technique of changing the viewpoint of a situation and replacing it with another viewpoint that fits the facts equally well but changes the entire meaning.

relapse The resumption of a pattern of substance use or dependency after a period of sobriety or abstinence.

relapse prevention A means of helping the chemically dependent individual maintain behavioral changes over a prolonged period of time.

religion An organized system of beliefs about the cause, nature, and purpose of life, often expressed through the belief in or worship of divine beings.

repression The involuntary exclusion of a painful, threatening experience. Begins in infancy and continues throughout life. Underlies all other defense mechanisms but also operates as its own defense mechanism.

residual symptoms Minor disturbances that may remain after an episode of schizophrenia but do not include delusions, hallucinations, incoherence, or gross disorganization.

resilience The ability to withstand physical, emotional, psychologic stress.

resistance The inability, whether conscious or unconscious, to accept change; the denial of new problems.

restrictive environment An environment that restricts activity of a client to help the client regain control of his or her behavior. The individual may be placed in open-door or closed-door seclusion during periods of extreme agitation, suicidal ideations, or threats of violence to oneself or others.

risk factors Certain identified internal characteristics or external influences that are present before a disorder occurs. An individual is more vulnerable to develop a disorder when these factors are present. Also see *protective factors*.

rites of passage Rituals such as puberty, marriage, birth, and death that facilitate maturational development; associated with life transition. These rites commonly consist of three stages: separation, transition, and incorporation.

roles Expected social behavior patterns generally determined by an individual's status in a particular group. Peplau identified four roles for the psychiatric mental health nurse: (1) resource person, (2) counselor, (3) surrogate, and (4) technical expert.

S

safety The sense of security developed within the therapeutic relationship when the responsibilities and expectations of each party are clearly defined. Safety develops from knowing the boundaries of a relationship and acting within them.

secondary gain Any benefit—such as personal attention, sympathy from others, or escape from unwanted responsibilities—that results from illness. Individuals with eating disorders may experience secondary gain when family or friends pay a great deal of attention to their eating behavior (e.g., preparing special meals or making special arrangements in an attempt to encourage them to eat).

secondary prevention Prevention efforts directed toward reducing the prevalence of mental disorders through early identification and treatment of problems. This stage occurs after the problem arises and aims at shortening the course or duration of the episode.

selective attention Focusing on only part of incoming stimuli or information.

self-actualization A concept developed by Maslow as an ongoing actualization of potentials, capacities, and talents as fulfillment of a mission and as a greater knowledge and acceptance of one's own intrinsic nature.

self-system Sullivan's term for the system that infants develop to cope with anxiety associated with the interpersonal process of need satisfaction and security. The individual develops self-appraisal as a result of significant others' responses to actions of the individual. Actions that cause anxiety result in "bad-me" self-appraisals. Actions that cause no anxiety result in "good-me" self-appraisals. Actions of disapproval cause severe anxiety, emotional withdrawal, and "not-me" self-appraisals.

severe and persistent This term is currently widely accepted and replaces the term *chronic* when referring to unremitting or frequently recurring symptoms of certain psychiatric disorders (schizophrenia) that continue to distress an individual and interfere with function throughout life.

severe and persistent mental illness A psychiatric disorder that persists over time with multiple and recurrences of severe and disabling symptoms.

sexual recidivism Chronic, repetitive acting out of sexual behaviors considered to be unacceptable that have or have not resulted in criminal conviction.

sexual response cycle The stages of desire, arousal, and orgasm.

sexual victimization The act of sexually aggressing on another person by deceitfulness or power, causing physical, emotional, psychologic, or spiritual injury.

sick role A set of social expectations that an ill person meets, such as (1) being exempt from usual social role responsibilities, (2) not being morally responsible for being ill, (3) being obligated to "want to get well," and (4) being obligated to seek competent help.

side effect An undesired nontherapeutic and often predictable consequence of medication. Frequently diminished with time. Contrast with adverse drug reaction.

sleep reversal A state in which normal sleeping patterns are reversed; the individual sleeps during the day and is active during the night.

SOAP note A problem-solving method nurses commonly use in health care settings to analyze relevant client problems and reduce lengthy charting. SOAP = Subjective, Objective, Assessment, Plannning.

sobriety The state of complete abstinence from alcohol or other drugs of abuse.

social learning The process by which children acquire the behaviors they need to survive and function in society. The behaviors result from repeated interactions in their environments.

social support The presence of other individuals who are able to give understanding, encouragement, and other assistance in life, especially during difficult times.

socialization The process of being raised within a culture and acquiring the characteristics of the given group.

somatic complaints Expressions of grief, depression, resentment, or other internal feelings that are manifested instead as bodily pain and discomfort. Often children, adolescents, and adults describe biologic symptoms for what are actually psychiatric disorders or dysfunctional responses to life crises.

somatization The conversion of mental states or experiences into bodily symptoms associated with anxiety.

spirituality The effort to find purpose and meaning in life through a search for the sacred.

splitting Keeping the positive and negative aspects of oneself or others separate from each other. An individual who uses the unconscious defense mechanism of splitting cannot tolerate ambiguity; therefore people, events, or ideas are either good or bad, right or wrong, black or white, but not gray.

stalking The act of stealthily pursuing another person; usually a compulsion.

standardized care plan A method used to deliver consistent quality care that features designated DSM and NANDA diagnoses and multidisciplinary input. Reduces the need to create new care plans for each client and provides more time for staff-client interactions. Plans can be individualized.

Standards of Care The professional activities the nurse performs during the six-step nursing process (assessment, diagnosis, outcomes, planning, implementation, and evaluation). Developed by the American Nurses Association.

static Fixed, stationary, unchanging. Opposite of dynamic.

stem cells Cells that have the complete genome intact but have not yet differentiated.

stereotypes To form an oversimplified, standardized opinion of a person or group of people that is often determined without adequate information.

stigma Social reproach. Attitudinal devaluation and demeaning by society of an individual or group of people with disabilities or disorders who are judged, labeled, alienated, and thought incapable of fulfilling valued social roles or contributing to society.

stress (1) A term that refers to both a stimulus and a response. It can denote a nonspecific response of the body to any demand placed on it, whether the causal event is negative (a painful experience) or positive (a happy occasion). (2) A state produced by a change in the environment that is perceived as challenging, threatening, or damaging to the person's dynamic equilibrium. (3) The wear and tear on the body over time. (4) Psychologic stress has been defined as all processes, whether originating in the external environment or within the person, that demand a mental appraisal of the event before the involvement or activation of any other system.

stress response The body's reaction to a significant stressor (physical, emotional, psychologic). The response is an attempt to adapt as in Selye's general adaptation syndrome.

subjectivity Emphasizing one's own moods, attitudes, and opinions in an interaction with another person.

substance A chemical or drug.

suicidal ideation The experience of suicidal thinking on a consistent basis, which is a risk factor for suicide and warrants close supervision in a secured environment.

suicide The act of taking one's own life.

suicidology The scientific and humane study of suicide/self-destruction.

sundowner's syndrome The confusion and irritation common in clients with dementia at the end of the day, probably resulting from general tiredness and an inability to process any more information after a long day of struggling to interpret their environment correctly.

superego The portion of the mind, differentiated from the ego, that contains the traditional values and taboos of society as interpreted by the child's parents and that becomes part of the self. Lies in the preconscious.

syntonic Pertaining to a state of stability.

T

tardive dyskinesia (TD) A syndrome of abnormal, involuntary movements occurring after months or years of treatment with neuroleptic drugs that block dopamine type 2 receptors. These movements are often described as oral, buccal, lingual, or masticatory, but they can occur throughout the body.

tasks in grief Tasks or activities common in the psychosocial experience of grieving. Accomplishing these tasks helps resolve grief.

taxonomy A classification of known phenomena under a hierarchical structure.

tertiary prevention Prevention efforts that have the dual focus of reduction of residual effects of the disorder and rehabilitation of the individual who experienced the mental disorder.

themes Repeated patterns of interactions the client experiences in relationships with the self or others.

therapeutic alliance A goal-oriented, purposeful relationship between a professional member of a treatment team and a client, in which each agrees to work together to help the client resolve problematic areas in the client's life. In nursing, this is the *nurse-client relationship.*

therapeutic communication Verbal and nonverbal communication that takes place between the nurse and client. The content signifies *what* is being discussed. The content has meaning and focuses primarily on the client's concerns. The process refers to all aspects of meta-communication, or *how* the client and nurse communicate and the intent of each message.

therapeutic milieu An environment designed to promote emotional health that is based on the assumption that the clients are active participants in their own lives and therefore need to be involved in the management of their behavior and environment.

therapeutic play Age-appropriate play activities that the nurse uses purposefully for assessment, intervention, and promotion of normal growth and development in children.

therapeutic relationship A personal relationship that is established to help one of the participants deal more effectively and maturely with some difficulty in life. It is a goal-directed, client-centered, and objective relationship.

thought blocking The abrupt interruption in the flow of thoughts or ideas resulting from a disturbance in the speed of associations.

tic A sudden, rapid, recurrent, nonrhythmic, stereotyped movement or vocalization that is considered irresistible but is often suppressible for short periods.

titration An incremental adjustment of medication dose to allow for tolerance to side effects. For example, many medications are administered in low doses, which may be slowly titrated to higher doses, to avoid untoward effects of the drug. Titration is also used to designate incremental release of a client from a locked unit to see whether the client is able to tolerate specified activities on the unlocked unit, or to go to dinner in the dining room off the locked unit, then return.

tolerance The need for greatly increased amounts of a substance used to achieve intoxication or the desired mind-altering effects or markedly decreased effects with continued use of the same amount of the substance.

transference The feelings or responses that a client has toward the nurse that are associated with someone significant in the client's life. Although transference may be a natural part of therapy, the nurse needs to be aware of it and manage it to avoid inappropriate behavior of the client toward the nurse.

transitional objects Objects that remind one of a significant person. For example, a man keeps a picture of his wife on his desk, which reminds him of her during work hours, or a child keeps pieces of a blanket he or she had as a baby to bring comfort in stressful moments.

triggers Any stimulus that evokes a response.

trust The reliance on the truthfulness or accuracy of the therapeutic relationship developed through the consistency of the nurse's words and actions.

U

unconditional positive regard The stance of the therapist modeling the unconditional acceptance of the client and based on the belief that the client is competent to direct himself or herself in his or her natural tendency to move forward toward integration.

unconscious suicidal intention A state outside of awareness during which persons engage in risk-taking behaviors that have a high likelihood of causing their deaths.

V

verbal communication Spoken or written words that compose the symbols of language.

vicarious learning Learning through imagining the experiences of others as if they are one's own.

victimizer Another term used to define a sex offender; may be used when discussing familial transmission of the paraphilia.

vigilance The ability to sustain attention over long periods of time.

violence Behavior that is physically, psychologically, or sexually harmful, injurious, or assaultive (e.g., child abuse, domestic violence, elder abuse, family violence).

W

Wernicke's center An area of the brain's dominant hemisphere that recognizes, recalls, and interprets words. May be affected in chronic alcoholism or severe malnutrition.

X

xenophobia A morbid fear of strangers and those who are not of one's own ethnic group.

Index

B